Textbook of Hyperbaric Medicine

About the Author

K.K. Jain, MD, is a neurosurgeon and has held fellowships and teaching positions at Harvard, UCLA, and the University of Toronto. He has been a visiting professor in several countries and served in the US Army with the rank of Lieutenant Colonel. He wrote the *Handbook of Laser Neurosurgery* based on his experience in microsurgery and lasers. He has been active in the field of hyperbaric medicine since 1976, starting with the application of this technique to stroke patients. The author of 15 books (including *Oxygen in Physiology & Medicine*, *Textbook of Gene Therapy*, and *Handbook of Nanomedicine*), Prof. Jain, in addition to his activities in biotechnology, serves as a consultant in hyperbaric medicine.

With contributions by

S.A. Baydin MD

Director General, Institute of Hyperbaric
Medicine and Techniques,
Post Box 853
Moscow, 119435 Russia
(Chapter 29, Pediatric Surgery)

J. Bookspan, PhD
Temple University and Jefferson Medical College,
Philadelphia, PA, USA
(Chapter 23, Headache)

T.M. Bozzuto, DO
Medical Director, Phoebe Wound Care & Hyperbaric Center
Phoebe Putney Memorial Hospital
Albany, GA, USA
(Chapter 41, United States)

F.K. Butler, Jr., MD
CAPT MC USN (Ret)
Chairman, Committee on Tactical Combat Casualty Care
Defense Health Board
Pensacola, FL, USA
(Chapter 32, Ophthalmology)

E.M. Camporesi, MD
Professor and Chairman, Dept. of Anesthesiology
SUNY, Syracuse, New York
(Chapter 38, Anesthesia)

C.E. Fife, MD
Associate Professor of Anesthesiology
Memorial Hermann Center for Hyperbaric Medicine
Houston, Texas 77030, USA
(Chapters 14, Chronic Lyme Disease; 23, Headache)

W.P. Fife, PhD
Professor of Hyperbaric Medicine (Emeritus)
Texas A & M University
College Station, Texas, USA
(Chapter 14, Chronic Lyme Disease)

P.G. Harch, MD
Director, Dept. of Hyperbaric Medicine
LSU School of Medicine at New Orleans
Harvey, LA, USA
(Chapters 19, Anoxia and Coma; 22, Cerebral Palsy; 44, Appendix)

P.B. James, MD
Professor Emeritus, Wofson Institute of Occupational Health
Medical School
Ninewells, Dundee, UK
(Chapters 10, Decompression Sickness; 21, Multiple Sclerosis; 44, Appendix)

H. Murphy-Lavoie, MD
Assistant Residency Director
Emergency Medicine Residency

Associate Program Director
Hyperbaric Medicine Fellowship
LSU School of Medicine/MCLNO
New Orleans, LA, USA
(Chapter 32, Ophthalmology)

R.A. Neubauer, MD†
Director, Ocean Hyperbaric Center
Fort Lauderdale, FL, USA
(Chapters 19, Anoxia and Coma; 21, Multiple Sclerosis; 22 Cerebral Palsy; 44, Appendix)

V. Neubauer
Ocean Hyperbaric Center
Fort Lauderdale, FL, USA
(Chapter 22, Cerebral Palsy)

M.H. Sukoff
Clinical Professor of Neurosurgery
University of California
Irvine, CA, USA
(Chapter 20, Neurosurgery)

H. Takahashi
Professor and Chairman
Department of Hyperbaric Medicine
University of Nagoya School of Medicine
Showa-Ku, Nagoya 466–8560
Japan
(Chapter 43, Japan)

K. Van Meter, MD
Chief, Section of Emergency Medicine
Clinical Professor of Medicine, Section of Emergency Medicine
LSU Health Sciences Center in New Orleans
Harvey, LA, USA
(Chapter 39, Emergency Medicine)

J.M. Uszler, MD
Professor of Nuclear Medicine
Santa Monica-UCLA Medical Center
Santa Monica, CA, USA
(Chapter 44, Appendix)

H.A. Wyatt, MD, PhD
Clinical Instructor of Medicine
LSU Health Sciences Center
Department of Medicine and Division of Hyperbaric Medicine
Marrero, LA, USA
(Chapter 37, Organ Transplants)

H. Yagi, MD
Director, Hyperbaric Medicine
Fukuoka Yagi Kosei-Kai Hospital
(2–21–25, Maidashi, Higashi-Ku,
Fukuoka, Japan
(Chapter 43, Japan)

Textbook of Hyperbaric Medicine

Fifth revised and updated edition

K. K. Jain, MD

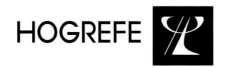

Library of Congress Cataloguing-in-Publication Data

is available via the Library of Congress Marc Database
under the LC Control Number 2008938004

National Library of Canada Cataloguing in Publication

Jain, K. K. (Kewal K.)
Textbook of hyperbaric medicine / K.K. Jain.—5th ed.

Includes bibliographical references and index.
ISBN 978-0-88937-361-7

1.Hyperbaric oxygenation. I.Title.

RM666.O83J35   2009   615.8'36   C2008-906643-X

PUBLISHING OFFICES
USA: Hogrefe Publishing, 875 Massachusetts Avenue, 7th Floor Cambridge, MA 02139
               Tel. (866) 823-4726, Fax (617) 354-6875, E-mail info@hogrefe.com
Europe: Hogrefe & Huber Publishers, Rohnsweg 25, 37085 Göttingen, Germany
               Tel. +49 551 49609-0, Fax +49 551 49609-88, E-mail hh@hogrefe.com

SALES AND DISTRIBUTION
USA: Hogrefe Publishing, Customer Service Department, 30 Amberwood Parkway,
               Ashland, OH 44805, Tel. (800) 228-3749, Fax (419) 281-6883, E-mail custserv@hogrefe.com
Europe: Hogrefe & Huber Publishers, Rohnsweg 25, 37085 Göttingen, Germany
               Tel. +49 551 49609-0, Fax +49 551 49609-88, E-mail hh@hogrefe.com

OTHER OFFICES
Canada: Hogrefe & Huber Publishers, 1543 Bayview, Toronto, Ontario, M4G 3B5
Switzerland: Hogrefe & Huber Publishers, Länggass-Strasse 76, CH-3000 Bern 9

Hogrefe & Huber Publishers
Incorporated and registered in Göttingen, Lower Saxony, Germany

Hogrefe Publishing
Incorporated and registered in the Commonwealth of Massachusetts, USA

Printed and bound in Germany
ISBN 978-0-88937-361-7

To my wife Verena and my children Eric, Adrian, and Vivien Jain
for their patience during the preparation of this work

Table of Contents

PART I: Basic Aspects

PART II: Clinical Applications

PART III: Appendix, Bibliography, Index

Foreword

James F. Toole, MD

Teagle Professor of Neurology
Director, Cerebrovascular Research Center
Wake Forest University School of Medicine, Winston-Salem, NC

Slowly but surely, hyperbaric medicine is becoming an established treatment modality for a variety of medical disorders, despite the rocky road that it has sometimes had to travel over the years. In some ways, I feel that the need for oxygen in medical treatments is akin to man's basic requirement for water and food, and I also think it is fair to say that the logic and utility of hyperbaric oxygen treatment now seem to be almost as undeniable as these basic requirements are.

It is certainly the case that, from time immemorial, remedies learned by trial and error have been handed down through the generations – with the result that many roots, berries, fruits, and leaves, as well as special waters containing minerals have been advocated throughout history for their curative powers. More recently, however, evidence-based medicine has come to the fore, demanding higher standards of evidence from basic and clinical/research trials and objective statistical results. One of the first instances of such objective studies in my lifetime was when Austin Bradford Hill and Richard Doll (Doll 2003) convinced colleagues to allocate patients with pulmonary tuberculosis randomly to prove the efficacy of streptomycin, although their trial followed a tradition started 200 years earlier by Linde, who provided citrus fruits aboard some, but not all ships in the British Navy to test whether they would prevent scurvy (Moberg & Chon 2000).

By means of prospective trials, it has been found that various "established" therapies can be detrimental for some diseases, while being clearly beneficial for others. This is precisely the case with hyperbaric medicine now: while a hyperoxic environment for newborn babies can lead to retrolental fibroplasia with blindness, there is also convincing evidence that hyperbaric treatments provide clear benefits in diseases such as various neurological disorders, stroke, cerebral ischemia, and wound healing. And, of course, those of us who have worked in high-altitude environments know the very short time window during which the human brain can function in hypoxic conditions. It never ceases to astonish me what a wide range of effects (beneficial or toxic) a seemingly innocuous substance such as oxygen can have in various circumstances.

By and large, the experts who have made such superb contributions to the *Textbook of Hyperbaric Medicine* are the world leaders in their fields. With their help, Dr. Jain has expanded his already outstanding book into a compendium of multi-authored chapters (containing over 2,000 references) covering areas of medicine as disparate as wound healing, gastrointestinal disorders, trauma, and obstetrics. Of particular interest in this edition are the extensive discussions of cerebral circulation and its disorders, as well as of stroke, diving accidents, and neurosurgery.

For an earlier edition, Dr. Jain enlisted a remarkable Foreword by Professor Edward Teller (see next page), who began by stating "Hyperbaric medicine is new and controversial" and that we live "in an age that has the habit of treating progress with suspicion," and then went on to pose the question, "But what is the innovator to do?" He also raised the age-old problem of the ethics of the double-blind trial, and cautioned us to be aware of the potential danger of high-pressure treatment for too long a period, in the same way that drug treatments at too high dosages bear clear risks. The field of hyperbaric medicine has indeed been subject to an at times intense debate, but much progress has been made since Professor Teller originally wrote his words (and will, I am sure, continue to be made in the future), on the basis of mutual respect, understanding, and cooperation, while also submitting beliefs to randomized trials.

Professor Teller wrote then: "It is not entirely impossible that, perhaps sometime in the next decade, professors of medicine will have difficulty in explaining why treatment with oxygen was not widely adopted much earlier." Reflecting today on these words by an elder statesman whose scientific observations went unheeded early on, we can safely conclude that the uphill battle for acceptance of hyperbaric oxygen as therapy now rests on a solid foundation. This solid foundation is described comprehensively and clearly within this outstanding text, in which the assembled experts provide a fair and balanced summary of the literature and evidence. And it also means that the "decade of HBO" to which Professor Teller indirectly referred has now come.

References

Doll R (2003). *The evolution of the controlled trial.* The Eighteenth John P. McGovern Award Lecture, delivered at the Thirty-Third Meeting of the American Osler Society, Edinburgh, Scotland, May 23.

Moberg CL, Chon ZA (Eds.). (1990). *Launching the antibiotic era. Personal accounts of the discovery and use of the first antibiotics.* New York: Rockefeller University Press.

Foreword to the Third Edition

Edward Teller[†]

Formerly Director Emeritus Lawrence Livermore National Laboratories, California & Senior Research Fellow Hoover Institution, Stanford University, Stanford, CA

Hyperbaric medicine is new and controversial. Indeed, since it is new, it must be controversial in an age that has the habit of treating progress with suspicion. But what is the innovator to do? If he applies a new and safe procedure to patients, and the procedure appears to be successful, his success might well be denigrated as anecdotal. Will he be allowed to run a double blind experiment in which half of the patients are denied the benefits of what appears to be a cure? It is an age-old problem that has grown sharper in the course of time.

Hyperbaric medicine grew out of the problems encountered by divers exposed to high pressures. The treatment of disturbances due to bubbles which develop during rapid decompression was the natural connection between high pressure and medicine. This limited application of a medical procedure is, of course, widely accepted. But its extension to counteract the damage due the air bubbles resulting from other causes, such as those accidentally introduced during medical treatment, is less generally recognized.

What is attempted in this book is a detailed and critical treatment of a large subject. If thorough discussion will lead to some consensus, the subject could grow very much larger. Indeed, oxygen, which in the form of hyperbaric oxygen (HBO) is called a drug, is the most natural of all drugs.

The first problem we must face is the danger of high pressure treatment used at excess pressure for too long a period, or in conjunction with the wrong kind of drug. Oxygen indeed has toxic effects. Furthermore, the delivery of the pressurized gas to the patient may be mishandled. A properly extensive discussion is devoted to such dangers, which are completely avoidable.

Perhaps the most natural use of HBO is to counteract carbon monoxide poisoning. The best known effect of carbon monoxide is to replace oxygen by being more firmly bound to hemoglobin. But, of course, high pressure oxygen can drive out the carbon monoxide and produce a cure in an understandable fashion.

A little harder to grasp is why pure oxygen at two atmospheres of pressure (which is ten times as concentrated as the natural occurrence) should have any general uses. Indeed, under normal circumstances, the hemoglobin in arterial blood is 97 percent saturated with oxygen. Are we exerting ourselves to supply the remaining 3 percent? The answer, of course, is no. Oxygen is also soluble in blood. At two atmospheres of pressure, oxygen can be dissolved into the plasma at several times normal levels, and can significantly improve tissue oxygenation. This is important because hemoglobin, while more eager to take up oxygen, is also more reluctant to part with it. The oxygen dissolved in the plasma, having a higher chemical potential, is pushed out from the capillaries and into the surrounding tissue. From there, it can spread small distances by diffusion.

Even in the blood itself, the dissolved oxygen may help the white blood cells in their phagocytic activity. Bacteria themselves may react in a variety of ways. It appears that many can use oxygen at normal pressures, but are damaged by oxygen at higher pressures. In the case of anaerobic bacteria, oxygen can act in a powerful way to stop the infection. In combination with other methods, HBO clearly appears effective in cases of gangrene.

But more is involved than the straightforward destruction of the pathogen. The natural healing process may also be assisted by the presence of oxygen. This obviously should be the case when hyperbaric treatment counteracts on oxygen deficiency. Many injuries involve the destruction of capillaries, the means of delivering oxygen. Under such circumstances, healing is itself tied to revascularization of the damaged tissue. But growth of the requisite capillaries is in turn tied to the oxygen supply. This relationship can explain why in the case of many slow healing wounds, HBO seems to have a strong positive effect. Very much more can and should be done to extend the study of the speed of healing to the more normal cases.

In the human body, 20 percent of the oxygen consumption occurs in 3 percent of the body mass: the brain. This is also the region most sensitive to a deficiency of oxygen, which can produce dramatic results. Indeed, surgical methods on the carotid artery are often used to relieve oxygen deficiency to the brain. It seems logical that in HBO we have a tool that can serve a similar purpose. This might be particularly important in the case of stroke, a high-ranking cause of death and disability. It is clearly worthwhile to explore whether and to what extent disability can be reduced or avoided by prompt use of hyperbaric treatment. If the blood supply to a small region of the brain is reduced, relief might come from the diffusion of oxygen into the ischemic region from neighboring capillaries.

For all new medical techniques, scientific evidence is demanded. Yet medicine is still partly an art, as well as a dramatically advancing science. Therefore in the complicated questions of life, disease, and recovery, it is sometimes hard to distinguish between the fight against the causes of a disease, and our efforts to aid toward the reassertion of overall health. There are good indications that HBO is helpful in many diseases, such as multiple sclerosis and osteomyelitis. One may mention these two applications because, in the former, earlier recognition of the disease made possible by the use of magnetic resonance imaging has made early treatment a better possibility, and seems to have given a real chance for help from HBO. In the latter case, osteomyelitis, the location of the disease is the bone, where oxygen is usually not amply available.

As members of the scientific community we are all naturally tempted to theorize, as long as a glimmer of a theory might be perceived. This book proceeds, however, along strictly step by step empirical lines. Case after case, the various pathologies are reviewed. In each situation, it is carefully stated to what extent the evidence merely indicates a conclusion, and to what extent the conclusion can be proved. In the present stage of HBO, it is a certainty that there will be considerable criticism. On the other hand, those who disagree are likely at the same time to disagree among themselves. I believe that the result will be not only critical reflection, but also more experimentation, more reviews, more understanding, and more progress. It is not entirely impossible that, perhaps sometimes in the next decade, professors of medicine will have difficulty in explaining why the treatment with oxygen was not widely adopted much earlier.

Preface to the Fifth Edition

K.K. Jain

American College of Hyperbaric Medicine

Almost 20 years have passed since the first edition of the *Textbook of Hyperbaric Medicine* was written, and since the publication of the 4th revised edition in 2004, there has been a considerable increase of research and development in applications of hyperbaric oxygen. Of the more than 1200 publications relevant to hyperbaric medicine during 2004–2008, approximately 300 have been selected and added to the list in this book, whilst a corresponding number of older references have been deleted to maintain the bibliography at 2000 entries. Several older publications have been retained for their historical interest, and some of these have indeed become classics.

There is an ever increasing use of hyperbaric oxygen for neurological disorders. Other areas of expansion include applications in ophthalmology and the chapter on this has been rewritten and expanded by Frank Butler and Heather Murphy-Lavoie. A new chapter by Alan Wyatt on the role

of hyperbaric oxygen in organ transplantation has been added as well as a chapter on the treatment of chronic lyme disease by William Fife and Caroline Fife.

Multimodality treatment is required in some complex disorders and hyperbaric oxygen has been combined with new advances in drug treatment and surgical procedures as well as with complementary medicine techniques such as acupuncture. As other new technologies such as those for manipulating stem cells develop, their interaction with hyperbaric oxygen is being studied. Hyperbaric oxygen may prove to be a useful adjunct to stem cell-based therapeutics and regenerative medicine.

I would like to thank the editorial staff at Hogrefe & Huber Publishers, particularly the Publishing Manager, Robert Dimbleby, for their help and encouragement during this revision.

Preface to the Fourth Edition

K.K. Jain

American College of Hyperbaric Medicine

The textbook has been revised in accordance with the progress made in hyperbaric medicine during the past four years. There were over 1000 publications relevant to hyperbaric medicine during 1999–2002. Approximately 200 of these were selected and a corresponding number of older references were deleted to keep the total number of references in the bibliography to 2000. The number of clinical trials for various applications in hyperbaric oxygen therapy has increased. These are included wherever the published results are available. As personalized medicine is developing, it will be applied to hyperbaric oxygenation as well. It is already obvious that patients require an individualized approach in hyperbaric therapy protocols. The dose of ox-

ygen, pressure, and duration of treatment need to be determined for each patient individually. It is difficult to reach any conclusions from clinical trials about a particular pressure of oxygen or even a range for a broad diagnostic category with many variants among patients that determine the response.

Applications in neurological disorders are developing further and space devoted to this area has been increased. A new chapter by Neubauer and Harch has been added on the treatment of cerebral palsy with hyperbaric oxygenation.

I wish to thank the publishing directors of Hogrefe Publishers and their Editor, Mr. Robert Dimbleby, for their help and encouragement throughout the period of revision.

Preface to the Third Edition

K.K. Jain

American College of Hyperbaric Medicine

Hyperbaric medicine continues to make progress. The textbook has been revised and expanded with inclusion of new contributors. We are fortunate to have an article from Prof. Hideyo Takahashi of Japan describing the state of development of hyperbaric oxygen therapy in Japan.

As in the previous edition, objective judgment has been exercised in deciding to include various reports and studies on this subject. There are more than 200 publications every year on hyperbaric medicine, and all the publications cannot be included in references. The bibliography already contains more than 2000 entries. Most of the older references have been retained because of their historical value.

Much of the original material still holds its value and has also been retained. Simply because no new work has been done in some areas does not mean that these indications for HBO are no longer valid. Research in hyperbaric medicine continues to be limited by lack of funding. However, the technique is available for clinical application in certain cases when the need arises and often a precedence in that area helps. Well-documented anecdotal reports have a teaching value, and this has been utilized in the textbook. This is particularly so in the case of emergency medicine and treatment of hypoxemic/ischemic encephalopathies, where it would be practically impossible to conduct controlled studies.

Much of the expansion of hyperbaric oxygen therapy is in the area of neurological disorders, which is reflected in the increased number of chapters devoted to this area. This application of hyperbaric oxygen holds the greatest promise for the future for diseases of the nervous system.

I wish to thank the publishing directors of Hogrefe & Huber and their Editor, Mr. Robert Dimbleby, for their help and encouragement throughout the period of preparation.

Preface to the Second Edition

K.K. Jain

American College of Hyperbaric Medicine

A great deal of progress has taken place in Hyperbaric Medicine since the publication of the first edition. This has necessitated a thorough revision of the book and inclusion of new contributors. Some of the outdated references were removed and new ones have been added, bringing the total about 1800 entries. I have tried to keep my judgment objective and this is helped by the fact I have no involvement in the political and financial aspects of hyperbaric medicine.

In spite of this critical revision and corrections, I am pleased to state that a great deal of the old stuff still holds its value. Use of hyperbaric oxygen therapy in neurological disorders continues to expand and required a chapter on neurosurgery, for which I was fortunate to have the collaboration of Dr. Michael Sukoff of the United States, who has done much of the pioneer work in this field. The chapter on pediatric surgery by Prof. Baydin from Russia is a useful new addition. With the inclusion of unpublished work on the role of neuropeptides in oxygen therapy (Prof. G.T. Ni) from China, the book is now truly international.

I wish to thank the publishing directors of Hogrefe & Huber Publishers for their help and encouragement throughout the period of revision. Countless other colleagues also helped and their names are too numerous to list here.

Preface to the First Edition

K.K. Jain

American College of Hyperbaric Medicine

This book goes considerably beyond the scope of the *Handbook of Hyperbaric Oxygen Therapy,* which was written by me, and published by Springer Verlag in 1988. In addition, with the many rapid developments in this field, the *Handbook* has already become remarkably outdated. Our use of the word "textbook" in the title of the present work is in keeping with the increasing worldwide recognition of this branch of medicine, and the need for a definite and inclusive source covering this body of knowledge, as it exists today.

In practice hyperbaric medicine of course involves mostly the use of hyperbaric oxygen, i.e., oxygen under pressure greater than atmospheric. As a result, this field overlaps with diving medicine in the areas of

- the effect of high pressure on the human body
- physical exercise under hyperbaric environments
- air embolism
- decompression sickness

I have made no attempt to intrude any further into diving medicine, as there are several excellent textbooks on that subject. In addition, the use of normobaric oxygen has been discussed elsewhere in a 1989 title by K.K. Jain, *Oxygen in Physiology and Medicine.*

I have written this current work in a textbook style, and there is more discussion on the pathophysiology of diseases and the rational basis of hyperbaric oxygen than in the *Handbook.* Extensive and up-to-date references have been assembled as an integral part of this project, and these total about 1,500.

The highlights of this present effort are the newly documented effectiveness of hyperbaric oxygen therapy in the rehabilitation of stroke patients, and the validation of these gains via the iofetamine scan technique. This same method has also been used to document the improvement in multiple sclerosis patients undergoing hyperbaric oxygen therapy.

In the preparation of this work I was considerably aided by the capable and cooperative management effort provided by the two directors of the Hogrefe & Huber publishing company. The execution of a project involving this degree of both scope and detail is certainly an exercise in teamwork between author and publisher, and it was a pleasure to have shaped the production in a creative and timely manner.

PART I:
BASIC ASPECTS

1

The History of Hyperbaric Medicine

K.K. Jain

This chapter reviews the historical relationship between hyperbaric therapy and diving medicine, recounting the important stages in the development of compressed gas technology and a few of the more interesting early attempts to utilize it for medical purposes. The sections involved are:

Hyperbaric Therapy and Diving Medicine

As is well known, the origins and development of hyperbaric medicine are closely tied to the history of diving medicine. While the attractions of the deep are easily understood, it was the various unpleasant physical consequences of venturing beneath the surface of the world's oceans that led directly to the many applications of compressed-gas therapy in modern medicine. Although scientifically based applications of hyperbaric technology are a relatively recent development, the use of compressed gas in medicine actually has ancient roots.

The origin of diving is not known, but it was recognized as a distinct occupation as far back as 4500 B.C. However, since humans can only hold their breath for a few minutes, unaided dives are limited to depths of less than about 30 meters. The first use of actual diving equipment to extend the limits of underwater activity is attributed in legend to none other than Alexander the Great, who, in 320 B.C., is said to have been lowered into the Bosphorus Straits in a glass barrel (see Figure 1.1), which purportedly gave him a secret weapon in the siege of Tyre.

Around the year 1500, Leonardo Da Vinci made sketches of a variety of diving appliances, without developing any for practical use. It was not until 1620 that the Dutch inventor Cornelius Drebbel developed the first true diving bell. His device was extremely limited, especially by its simple air supply that delivered air pressurized at only one atmosphere, but it was certainly the forerunner of all submersible vehicles.

In 1691 Edmund Halley, after whom the comet is named, advanced diving bell technology by devising a method of replenishing the air supply using weighted barrels (Smith, 1986). This was followed in the next two centuries by the development of compressed-air diving helmets and suits – which made it possible to remain under water for an hour or more.

Even though the duration of dives had been extended, divers were still limited to the same shallow waters as before. Undersea pioneers had quickly discovered the eardrum-rupturing effects of increasing water pressure. Those attempting to venture even deeper in diving bells also

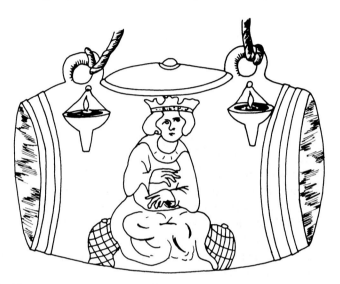

Figure 1.1
Alexander the Great was said to have been lowered into the Bosphorus Straits in a glass barrel. Note that the candles are lighted and if, indeed, Alexander went into this barrel, he was lucky to survive. The illustration is redrawn from a thirteenth century manuscript in the Burgundy Library in Brussels, and is reproduced courtesy of Dr. E. B. Smith (1986).

Table 1.1
Some Important Benchmarks in the History of Diving Medicine in Relation to Hyperbaric Medicine

4500 BC	Earliest records of breathholding dives for mother-of-pearl
400 BC	Xerxes used divers for work on ships and for salvaging sunken goods. Dives were for 2–4 min and to a depth of 20–30 m
320 BC	First diving bell used by Alexander the Great
300 BC	Aristotle described the rupture of the eardrum in divers
1670	Boyle gave the first description of the decompression phenomenon as "bubble in the eye of a snake in vacuum"
1620	Cornelius Drebbel developed a one-atmosphere diving bell, basically the forerunner of all modern submarines
1691	Edmund Halley improved bell technology by devising a method to replenish air supply in the diving bell
1774	Freminet, a French scientist, reached a depth of 50 ft (2.5 ATA) and stayed there for 1 h using a helmet with compressed air pumped through a pipe from the surface
1830	Cochrane patented the concept and technique of using compressed air in tunnels and caissons to balance the pressure of water in soil
1841	Pol an Watelle of France observed that recompression relieved the symptoms of decompression sickness
1869	Publication of *Twenty Thousand Leagues under the Sea,* a science fiction novel by Jules Verne; contains a description of diving gears with air reserves
1871	Paul Bert showed that bubbles in the tissues during decompression consist mainly of nitrogen
1920	Use of gas mixtures for diving (heliox); diving depth extended to 200 m
1935	Behnke showed that nitrogen is the cause of narcosis in humans subjected to compressed air above 4 ATA
1943	Construction of aqua lung by Cousteau; diving at 200 bar possible
1967	Founding of Undersea Medical Society, USA

quickly learned about the best-known medical problem associated with diving: decompression sickness. It was not until the middle of the nineteenth century that the effectiveness of countering decompression sickness with hyperbaric recompression was finally discovered (see Table 1.1). Although recompression in air was utilized first, hyperbaric oxygen (HBO) is now used, and this is the principal connection between diving medicine and the other forms of HBO therapy.

The Development of Hyperbaric Air Therapy

The first documented use of hyperbaric therapy actually precedes the discovery of oxygen. The British physician Henshaw seems to have used compressed air for medical purposes in 1662. The chamber he developed was an airtight room called a "domicilium," in which variable climatic and pressure conditions could be produced, with pressure provided by a large pair of bellows. According to Henshaw, "In times of good health this domicilium is proposed as a good expedient to help digestion, to promote insensible respiration, to facilitate breathing and expectoration, and consequently, of excellent use for the prevention of most afflictions of the lungs." There is, however, no account of any application of Henshaw's proposed treatment, and there were no further developments in the field of hyperbaric therapy for nearly two centuries.

In the nineteenth century there was a rebirth of interest in hyperbaric therapy in France. In 1834 Junod built a hyperbaric chamber to treat pulmonary afflictions using pressures of two to four absolute atmospheres (ATA). In 1837 Pravaz built the largest hyperbaric chamber of that time and treated patients with a variety of ailments. Fontaine developed the first mobile hyperbaric operating theater in 1877 (Figure 1.2), and by this time hyperbaric chambers were available in all major European cities. Interestingly, there was no general rationale for hyperbaric treatments, and prescriptions therefore varied from one physician to another. (In those days no methods were available to estimate the partial pressure of oxygen in blood, which at 2 ATA of air is about double that at sea level. In comparison, if pure oxygen is breathed at 2 ATA, the partial pressure of oxygen in the arterial blood is twelve times higher than normal.)

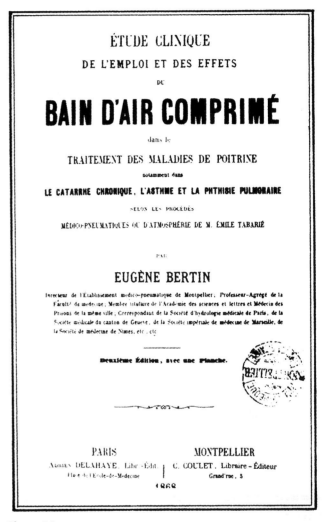

Figure 1.3
Title page of the 2nd edition (1868) of the book by Bertin on the treatment of diseases by compressed air.

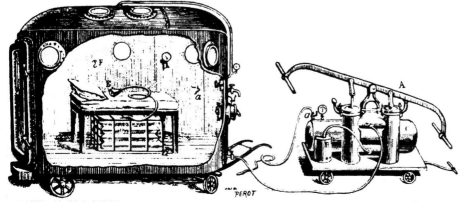

Figure 1.2
Fontaine's mobile operating room of 1877. Note the manual nature of the compressor apparatus and the anesthesia gas container and mask in the chamber. (Photo courtesy of Dr. Baixe, Toulon, France.)

During the second half of the nineteenth century, hyperbaric centers were advertised as being comparable to health spas. Junod referred to his treatment as *"Le Bain d'air comprimé"* (the compressed-air bath). In 1855 Bertin wrote a book on this topic (the title page is shown in Figure 1.3) and constructed his own hyperbaric chamber (Figure 1.4). The

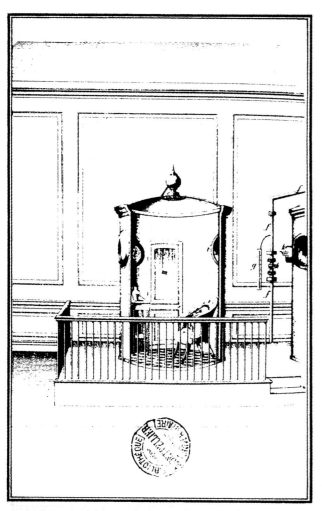

Figure 1.4
Hyperbaric chamber constructed by Bertin in 1874.

literature on hyperbaric medicine up to 1887 was reviewed by Arntzenius and contains a remarkable 300 references.

The first hyperbaric chamber on the North American continent was constructed in 1860 in Oshawa, Ontario, Canada, just east of Toronto. The first such chamber in the United States was built by Corning a year later in New York to treat nervous disorders. The chamber that received the most publicity, however, and was the most actively used, was that of Cunningham in Kansas City in the 1920s (Sellers, 1965). He first used his chamber to treat the victims of the Spanish influenza epidemic that swept the USA during the closing days of the First World War. Cunningham had observed that mortality from this disease was higher in areas of higher elevation, and he reasoned that a barometric factor was therefore involved. Cunningham claimed to have achieved remarkable improvement in patients who were cyanotic and comatose. In 1923, the first recorded hyperbaric chamber fire occurred at Cunningham's sanatorium. He had installed open gas burners under the tank to keep it warm in winter and someone turned the flame the flame too high so that it scorched the interior insulation. The patients were evacuated safely. However, one night a mechanical failure resulted in a complete loss of compression and all his patients died. This tragedy was a sobering lesson but ultimately did not deter Dr Cunningham. His enthusiasm for hyperbaric air continued, and he started to treat diseases such as syphilis, hypertension, diabetes mellitus, and cancer. His reasoning was based on the assumption that anaerobic infections play a role in the etiology of all such diseases. In 1928, in Cleveland, Cunningham constructed the largest chamber ever built – five stories high and 64 feet in diameter (Figure 1.5). Each floor had 12 bedrooms with all the amenities of a good hotel. At that time it was the only functioning hyperbaric chamber in the world.

As the publicity surrounding his treatments grew, Dr Cunningham was repeatedly requested by the Bureau of Investigations of the American Medical Association (AMA) to document his claims regarding the effectiveness of hyperbaric therapy. Apart from a short article in 1927, however, Cunningham made no efforts to describe or discuss his technique in the medical literature. He was eventually

Table 1.2
Landmarks in the History of Hyperbaric (Compressed) Air Therapy

1662	Henshaw used compressed air for the treatment of a variety of diseases
1834	Junod of France constructed a hyperbaric chamber and used pressures of 2–4 ATA to treat pulmonary disease
1837	Pravaz of France constructed the largest hyperbaric chamber of that time and used it to treat a variety of ailments
1837–1877	Construction of pneumatic centers in various European cities, e.g., Berlin, Amsterdam, Brussels, London, Vienna, Milan
1860	First hyperbaric chamber on the North American continent in Oshawa, Canada
1870	Fontaine of France used the first mobile hyperbaric operating theater
1891	Corning used the first hyperbaric chamber in the USA to treat nervous disorders
1921	Cunningham (USA) used hyperbaric air to treat a variety of ailments
1925	Cunningham tank was the only functional hyperbaric chamber in the world
1928	Cunningham constructs the largest hyperbaric chamber in the world; American Medical Association condemns Cunningham's hyperbaric therapy
1937	The Cunningham chamber is dismantled for scrap metal

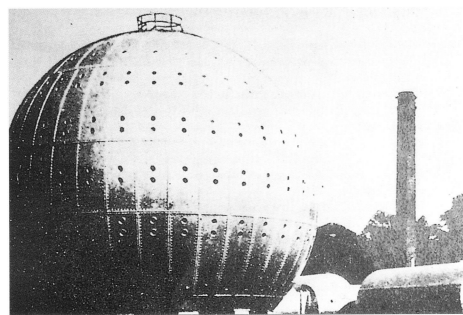

Figure 1.5
Cunningham's giant steel ball hyperbaric chamber built in 1928 in Cleveland, Ohio. It was six stories high and contained 72 rooms. (Photo courtesy of Dr. K.P. Fasecke.)

Table 1.3
Landmarks in the Development of Hyperbaric Oxygen (HBO) Therapy

1775	Discovery of oxygen by Priestley
1789	Toxic effects of oxygen reported by Lavoisier and Seguin, who discouraged use of HBO
1796	Beddoes and Watt wrote the first book on medical applications of oxygen
1878	Bert (father of pressure physiology) placed oxygen toxicity on a scientific basis; recommended normobaric but not hyperbaric oxygen for decompression sickness
1895	Haldane showed that a mouse placed in a jar containing oxygen at 2 ATA failed to develop signs of carbon monoxide intoxication.
1937	Behnke and Shaw first used HBO for treatment of decompression sickness
1938	Ozorio de Almeida and Costa (Brazil) used HBO for treatment of leprosy
1942	End and Long (USA) used HBO for treating experimental carbon monoxide poisoning in animals.
1954	Churchill-Davidson (UK) used HBO to enhance radiosensitivity of tumors
1956	Boerema (The Netherlands) father of modern hyperbaric medicine, performed cardiac surgery in a hyperbaric chamber
1960	Boerema showed life can be maintained in pigs in the absence of blood by using HBO
1960	Sharp and Smith become the first to treat human carbon monoxide poisoning by HBO
1961	Boerema and Brummelkamp used hyperbaric oxygen for treatment of gas gangrene; Smith *et al.* (UK) showed the protective effect of HBO in cerebral ischemia
1962	Illingworth (UK) showed the effectiveness of HBO in arterial occlusion in limbs
1963	First International Congress on Hyperbaric Medicine in Amsterdam
1965	Perrins (UK) showed the effectiveness of HBO in osteomyelitis
1966	Saltzman *et al* (USA) showed the effectiveness of HBO in stroke patients
1970	Boschetty and Cernoch (Czechoslovakia) used HBO for multiple sclerosis
1971	Lamm (FRG) used HBO for treatment of sudden deafness
1973	Thurston showed that HBO reduces mortality in myocardial infarction
1970s	Extensive expansion of hyperbaric facilities in Japan and the USSR
1980s	Development of hyperbaric medicine in China
1983	Formation of the American College of Hyperbaric Medicine (founder/president, late Dr. Neubauer of Florida)
1986	Undersea Medical Society (USA) adds the word hyperbaric to its name and is called UHMS. Reached a membership of 2000 in 60 countries
1987	Jain (Switzerland) demonstrated the relief of spasticity in hemiplegia due to stroke under hyperbaric oxygenation; HBO integrated with physical therapy
1988	Formation of the International Society of Hyperbaric Medicine
2001	The Undersea & Hyperbaric Medical Society established a clinical hyperbaric facility accreditation program in the USA.

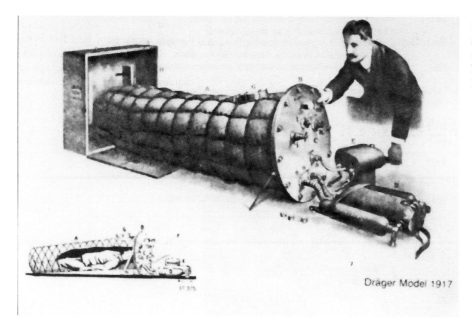

Figure 1.6
Sketch of the 1917 Dräger 2 ATA system for diving accidents, including oxygen breathing system. (Photo courtesy of Dr. Baixe, Toulon, France.)

censured by the AMA in 1928, in a report that stated: "Under the circumstances, it is not to be wondered that the Medical Profession looks askance at the 'tank treatment' and intimates that it seems tinctured much more strongly with economics than with scientific medicine. It is the mark of the scientist that he is ready to make available the evidence on which his claims are based."

Dr Cunningham was given repeated opportunities to present such evidence but never did so. A more detailed account of Cunningham's story and the history of hyperbaric medicine is to be found in Trimble (1974). The Cunningham chamber was dismantled for scrap in 1937, which brought to a temporary end the era of hyperbaric air therapy for medical disorders.

The Development of Hyperbaric Oxygen Therapy

Oxygen was not "discovered" until 1775, when the English scientist Joseph Priestley isolated what he called "dephlogis-ticated air." A more detailed history of the applications of oxygen since that time can be found in Jain (1989b). Although hyperbaric air had been used as early as 1662, oxygen was not specifically added to early hyperbaric chambers. The toxic effects of concentrated oxygen reported by Lavoisier and Seguin in 1789 were reason enough for hesitation to use it under pressure. Beddoes and Watt, who wrote the first book on oxygen therapy in 1796, completely refrained from mentioning the use of oxygen under pressure. Paul Bert, the father of pressure physiology, discovered the scientific basis of oxygen toxicity in 1878 and recommended normobaric, but not hyperbaric, oxygen for decompression sickness.

The potential benefits of using oxygen under pressure for the treatment of decompression sickness were first realized by Dräger, who in 1917 devised a system for treating diving accidents (Figure 1.6). For some unknown reason, however, Dräger's system never went into production. It was not until 1937 – the very year that Cunningham's "air chamber" hotel was demolished – that Behnke and Shaw actually used hyperbaric oxygen for the treatment of decompression sickness. The age of Hyperbaric Oxygen (HBO) therapy had finally arrived.

2 Physical, Physiological, and Biochemical Aspects of Hyperbaric Oxygenation

K.K. Jain

This chapter presents a basic scientific foundation detailing the important and interesting properties of oxygen, then surveys how these realities come into play under hyperbaric conditions. The sections involved are:

Introduction

Oxygen is the most prevalent and most important element on earth. A complete and in-depth discussion of the biochemical and physiological aspects of oxygen is available in Jain (1989b), but a brief description of how oxygen is transported and the basic physical laws governing its behavior will be useful for discussion in this book. The various terms frequently encountered in relation to oxygen include:

Partial pressure of a gas	p
Partial pressure of oxygen	pO_2
Partial pressure of oxygen in alveoli	pAO_2
Partial pressure of oxygen in arterial blood	paO_2
Partial pressure of oxygen in venous blood	pvO_2

Physical Basics

The atmosphere is a gas mixture containing by volume 20.94% oxygen, 78.08% nitrogen, 0.04% CO_2, and traces of other gases. For practical purposes air is considered to be a mixture of 21% oxygen and 79% nitrogen. The total pressure of this mixture at sea level is 760 millimeters of mercury (mmHg). Dalton's law states that in a gas mixture, each gas exerts its pressure according to its proportion of the total volume:

$$\text{partial pressure of a gas} = (\text{absolute pressure}) \times (\text{proportion of total volume of gas})$$

Thus, the partial pressure of oxygen (pO_2) in air is

$$(760) \times (21/100) = 160\,\text{mmHg}$$

Pressures exerted by gases dissolved in water or body fluids are certainly different from those produced in the gaseous phase. The concentration of a gas in a fluid is determined not only by the pressure, but also by the "solubility coefficient" of the gas. Henry's law formulates this as follows:

$$\text{concentration of a dissolved gas} = (\text{pressure}) \times (\text{solubility coefficient})$$

The solubility coefficient varies for different fluids and it is temperature-dependent, with solubility being inversely proportional to temperature. When concentration is expressed as volume of gas dissolved in each unit volume of water, and pressure is expressed in atmospheres, the solubility coefficients of the important respiratory gases at body temperature are as follows:

Oxygen:	0.024 ml O_2/ml blood atm pO_2
CO_2:	0.5 ml plasma/atm pCO_2
Nitrogen:	0.067 ml/ml plasma/atm pN_2

From this one can see that CO_2 is, remarkably, 20 times more soluble than oxygen.

Physiology of Oxygenation

The Oxygen Pathway

The oxygen pathway is shown in Figure 2.1. It passes from the ambient air to the alveolar air and continues through the pulmonary, capillary, and venous blood to the systemic arterial and capillary blood. It then moves through the interstitial and intracellular fluids to the microscopic points

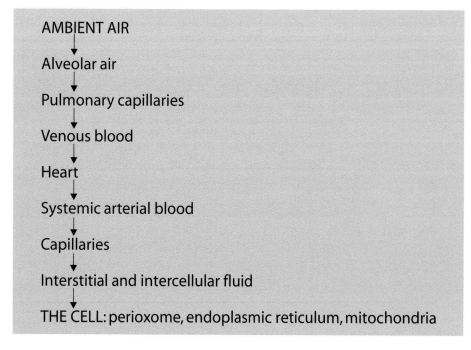

Figure 2.1
The oxygen pathway.

AMBIENT AIR
↓
Alveolar air
↓
Pulmonary capillaries
↓
Venous blood
↓
Heart
↓
Systemic arterial blood
↓
Capillaries
↓
Interstitial and intercellular fluid
↓
THE CELL: perioxome, endoplasmic reticulum, mitochondria

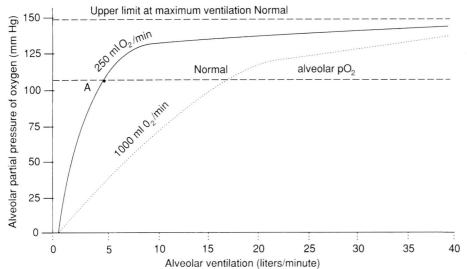

Figure 2.2
Effect of alveolar ventilation and rate on oxygen absorption from the alveoli on the alveolar pO_2.

of oxygen consumption in the perioxomes, endoplasmic reticulum, and mitochondria.

Ventilation Phase

Oxygen is continuously absorbed into the blood which moves through the lungs, and it thereby enters the systemic circulation. The effect of alveolar ventilation, and the rate of oxygen absorption from the alveoli on the pAO_2, are both shown in Figure 2.2.

At a ventilatory rate of 5 liters/min and oxygen consumption of 250 ml/min, the normal operating point is at A in Figure 2.2. The alveolar oxygen tension is maintained at 104 mmHg. During moderate exercise the rate of alveolar ventilation increases fourfold to maintain this tension, and about 1,000 ml of oxygen are absorbed per minute.

Carbon dioxide is being constantly formed in the body and discharged into the alveoli secretion is 40 mmHg. It is well known that the partial pressure of alveolar CO_2 (pCO_2) increases directly in proportion to the rate of CO_2 excretion, and decreases in inverse proportion to alveolar ventilation.

Transport Phase

The difference between pAO_2 (104 mmHg) and pvO_2 (40 mmHg), which amounts to 64 mmHg, causes oxygen to diffuse into the pulmonary blood. It is then transported, mostly in combination with hemoglobin, to the tissue capillaries, where it is released for use by the cells. There the oxygen reacts with various other nutrients to form CO_2, which enters the capillaries to be transported back to the lungs.

During strenuous exercise, the body oxygen requirement may be as much as 20 times normal, yet oxygenation of the blood does not suffer, because the diffusion capacity for oxygen increases fourfold during exercise. This rise results in part from the increased number of capillaries participating, as well as dilatation of both the capillaries and the alveoli. Another factor here is that the blood normally stays in the lung capillaries about three times as long as is necessary to cause full oxygenation. Therefore, even during the shortened time of exposure on exercise, the blood can still become nearly fully saturated with oxygen.

Normally 97% of the oxygen transported from the lungs to the tissues is carried in chemical combination with hemoglobin of red blood cells, and the remaining 3% in a dissolved state in plasma. It turns out that one gram of hemoglobin can combine with 1.34 ml oxygen from where it is removed continuously by ventilation. The normal concentration of hemoglobin is 15 g/100 ml blood. Thus, when hemoglobin is 100% saturated with oxygen, 100 ml blood can transport about 20 (i.e., 15×1.34) ml oxygen in combination with hemoglobin. Since the hemoglobin is usually only 97.5% saturated, the oxygen carried by 100 ml blood is actually 19.5 ml. However, in passing through tissue capillaries this amount is reduced by 14.5 ml (paO_2 40 mmHg and 75% oxygen saturation). Thus, under normal conditions, 5 (i.e. 19.5–14.5) ml of O_2 is transported to the tissues by 100 ml blood. On strenuous exercise, which causes the interstitial fluid pO_2 to fall as low as 15 mmHg, only 4.5 ml oxygen remains bound with hemoglobin in each 100 ml blood. Thus 15 (i.e. 19.5–4.5) ml oxygen is transferred by each 100 ml blood – three times the amount transferred under normal conditions. Since cardiac output can also increase up to six or seven times, for instance, in well-trained marathon runners, the end result is a remarkable 20-fold (i.e., $15 \times 6.6 =$ approx. 100; 100/5 = 20) increase in oxygen transport to the tissues. This is about the top limit that can be achieved.

Hemoglobin has a role in maintaining a constant pO_2 in the tissues and sets an upper limit of 40 mmHg. It usually delivers oxygen to the tissues at a rate to maintain a pO$_2$ of between 20 and 40 mmHg. In a pressurized chamber pO$_2$ may rise tenfold, but the tissue pO$_2$ changes very little. The saturation of hemoglobin can rise by only 3%, as 97% of it is already combined with oxygen. This 3% can be achieved at pO$_2$ levels of between 100 and 200 mmHg. Increasing the inspired oxygen concentration or the total pressure of inspired oxygen does not increase the hemoglobin-transported oxygen content of the blood. Thus, hemoglobin has an interesting tissue oxygen buffer function.

Shift of the Oxygen-Hemoglobin Dissociation Curve

Hemoglobin actively regulates oxygen transport through the oxygen-hemoglobin (oxyhemoglobin) dissociation curve which describes the relation between oxygen saturation or content of hemoglobin and oxygen tension at equilibrium. There is a progressive increase in the percentage of hemoglobin that is bound with oxygen as pO$_2$ increases. Bohr (1904) first showed that that the dissociation curve was sigmoid-shaped, leading Hill to postulate that there were multiple oxygen binding sites on the hemoglobin and to derive the following equation:

$$\left(\frac{\text{oxygen tension}}{\text{P50}}\right)^n = \frac{\text{oxygen saturation}}{100 - \text{oxygen saturation}}$$

where P$_{50}$ is the oxygen tension (in mmHg) when the binding sites are 50% saturated. Within the range of saturation between 15 and 95%, the sigmoid shape of the curve can

be described in the Hill coefficient and its position along the oxygen tension axis can be described by P$_{50}$ which is inversely related to the binding affinity of the hemoglobin for oxygen. The P$_{50}$ can be estimated by measuring the oxygen saturation of blood equilibrated to different levels of oxygen tension according to standard conditions and fitting the results to a straight line in logarithmic form to solve for P$_{50}$. The resulting standard P$_{50}$ is normally 26.3 mmHg in adults at sea level. It is useful for detecting abnormalities in the affinity of hemoglobin for oxygen resulting from hemoglobin variants or from disease. P$_{50}$ is increased to enhance oxygen unloading when the primary limitation to oxygen transport is peripheral, e.g., anemia. P$_{50}$ is reduced to enhance loading when the primary limitation is in the lungs, e.g., lung disease. The balance between loading and unloading is regulated by allosteric control of the P$_{50}$ and chemoreceptor control of ventilation which is matched to diffusing capacities of the lungs and the tissues. Optimal P$_{50}$ supports the highest rate of oxygen transport in health and disease.

A number of conditions can displace the oxyhemoglobin dissociation curve to the right or the left, as suggested in Figure 2.3.

Delivery of Oxygen to the Tissues

During transit from the ambient air to the cellular structures, the pO$_2$ of oxygen drops from 160 mmHg to a few mmHg in the mitochondria. This gradual drop is described as the "oxygen cascade" and is shown in Figure 2.4.

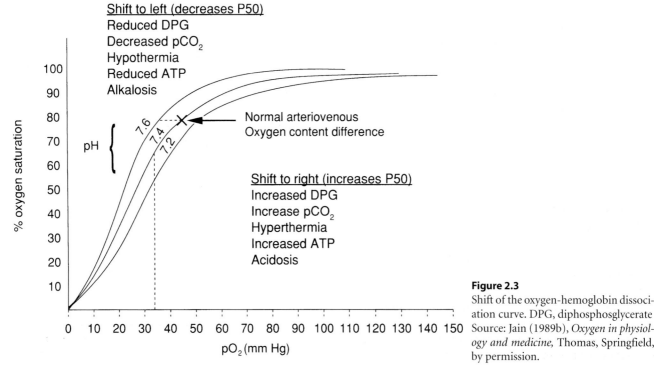

Figure 2.3
Shift of the oxygen-hemoglobin dissociation curve. DPG, diphosphosglycerate Source: Jain (1989b), *Oxygen in physiology and medicine,* Thomas, Springfield, by permission.

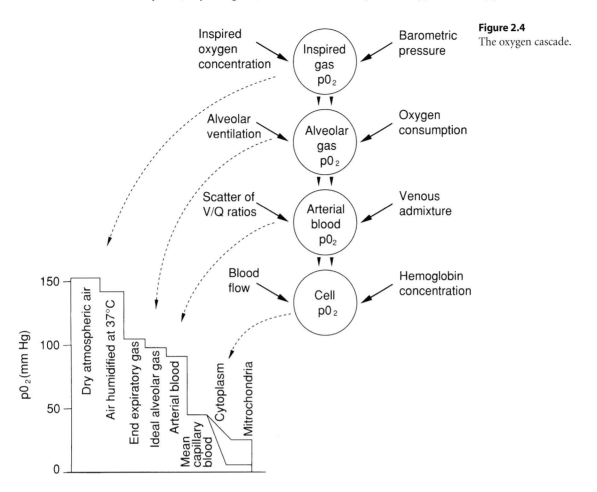

Figure 2.4
The oxygen cascade.

Oxygen Transfer at the Capillary Level

There is considerable resistance to oxygen transfer in the capillaries, and this is as significant as the resistance in the surrounding tissues.

Microvascular geometry and capillary blood flow are the most important factors responsible for regulating the oxygen supply to the tissues to meet the specific oxygen demands of organs such as the heart and brain. The tissues, of course, form the end point of the oxygen pathway. The task of the active transport system is to ensure an adequate end-capillary pO_2 so that passive diffusion of oxygen to the mitochondria is maintained.

Relation Between the Oxygen Transport and Utilization

The relationship between the transportation of oxygen and its utilization was first described long ago by Fick (1870). According to the Fick principle, oxygen consumption of the tissues (pO_2) is equal to the blood flow to the tissues (Q), multiplied by the amount of oxygen extracted by the tissue, which is the difference between the arterial and the mixed venous oxygen contents, $C(a–v)O_2$:

$$\text{Oxygen Consumption } (VO_2) = (Q) \times (C(a–v)O_2)$$

As the VO_2 of a given tissue increases, the normal response in the human body is to increase the local blood flow to the area, to maintain the local $(a–v)O_2$ content difference close to the normal range. A marked increase of $(a–v)O_2$, above 4–5 vol% is observed during physical exercise, as discussed further in Chapter 5. An increase of this magnitude in non-exercising individuals usually means an impaired circulation, inadequate to meet the increased demand of the tissues in some disease states, or it means that the oxygen content of the arterial blood is very low. The increased extraction of oxygen from the blood leads to a lower pO_2 compared to the normal level of 35–40 mmHg with O_2 saturation at 75%. Naturally the regional flow throughout the body is variable, and organs such as the heart and brain extract much more oxygen from the blood than do other organs. The brain makes up 2–3% of body weight but receives 15% of the cardiac output and 20% of the oxygen uptake of the entire body. Within the brain, cerebral blood flow and oxygen uptake vary according to the level of cerebral activity.

Oxygen Utilization in the Cell

The major site of utilization of molecular oxygen within the average cell is the mitochondria, which account for about 80%, while 20% is used by other subcellular organs, such as microsomes, nucleus, the plasma membrane, etc. Oxygen combines with electrons derived from various substrates to release free energy. This energy is used to pump H^+ ions from the inside to the outside of the mitochondria against an electrochemical gradient. As H^+ ions diffuse back, free energy is made available to phosphorylate adenosine diphosphate (ADP), and adenosine triphosphate (ATP) is generated.

Only a minute amount of oxygen is required for the normal intracellular chemical reactions to take place. The respiratory enzyme system is so geared that when tissue pO_2 is more than 1–3 mmHg, oxygen availability is no longer a limiting factor in the rate of chemical reactions. Under normal conditions, the rate of oxygen utilization by cells is controlled by the rate of energy expenditure within the cells, i.e., by the rate at which ADP is formed from ATP.

The diffusion distance from the capillary wall to the cell is rarely more than 50 μm, and normally oxygen can reach the cell quite readily. But, if pO_2 falls below the critical value of 1–3 mmHg, and if the cells are located farther away from the capillaries, the oxygen utilization is diffusion-limited and not determined by ADP. This is particularly true for cerebral white matter, which is very sensitive to hypoxia as well as hyperoxia.

Effect of Blood Flow

Since oxygen is transported to the tissues in the bloodstream, interruption of blood flow means that the amount of available oxygen to the cells also falls to zero. Under these conditions, the rate of tissue utilization of oxygen is blood-flow limited.

Effect of Oxygen-Hemoglobin Reaction on Transport of CO₂

This response, known as the Haldane effect, results from the fact that the combination of oxygen with hemoglobin causes it to become a stronger acid. This displaces CO_2 from the blood in two ways:

- When there is more acid, hemoglobin has less of a tendency to combine with CO_2 to form carbhemoglobin. Much of the CO_2 present in this form in the blood is thus displaced.
- The increased acidity of the hemoglobin causes it to release an excess of H^+ ions and these, in turn, bind with bicarbonate ions to form carbonic acid which then dissociates into water and CO_2, which is released from the blood into the alveoli.

Thus in the presence of oxygen, much less CO_2 can bind.

The Haldane effect is far more important in promoting CO_2 transport than the Bohr effect on the transport of oxygen. The combined Bohr-Haldane effect on oxygen transport is more important than on pH or CO_2 transport. Equations have been described for predicting the limits of the rates of oxygen supply to the cells of living tissues and organs. It is possible to delineate the mechanisms by which molecular oxygen is transported from the red cells while being carried in the bloodstream longitudinally through capillaries into the moving plasma, and thence radically out and through the capillary wall into the surrounding tissues for tissue cell respiration.

Autoregulation of the Intracellular pO2

Intracellular pO_2 has not as yet been measured in humans, simply due to the lack of a suitable device for doing so. Such studies have been carried out in experimentally using microelectrodes implanted in the giant neurons of aplysia (500 μm–1 mm), and comparing it with the extracellular pO_2 (EpO_2). At an EpO_2 value of +20 mmHg, the IpO_2 showed a stable value of between 4.5 and 8 mmHg. At between 10 to 50 mmHg EpO_2, IpO_2 is kept fairly constant by "autoregulation." A simple, minimally invasive method for the analysis of intracellular oxygen in live mammalian cells is available. Loading of the cells with the phosphorescent oxygen-sensing probe, MitoXpress (Luxcel Biosciences Ltd, Cork, Ireland), is achieved by passive liposomal transfer or facilitated endocytosis, followed by monitoring in standard microwell plates on a time-resolved fluorescent reader (O'Riordan et al 2007). Phosphorescence lifetime measurements provide accurate, real-time, quantitative assessment of average oxygen levels in resting cells and their alterations in response to stimulation.

Hyperbaric Oxygenation

Theoretical Considerations

Hyperbaric oxygenation (HBO) involves the use of oxygen under pressure greater than that found on earth's surface at sea level. Units commonly used to denote barometric pressure include:

mmHg	millimeters of mercury
in Hg	inches of mercury
psi	pounds per square inch

Table 2.1
Comparison of Pressure Units in Range Encountered in Hyperbaric Therapy

ATA	Absolute mmHg (torr)	pressures (bar) Pa	fsw	Gauge pressures msw	psi	atm
1	760	1.013	101.3	0	0	0	0
1.5	1140	1.519	151.9	16	5.16	7.35	0.5
2	1520	2.026	202.6	33	10.32	14.7	1
2.5	1900	2.532	253.2	50	15.48	21.05	1.5
3	2280	3.039	303.9	66	20.64	29.4	2
4	3040	4.052	405.2	99	30.97	44.0	3
5	3800	5.065	506.5	132	41.29	58.7	4
6	4560	6.078	607.8	165	51.61	73.3	5

Pa, kilo Pascal; Pascal (Newton per square meter) is the SI unit of choice.

Table 2.2
Range of Partial Pressures in Hyperbaric Therapy

Total pressure ATA	mmHg	Oxygen pressure ATA	mmHg
1	760	0.21	159.7
1.5	1140	0.31	239.4
2	1520	0.42	319.2
2.5	1900	0.53	394.0
3	2280	0.63	478.8
4	3040	0.84	638.4
5	3800	1.05	798.0
6	4560	1.26	957.6

Table 2.3
Ideal Alveolar Oxygen Pressures

Total pressure		pAO_2 breathing air	pAO_2 breathing 100% O_2
ATA	mmHg	mmHg	mmHg
1	760	102	673
1.5	1140	182	1053
2	1520	262	1433
2.5	1900	342	1813
3	2280	422	2193
4	3040	582	O_2 not adminis-
5	3800	742	tered at pressures
6	4560	902	> 3 ATA

Table 2.4
Effect of Pressure on Arterial O_2

Total pressure ATA	mmHg	Ideal dissolved oxygen content (vol%) Breathing air	Breathing 100% O_2
1	760	0.32	2.09
1.5	1140	0.61	3.26
2	1520	0.81	4.44
2.5	1900	1.06	5.62
3	2280	1.31	6.80
4	3040	1.80	O_2 not adminis-
5	3800	2.30	tered at pressures
6	4560	2.80	> 3 ATA

Values assume arterial pO_2 = alveolar pO_2 and that hemoglobin oxygen capacity of blood is 20 vol%.

kg/cm^2 kilograms per square centimeter
bar   bar
fsw, msw feet or meters of sea water
atm   atmospheres
ATA   atmospheres absolute

The only absolute pressures are those measured by a mercury barometer. In contrast, gauge pressures are a measure of difference between the pressure in a chamber and the surrounding atmospheric pressure. To convert pressure as measured by a gauge to absolute pressure (ATA) requires addition of the barometric pressure. A guide to these conversions is shown in Table 2.1. The range of partial pressures of oxygen under HBO is shown in Table 2.2, and the ideal alveolar oxygen pressures are shown in Table 2.3.

Boyle's well-known law states that if the temperature remains constant, the volume of a gas is inversely proportional to its pressure. Therefore, normal or abnormal gas-containing cavities in the body will have volume changes as HBO therapy is applied.

Density

As barometric pressure rises there is an increase in the density of the gas breathed. The effect of increased density on resting ventilation is negligible within the range of the 1.5–2.5 ATA usually used in HBO. However, with physical exertion in patients with decreased respiratory reserves or respiratory obstruction, increased density may cause gas flow problems.

Temperature

The temperature of a gas rises during compression and falls during decompression. According to Charles' law, if the volume remains constant, there is a direct relationship between absolute pressure and temperature.

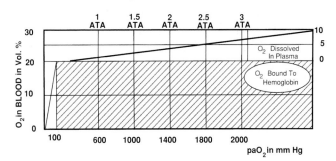

Figure 2.5
Oxygen uptake curve under HBO in humans.

Effect of Pressure on Oxygen Solubility in Blood

Only a limited amount of oxygen is dissolved in blood at normal atmospheric pressure. But, under hyperbaric conditions, as seen in Table 2.4, it is possible to dissolve sufficient oxygen, i.e., 6 vol% in plasma, to meet the usual requirements of the body. In this case oxyhemoglobin will pass unchanged from the arterial to the venous side because the oxygen physically dissolved in solution will be utilized more readily than that bound to hemoglobin. The typical arterial oxygen uptake under HBO is shown in Figure 2.5. Here the usual oxygen dissociation curve has been extended to include increases in oxygen content as a result of inspiring oxygen up to 3 ATA. The pO_2 simply rises linearly with rise of pressure.

Effect of HBO on Capillary Oxygen Pressure Drop

The oxygen extraction by average tissues of 5 vol% results in a remarkable pressure drop of 60 (100 down to 40) mmHg from the arterial end to the venous end of the capillary. At 2,000 mmHg the oxygen content is approximately 25 (20+5) vol%. The extraction of 5 vol% in this case causes a pressure drop of about 1,900 mmHg. Each of the differences in pO_2 represents the same number of oxygen molecules, in the first case carried by the hemoglobin and in the second case by the plasma. The metabolic requirement of the cells can ultimately be expressed as a certain number of molecules of oxygen per minute.

HBO and Retention of CO_2

When HBO results in venous blood being 100% saturated with oxygen, there is a rise in blood pCO_2 and a shift of pH to the acid side. This is due to loss of hemoglobin available to transport CO_2. This affects only the 20% of the venous content of CO_2 which is transported by hemoglobin. Excess CO_2 is transported by the H_2CO_3/HCO_3 mechanism, as well as by entering into physical solution in plasma. The

elevation of cerebral venous pCO_2 is of the order of 5–6 mmHg when venous hemoglobin is 100% saturated with oxygen. CO_2 does not continue to rise in venous blood and the tissues as long as the blood flow remains constant, and presents no major problems.

Tissue Oxygen Tension under HBO

Various factors relating to tissue oxygen tension under HBO are:

- Arterial pO_2 is the maximum pO_2 to which any tissue will be exposed, and plays a major part in determining the pO_2 diffusion gradient driving oxygen into the tissues. Arterial pO_2 depends on the inspired pO_2.
- Arterial pO_2 content is the total amount of oxygen available. It depends on the inspired oxygen and the blood hemoglobin level.
- Tissue blood flow regulates the delivery of oxygen to the tissues.
- Tissue oxygen levels vary according to utilization of the available oxygen.

In a *typical* tissue, arteriovenous oxygen difference rises to 350 mmHg when 100% oxygen is breathed at 3 ATA. If the blood flow to the tissues is reduced by half, the corresponding values of capillary pO_2 will be 288 mmHg and 50 mmHg. But, of course, the oxygen requirement of different tissues varies. For example, the needs of cardiac muscle are ten times that of the skin.

Another factor is the vasoconstricting effect of HBO, which reduces the blood flow. Effective cellular oxygenation can be accomplished at very low rates of blood flow when arterial pO_2 is very high.

General Effects of HBO on the Healthy Human Body

The important general effects of hyperoxia on a healthy human body are listed in Table 2.5. The effects vary according to the pressures used, the duration of exposure, and the health of the subject. Unless otherwise stated, HBO refers to the use of 100% oxygen. The effects of HBO on each system, both in health and in disease, will be discussed in chapters dealing with disorders of those systems. As an introduction, some important effects are described here briefly.

Table 2.5
Effects of Hyperoxia

I. Oxygen transport and metabolism
   1. Inactivation of the hemoglobin role in oxygen and CO_2 transport
   2. The biological burning of normal oxygen metabolism

II. Respiratory system
   1. Suppression of carotid and aortic bodies with depression of ventilation
   2. Washout of N_2 with increased susceptibility to lung collapse

III. Cardiovascular system
   1. Bradycardia
   2. Decreased cardiac output and decreased cerebral blood flow

IV. Peripheral vessels
   1. Vasoconstriction of peripheral blood vessels: brain, kidney, eye
   2. Increased peripheral resistance

V. Metabolic and biochemical
   1. Increase of CO and H ions with decrease of PH in tissues
   2. Inhibition of cell respiration
   3. Inhibition of enzymatic activity: enzymes containing SH group
   4. Increase of free radical production

Cardiovascular System

The most important study on this subject is that by Bergö (1993) which was conducted on awake rats exposed to 100% oxygen at pressures ranging from 1–5 ATA. The cardiovascular observations were made as a background to the study of the effect of HBO on cerebral blood flow. Some of the conclusions drawn were as follows:

1. Increase of systolic blood pressure with fall of diastolic pressure. Although pulse pressure was increased, the mean arterial blood pressure remained constant.
2. Decrease of heart rate and cardiac output.
3. The number of cardiac arrhythmias increased with rising oxygen pressures and exposure duration.
4. Increase of peripheral vascular resistance

In human patients, HBO results in a decrease in cardiac output (CO), due to bradycardia, rather than a reduction in stroke volume. Blood pressure remains essentially unchanged. Blood flow to most organs falls in proportion to the fall of cardiac output except to the right and the left ventricles of the heart. There is no impairment of the function of any of these organs because the raised pO_2 more than compensates for the reduction of the blood flow. Vasoconstriction may be viewed as a regulatory mechanism to protect the healthy organs from exposure to excessive pO_2. Usually the vasoconstrictor response does not take place in the hypoxic tissues.

Dermal blood flow has been shown to decrease as a response to hyperoxia; it has been measured by laser Doppler flowmetry. It was also demonstrated that the reduction of blood flow did not occur in the vicinity of a chronic skin ulcer and that the vasoconstrictor response was restored after the ulcer had healed.

HBO is considered to modify fibrinolytic activity in the blood. To clarify the stage of fibrinolytic activation by HBO exposure, Yamami et al (1996) examined its alterations in human during and after the HBO exposure. Eight healthy female volunteers breathed oxygen at 284 kPa (2.8 ATA). Blood samples were collected before compression, shortly after compression to the pressure 284 kPa, shortly before the start of decompression, shortly after decompression, and then again 3 hours after decompression. The euglobulin fibrinolytic activity (EFA) and, the activities and antigens of both tissue-type plasminogen activator (t-PA) and plasminogen activator inhibitor-1 (PAI-1) were estimated. The PAI-1 activity and PAI-1 antigen showed significant decrease after compression to a pressure 284 kPa, before the start of decompression, and after decompression. The EFA level and t-PA activity rose significantly shortly after decompression, and 3 hours later returned on baseline. These findings suggest that fibrinolytic activity is elicited after HBO rather than during HBO.

Respiratory System

Hyperoxia suppresses the respiratory reactivity to CO_2. After an initial depression of respiration, there is hyperventilation. HBO reversibly depresses the hypoxic ventilatory drive, most probably by a direct effect on the carotid CO_2 chemoreceptors.

Usually there are no differences between forced vital capacities (FVC) and maximal expiratory flows before and after hyperbaric oxygen exposure while breathing dry or humidified oxygen. However, decreases in mean expiratory flow with steady FVC have been reported after 14 days of daily hyperbaric therapy (0.24 MPa) with although 80% of the patients were symptom free and remained so 1 year after the study (Mialon et al 2001). This toxicity is clinically insignificant in subjects free of inflammatory lung diseases. HBO therapy, though safe, is not entirely without effect on the lungs.

Nervous System

Vasoconstriction and reduced cerebral blood flow do not produce any clinically observable effects in a healthy adult when pressures of 1.5 to 2.5 ATA are used. Pressures higher than 3 ATA for prolonged periods can lead to oxygen convulsions as a result of oxygen toxicity. The effects of HBO are more pronounced in hypoxic/ischemic states of the brain. HBO reduces cerebral edema and improves the function of neurons rendered inactive by ischemia/hypoxia. The improvement of brain function is reflected by the improved electrical activity of the brain. The effect of HBO on cerebral blood flow is discussed in Chapter 17.

Microcirculation

HBO improves the elasticity of the red blood cells and reduces platelet aggregation. This, combined with the ability of the plasma to carry dissolved oxygen to areas where RBCs cannot reach, has a beneficial effect on the oxygenation of many hypoxic tissues in various circulatory disorders.

Biochemical Effects of HBO

Biochemical Marker of HBO

Urine methylguanidine (MG) which is known as a uremic toxin is synthesized from creatinine. Urine MG/urine creatinine/serum creatinine ratio is used as an index of MG synthesis rate which has been shown to increase during HBO therapy in human subjects and can be used as a marker of active oxygen products in vivo (Takemura *et al* 1990).

Effect of HBO on the Acid-Base Balance

Increased partial pressure of oxygen in the blood disturbs the reduction of oxyhemoglobin to hemoglobin. Of the alkali that neutralizes the transported CO_2, 70% originates from the hemoglobin. As a result of HBO and due to increased solubility of CO_2, there is retention of CO_2 leading to a slight rise of H^+ ions in the tissues.

HBO reduces excess lactate production in hypoxic states, as well as during exercise. This important subject is discussed extensively in Chapter 5.

Effect of HBO on Enzymes

Cyclo-Oxygenase Inactivation. This results in decreased production of prostacyclin by hyperoxic tissues. A study was made in human umbilical arteries by Yamaga *et al* (1984) who showed that brief exposure of arteries to hyperoxia resulted in a 30% decrease in activity of cyclo-oxy-genase, in contrast to a 49% increase in its activity throughout the hypoxic arterial segments.

Heme oxygenase (HO). This enzyme catalyzes the rate-limiting step in the oxidative degradation of heme to biliverdin. The isoform HO-1 is inducible by a variety of agents causing oxidative stress and has been suggested to play an important role in cellular protection against oxidant-mediated cell damage. A low-level overexpression of HO-1 induced by HBO exposure provides protection against oxidative DNA damage by further exposures to HBO (Rothfuss & Speit 2002).

Tyrosine Hydroxylase. Increased oxygen saturation of this enzyme leads to increased turnover of catecholamines..Hyperoxia inhibits phenylalanine and tyrosine hydroxylase.

Succinic Dehydrogenase (SDH) and Cytochrome Oxidase (CCO). These enzymes are activated by HBO. Their levels decline in the liver and kidneys of patients with intestinal obstruction. HBO after surgery led to the normalization of the levels of these enzymes.

Effect of HBO on Free Radical Production

The role of hyperbaric oxygen (HBO) therapy in free radical-mediated tissue injury is not clear. HBO has been shown to enhance the antioxidative defense mechanisms in some animal studies, but HBO has also been reported to increase the production of oxygen free radicals. Hyperoxia causes an increase in nitric oxide (NO) synthesis as part of a response to oxidative stress. Mechanisms for neuronal nitric oxide synthase (nNOS) activation include augmentation in the association with Hsp90 and intracellular entry of calcium (Thom *et al* 2002).

Effect of HBO on Cerebral Metabolism

The most important metabolic effects of HBO are on the brain. Most of the investigations of this topic have been prompted by the problem of oxygen toxicity. It is believed that the preconvulsive period of oxygen toxicity is characterized by alterations in several interrelated physiological functions of the brain, such as electrical activity, blood flow, tissue pO_2, and metabolic activity. The relation of these changes to the development of oxygen-induced convulsions has not yet been clarified. Nonetheless, several interesting observations have been made as a result of these studies which throw some light on the effect of HBO on cerebral metabolism in the absence of clinical signs of oxygen toxicity. Most of the cerebral metabolic studies are now done on human patients with various CNS disorders. Use of brain imaging in metabolic studies is described in Chapters 17, 19, and 44.

Glucose Metabolism

Studies on regional cerebral glucose metabolic rate (rCMRgl) in rats after exposure to pressures of 1, 2, and 3 ATA. show that the degree of central nervous system effects of HBO depend upon the pressure as well as the duration of exposure. Increased utilization of glucose in some neuronal structures precedes the onset of central nervous system manifestations of oxygen toxicity. Exposure of rats to 100% oxygen at 3 ATA causes an increase in rCMRgl, and this is related to the oxygen-induced preconvulsive pattern of the electrocorticogram.

In cats HBO (3 ATA for 60 min), has a definite effect on the glycerophosphate shuttle mechanism following acute blood loss. HBO stimulates the mitochondrial glycerol-3-phosphate dehydrogenase in the sensorimotor cortex and the medulla oblongata, providing glycerol-3-phosphate dehydrogenation. There is activation of the cytoplasm hydrogen delivery to the mitochondrial respiratory chain. In addition, there is prevention of a rise in glycerol-3-phosphate and NADH levels, as well as inhibition of glycerol-3-phosphate dehydrogenase, which limits lactate production.

Energy metabolism has also been found to be highly sensitive to raised pressures of oxygen, which can reduce the formation of ATP molecules considerably.

Ammonia Metabolism

Following injury to the brain, the activity of glutaminase increases sharply, providing a release of ammonia from glutamine and a rise in transcapillary transfer of ammonia into the brain tissue from the blood. At the same time there is activation of glutamate formation pathways under the effect of glutamine dehydrogenase, and decrease of glutamine formation due to inhibition of glutamine synthase. This also leads to a decrease in the amount of α-ketoglutarate. HBO at 3 ATA for 60 min prevents ammonia toxicity from increasing in the dehematized brain. The toxic effects of ammonia ions on the brain are eliminated via:

- stimulation of the activity of the mitochondrial GDG providing glutamate formation from α-ketoglutarate
- binding of ammonia with glutamate resulting in glutamine formation
- a decrease of glutaminase activity inhibiting the process of deaminization of glutamine – a potential source of ammonia
- transcapillary discharge of ammonia in the form of glutamine from the brain to the blood

Effect of HBO at Molecular Level

Effect on DNA

Dennog et al (1996) have investigated the DNA-damaging effect of HBO with the alkaline version of the single cell gel test (comet assay). Oxidative DNA base modifications were determined by converting oxidized DNA bases to strand breaks using bacterial formamidopyrimidine-DNA glycosylase (FPG), a DNA repair enzyme, which specifically nicks DNA at sites of 8-oxo-guanines and formamidopyrimidines. HBO treatment under therapeutic conditions clearly and reproducibly induced DNA damage in leukocytes of all test subjects investigated. Increased DNA damage was found immediately at the end of the treatment, while 24 h later, no effect was found. Using FPG protein the authors detected significant oxidative base damage after HBO treatment. DNA damage was detected only after the first treatment and not after further treatments under the same conditions, indicating an increase in antioxidant defenses. DNA damage did not occur when the HBO treatment was started with a reduced treatment time which was then increased stepwise. Speit et al (1998) have shown that HBO-induced DNA strand breaks and oxidative base modifications are rapidly repaired, leading to a reduction in induced DNA effects of > 50% during the first hour. A similar decrease was found in blood taken immediately after exposure and post-incubated for 2 h at 37°C in vitro and in blood taken and analyzed 2 h after exposure, suggesting similar repair activities in vitro and in vivo. When the same blood samples showing increased DNA damage after HBO in the comet assay were analyzed in the micronucleus test, no indications of induced chromosomal breakage in cultivated leukocytes could be obtained. The results suggest that the HBO-induced DNA effects observed with the comet assay are efficiently repaired and are not manifested as detectable chromosome damage.

Conclusions

The practical significance of many of the general effects of HBO is not clear. The study of the effects on cerebral metabolism was motivated by a search for the mechanism of oxygen-induced seizures. High pressures such as 6 ATA have been used which have no clinical relevance; the pressures for treatment of cerebral disorders usually do not exceed 2 ATA. The optimal pressure for treating patients with brain injury is 1.5 ATA. The cerebral glucose metabolism is balanced at this pressure. Raising the pressure even only to 2 ATA has unfavorable effects.

Generally HBO therapy is safe and well tolerated by humans at 1.5–2 ATA. The duration of exposure and the percentage of oxygen also have a bearing. No adverse effects are seen at 1.5 ATA for exposures up to 40–60 min.

3 Effects of Diving and High Pressure on the Human Body

K.K. Jain

This chapter examines physiological responses to variations in environmental pressure. In addition to detailing effects on specific body systems, the symptoms and treatments related to a variety of pressure-induced medical conditions are presented. The sections involved are:

Physical Effects of Pressure

When human beings descend beneath the surface of the sea, they are subjected to tremendous pressure increases. To keep the thorax from collapsing, air must be supplied under high pressure, which exposes the blood in the lungs to extremely high alveolar gas pressures. This is known as hyperbarism. Workers in caissons, for example, must work in pressurized areas.

Relation of Sea Depth to Pressure. A vertical column of sea water 33 feet (approximately 10 m) high exerts the same absolute pressure as that of the atmosphere at sea level (760 mmHg, as measured by a mercury barometer) and referred to as 1 ATA or 1.013 bar. Therefore, a person 33 feet beneath the surface of the sea is exposed to a pressure of 2 ATA (1 ATA caused by the weight of the water and 1 ATA by the air above the water) and a dive to 66 feet involves exposure to pressure of 3 ATA. Studies in diving medicine may refer to a dive to so many feet or the diver being subjected to so many ATA or bar. Similar terms are used to described simulations in hyperbaric chambers.

Effect of Depth on Volume of Gases. Boyle's law states that the volume to which a given quantity of gas is compressed is inversely proportional to the pressure. Thus 1.0 L of air at sea level is compressed to 0.5 L at 10 m (33 feet).

The effects of pressure on the human body vary according to the following factors:
1. Total pressure
2. Duration of exposure to pressure
3. State of activity of the diver resting or exercising
4. Temperature
5. Drugs in the body
6. Gas mixtures used
7. Rate of descent

Effects of Pressure on Various Systems of the Body

Hematological and Biochemical Effects

A 14-day exposure to 5.2% oxygen and nitrogen at pressure of 4 ATA has been shown to cause hemoconcentration with slight elevation of Hb, Hct, RBC, plasma proteins, and cholesterol because of a decrease of plasma volume with diuresis. Loss of intracellular fluid has been observed, but this reverses partially during the postexposure period. Weight loss has been observed in divers compressed to 49.5 ATA (488 msw) in He-oxygen environments. This loss was shown to be 3.7 to 10.2 kg in 14 days of hyperbaric exposure.

Diuresis occurs in practically all saturation dives and is associated with natriuresis at pressures greater than 31 ATA. Three mechanisms may be involved in the development of this diuresis):

- Inhibition of ADH release
- Inhibition of tubular reabsorption of NA^+ (pressure inhibits active transcapillary transport of NA^+)
- Inhibition of hydrostatic action of ADH on the tubules

Fluid loss induced by diving and/or weightlessness might also add substantially to the pressure-induced diuresis. Because the sense of thirst is impaired in hyperbaric environments, and the resultant fluid imbalance reduces performance of divers, counter measures against fluid loss should be taken during operational saturation diving.

Effect on Ammonia Metabolism

Long-term exposure to hyperbaric conditions has been shown to increase blood urea in US Navy divers. This is interpreted as evidence of hyperammonemia, because urea is formed with ammonia buffering.

Effect on Blood Cells and Platelets

Increase of neutrophils, blood platelets and fibrinogen concentration in the blood plasma immediately after diving is of temporary character, being a typical reaction observed during diving (Olszanski et al 2002). The values usually return to normal spontaneously. Environmental stress such as cold water may contribute to platelet activation, which plays an important role in the pathogenesis of prethrombotic states and thus may be responsible for decompression illness during compressed air diving.

Changes in the Respiratory System and Blood Gases

Breathing mixtures with normal oxygen content at pressures up to 60 bar produces moderate changes in respiration, compared with the pattern of respiration at normal ambient pressure. At pressures over 80 to 100 bar, oxygen transport is likely to be compromised by changes in hemoglobin affinity. Breathing high concentrations of oxygen (pO_2 over 500 mbar) leads to retention of CO_2 in the tissues, which, in turn, leads to hyperventilation. However, if the subject is exercising, reduced chemoreceptor activity leads to impaired alveolar ventilation.

Rapid changes in environmental pressure produce an inequality between inspiratory and expiratory volumes; compression causes hypercapnia while decompression causes hypocapnia. The following influence the respiratory effects of pressure:

- Position of the diver. The upright position causes less dyspnea than the prone position.
- Physical activity, which increases the tendency for CO_2 accumulation
- Gas density. The higher the density of the gas mixture breathed the greater the airway resistance is; it therefore requires more energy to breath denser mixtures.

If the diver uses a face mask, the breathing gas should provide a static lung load of approximately 0 to +10 cm of water (0 to 0.01 ATA) regardless of the diver's orientation in the water. The increased ventilation observed in experimental animals breathing He-oxygen mixtures at extremely high pressures (up to 10 MPa) is responsible for fatigue of the respiratory muscles, and may lead to ventilatory failure.

Adaptation has been shown to occur during a 14-day exposure to a high nitrogen pressure environment of 4 ATA with naturally inspired oxygen tensions. This modification of respiratory control is exemplified by a diminished ventilatory response to CO_2. The diminished response is more likely related to the density of respiratory gas than to the narcotic influence of the respired nitrogen.

Multiple diving exposures affect both the vital capacity and the forced rotatory flow rate of smaller lung volumes. This is evidence for the narrowing of the airways that may be secondary to diving-induced loss of elasticity of the lung tissue. A longitudinal study of lung function in military oxygen divers showed that substantial exposure to elevated oxygen partial pressure while diving is not associated with an accelerated decline in lung function (Tetzlaff *et al* 2005). Factors other than hyperoxia (e.g., venous gas microemboli and altered breathing gas characteristics) may account for the long-term effects that have been found in professional divers.

Hypoxic states usually do not occur in divers, but the response of divers to hypoxia is the same as that of nondivers. The effects of repeated acute exposures to breathing 100% oxygen at pressure – such as those encountered during oxygen diving – may affect the peripheral oxygen chemosensors.

Effects on the Cardiovascular System

Exposure to hyperbaric environments has been shown to cause a variety of disturbances in the electrical activity of the mammalian heart. Arrhythmias under these conditions are considered to be the result of an increase in parasympathetic tone. Increased hydrostatic pressure also decreases excitability and conduction through direct effects on the myocardial cell membrane. Hyperbaric exposure alters cardiac excitation-contraction coupling in anesthetized cats during He-oxygen dives to 305 msw.

Some conclusions of the studies of the effects of moderate hyperbaric exposure on the rat heart are as follows:

1. Cardiac contractility is increased during hyperbaric exposures despite administration of calcium and sodium channel blockers, thus reducing the possibility of involvement of these channels in the mechanism of this effect. Starling's mechanism or neurotransmitter involvement was also excluded.
2. Repeated hyperbaric exposures causes hypertrophy of the heart
3. Left ventricular pressure increased at 5 bar and the degree of rise varied with the breathing gases used.
4. Heart rate remained unchanged in all normoxic experiments.

Doppler-echocardiographic studies in healthy divers indicate that circulating gas bubbles are associated with cardiac changes, suggesting a right ventricular overload and an impairment of ventricular diastolic performance. Postdive humoral and hematologic changes are consistent with the hypothesis that "silent" gas bubbles may damage pulmonary endothelium and activate the reactive systems of the human body.

The increased environmental pressure seems responsible of the hemodynamic rearrangement causing reduction of cardiac output seen in diving humans because most of changes are observed during diving (Marabotti *et al* 2008), Left ventricular diastolic function changes suggest a constrictive effect on the heart possibly accounting for cardiac output reduction.

Changes in the Endocrine System

The following changes in the endocrine function can occur as a result of hyperbaric exposures exceeding 4 ATA (30 msw) while breathing 6.2% nitrogen in oxygen:

1. Increase in the circulating levels of epinephrine, norepinephrine, and dopamine
2. Decrease in ADH secretion without a change in aldosterone excretion
3. Severe hyperbaric conditions associated with deep dives have a profound effect on male reproductive function due to fall in the quality of semen and oligozoospermia.
4. Decrease of thyroxine levels in the blood
5. Increase in the insulin and angiotensin I level in plasma
6. Increase in the circulating concentration of atrial naturetic factor (ANF, a diuretic hormone). This may explain the diuresis observed in divers. The endocrine reactions as well as the accompanying reductions in cognitive performance in divers, however, may be the result of emotional reactions to the dive rather than the direct effect of nitrogen narcosis.

Effect on the Skeletal System

Dysbaric osteonecrosis is a type of avascular necrosis caused by ischemia and subsequent infarction of bone. This usually involves the head of the femur. The disruption of blood flow in bone has been attributed to the formation of nitrogen bubbles as a result of diving but blood pressure at the femoral head has been shown to be reduced by prolonged exposure to compressed air. Dysbaric osteonecrosis has been reorted in 25% of workers who perform in high-pressure environments (Cimsit *et al* 2007).

Effects of High Pressure Environments on the Nervous System

Neuropsychological Effects

Scuba diving was shown to have adverse long-term neuropsychological effects only when performed in extreme conditions, i.e. cold water, with more than 100 dives per year, and maximal depth below 40m (Slosman *et al* 2004). Deterioration of both mental and motor function has been reported in dives to 10 and 13 ATA – while breathing air and at rest.

Hyperbaric air at 7 ATA does not impair short-term or long-term memory in test subjects, but long-term memory is impaired at 10 ATA, although it recovers on switching to an 80/20 He-oxygen mixture.

A study of non-saturation construction divers did not reveal clear evidence of neuropsychological deficit due to repeated diving but it is suggested that the prolonged reaction time can be ascribed to extensive non-saturation diving (Bast-Pettersen 1999). Middle-aged divers who are exposed to critical depths of more than 60 msw, have navigational problems and the number of brain lesions detected on MRI can be related to the number of hyperbaric exposures (Leplow *et al* 2001).There is a belief among occupational divers that a "punch drunk" effect is produced by prolonged compressed air diving. Most of the studies on this topic have serious limitations in statistical analysis and use of control groups. Dementia is recognized as a complication of severe hypoxia, cerebral embolism, or cerebral decompression sickness, but temporary neurological insults experienced by divers breathing compressed air are not translated into hard evidence of brain damage.

Nitrogen Narcosis

Behnke noted in 1935 that humans subjected to compressed air above 5 ATA exhibited symptoms similar to alcohol intoxication. As the symptoms were immediate in onset and did not occur when He-oxygen mixtures were used, Behnke concluded that nitrogen was the causal agent. Since then many investigators have studied this phenomenon which Cousteau calls "l'ivresse des grandes profondeurs" or "rapture of the depths." The symptoms of nitrogen narcosis are euphoria, dulled mental ability, difficulty in assimilating facts, and quick decision-making.

Many suggestions have been made to explain the narcotic effects of inert gases, but the most satisfactory explanation seems to be the degree of lipid solubility. Auditory evoked potential studies ave been used to assess the degree of narcosis induced by diving and indicate that nitrogen is the major cause of compressed air narcosis and that oxygen does not have a synergistic effect with nitrogen. Some of the noble gases which have been substituted for nitrogen also tend to cause some narcosis, but to a much lesser degree. Nitrogen and a raised CO_2 tension in the tissues as a result of hypoventilation and impaired CO_2 elimination are the causes of narcosis, but they can also cause a deterioration in the performance of the affected diver. Increasing the oxygen partial pressure and the density of the breathing mixture causes retention of the carbon dioxide in the cerebral tissues and synergistically potentiates the nitrogen narcosis.

Most of these studies were carried out under hyperbaric conditions although nitrous oxide is known to be an inducer of narcosis at atmospheric pressure as well. One study has compared two narcotic environments; a normobaric narcosis under several percentages of nitrous oxide, and an hyperbaric narcosis under 0.9 MPa of Nitrox in rats that hat to press a lever to get rewarded (Turle-Lorenzo *et al* 1999). The results showed significant performance decreases: the number of pressed lever are reduced by 50% under Nitrox and by 70% under N_2O. Nitrous oxide could thus be considered as a normobaric model of hyperbaric narcosis.

Effects of anesthetics and high pressure nitrogen can be compared. Conventional anesthetics, including inhalational agents and inert gases, such as xenon and nitrous oxide, interact directly with ion channel neurotransmitter receptors. However, there is no evidence that nitrogen, which only exhibits narcotic potency at increased pressure, may act by a similar mechanism; rather nitrogen at increased pressure might interact directly with the GABA(A) receptor (David *et al* 2001). Repetitive exposures to nitrogen narcosis produce a sensitization of postsynaptic N-methyl M-D-Aspartate receptors on dopaminergic cells, related to a decreased glutamatergic input in substantia nigra pars compacta (Lavoute *et al* 2008). Consequently, successive nitrogen narcosis exposures disrupt ion channel receptor activity revealing a persistent nitrogen-induced neurochemical change underlying the pathologic process.

Diving deeper than 100 m cannot be done breathing air, as the nitrogen contained in such a mixture becomes narcotic at pressures greater than 6 ATA. In order to avoid nitrogen narcosis, mixtures of helium and oxygen (heliox) are used, and this permits dives beyond 100 m.

High Pressure Neurological Syndrome

This subject has been reviewed in detail elsewhere (Jain 1994; Jain 2009a). High pressure neurological syndrome (HPNS) is a condition encountered in deep diving beyond a depth of 100 m which is made possible by breathing of special gas mixtures such as helium and oxygen (heliox). It is characterized by neurological, psychological, and electroencephalographic abnormalities.

Clinical features of HPNS have been reviewed by several authors and can be summarized as follows:

I. Symptoms
  1. Headache
  2. Vertigo
  3. Nausea
  4. Fatigue
  5. Euphoria
II. Signs
  A. Neurological
    1. Tremor
    2. Opsoclonus
    3. Myoclonus
    4. Dysmetria
    5. Hyperreflexia
    6. Sleep disorders
    7. Convulsions (only in experimental animals)
  B. Neuropsychological
    1. Memory impairment
    2. Cognitive deficits
III. Electroencephalographic disturbances

Pathophysiology of HPNS

HPNS is primarily a result of excessive atmospheric pressure on different structures in the central nervous system. The rate of compression influences the manifestations of HPNS; a faster rate of compression increases the intensity of HPNS and decreases the pressure threshold for the onset of symptoms. The manifestations persist during a stay at a constant depth and decrease during decompression. The symptoms usually subside after the pressure is normalized, but some of these, such as lethargy, may linger on for days. In some cases, complaints such as memory disturbances take several months to resolve. Eventually all of the divers who experience only HPNS recover. There is no evidence of permanent neurological sequelae or histopathological changes in the brain resulting from HPNS.

Sensitivity of the nervous system to high pressures may be compensated by a physiological adaptive response. Synaptic depression that requires less transmitter turnover may serve as an energy-saving mechanism when enzymes and membrane pumps activity are slowed down at pressure (Talpalar & Grossman 2006). Lethargy and fatigue, as well as reduction in cognitive and memory functions, are compatible with this state. Maladaptation to high pressure may lead to a pathophysiological response, i.e., HPNS. Some of the neurological signs may be an unmasking of previously silent brain lesions as a result of DCS. Various neurological manifestations appear at different depths. Tremor is seen at 200 to 300 m, myoclonus at 300 to 500 m, and EEG abnormalities are noted at 200 to 400 m.

Psychotic-like episodes in divers exposed to high pressure have been attributed to either the HPNS, confinement in pressure chamber, the subject's personality, or the addition of nitrogen or hydrogen to the basic helium-oxygen breathing mixture used for deep diving. Alternatively, it is suggested that these disorders are in fact paroxysmal narcotic symptoms that result from the sum of the individual narcotic potencies of each inert gas in the breathing mixture. This hypothesis has been tested against a variety of lipid solubility theories of narcosis and the results clearly support the hypothesis that there are cellular interactions between inert gases at raised pressure and pressure itself.

Role of Neurotransmitters in the Pathogenesis of HPNS

Various neurotransmitters and amino acids have been implicated in the pathogenesis of HPNS: GABA, dopamine, serotonin (5-HT), acetylcholine, and glutamate. Conclusions from various studies on this subject are:

1. Various neurological and behavioral disturbances of HPNS are regulated by different mechanisms in the same areas of the brain.
2. Neurotransmitter interactions in HPNS differ in various parts of the brain.
3. The biochemical substrates for epileptic and HPNS-associated convulsions are different, for example, adenosine compounds protect against epilepsy but not against HPNS seizures.

The motor symptoms of HPNS are attributed to changes in neural excitability at spinal and midbrain levels. Serotonin may be implicated in hyperbaric spinal cord hyperexcitability. Quinolinic acid and kynurenine are metabolites of 5-HT that have been proposed as endogenous convulsants. The precise balance between these two may be an important determinant of onset of HPNS.

The clinical features of serotonin syndrome are changes in mental status, restlessness, myoclonus, hyper-reflexia, shivering, and tremor. Behavioral changes in rats exposed to pressure resemble serotonin syndrome and are consistent with the activation of 5-HT receptor subtype 1A.

Prevention and Management of HPNS

Measures for the prevention and management of HPNS are as follows:

1. Reduction of the speed of compression
2. Modifications and additions to breathing gas mixtures: addition of nitrogen or hydrogen to heliox
3. Anesthetics
4. Barbiturates
5. Anticonvulsant drugs
6. Non-anesthetic compounds

A promising pharmacological approach is based on the resemblance of HPNS to serotonin syndrome. 5-HT$_{1A}$ receptor antagonists may provide a promising approach to prevent HPNS.

Headaches in Divers

Headaches in divers are uncommon include benign causes such as exertion, cold stimulus, migraine, and tension as well as serious causes such as decompression sickness, air embolism and and otic or paranasal sinus barotrauma (Cheshire & Ott 2001). Inadequate ventilation of compressed gases can lead to carbon dioxide accumulation, cerebral vasodilatation, and headache. A case of an cerebral aneurysm rupture associated with barotrauma has been reported (Reichardt et al 2003). It is unclear whether volume expansion of trapped air, the blood pressure increase associated with barotrauma, or systemic vasodilation caused the aneurysm to rupture in this case. Correct diagnosis and appropriate treatment require a careful history and neurologic examination as well as an understanding of the unique physiologic stresses of the subaquatic environment.

Central Nervous System (CNS) Lesions in Divers

Decompression sickness is described in Chapter 10. Amateur divers may, however, have small CNS lesions which may accumulate with time. A controlled study on amateur divers, showed that hyperintense lesions of the subcortical white matter as demonstrated on MRI scan, are more common in divers than in normal controls (Reul et al 1995). These results differ from studies on saturation divers who have fewer such lesions than control subjects, even though neurological manifestations are more common among divers. Professional saturation diving involves breathing of helium/oxygen mixtures rather than compressed air as in the case of amateur divers. It is possible that MRI lesions in amateur divers are due to intravascular gas microbubbles. The only direct evidence for this is the demonstration by fluorescein angiography of pathological changes in the retinal microvasculature of divers even when they have not experienced decompression sickness.

Microbubble Damage to the Blood-Brain Barrier

Myelin damage has been discovered at the autopsy of divers with no recorded incidence of neurological decompression syndrome during life. Hyalinization of cerebral vessels has also been described in divers. Subtle neuropsychological changes in divers have not always been correlated with any pathology in the brain.

James and Hill (1988) have proposed that as divers undergo decompression microbubbles (15 ± 5 mm) pass the pulmonary filter into the cerebral arterial circulation and impair the blood-brain barrier, leading to extravasation of protein and focal cerebral edema. This can account for the myelin damage and cerebral vascular pathology in divers. This observation has important implications in the pathophysiology and management of some CNS disorders such as multiple sclerosis.

Effect of Pressure on the Peripheral Nerve Conduction Velocity

Moderate pressure has been shown to increase nerve conduction velocity and amplitude in experimental animals, whereas high pressures depress these parameters. Various studies of nerve conduction velocities of divers at depth have concluded:

1. There is no significant correlation between slow sensory conduction and hyperbaric pressure.
2. Distal motor latencies increase with increases in hyperbaric pressure as well as with decreases in ambient temperature.
3. The effect of pressure is independent of the temperature
4. No significant changes were detected in the main nerve trunk proximal to the wrist, or in the F-wave response.
5. The effect on peripheral nerves may contribute to the reduced work capacity of divers at depth.

Effect of Hyperbaric Pressure on Autonomic Nerve Functions

Autonomic nerve functions under severe hyperbaric pressure were evaluated by measuring heart rate variability and catecholamine excretion rate in 16 normal volunteers in submarine experimental facilities simulating conditions 330 m below sea level (Kurita et al 2002). HRV and urinary catecholamine levels were evaluated to assess sympathetic and parasympathetic tone. There was significant negative correlation between HRV and urinary catecholamine levels. Evaluation of autonomic nerve functions under hyperbaric conditions by measuring HRV was shown to be a useful method. Thus, the present results indicate that the autonomic nerve functions of people who work under deep-sea conditions can be evaluated adequately by measuring HRV.

Hearing and Vestibular Impairment in Hyperbaric Environments

Hearing loss in professional divers is well known. A general etiological classification of hearing loss that is associated with hyperbaric environments is shown in Table 3.1. The hearing threshold in water appears to be 20 to 60 dB higher than in air. In the hyperbaric chamber, application of pressure on the middle ear or the external ear causes temporary impairment of hearing – especially in the low frequency range. At 4 to 11 ATA in hyperbaric air the threshold of hearing is raised to 30 to 40 dB – proportional to the pressure. In a heliox environment at 31 ATA, the hearing loss does not exceed 30 to 40 dB. The conclusions of a study by Farmer *et al* (1971) on this subject are:

- Humans with patent Eustachian tubes, exposed to hyperbaric heliox conditions, develop a conductive hearing loss related to depth.
- After 6 days of exposure at a depth of 600 ft, there is less variation in the hearing levels and a greater loss in the lower frequencies.
- Sensory-neural auditory functions, as measured by sensory acuity levels and frequency differences, are not altered by hyperbaric heliox exposures up to 19.2 ATA.
- The conductive hearing loss is assumed to be the result of an increased impedance of the middle ear transformer in the denser atmosphere plus an upward shift in the ear resonance frequency in a helium atmosphere

Damage to the Middle Ear and Inner Ear in Diving

The pressure changes that are encountered in diving can cause damage to the ear in at least three distinctly different ways:

- Middle ear barotrauma of descent
- Middle ear barotrauma as a manifestation of pulmonary barotrauma during ascent
- Inner ear barotrauma

Middle ear barotrauma occurs during descent when there is a failure to equalize the middle ear and the ambient pressures by means of the Eustachian tube. When this occurs, there may be bleeding in the middle ear and even rupture of the ear drum. Forceful autoinflation of the middle ear (Valsalva maneuver) during descent may cause rupture of the round window membrane and leakage of perilymph into the middle ear. Damage to the inner ear may occur by decompression sickness, that is, release of dissolved nitrogen bubbles during ascent from a deep dive. It can lead to hearing loss and dizziness. This damage is usually unilateral and can be reversed with prompt recompression procedure, including HBO therapy. Barotrauma of the ear has been shown to be preventable by myringotomy (puncture of the tympanic membrane) before the dive.

Money *et al* (1985) examined the temporal bones of divers who died of unrelated causes, but had a history of barotrauma of the ears. Their classical findings, shown in Figures 3.1 and 3.2, are very similar to experimental findings in monkeys subjected to barotrauma. They also found new bone formation in the inner ear following decompression sickness and consider that it may have been responsible for the late onset of hearing deficits.

Professional diving may cause a more rapid deterioration of high frequency hearing loss than is seen in the general population. An audiometric survey of abalone divers showed that over 60% of them suffered from high frequency deafness unacceptable by the Australian standards. The hearing loss was unilateral in one-half of the cases and bilateral in the rest (Edmonds 1985).

Wilkes *et al* (1989) subjected minipigs to a compression-decompression profile that was considered to be safe for compressed air workers. There was loss of hearing as well

---

Table 3.1
Hearing Loss Related to Hyperbaric Environments: An Etiological Classification

Conductive
Hearing acuity under hyperbaric conditions
    Under water
    Hyperbaric chamber
Obstruction to the external ear
Tympanic membrane perforation
    Middle ear barotrauma of descent
    Shock wave
    Forceful autoinflation
Middle ear cleft
    Middle ear barotrauma of descent
    Otitis media
    Forceful autoinflation

Sensorineural
Inner ear barotrauma
Otologic problems occurring at depths
Otologic decompression sickness
Noise-induced deafness

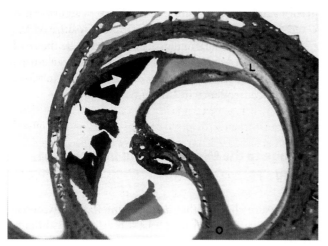

Figure 3.1
Blood in the middle turn of the cochlea (*white arrow*) in a diver following decompression sickness. Postmortem examination.
L: spiral ligament
O: osseous spiral lamina

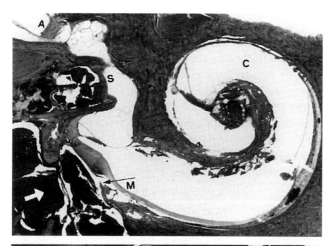

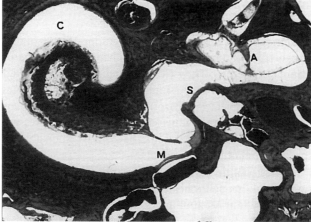

Figure 3.2 a, b
Middle and inner ears, left (**top**) and right (**bottom**) of a diver who died underwater from unknown causes. Left ear has the round window membrane (**M**) ripped (**black arrow**) and the middle ear is filled with blood (**white arrow**). C, cochlea; A, lateral ampullary crista; S, footplate of stapes. (Photos courtesy of Dr. K.E. Money, reproduced from Money *et al* 1985).

as loss of hair cells in the cochlea of all the compressed animals.

Vertigo and Diving

Because of the close anatomical relationship between the hearing organ and the vestibular apparatus, vestibular disorders like dizziness and vertigo are frequently associated with barotrauma of the ear. Inner ear barotraumas and decompression sickness may cause acute vestibular symptoms in divers. The result may be irreversible damage to the vestibular end organs or their central connections. An etiological classification of vertigo in divers is shown in Table 3.2.

In a survey of divers and non-diver controls, the prevalence of dizziness (28%), spinning vertigo (14%), and unsteady gait (25%) was significantly higher in divers than controls (Goplen *et al* 2007). These symptoms were strongly associated with a previous history of DCS, particularly type I, which was reported by 61% of the divers. Symptoms were less strongly associated with the number of dives. In divers with dizziness, the prevalence of abnormal postural sway, nystagmus, canal paresis, or pathological smooth pursuit was 32%,

Table 3.2
Vertigo in Diving: An Etiological Classification

Due to Unequal Vestibular Stimulation
1. Caloric
   Unilateral external auditory canal obstruction
   a) Cerumen
   b) Otitis externa
   c) Miscellaneous causes
   Tympanic membrane perforation
   a) Shock wave
   b) Middle ear barotrauma of descent
   c) Forceful autoinflation
2. Barotrauma external and/or middle ear
   a) External ear barotrauma of descent
   b) Middle ear barotrauma of descent
   c) Middle ear barotrauma of ascent
   d) Forceful inflation
3. Inner ear barotrauma
   a) Fistulas of the round window
   b) Fistulas of the oval window
4. Decompression sickness
   a) Peripheral decompression sickness
   b) Central decompression sickness
5. Air embolism
6. Miscellaneous causes

Due to Unequal Vestibular Responses
1. Caloric
2. Barotrauma
3. Abnormal gas pressures
4. Sensory deprivation

(According to Caruso *et al* 1977)

9%, 7%, and 11%, respectively. Among the reasons for the high prevalence of vestibular symptoms among the divers, the high exposure to DCS is probably an important factor.

Inert gas narcosis may lead to balance disturbances and nystagmus.) Velocity of the slow component of the vestibular ocular reflex, as determined by electronystagmography (ENG) increases by 50% after inhalation of 25% nitrous oxide. Caloric tests conducted during saturation dives to 450 msw (4.6 mPa) while breathing trimix do not show any significant nystagmus upon ENG.

Taste Sensation Under High Pressure

Significant changes in taste sensation have been shown to occur on exposure to heliox at 18.6 ATA. These changes include:

- Increased sensitivity to sweetness
- Increased sensitivity to bitter taste
- Decline of sour sensitivity
- Decrease of salt sensitivity

Effect of High Pressure on Effect of Drugs

The efficiency of a number of drugs is affected by pressure – usually manifested as a decrease in activity – but the results may be unpredictable. High pressure has been reported to reduce the efficiency of drugs which act on cell membranes, such as anesthetics, tranquilizers, and narcotics. This effect is ascribed to the pressure changes affecting the cell membrane itself. The major enzyme involved in drug metabolism is cytochrome P-450 which is bound to the cell membrane. The effect of pressure on the membrane may be differential. The so-called "pressure of anesthesia" may be due to an antagonism, not only on a pharmacological level, but also on a physiological level via increased sensory feedback under high pressure.

Dimenhydrate (Pharmacia's Dramamine), an antihistamine, often is taken by divers to control seasickness. Its effects in the hyperbaric environment have been poorly studied, although decrements in learning were reported. One study has shown that dimenhydrate adversely affects mental flexibility and that depth adversely affects memory (Taylor *et al* 2000). It is likely that these effects in combination increase the risk to scuba divers. Divers who suffer from severe seasickness may have to take dimenhydrate to avoid the miseries of this condition, but they would be wise to incorporate extra margins of safety into planning dives.

Information on the manner in which high pressure affects the drug disposition in the body is scarce.

Conclusions

Important effects of pressure on the human body have been reviewed. This may be of interest to physicians who treat complications of diving with HBO. For those interested in diving medicine, several excellent texts are available including that by Bennett and Elliot (2003). The most important effect of high pressure is on the nervous system. This should be distinguished from oxygen toxicity. The major complication of diving, decompression sickness, is discussed in Chapter 10 and cerebral air embolization is described in Chapter 11.

4 Physical Exercise Under Hyperbaric Conditions

K.K. Jain

This chapter investigates the role of exercise under normoxic and hyperbaric conditions, as well as the impact of greatly reduced supplies of oxygen. These results help set the stage for later detailed analyses of the strengths and limits of HBO therapy itself. The main sections of this chapter are:

Introduction

Oxygen plays an important role in exercise physiology, and this extensive subject was discussed in an earlier book (Jain 1989b). The following brief account of what happens during exercise under normoxic conditions serves as an important introduction to the effects of hyperbaric conditions on physical exercise.

The dynamic transition among different metabolic rates of V O2 (V O2 kinetics), initiated, for example, at exercise onset, provides a unique window into understanding metabolic control. Because of interfiber type differences in O2 supply relative to V O2, the presence of much lower O2 levels in the microcirculation supplying fast-twitch muscle fibers, and the demonstrated metabolic sensitivity of muscle to O2, it is possible that fiber type recruitment profiles might help explain the slowing of V O2 kinetics at higher work rates and in chronic diseases (Poole et al 2008).

Oxygen demands on the body can of course increase dramatically during exercise. Our normal oxygen consumption of about 150 ml/min might rise to 1000 ml/min during moderate exercise, even though alveolar pO_2 is maintained at 104 mmHg. This situation is achieved by a fourfold increase of alveolar ventilation. During strenuous physical activity, such as a marathon race, the body's oxygen requirements may be 20 times normal, yet oxygenation of the blood does not suffer. There is, however, tissue hypoxia in some of the working muscles and strenuous exercise may be considered as a hypoxic episode. The response to physical exercise is outlined in Table 4.1. Physical activity, in the form of voluntary wheel running, induces gene expression changes in the brain. Animals that exercise show an increase in brain-derived neurotrophic factor, a molecule that increases neuronal survival, enhances learning, and protects against cognitive decline. Microarray analysis of gene expression provides further support that exercise enhances and supports brain function.

Exercise Under Hypoxia

Some decline in pO_2 may occur during intensive exercise, particularly in individuals with high $VO_{2\,max}$. Whether this can be termed "hypoxia" or not is controversial. Exercise is not considered to be hypoxia unless the pO_2 falls below the critical level of 40 mmHg. Exercise is hypoxic under the following circumstances:

- Exhausting exercise by normal individuals in normoxic environments
- Exercise at high altitudes
- Exposure to carbon monoxide in the atmosphere
- In patients with chronic obstructive pulmonary disease.

Table 4.1
Effects of Physical Exercise on the Human Body

System	Acute Effects (in untrained subjects)	Effects of Chronic Dynamic Exercise
Cardiovascular	Tachycardia Rise of cardiac output from 5 to 30 l/min	Bradycardia Increase of stroke volume of the heart Increase of heart size Increase of myocardial capillary to fiber ratio
Respiratory	Rise of alveolar ventilation linearly with rise of O_2 uptake Increased work of respiratory muscles, using up 10% of total O_2 uptake	Increase of number of alveoli available for O_2 exchange Increase of extraction fraction of (a-v) O_2 difference
Blood	Hemoconcentration due to fluid loss Reduction of O_2 saturation (5%) Rise of ammonia and lactate	Increase of hemoglobin Increase of 2,3-diphosphoglycerate Less accumulation of ammonia and lactate
Metabolism		Raised anaerobic thresholds Increased utilization of FFA Increased intracellular pools of ATP and phosphocreatine
Skeletal muscle		Increase of maximal blood flow rate Increase of mitochondrial volume and oxidative enzymes Increase of capillary density
Brain		Increase of cerebral blood flow Increase in brain-derived neurotrophic factor Enhances leaning and prevents cognitive decline.

Table 4.2
Effects on the Human Body of Exercise Under Hypoxic Conditions

Cardiovascular System
– Increase of cardiac output and muscle blood flow compared with normoxic conditions)

Respiratory System
– Increase of ventilation
– Increase in oxygen consumption
– No appreciable change in alveolar and arterial CO_2 transport

Metabolic
– Increase of "excess lactate"
– Increase of ammonia formation

The effects of physical exercise under hypoxic conditions are shown in Table 4.2.

The main changes in chronic hypoxia in relation to exercise are:

1. Decrease in arterial saturation (due to a fall of inspired oxygen pressure)
2. Decrease in maximal cardiac output (due to a fall of maximal heart rate)
3. Increase in hemoglobin concentration
4. Decrease in the maximal oxygen flow through muscle capillaries
5. Change in respiratory potential of the muscles due to loss of oxidative enzymes.

Exercise in Hyperbaric Environments

The study of human work performance in hyperbaric environments is important for evaluating the effects of diving on the human body. The effects of physical exercise while diving depend upon the following key factors:

1. Pressure to which the diver is subjected
2. Composition of the breathing mixture
3. Type of activity e.g., swimming, walking underwater, or operating a machine
4. Body posture, e.g., vertical or prone
5. Ambient temperature.

The increase of VO_2 under hyperbaric conditions corresponds to the rise in oxygen needs. The oxygen consumption during a standard exercise at 5 ATA of air is higher than at 1 ATA. The main reason for this is the increase of respiratory resistance due to a rise of gas density. Whereas the total oxygen consumption at 1 ATA comprises 81.5%

of the total oxygen needs, this value decreases to 73.9% at 5 ATA. Factors that limit work capacity at depth include:

1. Increased respiratory resistance to breathing dense gases
2. Increased energy cost of ventilation
3. Carbon dioxide retention
4. Dyspnea
5. Adverse cardiovascular changes.

Exercise in hyperbaric environments depresses the heart rate. Part of this depression is due to the effects on the heart of a rise in the partial pressure of oxygen, both directly and via the parasympathetic efferents. In addition, other factors such as gas density, high inert gas pressure, or hydrostatic pressure may interfere with sympathetic stimulation of the heart.

A reduction of ventilation and bradycardia during exercise under 2 ATA in air has been attributed to the increase in gas density.

Hyperbaric conditions are known to increase the subjective feeling of fatigue in divers. there is a decrease of vigilance and a subjective feeling of change in the body functions of divers who undergo saturation dives to simulated pressures of 40 ATA. This feeling is more pronounced during compression and saturation, and decreased during compression.

Exercise Under Hyperoxia

Hyperoxia here refers to the use of raised oxygen fractions in the inspired air, but at a pressure not higher than 1 ATA.

The results may vary according to the method used to achieve hyperoxia, i.e., whether the hyperoxia is achieved

Table 4.3
Effect on the Human Body of Physical Exercise Under Hyperoxic Conditions

1. Cardiovascular response
   a) Variable decrease of heart rate
   b) Decrease of blood flow to the exercising limb to offset the raised O_2 tension
2. Pulmonary function
   a) Reduction of pulmonary ventilation
   b) Decrease of oxygen consumption compared with exercise under normoxia
3. Biochemical
   a) H^+ ion concentration is higher than during exercise under normoxia
   b) Reduction of excess lactate
4. Energy metabolism
   a) Decreased rate of glucose utilization and lactate production
   b) Shift of respiratory quotient toward fat metabolism, thus lowering RQ

by breathing a gas with high fractional concentration of oxygen at sea level, or by the study being carried out in a pressure chamber. The response to exercise at a given arterial pO_2 is not the same under these two conditions. Performance increases with increasing pO_2 under both conditions, but in hyperbaric studies performance levels were somewhere between 200 and 400 mmHg. In hyperoxia at 1 ATA, performance increases continuously as pO_2 increases. Increased gas density in the hyperbaric environment increases the work of breathing and compromises performance at high pressures. The effects of hyperoxia on exercise and the possible mechanisms involved are listed in Table 4.3. Cardiovascular function during exercise under hypoxia is described in Chapter 24.

Exercise studies on healthy volunteers have shown that leg $VO_{2\,max}$ is limited by oxygen supply during normoxia but it does not increase during hyperoxia in proportion to either the femoral venous pO_2 or mean leg capillary pO_2.

Physical Exercise Under Hyperbaric Conditions

General Effects

The effects of physical exercise under hyperbaric oxygenation (HBO) are often quite difficult to evaluate, due to the variable interaction of three factors: oxygen, pressure, and exercise. The effects of these factors are better known when applied individually. HBO at 1.5 ATA accentuates some of the effects of normobaric hyperoxia, but higher pressures may cancel some of the advantages of HBO such as reduction of the metabolic complications of exhausting physical exercise. Most of the studies on this topic have concentrated on the metabolic aspects, particularly the lactate accumulation in the blood, which can be easily measured.

A decrease of ventilation and some bradycardia is usually observed while exercising under HBO conditions. $VO_{2\,max}$ increases by 3% during exercise while breathing 100% O_2 at 1 ATA, but does not increase further when the pressure is raised to 3 ATA. There are no changes in oxygen consumption or oxygen extraction during exercise under HBO at 2 ATA, as compared with exercise while breathing normobaric air.

The (a–v)O_2 difference is the same in healthy young volunteers whether they exercise breathing normal air or under HBO at 3 ATA (pAO_2 1877 mmHg). It appears probable, therefore, that the maximum oxygen uptake in active muscles does not increase when the arterial oxygen content is increased. Thus, the maximum oxygen uptake in an active muscle seems not to be limited by the blood flow to the muscle or the oxygen diffusion from the blood to the interior of the muscle cell, but rather by the oxygen utilization system inside the cell.

Effect on Lactate Production and Clearance

Studied of the effect of HBO (3 ATA) on excess lactate production during exercise in dogs show that the values of excess lactate are much lower than those observed during previous exercise by the same animals at 1 ATA while breathing air. If exercise is conducted under HBO first, not only is the excess lactate low, but it remains so during subsequent exercise at 1 ATA breathing air 45 min later. Three mechanisms for this effect are:

- Oxygen provided to the exercising muscles during hyperoxia is sufficient to lower the excess lactate formation. It counteracts the hypoxia that usually results while exercising at atmospheric pressure, and is responsible for the production of lactic acid.
- There is increased removal of excess lactate as a result of stimulation of the oxidative enzymatic process.
- HBO produces inhibition of glycolytic sulfhydryl enzymes. This results in an improvement of glycolysis, and therefore in lowered lactate formation. Such an inhibitory effect could well persist for up to 45 min and explain the continual decrease of excess lactate after HBO exposure when exercise under atmospheric air followed.

The myocardium and liver of dogs exercised under 3 ATA HBO can eliminate the increased amount of lactate at the expense of glucose consumption.

Studies of the blood chemistry parameters in healthy adult volunteers who exercised while breathing air, normobaric oxygen, and oxygen at 1.5 ATA revealed that in the rest period following exercise, uric acid, lactate, and pyruvate decreased significantly compared with the levels after exercise without HBO. The drop in the level of ammonia was less. However, the ammonia levels 1 min and 15 min after exercise under HBO were much lower than the corresponding values during exercise while breathing normobaric oxygen (see Figure 4.1). Lactate levels immediately after exercise (1–20 min) were lower during exercise while breathing oxygen than during exercise in room air. Lactate levels were lower during exercise under HBO than they had been 1, 5, 10, and 15 min previously after exercise, breathing normobaric oxygen. The rise of excess lactate was less after ergometry under HBO than after ergometry under oxygen breathing. The excess lactate (XL) was calculated according to the formula:

$$XL = (Ln - Lo) - (Pn - Po)\frac{Lo}{Po}$$

where Lo is the resting and Ln the exercise blood lactate, and Po and Pn are the resting and exercise blood pyruvate values, respectively. There was a fall of glucose during exercise under HBO, suggesting inhibition of glycolysis, which is a contributory factor to the rise in the level of ammonia. Inhibition of glycolysis should lead to diminu-

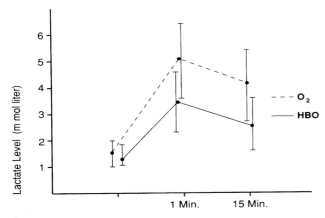

Figure 4.1
Effect of physical exercise on lactate levels under normobaric oxygenation (---O₂) and hyperbaric oxygenation (—HBO). Arterial blood lactate levels were determined before treadmill exertion as well as 1 min and 15 min following the completion of exercise.

tion of uricemia. Whether there is stimulation or depression of the Krebs cycle at 1.5 ATA HBO remains to be determined. But in any case, the tendency of ammonia levels to fall is striking. These findings tend to support the hypothesis that more glycogenic amino acids go into the citric acid cycle than does α-ketoglutaric acid.

Effect of Exercise on Ammonia Metabolism

Lactate accumulation is well known as a factor in causing fatigue and limiting the capacity for physical exertion. However, the role of ammonia in causing fatigue is not quite so clear.

At rest skeletal muscle is consistently an ammonia consumer with a clearance of approximately 0.3 mmol/kg wet wt/min by resting muscle. Assuming that the body is 40% muscle, there is 8 mmol/min uptake by the resting muscle. Ammonia levels are known to rise steeply following muscular exertion, but they decline spontaneously in a short time in healthy adults. Hyperammonemia of exercise is due mainly to a release of ammonia from muscles during the recovery phase. As muscle pH returns to the resting level, more ammonia diffuses from the muscle into the blood. If the ammonia levels do not subside promptly, untoward effects may be experienced by a person doing exhaustive physical exercise. This is likely to happen in untrained persons with neurological disorders. Healthy young athletes usually do not suffer from "ammonia hangover."

Ammonia levels are lower in those exercising under HBO compared with those exercising under normobaric conditions. The mechanism by which HBO lowers ammonia levels in the blood is not clear. Ammonia is formed in the body by deamination of amino acids where the amino group is transferred to α-ketoglutaric acid, which becomes glutamic acid and may release ammonia again. Most of the ammonia is removed from the blood by conversion to urea in the liver. HBO has been shown to lower blood ammonia in hepatic encephalopathy (see Chapter 26). Blood urea can be lowered in volunteers exercising under HBO, an effect attributed to inhibition of glycolysis.

Effect of HBO on Antioxidant Enzyme Skeletal Muscle

In skeletal muscle the activity of the enzymatic antioxidants superoxide dismutase (SOD), glutathione peroxidase (GPx), and catalase (CAT) is regulated in response to generation of reactive oxygen species (ROS). Increased activity of these enzymes is observed after repeated bouts of aerobic exercise, a potent stimulus for intracellular ROS production. Although ROS formation in response to vigorous physical exertion can result in oxidative stress, ROS also play an important role as signaling molecules (Niess and Simon 2007). ROS modulate contractile function in unfatigued and fatigued skeletal muscle. Furthermore, involvement of ROS in the modulation of gene expression via redox-sensitive transcription pathways represents an important regulatory mechanism, which has been suggested to be involved in the process of training adaptation.

HBO inhalation also stimulates intracellular ROS production although the effects of HBO on skeletal muscle SOD, GPx and CAT activity have not been studied. In adult male rats acute HBO inhalation at 3 ATA reduced catalase activity by approximately 51% in slow-twitch soleus muscles (Gregorevic et al 2001). Additionally, repeated HBO inhalation (twice daily for 28 days) increased Mn^{2+}-superoxide dismutase activity by approximately 241% in fast-twitch extensor digitorum longus muscles. Thus both acute and repeated HBO inhalation can alter enzymatic antioxidant activity in skeletal muscles.

Physical Exercise in Relation to Toxic Effects of HBO

The toxic effects of oxygen are not usually seen during HBO below pressures of 3 ATA. Concern has been expressed that physical exercise may predispose patients to oxygen toxicity.

Breathing oxygen at 2 ATA during exercise lowered ventilation and restores arterial pH and pCO_2 toward resting levels. There is either a slight elevation of cerebral blood flow or a diminished rate of cerebral oxygen consumption during exercise while breathing oxygen at 2 ATA, without gross elevation of cerebral venous pO_2.

Physical exercise is accompanied by a rise in body temperature that may increase the possibility of oxygen toxicity. In the hyperbaric chamber, the temperature is usually controlled and this factor is eliminated. Peripheral vaso-constriction usually limits blood flow and oxygen delivery under hyperoxia, but exercise may have a vasodilating effect which might allow exposure of the tissues to high oxygen concentrations.

Conclusions

Although HBO reduces the biochemical disturbances resulting from physical exertion, it has not been shown that HBO extends human physical performance. The duration of time to physical exhaustion does not decrease in the hyperbaric chamber. Unlike other methods that elevate oxygen content of the blood, acute HBO exposure appears to have no significant effect on subsequent high-intensity running or lifting performance (Rozenek *et al* 2007). However, HBO, by facilitating biochemical recovery after exhaustive exercise, may shorten the recovery time from exhaustion. Further studies need to be done on this topic to determine the role of HBO in the training of athletes. The current knowledge may also help in using HBO for the rehabilitation of patients with neurological disability, such as hemiplegia and paraplegia, as HBO may enable these patients to undertake more strenuous exercise than possible for them under normobaric conditions.

5 Hypoxia

K.K. Jain

Tissue hypoxia plays an important role in the pathogenesis of many disorders, particularly those of the brain. Correction of hypoxia by hyperbaric oxygenation is, therefore, an important adjunct in the treatment of those disorders. This chapter looks at:

Introduction

The term "hypoxia" generally means a reduced supply of oxygen in the living organism. In contrast, "anoxia" implies a total lack of oxygen, although the word is sometimes used as a synonym for hypoxia. It is difficult to define hypoxia precisely, but it may be described as a state in which aerobic metabolism is reduced by a fall of pO_2 within the mitochondria. In this situation, the partial pressure of oxygen, which in dry air is 160 mmHg, drops to about 1 mmHg, by the time it reaches the mitochondria of the cell. Below this value aerobic metabolism is not possible.

The subject of hypoxia has been dealt with in detail elsewhere (Jain 1989b). A few important aspects should be discussed here because relative tissue hypoxia is frequently the common denominator of many diseases that are amenable to HBO therapy.

Pathophysiology of Hypoxia

Within the cell, 80% of the total oxygen consumption is by mitochondria, and 20% by a variety of other subcellular organs. The biochemical reactions in these locations serve a variety of biosynthetic, biodegradative, and detoxificatory oxidations. Some of the enzymes involved in the synthesis of neurotransmitters have low affinities for oxygen and are impaired by moderate depletions of oxygen. Some of the manifestations of oxygen depletion are related to "transmitter failure" (decreased availability of transmitter), rather than bioenergetic failure. The disturbances that lead to decreased oxygen supply could operate at any of the three phases mentioned in Chapter 2, i.e.,

- The respiratory phase,
- The phase of oxygen transport, or
- The phase of oxygen use by the tissues.

Hypoxia can potentiate injury due to oxidative stress. The proposed sequences are shown in Figure 5.1.

Effect of Hypoxia on Cellular Metabolism

Hypoxia depresses mitochondrial oxidative phosphorylation. Creatine phosphorylase is released, as evidenced by sarcolemmal damage during hypoxia. This process is considered to be calcium-mediated, because calcium channel blockers protect the cell from hypoxic damage.

A rapid decline in ATP levels under hypoxic conditions may cause an increase in calcium flux into the cytosol because of inhibition of the calcium pump in the plasma membrane, mitochondria, and endoplasmic reticulum. Alternatively, ATP may be metabolized to hypoxanthine, a substrate for superoxide anion formation.

Barcroft (1920) classified hypoxia as follows:

- Hypoxic: includes all types of hypoxia in which not enough oxygen reaches the alveoli
- Anemic: caused by inadequate hemoglobin or abnormal hemoglobin, so that not enough oxygen can be transported to the tissues
- Stagnant or circulatory: blood flow is inadequate to carry the oxygen to the tissues.
- Histotoxic: the tissues cannot use the oxygen even though it reaches the tissues in adequate quantities.

The causes of hypoxia are shown in Table 5.1.

General Impact of Hypoxia

The effects of hypoxia vary in accordance with its cause, whether the situation is acute or chronic, and also with the overall state of health of the individual in question.

Cellular hypoxia may develop in multiple organ failure syndrome because of the increased oxygen demand at the tissue level and/or because the ability to extract oxygen at the cellular level is decreased. Restoration of oxygen transport and metabolic support are important components of treatment.

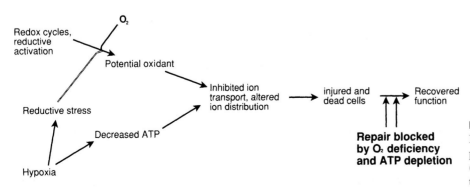

Figure 5.1
Proposed sequence in which hypoxia potentiates injury due to oxidative stress (Jones 1985, by permission of the author).

Table 5.1
Causes of Hypoxia

I. Inadequate oxygenation in the lungs
1. Deficient oxygen in the atmosphere: high altitudes, closed spaces
2. Hypoventilation:
   a) Respiratory muscle paralysis or weakness due to neuromuscular or neurological diseases
   b) Extreme obesity
   c) Central depression of respiration due to the effect of sedatives, narcotics or anesthetic
3. Pulmonary disorders:
   a) Chronic obstructive pulmonary disease, such as: chronic bronchitis and emphysema, hypoxic cor pulmonale
   b) Restrictive lung disease: adult respiratory distress syndrome, chest injuries, deformities of the chest and the thoracic spine
4. Sleep disordered breathing: Sleep apnea, snoring, nocturnal hypoxia
5. Increased demand of tissues beyond normal supply (relative hypoxia): Exercise, inflammation, and hyperthermia

II. Inadequate transport and delivery of oxygen
1. Carriage of oxygen combined with hemoglobin:
   a) Anemia; reduced RBC
   b) Reduced effective hemoglobin concentration: COHb, MetHb, etc.
2. Increased affinity of hemoglobin for oxygen:
   a) Reduced DPG in RBC
   b) Reduced temperature
   c) Increased pH of blood
3. Circulatory disorders:
   a) Global decrease of cardiac output
   b) Systemic arteriovenous shunts; right to left cardiac shunts
   c) Maldistribution of cardiac output; regional circulatory disturbances
4. Disturbances of hemorrheology and microcirculation:
   a) Increased viscosity
   b) RBC disease: decreased surface, stiff cell membrane, etc.

III. Capability of tissue to use oxygen is inadequate
1. Cellular enzyme poisoning: cytochrome P-450 and a3 cytochrome oxidase
2. Reduced cellular enzymes because of vitamin deficiency

(Reproduced from K.K. Jain: *Oxygen in Physiology and Medicine*. Thomas, Springfield, Illinois 1989b. By permission of the publisher).

Respiratory Function

Hypoxia initially leads to an increase in the respiratory rate, but later the rate is decreased. It remains controversial whether there is depression of the respiratory center, decreased central chemoreceptor pCO_2, or both. Respiratory depression is likely due to a fall in tissue pCO_2 resulting from an increase in blood flow caused by hypoxia.

In hypoxia caused by hypoventilation, CO_2 transfer between alveoli and the atmosphere is affected as much as oxygen transfer, and hypercapnia results, i.e., excess CO_2 accumulates in the body fluids. When alveolar pCO_2 rises above 60–75 mmHg, dyspnea becomes severe, and at 80–100 mmHg stupor results. Death can result if pCO_2 rises to 100–150 mmHg.

Cardiovascular System

Circulatory responses to hypoxia have been studied mainly in the laboratory animals and a few conclusions that can be drawn are as follows:

- The local vascular effect of hypoxic vasodilation is probably common to all but the pulmonary vessels. It is strongest in active tissues (heart, brain, working skeletal muscle) that are dependent on oxygen for their metabolism.
- A chemoreceptor reflex produces an increase in cardiac contractility as well as selective vasoconstriction that supports arterial pressure and some redistribution of cardiac output.
- The overall response to hypoxia involves an increase in cardiac output and selective vasodilation and vasoconstriction in an attempt to maintain oxygen delivery and perfusion pressure to all organs.

General Metabolic Effects

The following disturbances have been observed as a result of experimental hypoxia produced in animals:

- Appearance of excess lactate in the blood
- Appearance of 2,3-DPG in the blood of animals exposed to hypoxia of high altitudes
- Higher plasma levels of corticosterone, leading to neoglucogenesis
- Decrease of long-chain unsaturated fatty acids in the blood sera of rats adapted to hypoxia

Effects of Hypoxia on the Brain

Although any part of the body can be affected by hypoxia, the effects are most marked on the cells of the central nervous system, for the following key reasons:

- The brain has unusually high resting energy requirements, which can only be met by oxidative breakdown of the exogenous substrate. Anaerobic production of energy by glycolysis is not adequate to maintain normal brain function.
- The brain cannot store oxygen. Its energy reserves are

low and usually it cannot tolerate anoxia (due to lack of circulation) for more than 3 min.

- The brain, unlike muscle tissue, is incapable of increasing the number of capillaries per unit of volume.
- Neurons have a poor capacity to recover or regenerate after dysoxia.

Cerebral Metabolism

Basic Considerations

Cerebral metabolism, particularly that of oxygen, is closely tied in with cerebral blood flow (CBF). The brain, although it makes up only 2% of the body weight, consumes 20% of the oxygen taken in by the body and receives 15% of the cardiac output. This is a remarkably high oxygen consumption, considering that the brain, unlike the heart muscle, does not perform any physical work.

Cerebral metabolism is depicted by another term, glucose oxidation quotient (GOQ). It denotes the ratio:

$$\text{AVD of Glucose} - \text{AVD of Lactate (in mg/dl)} :$$
$$\text{AVD Oxygen (in vol\%)}$$

where AVD is the arterio-venous difference. Normally this value is 1.34, because 1.0 ml of oxygen oxidizes 1.34 mg of glucose.

Cell energy metabolism is simply a balance between use of adenosine triphosphate (ATP) during the performance of work and its resynthesis in anabolic sequence, which provides the energy required to rephosphorylate adenosine diphosphate (ADP). The resulting energy metabolism is depicted by the following equations:

Energy utilization:
$$ATP + H_2O > ADP + \text{Phosphate} + \text{energy}$$

Energy production:
$$ADP + \text{Phosphate} + \text{energy} \rightarrow ATP + H_2O$$

The brain produces about as much CO_2 as it consumes in oxygen; i.e., the respiratory quotient is close to 1.0. On a molar basis, the brain uses a remarkable six times as much oxygen as glucose. Glucose is normally the sole substrate and is completely utilized.

The rate of electron transport, and thereby of oxygen use, is determined by the rate of consumption of ATP and the rate of accumulation of ADP and P_i. Most studies in humans have shown that oxygen consumed accounts for only 90%–95% of the glucose extracted, leading to the view that 5%–10% of the glucose extracted by the brain is metabolized to lactic acid. The cause of this is not known, but it may be an "emergency metabolic exercise" by the brain.

Pathways of cerebral metabolism (glycolysis, the citrus cycle, and the GABA pathway) are shown in Figure 5.2.

Glycolysis includes a series of enzymatic reactions by which the cytoplasmic glucose is built into 2 molecules of lactate. Thus no oxygen is necessary, but nicotinamide adenine dinucleotide (NAD^+) is required. In all, glycolysis produces 2 molecules of NADH and ATP from each molecule of glucose. Under aerobic conditions, pyruvate is decarboxylated oxidatively:

$$\text{pyruvate} + CoA + NAD^+ \rightarrow \text{acetyl CoA} + NADH + CO_2$$

Acetyl CoA is transported in the mitochondria and goes into the citrus cycle; NADH is oxidized through mitochondrial electron transfer. Pyruvate and several other products of intermediate metabolism are oxidized through the citrate cycle, whereby the hydrogen of NAD^+ and flavine adenine dinucleotide (FAD) is carried over by substrate specific dehydrogenases. In summary, the balance of the cycle is:

$$\text{acetyl CoA} + NAD^+ + FAD + GDP + P_i + 2 H_2O \rightarrow 3 NADH$$
$$+ FADH_2 + GTP + 2 CO_2 + 2 H^+CoA$$

where lactate is the end product of the glycolytic reaction, we obtain:

$$\text{glucose} + 2 ADP + 2 P_i \rightarrow 2 ATP + 2 \text{ lactate}$$

If we add up all ATP formed from the oxidation of 1 molecule of glucose, we find the following balance:

$$\text{glucose} + 6 CO_2 + 38 ADP + 38 P_i > 6 CO_2 + 44 H_2O + 38 ATP$$

Thus the complete oxidation of a glucose molecule provides 19 times as much ATP as anaerobic glycolysis.

The key enzyme for the regulation of the rate of glycolysis is phosphofructokinase, which is activated by P_i, adenosine monophosphate (AMP), cyclic AMO (cAMP), ADP, and ammonia. It is inhibited by ATP and citrate.

Glucose degradation is partly regulated by glucose availability. In the presence of glucose, norepinephrine-induced glycogenolysis is blocked despite elevations in cAMP.

On the whole, the brain energy turnover is 7 molecules/min. One molecule of ATP contains 29.7 kJ of energy.

It is postulated that the relative concentration of adenine nucleotide, also expressed as energy charge (EC), has the most important metabolic regulatory effect:

$$\frac{EC + ATP + \frac{1}{2}ADP}{AMP + ADP + ATP}$$

Under physiological conditions this quotient generally has a value between 0.85 and 0.95, and this value falls significantly in cerebral ischemia.

The GABA Shunt

It has been shown that 10% of the carbon atoms from pyruvate molecules are metabolized via the GABA shunt. When coupled with the aspartate aminotransferase (AST) reaction, aspartate formation results:

$$\text{glutamate} + \text{oxaloacetate} > \text{aspartate} + \alpha\text{-ketoglutarate}$$

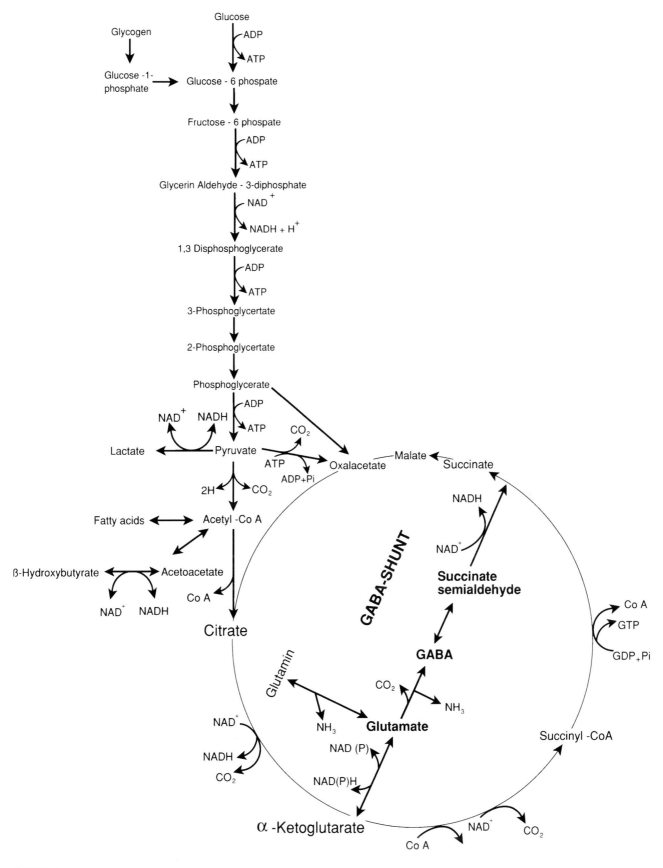

Figure 5.2
Glycolytic pathway, critic acid cycle, and GABA shunt.

Two associated reactions give rise to the formation of glutamine and alanine:

$$glutamate + NH_3 + ATP \rightarrow glutamine + ADP + P_i$$
$$pyruvate + glutamate \rightarrow \alpha\text{-ketoglutarate} + alanine$$

The GABA shunt pathway and its associated reactions allow the synthesis of glutamate, GABA, aspartate, alanine, and glutamine from ammonia and carbohydrate precursors. They have two main functions: detoxification of ammonia, and resynthesis of amino acid transmitters that are lost from neurons during functional activity.

Pyruvate and the Citric Acid Cycle

Under some conditions pyruvate can be introduced into the citric acid cycle via pyruvate decarboxylase or malate dehydrogenase. Pyruvate dehydrogenase is an intramitochondrial enzyme complex that catalyzes the conversion of pyruvate into acetyl CoA and CO_2. The proportion of pyruvate dehydrogenase in active form in the brain mitochondria changes inversely with changes in mitochondrial energy charge. Normally there is a slight excess of pyruvate dehydrogenase in comparison with pyruvate flux, as the brain usually depends on carbohydrate utilization.

Cerebral Metabolism During Hypoxia

During tissue hypoxia, molecular oxygen or the final receptor of hydrogen is reduced. This results in diminution in the amount of hydrogen which can reach the molecular oxygen via the respiratory chain. As a sequel, not only is the oxidative energy production reduced, but the redox systems are shifted to the reduced side with ensuing tissue acidosis.

The reduction of oxidative ATP formation leads to an increase of nonoxidative energy production, i.e., by glycolysis due to decrease of the ATP/AMP quotient. The increased glycolysis results in an accumulation of pyruvate and NADH within the cytoplasm of the cell. Since triose phosphate dehydrogenase is an enzyme of glycolysis dependent on NAD, the activity of this enzyme, and thus of the glycolytic pathways, requires NAD within the cytoplasm for maintenance of the cell function.

Under hypoxic conditions NAD is provided within the cytoplasm by means of the following reaction catalyzed by lactate dehydrogenase:

$$pyruvate + NADH \rightarrow lactate + NAD$$

This causes a reduction of intracellular pyruvate and NADH concentration, and a supply of NAD and lactate. Whereas lactate, the final product of glycolysis, is bound, NAD is made available as hydrogen receptor to the triose phosphate dehydrogenase. This is how glycolysis, with its relatively low energy production, may be maintained even under hypoxic conditions. This biochemical process is extremely valuable for the structural conservation of the neurons under hypoxic conditions.

Hypoxia also disturbs the acid-base balance of the tissues by an increase of H^+ ion concentration and an excess of lactate as a result of intensified glycolysis. It affects the cytoplasmic NADH/NAD as well as lactate/pyruvate ratios, as expressed in the following equation:

$$\frac{lactate}{pyruvate} \times \frac{K}{H} = \frac{NADH}{NAD}$$

where K is an equilibrium constant. The redox system is shifted to the reduced side. There is increased pyruvate concentration, which, however, falls short of the increase in lactate.

In total anoxia the glycolysis increases four to seven times. There is decrease of glucose, glucose-6-phosphate, and fructose-hexose phosphate, and an increase of all substrates from fructose diphosphate to lactate. These changes can be interpreted as resulting from facilitation of phosphorylation of glucose to fructose-hexose phosphate.

Studies with labeled glucose uptake in the brain under hypoxic conditions show that the hippocampus, the white matter, the superior colliculi, and the geniculate bodies are the areas most sensitive to the effects of hypoxia. The rela-

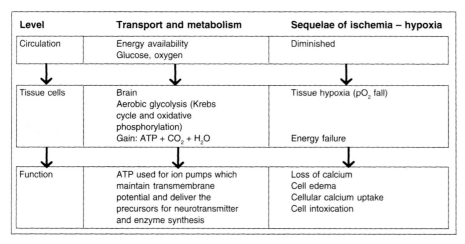

Level	Transport and metabolism	Sequelae of ischemia – hypoxia
Circulation	Energy availability Glucose, oxygen	Diminished
Tissue cells	Brain Aerobic glycolysis (Krebs cycle and oxidative phosphorylation) Gain: ATP + CO_2 + H_2O	Tissue hypoxia (pO_2 fall) Energy failure
Function	ATP used for ion pumps which maintain transmembrane potential and deliver the precursors for neurotransmitter and enzyme synthesis	Loss of calcium Cell edema Cellular calcium uptake Cell intoxication

Figure 5.3
A three-stage model of ischemic-hypoxic disturbances of the brain.

tively greater sensitivity of the white matter to hypoxia may lead to an understanding of the white matter damage in postanoxic leukoencephalopathy and its possible prevention with HBO. The relative paucity of capillaries in white matter may predispose them to compression by edema.

Anoxia and hypoxia have different effects on the brain. In hypoxia, the oxidative metabolism of the brain is impaired but not abolished. A three-stage model of ischemic hypoxic disturbances of the brain is shown in Figure 5.3.

Changes in Neurotransmitter Metabolism

The following changes in neurotransmitter metabolism during hypoxia are particularly significant:

Synthesis of acetylcholine is impaired by hypoxia. Decrease of acetylcholine following cerebral hypoxia correlates with impairment of memory and learning processes. Indirect evidence for this includes the ameliorating effect of cholinergic drugs in cerebral insufficiency due to hypoxia.

Reduction of brain catecholamines. Norepinephrine, epinephrine, and dopamine are synthesized by a combination of tyrosine and oxygen. Hypoxia limits this biosynthesis; the turnover of 5-HT is reduced. A reduction has also been observed in the synthesis of glucose-derived amino acids.

Disturbances of CBF Regulation

In the normal person CBF remains constant in spite of variations in blood pressure up to a certain extent by virtue of autoregulation. This reflects an inherent capacity of the brain to regulate the circulation according to its requirements. The arteries and arterioles contract when the blood pressure rises, and dilate when the blood pressure falls. Hypoxia impairs and blocks this critical mechanism; indeed, there may be marked vasodilatation in the hypoxic brain. Thus, the blood supply of the affected brain region is dependent upon the prevailing blood pressure. The disruption of autoregulation accompanied by focal ischemia and peripheral hyperemia is called the "luxury perfusion syndrome." Following hypoxia, CBF increases as much as twofold initially, but the blood flow increase is blunted somewhat by a decreasing arterial Pco2 as a result of the hypoxia-induced hyperventilatory response (Xu & Lamanna 2006). After a few days, however, CBF begins to fall back toward baseline levels as the blood oxygen-carrying capacity is increasing due to increasing hemoglobin concentration and packed red cell volume as a result of erythropoietin upregulation. By the end of 2 weeks of hypoxic exposure, brain capillary density is increased with resultant decreased intercapillary distances. The relative time courses of these changes suggest that they are adjusted by different control signals and mechanisms.

Disturbances of Microcirculation

In the hypoxic brain there is aggregation of thrombocytes regardless of the etiology of hypoxia. This is followed by aggregation of red cells, and the phenomenon of "sludging" in the blood. This is aggravated by a reduction of velocity in the blood flow and can result in stasis with its sequelae, such as extension of the area of infarction.

Disturbances of the Blood-Brain Barrier

The hypoxic brain tissue is readily affected by disturbances of the permeability of the blood-brain barrier (BBB) and the cell membranes, because the energy-using mechanisms are dependent upon the integrity of these membranes. Disturbances of the BBB impair the active transport of substances in and out of the brain tissues. This may particularly affect glucose transport to the neurons during its metabolism. The oxygen deficiency can also result in a secondary disturbance of the utilization of the substrate.

Cerebral Edema

A further sequel of BBB damage is cerebral edema. Although injury to the brain contributes to the edema, the loss of autoregulation is also an important factor. The rise

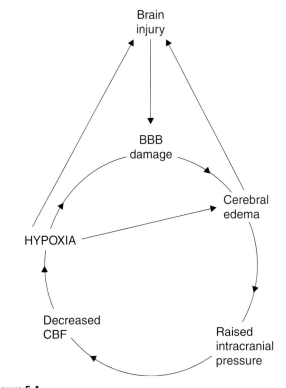

Figure 5.4
Hypoxia as a central factor in edema due to brain injury.

of intracapillary pressure leads to seepage of fluid into the extracellular space. The edema impairs the oxygen supply to the brain and leads to an increase of intracranial pressure and a decrease of CBF. Hypoxia which complicates a brain injury is a dreaded phenomenon, and represents a decisive factor in the outcome of the illness. Hypoxia is the central factor in the vicious circle shown in Figure 5.4.

Effect of Hypoxia on the Electrical Activity of the Brain

The electrical activity of the neurons in the human CNS is remarkably sensitive to hypoxia. EEG activity is attenuated after 10–30 s, and evoked potentials are depressed within 1–3 min of hypoxia. Little is known of the important mechanisms underlying these effects.

Disappearance of EEG activity with hypoxia and reappearance on oxygenation are related to the creatine phosphate (CrP)/creatine (Cr) quotient, pointing to a close functional relationship between brain energy potentials and EEG activity. Computer analysis of EEG in induced hypoxia in human subjects shows that both the mean frequency and the mean amplitude closely reflect the degree of hypoxia.

Electrocerebral silence occurs when cerebral venous pO_2 reaches 20 mmHg, or after only 6 s of total anoxia.

Disturbances of Mental Function in Cerebral Hypoxia

McFarland *et al* (1944) demonstrated that oxygen deprivation, whether induced by high altitude or CO poisoning, leads to loss of capacity of sensory perception and judgment. The subjects recovered when oxygen supply was resumed. Some important causes of hypoxia that lead to impairment of mental function are:

- Chronic carbon monoxide poisoning
- High altitudes; climbing peaks over 8000 m without supplemental oxygen
- Sleep disordered breathing
- Chronic obstructive pulmonary disease

Hypoxia has been considered a causal factor in the decline of intellectual function in the elderly. Cerebral symptoms appear at even a moderate degree of hypoxic hypoxia, demonstrating that certain higher functions are very sensitive to restriction of the oxygen supply, as suggested in Figure 5.5. Delayed dark adaptation has been reported at alveolar oxygen tensions of 80 mmHg, but abnormalities in psychological tests do not occur until alveolar pO_2 is reduced below 50 mmHg, and gross deterioration of mental functions appears only below alveolar pO_2 values of 40 mmHg.

Schlaepfer *et al* (1992) have shown that a mild and rapid hypoxic challenge, by breathing 14.5% oxygen or rapid ascent by helicopter to a mountain peak 3450 m high, may

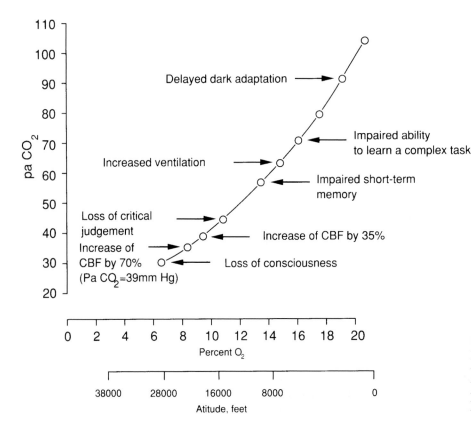

Figure 5.5
Influence of inspired oxygen concentration on alveolar pO_2 in man, with symptoms of and physiological responses to hypoxia (Siesj *et al* 1974, by permission of the author).

improve a simple measure of cognitive performance. Effects of hypoxia vary according to the mode of induction, severity, and duration.

Structural Changes in the Brain After Hypoxia

Patients who recover following resuscitation for cardiopulmonary arrest may not show any structural changes demonstrable by imaging studies. Patients with a residual vegetative state usually develop cerebral atrophy with decrease of rCBF and oxygen consumption. In the subacute phase these patients may show white matter lucencies on CT scan. PET findings (decrease of rCBF and rCMRO), weeks after the ischemic-hypoxic insult, correlate with the neuropsychiatric deficits due to cardiopulmonary arrest.

Conditions associated with Cerebral Hypoxia

Various conditions associated with cerebral hypoxia are shown in Table 5.2. Pathophysiology and management of these are discussed in various chapters of this book.

Table 5.2
Conditions Associated with Cerebral Hypoxia

- Air embolism
- Carbon monoxide poisoning
- Cardiac arrest
- Cyanide poisoning
- Decompression sickness involving the brain
- Drowning
- Fat embolism
- Severe head injury
- Strangulation
- Stroke

Assessment of Hypoxic Brain Damage

Various abnormalities demonstrated on brain imaging are described in Chapters 17 and 19. Delayed hypoxic changes are likely to manifest by changes in basal ganglia. The classical example of hypoxic brain damage is that after cardiac arrest. Hypoxic brain damage after cardiac arrest can be estimated by measurements of concentrations of serum S-protein which is an established biomarker of central nervous system injury. It is a reliable marker of prediction of survival as well as of outcome.

Role of HBO in the Treatment of Hypoxic States

Hypoxia due to inadequate oxygenation in the lungs, either from extrinsic factors or owing to pulmonary disease, can usually be corrected by oxygen. The role of HBO in pulmonary disorders is discussed in Chapter 28. The major applications of HBO are in conditions with inadequate transport and delivery of oxygen to the tissues, or inadequate capacity of the tissues to use oxygen. The uses of HBO in the treatment of circulatory disturbances and tissue edema are discussed in other chapters: myocardial ischemia in Chapter 24, CO poisoning in Chapter 12, stroke in Chapter 18, and global ischemia/anoxia and coma in Chapter 19.

Neurons can tolerate between 20 and 60 min of complete anoxia without irreversible changes. Following these severe insults, neurons regain the ability to synthesize protein, produce ATP, and generate action potentials. HBO can facilitate this recovery process.

The most significant effects of hypoxia are on the brain, and a review of the metabolic effects leads to the rationale of HBO therapy in hypoxic conditions of the brain, particularly those due to cerebrovascular ischemia.

Hypoxia is also a common feature of the tumor microenvironment and a major cause of clinical radioresistance. Role of HBO in enhancing cancer radiosensitivity is discussed in Chapter 36.

The Role of Nitric Oxide Synthase in the Effect of HBO in Hypoxia

The adhesion of polymorphonuclear leukocytes to endothelial cells is increased following hypoxic exposure and is reduced to control levels following exposure to HBO (Buras *et al* 2000). In experimental studies, HBO exposure induced the synthesis of endothelial cell nitric oxide synthase (eNOS). The NOS inhibitor nitro-L-arginine methyl ester attenuated HBO-mediated inhibition of intercellular adhesion molecule-1 (ICAM-1) expression. These findings suggest that the beneficial effects of HBO in treating hypoxic injury may be mediated in part by inhibition of ICAM-1 expression through the induction of eNOS.

Possible Dangers of HBO in Hypoxic States

Although it appears logical that HBO would be useful in hypoxic states, some concern has been expressed about the free radical damage and damage to the carotid bodies which impairs hypoxic ventilatory drive.

Free Radicals. Hypoxia can potentiate tissue injury due to oxidative stress and free radicals and there is theoretical concern that oxygen given in hypoxia may cause further cell damage. The counter argument is that correct of hypoxia by HBO would reduce the free radical formation resulting from hypoxia. Although the concept of oxygen toxicity at reduced oxygen tensions is a paradox, it cannot be dismissed. It is conceivable that partial lack of oxygen, by impeding electron acceptance at the cytochrome oxidase step, increases the "leak current," i.e., free radical formation. This subject is discussed further in Chapter 6 (oxygen toxicity).

Damage to Carotid Bodies. The carotid body chemosensory response to hypoxia is attenuated following prolonged exposure to normobaric hypoxia in the cat and is attributed to generation of free radicals in the carotid bodies. Torbati *et al* (1993) conducted further studies on the cat using exposure to 5 ATA and observed the diminution of chemosensory responsiveness to hypoxia within 2 hours which was not considered to be due to lack of neurotransmitters. Ultrastructural changes in the carotid bodies(increased number of mitochondria in the glomus cells) after HBO exposure could be explained by the oxidative stress.

6

Oxygen Toxicity

K.K. Jain

Prolonged exposure to oxygen at high pressure can have toxic effects, particularly on the central nervous system, but at pressures used clinically it does not pose a problem. The main topics discussed here are:

Introduction

Priestley (1775, see Chapter 1), the discoverer of oxygen, theorized about the effects of hyperoxia in this charming passage:

We may also infer from these experiments, that though pure dephlogisticated air might be very useful as a medicine, it might not be so proper for use in the healthy state of the body: for, as a candle burns out much faster in dephlogisticated than in common air, so we might, as might be said, live out too fast, and the animal powers be too soon exhausted in this pure kind of air. A moralist, at least, may say that the air which nature has provided for us is as good as we deserve.

Paul Bert (1878, see Chapter 1) was the first to actually document the toxicity of oxygen. He conducted experiments to test the effects of hyperbaric oxygen (HBO), not only on himself but also on other life forms. Indeed, seizures resulting from the toxicity of oxygen to the central nervous system are still referred to as the "Paul Bert effect." Although his work is a classic, Bert completely missed pulmonary toxicity as an effect of normobaric oxygen. This was later discovered by Lorraine Smith (1899) and is fittingly referred to as the "Lorraine Smith effect." Bean (1945) studied the toxic effects of continuous exposure to HBO beyond the point of seizures, to irreversible neurological damage and eventual death; this problem is now widely known as the "John Bean effect."

Behnke *et al* (1936) carried out a variety of experiments in human subjects to show the effects of oxygen toxicity. As a result of these earlier studies it became generally accepted that a 3-h exposure at 3 ATA and a 30- to 40-min exposure at 4 ATA were the limits of safe tolerance by healthy human adults. It is now generally accepted that HBO at 3 ATA affects primarily the nervous system, while the respiratory system is affected independently at 2 ATA. There is a vast amount of literature on basic mechanism of oxygen toxicity (Bean 1945; Balentine 1982).

This chapter describes mainly the toxic effects of HBO.

Normobaric hyperoxia, which usually leads to pulmonary oxygen poisoning, has been dealt with in detail elsewhere (Jain 1989a).

Pathophysiology of Oxygen Toxicity

The molecular basis of CNS as well as pulmonary oxygen poisoning, involves generation of reactive oxygen species (ROS). This has been known as the free radical theory of oxygen poisoning. The basis of this theory, for the CNS oxygen toxicity, is that an increased generation of ROS during HBO may ultimately lead to alterations in cerebral energy metabolism and electrical activity due to membranes lipid peroxidation, enzyme inhibition, and/or enzyme modulation. Although HBO-induced generation of ROS could directly alter the functions of various SH-containing enzymes, membrane-bound enzymes and structures as well as the nucleus, the physiological effects of HBO may also indirectly cause hypoxic-ischemia, acidosis, anemia, and hyperbilirubinemia.

At higher pressures of oxygen, events in the brain are a prelude to a distinct lung pathology. The experimental observation that CNS-mediated component of lung injury can be attenuated by selective inhibition of neuronal nitric oxide synthase (nNOS) or by unilateral transection of the vagus nerve has led to the hypothesis that extrapulmonary, neurogenic events predominate in the pathogenesis of acute pulmonary oxygen toxicity in HBO, as nNOS activity drives lung injury by modulating the output of central autonomic pathways (Demchenko *et al* 2007).

Free Radical Mechanisms

Oxygen free radicals are products of normal cellular oxidation- reduction processes. Under conditions of hyperoxia, their production increases markedly. The nature of the ox-

---

Table 6.1
Animal Experimental Studies of the Effect of HBO on Brain Lipoperoxide Levels

Authors and year	Pressure	Effects
Zirkle *et al* (1965)	4 ATA	Clinical level of CNS toxicity correlated with elevated lipoperoxide content; convulsions were considered to be due to raised AChE (acetylcholinesterase) activity
Galvin (1962)	2 ATA	Cerebral peroxide level not elevated; no difference in the peroxide level between convulsing and nonconvulsing animals
Jerrett *et al* (1973)	5 ATA	H_2O_2 levels were elevated except in those animals given supplemental α-tocopherol
Yusa *et al* (1987)	3 ATA	Rise of H_2O_2 level in brain by 300% when symptoms of CNS toxicity became apparent
Torbati *et al* (1992)	5 ATA	Direct demonstration of reactive oxygen species before onset of CNS convulsions

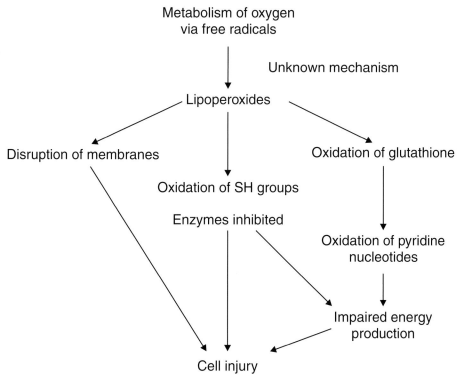

Metabolism of oxygen
via free radicals

Unknown mechanism

Lipoperoxides

Disruption of membranes

Oxidation of glutathione

Oxidation of SH groups

Enzymes inhibited

Oxidation of pyridine
nucleotides

Impaired energy
production

Cell injury

(Altered membranes, impaired mitochondria, impaired neurotransmission,
inhibition of nuclear function and/or protein synthesis)

Cell death

Figure 6.1
Summary of the hypothesis of oxygen toxicity. SH = sulfhydryl. (Reproduced from Chance and Boveris 1978, by permission.)

ygen molecule makes it susceptible to univalent reduction reactions in the cells to form superoxide anion (O_2^-) a highly reactive, cytotoxic free radical. In turn, other reaction products of oxygen metabolism, including hydrogen peroxide (H_2O_2), hydroxyl radicals ($OH\cdot$), and singlet oxygen ($^1O_2$), can be formed. These short-lived forms are capable of oxidizing the sulfhydryl (SH) groups of enzymes, interact with DNA, and promote lipoperoxidation of cellular membranes. Animal studies showing the effect of HBO in raising the cerebral peroxide content and correlating it with CNS toxicity are listed in Table 6.1.

Boveris and Chance presented an excellent unifying concept of the mechanism of oxygen toxicity in 1978, which is a classic now. H_2O_2 generation as a physiological event has been documented in a variety of isolated mitochondria and is rapidly enhanced by hyperoxia. Superoxide ions, generated submitochondrial fractions, are the source of H_2O_2 (Boveris & Chance 1978). This hypothesis is shown in Figure 6.1. As a primary event, the free radical chain reactions produce lipoperoxidation. Lipoperoxides, in turn, will have disruptive effects on the structure of the biomembranes, inhibit enzymes with SH groups, and shift the cellular redox state of glutathione toward oxidation. This will be transmitted through the secondary events to pyridine nucleotides, with the mitochondrial NADH oxidation resulting in

impaired energy production. Enzyme inhibition, altered energy production, and decrease or loss of function may be consequences of either increased peroxides or a decline in the antioxidant defence.

Although increased generation of ROS before the onset of HBO-induced convulsions has been demonstrated in conscious rats, their production in association with oxygen toxicity has not been demonstrated satisfactorily in human subjects. There are increased electron spin resonance signals from blood of persons exposed to HBO but these return to normal within 10 min of cessation of exposure to HBO.

Pathology of Oxygen Toxicity

The pathology of oxygen toxicity has been documented comprehensively in a classical work on this topic (Balentine 1982). The various manifestations of oxygen poisoning are summarized in Figure 6.2. It is well known that the development of pulmonary and CNS toxicity depends upon the partial pressure and the duration of exposure, as shown in Figure 6.3. Fortunately, the early effects of poisoning are completely reversible, but prolonged expo-

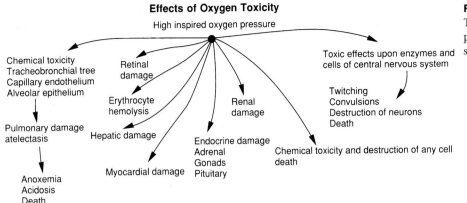

Effects of Oxygen Toxicity

High inspired oxygen pressure

Chemical toxicity
Tracheobronchial tree
Capillary endothelium
Alveolar epithelium

Pulmonary damage
atelectasis

Anoxemia
Acidosis
Death

Retinal
damage

Erythrocyte
hemolysis

Hepatic damage

Myocardial damage

Renal
damage

Endocrine damage
Adrenal
Gonads
Pituitary

Chemical toxicity and destruction of any cell
death

Toxic effects upon enzymes and
cells of central nervous system

Twitching
Convulsions
Destruction of neurons
Death

Figure 6.2
The effects of oxygen poisoning. (Reproduced from Clark 1974, by permission.)

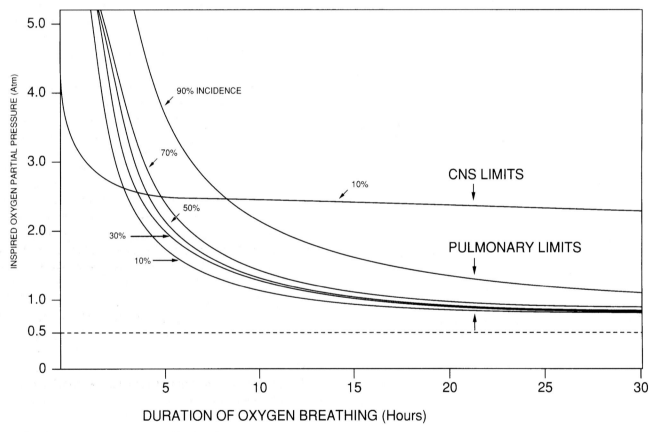

PULMONARY OXYGEN TOLERANCE CURVES IN NORMAL MEN
(BASED ON 4% DECREASE IN VITAL CAPACITY)

90% INCIDENCE

70%

10%

CNS LIMITS

50%

PULMONARY LIMITS

30%

10%

INSPIRED OXYGEN PARTIAL PRESSURE (Atm)

DURATION OF OXYGEN BREATHING (Hours)

Figure 6.3
Individual variation in susceptibility to oxygen poisoning. Curves designated as pulmonary limits are inspired pO_2 exposure duration relationships for occurrence of one or more neurologic signs and symptoms listed in Table 6.5. (From Clark JM, Fischer AB: Oxygen toxicity and extension of tolerance in oxygen therapy. In Davis JC, Hunt TK (Eds.): Hyperbaric oxygen therapy, Bethesda, MD, Undersea and Hyperbaric Medical Society 1977. By permission.)

sure first lengthens the recovery period and then eventually produces irreversible changes. Many organs have been affected in experimental oxygen toxicity studies of long exposure to high pressures – a situation that is not seen in clinical practice.

High-pressure oxygen leads to increased pyruvate/lactate and pyruvate malate redox couples, as well as to a de-

crease in the incorporation of phospholipid long-chain fatty acid and pyruvate into the tissue lipid. During recovery from the effects of high-pressure oxygen these changes are reversed. These data indicate that oxygen poisoning of tissues is not the result of an inhibition of carbohydrate metabolism, but instead may result from the formation of toxic lipoperoxides.

The power expression for cumulative oxygen toxicity and the exponential recovery have been successfully applied to various features of oxygen toxicity at the Israel Naval Medical Institute in Israel (Arieli *et al* 2002). From the basic equation, the authors derived expressions for a protocol in which PO_2 changes with time. The parameters of the power equation were solved by using nonlinear regression for the reduction in vital capacity (DeltaVC) in humans:

$$DeltaVC = 0.0082 \times t_2\ (PO_2/101.3)(4.57)$$

where t is the time in hours and PO_2 is expressed in kPa.

The recovery of lung volume is:

$$DeltaVC(t) = DeltaVC(e) \times e(-(-0.42 + 0.00379\ PO_2)t)$$

where DeltaVC(t) is the value at time t of the recovery, DeltaVC(e) is the value at the end of the hyperoxic exposure, and PO_2 is the prerecovery oxygen pressure.

Data from different experiments on CNS oxygen toxicity in humans in the hyperbaric chamber were analyzed along with data from actual closed-circuit oxygen diving by using a maximum likelihood method. The parameters of the model were solved for the combined data, yielding the power equation for active diving:

$$K = t_2\ (PO_2/101.3)(6.8),$$

where t is in minutes.

It was suggested that the risk of CNS oxygen toxicity in diving can be derived from the calculated parameter of the normal distribution:

$$Z = [\ln(t) - 9.63 + 3.38 \times \ln(PO_2/101.3)]/2.02$$

The recovery time constant for CNS oxygen toxicity was calculated from the value obtained for the rat, taking into account the effect of body mass, and yielded the recovery equation:

$$K(t) = K(e) \times e(-0.079t)$$

where K(t) and K(e) are the values of K at time t of the recovery process and at the end of the hyperbaric oxygen exposure, respectively, and t is in minutes.

Pulmonary Oxygen Toxicity

This is usually a manifestation of prolonged exposure (more than 24 h) to normobaric 100% oxygen, as well as during exposure to HBO from 2 to 3 ATA O_2 in human and experimental animals. The pathology and pathophysiology of pulmonary oxygen toxicity are described in more detail elsewhere (Jain 1989b). The major mechanism by which HBO produces lung injury in rabbits is by stimulating thromboxane synthesis. Lung injury induced by free radicals has been demonstrated in an animal model of smoke inhalation, and the free radicals clear up after

about an hour. Normobaric 100% oxygen given for one hour does not increase the level of free radicals in this model, but HBO at 2.5 ATA does so.

Acute changes in the lungs resulting from oxygen toxicity consist of alveolar and interstitial edema, alveolar hemorrhages, and proteinaceous exudates. This is followed by an inflammatory reaction. Further prolonged exposure to oxygen leads to a proliferative phase, which includes proliferation of type II epithelial cells and fibroblasts, followed by collagen deposits. Healing may occur after discontinuance of oxygen exposure, but areas of fibrosis and emphysema may remain. In patients with heart failure or in patients with reduced cardiac ejection fractions, HBO may contribute to pulmonary edema by increasing left ventricular afterload, increasing oxidative myocardial stress, decreasing left ventricular compliance by oxygen radical-mediated reduction in nitric oxide, increasing pulmonary capillary permeability, or by causing pulmonary oxygen toxicity (Weaver & Churchill 2001).

Repeated exposure to HBO at intervals insufficient to allow total recovery from pulmonary oxygen toxicity may lead to cumulative effects. The progression of toxicity can be monitored by serial pulmonary function studies. The concept of a "unit pulmonary toxic dose" (UPTD) has been developed (Bardin & Lambertsen 1970), and this allows comparison of the pulmonary effects of various treatment schedules of HBO (Table 6.2). The UPTD is designed to express any pulmonary toxic dose in terms of an equivalent exposure to oxygen at 1 ATA. It is only an arbitrary measure and does not allow for the recovery between HBO exposures. For example, 10 HBO treatments at 2.4 ATA for 90 min each would give the patient a UPTD of more than 200 and would indicate significant pulmonary toxicity with a 20% reduction in vital capacity. In practice, however, no clinical evidence of pulmonary toxicity is seen with this schedule. There is no significant impairment of pulmonary diffusing capacity in divers who have been intermittently exposed to HBO at 4 ATA for years.

Prolonged exposure to elevated oxygen levels is a frequent and important clinical problem. Superoxide dismutase (SOD) and catalase, the major intracellular antioxidant enzymes, cooperate in the detoxification of free oxygen radicals produced during normal aerobic respiration. Therapeutic approaches designed to deliver SOD or catalase to these intracellular sites would be useful in mitigating the pulmonary oxygen toxicity. A number of approaches to deliver these enzymes have not been successful. Adenovirus-mediated transfer to lungs of both catalase and SOD cDNA has been shown to protect against pulmonary oxygen toxicity. Distal airway epithelial cells, including type II alveolar and nonciliated bronchiolar epithelial cells, are important targets for oxygen radicals under the hyperoxic condition. The accessibility of these distal airway epithelial cells to *in vivo* gene transfer through the tracheal route of administration, suggests the

Table 6.2
Cumulative Pulmonary Oxygen Toxicity Indices for Commonly Used Oxygen Therapy Tables (Bardin & Lambertsen 1970)

Therapy table	UPTD[a]
• Chronic osteomyelitis/radionecrosis	
120 min oxygen at 33 fsw	300
90 min oxygen at 45 fsw	270
• Anaerobic infection	401
45 min oxygen/15 min air/45 min oxygen at 60 fsw	
45 min oxygen at 60–0 fsw with 8 min at 20 fsw and 27 min at 10 fsw	
• CO intoxication	445
45 min oxygen at 60 fsw	
30 min oxygen at 60–30 fsw	
15 min air/60 min oxygen at 30 fsw	
30 min oxygen at 30–0 fsw	
• USN 6	645
• USN 6 extended	
20 min oxygen/5 min air at 60 fsw	718
15 min air/60 min oxygen at 30 fsw	787
20 min oxygen/5 min air at 60 fsw and 15 min air/60 min oxygen at 30 fsw	860
• USN 6A	690
• USN 6A extended	
20 min oxygen/5 min air at 60 fsw	763
15 min air/60 min oxygen at 60 fsw	833
20 min oxygen/5 min air at 60 fsw and 15 min air/60 min oxygen at 30 fsw	906
• IFEM 7A (air and oxygen)	1813
• IFEM 7A alternating 50/50 Nitrox with air 30 min on/30 min off from 100–70 fsw	2061

UPTD value indicates duration (min) of oxygen breathing at 1.0 ATA that would cause equivalent degree of pulmonary intoxication (measured as decrease in vital capacity)

potential for *in vivo* transfer of MnSOD and extracellular SOD genes as a future approach in the prevention of pulmonary oxygen toxicity (Tsan 2001).

Oxygen-Induced Retinopathy

Retrolental fibroplasia is considered to be an oxygen-induced obliteration of the immature retinal vessels when 100% oxygen is given to premature infants. A recent study showed that oxygen therapy for more than 3 days, in infants delivered following 32–36 weeks of gestation, was not associated with an increased risk of retinopathy of prematu-

rity (Gleissner *et al* 2003). HBO (2.8 ATA, 80% oxygen) given to premature rats does not result in retinopathy, whereas control animals given normobaric 80% oxygen developed retinopathy. This topic is discussed further in Chapter 32.

Factors that Enhance Oxygen Toxicity

Various factors which enhance oxygen toxicity are listed in Table 6.3. Combining HBO with the substances listed, together with morbid conditions such as fever, should definitely be avoided.

Mild hyperthermia (38.5 °C) has been used therapeutically for a number of conditions. An increase of temperature increases oxygen uptake by body tissues. Hyperthermia may thus be expected to enhance oxygen toxicity. Transient biochemical side effects of mild hypothermia such as hyperammonemia can be inhibited by HBO, but this combination should be used cautiously to avoid oxygen toxicity.

It is generally believed that high humidity enhances oxygen toxicity as manifested by lung damage and convulsions. This has been experimentally verified in rodents exposed to HBO (515 to 585 kPa) under conditions of low humidity as well as 60% relative humidity.

Physical exercise definitely lowers the threshold for CNS oxygen toxicity in the rat over the entire range of pressures from 2 to 6 ATA. This observation should be kept in mind in planning physical exercise in hyperbaric environments (see Chapter 4). Various enzymes inhibited by hyperoxia are shown in Table 6.4. This may explain how hyperoxia leads to oxygen toxity.

Glutathione reductase is an integral component of the antioxidant defence mechanism. Inhibition of brain glutathione reductase by carmustine lowers the threshold for seizures in rats exposed to HBO.

Table 6.3
Enhancers of Oxygen Toxicity

• Gases	Disulfiram
Carbon dioxide	Guanethidine
Nitrous oxide	• Trace metals
• Hormones	Iron
Insulin	Copper
Thyroid hormones	• Morbid conditions
Adrenocortical hormones	Fever
• Neurotransmitters	Vitamin E deficiency convulsions
Epinephrine and norepinephrine	
• Drugs and chemicals	Congenital spherocytosis
Acetazolamide	• Physiological states of increased metabolism
Dextroamphetamine	Physical exercise
NH_4Cl	Hyperthermia
Paraquat	Diving
Aspirin	

Table 6.4
Enzymes Inhibited by Hyperoxia at 1–5 ATA

1. Embden-Meyerhof pathway
   Phosphoglucokinase
   Phosphoglucomutase
   Glyceraldehyde-phosphate-dehydrogenase*
2. Conversion of pyruvate to acetyl-CoA
   Pyruvate oxidase
3. Tricarboxylic acid cycle
   Succinate dehydrogenase*
   α-ketoglutarate dehydrogenase*
   Malate dehydrogenase*
4. Electron transport
   Succinate dehydrogenase*
   Malate dehydrogenase*
   Glyceraldehyde-phosphate dehydrogenase*
   DPNH dehydrogenase*
   Lactate dehydrogenase*
   Xanthine oxidase
   D-Amino acid oxidase
5. Neurotransmitter synthetic enzymes
   Glutamic acid decarboxylase
   Choline acetylase
   Dopa decarboxylase
   5-HTP decarboxylase
   Phenylalanine hydroxylase
   Tyrosine hydroxylase
6. Proteolysis and hydralysis
   Cathepsin
   Papain
   Unspecified proteases and peptidases
   Unspecified in autolysis
   Arginase
   Urease
   Ribonuclease
7. Membrane transport
   NA^+, K^+-ATPase$^+$
8. Molecular oxygen reduction pathway
   Catalase
9. Others
   Acetate kinase
   Cerebrosedase
   Choline oxidase
   Fatty acid dehydrogenase
   Formic acid dehydrogenase
   Glutamic dehydrogenase
   Glutamic synthetase
   Glyoxylase
   Hydrogenase
   Isocitrate lyase
   Malate syntase
   Myo kinase (adenylate kinase)
   Phosphate transacetylase
   Transaminase
   Zymohexase (aldolase)

*Asterisks indicate enzymes containing essential sulfhydryl (SH) groups, emphasized as being inactivated by oxidation of these groups.

Central Nervous System Oxygen Toxicity

Effect on Cerebral Metabolism

Disturbances of cerebral metabolism resulting from hyperoxia have been described in Chapter 2. HBO at 2 ATA has been shown to stimulate rCMRGl slightly, but does not result in any toxic manifestations. Oxidative metabolism of the brain is usually not affected by pressures up to 6 ATA. In the primary rat cortical culture, HBO exposure to 6 ATA for 30, 60, and 90 min increased the lactate dehydrogenase (LDH) activity in the culture medium in a time-dependent manner (Huang *et al* 2000). Accordingly, the cell survival was decreased after HBO exposure. Pretreatment with the NMDA antagonist MK-801 protected the cells against the HBO-induced damage. The protective effect was also noted in the cells pretreated with L-N(G)-nitro-arginine methyl ester, an NO synthase inhibitor. These results suggest that activation of NMDA receptors and production of NO play a role in the neurotoxicity produced by HBO exposure.

There is no evidence that seizures are related to oxidative metabolic changes. However, increase of glucose utilization precede the onset of electrophysiological manifestations of CNS oxygen toxicity). Increased nitric oxide (NO) production during prolonged HBO exposure is responsible for escape from hyperoxic vasoconstriction in cerebral blood arterioles. The finding suggests that NO overproduction initiates CNS oxygen toxicity by increasing rCBF, which allows excessive oxygen to be delivered to the brain (Demchenko *et al* 2001). The hypothetical pathophysiologic pathways leading to acute and chronic CNS oxygen toxicity are illustrated in Figure 6.4.

Effect on Neurotransmitters

Neurotransmitters have been shown to be downregulated under hyperbaric hyperoxia (Courtiere *et al* 1991). With the recognition of nitric oxide (NO) as a neurotransmitter, its relationship to hyperia has been studied. Experimental studies of Zhang *et al* (1993) showed that rats can be protected against oxygen toxicity by a combination of a monoamine oxidase inhibitor and a nitric oxide (NO) synthase inhibitor. Their data showed that protection against oxygen toxicity by these agents is not related to the preservation of the GABA pool. They found that oxygen-dependent noradrenaline metabolism and NO synthesis appear to be inactive during oxygen neurotoxicity. Oury *et al* (1992) consider NO to be an important mediator in oxygen neurotoxicity and suggest that extracellular superoxide dismutase increases oxygen neurotoxicity by inactivation of NO.

Exposures to HBO at 2 and 2.8 ATA stimulated neuronal NO synthase (nNOS) and significantly increased steady-state

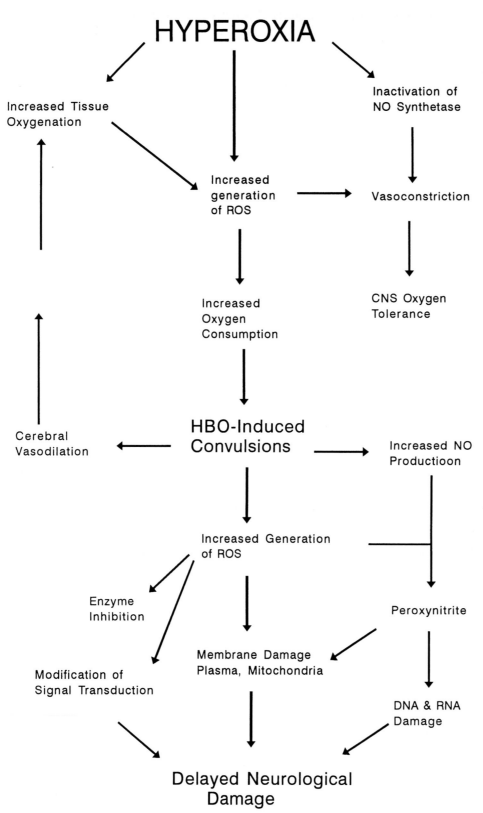

Figure 6.4
Basic mechanisms of CNS oxygen toxicity. ROS = reactive oxygen species, NO = nitric oxide (by D. Torbati, PhD).

(Thom *et al* 2003). At both pressures, elevations in NO concentration were inhibited by the nNOS inhibitor 7-nitroindazole and the calcium channel blocker nimodipine. Infusion of superoxide dismutase inhibited NO elevation at 2.8, but not 2 ATA HBO. Hyperoxia increased the concentration of NO associated with hemoglobin. These findings highlight the complexity of oxidative stress responses and may help explain some of the dose responses associated with therapeutic applications of hyperbaric oxygen.

Ammonia and Amino Acids

Single seizures induced in rats subjected to HBO at 6 ATA have been shown to be associated with accumulation of ammonia and alterations in amino acids in the brain, with the greatest changes taking place in the striatum (Mialon *et al* 1992). These changes were considered to be caused by an increase in oxidative deamination or possibly the result of glial failure to capture released amino acids. The subsequent imbalance between the excitatory and inhibitory mediators in the striatum was offered as an explanation of the recurrence of seizures in animals maintained on HBO.

Changes in the Electrical Activity of the Brain and Seizures

Conscious rats and rabbits exposed to HBO usually demonstrate an increased EEG slow wave activity which eventually develops into bursts of paroxysmal electrical discharges. These electrical events precede the onset of visible HBO-induced convulsions, and therefore were suggested as an early signs of CNS oxygen toxicity in experimental animals. *In vitro* studies with HBO also show changes in neuronal electrical activity, which may be associated with seizures.

The seizure associated with HBO usually occurs toward the end of the oxygen exposure while the patient is being decompressed. It is a violent motor discharge with a brief period of breathholding. In such cases, therefore, decompression should be temporarily halted until the seizure is over; otherwise there could be rupture of lung alveoli.

Oxygen-induced seizures are not a contraindication for further HBO therapy. Further HBO treatments may be carried out at lower pressures and shorter exposures. Anticonvulsant medications are usually not indicated, but may be used. In animal experiments Carbamazepine (Reshef *et al* 1991) and vigabatrin (Tzuk *et al* 1991) have been found to be effective in preventing HBO-induced convulsions. Acupuncture has been claimed to protect against oxygen-induced convulsions by increasing GABA in the brain levels (Wu *et al* 1992).

Epilepsy has been listed as a contraindication for using HBO therapy. This is based on the assumption that oxy-gen is liable to precipitate a seizure in an epileptic patient and such an event in a chamber might be detrimental to the patient. Seizures in epileptic patients are rare during HBO therapy where pressures less than 2 ATA are used. There is no published study that reexamines this issue. The question therefore still arises: is HBO really dangerous for an epileptic? If epilepsy is included in the contraindications for HBO, patients with head injuries and strokes who happen to have seizures would be deprived of the benefit of HBO therapy. The mechanism of epilepsy in such patients is different from that of an oxygen-induced convulsion. It has even been shown that EEG abnormalities in stroke patients improve with HBO treatment (Wassmann 1980). It is possible that HBO may abort a seizure from a focus with circulatory and metabolic disturbances by correcting these abnormalities. Seizures are extremely rare and no more than a chance occurrence during HBO sessions at pressures between 1.5 and 2 ATA even in patients with a history of epilepsy.

Neuropathology

In experimental studies, there is no damage to the CNS of rats exposed to HBO until the pressure exceeded 4 ATA. The brain damage is increased by CNS-depressant drugs, increase of pCO_2, acetazolamide, and NH_4Cl. Permanent spastic limb paralysis has been observed in rats (the John Bean effect) after repeated exposure to high oxygen pressures (over 5 ATA). There is selective necrosis of white matter both in the spinal cord and the brain, and this is considered to be the effect of hyperoxia. HBO-induced rat brain lesions, examined by electron microscopy, show two types of nerve cell alterations: (1) type A lesions characterized by pyknosis and hyperchromatosis of the nerve cells, vacuolization of the cytoplasm, and simultaneous swelling of the perineural glial processes; (2) type B lesions are characterized by lysis in the cytoplasm and karyorrhexis.

Manifestations of CNS Oxygen Toxicity

Signs and symptoms of CNS oxygen toxicity are listed in Table 6.5.

Clinical Monitoring for Oxygen Toxicity

The most important factor in early detection of oxygen toxicity is the observation of signs and symptoms. For monitoring pulmonary function, determination of vital capacity is the easiest and most reliable parameter, as it is reduced before any irreversible changes occur in the lungs. EEG

Table 6.5 **Signs and Symptoms of CNS Toxicity**	
Facial pallor	Acoustic symptoms
Sweating	Music
Bradycardia	Bell ringing
Choking sensation	Knocking
Palpitations	Unpleasant olfactory sensations
Epigastric tensions	Unpleasant gustatory sensations
Sleepiness	Respiratory changes
Depression	Panting
Euphoria	Grunting
Apprehension	Hiccoughs
Changes of behavior	Inspiratory predominance
Fidgeting	Diaphragmatic spasms
Disinterest	Severe nausea
Clumsiness	Spasmodic vomiting
Visual symptoms	Vertigo
Loss of acuity	Fibrillation of lips
Dazzle	Lip twitching
Lateral movement	Twitching of cheek and nose
Decrease of intensity	Syncope
Constriction of visual field	Convulsions

Table 6.6
Factors Protecting Against Generalized Oxygen Toxicity

Antioxidants, free radical scavengers, and trace minerals
   allopurinol
   ascorbic acid
   glycine
   magnesium
   selenium
   superoxide dismutase, SOD
   tyloxapol
   vitamin E
Chemicals and enzymes modifying cerebral metabolism
   arginine
   coenzyme Q10 and carnitine
   gamma-aminobutyric acid, GABA
   glutathionehemocarnisine
   interleukin-6
   leukotriene B$_4$ antagonist SC-41930
   paraglycine and succinic acid
   sodium succinate and glutamate
Drugs
   adrenergic-blocking and ganglion-blocking drugs
   barbiturates
   BCNU
   chlorazepate
   diazepam
   ergot derivatives: lisuride and quinpirole
   isonicotinic acid hydrazide
   levodopa
   lithium
   milecide
   MK-801 (a competitive NMDA receptor antagonist)
   neuroleptics: chlorpromazine, thorazine
   propranolol
Intermittent exposure to HBO
   acclimatization to hypoxia
   interposition of air-breathing periods
Endocrine factors
   adrenalectomy
   hypophysectomy
   thyroidectomy
Gene therapy

tracings do not show any consistent alterations before the onset of seizures and are not a reliable method of early detection of oxygen toxicity.

Decrease in [9,10–^{3}H] oleic acid incorporation by human erythrocytes detected *in vitro* after HBO exposure *in vivo* may reflect an early event in the pathogenesis of oxygen-induced cellular injury and may be a useful monitoring procedure.

An increase in CBF velocity (BCFV) precedes onset of symptoms of oxygen toxicity during exposure to 280 kPa oxygen, which may be followed by seizure (Koch *et al* 2008). At rest a delay of approximately 20 min precedes the onset of CNS oxygen toxicity and seizure can be aborted with timely oxygen reduction.

Protection Against Oxygen Toxicity

Various agents and measures for prevention or treatment of oxygen toxicity are listed in Table 6.6; these are mostly experimental. The most promising agents are the antioxidants. The use of vitamin E (tocopherol) is based on the free-radical theory of oxygen toxicity. It has been used to protect premature infants (who lack vitamin E) against oxygen toxicity. Dietary supplementation with selenium and vitamin E, which increase the cerebral as well as extracerebral GSH content, does not protect rats against the effect of HBO by delaying the onset of first electrical discharge (Boadi *et al* 1991). However, such diets may still be advantageous in promoting recovery and reversal of toxic process, as occurs between consecutive HBO exposures or during intermittent oxygen exposure (Bleiberg & Kerem 1988).

Not all of the dietary free-radical scavengers are effective in counteracting oxygen toxicity. In animal experiments, no correlation was found between *in vitro* inhibition of lipid peroxidation and *in vivo* protection against oxygen toxicity.

Hypothermia has been considered to be a protector against oxygen toxicity, but HBO at 5 ATA induces hypothermia in mice, and this has little protective effect against convulsions.

Every clinician who treats patients should be aware of oxygen toxicity, although it is rare. At pressures of 1.5 ATA, even prolonged use in patients with cerebrovascular disease has not led to any reported case of oxygen toxicity. It should not be assumed that experimental observations regarding oxygen toxicity under hyperbaric conditions are applicable to normobaric conditions.

Whereas disulfiram protects against hyperbaric oxygen, it potentiates the toxicity of normobaric oxygen in rats. Ascorbic acid is also a free radical scavenger and protects against oxygen toxicity, but large doses of this vitamin may prove counterproductive in treating oxygen toxicity if the reducing enzymes are overloaded. An oxidized ascorbate might actually potentiate oxygen toxicity through lipoperoxide formation. Mg^{2+} has a double action against the undesirable effects of oxygen. It is a vasodilator and also a calcium blocker and protects against cellular injury. Magnesium sulfate suppresses the electroencephalographic manifestations of CNS oxygen toxicity and an anticonvulsant effect has been demonstrated in rats exposed to HBO at 6ATA. A prophylactic regimen of 10 mmol Mg^{2+} 3 h before a session of HBO and 400 mg of vitamin E daily, starting a couple of days before the HBO treatment, is useful in preventing oxygen toxicity, but no controlled study has been done to verify the efficacy of this regime.

The detoxifying function of cytochrome c to scavenge ROS in mitochondria has been confirmed experimentally (Min & Jian-xing 2007). A concept of mitochondrial radical metabolism is suggested based on the two electron-leak pathways mediated by cytochrome c that are metabolic routes of oxygen free radicals. The main portion of oxygen consumed in the electron transfer of respiratory chain is used in ATP synthesis, while a subordinate part of oxygen consumed by the leaked electrons contributes to ROS generation. The models of respiratory chain operating with two cytochrome c-mediated electron-leak pathways and a radical metabolism of mitochondria accompanied with energy metabolism are helpful in understanding the pathological problems caused by oxygen toxicity

Distal airway epithelial cells, including type II alveolar and nonciliated bronchiolar epithelial cells, are important targets for O_2 radicals under the hyperoxic condition. The accessibility of these distal airway epithelial cells to *in vivo* gene transfer through the tracheal route of administration, suggests the potential for *in vivo* transfer of MnSOD and extracellular SOD genes as a future approach in the prevention of pulmonary O_2 toxicity (Tsan 2001).

Extension of Oxygen Tolerance

Tolerance to oxygen primarily means tolerance to the toxic effects, because the physiological effects have no prolonged consequences. This subject has been discussed in detail by Lambertsen (1988). He considers a positive emphasis on extending oxygen tolerance as desirable, as opposed to a restrictive fear of oxygen poisoning. The following are compiled from his comments regarding extension of oxygen tolerance.

Tolerance Extension by Adaptation

At low levels of atmospheric hyperoxia, some forms of true protective adaptation appear to occur, such as that related to changing antioxidant defenses in some tissues. At higher oxygen pressures, some adaptation could conceivably occur in some cells of the intact human being with progressive and severe poisoning in other cells. At very high oxygen pressure, rapid onset of poisoning would make adaptation inadequate and too late.

Tolerance Extension by Drugs

A pharmacological approach, such as that of providing free radical scavengers, will attain broad usefulness only if the drug can attain the free permeability of the oxygen molecule. The drug should reach the right location at the right time, and remain effective there in the face of continuous hyperoxia, without itself inducing any toxic effects. There is no such ideal drug available at present.

Tolerance Extension by Interrupted Exposure to Oxygen

Interruption of exposure to HBO is known to extend the safe exposure time. In experimental animals, intermittent exposure to HBO postpones the gross symptoms of oxygen toxicity along with changes in enzymes, such as superoxide dismutase, in the lungs (Harabin *et al* 1990). Species differences were noted in this study; biochemical variables were more pronounced in guinea pigs than in rats.

There is no accepted procedure for quantifying the recovery during normoxia. A cumulative oxygen toxicity index – K, when K reaches a critical value (Kc) and the toxic effect is manifested, can be calculated using the following equation:

$$K = t_2e \times PO_2c$$

where t(e) is hyperoxic exposure time and PO_2 is oxygen pressure and c is a power parameter.

Recovery during normoxia (reducing K) is calculated by the following equation

$$K_2 = K_1 \times e[-rt(r)]$$

where t(r) is recovery time, r being the recovery time constant.

A combination of accumulation of oxygen toxicity and its recovery can be used to calculate central nervous system oxygen toxicity. Predicted latency to the appearance of the first electrical discharge in the electroencephalogram, which precedes clinical convulsions, was compared to measured latency for seven different exposures to HBO, followed by a period of normoxia and further HBO exposure (Arieli & Gutterman 1997). Recovery followed an exponential path, with r = 0.31 (SD 0.12) min (−1). Calculation of the recovery of the CNS oxygen toxicity agreed with the previously suggested exponential recovery of the hypoxic ventilatory response and was probably a general recovery process. The authors concluded that recovery can be applied to the design of various hyperoxic exposures.

Inclusion of air breaks in prolonged HBO treatment schedules is a recognized practice. The return to normobaric air between HBO sessions may lead to low pO_2 seizures, which are also described as a "switch off" phenomenon. However, much research still needs to be done to find the ideal schedules to extend oxygen tolerance.

Effect of HBO on the CNS of Newborn Mammals

Newborn mammals are extremely resistant to the CNS effects of HBO compared to adults. Indirect evidence indicates that HBO in newborn rats induces a persistent cerebral vasoconstriction concurrently with a severe and maintained reduction in ventilation. The outcome of these exposures may be as follows:

- Extension of tolerance to both CNS and pulmonary oxygen toxicity,
- Creation of a hypoxic-ischemic condition in vulnerable neuronal structures, and
- Impairment of circulatory and ventilatory responses to hypoxic stimuli on return to air breathing, with subsequent development of a hypoxic-ischemic condition.

These events may set the stage for development of delayed neurological disorders.

Conclusion and Directions for Future Research

The exact mechanism underlying oxygen toxicity to the CNS is not known, but the free radical theory appears to be the most likely explanation. The role of nitric oxide in the effect of HBO has also been established. Fortunately, CNS oxygen toxicity is rare because most HBO treatments are carried out at pressures below 2.5 ATA, and the duration of treatment does not exceed 90 min. Nevertheless, a physician treating patients with HBO must be aware of oxygen toxicity. There is no rational prevention or treatment, but free radical scavengers are used in practice to prevent the toxic effects of oxygen. Until a better understanding of the mechanism of oxygen toxicity and better methods of treatment are available, use of the free radical scavengers that are available appears to be a reasonable practice, particularly when these are relatively nontoxic. In situations where prolonged exposures to HBO are required, the benefits of treatment versus the risks of oxygen toxicity should be carefully weighed.

The chemiluminescence index, which is a measure of tissue lipid peroxidation indicates individual sensitivity of the body to HBO. Such a technique would enable the prediction of the effectiveness of HBO treatment as well as control its duration. Oxygen toxicity can also be exploited for therapeutic purposes. One example of this is the use of HBO as an antibiotic. Induced oxygen toxicity by HBO with protection of the patient by free radical scavengers should be investigated as an adjunctive treatment for AIDS, because the virus responsible for this condition has no protective mechanisms against free radicals. Since induction of antioxidative defence mechanisms has been determined after HBO exposure, a modified treatment regimen of HBO therapy may avoid genotoxic effects (Speit et al 2002).

The methods for estimating free radicals are still cumbersome and not in routine use. More practical methods should be developed as a guide to the safe limits of HBO therapy.

The molecular basis of oxygen toxicity should be sought at the cellular and organelle levels. Simultaneous monitoring of cerebral, electrical, circulatory, and energy-producing functions is a useful tool for determining the safety margins of HBO, as well as for tracing the primary mechanisms of oxygen toxicity in the CNS.

Mammalian cell lines have been shown to develop tolerance to oxygen by repetitive exposure to HBO at 6 to 10 ATA for periods up to 3 h. Repeated screening of various cell lines may lead to the discovery of oxygen-resistant cell types, which might provide an insight into the factors inherent in the development of oxygen tolerance.

The latest approach to counteract pulmonary oxygen toxicity is gene therapy by viral-mediated transfer SOD and catalase to the pulmonary epithelium. This appears to be the most promising method of delivery of these enzymes.

7 Hyperbaric Chambers: Equipment, Technique, and Safety

K.K. Jain

Tremendous improvements have been made in hyperbaric chambers and ancillary equipment to provide a safe place for HBO treatments. The following main topics are discussed here:

Equipment Used in Hyperbaric Medicine

Introduction

The main facility required for hyperbaric medicine is of course the hyperbaric chamber itself. This is essentially a chamber constructed to withstand pressurization, so that oxygen can be administered inside at pressures greater than at sea level. The size, shape, and pressure capabilities of the designs chambers vary considerably. The technical details of each model now available are provided by the manufacturers, and a classification of various types of chambers is shown in Table 7.1.

Table 7.1
Types of Hyperbaric Chambers

1. Monoplace
2. Multiplace or "walk-in" chambers
3. Mobile or portable
   Monoplace: transportable by air, sea, or land
   Multiplace: chamber can be driven from place to place
4. Chambers for testing and training divers
5. Small hyperbaric chambers
   for neonates
   for animal experiments

Monoplace Chambers

Monoplace chambers are the most commonly used; in most of them the pressure cannot be raised over 3 ATA. The patient can be transferred into this chamber on a gurney, and the chamber is filled with oxygen under pressure. There are two types of oxygen flow mechanisms:

- Constant purging: This type has a fixed rate of oxygen flow through the chamber and out again to the external environment.
- Recycling: This type recycles all or a portion of the gases, which are used again after they are properly cleaned and unwanted CO_2 and water vapor are absorbed. Communication with the patient is through an intercom.

Advantages

The monoplace chamber has the following advantages:

1. Handling of patients individually; privacy and, in case of infection, isolation.
2. Ideal for intensive care; no transfer or interruption of medical treatment needed, patient can stay in chamber.
3. Face mask not required; no danger of oxygen leak; comfortable.
4. Ideal for patients confined to bed in acute stage of illness or injury, e.g., paraplegics.
5. Easy to observe patient.
6. No special decompression procedures required.
7. Economy of space and cost; can be easily moved and placed anywhere in hospital.
8. Fewer operators required.

Disadvantages

The disadvantages of monoplace chambers are:

- There is a potential fire hazard in an oxygen-filled environment.
- Direct access to the patient is very limited, except in the case of modified chambers with a side room for the attendant (Reneau dual compartment).
- Physical therapy cannot be carried out in the limited space.
- It is difficult to provide an "air brake" for a patient with decompression sickness unless the patient is conscious, cooperative, and able to put on a mask himself.

This design is ideal for the care of a patient who does not required the presence of medical personnel in the chamber. Most of the essential body functions can be monitored externally, and even the respirator can be controlled from outside the chamber.

A Sechrist monoplace chamber, in common use in the USA, is shown in Figure 7.1. The design of a monoplace chamber for an acute care facility or an intensive care unit is shown in Figure 7.2. An example of a small 1-man portable chamber is the Hyperlite folding hyperbaric chamber (SOS Ltd, London, UK) shown in Figure 7.3. It is made of modern lightweight material and can be easily pressurized on site and then transferred under pressure to and into virtually any therapeutic facility. It is suitable for diving complications, trauma and other emergency indications for HBO. It may be useful for the emergency treatment of acute stroke.

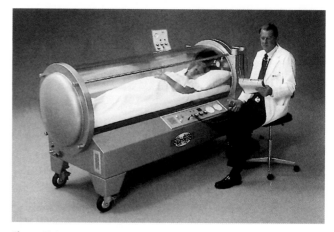

Figure 7.1
The Sechrist monoplace hyperbaric chamber.

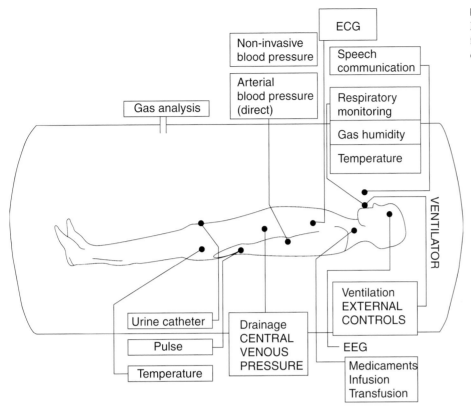

Figure 7.2
Monitoring and routine care functions for acute medical care in a monoplace chamber.

ECG

Non-invasive blood pressure

Speech communication

Arterial blood pressure (direct)

Respiratory monitoring

Gas analysis

Gas humidity

Temperature

VENTILATOR

Urine catheter

Pulse

Temperature

Drainage CENTRAL VENOUS PRESSURE

Ventilation EXTERNAL CONTROLS

EEG

Medicaments Infusion Transfusion

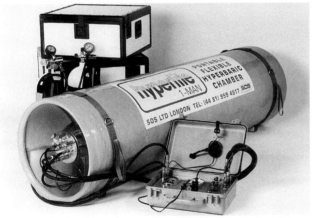

Figure 7.3a
The Hyperlite 1-man portable hyperbaric chamber (photos courtesy of SOS Ltd, London, UK).

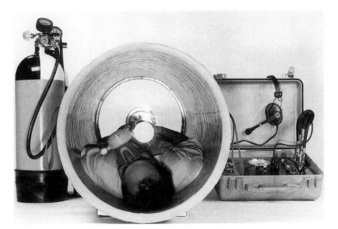

Figure 7.3b

Another transportable chamber which is in development is the Gamow bag which can be carried as a back pack and pressurized when required. It has been found to be useful for treating high altitude illness. The pressure limit of the original bag is set at 2 psi because of the fragility of the fabric. However, improvement of the hardware to make the bag capable of withstanding higher pressures has made it possible to perform standard HBO therapy with the newly devised portable chamber, the Chamberlite 15. In this study, the safety of the new bag was examined using healthy human volunteers, and the bag was shown to be usable in clinical emergency cases, such as CO intoxication and decompression sickness (Shimada *et al* 1996). The effectiveness of emergency hyperbaric oxygen therapy was also examined using the CO intoxication model of the rat. Evidence suggested that HBO was especially beneficial if applied during the first 30 min of rescue work. It was concluded that the transportable chamber was a promising emergency tool for CO intoxication. This bag can be considered for HBO treatment of acute stroke patients during transport to a medical center.

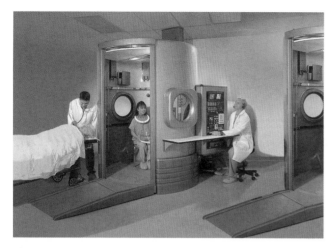

Figure 7.4

A pair of OxyHeal 2000 Class A multiplace hyperbaric chambers. These 3 ATA chambers accommodate four occupants. All BIBS gases can be controlled internally or externally. An extension tube permits the introduction of supine patients. Low voltage automated devices with manual back-ups control treatments. (Photo courtesy of OxyHeal Health Group, La Jolla, CA 92038, USA.)

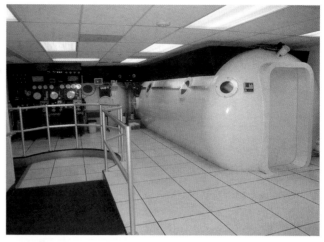

Figure 7.5

OxyHeal 4000 Class A Multiplace hyperbaric chamber. A 3-lock, 6 ATA, 18-patient horizontal cylinder hyperbaric chamber system at Presbyterian/St. Luke's Hospital in Denver, Colorado, USA. This chamber performs a significant number of critical care treatments annually. (Photo courtesy of OxyHeal Health Group, La Jolla, CA 92038, USA.)

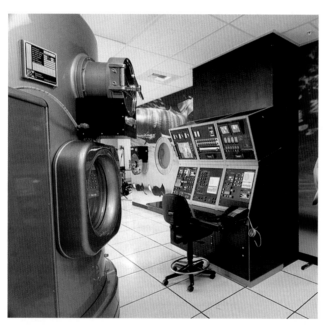

Figure 7.6a

OxyHeal 5000 Rectangular Chamber. The 3 ATA hyperbaric chamber complex adjoining the Regional Burn Center at the University Medical Center, Las Vegas, Nevada, USA. The complex consist of a large two-lock rectangular geometry Class A hyperbaric chamber designed to accommodate 12-patients and to perform critical care. The OxyHeal 2000, shown in the foreground, is used to enable routine hyperbaric treatments when the larger chamber is performing critical care treatments. The chamber complex Control Console operates both hyperbaric systems.

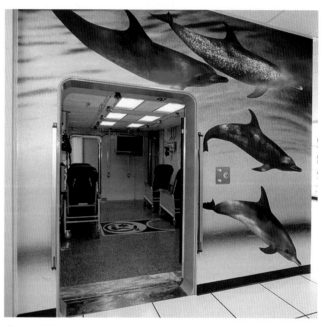

Figure 7.6b

OxyHeal 5000 Rectangular Chamber Interior. The view shows non-dedicated seating, large entertainment screen and floor level doors large enough to roll a hospital bed into. Underwater scene murals are applied in order to reduce patient anxiety. (Photo courtesy of OxyHeal Health Group, La Jolla, CA 92038, USA.)

Multiplace Chambers

Multiplace chambers are used for simultaneous treatment of a number of patients. The capacity varies from a few to as many as 20 patients. The chamber is filled with air and breathing is done via a mask covering the mouth and nose. Modern chambers of this type are fitted with a comprehensive gas supply and monitoring systems; the gas composition in the chamber is monitored and corrected, particularly if there are oxygen leaks from the masks. The atmosphere is air-conditioned for humidity as well as temperature. Examples of multiplace hyperbaric chambers manufactured in the USA are:

- Dual OxyHeal 2000 Hyperbaric chamber (OxyHeal Health Group). A pair of Class A multiplace hyperbaric chambers accommodate four occupants (Figure 7.4).
- OxyHeal 4000 Multiplace hyperbaric chamber (OxyHeal Health Group). A 3-lock, 6 ATA, 18-patient horizontal cylinder Class A hyperbaric chamber system is used for critical care treatments (Figure 7.5).
- OxyHeal 5000 Rectangular Chamber (OxyHeal Health Group). The 3 ATA hyperbaric chamber complex Class A hyperbaric chamber is designed to accommodate 12-patients and to perform critical care (Figure 7.6).

Advantages

The advantages of multiplace chambers are as follows:

1. Simultaneous treatment of a large number of patients is possible.
2. They are essential for treatment that requires presence of a physician and special equipment, as in an operating room.
3. There is reduced fire hazard.
4. Physical therapy can be performed in the chamber.
5. Pressure can be raised to 6 ATA for special situations in air embolism and decompression sickness.

Multiplace hyperbaric chambers can be used to deliver patient care with enormous flexibility. Standard critical care techniques, such as mechanical ventilation, endotracheal suctioning, hemodynamic monitoring, blood gas measurement, and emergency therapy such as cardiopulmonary resuscitation, including defibrillation and cardioversion, can all be performed inside a multiplace chamber. The multiplace chamber can be considered an extension of the intensive care unit. This flexibility is accompanied by increased complexity of chamber operation. Defibrillation plays a crucial role in the resuscitation of patients from acute life-threatening cardiac dysrhythmias causing cardiac arrest. Concerns over safety and function of defibrillators under pressure have so far prevented their routine use in clinical hyperbaric chambers. Now increasing numbers of unstable and critically ill patients are being treated in such facilities.

Minor surgical procedures can be performed in the usual multiplace hyperbaric chamber, but major surgery such as heart surgery requires a specially designed chamber. There are many such chambers in existence in the USSR and Japan, but few in Europe (Graz & Amsterdam). The hyperbaric chamber with an operating room located at the University of Nagoya, Japan, is shown in Figure 7.7.

There are some technical problems of surgery in a hyperbaric chamber as some types of equipments cannot be operated in a chamber, e.g., electrocoagulation for hemostasis.

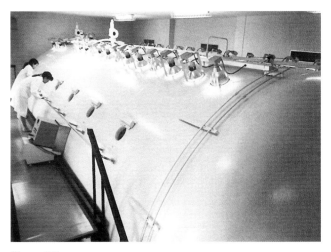

Figure 7.7a
Large hyperbaric chamber at the University of Nagoya, Japan, outside view.

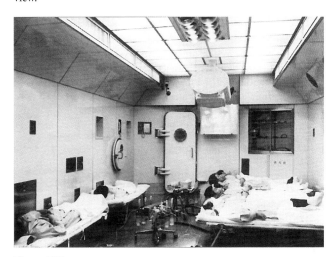

Figure 7.7b
Inside view. Operations can be carried out in this chamber.

Mobile Multiplace Hyperbaric Chambers

The first mobile multiplace chamber was constructed in the form of a bus in Nagoya, Japan, but it is no longer in use. Other mobile chambers are now available, in various locations throughout the world. An OxyHeal 4000 triple lock, 6 ATA, 18-patient mobile hyperbaric chamber (OxyHeal Health Group) resides within the over-the-road trailer. This chamber complex is now permanently installed on a roof of the Hermann Hospital in Houston, Texas, USA, where it has been in continuous operation since 1990. An OxyHeal 4000 dual lock, 6 ATA, 12-patient hyperbaric chamber (OxyHeal Health Group), shown in Figure 7.8 is placed next to the emergency department of Advocate/Lutheran General Hospital in Park Ridge, Illinois, USA. This was one of the first American hospitals to perform hyperbaric surgeries and the hyperbaric center there has been in continuous operation since the early 1960s.

Advantages

The advantages of the mobile chamber are:

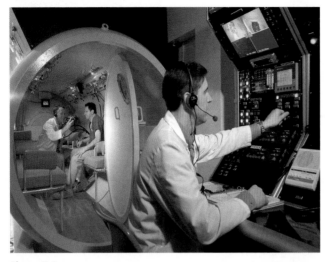

Figure 7.8
Mobile Hyperbaric System Interior. An OxyHeal 4000 dual lock, 6 ATA, 12-patient hyperbaric chamber inside a 52' over-the-road trailer, installed adjoining the Emergency Room at Advocate/Lutheran General Hospital in Park Ridge, Illinois, USA. (Photo courtesy of OxyHeal Health Group, La Jolla, CA 92038, USA.)

- It can be moved where needed. It can function, for instance, in the parking lot of a hospital.
- It is comfortable and safe.
- It is ideal for clinical use as well as for research.
- It is suitable for use in military medicine. It can be moved to the base hospital in case of war. It can also be transported by air and sea.

Special Uses

The mobile chamber has various special uses:

- Sports physiology and physical therapy research. A treadmill is placed in the chamber and all the necessary investigations can be done while the patient exercises in the chamber.
- Treatment of patients with cerebrovascular insufficiency, myocardial ischemia, and peripheral vascular disease.
- "Brain jogging" mental exercises and psychological testing can be performed in the chamber during HBO administration or immediately afterward in the anteroom. This is useful in the treatment and assessment of patients with cognitive deficits.
- Emergency treatment of the patient can be carried out during long-distance transport in the chamber.

a)
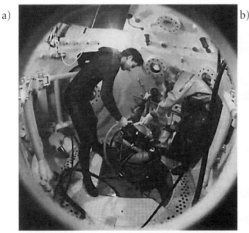

b)
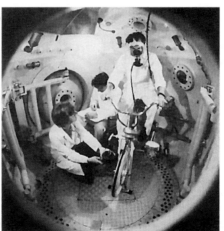

Figure 7.9a-e
Combined treatment and diver testing hyperbaric chamber at the University Hospital, Zurich, Switzerland (a) Diving testing; (b) exercise testing; (c) a patient being transferred into the chamber on a special device; (d) patients being treated inside the chamber – note the oxygen tents used by the patients; (e, next page) overall view. This chamber can be used for simulating dives to depths of 1000 m and high altitude simulation up to 10,000 m (Photos courtesy of Dr. B. Schenk, Head of Operations, Hyperbaric Laboratory, University Hospital, Zurich).

c)
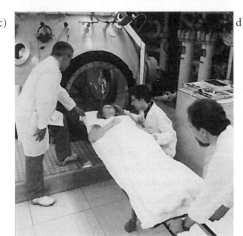

d)
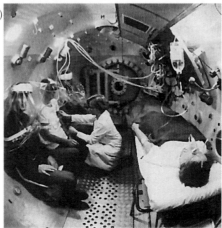

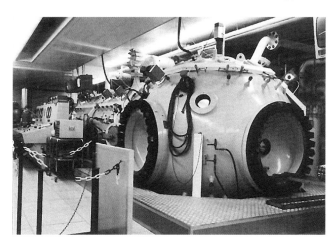

Figure 7.9e

Hyperbaric Chambers for Diving Medicine

Diving chambers are used for testing and training divers with simulated depths. These facilities can be combined with hyperbaric chambers for patient treatment in a hyperbaric center. An example of this is shown in Figure 7.9.

Small Hyperbaric Chambers

Hyperbaric chambers have been constructed for use in experiments with small animals. Small portable chambers are available for resuscitation of newborns. A specially designed chamber for animal experiments is shown in Figure 7.10. OxyCure 3000 Hyperbaric Cellular Incubator (Oxy-Heal Health Group) is a class C chamber with controls for the pressure, gases, temperature and humidity shown in Figure 7.11. It is used in cellular studies and to induce autologous stem cell replication.

Selection of a Hyperbaric Chamber

A classification of hyperbaric chambers according to pressure, size, and uses is shown in Table 7.2. Most of the indications (90%) can be covered by chambers of types I and II. Pressure up to 2.5 ATA is not only the upper limit for most applications, it is also the starting point for compulsory inspection by the technical inspection agency (TÜV) in Germany. This classification may help the manufacturer as well as the consumer to choose a chamber within a certain category. It would be uneconomical to make all the chambers capable of withstanding a pressure of 6 ATA. Two indications for which pressures of 6 ATA have been used in the past, i.e., decompression sickness and air embolism, are being reassessed. For both these conditions, the highest pressures required may not exceed 3 ATA, as discussed in Chapters 10 and 11.

The hyperbaric chamber is a durable piece of equipment

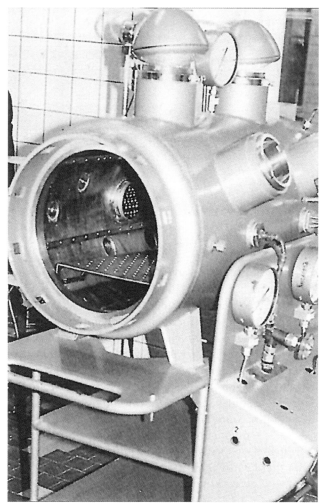

Figure 7.10
A hyperbaric chamber for animal experiments at the All Union Center for Surgical Research, Moscow.

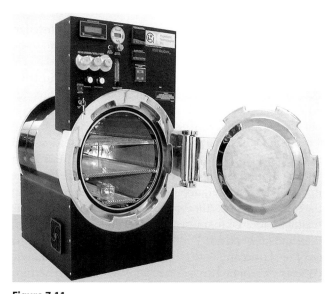

Figure 7.11
OxyCure 3000 Hyperbaric Cellular Incubator for cellular studies. Acknowledgment: Photo courtesy of OxyHeal Health Group, La Jolla, CA 92038, USA.

Table 7.2
Classification of Hyperbaric Chambers According to Use and Pressure

Type	Pressure	Type	Typical indications
I	Up to 1.5 ATA	Mobile and multiplace	Ischemic disorders: cerebral, cardiac, peripheral-vascular: adjuvant to physical therapy and sports medicine; adjuvant to survival of skin flaps; acoustic trauma
II	Up to 2.5 ATA Up to 3.0 ATA	Monoplace and portable	Gas gangrene Burns Crush injuries of extremities Emergency treatment of decompression sickness
III	Up to 6.0 ATA	Multiplace	Air embolism Decompression sickness

and many old chambers are still performing well. The safety record has been good. However, as in any other technology, there is constant evolution and improvement. The latest addition to the hyperbaric chamber family is the mobile multiplace chamber. This chamber gives us an ideal opportunity to conduct further investigations in the field of rehabilitation and sports medicine. Another advantage of the mobile chamber is that the equipment can be moved to any desired location at short notice with no necessity for installation procedures. Hyperbaric chambers are still expensive, and the number of chambers available is not adequate to treat all the patients who would potentially benefit from HBO therapy. In this situation, the mobile hyperbaric chamber is an economical proposition.

Technique of Hyperbaric Oxygenation

The schedules of pressure for different diseases are listed in the appropriate chapters. We restrict ourselves here to some general comments about technique.

The hyperbaric technician follows the prescribed instructions from the hyperbaric physician about the pressure, duration, and frequency of treatment. Most of the treatments at our hyperbaric center are given at pressures between 1.5 and 2.5 ATA, and the usual duration of a hyperbaric session is 45 min. Of this 10 min are required for compression and 5 min for decompression if pressures of 1.5 ATA are used. Thus, the maximal oxygen saturation is maintained for about 0.5 h. In the case of infections, the treatment duration is doubled. The treatment sessions for most chronic conditions are given daily, including weekends. For the multiplace chamber, patients are grouped according to indications. For example, all stroke patients are grouped to go in the same session and are accompanied by a physiotherapist or a physician if a research project is involved. The technician keeps a complete log of the session and the data can be recorded and reproduced by computer. Compression and decompression are quite smooth,

and if the patient complains of any discomfort such as ear pain, the procedure can be halted. In case of a more severe problem, the affected patient can be moved to the anteroom of the multiplace chamber and decompression started while the treatment of the remaining patients is continued in the main chamber with the door between the two chambers locked.

In the case of a monoplace chamber, oxygen is introduced into the chamber at the start while pressure is raised. In the multiplace chamber, oxygen masks are used and oxygen inhalation is started only when the chamber has been pressurized to the desired level.

Oxygen partial pressures are not measured routinely, but only for research purposes or in some special cases. Most of the measured values of paO_2 are around 1000 mmHg at 1.5 ATA.

Table 7.3
Ancillary Equipment for the Hyperbaric Chamber

1. Oxygen masks and hoods
2. Respirators and ventilators
3. Miscellaneous equipment for treatment
   Cardiopulmonary resuscitation apparatus
   Endotracheal tubes
   Suction equipment
   Intravenous infusions
4. Equipment for diagnosis
   Basic medical examination tray
   Transcutaneous oxygen measurement
   EEG
   ECG
   Blood gases and hemorrheology equipment
   Intracranial pressure and CSF oxygen tension monitors
   Blood pressure measurement cuff
5. Neurological assessment equipment
   Ophthalmoscope
   Dynamometer to measure spasticity
6. Equipment for exercise: treadmill
7. Therapeutic equipment such as cervical traction for cervical spine injuries

Ancillary Equipment

Various types of ancillary equipment are listed in Table 7.3.

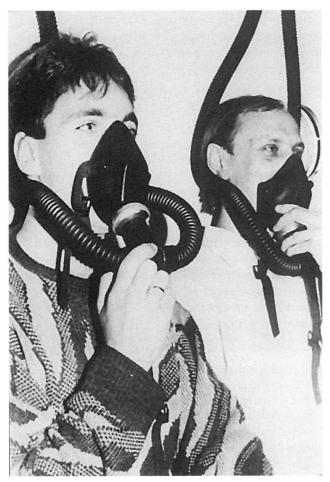

Figure 7.12
Oxygen masks for use in hyperbaric chambers.

Oxygen Masks and Hoods

Oxygen masks are required only in the multiplace hyperbaric chambers. The mask should fit tightly and not allow any leakage of oxygen. The US Air Force aviator's mask, when properly fitted, has end-inspired oxygen levels of 96.9–99%, and paO_2 of 1640 mmHg is reached at 2.4 ATA. One type of mask in common use is shown in Figure 7.12. The masks are made of rubber or silicon and can be cleaned and disinfected easily. Headbands of the masks can be placed easily. Oxygen hoods and oxygen tents have been used as an alternative to the masks and are particularly useful in patients with head and neck lesions.

Respirators and Ventilators

Various ventilators found to be effective in hyperbaric environments at pressures up to 6 ATA are:

- The Sechrist model 500A mechanical ventilator, shown in Figure 7.13, for use with the Sechrist monoplace chamber. Patients with respiratory failure can be placed in it and it will compensate for changes in pressure inside the chamber. Its specifications are shown in Table 7.4.
- The Penlon Oxford ventilator: this is a bellows type, volume-set, timed-cycle device and is used at some medical facilities.
- The Siemens Servo ventilators – sophisticated, volume-set, timed-cycle devices used in intensive care units.
- The Monaghan 225 ventilator is driven by compressed air rather than oxygen. At 1 ATA, this ventilator delivers between 35 and 40 l of the gas/min to the patient. Although this ventilator functions satisfactorily, gas delivery drops to 18 l/min, still adequate for the majority of patients.

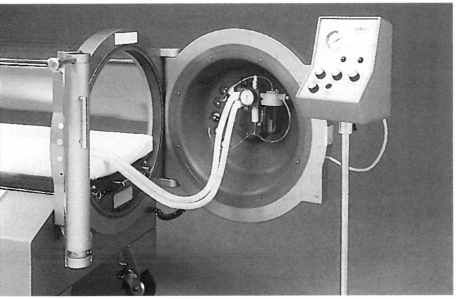

Figure 7.13
Sechrist Model 500A Mechanical Ventilator for the Sechrist monoplace hyperbaric system. (Photo courtesy of Sechrist Industries Inc, Anaheim, California.)

Table 7.4
Specifications of the Hyperbaric Ventilator, Model 500A (Sechrist)

Principals of function	Automatic adjustment of delivery pressure of ventilation to variations of pressure in the hyperbaric chamber
Regulating system	2 components: breathing circuit in the chamber and control module outside the chamber
Respiratory frequency	8–30 breaths/min
Respiratory minute vol.	0–15 l/min at 3 ATA
Tidal volume range	0–1.5 l at 3 ATA
Breathing time relationship (inspiration: expiration)	1:5–3.5:1
Respiratory flow range	0–100 l/min at ambient. 0–60 l/min at 3 ATA
Inspiratory pressure limit	20–80 cm water

The desirable features of a ventilator for hyperbaric environments are:

- No electrically driven components.
- Volume and rate remain stable with all changes in pressure.
- Low oxygen bleed into the chamber to prevent contamination of the air inside.
- Continuous flow in intermittent mandatory ventilation is superior to a demand valve, as it minimizes the inspiratory work and maintains a constant airway pressure.

Diagnostic Equipment

Basic medical diagnostic equipment such as reflex hammers, stethoscope, and ophthalmoscope should be available in the chamber.

Transcutaneous oxygen tension

Transcutaneous oxygen tension ($tcpO_2$) measurement is a noninvasive technique for measuring oxygen tension of the tissues by means of an electrode taped on the skin. It cannot be used in the monoplace chamber, as the electrodes are electrically heated and constitute a fire hazard. The results of measurements of $tcpO_2$ in volunteers breathing air and HBO up to 4 ATA show close correlation with pO_2 values measured directly in blood from arterial puncture inside the hyperbaric chamber. In patients with various degrees of peripheral vascular occlusive disease, the $tcpO_2$ are significantly lower than in control subjects.

ECG and EEG

ECG and EEG pose no special problems and should be standard in chambers for treating patients with cerebrovascular insufficiency. Changes in the signal quality of ECG can occur with high pressures. EEG power spectrum recording can be performed quite satisfactorily in the hyperbaric chamber. Somatosensory evoked potential studies can also be conducted.

Blood Gases

Blood gases should ideally be determined inside the chamber due to the problem of release of gases if the sample is brought outside to sea-level pressure. Several blood gas analysis systems have been modified to function inside the hyperbaric chamber. Blood samples of gases can also be analyzed at the pressure of measurement with specially calibrated equipment. The ratio of arterial to alveolar pO_2 (a/A ratio) is a constant, independent of the inspired oxygen concentration. This is also true at elevated atmospheric pressure, in healthy volunteers as well as patients. It is possible to predict the paO_2 at 3 ATA from the values obtained at 1 ATA.

Glucose Monitoring Devices

Diabetic patients may experience fluctuations in blood glucose levels during HBO treatment for ischemic non-healing wounds. Therefore, whole blood glucose levels should be monitored during treatment. Most of the currently marketed glucose monitoring devices (glucometers) measure glucose with glucose oxidase- or glucose dehydrogenase-based methods. Glucose dehydrogenase methods do not utilize oxygen but inaccuracies have been reported between measurements at ground level and at 2.36 ATA (Price et al 1995). Glucose oxidase-impregnated reagent strips are are affected because both high and low pressures of oxygen interfere with enzymatic reactions involved which utilize oxygen.

Miscellaneous Medical Equipment

Basic cardiopulmonary resuscitation equipment should be available in the chamber. Endotracheal tubes and Foley catheter cuffs should be inflated with water or saline instead of air. Suction can be generated in the chamber by compressed air or made available from outside through a pressure reduction regulator. Special injection kits for intravenous infusion are available from the manufacturers for use in their chambers. In the case of monoplace chambers, special precautions are necessary when running an intravenous infusion because of the difference between chamber pressure and external pressure. A treadmill motor can be placed under the hyperbaric chamber and the motion transmitted by a shaft through the floor of the chamber (Figure 7.10).

Pleural suction drainage systems can be dramatically affected by pressure change, but can be used safely in a hyperbaric environment provided that the following precautions are taken (Walker *et al* 2006):

- Suction should not be applied during pressurization.
- Pressurization needs to be slow, 10 kpa/min or less.
- Suction must be applied during depressurization if there is an air leak of 5/min or greater coming from the patient, otherwise suction is not essential.
- Hyperbaric compatibility should be tested before use.

Monitoring of Patients in the Hyperbaric Chamber

Patients and attendants in the chamber can be monitored by any of the following means:

- Visual. Direct view into a monoplace chamber; closed circuit TV in the multi-place chamber.
- Auditory. For both monoplace and multiplace chambers; several two-way communication systems are available for this purpose.
- Use of diagnostic and monitoring equipment both inside and outside the chamber; direct observation by the accompanying attendants in case of multiplace chambers.

The level of monitoring depends on the severity and type of illness. With critically ill patients, the routine monitoring in the ICU can be continued into the chamber. In patients not requiring medical attention by contact, most of the essential monitoring can be done in a suitably equipped hyperbaric chamber, such as the Dräger HTK 1200 monoplace chamber. Some of the problems of monitoring head-injured patients in the monoplace chamber are:

1. If the arterial blood pressure is monitored by an indwelling radial artery catheter, a pressure infuser should be used to keep the line flushed open with a heparinized solution. Any obstruction of the catheter during pressure changes may dampen the wave form or flatten it.
2. Central venous pressure can be measured by connecting the line to a transducer and a monitoring module.
3. Swan-Ganz catheter. Pulmonary artery pressures can be monitored during HBO therapy; satisfactory wave forms are obtained without significant changes in the pulmonary artery pressure.
4. For EEG monitoring, the electrodes should be attached

prior to entry to the chamber, and the collodion should be allowed to dry because when wet, it is flammable. Properly placed electrodes can stay in position for up to 5 days.
5. The cuffs of the endotracheal tubes should be filled with sterile normal saline during HBO. After the treatment, the saline is removed and replaced by air.
6. Arterial blood gas analysis. Arterial blood gas samples can be aspirated from the arterial line for analysis during HBO treatment. Transcutaneous oxygen monitoring cannot be done in a monoplace chamber because the electrode presents a fire hazard.

Miscellaneous Special Diagnostic Procedures

Intracranial pressure monitoring is important in patients with head injuries and cerebral edema. The Richmond subarachnoid bolt system connected to a standard arterial pressure transducer located inside the chamber with electrical leads passing through the walls is satisfactory. Intracellular current passage and recording inside a hyperbaric chamber can be carried out without danger of fire by using using glass microelectrodes and micromanipulators.

The cerebrospinal fluid (CSF) reflects the oxygen tension of the brain. CSF examination by cistern puncture or after removal from an Ommaya CSF reservoir may give an idea of the state of oxygenation of the brain tissues. This is important, as there is no satisfactory practical method of measuring cerebral blood flow in the hyperbaric chamber.

Safety in the Hyperbaric Chamber

Operational Safety

Safety is a very important consideration in the construction of hyperbaric chambers. Loss of chamber structural integrity can result in rapid decompression and decompression sickness. Most chambers in the United States are constructed according to the requirements of the ASME Boiler and Pressure Vessels Code, as amplified by ANSI-ASME PUHO (Sect. VIII, Div. 1, American Society of Mechanical Engineers, New York). A chamber built according to these standards can be expected to give years of reliable service, if it is properly maintained.

The windows of a hyperbaric chamber are usually made of acrylic plastic because it is easily formed and gives ample warning of impending failure. These materials are subject to corrosion and alcohol-based solutions should not be used for cleaning windows. Acrylic is subject to damage by heat and nuclear radiation.

Essential controls and monitors for a hyperbaric chamber should be provided with an emergency power source in the event of loss of power, and the transfer from normal to emergency power should be automatic.

Atmospheric Control

This refers to maintenance of a safe atmosphere inside the chamber. Contamination of the atmosphere is possible by products carried into the chamber. The hyperbaric chamber is pressurized by one of three methods:

- compressed gas directly from a compressor,
- compressed gas from a pressurized accumulator,
- gas from a cryogenic supply system through a suitable vaporizer.

Large multiplace chambers are pressurized by compressed air from an accumulator that acts as a buffer in the event of compressor failure or loss of electric power. Pressurized air, regardless of the source, should be checked periodically for composition and purity. Sufficiently clean air can be provided by locating the air intake away from sources of pollution and providing suitable absorbers for pollutants. Safety standards for the composition of chamber air are given in Table 7.5.

Table 7.5
Recommended Maximum Values for Contaminants in Hyperbaric Air (from Hamilton and Sheffield 1977, by permission)

- Oxygen: 20%–22% by volume
- Carbon dioxide: 1000 ppm by volume (0.10%)
- Carbon monoxide: 20 ppm by volume (0.002%)
- Gaseous hydrocarbons (methane, ethane, etc.): 25 ppm by volume (0.0025%)
- Halogenated solvents: 0.2 ppm by volume (0.00002%)
- Oil and particulate matter: 0.005 mg/l, weight/volume
- Total water: 0.3 mg/l, weight/volume
- Odor: None objectionable or unusual

Masks and Breathing Control System

The breathing control system is also referred to as BIBS (built in breathing system) in a multiplace chamber. It provides a safe and secure source of breathing gas in case of contamination of the chamber atmosphere. The masks for supplying oxygen are supplied by an overhead dumping system where the exhaled breath is directed out of the chamber. The masks should fit well. Oxygen leaking from the masks not only reduces the effectiveness of the treatment but also raises the oxygen concentration of the chamber air above accepted levels and should not exceed 23 vol%. The expired gases are removed directly by a so called "overboard dumping system." In the case of hoods, special attention is required to CO_2 removal and prevention of excessive humid-

ity. The oxygen supply to the mask should be humidified to prevent the irritating effect of oxygen.

Fire Safety in the Chamber

Prior to 1970, there were no national fire safety standards for clinical hyperbaric chambers in the United States. Fire prevention was a matter left to common sense of the operators. Considering the widespread use of hyperbaric oxygen therapy, the record of fire safety in hyperbaric chambers has been good. The first hyperbaric chamber fire occurred in 1923 in Cunningham's chamber in in the United States (see Chapter 1). There have been a total of 25 fires in clinical hyperbaric chambers worldwide from 1923 to 1996 (Sheffield & Desautels 1997, 1998). The review by these authors was based on reports in the literature as well as the Chambers Experience and Mishap Database of the Undersea and Hyperbaric Medical Society. During the 73-year period reviewed, there were 91 human fatalities associated with 40 fires in pressure-related chambers of all types including diving bells, decompression chambers and pressurized Apollo Command Module. There were 60 deaths in 21 clinical hyperbaric chamber fires. No death occurred in clinical hyperbaric chambers in the United States. Most of the deaths prior to 1980 were associated with electrical ignition inside the chamber but after this period the reported source of ignition has usually been a prohibited source of ignition carried by an occupant inside the chamber. All fatal fires occurred in enriched oxygen environments and only reported survivors were in chambers pressurized with air.

The first fire in a clinical monoplace chamber was reported in Japan in 1967 and three more occurred in in the following years; all were initiated by hand warmers. Tobin (1978) reported an explosion due to static electricity while a patient was having cobalt irradiation under HBO at 3 ATA in a monoplace chamber. The patient developed a lung rupture due to explosive decompression but survived. From 1976 to 189, static electricity was considered to be the cause of seven fires resulting in five deaths in monoplace chambers filled with pure oxygen. Static charge stored in the fiberglass tray was considered to be the initiating factors and these trays were replaced with stainless steel trays. Strict guidelines to this effect as well as for grounding were laid down by the National Fire Protection Association of the United States and no such incidents have been reported since then.

Another accident occurred in 1987 in Naples, when a child died in a fire in a monoplace chamber. The child was playing with a toy pistol that may have caused the ignition. The accident was attributed to the laxity of the attendant in allowing the child to take a toy into the chamber. No prompt measures were taken to rescue the child, who was practically incinerated.

The first occurrence of a fire in a multiplace chamber was reported by Youn *et al* (1989). It was precipitated by an externally heated microwave blanket introduced through the safety lock. The fire was rapidly extinguished with a central deluge system. A second mishap occurred in Milan Italy in 1997 when a fatal explosion occurred in a multiplace chamber with 11 deaths. A gas operated hand warmer was the likely trigger and it is likely that the chamber was pressurized with oxygen rather than air as explosive fire would not occur in a chamber pressurized with air. There have been no fires reported in hyperbaric chambers during the past five years.

Fatal hyperbaric fires are usually caused by a combination of factors: abundance of combustible materials, high oxygen levels, faulty electrical components, inadequate fire extinguishing equipment and lack of vigilance for carriage of prohibited items into the chamber. Emphasis should be placed on the prevention, detection, and elimination of known and suspected fire hazards in a hyperbaric chamber. Fire is more of a hazard in a monoplace chamber because it is filled with 100% oxygen.

The following measures should be taken to prevent fire in a monoplace chamber:

- There should be no electrical equipment inside the chamber. All leads for diagnostic equipment should be connected to instruments outside the chamber. All ignition sources inside the chamber should be eliminated.
- There should be no nylon garments inside the chamber.
- The patient should not use an oil-based or volatile cosmetic (facial cream, body oil, or hair spray) before a hyperbaric session.
- In case of fire, prompt decompression should be performed and the chamber opened. Fire precautions should be continued outside the chamber until the oxygen soaked into the garment or the mattress under the patient has dissipated.

For multiplace hyperbaric chambers, guidelines of the U. S. National Fire Protection Association should be followed (NFPA-56D dealing with hyperbaric facilities, and NFPA-53M dealing with fire hazards in oxygen-enriched environments 1987). The standards include the following basic points:

- All equipment should be designed and tested to be intrinsically safe for hyperbaric conditions, i.e. it must be pressure tested and spark proof.
- All wiring and fixed electrical equipment must comply with NFPA-70, National Electrical Code, Article 500, Class I, Division I.
- All equipment, circuits included, must be waterproof, explosion proof, and from the chamber's sprinkler system.

The following additional measures should be taken in multiplace chambers:

1. No volatile or flammable liquid should be allowed inside the chamber.
2. Lubricants for mechanical devices inside the chamber should be of the halogenated polymer hydrocarbon type. All combustible lubricants should be avoided.
3. Electric motors should be replaced by air-driven or hydraulic motors.
4. Oxygen concentration in the chamber must be kept below 23%. If it goes over 25%, the oxygen supply should be shut off until the source of the leak is found.
5. Fire-detecting systems, manual or automatic, should be installed. The latter should have a safeguard for false alarms.
6. A fire extinguishing system should be provided. Pressurized water should be supplied by a built-in flooding system with additional hand-held hoses. Fire drill and escape procedures should be practiced periodically.

NFPA 99, Chapter 19, has specific guidance for fire extinguishing systems in class A (multiplace) chambers (National Fire Protection Association 1996). The important points are:

- Fire extinguishing systems must be capable of activation from inside or outside of chambers.
- Water is the extinguishing element of choice.
- Each member of the hyperbaric team should be trained in activating the chamber fire extinguishing system.
- NFPA has no guidelines on extinguishing fires in monoplace pure-oxygen chambers as fires in this atmosphere are not survivable.

Use of Portable Hyperbaric Chambers in Patient's Rooms

It is safe to use a portable hyperbaric chamber in a patient's room in a hospital provided all the precautions for an oxygen rich environment are observed and adequate technical supervision is provided.

Particular measures to be taken are:

1. All combustible material should be removed from the room
2. Electrical appliances should be placed at least 5 ft (1.5 m) away from areas where the oxygen concentration is greater than 23.5%.
3. All personal items likely to produce static discharges should be removed from the patient.

Regulatory Issues Relevant to Hyperbaric Medicine

There does not appear to be clearcut single authority for regulating hyperbaric medicine in any country. In the United States, the local fire marshal's office enforces the safety regulations of the National Fire Protection Association. The Food and Drug Administration (FDA), which is the main regulatory authority for pharmaceuticals and medical devices, had a rather background role in clinical hyperbaric medicine in the past but it is becoming more significant now. Oxygen is classified as a drug by the FDA. Therefore, both its application and the devices used to administer it fall under FDA's jurisdiction. Hyperbaric chambers are medical devices used for the administration of oxygen and are subject to FDA control which applies to all medical devices which entered into use since 1976. Hyperbaric chambers constructed prior to 1976 are not subject to FDA control.

Medical devices are divided by the FDA into three classes with differing levels of FDA involvement according to the class:

- **Class I:** General controls. These are simple devices where performance is not much of a concern, such as tongue depressors. Notification of intention to market the device is required under Section 510 (k) of the Safe Medical Device Amendments enacted in 1976. FDA clearance of the Premarket Notification (hence the term 510K) is required prior to marketing the device or placing it for commercial distribution.
- **Class II:** Special controls. These are complex devices where performance is a concern, but at a somewhat general level. Class II devices must comply with general controls and the requirement of some applicable standards. A 510K Pre-market Notification to the FDA is required. FDA clearance of the Pre-market Notification is required prior to marketing the device or placing it in commercial distribution.
- **Class III:** Pre-market approval. These are generally devices that are directly related to patient life support with a substantial risk of injury in the event of malfunction. An example is a cardiac pacemaker. Pre-market approval by the FDA is required. The resulting design and manufacturing controls are very strict.

Hyperbaric chambers are considered to be class II devices and the applicable industry standard is NFPA 99, Chapter 19 and "Safety Standard for Pressure Vessels for Human Occupancy (PVHO-1)" issued by the Safety Code Committee of the ASME.

All classes of medical devices are subject to the FDA's **Good Manufacturing Practice** (GMP) regulations. These are similar to the international quality assurance regulations (ISO 9000, ISO 9001, etc) that have come into widespread use in recent years. The main requirements are:

- As established design for the product (e.g., drawings) approved by some reasonable person.
- Production in accordance with the design
- Testing to confirm performance in accordance with design requirements
- Receipt control and inspections of incoming materials
- Established procedures for resolving problems and customer complaints
- Production documentation sufficient to maintain accountability and to confirm that the above requirements are being met.
- The manufacturing establishment and the product must be registered annually with the FDA.

Conformance with the FDA's rules as they apply to the manufacture of hyperbaric chambers is usually not difficult in a technical sense. However, it does require a commitment to procedural controls that can be difficult to maintain.

"Labeling" is interpreted by the FDA to mean just about everything the manufacturer says about what the device can be used for and how it can be used. In case of oxygen, the recognized claims are the indications recommended by the Undersea and Hyperbaric Medical Society.

Adultered devices are prohibited by the FDA. This term applies to devices that are:

- Built in an unregistered establishment
- Built without a cleared 510K Premarket Notification
- Altered or otherwise not built in accordance with the approved design

Avoidance of appearance of endorsement of products. Manufacturers are not permitted to refer to their FDA 510K Premarket notification nor resulting FDA clearance in advertising in any published literature. However, a manufacturer can respond to a request from a potential customer regarding whether or not a manufacturer has a cleared 510K Pre-market Notification for a specific device.

Regulation of hyperbaric chambers varies in other countries. A European code of good practice for hyperbaric oxygen therapy represents the harmonized European view on safety in therapeutic hyperbaric facilities and can be used as a reference document for European countries for guidelines, regulations, and standards in hyperbaric medicine (Kot *et al* 2004). One of the countries with very strict technical regulations is Germany where a certificate from an organization called TÜV (Technischer Überwachungsverein) is required before a hyperbaric chamber can be approved for use. Guidelines for quality control of laid down by GTÜM (Gesellschaft für Tauch- und Überdruckmedizin e.V.) which is an organization for diving and hyperbaric medicine. Germany has an excellent record of safety in hyperbaric medicine and no mishaps have occurred in recent years. Currently all the hyperbaric chambers approved for use in Germany are multiplace and monoplace chambers are not allowed because of the fire hazard.

Staffing of Hyperbaric Facilities

All personnel employed in hyperbaric facilities should, of course, be properly trained, and familiar with all relevant safety precautions and decompression procedures.

Paramedical personnel are hyperbaric technicians and nurses. The technicians are mostly concerned with the operation and safety of the chamber but they should also have an elementary knowledge of hyperbaric medicine. Nurses are concerned mostly with the care of the patients before, during, and after HBO treatments. Although they are expected to have a fair medical knowledge of conditions treated by HBO, they should also be familiar with the operation of the hyperbaric chambers. The role of nurses in hyperbaric medicine has been reviewed elsewhere (Leifer 2001)

The occupational health and safety of hyperbaric attendants is an important issue for staff of hyperbaric medicine units. The reported incidence of DCI in attendants ranges from 0.01% to 1.3%. This is mostly related to depth of pressure exposure. DCI can be prevented by oxygen breathing and rotation of attendants. Ear trauma is a frequent complaint. No complaints have been reported from physical therapists carrying out treatments on patients at 1.5 ATA on a daily basis for several weeks. The health and safety record of hyperbaric chamber attendants has been very good with one death reported.

Conclusions

There is a great variety of hyperbaric chambers available and the hyperbaric physician has to choose the equipment best suited to the needs of his unit and according to the financial resources. The choice of ancillary equipment also depends upon the requirements. In general, the operation of hyperbaric chambers is safe if the safety precautions are followed. There is still room for improvement in the technical devices for monitoring the patients during hyperbaric treatment.

The basic technology for hyperbaric chambers is well established, though innovations continue to be made according to requirements. Gas supplies, the chamber hulls, control systems, monitoring equipment, and safety devices are constantly being adapted according to the most recent technical developments. Subtypes of hyperbaric chambers such as those for treatment or training or experimental use require different technical devices. Alarm as well as technical monitoring systems, fire-fighting equipment, and pressure locks are absolute requirements for any hyperbaric chamber. In chambers used for therapeutic purposes, facilities for invasive as well as noninvasive patient monitoring need to be ensured.

8 Indications, Contraindications, and Complications of HBO Therapy

K.K. Jain

In this chapter we summarize the literature and present a synthesis regarding:

Table 8.1
Uses of HBO Approved by the Undersea and Hyperbaric Medical Society

- Air or gas embolism
- Carbon monoxide poisoning and carbon monoxide poisoning complicated by cyanide poisoning
- Clostridial myonecrosis (gas gangrene)
- Crush injury, the compartment syndrome, and other acute traumatic ischemias
- Decompression sickness
- Enhancement of healing in selected problem wounds
- Exceptional anemia resulting from blood loss
- Necrotizing soft tissue infections (of subcutaneous tissue, muscle, or fascia)
- Refractory osteomyelitis
- Intracranial abscess
- Radiation tissue damage (osteoradionecrosis)
- Compromised skin grafts and flaps
- Thermal burns

Indications

Indications for hyperbaric oxygen (HBO) therapy vary in different countries and are described in Chapter 43. The indications approved by the Undersea and Hyperbaric Medical Society (Table 8.1) are very limited and rely on the proof of efficacy of HBO by controlled studies. A summary of indications is shown in Table 8.2. The table lists all the conditions where HBO has been shown to be useful, although, to date, few of these have been proven by controlled studies.

Contraindications

Contra-indications for HBO therapy are shown in Table 8.3.

Pneumothorax. The only absolute contraindication for HBO is untreated pneumothorax. Surgical relief of the pneumothorax before the HBO session, if possible, removes the obstacle to treatment.

The contraindications listed below are not absolute but relative. The potential benefits should be weighed against the condition of the patient and any ill-effects that may occur.

Upper Respiratory Infections. These predispose to otobarotrauma and sinus squeeze.

Emphysema with CO_2 Retention. Patients with this problem may develop pneumothorax due to rupture of an em-

Table 8.2
Summary of International Indications for HBO

1. Decompression sickness
2. Air embolism
3. Poisoning: carbon monoxide, cyanide, hydrogen sulfide, carbon tetrachloride
4. Treatment of certain infections: gas gangrene, acute necrotizing fascitis, refractory mycoses, leprosy, osteomyelitis
5. Plastic and reconstructive surgery:
   - for nonhealing wounds
   - as an aid to the survival of skin flaps with marginal circulation
   - as an aid to reimplantation surgery
   - as an adjunct to the treatment of burns
6. Traumatology: crush injuries, compartment syndrome, soft tissue sports injuries
7. Orthopedics: nonunion of fractures, bone grafts, osteoradionecrosis
8. Peripheral vascular diseases: shock, myocardial ischemia, aid to cardiac surgery
9. Peripheral vascular disease: ischemic gangrene, ischemic leg pain
10. Neurological: stroke, multiple sclerosis, migraine, cerebral edema, multi-infarct dementia, spinal cord injury and vascular diseases of the spinal cord, brain abscess, peripheral neuropathy, radiation myelitis, vegetative coma
11. Hematology: sickle cell crises, severe blood loss anemia
12. Ophthalmology: occlusion of central artery of retina
13. Gastro-intestinal: gastric ulcer, necrotizing enterocolitis, paralytic ileus, pneumotoides cystoides intestinalis, hepatitis
14. For enhancement of radiosensitivity of malignant tumors
15. Otorhinolaryngology: sudden deafness, acute acoustic trauma, labyrinthitis, Meniere's disease, malignant otitis externa (chronic infection)
16. Lung diseases: lung abscess, pulmonary embolism (adjunct to surgery)
17. Endocrines: diabetes
18. Obstetrics: Complicated pregnancy – diabetes, eclampsia, heart disease, placental hypoxia, fetal hypoxia. Congenital heart disease of the neonate
19. Asphyxiation: drowning, near hanging, smoke inhalation
20. Aid to rehabilitation: spastic hemiplegia of stroke, paraplegia, chronic myocardial insufficiency, peripheral vascular disease.

Table 8.3
Contraindications for HBO Therapy

Absolute
- Untreated tension pneumothorax

Relative
- Upper respiratory infections
- Emphysema with CO_2 retention
- Asymptomatic air cysts or blebs in the lungs seen on chest X-ray
- History of thoracic or ear surgery
- Uncontrolled high fever
- Pregnancy
- Claustrophobia (see complications of HBO)

physematous bulla during HBO. Pretreatment x-rays of the chest should be taken to rule this out.

Air Cysts or Blebs in the Lungs Seen on Chest X-Ray. These may predispose to pulmonary barotrauma by causing air trapping during HBO treatment. A survey was conducted to determine how patients were evaluated for pulmonary blebs or bullae in different hyperbaric centers (Toklu *et al* 2008). Of the 98 centers that responded to a questionnaires, sixty-five (66.3%) reported that they applied HBO to the patients with air cysts in their lungs. X-ray was the most widely used screening method for patients with a history of a lung disease. The prevalence of pulmonary barotrauma in theses centers was quite low at 0.00045%.

History of Thoracic Surgery or Ear Surgery. The patient should be thoroughly evaluated before HBO therapy is considered.

Uncontrolled High Fever. Fever predisposes to seizures. If HBO therapy is indicated for an infection with fever, the temperature should be lowered before therapy is commenced.

Pregnancy. There is animal experimental evidence that exposure to HBO during early pregnancy increases the incidence of congenital malformations. However, if a pregnant woman is poisoned with CO_2 the primary consideration is to save the mother's life. Exposure to HBO later in pregnancy appears to have no adverse effects. If the mother's life is threatened, for example in CO poisoning, she should receive HBO therapy as this has priority over consideration for the fetus. Many successful HBO treatments have been carried out during pregnancy without any danger to the fetus (see Chapter 33).

The following conditions have been considered to be contra-indications previously but are not supported by evidence. Several patients have been treated by use of HBO with aggravation of these conditions.

Seizure Disorders. Patients CNS disorders such as stroke may suffer seizures as a manifestation their primary disorder. However, seizures are rare during HBO sessions for neurological indications where the pressures do not exceed 1.5 ATA. If the disorder is due to a focal cerebral circulatory disorder or hypoxia, HBO should help to reduce the tendency toward seizures. Wong and Zhao (1994) treated 100 epileptic children with HBO and reported improvement in control of seizures in 68% and cognitive function in 38%. They were able to reduce the amount off antiepileptic drugs and there was no aggravation of seizures.

Malignant Disease. There is some concern regarding the effect of HBO on tumor growth because HBO is used as an adjunct to radiotherapy and also for the treatment of radiation necrosis in patients who may have residual cancer. This topic is discussed in Chapter 16 where it is concluded that malignant disease is generally not considered to be a contra-indication for HBO therapy.

Complications of Hyperbaric Oxygenation

Some of the complications of HBO therapy are listed in Table 8.4.

Table 8.4
Complications of Hyperbaric Oxygen Therapy

- Middle ear barotrauma
- Sinus pain
- Myopia and cataract
- Pulmonary barotrauma
- Oxygen seizures
- Decompression sickness
- Genetic effects
- Claustrophobia

Middle Ear Barotrauma. This is the commonest reported complication of HBO but the incidence varies in different series. A review of 1505 patients who underwent 52,758 2-h HBO treatment sessions showed that patients had to be removed from the hyperbaric chamber during treatment on 198 occasions (0.37%) because of an inability to equalize middle ear pressure; the sessions were resumed after treatment and training (Davis 1989). In 11,376 HBO therapy sessions within a multiplace chamber in an orthopedic clinic, more than 17% of all patients experienced ear pain or discomfort as an expression of problems in equalizing the middle ear pressure (Plafki *et al* 2000). Most episodes were not related to a persistent eustachian tube dysfunction since they only occurred once. Barotraumatic lesions on visual otological examinations (ear microscopy) were verified in 3.8% of all patients. Patients with sensory deficits involving the ear region need special attention, because they seem to be at risk for rupture of the tympanic membrane (three cases documented).

The Eustachian tube openings in the nasopharynx are slit-like, and the patient may have difficulty in equalizing the middle ear pressure with that of outside air during compression. Most patients can learn to remedy this by Frenzel's maneuver which consists of pinching the nose, closing the mouth, and pushing the tongue against the soft palate to force air through the Eustachian tubes into the middle ears. This complication can lead to permanent hearing loss and vertigo. Unconscious patients and infants present a special diagnostic challenge because of difficulties in communicating pain and equalizing pressure across the ears. The slow compression method of HBO has proved to be safer as well as better than the standard compression technique and reducres the incidence of middle ear barotrauma (Vahidova *et al* 2006).

The use of nasal decongestants is considered to be helpful. However, in a prospective, parallel, double-blind, randomized trial, there was no significant difference in the occurrence of ear discomfort in those receiving the decongestant oxymetazoline from those receiving spray of distilled water (Carlson *et al* 1992). This study suggests that topical decongestants may not be effective in preventing middle ear barotrauma. Capes and Tomaszewski (1996) carried out a phone survey to all hospital-based HBO centers in the United States concerning routine practice for middle ear barotrauma prophylaxis. Results indicate that more than a fifth of centers always do routine prophylactic myringotomies on intubated patients (30 of 126) and infants (19 of 86). Less than half of centers never performed the procedure as routine prophylaxis. A third of centers (49 of 145) routinely administered prophylactic drugs before HBO treatment. Topical nasal decongestants, particularly oxymetazoline, were preferred to systemic oral medications. These results show that there is great variance in clinical practice with regard to middle ear barotrauma prophylaxis among US HBO centers.

Clements *et al* (1998) reviewed 45 patients referred to a department of otolaryngology for inability to tolerate hyperbaric oxygen therapy. All patients underwent bilateral myringotomy and tube placement. Seventeen (38%) of these patients experienced complications, with most having more than one. Most complications occurred after conclusion of hyperbaric oxygen therapy. Otorrhea was most common, occurring in 13 patients (29%) and persistent tympanic membrane perforations occurred in 7 patients (16%). This rate of complications is higher than reported for placement of tympanostomy tubes in other patient populations. Coexisting illness, such as diabetes mellitus, may contribute to the development of complications in patients undergoing hyperbaric oxygen therapy. Alternative methods of tympanostomy, with emphasis on shorter duration of intubation, should be considered in this patient population.

In a prospective study, Fernau *et al* (1992) measured the changes in Eustachian tube function before and after HBO treatment in 33 adult patients by 9-step inflation-deflation test of Bluestone. Fifteen of these (45%) had evidence of Eustachian tube dysfunction after the treatment was initiated and all of them complained of a sensation of fullness in the ears. Thirteen of these patients (87%) developed serous otitis media and 7 (47%) required tympanostomy tubes. Patients with history of Eustachian tube dysfunction after first HBO treatment were found to be at greater risk of developing serous otitis media with subsequent treatments.

Unconscious patients are more likely to show barotrauma in the middle ear due to obvious inability to equalize pressure changes.

Sinus Pain. Sinus block during pressurization may produce severe pain, particularly in the frontal sinuses. If a patient has upper respiratory infection, the HBO treatment should be postponed, or, if it is urgently required, the patient should be given decongestant medication and the compression performed slowly.

Myopia and Cataract. Myopia is a reversible complication of acute exposure to HBO and cataract is a complication of chronic long-term exposure. These are discussed further in Chapter 32.

Pulmonary Barotrauma. Incidence of pulmonary barotrauma is quite low and most series with treatments under 2ATA do not report any cases. However, overinflation with pressure may lead to lung rupture, which may present as an air embolus, mediastinal emphysema, or tension pneumothorax. Pneumothorax in a patient under HBO treatment is a serious complication. In a multiplace chamber the physician should auscultate the patient, although the lung sounds are difficult to hear. Lung rupture may be suspected from the symptoms – sudden stabbing chest pain and respiratory distress. Tracheal shift and asymmetrical movements of the chest may be the only signs on physical examination. Decompression should be halted and thoracentesis performed. Plainly, this complication is more difficult to detect and to treat if it happens in a monoplace chamber.

Murphy *et al* (1991) reported three comatose patients who developed tension pneumothorax while receiving HBO therapy for CO poisoning. Each patient was intubated and received closed chest compressions for cardiac massage prior to HBO session. There was no evidence of pneumothorax prior to HBO therapy and tension pneumothorax was detected after decompression. These authors recommended serial physical examinations, arterial blood gas determinations, and chest radiographs in patients with a high index of suspicion of this complication in the setting of emergency HBO therapy.

Oxygen Seizures. Seizures as a manifestation of oxygen are described in Chapter 6. In a series of 80,000 patient treatments with HBO, only two seizures were documented, yielding an incidence of 2.4 per 100,000 patient-treatments and both cases occurred in a multiplace chamber pressurized to 2.4 ATA with O2 delivered by mask for three × 30 min with 5-min air breaks (Yildiz et al 2004). Use of pressure at 1.5 ATA does not lead to any oxygen-induced seizures when the duration of treatment was kept below one hour. If a seizure occurs in a multiplace chamber, the oxygen mask should be removed; this will invariably stop the seizure. If not, 60–120 mg of phenobarbital should be given. The chamber pressure should not be changed: sudden decompression of the chamber during a seizure can cause lung rupture. Decompression can be carried out after the seizure stops.

Decompression Sickness. This occurs only when high pressures are used and decompression is sudden. It is more likely to occur in the attendants in the hyperbaric chamber who breathe air. Decompression sickness (DCS) occurs rarely during therapeutic compression to 6 ATA in air embolism cases. Richter *et al* (1978) reported an incident that occurred in Hanover, FRG. Twenty elderly patients were receiving HBO in a multiplace chamber at 4 ATA. One patient developed air embolism after 1 h when decompression was started during the first dive. During the second dive, at about 5 h, the chamber door was opened with a sudden explosive reduction of pressure. Five patients died of DCS. This was the first report of fatal accident involving DCS in a hyperbaric chamber. There are no reports of such a complication in recent years.

Genetic Effects. Treatment of cells with HBO can result in generation of reactive oxygen species and induction of DNA damage. Cytogenetic data obtained from peripheral blood of patients who were treated with HBO at 1.5–2 ATA for 40 min daily for 10 days showed significant increase of chromosome aberrations. These were considered to be mainly caused by chromatid and chromosome breaks and showed individual variations. These results indicate that HBO may have an indirect effect on the genetic apparatus of the human somatic cells. High quantity of chromosome breaks in cells of somatic tissues is an adaptive reaction of the organism to HBO.

Exposure to 100% oxygen at a pressure of 1.5 ATA for a total of 1 h has been shown to induce DNA damage in the alkaline comet assay with leukocytes from test subjects. Under these conditions, HBO does not lead to an induction of gene and chromosome mutations. Because of known toxic effects, exposure of humans to HBO is limited, and possible genetic consequences of HBO cannot be completely evaluated *in vivo*. HBO treatment of cell cultures is a suitable model for investigating the relationship between oxygen-induced DNA lesions and the formation of gene- and chromosome mutations. The results of one study indicate that HBO induces sister chrmatid exchange and that lymphocytes retain increased sensitivity to the genotoxicity of mitomycin C one day after completing the HBO (Duydu *et al* 2006).

Claustrophobia. This is often referred to as a complication of or contraindication for hyperbaric therapy, and some patients decline or discontinue treatment for this reason. Claustrophobia is relatively common in the general population and some of the claustrophobic individuals may require HBO treatments. Claustrophobia can be a manifestation of anxiety due to confinement in a closed space and unfamiliar surroundings. It is more likely to be experienced in a small monoplace or portable chamber and less likely in a large multiplace chamber with easy communication to the outside. Hillard (1990) reported the case of a patient who refused HBO treatment because of her claustrophobia. After an intensive two-week treatment of her phobia, she underwent HBO treatments successfully.

Anxiety reactions. There are several reports in the literature of anxiety reactions in patients undergoing HBO treatment. Anxiety levels of patients undergoing HBO treatments can be assessed by Spielberger State-Trait inventory Questionnaire. There is an increase in magnitude of anxiety with a new treatment but this decreases after the treatment. It is important to communicate with the patient and explain the procedure with reassurance. Larger studies on this topic would be useful.

Complications in critically ill patients. Patients are more likely to have a complication during HBO treatment if they are critically ill, unconscious or intubated. Keenan *et al* (1998) reviewed thirty-two children were treated with HBO while mechanically ventilated: 21 had necrotizing infections, 9 had CO poisoning, and 2 had iatrogenic arterial air embolism. Complications or events occurring during HBO therapy included hypotension (63%), bronchospasm (34%), hemotympanum (13%), and progressive hypoxemia (6%).

Coincidental Medical Events in the Hyperbaric Chamber

A medical event may take place in the hyperbaric chamber and may not have any relation to the HBO therapy. Often such events are mistakenly attributed to HBO therapy. Reported coincidental events include the following:

1. Stroke
2. Myocardial infarction patients with known atherosclerotic disease and other risk factors for heart disease.
3. Focal seizures in patients with a history of epilepsy or intracranial lesions.

Precautions in Selection of Patients for HBO Treatment

In emergency situations, it is not possible to select patients and sometimes a risk has to be taken. For elective treatments, the patients should be screened carefully. History-taking should include information of any chest or ear operations.

Examination of the patient should include the following:

- Chest x-ray
- Pulmonary function testing
- Examination of the ear drums

In many other conditions, the decision should be made on an individual basis. Particular attention should be paid to the following two situations:

1. Large skull defects. In a patient with a large skull defect following surgery, HBO treatments should be avoided if the scalp flap is caved in.
2. Implanted devices.
   - Cardiac pacemakers. If the patient is wearing a cardiac pacemaker, it should be ascertained that it is one of the newer models that are pressure proof. Failure of temporary cardiac pacemakers has been reported under HBO. They recommended the use of permanent hermetically sealed pacemakers, which function quite well under hyperbaric conditions. In a recent review all pacemakers were reported to be adequate to treatment depths below 3 ATA (Simmons 1998).
   - Intrathecal pumps are used for administration of drugs directly into the intrathecal space of the spinal canal for relief of spasticity or pain. Baclofen infusion pump is used in paraplegic patients with spinal cord spasticity. These patients may be treated by HBO for decubitus ulcer. Akman *et al* (1994) reported a patient who developed retrograde leakage of CSF into the pump reservoir while undergoing HBO treatment at 2 ATA. There is no adverse effect of this except for the dilution of the medication in the pump. Tests by the manufacturers of these pumps have not shown any collapse of the pump although the pumps do not function during the exposure to high atmospheric pressure. This information may be important if spasticity is to be treated with HBO.

Increase of pain during HBO treatment was reported in another patient receiving morphine via an intrathecal pump (Baker 1992). Presumably the device did not function during the hyperbaric exposure.

Conclusions

Generally speaking, no serious complications are associated with moderate pressure HBO treatment, but some complications may be related to the primary disease treated. Contraindications should be noted and precautions taken during treatment of those with risk factors for complications. Some implanted devices used in treatment of patients may not function properly in hyperbaric chambers.

9 Drug Interactions with Hyperbaric Oxygenation

K.K. Jain

Interactions of HBO with other drugs should be recognized for prevention of adverse reactions as well as for enhancement of therapeutic effects. This chapter looks at:

Oxygen as a Drug

When oxygen is breathed in concentrations higher than those found in the atmospheric air, it is considered to be a drug. By this definition, hyperbaric oxygen (HBO) is definitely a drug and it can interact with other drugs. It is important to be aware of these interactions in patients who are receiving other drugs, for HBO can either potentiate or reduce the effects of other drugs. Conversely, there are also drugs that reduce or potentiate the effects of HBO. These correspond to protectors against and enhancers of oxygen toxicity, respectively, as discussed in Chapter 6.

Many drugs, including nonprescription drugs, have undesirable side effects that may be modified in the hyperbaric environment. Some drug effects are potentiated and some are antagonized; some agents produce entirely different effects than those observed in normobaric environments.

Drugs Affecting the Central Nervous System (CNS)

Anesthetics. The interactions of anesthetics with HBO is discussed Chapter 38, but some of the drugs used are reviewed briefly here, due to their importance in many aspects of the current topic.

CNS Stimulants. CNS stimulants such as amphetamines interact unfavorably with HBO. And, notably, excessive coffee drinking in those who are susceptible to caffeine may also predispose to oxygen toxicity.

Ethanol. Hyperbaric air has a synergistic effect with ethanol and increases the sleeping time in mice. This may explain the increased susceptibility to the effects of compression and decompression of those who have imbibed alcohol. There are no special ill effects of HBO on patients who suffer carbon monoxide poisoning while they are inebriated. There is no evidence that HBO accelerates the metabolism of "sobering up" in alcoholics.

Narcotic Analgesics. Narcotic drugs generally depress respiration by reducing the reactivity of medullary centers to CO_2. This, combined with the depressing effect of HBO on respiration, can lead to a rise in $paCO_2$, which causes vasodilatation and enhances oxygen toxicity.

Pharmacokinetics of meperidine in dogs breathing air at 1 ATA is not altered under HBO at 2.8 ATA, or breathing air at 6 ATA. The findings in dogs cannot, of course, be extrapolated to humans, as the two species handle drugs very differently. The action of morphine also is unchanged by HBO.

Pentobarbital. It has been mentioned in Chapter 3 that pentobarbital anesthesia can be reversed in rats under atmospheric pressure. Attempts to distinguish between the two possible causes of this reversal – changes in the drug disposition and changes in drug-receptor interaction – by studying the pharmacokinetics of pentobarbital in dogs exposed to HBO shows no significant effect of HBO on total plasma clearance, volume of distribution, or elimination half-life of pentobarbital. This rules out changes in drug disposition as a cause of reversal of central nervous system (CNS) depression by pentobarbital.

Scopolamine. This is an anticholinergic compound used widely for management of motion sickness and may be used concomitantly with HBO, particularly in divers. Bitterman *et al* (1991) tested the interaction of scopolamine with HBO at 5 ATA in rats. The duration of the latent period preceding the onset of hyperoxic convulsions was not altered. However, the visual and cardiovascular side effects of the drug should be taken into consideration when scopolamine is used in combination with HBO.

Interaction of HBO with Various Drugs

Antimicrobials

HBO increases the permeability of the blood-brain barrier (BBB), as described in Chapter 2. This has led to the investigation of HBO as an enhancer of the penetration of some antibiotics across the BBB into the cerebrospinal fluid (CSF) in order to increase their effectiveness in meningitis.

Aminoglycoside Antibiotics. CSF transfer of the aminoglycoside antibiotic tobramycin is not altered under HBO in rabbits, and HBO has no significant effect on the CSF concentration of this agent. CO_2, which is known to damage BBB, more than doubles the CSF:blood ration for tobramycin. Pharmacokinetics of gentamicin does not change in healthy volunteers exposed to HBO.

Sulfonamides. Increase of oxygen tension has a synergistic bactericidal effect with sulfonamides rather than the usual bacteriostatic action. HBO and antibiotic synergism are discussed in Chapter 13.

Mafenide acetate (Sulfamylon), an antibacterial agent used in burn patients, is a carbonic anhydrase inhibitor and tends to promote CO_2 retention and vasodilatation. This substance must be removed from patients before they are placed in a hyperbaric chamber for HBO treatment.

Antineoplastics

The role of HBO in enhancing cancer radiosensitivity is discussed in Chapter 36. Interaction of HBO with some antineoplastic agents will be described here.

Exposure of cancer cells to HBO at 3 ATA for 2 h produced inhibition of DNA synthesis or mitosis. Simultaneous exposure to HBO and adriamycin results in decreased cytotoxicity. However, exposure to adriamycin 2–8 h before or after HBO produces an increase in the drug effect. Cytotoxicity increases when cells were exposed to HBO before, during, or after nitrogen mustard administration.

HBO enhances the chemotherapeutic effect of doxorubicin both in cell culture and in the rat model (Petre et al 2003). HBO reduces the rate of misonidazole metabolism, thus increasing the concentration of this substance in tumors, which enhances radiosensitivity. However, doxorubicin is regarded as a contraindication for concomitant use with HBO therapy because of the increased risk of cardiotoxicity. An experimental study has shownb that HBO exposure does not potentiate doxorubicin-induced cardiotoxicity in rats, but confers cardioprotection against doxorubicin, which warrants further investigation (Karagoz et al 2008).

Cardiovascular Drugs

Adrenomimetic, Adrenolytic, and Ganglion-Blocking Agents. Under HBO, there is a considerable reduction of hypotensive effect of α- and β-blockers, ganglion blockers, and b-adrenomimetics, and elimination of the effects of central adrenomimetics. The pressor effects of the directly and particularly of the indirectly acting a-adrenomimetics, as well as the cardiotropic effects of β-adrenoblockers, are potentiated. Therefore, these drugs should be given after but not before the HBO session.

Digitalis/Digoxin. HBO has been reported to decrease the effectiveness of cardiac glycosides. There is some evidence that HBO may reduce the toxic effects of digitalis.

Antianginal drugs. The effect of a single HBO session (1.5 ATA, duration 40 min), in combination with antianginal drugs, has been investigated in patients with ischemic heart disease and angina pectoris of effort, NYHA functional class II-III. HBO reduces the degree of indirect hemodynamic effect of nifedipine, potentiates negative chronotropic, and inotropic effects of propranolol – but has no impact on the degree of hemodynamic effect of depot-glycerol trinitrate.

Heparin. Heparin-treated animals exposed to HBO develop pulmonary hemorrhages as a result of interactions of the anticoagulant effect of heparin and oxygen-induced pulmonary lesions. The pressures and exposure times in experimental studies are much longer than those used clinically and these observations are not applicable to humans. However, since heparin has been used as an adjunctive measure in patients undergoing HBO treatments, this potential complication should be kept in mind, although none has been reported in patients on heparin undergoing HBO treatments.

Interaction of HBO with Miscellaneous Drugs

Insulin. The dosages of insulin required in diabetes are decreased during HBO therapy and should be readjusted.

Losartan. Addition of HBO therapy to losartan, an angiotensin receptor blocker, increases the drug efficacy and has significant benefits in the management of proteinuria (Yilmaz et al 2006).

Reserpine and Guanethidine. Reserpine and guanethidine have been shown to interact unfavorably with HBO.

Salicylates. There is a significant increase in salicylate clearance in dogs at 2.8 ATA. There are no studies in humans.

Theophylline. There are no effects of HBO (2.8 ATA) on the pharmacokinetics of theophylline in the dog. There are no studies in humans.

Practical Considerations of Drug Administration During HBO Therapy

The mechanical effect of the pressure on the drug containers should be taken into consideration. Drugs stocked in a multiplace chamber and subjected to repeated compression and decompression should be put into pressure-proof containers. There are no problems of explosion with small vials when pressures are below 3 ATA. Multidose rubber top vials should be used only once in a hyperbaric chamber because of possible contamination while withdrawing a drug. Precautions for intravenous infusions are discussed in Chapter 7.

Drugs that Enhance Oxygen Toxicity

Acetazolamide. Acetazolamide is a carbonic anhydrase inhibitor that prevents oxygen-induced vasoconstriction and increases blood flow under HBO. This predisposes the brain to the toxic action of oxygen. Acetazolamide should not be used at pressures greater than 2 ATA.

CNS Stimulants. See section on CNS drugs.

Disulfiram. This drug is used in alcohol aversion therapy. It may potentiate oxygen toxicity via *in vivo* reduction to diethyldithiocarbamate and subsequent inhibition of superoxide dismutase.

Thyroid Extract. Thyroid or thyroid extract given to experimental animals under HBO enhances the toxic effects of oxygen. The increase of metabolic rate is thought to predispose to oxygen-induced convulsions. It is a reasonable assumption that this would also occur in humans).

Drugs that Protect Against Oxygen Toxicity

This topic has been discussed in Chapter 6 and a list of drugs that protect against oxygen toxicity is given in Table 6.6.

Anticonvulsants. Phenytoin (Dilantin) and diazepam (Valium) are used to prevent seizures, and do not have any protective effect against oxygen toxicity as such. Barbiturates are also used as antiepileptics, and may have a protective effect against oxygen toxicity. But the disadvantage of using barbiturates is that they are respiratory depressants. Diazepam (Valium) is used to prevent and control seizures of nonhyperbaric origin. The dosage is 5–50 mg given slowly by intravenous injection. It may also lead to respiratory depression. Lorazepam is similar in action to diazepam but requires one-fifth the dose. If phenytoin is used, care should be taken not to use high pressures of oxygen for long periods: CNS toxicity may occur without the warning signs of seizures. Carbamazepine has been found to be useful for the prevention of CNS toxicity during HBO therapy of epilepsy-prone patients.

Ergot Derivatives. Two ergot derivatives lisuride and quinpirole have been shown to antagonize convulsions in mice induced by HBO at 5 ATA. This protection was found to about 50% of that obtained by diazepam. There is no report of use of any ergot derivatives in patients for this purpose.

Magnesium. Mg ion compounds are substances with antioxidant and vasodilating effects and therefore reduce oxygen toxicity. A single dose of 10 mmol of magnesium sulfate can be given 3 h before a HBO session.

Phenothiazines. Chlorpromazine is considered to be protective against oxygen toxicity.

Propranolol. L-propranolol has been shown to protect mice against HBO-induced seizures (Levy *et al* 1976). There have been no reports of clinical application of this effect.

Vitamin E. Vitamin E is believed to protect against oxygen toxicity by counteracting the oxygen free radicals. A dose of 400 mg daily should be given to patients scheduled for HBO therapy starting 2 days before the therapy.

Conclusions

Drug interactions with HBO represent an important subject, but there is a lack of studies for many of the commonly used medications. Animal studies cannot always be applied to humans. Therefore, studies of the pharmacokinetics of commonly used drugs in patients receiving HBO should be carried out and an authoritative drug incompatibility list compiled; such a list would be incorporated in various pharmacopoeias and displayed in hyperbaric treatment facilities. A careful history should be taken of drug use by patients and caution should be exercised in the use of drugs known to interact with oxygen.

PART II:
CLINICAL APPLICATIONS

10 Decompression Sickness

P.B. James and K.K. Jain

Early recompression with HBO is a recommended treatment for decompression sickness. This chapter looks at:

Introduction

Decompression sickness (DCS) is one form of dysbarism, which is a general term applied to all pathological changes secondary to altered environmental pressure. Other forms are pulmonary barotrauma and also aseptic bone necrosis, which is likely to be a form of decompression sickness. DCS is caused by gas phase formed by a sufficiently rapid reduction of environmental pressure to cause supersaturation of the gases dissolved in the tissues. The principle component is most usually nitrogen, but when helium and oxygen mixtures are used it is helium. DCS is also described by the terms, caisson disease, "the bends" (joint pains), "the chokes" (pulmonary symptoms), the "staggers" (vestibular symptoms) and "hits" (spinal cord symptoms). DCS occurs in divers and also in those who work in compressed-air as in caissons and tunnels. It can also result from a reduction of normal barometric pressure, such as in a hypobaric chamber, and in aircraft at altitudes in excess of 5000 meters even when oxygen is breathed. It complicates flight in some high altitude military aircraft and may occur when astronauts don suits for undertaking extravehicular activity. Bubble formation may also be a component of altitude sickness in climbers making a rapid ascent. At sea level almost 1 liter of nitrogen is dissolved in the body. A little less than one-half of this is dissolved in water and a little more than one-half in the fat, which constitutes only 15% of the normal male body – nitrogen is five times more soluble in fat than in water. In diving the additional amount of nitrogen that dissolves in the body depends upon the depth and the duration of a dive. For steady state conditions the volume of nitrogen that is liberated returning from 10 m to normal barometric pressure is 2 liters. A helium and oxygen exposure to the same conditions would result in only 1 liter of gas dissolved with the difference being mainly due to the lower solubility of the gas in fat. However on resumption of air breathing at 1 ATA the elimination of helium is very rapid. To achieve steady state at a particular pressure – often known as saturation – requires many hours and the time required in greater for nitrogen than for helium. The formulation of decompression tables is generally based on methods introduced by Haldane from his observation that decompression sickness is rare when the absolute pressure is halved. However he warned against the extrapolation of this principle to pressures above 6 ATA. Figure 10.1 shows the approximate half-lives of nitrogen in various tissues. However the demonstration of gas formation in tissues after a decompression halving the absolute pressure indicates that this method is empirical and can only be used as a guide in decompression table formulation. After achieving steady state conditions in air diving the central nervous system has a high concentration of nitrogen because of the high solubility of the gas in lipids. Using helium the amount dissolved under equivalent steady state conditions

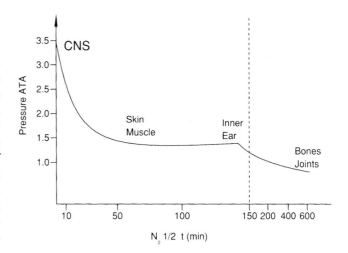

Figure 10.1
Half-life of nitrogen in various tissues.

is much less because of the lower solubility of the gas in fat. Commercial diving expanded dramatically with the exploration for offshore oil and gas and the experience gained has influenced practice in both military and amateur diving. For depths in excess of 50 msw "saturation" techniques have been developed where divers live at constant pressure in a helium and oxygen environment (heliox), using a bell to transfer to the water. Attempts to use nitrox for saturation dives have not been commercially successful. Operational dives have been undertaken to 450 msw using heliox and experimental dives to 523 msw, using mixtures of hydrogen, helium and oxygen. The inclusion of hydrogen reduces gas density and the work of breathing and also ameliorates the effects of the high pressure on nervous system function. These symptoms are known as the high pressure nervous syndrome (see Chapter 3).

Recently several physicians have proposed a new term for describing disorders resulting from decompression: decompression illness (DCI) which is proposed to encompass disorders previously known as DCS and AGE (arterial gas embolism). The reason given for the new proposal is that the etiology of decompression disorders is difficult to define and that DCS and AGE are difficult to separate from each other. This proposal is not widely accepted and we will be using the traditional terms: DCS and arterial gas embolism (see Chapter 11).

Pathophysiology

Bubble Formation

The elimination of the excess "inert" gas taken up during a dive ultimately depends upon the transfer of gas from blood to the respired gas in the lungs. All decompression tables assume that blood passing through the lungs is

Pressure Outside Body

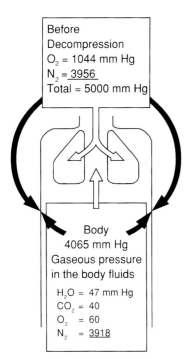

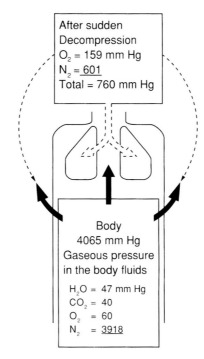

Figure 10.2
Bubble formation after decompression due to great excess of intrabody pressure shown at right.

equilibrated with the partial pressure of the gas being respired, but because of ventilation/perfusion mismatch in the lung this cannot be the case and some supersaturated blood must achieve the systemic circulation on decompression. Decompression sickness can follow repeated breathhold dives because the elevation of the partial pressure of the nitrogen in the air compressed in the lungs is reflected in an increase in the plasma and tissue nitrogen content. Cerebral symptoms have been associated with multiple breathhold dives. Decompression beyond the unsaturation associated with the metabolic use of oxygen (the oxygen window) produces supersaturation and risks the emergence of dissolved gas from solution. The formation of gas phase can be imaged in tissue planes in, for example, muscle, using ultrasound. The principle component is the diluent gas present, but oxygen, carbon dioxide and water vapor also contribute to the gas volume. Gas formation is believed to depend on the presence of gas micronuclei, which are very small quantities of undissolved gas and the formation of gas bubbles may occur very rapidly. It is universally agreed that the formation of gas is the initial event in the etiology of DCS. The principles underlying bubble formation are shown in Figure 10.2. There is considerable evidence that gas formation in the tight connective tissue of tendon is responsible for the classical joint pain of the "bends". Investigations using radiographs in aviators decompressed to altitude has demonstrated gas phase in the ligaments and tendons of the knee and these observations are relevant to those seen in decompression after exposure to hyperbaric environ-

ments. Sequential perfusion has been observed in connective tissue and this intermittent perfusion is probably a major factor in gas formation in this and other tissues, because a tissue will take up gas when it is perfused, but release of gas will be limited if the microcirculation closes during decompression. The gas exchange will then be diffusion, not perfusion. Also, because the oxygen contained in the area of tissue will be metabolized, there may be a reduction in the inherent unsaturation as more nitrogen is absorbed.

Intravascular bubbles are often detectable in the pulmonary artery during or after decompression. The timing is dependent on the nature of the dive. For example, circulating bubbles may be detected during the decompression from heliox saturation dives, but in air diving they are generally only detectable after decompression has been completed. The principles underlying bubble formation are shown in Figure 10.2.

Electron microscopy studies of human tissues from fatal cases of DCS have shown that each bubble is covered with an osmiophilic, nonhomogeneous coat of a flocculent material that is associated with an electrokinetic zonal activity. This surface coat reduces the rate of nitrogen elimination via the blood-lung barrier when bubbles are trapped in the pulmonary capillaries. Bubbles induce changes in vascular permeability and in severe decompression sickness this may precipitate hypovolemic shock and a reversible blood sludging. In addition to formation of bubbles in tissues, humoral agents may be released from tissues secondary to trauma caused by expanding gas. Intra-arterial bubble formation occurs only if there is a very sudden decompression from a high pressure exposure. DCS generally increases in severity as the free gas in the body becomes more abundant. Exercise increases the elimination of gas but, may also increase the release of gas in tissues and bubbles into the circulation. Lynch *et al* (1985) studied the origin and time course of gas bubbles following rapid decompression in hamsters. Their data indicated that bubbles first form on the venous side of the circulation and then, if they exceed a certain number, move through the pulmonary circulation into the systemic circulation. It is accepted that there is a threshold for the transpulmonary passage of emboli. The transfer of bubbles into the systemic circulation may also occur through an atrial septal defect. The location and extent of bubble formation depends upon the severity of the supersaturation and the solubility of the diluent gas. Only in very severe experimental situations have bubbles been found intracellularly, in the anterior chamber of the eye, or in the cerebrospinal fluid. Diving using only oxygen as the respired gas is employed in the armed forces. Although it is not associated with bubble formation, it carries the risk of acute oxygen toxicity manifest by convulsions which may lead to drowning. Oxygen enriched air mixtures are used to reduce the risk of decompression sickness or extend bottom time and are becoming popular in amateur diving. They do not eliminate the risk of DCS and, again, because there is a very real risk of convulsions from oxygen toxicity, a full face mask or helmet should be used.

Pulmonary Changes

The first attempt to detect bubbles using ultrasound found them present in the inferior vena cava in a pig during decompression at 4 ATA after an exposure to compressed air at a pressure of 6 ATA for an hour (Gillis *et al* 1968). Human studies have used transcutaneous ultrasonic detectors which are much less sensitive than implanted devices. Bubbles can be detected in the pulmonary artery in the majority of divers after significant dives, but they generally do not produce symptoms. Experimental studies have shown that venous bubbles can cross the lungs of anesthetized dogs when driving pressures are high enough to overcome the normal filtering function of the lungs. Bubbles trapped in the lung may also cross the pulmonary circulation as a result of the reduction in their size on compression. Before decompression tables were formulated, pulmonary decompression sickness – the "chokes" – often proved fatal and the events have been followed in experimental animals. The pulmonary changes are accompanied by hypoxemia, pulmonary hypertension, and respiratory distress. These features are shared by other microembolic syndromes as, for example, fat embolism, and are examples of the (adult) respiratory distress syndrome. Noncardiac pulmonary edema has been found to be the principal response of the lung to decompression stress and the precipitating event is a large number of microbubbles arriving in the lung. Peribronchial edema has also been described.

Pulmonary barotrauma may occur in divers because an increase in the volume of gas entrapped in the lungs during ascent, leading to alveolar rupture, entry of the gas into systemic circulation via the pulmonary veins, and systemic air embolism (see Chapter 11). The gas may track around the vessels, leading to mediastinal emphysema. Rupture of peripheral alveoli may lead to pneumothorax. Pulmonary barotrauma is much more common in amateur divers using self-contained breathing apparatus (SCUBA) than professional divers, because of panic or the exhaustion of their gas supply. When arterial gas embolism occurs as a result of a rapid ascent at the end of a dive it is complicated by the excess of nitrogen in the tissues.

Bubble-Induced CNS Injury

Large and numerous bubbles may enter the cerebral circulation in arterial gas embolism associated with pulmonary barotrauma and cause gross obstruction to flow and ischemia. However, in contrast, bubbles formed on decompression are small, generally measuring about 25 microns on the surface. As with solid micro-emboli, the diameter of microbubbles is a critical factor in their behavior in the circulation, but the size of gaseous emboli depends on the absolute pressure. Ischemia is a major factor in bubble-induced CNS injury in decompression sickness. In experiments using labeled granulocytes, ischemia activates the chemotaxic process at an early stage and that granulocytes may be involved in CNS injury. Ischemia is conventionally associated with vascular occlusion, but gas embolism also causes endothelial damage and in the CNS this involves opening of the blood-brain barrier and edema. This has also been produced by the transit of microbubbles without initial being associated with ischemia (Hills & James 1991). Opening the blood-brain barrier causes the extravasation of plasma proteins which triggers the complement cascade. This induces the inflammatory cascade and ischemia only develops when focal edema causes compression of the microcirculation. Pearson *et al* (1992) observed bubbles in the cerebral circulation which preceded changes in evoked potentials in an experimental model. Blood complement also induces granulocyte clumping in DCS. The result of these interactions between blood and the damaged tissues may well be a major determinant of the extent of neuronal recovery following focal blood brain barrier disturbance and ischemia in the CNS. Fat embolism may also occur on decompression sickness and even cause death from an acute disseminated encephalitis. Fat emboli being fluid also cross the lung filter and cause cerebral edema because of damage to the blood-brain barrier. The protein leakage and edema leads to focal demyelination with relative preservation of axons.

The nutrition of areas of the white matter of both the cerebral medulla and the spinal cord depends on long draining veins which have been shown to have surrounding capillary free zones. Because of the high oxygen extraction in the microcirculation of the gray matter of the central nervous system, the venous blood has low oxygen content. When this is reduced further by embolic events, tissue oxygenation may fall to critically low levels, leading to blood-brain barrier dysfunction, inflammation, demyelination and eventually, axonal damage. These are the hallmarks of the early lesions of multiple sclerosis where MR spectroscopy has also shown the presence of lactic acid. Significant elevation of the venous oxygen tension requires oxygen to be provided under hyperbaric conditions. Arterial tension is typically increased ten-fold breathing oxygen at 2 ATA, but this results in only a 1.5-fold increase in the cerebral venous oxygen tension. The treatment of DCS, and both animal and clinical studies, have confirmed the value of oxygen provided under hyperbaric conditions in the restoration and preservation of neurological function in the "perivenous" syndrome (James 2007).

An alternative mechanism by which bubbles may generate CNS injury is their nucleation within the white matter. Bubbles are seen in the myelin sheaths on the rapid decompression of experimental animals from high pressures. Autochthonous (formed in situ) bubbles have been shown to traumatize neurons at the site of nucleation and compress adjacent ones and this is one mechanism which can explain the sudden onset of symptoms. However the conditions used in these experiments are much more extreme than in most cases of human decompression sickness. Because of the need for a reliable animal model and to avoid the unpredictability of decompression sickness which characterizes human dives very extreme conditions and often double exposures have been used.

The most obvious disability from neurological (Type 2) DCS in diving is paraplegia due to the involvement of the spinal cord, but this is a rare complication of hypobaric decompression, indicating the importance of bubble size and tissue gas loading. Most divers with spinal cord symptoms when questioned actually admit to symptoms which indicate disturbed brain function. Three mechanisms have been postulated to explain the pathophysiology of spinal cord lesion:

- Arterial bubble embolism
- Epidural venous obstruction leading to infarction
- Autochthonous bubbles

The paramount difficulty is the attribution of spinal cord decompression sickness to arterial embolism has been the failure to recognize a natural disease of the spinal cord due to arterial microembolism. However this has been answered by the recognition that multiple sclerosis (MS) may be due to subacute fat embolism and retinal changes occur in both decompression sickness and MS. In MS as in decompression sickness the clinical presentation is dominated by symptoms affecting the spinal cord which can be described as a transverse myelitis. Late deterioration has been described thirteen years after spinal cord decompression sickness. In both conditions focal cranial nerve problems, such as optic neuritis and oculomotor palsies have been described and vestibular damage may leave permanent nystagmus. Epidural venous obstruction generally leads to central infarction of the cord and not the characteristic focal changes seen in the decompression sickness. Gas or edema may cause ischemia in the cord because of an increase in the internal pressure due to non-elasticity of the pia mater (Hills & James 1982).

Unfortunately, fibrocartlilaginous embolism has been overlooked in the debate about the mechanism of neurological decompression sickness. Material from the nucleus pulposus of spinal disks can cause embolic damage to the nervous system and the first case was described in 1961 (Naiman et al 1961). Although retrograde venous flow has been suggested as the mechanism, the post-mortem finding of a 200 micron fibrocartilage embolus in the middle cerebral artery of a 17-year-old girl (Toro-Gonzalez et al 1993) has demonstrated beyond doubt that system embolization does occur. As in decompression sickness material may gain access to the systemic circulation by transpulmonary passage, or through an atrial septal defect. The girl, who had collapsed while playing basketball, died of myocardial infarction, and emboli were found in the coronary arteries. The size range of emboli, from 20 to 200 microns, indicates that the microcirculation of the lung may be sizing the material. The mechanism has been described in other mammals, where it is now regarded as a relatively common cause of neurological symptoms. The cases described include an 11-day-old lamb (Jeffrey & Wells 1986).

Changes visible with both light and electron microscopes are seen in the spinal cords of animals subjected to severe experimental DCS. The finding of widened myelin sheaths showing a banded pattern of myelin disruption may be compatible with autochonous gas, but similar patterns are seen in experimental allergic encephalomyelitis due to edema.

Divers may be at risk of long-term CNS damage from non-symptomatic hyperbaric exposure. The effect of severe, controlled hyperbaric exposure was investigated on goats exposed to various dive profiles over a period of 5 years, with some experiencing DCS (Blogg et al 2004). MRI was done and the animals were then sacrificed for neuropathological examination the brain and spinal cord. No significant correlation was found between age, years diving, DCS or exposure to pressure with MRI-detectable lesions in the brain, or with neuropathological lesions in

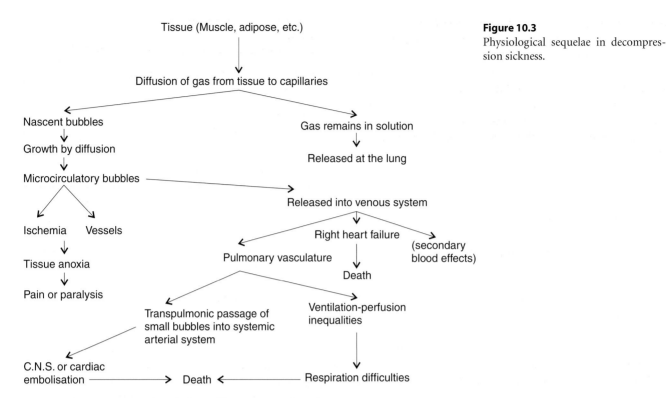

Figure 10.3
Physiological sequelae in decompression sickness.

the brain or spinal cord. However, spinal scarring was noted in animals that had suffered from spinal DCS.

Changes in Blood

Even asymptomatic decompression of sufficient severity can be associated with a reduction of the number of circulating platelets by one-third during a 24-h period following a severe dive. A smooth muscle-activating factor released during decompression may potentiate other bioactive amines, such as bradykinin, serotonin, and histamine, which are known to be involved in shock caused by rapid decompression. Hyperagglutinability of the platelets is important in the pathogenesis of DCS. This phenomenon may be based on production of metabolites of arichodonic acid and prostaglandin-like compounds.

Adhesion of platelets to the surfaces of bubbles and formation of platelet aggregates have been shown by scanning electron microscopy. Other platelet agonists like ADP, epinephrine, and serotonin, which may be present in vivo, accelerate this interaction, and the platelet antagonists have been shown to depress platelet aggregation. These factors may delay gas resolution on recompression.

Dysbaric Osteonecrosis

Dysbaric osteonecrosis (DON) has been reported in humans and experimental animals after a single hyperbaric air exposure with inadequate decompression. It is usually considered to be the result of gas bubbles entering the end arteries in the bone, and is seen most commonly in compressed-air workers.

Jones *et al* (1993) hypothesize that DON does not result from primary embolic or compressive effects of the nitrogen bubbles on the osseous vasculature. These authors report the presence of gas bubbles in the fatty marrow of the femoral and humeral heads and lipid and platelet aggregates were found on the surface of marrow bubbles. Fibrin platelet thrombi were found in systemic vessels, suggesting that injured marrow adipocytes can release liquid fat, and this fat embolism causes the release of thromboplastin, and other vasoactive substances that can trigger systemic intravascular coagulation and DON.

Role of Free Radicals

There is increasing awareness of the role of oxygen-derived free-radicals in reperfusion injury. However occlusion of flow is more a feature of air embolism rather than decompression sickness, the latter being associated with increased vascular permeability and inflammation. After the first phase of DCS caused by the mechanical action of bubbles, the symptoms in the second phase may result from oxygen-free radicals associated with ischemia and hypoxia. It has been recognized since the introduction of the minimal recompression tables using 100% oxygen at 2.8 ATA (US Navy Manual 1970) that these procedures could be associated with worsening and oxygen toxicity with free radical formation may be a component in this deterioration. However, it is universally recognized that recompression treatment should be carried out as quickly as possible and that recompression with the additional use of heparin, superoxide dismutase and catalase does not improve the outcome of severe DCS in experimental animals.

A schematic of the pathogenesis of the forms of DCS is shown in Figure 10.3.

Clinical Features

Decompression Sickness in Diving

Haldane (1907) classified DCS into three categories: Type I, joint pain; Type II, systemic symptoms or signs, caused by the involvement of the CNS or the cardiopulmonary systems; and Type III, characterized by convulsions and death. The first two parts of the classification are still the accepted standard internationally.

The clinical features of DCS are shown in Table 10.1. DCS is a disease that manifests itself in a variety of organ systems. However studies of both compressed air workers and divers have shown that Type I DCS is the most common presentation, but the nature of the dive is important. For example, mild joint pains are not unusual during heliox saturation decompressions but Type II symptoms are extremely rare. In surface decompression procedures Type II DCS is more common and on deep dives presents more frequently than Type 1 symptoms. It is obvious that joint pain is easier for a diver to recognize than symptoms affecting the nervous system.

The majority of divers who have undertaken surface-orientated dives experience symptoms within 3 h of surfacing, although the onset of symptoms may be delayed for as long as 35 h. In air diving nearly one-half of the cerebral cases become apparent within 3 min of surfacing, and a similar proportion of spinal cases also become apparent within 3 min of surfacing.

The most serious sequelae are those involving the CNS: neurologic manifestations of DCS comprise symptoms from the cerebral hemispheres, the spinal cord, as well as vestibular disturbances (Jain 2009i). The most common area involved is the lower thoracic segments spinal cord, but the level can vary from C4 to L1. In air diving with in-water decompression CNS involvement occurs in 25% of DCS cases. Late deterioration of spinal cord function has been described thirteen years after an episode of decompression sickness (Dyer & Millac 1996). Other neurologic syndromes may also occur. Some divers develop evidence of acute cerebral hemisphere dysfunction, such as hemiparesis, aphasia, or hemianopsia. Memory loss, convulsions, and even coma can occur.

Table 10.1
Signs and Symptoms of Decompression Sickness (DCS)

Type 1 DCS: Limb and joint pains (bends), skin rash
Type II DCS
Neurological
1. Cerebral
   – visual disturbances
   – aphasia
   – hemiplegia
   – memory loss
   – convulsions
   – coma
2. Spinal ("hit")
   – sensory disturbances of extremities: paresthesias, numbness
   – weakness, difficulty in walking
   – bladder dysfunction
   – paraplegia or quadriplegia
3. Vestibular disturbances ("staggers")
   – nystagmus
   – vertigo
Pulmonary ("chokes")
1. Dyspnea
2. Hyperventilation
3. Chest pain
4. Acute respiratory distress syndrome (ARDS)
Cardiac
1. Tachycardia
2. Cardiac arrhythmias

Repetitive breath-hold diving can lead to accumulation of nitrogen in blood and tissues, which may give rise to DCS. MRI in four professional Japanese breath-hold divers (Ama) with histories of diving accidents showed cerebral infarcts localized in the watershed areas of the brain (Kohshi et al 2005). A survey conducted on their island revealed that many Ama divers had experienced stroke-like events. A clinical feature of DCS in breath-hold diving is that the damage is limited to the brain. Although the mechanisms of brain damage in breath-hold diving are unclear, nitrogen bubbles passing through the lungs or the heart so as to become arterialized are most likely to be the causative factor.

Cardiac arrhythmias (premature ventricular contractions) have been reported in DCS. Pulmonary symptoms occur in about 2% of cases. Noncardiogenic pulmonary edema is an uncommon manifestation of Type II DCS. It usually occurs within 6 h of a dive and is believed to be caused by microbubbles in the pulmonary circulation. Shock is rare in DCS but may follow severe dives.

Altitude Decompression Sickness

Altitude DCS is usually seen in aviators at an altitude of 6098 m (20,000 ft), but it may occur at lower altitudes in those with risk factors for DCS. A case of DCS with rapid decompression at 2439 m (8000 ft) and a good response to recompression therapy has been reported by Rudge (1990a). A review of 133 cases from the United States Air Force by Wirjosemito et al (1989) showed that the most common manifestations were joint pain (43.6%), headaches (42.1%), visual disturbances (30.1%), limb paresthesias (27.8%), and mental confusion (24.8%). Spinal cord involvement, chokes, and unconsciousness were rare. HBO treatment was successful in 97.7% of the cases, and residual deficits were noted in only 2.3% of the cases. Altitude-related DCS can present with a wide variety of symptoms in the same patients, such as nausea, headache, fatigue, and respiratory difficulty, which can be misdiagnosed as viral illness. Rudge (1991) reported two such patients in whom the symptoms resolved following recompression with HBO, thus confirming the diagnosis of DCS.

Cerebral hypoxia is usually not a feature of diving-related DCS, but explains the greater severity of the cerebral presentations at altitude DCS. Sheffield and Davis (1976) used HBO in the treatment of a pilot who underwent rapid decompression from 753 hPa (2348 m altitude) to 148 hPa. The pilot lost consciousness in 5 to 8 s. Supplemental oxygen was given after a delay of 6 to 8 min. On the ground the pilot was blind and disoriented and remained so for the next 6.5 h until HBO therapy was started. The pilot eventually recovered with no neurological deficits. Davis et al (1977) reviewed 145 cases of altitude DCS and recommended immediate compression to 2.8 ATA and a series of intermittent oxygen-breathing and air-breathing periods during the subsequent slow decompression. The US Air Force has modified the US Navy procedure Table 6.

Optic atrophy has been reported in a parachutist after repeated hypobaric exposures (Butler 1991) and vision improved with recompression and HBO therapy.

After a review of 233 cases treated at the USAF School of Aerospace Medicine, Rudge and Shafer (1991) concluded that, as in diving, the treatment of altitude DCS with compression therapy is most useful when it is begun as early as possible. The greater the delay in treatment, the longer the symptoms of DCS persist and the greater the rate of residual symptoms.

Another manifestation at altitude is acute mountain sickness (AMS), which usually occurs in individuals ascending above 3000 m without adequate acclimatization. The clinical signs and symptoms of AMS include headache, nausea, irritability, insomnia, dizziness, and vomiting. In some individuals AMS may proceed to cerebral edema and/or pulmonary edema. Cerebral edema is considered to be secondary to hypoxic cerebral vasodilation and elevated capillary hydrostatic pressure, but it cannot be ruled out that bubbles may be a contributing factor. These events elevate peripheral sympathetic activity that may act in concert with pulmonary capillary stress failure to cause pulmonary edema but again pulmonary entrapment of bubbles offers an alternative explana-

tion. Oxygen breathing and descent from altitude are proven effective measures for AMS and a portable hyperbaric chamber has been found to be useful. During acute ascent in the Alps, an early 3-hr pressurization of unacclimatized subjects using air was shown to slightly delay the onset of AMS, but did not prevent it or attenuate its severity on presentation (Kayser et al 1993).

Extravehicular activity during missions on space stations and to establish a permanent presence on the Moon carry a risk of DCS because of the reduction of pressure required to use space suits. Loss of pressure from a space suit would be rapidly fatal unless immediate recompression is carried out and it has been suggested that space stations and lunar missions should include a hyperbaric treatment capability.

Ultrasonic Detection of Bubbles

It is of course not possible in conventional diving to use ultrasonic monitoring, but it has been used to develop and monitor decompression procedures. Gillis et al (1968) were the first to describe bubbles on decompression experimentally. Spencer (1976) used ultrasound to detect venous gas emboli in divers and stated that in these experiments no bends developed prior to detection of bubbles over the precordium. However Powell et al (1983) noted that during decompression with elevated oxygen, precordially determined bubbles at depth were predictive of limb pain in only 50% of cases. Seventy percent of the divers encountered bends without detectable bubbles. The amplitude of the Doppler-detected pulmonary artery flow sound, however, increased, and it was suggested that this may have indicated the presence of numerous microbubbles.

Pulse-echo ultrasound imaging techniques have been used to study the formation of bubbles. These can monitor the extent of bubble formation during decompression with a view to predicting symptoms. The results of such studies confirm that:

- A threshold of supersaturation for bubble formation exists
- The earliest bubbles are intravascular
- There is usually an accumulation of stationary bubbles before precordial bubbles are detected and symptoms of Type 2 DCS develop.

Diagnosis

DCS is rare unless the patient has been exposed to pressures greater than 2 ATA although cases have been described from long exposures to lesser pressures. The diagnosis can be made on the basis of history and clinical features and it is essential to stress that if a significant dive has been undertaken then the presumption must be made that the symptoms are due to decompression sickness not natural disease.

The differential diagnosis of neurological DCS, particularly in atypical cases, should include multiple sclerosis. A case is reported of clinically definite multiple sclerosis presenting as neurological decompression sickness 3 weeks following SCUBA dive (Jan & Jankosky 2003). There was no improvement with HBO treatment, and further evaluation led to the diagnosis of multiple sclerosis.

Recompression has been advocated as a definitive test for DCS, and providing it is undertaken immediately it is a valuable guide. However immediate recompression is usually only possible in commercial diving operations where in most cases a chamber is on site. In Type 1 DCS a small increase in pressure may resolve the pain and on decompression it may recur in the same site suggesting a mechanical origin. In general, the higher the pressure of the onset of pain the greater the pressure increase that is required for its resolution indicating a relationship to gas volume. With CNS symptoms, as bubbles induce tissue hypoxia by interfering with blood flow it may be difficult to determine if improvement is due to a reduction in gas volume with pressure, or the resolution of edema and hypoxia from the use of a high partial pressure of oxygen.

In general laboratory tests are not helpful in decompression sickness, but several have been used in experimental animal studies and some human laboratory dives.

Fibrinogen Degradation Products Test

The fibrinogen degradation products test reflects disseminated intravascular coagulation or agglutination. The diagnostic value of this test in the absence of clinical information is questionable.

Bone Scanning

A Tc 99 bone scan has been shown to be positive as early as 72 h after the traumatic insult in a patient with joint pain Type 1 DCS. This test, however, like epidemiological studies, has not shown a relationship between symptoms of DCS and the sites of bone lesions.

X-rays

Bone necrosis due to decompression may be detectable using X-rays, but it may take 6 months or longer for the radiological changes to appear. More than 10% of men who have been diving for 12 or more years have some bone necrosis and the proportion is much higher in compressed-air workers. The most frequent sites are the head of the humerus, the lower part of the shaft of the femur, and the upper end of the tibia.

Imaging

Abnormalities detected in CT scans of patients who have symptoms of neurological involvement after decompression and are treated by recompression frequently cannot be correlated with clinical manifestations. Therefore, CT scan is not a cost-effective method for post-treatment evaluation in DCS. As CT is a method of densitometry is not surprising that it has failed to reveal useful information and it has been superseded by magnetic resonance imaging (MRI), which has much greater soft tissue resolution. Medullar lesions after scuba diving have also been demonstrated using MRI (Sparacia *et al* 1997). MRI can be useful in follow-up studies and in early diagnosis of DCS when symptoms do not fit the classic picture or loss of consciousness occurs during surfacing (Aksoy 2003).

Electrophysiological Studies

EEG has been a useful technique to monitor the effect of recompression in cerebral disturbance in experimental animals and somatosensory evoked potentials have also shown abnormalities when the spinal cord is involved in DCS.

Neuropsychological Assessment

Neuropsychological assessment cannot be used as a test in acute decompression sickness because it requires considerable time and expertise. However, cognitive impairment can be detected by neuropsychological testing, even in the absence of neurological signs. Monitoring of the recovery of neurological deficits following HBO therapy can be demonstrated by using this method.

Treatment

Emergency Management and Evaluation

In amateur divers there may be problems in the differentiation of air embolism and decompression sickness on the history because they may run out of gas and make a rapid ascent. Barotrauma is exceptionally rare in altitude excursions and also in commercial divers who usually have an unlimited supply of gas provided from the surface. It is also less likely to occur at the greater depths achieved in bell diving, because the volumetric change is less for a given pressure change with increasing depth. It is important to recognize that barotrauma can occur on rapid ascent from a depth of a few meters. However, the essentials of therapy are the same for both air embolism and decompression sickness, that is, after ensuring a clear airway and using cardiopulmonary resuscitation when necessary, a diver must be given 100% oxygen as soon as possible and transferred to a chamber. The treatment of air embolism is described in Chapter 11. The Diver Alert Network (DAN) provides a 24 hr hotline in the USA and internationally for advice regarding the management of diving accidents.

Recompression and HBO Treatment

The objectives of recompression are:

• To reduce bubble volume
• To redistribute and redissolve gas
• To reduce tissue edema and hypoxia

The joint pain of Type I DCS resulting from in surface orientated diving generally resolves rapidly with prompt rapid recompression. In very rare cases there may be an initial increase in the pain which is thought to be due to a "squeeze." Many cases will improve breathing oxygen at the surface and it is important to note that no sequelae have been described from this presentation of DCS. It is important to ensure that the patient does not have neurological symptoms and as a neurological examination is difficult and unreliable in the presence of pain and reliance must be placed on the patient's account of their symptoms. Even 100% oxygen at normal atmospheric pressure is also of value in Type II DCS but it must be emphasized that a tight fitting mask must be used to ensure that there is minimal dilution of the oxygen by air. Fluids can be given by mouth if the patient is not nauseated, otherwise intravenous fluid therapy should be used.

Recompression has been established as the definitive treatment for DCS and was first introduced in compressed-air working where traditionally air was used. However recompression breathing air is accompanied by the respiration of additional nitrogen and problems with air recompression tables led to the development of recompression to 2.8 ATA breathing oxygen. This became standard practice following the development of Tables 5 and 6 by the US Navy in 1970. This pressure reduces the volume of any gas present by almost a third and has the advantage of counteracting the hypoxic/ischemic effects of DCS, particularly those on the CNS. The limitation of oxygen breathing is that it cannot be undertaken at pressures higher than 2.8 ATA because of oxygen toxicity. Although rare, convulsions do indeed occur at 2.8 ATA using US Navy procedures. The more complex procedures necessary in commercial diving are beyond the scope of this text, but recompression and increased partial pressures remain the cornerstones of therapy.

For type I DCS (joint pain only), USN Table 5 may be used, as shown in Figure 10.4. The schedule is 135 min in length and has 5-min breaks before beginning the ascent from 60 fsw (2.8 ATA). However it must be emphasized that if pain does not resolve or Type II symptoms are present USN Table 6 must be used and many centers have ceased using Table 5 because of the relapse rate and failure to recognize underlying neurological problems. If symptoms of joint pain do not respond within 10 min of oxygen breathing at 2.8 ATA, USN Table 6, that is the schedule shown in Figure 10.5, should be used. Three sessions of 20 minutes oxygen breathing are undertaken at 2.8 ATA interspersed by 5 minute air breaks. The 150-min period at 30 fsw (1.9 ATA) is divided into alternating periods of 60-

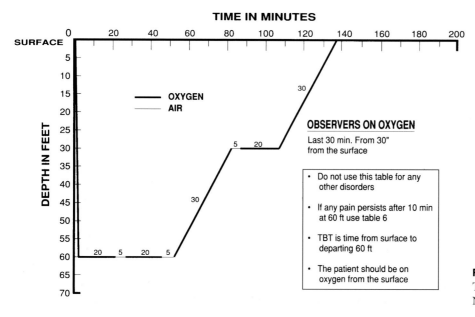

Figure 10.4
The US Air Force modification of US Navy treatment Table 5.

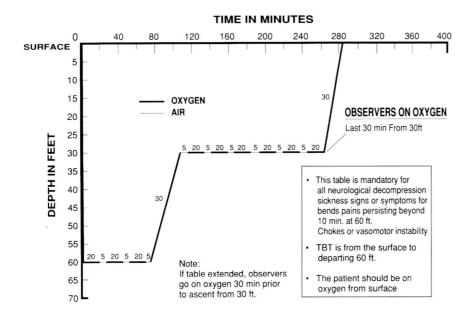

Figure 10.5
The US Air Force modification of the US Navy treatment Table 6.

min of oxygen breathing with two 15 minute periods of air breathing. The total length of this schedule is 285 min, and it may be extended by 100 min if necessary. The US Air Force has produced modifications of these tables for use in altitude decompression sickness.

As an alternative, the flow chart (Figure 10.6) should be consulted. If a COMEX 30 schedule is to be followed, the information is given in Tables 10.2 and 10.3. The gas of preference for this schedule is 50/50 helium and oxygen as much less satisfactory results have been obtained using a 50/50 nitrogen/oxygen mixture. USN Table 6A (1979) is intended for use when it is unclear whether the symptoms are due to air embolism or decompression sickness. Lee *et al* (1988) have modified this table by adding three or more stops from 165 feet to 60 feet. With this approach the total cure rate has been 72%, a substantial improvement over their first recompression response of 37.9%.

Management of Altitude Decompression Sickness

Altitude decompression sickness is treated with hyperbaric therapy has usually been treated the same manner as diving DCS. Expanding space operations and higher flying, more remotely placed military aircraft have stimulated a re-examination of this paradigm. Butler *et al* (2002) prospective treated 12 patients with a new treatment table. USAF Treatment Table 8 (TT8) consists of 100% oxygen delivered at 2 ATA for four 30-min periods with intervening 10-min air breaks (a total oxygen dose of 2 h). Treatment was successful in 9 of 10 cases with Type I altitude DCS. One failure with a recurrence of elbow pain required further therapy. Two patients were treated for Type II altitude DCS with one failure (incomplete clearance of sensory deficits and weak-

ness in the shoulder) requiring further therapy. Although TT8 had two failures, its successes suggest that a new protocol using TT8 for the treatment of altitude decompression sickness is viable but requires further clinical trials.

Management of Neurological Manifestations of Decompression Sickness

Spinal Cord DCS

The response of spinal cord DCS to HBO therapy depends upon the pathophysiology of the lesions. Magnetic resonance imaging (MRI) of the spinal cord should be performed, which may reveal demyelination and also show dorsal white matter lesions typical of venous infarction (Kei *et al* 2007). Cases with short latency may have direct neuronal damage and hemorrhage present. In general such cases require more HBO treatments, and fare less well than those with DCS of late onset. In the latter case, ischemia contributes to neurological deficits and is responsive to HBO treatments. Improvement in MRI findings is not associated with improved clinical status, suggesting that delayed damage subsequent to initial spinal cord lesions may affect the clinical course (Yoshiyama *et al* 2007). HBO therapy was shown by the US Navy to be more effective than the air recompression tables and this has been confirmed in spinal cord DCS.

Helium and oxygen mixtures have been extensively used in recompression therapy in commercial diving (James 1981). The treatment of spinal cord DCS with helium saturation has significant advantages when there has been no clear improvement in neurological status after three 20-min sessions of 100% oxygen at 2.8 ATA. Helium has the

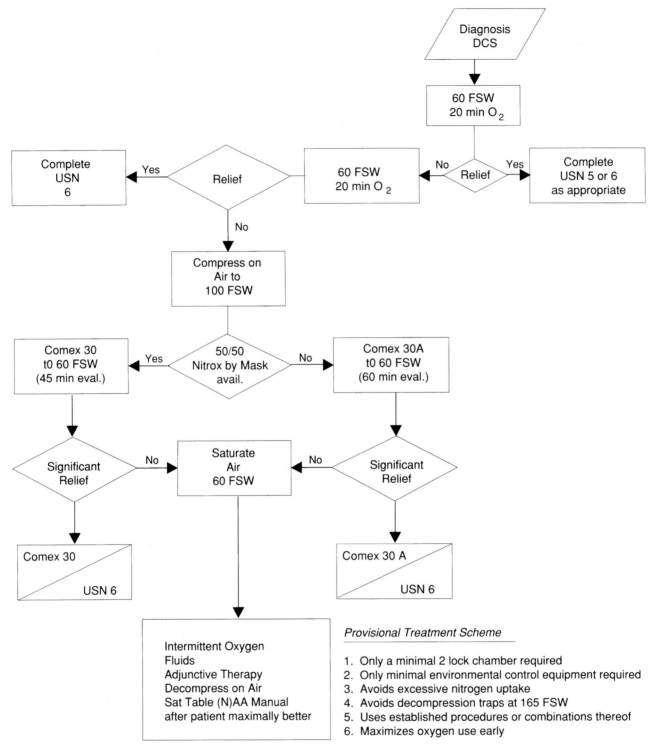

Figure 10.6
Flow chart for decision-making in decompression sickness.

advantage of increasing the rate of nitrogen elimination from the tissues. Kol *et al* (1993) have used helium in cases of spinal cord injury in DCS following air diving. They treated six cases using Comex-30 oxy-helium tables initially and some had additional HBO therapy. Five of these patients made full recoveries and 2 had mild residual neuro-

logical deficits. In one case a US Navy Table 6 had failed, but the patient recovered dramatically on recompression to 30 msw breathing a 50/50 helium and oxygen mixture 24 hours later on Comex 30.

HBO at lower pressure (2 ATA) can be a useful tool in the treatment of acute and subacute phases of CNS ischemia and continued treatment is now recommended by the US Navy.

Aharon-Peretz *et al* (1993) reviewed their experience in treating 68 sports divers with spinal cord DCS at the Israeli Naval Medical Institute over a period of 16 years. Hydration and 100% oxygen breathing were used until the patients reached the hyperbaric chamber. All patients received recompression therapy based on US Navy treatment tables using oxygen, except for six who were treated on Comex Treatment Table CX-30, which uses a 50/50 helium and oxygen mixture in addition to oxygen. Full recovery was achieved in 79% of these patients. Ball (1993) reviewed 49 cases of spinal DCS from a US naval station and classified them according to severity and time to recompression with oxygen. Delay in treatment was found to worsen the outcome for severely injured divers. Residual severity after all treatments was correlated with the severity after first treatment. Retreatment did not alter the outcome in these patients.

Inner Ear Disturbances

Inner ear disturbances are unusual in air diving but may follow a switch from heliox to air in mixed gas diving. In this situation the problem may reside in the inner ear, the brain stem or the cerebellum. Hearing loss is also an unusual manifestation of decompression sickness and in the absence of other manifestations of DCS, it is difficult to distinguish it from middle and inner ear barotrauma. Once the diagnosis is established, immediate recompression with HBO may result in complete recovery of hearing (Talmi *et al* 1991). These disturbances can be treated with vasodilators, anti-inflammatory agents, and HBO. The last is a useful adjunct even if applied after a delay.

Facial Baroparesis

Ischemic neuropraxia of the facial nerve occurs during decompression if impaired Eustachian tube function causes the overpressure to persist in the middle ear in a person with a deficient facial canal; it is not a common event. The importance of recognition of this complication lies in differentiating it from DCS of the CNS and avoiding prolonged recompression therapy. There is no definite treatment, but HBO may be used, as this approach has been found useful in cases of Bell's palsy (see Chapter 19).

Retinal and Optic Nerve Sequelae

This is a rare complication of DCS. A case has been reported in a fisher-diver who presented with loss of vision, but recovered after HBO treatments even though the therapy was started after a delay of two weeks (Hsu *et al* 1992).

Late Sequelae of DCS

Divers who have had episodes of DCS are more liable to be hospitalized in the following years. These admissions may be due to late sequelae of DCS some of which are:

1. Persistent joint and limb pains.
2. Aseptic necrosis of bone. The cause of aseptic necrosis of bone, which is a late manifestation of DCS, is not known. It may be the result of damage to the endothelium or the capillaries supplying blood to the bone (see Chapter 29).
3. Motor disorders.
4. Peripheral neuropathy.
5. Patients who have suffered DCS have a higher incidence of vascular diseases.
6. Neuropsychological deficits

Monoplace vs Multiplace Chambers

Most recompression facilities available to divers are two compartment multiplace chambers. The use of monoplace chambers for DCS has been controversial, because examination of the casualty is not possible and most cannot be compressed beyond 3 ATA. However compression to 6 ATA is unnecessary in DCS following surface-orientated diving, especially when treatment is delayed. Monoplace chambers can be used for the treatment of DCS under the following circumstances:

- Diving accident victims who arrive at a hyperbaric facility where only a monoplace chamber is available should be accepted for treatment.
- Monoplace chambers should be equipped to provide air breaks using a mask and an external source of compressed-air to allow USN Tables 5 and 6 to be followed.

Air breaks are possible in a Sechrist model 2500-B monoplace chamber and the equipment is easily fitted into other monoplace designs.

Use of Oxygen vs Other Gas Mixtures

Oxygen treatment has disadvantages, because it cannot be used at pressures greater than 2.8 ATA because of oxygen toxicity and air breaks are therefore used at this pressure. In fact, convulsions may occur after even 20 minutes at this pressure and there may also be severe vasoconstriction which may cause worsening of symptoms. Because of the fire hazard raised by pure oxygen, compressed air is still commonly used for the treatment of DCS in workers in compressed-air working, but the results are inferior to those obtained using oxygen treatment. Oxygen treat-

Table 10.2
Therapeutic Table: COMEX 30A

Depths (Meters)	Time (min)	Gas Breathed Patient	Attendant	Total Time (min)
30	40	50/50	Air	40
30 to 24	5	Air	Air	45
(5 min/m)	25	50/50	Air	40
24	5	Air	Air	75
24	25	50/50	Air	100
24 to 18	5	Air	Air	105
(5 min/m)	25	50/50	Air	130
18	5	Air	Air	135
18	25	O$_2$	Air	160
18	5	Air	Air	165
18	25	O$_2$	Air	190
18 to 12	5	Air	Air	195
(5 min/m)	25	O$_2$	Air	220
12	10	Air	Air	230
12	45	O$_2$	Air	275
12	10	Air	Air	285
12	45	O$_2$	O$_2$	330
12	10	Air	Air	452
12	45	O$_2$	O$_2$	385
12	10	Air	Air	395
12 to surface	24	O$_2$	O$_2$	419
(Rate = 2 min/m)				

Table 10.3
Therapeutic Table: COMEX 30A

Depths (Meters)	Time (min)	Gas Breathed Patient	Attendant	Total Time (min)
30	60	Air	Air	60
30 to 24 (1 min/m)	6	Air	Air	66
24 to 21 (20 min/m)	60	Air	Air	126
21 to 18 (22 min/m)	66	Air	Air	192
18 to 15 (24 min/m)	72	Air	Air	264
15 to 12 (26 min/m)	78	Air	Air	342
(2 tablets 5 mg Valium on arrival at 12 m)	18			
12	10	Air	Air	352
12	40	O$_2$	O$_2$	392
12	10	Air	Air	402
12	40	O$_2$	O$_2$	442
12	10	Air	Air	452
12	40	O$_2$	O$_2$	492
12	5	Air	Air	497
12 to surface	24	O$_2$	O$_2$	521
(Rate = 2 min/m)				

ment in recompression has the following advantages over air:

- A large gradient for nitrogen elimination
- No further addition of nitrogen
- Tissue oxygenation is improved even without full restoration of blood flow
- Reduced blood sludging
- Improved WBC filterability

In commercial diving it is essential to avoid the use of compressed-air in the recompression therapy of helium and oxygen mixture divers because the addition of nitrogen may cause dramatic worsening of symptoms and even death because of gas countertransport (James 1981). For cases presenting after surfacing the oxygen tables may be used but for deeper recompression therapy helium and oxygen mixtures must be used. This practice has now been incorporated into US Navy procedures (USN Manual 1993). Considerable commercial experience has been gained in the use of 50/50 heliox on the Comex 30 table for both air and heliox divers (Table 10.2). In contrast to oxygen at 2.8 ATA no cases of deterioration in divers have been recorded using heliox in recompression therapy. This is now fully supported by extensive animal experimentation with direct observation of bubbles in tissue. The only contrary experimental data has been from a severe experimental models where following the use of heliox a tran-

sient in pulmonary arterial pressure was seen. However this has not been a problem in the therapy of human decompression sickness and James (1988) has stated that the advice first given by the US Navy in 1959 to use helium-oxygen mixtures is still current in the US Navy. Helium and oxygen mixtures can be used in place of air on any of the USN air recompression tables and are the preferred choice for recompression beyond 2.8 ATA.

Role of Drugs

1. IV Saline The only effective "drug" intervention proven to be effective in decompression sickness is rehydration. Wells (1978) demonstrated a reversal of the sludging of blood. His studies failed to demonstrate benefit from other plasma expanders and the Dextrans may provoke allergic reactions.
2. Steroids. As in spinal cord injury there is evidence that steroids may be beneficial when edema is present.
3. Intramuscular diclofenac sodium, a nonsteroidal anti-inflammatory agent, has been used to relieve the residual pain of DCS.
4. Lidocaine, a sodium-channel-blocking agent used clinically as an antiarrhythmic and local anesthetic, can be used as a neuroprotective agent in DCS. Clinical evidence of efficacy in DCS is limited to anecdotal reports. Expeditious administration of lidocaine may be justified

in severe neurologic DCS after patient counseling and consent.

5. Nitric oxide (NO)-donating agents. This is based on the hypothesis that exogenous NO administration or pharmacological up-regulation of NO may reduce DCS risk and severity by decreasing bubble formation, reduction of bubble-mediated inflammatory and coagulation cascades and protection of endothelial integrity (Duplessis & Fothergill 2008). Some of these effects can be achieved by statins, which are approved for treatment of hypercholesterolemia. Statin-mediated lipid reduction may reduce bubble generation via alterations in plasma rheology and surface tension. Use of NO-donor medications such as isosorbide mononitrate and nitroglycerine should be investigated for te treatment of DCS.

6. Lekotrienes. Zafirlukast and zileuton, which are 5-lipoxygenase inhibitors, can reduce inflammatory responses to DCS in rats (Little & Butler 2008).

Hydration of the patient is very important, but saline or balanced electrolyte solution should be used rather than 5% dextrose solution, which may aggravate CNS edema.

Platelet antagonists such as aspirin can reduce platelet aggregation surrounding microbubbles. Substances that increase the intracellular levels of cyclic AMP seem most promising in this respect. There has been no significant human experience with heparin which may promote hemorrhage. In experimental animals perfluorocarbon emulsion (FC-43) combined with 100% oxygen breathing has been shown to provide hemodynamic and neurological protection in DCS. On balance it seems unlikely that pharmacological strategies will become available for the management of DCS and reliance must be placed on early recompression therapy with high partial pressures of oxygen and helium oxygen mixtures.

Importance of Early Treatment

The importance of early treatment has been established beyond dispute in military and commercial diving experience and has been emphasized by Bayne (1978). Fifty consecutive cases of DCS in US Navy divers were reviewed after recompression therapy. There was no mortality or obvious morbidity. The common factors in these cases were as follows:

1. Medical screening and conditioning were strict.
2. Physicians and divers were acquainted with the signs and symptoms.
3. The interval between onset of symptoms and recompression was short.
4. There was aggressive diagnostic and therapeutic use of HBO.
5. There was judicious use of adjunctive measures such as intravenous fluids and dexamethasone.

Immediate hyperbaric treatment is the main factor in ensuring complete recovery from severe DCS.

Once DCS is treated, current guidelines recommend an observation period of at least 6 h for patients with neurological symptoms in case of relapse. Surveys have shown a symptom relapse rate as high as 38.5%, with half of those occurring in the first 24 h. A short-term observation unit is recommended for monitoring of these patients. A retrospective study of patients presenting with DCS at a major hyperbaric facility showed that of 102 consecutive patients with DCS who receiving HBO, 42 (41.2%) had neurological sequelae; 10 required more than one treatment for refractory symptoms or relapse; 38 received up to three treatments, which can be done within the time requirements of short-term observation (Tempel et al 2006). Therefore, short-term observation units would provide a safe and efficient disposition for patients after receiving HBO.

Delayed Treatment

Patients with residual symptoms of DCS who present several days following the exposure, can also benefit from HBO treatment, with complete resolution of their symptoms. Therefore, DCS cases should be treated with HBO whenever they are seen, even as late as 2 weeks days after the first symptoms.

A transportable recompression rescue chamber (TRRC) has been suggested as an alternative to delayed treatment TRRC for one person can be used for the rapid initiation of treatment and evacuation in severe scuba-diving accidents. This chamber has also been used for evacuation, although a two-compartment chamber (one compartment for the victim and one for the attendant) is better.

There is some risk is involved in transport as gas bubbles may expand as altitude is increased in an aircraft and hypoxia will be worsened. However some aircraft can maintain sea level conditions at altitude and the Swiss air-rescue service can transport a monoplace hyperbaric chamber in a helicopter. The ideal transportable hyperbaric chamber should be two compartment and fully equipped for ancillary treatment. Some chambers are available for surface transport and can be modified and fitted into a boat or a helicopter so that the patients can be treated while they are being transported to a regular medical facility for further care.

Treatment of Residual Neurological Injury and SPECT Brain Imaging in Type II DCS

The first DCS case where HMPAO – SPECT brain imaging was used to identify viable brain tissue and document the response to HBO at pressures lower than those used conventionally for the treatment of DCS was reported by

Harch *et al* (1993). Since then a total of 13 divers who had type II DCS or cerebral arterial gas embolism were managed by this approach (Harch *et al* 1994a). HMPAO-SPECT scans were done after test exposure to HBO at 1.5 or 1.7 ATA for 90 min. The initial scans were abnormal in all cases. "Tailing" HBO treatments at low pressures (1.5–2 ATA) were continued with primary HBO treatment for DCS in 9 of these and 4 with delays of 4 to 86 days. Neurological improvement was correlated with improvements shown on SPECT scans. A case history with illustrations of SPECT is shown in Appendix 2. This approach has now been adopted by the US Navy and it is essential to recognize that this therapy is addressing hypoperfusion due to edema by utilizing the vasoconstrictive properties of oxygen at increased dosage and is not directed at persisting gas phase.

Risk Factors for DCS

The following risk factors for DCS have been recorded for air diving:

1. Obesity. Obesity increases the risk of DCS. Divers who are more than 20% in excess of ideal weight, according to standard tables, should be prohibited from diving until they have reduced their weight to acceptable levels.
2. Early, retrospective reports of the incidence of altitude decompression sickness (DCS) during altitude chamber training exposures indicated that women were more susceptible than men. In a recent study, no differences in altitude DCS incidence were observed between the sexes (Webb *et al* 2003). Women are at a higher risk of developing altitude-related DCS during their menstrual periods.
3. Sensitivity to complement fixation. Individuals who are more sensitive to complement activation by alternate pathways are more susceptible to DCS.
4. High serum cholesterol levels and hemoconcentration predispose to bubble formation.
5. Moon *et al* (1989) examined 37 patients with a history of DCS, using bubble contrast, two-dimensional echocardiography, and Doppler imagery. Bubble contrast showed right-to-left shunting through the patent foramen ovale in 11 (37%) of these patients, as compared with a 5% incidence in 176 healthy volunteers detected using the same technique. Persons with a patent foramen ovale and a cardiac right-to-left shunt have an increased risk of developing neurologic complications even after recreational scuba diving in shallow water (Schwerzmann & Seiler, 2001). The presence of a foramen ovale,

therefore, is a risk factor for the development of DCS in divers, because it allows the passage of venous emboli into the systemic circulation. The fetus may be at risk of DCS in a pregnant diver. The pulmonary filter is not functioning in the fetus and the bubbles generated by either the fetal or the placental tissues will pass through the foramen ovale into the fetal arterial circulation, where they can proceed to embolize the brain, the spinal cord, and other organs.

6. A prolonged stay under pressure followed by rapid decompression.
7. Heavy exercise or other stress at depth.
8. Flying after diving and a rapid ascent to high altitude.

Several decompression tables, some of them computerized, are available for the guidance of divers. Essentially all calculations assume that the additional gas taken up remains in solution and gas equilibrates in the lung to ambient conditions. Both of these assumptions are now known to be untrue. In effect decompression tables contrive to minimize bubble formation and allow the safe elimination of the bubbles formed.

The hypothesis that number of bubbles evolving during decompression from a dive, and therefore the incidence of DCS, might be reduced by pretreatment with HBO, has been tested in rats (Katsenelson *et al* 2007). HBO pretreatment was shown to be equally effective at 304, 405 or 507 kPa, bringing about a significant reduction in the incidence of DCS in rats decompressed from 1,013 kPa. this method has not yet been tested in humans.

Conclusions

The evidence is now conclusive that gas phase forms during most decompressions and adherence to published "no-decompression" limits or decompression tables does not eliminate the risk of decompression sickness. Air diving beyond 30 msw (4 ATA) is associated with a greatly increased risk of decompression sickness.

Early recognition and prompt management of a patient with DCS is essential and early recompression treatment reduces the incidence of late complications. Recompression with a high partial pressure of oxygen is recommended for the initial treatment and US Navy tables 5 and 6 are the most widely used in surface-orientated diving. When required, further recompression should be undertaken using helium and oxygen mixtures. Adherence to good diving practice and the recognition of risk factors for DCS are important to reduce the incidence of this disease.

11 Cerebral Air Embolism

K.K. Jain

HBO is the most effective treatment of air embolism; it reduces the size of air bubbles and counteracts the secondary effects. This chapter on cerebral air embolism examines:

Causes

The introduction of air into the venous or the arterial system can cause cerebral air embolism leading to severe neurological deficits. The first known recognition of arterial air embolism was reported by Morgagni in 1769, and later, in 1821, Magendie described the consequences of pulmonary overinflation leading to arterial gas embolism. The most common causes reported in the literature are iatrogenic, the embolism occurring as a result of invasive medical procedures or surgery. Less commonly, air embolism occurs in divers undergoing rapid decompression and in submarine escape. Causes of air embolism are shown in Table 11.1.

Table 11.1
Causes of Air Embolism

A. Sudden decompression or ascent in diving and submarine escape
- Pulmonary barotrauma – "burst lung" in divers
- Rapid decompression in an altitude chamber for flight training

B. Trauma
- Cardiopulmonary resuscitation in patients with undetected lung injury
- Head and neck injuries
- High-altitude accidents

C. Iatrogenic
1. Diagnostic and minor procedures
- Intravenous fluids and central venous pressure (CVP) lines
- Arterial lines for blood and medication infusion
- Angiography: diagnostic and therapeutic catheterization of blood vessels
- Mechanical positive pressure ventilation
- Air contrast salpingogram
- Air insufflation with pneumatic otoscope
- Needle biopsy of the lung
- Hemodialysis
- Gastrointestinal endoscopy
2. Intraoperative complications
- Neurosurgical operations in the sitting position: tear into veins in the posterior fossa or the cervical spinal canal
- Cardiac surgery: open heart surgery with extracorporeal circulation
- Vascular surgery: carotid endarterectomy with shunt
- Thoracic surgery: opening of pulmonary veins at subatmospheric pressures
- Endobronchial resection of lung tumor using Neodymium-YAG laser
- Pelvic surgery in Trendelenburg position. Operative hysteroscopy with laser
- Cesarian section

D. Miscellaneous and rare causes
- Faulty abortion
- Orogenital sex during pregnancy
- Inhalation of helium directly from a pressurized helium tank.
- Ingestion of hydrogen peroxide solution

There are approximately 20,000 cases of air embolism per year in the USA. The exact incidence of various causes is difficult to determine, as not all cases are reported in the literature. An excellent review of the topic is presented elsewhere (Hodics & Linfante 2003). Some victims recover spontaneously. This review concerns those cases where hyperbaric treatment was used.

The incidence of air embolism during cardiopulmonary bypass operations is 0.1%. The actual prevalence may be higher because several such complications are not recognized and reported. Air enters the venous system in 30%–40% of the patients undergoing neurosurgical operations in the sitting position. Air embolism can occur during neuro-angiographic interventional procedures such as aneurysm coiling embolization and carotid stent placement but overall incidence during diagnostic neuroangiographic procedure is very low in the order of 0.08% (Gupta *et al* 2007).

Mechanisms

In iatrogenic cases the air is either sucked into the veins with negative pressure or introduced into the veins or arteries under pressure. The lung is usually an effective filter for air bubbles greater than 22 μm in diameter when air is injected slowly. A bolus injection of air more than 1.5–3 ml/kg exceeds the filter capacity of the lungs and produces embolization through the left heart into the arterial circulation until it blocks arterioles 30–60 μm in diameter. Air has a large surface tension at the blood-air interface and the globules of air cannot be deformed enough to navigate the capillaries.

A patent foramen ovale occurs in 20% to 35% of the normal adult population and in one out of ten of these is at risk of having arterial air embolism when air enters the venous system inadvertently. The exact prevalence rate of functional right to left atrial shunt in the healthy adult population, however, is unknown. In the absence of such a shunt, venous air must first traverse the pulmonary vasculature in order to enter the cerebral circulation.

In pulmonary barotrauma, lung volumes expand during rapid ascent. When alveolar pressure exceeds 80–100 mmHg, air can be forced into pulmonary capillaries. Alveoli may rupture into the pleural space, causing pneumothorax, or into the pulmonary veins, where the embolus may traverse the left side of the heart to enter the aorta and may ascend the carotid arteries to the cerebral circulation, as the diver is usually upright during ascent.

Pathophysiology

Air emboli lodge distally in the smaller arteries and arterioles of the brain and obstruct the flow of blood. The result is ischemia, hypoxia, and cerebral edema. Even when the bubble is dissolved, a "no reflow" phenomenon may occur in the damaged tissues. The bubble acts as a foreign body and starts a number of biochemical reactions in the blood. Platelets are activated and release vasoactive substances including prostaglandins. The bubble may damage the endothelial cells of the vessel wall by direct contact. Margination and activation of leukocytes follows, and may cause a secondary ischemia. If the bubble persists, it is surrounded by platelets and fibrin deposit, which may prevent dislodging of the bubble. Although the potential of large bubbles to cause cerebral injury is not disputed, there is controversy over the significance of exposure to small bubbles in cardiac surgery. It is known that postsurgical neuropsychological deficits do correlate positively with the number of emboli to which patients are exposed; to date, however, the technology for distinguishing between gaseous and particulate emboli or for sizing emboli accurately is not readily available (Mitchell & Gorman 2002).

Air bubbles injected directly into the cerebral circulation of experimental animals can open the blood-brain barrier. The barrier, however, repairs itself within a few hours. Ischemic hypoxia produced by air embolism is not severe enough to produce gross cerebral infarction, but produces necrosis of the deep cortical layers at the gray-white matter junction.

There may be segmental arterial vasospasm followed by dilatation, and some of the air may escape from the arteries into the veins via capillaries. As a result of arterial obstruction regional cerebral blood flow (rCBF) declines and EEG activity may cease in the affected region. The changes are typical of cerebral ischemia, but the blood-brain barrier permeability increases immediately after air embolism, in contrast to vascular occlusion from other causes, where the onset is delayed. Focal ischemia of short duration does not lead to cell loss, and the processes causing deterioration are potentially reversible. The other potentially reversible process that occurs in the tissues is cerebral edema. Although the brain is the major concern in arterial embolism, the coronary arteries may occasionally be involved.

Animal brain models of cerebral arterial gas embolism may be useful in comparing the effectiveness of various recompression schedules. Murrison (1993) has reviewed various animal models for neurophysiological investigations of pathophysiology of central nervous system (CNS) damage in arterial gas embolism. Most of these studies involve injection of air into cerebral vasculature. Secondary CNS deterioration may be may be due to endothelial damage or change in blood constituents rather than mechanical bubble action and may explain the failure of recompression therapy in such cases. The results of these animal studies cannot be extrapolated to humans.

Clinical Features

Clinical manifestations, essentially neurological or cardiovascular disorders vary greatly. The clinical features of air embolism depend on the patient's posture, the route of entry of air, the volume of air, the size of the bubbles, and the rate of entry of air. If the patient is reclining, air is more likely to enter the coronary arteries, whereas it is more likely to enter the cerebral arteries if the patient is upright. Neurological sequelae have been estimated to occur in 19 to 50% of the patients with cerebral air embolism.

Signs and symptoms of air embolism in divers may not be clear-cut. In 50% of such cases, dysbaric air embolism was found to be part of dysbarism syndrome including decompression sickness. A sudden change in sensorium is the most common symptom and ranges from disorientation to coma. Focal neurological deficits such as hemiplegia or monoplegia may occur, according to the location of the lesions. Respiratory arrest and seizures are less common. A shock-like state may occur with massive embolism. Associated symptoms may be those of pneumothorax (in pulmonary barotrauma) or myocardial ischemia. Liebermeister's sign, i.e., the presence of areas of pallor on the tongue after air embolism, may be found.

Diagnosis

The diagnosis of air embolism is based on a careful consideration of the patient's history and neurological findings. In cases of sudden decompression with neurological deficit, the diagnosis is easier. During surgical procedures monitored by doppler ultrasound, air embolization is detected at an early stage and appropriate measures can be taken to stop further air entering the blood vessels. Transcranial doppler studies show that microscopic cerebral artery air emboli are present in virtually all patients undergoing cardiac surgery. Microbubbles can be detected with two-dimensional echocardiography, which is often used for this purpose during open heart and bypass surgeries (Kearney et al 1997). EEG monitoring is also useful for early detection of acute cerebral dysfunction.

Subtle changes in mental function may be a major manifestation even in the absence of other objective neurological signs. CT scan offers a possibility of diagnosis of subclinical lesions of the brain. Air bubbles may also be seen on fundoscopic examination. Air may be seen in the cerebral arteries during a neurosurgical operation, or air can be demonstrated in a specimen of arterial blood. A high index of suspicion is very important in diagnosis. Under suspicious circumstances air embolism should be assumed present unless otherwise proven. In some cases the diagnosis is proven only after successful response to hyperbaric therapy.

In air embolism associated with diving, there is muscle injury and elevated serum creatine kinase which a marker of the severity of this complication (Smith & Neuman 1994).

Treatment

Emergency measures include administration of 100% oxygen, using a closely fitting mask, and transport of the patient to a hyperbaric facility. If transport by air is unavoidable, the patient should travel in a pressurized cabin, and the aircraft should stay at a low altitude. A bolus dose (10 mg) of dexamethasone may be given to prevent cerebral edema. Oxygen serves to reduce the size of the air bubble by depletion of nitrogen and also counteracts the hypoxia and ischemia of the surrounding brain tissue.

The important consideration in treatment of cerebral air embolism is preparedness and anticipation. Procedures with a known risk of air embolism should not be performed far away from a hyperbaric facility, and a hyperbaric chamber should be available in institutions that conduct open heart surgery. Time is the more important element in management – the shorter the delay, the better the outcome. Emboli large enough to produce symptoms require immediate treatment because of the risk of "gas lock" in the right side of the heart and subsequent circulatory failure (Jørgensen et al 2008).

The generally accepted treatment of air embolism is immediate compression to 6 ATA air for a period of not more than 30 min followed by ascent to 2.8 ATA with oxygen. The rationale of this approach is as follows:

1. Compression of the bubbles reduces their size. According to Boyle's law, the volume of a gas is inversely proportional to the pressure exerted on the gas. Compression to 6 ATA would reduce the size of a bubble to one-sixth, or approximately 17%, of its original size (Table 11.2). The reduction of the surface area of the bubble to 30% reduces the inflammatory effect of the bubble-blood interface.

Table 11.2
Relative Volume and Surface Area of a Bubble with Compression

Pressure (ATA)	Relative volume (%)	Relative surface area (%)
1	100	100
2.8	35	50
6	17	30

2. Delivery of high levels of oxygen is important to counteract the ischemic and hypoxic effects of vascular obstruction. Breathing oxygen (100%) at 2.8 ATA leads to an arterial pO_2 level of 1800 mmHg. At this pressure 6 ml oxygen is dissolved in 100 ml plasma.
3. Fick's law can be applied to relate the rate of nitrogen diffusion to the concentration gradient between the bubble and the surrounding tissue. Oxygen at 100% concentration improves the diffusion of nitrogen from the bubble.
4. Cerebral edema associated with cerebral air embolism is decreased by HBO.
5. Vasoconstriction induced by HBO inhibits air embolus redistribution. This is possible because the reactivity of the cerebral arteries is not impaired in cerebral air embolism (Gordman & Browning 1986).

The first experimental study employing hyperbaric therapy was conducted by Meijne et al (1963). They injected air into the carotid arteries of rabbits and showed a remarkable improvement in the survival rate of the animals treated with HBO. Leitch et al (1984a–d) carried out a series of experimental studies to reassess the hyperbaric treatment of air embolism. They tested the question, "Is there a benefit in beginning treatment at 6 ATA?" in dog models of air embolism treated at various pressures. The effectiveness of the treatment was assessed by sensory evoked potentials (SEP) and CBF. It was concluded that there was no advantage in using air at 6 ATA prior to treatment with oxygen at 2.8 ATA. The data showed that clearance of air is probably independent of pressure past the threshold of 2 ATA and is certainly hastened by oxygen. Approximately 8 min were required to clear the embolism. A number of air-treated dogs had redistribution of air embolism after initial decompression and concomitant reduction of CBF. More recently, McDermott et al (1992) carried out a study of various pressure schedules in experimental feline arterial air embolism with assessment of severity by cortical SEP. They found no additional benefits of initial treatment at 6 ATA as compared to 2.8 ATA.

Transcranial doppler studies show that microscopic cerebral artery air emboli (CAAE) are present in virtually all patients undergoing cardiac surgery. Massive cerebral arterial air embolism is rare. If it occurs, HBO is recommended as soon as surgery is completed. Dexter and Hindman (1997) have used a mathematical model to predict the absorption time of air embolus, assuming that the volumes of clinically relevant air emboli vary from 10^{-7} to at least 10^{-1} ml. Absorption times are predicted to be at least 40 h during oxygenation using breathing gas mixtures of fraction of inspired oxygen approximately equal to 40%. When air emboli are large enough to be detected by CT, absorption times are calculated to be at least 15 h. Decreases in cerebral blood flow caused by the air emboli would make the absorption even slower. Analysis of these authors suggests that if the diagnosis of massive

Table 11.3
Examples of Applications of HBO for Cerebral Air Embolism

Authors and year	No. of cases	Cause	Pressure used	Results and comments
Davis et al (1990)	1	Cesarian section	Table 6	HBO treatment started 8 hours after onset with impairment of consciousness and left hemiplegia. Recovered with minimal neurological deficit.
Armon et al (1991)	1	Open heart surgery	Table 6A	HBO treatment was started 30 hours after the incident with coma, decerebrate rigidity and seizures. Recovered with minimal residual neurological deficits at 14 months follow-up.
Kol et al (1993)	6	Cardiopulmonary by-pass	Table 6A	2 died 2 partial recovery 2 full recovery
Rios-Tejada et al (1997)	1	Decompression at flight level 280 (28,000 ft) in an altitude chamber.	Table 6A (extended) +3 HBO sessions at 2 ATA/90 min	Complete recovery from left hemiplegia.
Droghetti et al (2002)	1	Paradoxical air embolism during percutaneous nephrolithotripsy in the prone position.	Table 6	Patient presented neurological deficits 8 hours later, when HBO treatment was started. Full recovery.
Wherrett et al (2002)	1	Diagnostic bronchoscopy in a patient with previous lobectomy for bronchogenic carcinoma.	Modified Table 6	Treated 52 h after the event. Discharged after fully recovery 1 week later.

CAAE is suspected, CT should be performed, and consideration should be given to HBO therapy if the emboli are large enough to be visualized, even if patient transfer to a HBO facility will require several hours.

Some authors recommend supportive care as the primary therapy for venous gas embolism, while HBO therapy in addition to supportive care is the first line of treatment for arterial gas embolism (Fukaya & Hopf 2007). The criterion for use of HBO is clinical manifestation, particularly neurological and not the source of air embolism.

Clinical Applications of HBO

Clinical applications of HBO for air embolism during the past decade are shown in Table 11.3. If we consider the overall mortality of air embolism without hyperbaric treatment as 30%, these results represent a remarkable improvement. A controlled prospective study has shown that mortality can be reduced to 14% if hyperbaric oxygen therapy is given within 12 hours of the accident (Bacha et al 1996). Treatment appears to be ineffective after irreversible damage has already been done.

HBO has been used successfully in cases of air embolism as a complication of open heart surgery, endoscopy (Raju et al 1998) and transthoracic percutaneous thin-needle biopsy (Regge et al 1997). The usual schedule of hyperbaric treatment is US Air Force Modification of US Navy Table 6 (Figure 10.5; Chapter 10). The initial approach is to compress the patient to 6 ATA. After 30 min, decompression is carried out to 2.8 ATA.

Ancillary Treatments

The following treatments have been used in addition to hyperbaric therapy.

Antiplatelet Drugs. These have been used to counteract the platelet aggregation associated with air embolism. The use of heparin as anticoagulant is considered risky due to the danger of hemorrhage in infarcted areas. Patients who are already on heparin have a better prognosis after air embolism than those who are not anticoagulated. This is particularly noted during cardiopulmonary bypass for cardiac surgery. Oral aspirin is safer but takes about 30 min to act after ingestion.

Steroids. These have been used to prevent cerebral edema. Delayed cerebral edema can occur after initially good results from recompression following air embolism. Steroids should be administered cautiously during HBO as they may accelerate the development of oxygen toxicity.

Hemodilution. Hematocrit has been shown to have a relation to the infarct size in vascular occlusion, and many cases of air embolism display hemoconcentration. Hemodilution, e.g., by dextran-40, is indicated. Lowering of hematocrit also causes a reduction in oxygen-carrying capacity, but this is more than adequately compensated by HBO.

Control of Seizures. An anticonvulsant medication may be required for control of seizures. Prophylactic use of lidocaine not only controls seizures but also reduces infarct size and prevents cardiac arrhythmias associated with air embolism.

Measures to Improve Cerebral Metabolism. Loss of blood supply causes immediate reduction of neuronal pools and increased production of lactate. The total energy available is reduced. Increased blood glucose levels are associated with increased lactate production by the ischemic brain and increase in infarction. The control of blood glucose, therefore, is important after air embolism and routine use of intravenous dextrose should be avoided. There is evidence that HBO serves to normalize the cerebral metabolism (see Chapter 17) and also lowers blood glucose.

Hyperbaric Treatment in Special Situations

Cerebral Edema

The following example is given to illustrate the special use of HBO in cerebral edema. Thiede and Manley (1976) reported a patient with air embolism who responded to initial compression to 6 ATA but deteriorated into coma and decerebrate posturing during decompression at 1.9 ATA. There was increased intracranial pressure, indicating cerebral edema. The patient was given repeated HBO treatments twice daily at 2.8 ATA (100% oxygen) and recovered completely. HBO in this case was doubly indicated – for air embolism as well as for cerebral edema.

Cardiovascular Surgery

Calverley *et al* (1971) reported air embolism during cardiac catheterization in a 4-month-old infant with ventricular septal defect. A quantity of 10 ml air was inadvertently injected into the right ventricle. Anesthesia was terminated and air compression was done to 6 ATA 35 min after the episode. Decompression was started after a further 15 min and completed in 5 h. No oxygen was given. The infant made a good recovery and the planned cardiac surgery was carried out. Calverley *et al* made an important observation about nitrous oxide anesthesia: if air embolism occurs during this type of anesthesia, nitrous oxide diffuses rapidly into enclosed pockets of gas, causing an increase in pressure (or an increase in volume if the surrounding tissues permit). The authors recommended that nitrous oxide anesthesia should be discontinued if air embolism occurs.

HBO has been used to treat patients with extensive neurological deficits from air emboli during open heart surgery. Treatment is usually not started until after completion of surgery, but is still effective. Some complicated operations in cardiac surgery and neurosurgery cannot be aborted because of air embolism. In such cases, compression treatment can be started after completion of the operation.

Huber *et al* (2000) reported a case of a 5-year-old girl who suffered a massive arterial air embolism during surgical closure of an atrial septal defect. They successfully treated a proven arterial air embolism with intraoperative (retrograde cerebral perfusion) combined with postoperative procedures (deep barbiturate anesthesia and HBO). At discharge the girl had fully recovered from the initial neurologic defects.

Hypothermia has been used in cardiac surgery for cerebral protection. Patients who suffer massive air embolism during cardiopulmonary bypass can be treated by using a combination of hypothermia and HBO with good results. According to Charles' law, the volume of a gas varies according to temperature. Theoretically hypothermia is expected to decrease the size of the gas bubbles and should be beneficial in air embolism. Animal experimental studies are required to determine if HBO and hypothermia complement one another in air embolism.

Neurosurgery

Air embolism following posterior fossa surgery in the sitting position can be promptly treated by recompression according to the standard schedule. The patients usually recover without neurological deficits.

Pulmonary Barotrauma

Leitch and Green (1987) reviewed treatment of 89 cases of air embolism due to pulmonary barotrauma in divers. There was a 65% success rate with hyperbaric treatments, and one of the victims had a relapse. The authors concluded that although most cases would recover with oxygen at 2.8 ATA, there was no reason to alter the established technique of initial compression with air to 6 ATA prior to HBO at 2.8 ATA. Air embolism associated with pulmonary barotrauma during rapid decompression in an altitude chamber has been managed by the use of treatment table 6A (Rudge 1992).

Pulmonary barotrauma with air embolism has been reported as a complication of HBO therapy for a non-healing ulcer of the foot (Wolf *et al* 1990). Pneumothorax has been reported as a complication of recompression therapy for cerebral arterial gas embolism associated with diving (Broome & Smith 1992).

In an unusual presentation of cerebral air embolism, a patient became unresponsive and developed subcutaneous emphysema during the direct insufflation of oxygen into the right middle lobe bronchus (Wherrett *et al* 2002). An endotracheal tube and bilateral chest tubes were immediately placed with resultant improvement in the oxygen saturation. However, the patient remained unresponsive with extensor and flexor responses to pain. Later, there was seizure activity requiring anticonvulsant therapy. CT scans of the head and cerebral spinal fluid examination were negative, though the electroencephalogram was abnormal. A CT of chest showed evidence of barotrauma. 52 hours after the event, a presumed diagnosis of cerebral air embolism was made, and the patient was treated with HBO using a modified US Navy Table 6. 12 hours later he had regained consciousness and was extubated. He underwent two more HBO and was then discharged from hospital 1 week after the event, fully recovered. Although HBO was started after significant delay, the patient made a good recovery.

Air Embolism During Invasive Medical Procedures

Catron *et al* (1991) used HBO to treat two patients with cerebral air embolism resulting from invasive medical procedures. Both patients recovered without any evidence of damage on clinical examination and MRI.

Cerebral Air Embolism During Obstetrical Procedures

Two cases of cerebral air embolism occurring during cesarian section were treated successfully with the use of HBO (Sadan *et al* 1991; Davis *et al* 1990). Air embolism manifested by cortical blindness was reported in a patient following induced abortion by means of intra-amniotic hypertonic saline instillation and the patient made a complete recovery after treatment with HBO (Weissman *et al* 1989). Venous air embolism is likely during cesarian section as air enters uterine sinuses, particularly if the placenta separates before delivery as in the case of placenta previa (Davis *et al* 1990).

Cerebral Air Embolism Due to Orogenital Sex During Pregnancy

Twelve cases of this type have been reported in the literature; only one of them survived. Two cases have been treated successfully using HBO (Bray *et al* 1983; Bernhardt *et al* 1988).

Cerebral Embolism Due to Hydrogen Peroxide Poisoning

Hydrogen peroxide can produce acute gas embolism. There is a case report of an adult who suffered an apparent stroke shortly after an accidental ingestion of concentrated hydrogen peroxide (Mullins & Belltran 1998). Complete neuro-

logic recovery occurred quickly following HBO treatment. In another case report, a patient developed cerebral air embolism a short time after ingestion of a small amount of hydrogen peroxide manifested by hematemesis, left sided hemiplegia, confusion, and left homonymous hemianopsia. Initial laboratory studies, chest x-ray, and brain CT were normal. MRI demonstrated areas of ischemia and 18 h hours after arrival, the patient underwent HBO treatment with complete resolution of symptoms (Rider *et al* 2008). Of the seven reported cases of air embolism from hydrogen peroxide that did not undergo HBO, only in one patient was there a report of symptom resolution. HBO can be considered as the definitive treatment for gas embolism from hydrogen peroxide ingestion as with all other causes of acute gas embolism.

Pediatric Air Embolism

Van Rynen *et al* (1987) reported successful treatment of cerebral air embolism in a 3-month-old infant who had undergone a palliative closed heart operation. The treatment was conducted in a Reneau monoplace chamber using initial recompression to 6 ATA. The infant made a good recovery.

Relapse Following Spontaneous Recovery

In cases of spontaneous redistribution of air bubbles, a period of apparent recovery is frequently followed by relapse. The etiology of relapse appears to be multifactorial and is chiefly the consequence of a failure of reperfusion. Prediction of who will relapse is not possible, and any such relapse carries poor prognosis. It is advisable, therefore, that air embolism patients who undergo spontaneous recovery be promptly recompressed while breathing oxygen (Clark *et al* 2002). Therapeutic compression serves to antagonize leukocyte-mediated ischemia-reperfusion injury; to limit potential re-embolization of brain blood flow, secondary to further leakage from the original pulmonary lesion or recirculation of gas from the initial occlusive event; to protect against embolic injury to other organs; to aid in the resolution of component cerebral edema; to reduce the likelihood of late brain infarction reported in patients who have undergone spontaneous clinical recovery; and to prevent decompression sickness in high gas loading dives that precede accelerated ascents and omitted stage decompression.

Delayed Treatment

Air embolism should be treated as quickly as possible after it is detected. This is not always possible and several cases receive delayed treatment. HBO treatments have led to recovery in cases of air embolism with severe neurological deficit where treatment was delayed for 24 h. In a subgroup of 5 patients with air embolism secondary to cardiopulmonary bypass accidents, pulmonary barotrauma induced by mechanical ventilation and central vein catheterization, significant recovery was noted even when treatment was started 15 to 60 h after the event (Bitterman & Melamud 1993). Full recovery was reported in a case of hemodialysis associated venous air embolism, where HBO treatment was commenced 21 h after the event when the patient already appeared to be decerebrate (Dunbar et al 1990).

Conclusions

Hyperbaric treatment has been proven to be unquestionably indicated for the treatment of air embolism with neurological deficits. The conventional methods of treatment, such as posturing the patient in certain ways, aspirating the air, providing normobaric oxygen, closed chest massage, and steroids, have not been adequate to manage this problem. The consensus concerning the pressure favors the retention of 6 ATA initial compression with air. If the patient's condition does not permit exposure to this high pressure or the chamber immediately available cannot provide this pressure, 100% oxygen at 2.8 ATA would be acceptable as an alternative, particularly when only a monoplace chamber is available. The diagnosis of air embolism cannot always be made with certainty. There is need to improve technologies for early detection of air bubbles. It is acceptable to treat the patient with compression if air embolism is suspected, and the response to compression may be diagnostic in such cases. Early treatment provides better results than late treatment but HBO treatment should be considered at any stage the patient presents.

Considering that air embolism is a complication of medical and surgical procedures, it stands to reason that hyperbaric chambers should be available at clinics that perform such procedures. Open heart surgery, certainly, should not be done in a hospital that does not have a hyperbaric chamber.

12 Carbon Monoxide and Other Tissue Poisons

K.K. Jain

Hyperbaric oxygenation is a recognized treatment for carbon monoxide (CO) poisoning and has a supplemental role in the treatment of some other tissue poisons. Important sections in this chapter are:

Classification of Tissue Poisons

This chapter deals mainly with the role of hyperbaric oxygenation in the treatment of carbon monoxide (CO) poisoning; several other tissue poisons that have been treated with HBO are also discussed. Classification of these poisons by their mode of action is shown in Table 12.1.

Table 12.1
Classification of Tissue Poisons Where HBO Has Been Used Successfully
1. Action by combination with cytochrome α_3 oxidase and P-450
– Carbon monoxide
– Hydrogen sulfide
2. Hepatotoxic free radical formation mediated by P-450
– Carbon tetrachloride
3. Drug-induced methemoglobinemias
– Nitrites
– Nitrobenzene

Carbon Monoxide Poisoning

Historical Aspects of CO Poisoning

Human beings have been exposed to CO ever since they have made fire inside sheltered caves. In 300 BC, Aristotle stated that "coal fumes lead to heavy head and death." Obviously, this was a reference to CO poisoning. Claude Bernard showed in 1857 that CO produces hypoxia by reversible combination with hemoglobin (Bernard 1857); and in 1865, Klebs described clinical and pathologic findings in rats exposed to CO (Klebs 1865). The classical bilateral lesions of the globus pallidus and diffuse subcortical demyelination were described and correlated with psychic akinesia by Pineas (1924), and with parkinsonism by Grinker (1925).

In 1895, Haldane showed that rats survived CO poisoning when placed in oxygen at a pressure of 2 atmospheres (Haldane 1895). The effectiveness of hyperbaric oxygen in experimental CO poisoning in dogs and guinea pigs was demonstrated in 1942 (End & Long 1942). In 1960, hyperbaric oxygen was first used successfully in treating human cases of CO poisoning (Smith & Sharp 1960).

Biochemical and Physical Aspects of CO

This subject has been dealt with in detail by Jain (1990), and it will be briefly reviewed here with more recent findings.

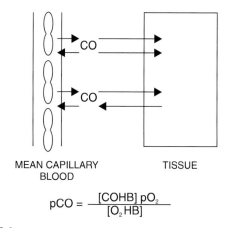

$$pCO = \frac{[COHB]\ pO_2}{[O_2HB]}$$

Figure 12.1
Mean tissue CO tension is equal to the mean CO tension in capillary blood. CO tension in mean capillary blood depends on the parameters listed in the Haldane equation depicted in this figure (after Coburn 1970).

CO Body Stores

Most of the body deposits of CO are found in the blood chemically bound to Hb. However, 10 to 15% of the total body content of CO is located in extracellular space, probably in combination with myoglobin (Mb).

The combination of Hb with CO is governed by Haldane's law. Accordingly, when a solution containing Hb is saturated with a gas mixture containing oxygen and CO_2, the relative proportions of the Hb that combine with the two gases are proportional to the relative partial pressures of the two gases (Figure 12.1), allowing for the fact that the affinity of the CO for Hb is 240 times greater than that of O_2. This is expressed by the equation:

$$\frac{COHb}{O_2Hb} = K \times \frac{pC=_2}{pO_2}$$

where K is 240.

The rate of formation of COMb can also be expressed by the Haldane equation, except that the estimated value of the constant K is then 40. Apparently Mb is involved in the oxygen transport mechanism and is ready to deliver oxygen when needed. Examination of O_2Hb and O_2Mb dissociation curves reveals that, at pO_2 less than 60 mmHg, O_2 has greater affinity for Mb than for Hb.

Biochemical Effects of CO on Living Organisms

Carbon monoxide inhibits oxygen transport, availability, and utilization; its biochemical effects are summarized in Table 12.2. CO lowers the oxygen saturation in direct proportion to the COHb concentration, thus blocking oxygen transport from the lungs to the tissues. The binding of one or more CO molecules to Hb also induces an allosteric modification in the remaining heme group, distorting the oxygen dissociation curve and shifting it to the left. Tissue

Table 12.2
Biochemical Effects of Carbon Monoxide

1. Effects on the blood
   - Increase of the carboxyhemoglobin level
   - Shift to the left of the oxygen dissociation curve
   - Rise of the lactate level
2. Action at the cellular level
   - Inhibition of cytochrome α_3 oxidase P-450

influenced by 2,3-DPG, which is located inside the red blood cells (RBC). When 2,3-DPG levels rise, for example, in anaerobic glycolysis, hypoxia, anemia, and at high altitudes, affinity of the oxygen for Hb is reduced.

Inhibition of the Utilization of Oxygen by CO

Until recently it was believed that the sole effect of CO was to produce COHb, which blocks oxygen transfer to the cells. Warburg had already demonstrated in 1926 that CO competes with oxygen for the reduced form of cytochrome a3 oxidase, which is the terminal enzyme of the cellular respiratory chain. The possibility that CO is directly cytotoxic is borne out by in vitro demonstration of CO interactions with non-Hb hemoproteins. Reduced cytochrome a3 (cytochrome c oxidase) and cytochrome P-450 bind sufficient CO to inhibit their function in vitro. The possibility that CO inhibits mitochondrial electron transport in vivo is interesting because of the close relationship between the respiratory chain function and the cellular energy metabolism (Figure 12.2). These basic mechanisms have been

anoxia is thus far greater than would result from the loss of oxygen-carrying capacity alone. A concentration of 0.06% of CO in the air is enough to block one-half of the Hb available for oxygen transport. The manner of CO combination with Hb differs appreciably from that of oxygen at high levels of CO saturation, but is virtually the same at low levels of CO saturation.

Important factors that influence the accumulation of COHb are pH, pCO₂, temperature, and 2,3-DPG (diphosphoglycerate). The affinity of oxygen for the Hb is strongly

Mitochondrial Respiratory Chain

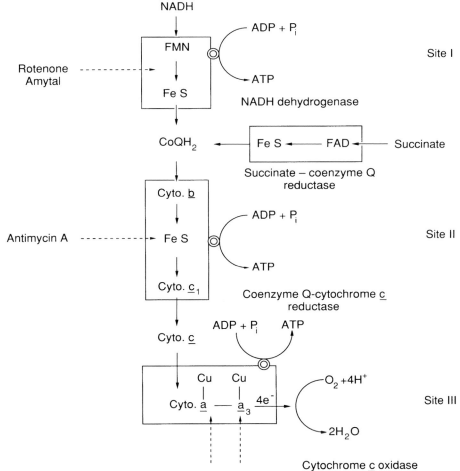

Figure 12.2
The mitochondrial respiratory chain indicating sequence of electron transport, three sites of energy coupling (oxidative phosphorylation), and location of action of CO (Piantadosi 1987).

confirmed by Chance *et al* (1970). CO combines with cytochrome a3 oxidase, and cytochrome P-450, thus blocking cellular oxidation and causing cellular hypoxia. Organs with high metabolic rate, such as the heart and brain, are particularly affected by CO. Cytochrome prefers oxygen to CO by a factor of 9:1, and this may explain the disparity between COHb levels and the clinical effects. This also explains the beneficial effect of HBO therapy. CO alters brain metabolism in vivo independently of the COHb-related decreases in oxygen delivery.

In conclusion, it can be stated that CO poisoning is highly complex, and a great deal more is involved than simple production of COHb. Formation of carboxycytochrome oxidase has been postulated to act as a toxin by blocking cellular use of oxygen. The half-life of CO bound with cytochrome a3 oxidase is not known. More research is needed to determine this value, as it may be an important factor in the genesis of late sequelae of CO poisoning, and it may also provide a rational basis for determining the duration of treatment by oxygen therapy.

Epidemiology

CO is the leading cause of death by poisoning in the United States. More than 4000 persons die annually from CO poisoning and 10,000 receive emergency treatment for exposure to CO fumes. In addition to this, CO accounts for more than half of the approximately 12,000 annual fire-associated deaths. In Korea, the incidence of CO poisoning in households using charcoal briquettes for heating and cooking was 5.4% to 8.4% as shown in a survey of four major cities (Cho *et al* 1986). There are no figures available for a much larger number of sufferers from occult CO poisoning.

Table 12.3
Causes of CO Poisoning

1. Endogenous
Hemolytic anemias (rise of COHb to 4%–6%)

2. Exogenous
A. Natural environments
   – Microbial activity in plant life
B. Artificial
   – Automobile exhaust
   – Defective domestic appliances for heating and cooking
   – Industrial plant exhausts
   – Mining accidents
   – Fires
C. Indirect
   – Poisoning by methylene chloride (paint-stripping solvent) due to its conversion to CO *in vivo*
D. Cigarette smoking
   – Active smoking
   – Passive smoking

Causes of CO Poisoning

CO is present universally, but clinically manifest poisoning occurs only when critical levels are exceeded. Various causes for this are listed in Table 12.3. Endogenous CO is unimportant because the values seldom exceed 3% COHb. The most important sources of CO poisoning are exogenous.

Sources of CO Poisoning

The commonest source of CO poisoning in industrialized urban areas of Western countries is automobile exhausts. They contain 6 to 10% CO and are responsible for 90% of the CO content of the atmosphere of a city. Frequently such fatal poisoning occurs in a closed garage with the car engine running, a common method of suicide. There are approximately 2300 such suicides annually in the USA.

At busy city intersections, CO concentrations as high as 0.03% have been measured. A pedestrian on a street with heavy automobile traffic is exposed to CO. A concentration of 20 to 40 mg/ml can raise COHb 1.5- to 2-fold within 1 h. Jogging in this environment increases the CO intake and further raises the COHb. Persons doing manual work on streets with heavy automobile traffic can suffer a rise of COHb to toxic levels. Jogging in Central Park in New York City can be more dangerous than walking or just standing around. Smoking in such environments further aggravates CO intoxication and COHb levels of 13% can be reached.

After the garage, the kitchen is the most dangerous place and a frequent site of CO poisoning. Cooking gas usually contains 4 to 14% CO. If not burned properly (as in a defective oven or stove), CO can leak into the room. Other sources of danger in the house are space-heating systems, such as a gas boiler. In Korea, household appliances are the commonest source of CO poisoning, open wood or coal-burning furnaces being the most frequent culprits.

Even though natural gas has been substituted for coal gas, 1000 persons still die annually in England and Wales as a result of CO poisoning from this source. Although natural gas burns more efficiently and cleanly than other forms of fuel, it is also the most potentially lethal if combustion is incomplete and is responsible for most of the deaths from domestic CO poisoning in the US. Incomplete combustion of other fuels such as charcoal and wood can also release CO, which can be trapped inside the building if the chimney is clogged. CO poisoning is more likely to occur in houses that are insulated and airtight to conserve energy.

Exhausts of many industrial plants, mills, and workshops contain CO. Risks are particularly high in blast furnaces and coal mines. Explosives can emit as much as 60% CO. Smoke contains CO, and smoke inhalation injury is usually associated with CO intoxication. Wood and paper fires contain 12% CO. Firefighters are particularly at risk from CO poisoning. COHb levels of 50% have been found in those dying within 12 h of receiving burns, implicating CO as the main culprit.

Pathophysiology of CO Poisoning

CO binding to myoglobin. It has been known for decades that death from CO poisoning is caused by hypoxia resulting from displacement of oxygen from the Hb. The mechanism of this, however, is not straightforward. Oxygen is stored in myoglobin and this is made possible by the crooked angle at which oxygen binds to the protein. CO, which prefers to sit upright, competes with for space with oxygen in this molecular shuttle. When myoglobin's structures forces CO to lie on its side, it is excluded. This classical view has been challenged by the work of Lim *et al* (1995) with spectroscopic techniques which provides evidence that a nearly perpendicular CO fits comfortably in myoglobin and that forced bending has little to do with CO exclusion. The reason is more likely that the unbound CO is pinned on its side near the binding site and little binding takes place.

Both CO and oxygen bind to an iron atom in the middle of the ring-shaped portion of myoglobin known as the heme group. Heme when isolated in experiments, binds to CO 10,000 times as strongly as it does to oxygen but when embedded in myoglobin, it binds only 20–30 times as strongly as oxygen. This led the authors to conclude that protein must be doing something to suppress CO relative to oxygen.

CO-induced hypoxia. Although the toxic effect of CO is postulated to be at the cellular level, by formation of carboxycytochrome oxidase, CO poisoning is primarily a hypoxic lesion caused by the replacement of OHb by COHb. These authors compared the effect in dogs of anoxia induced by 0.5% CO ventilation with that induced by breathing low oxygen mixtures. They found no significant differences in oxygen consumption or oxygen extraction in the two sets of animals who were subjected to equal reduction of arterial OHb, although the mode of desaturation was CO poisoning in one group.

The term CO-hypoxia implies that there is inhibition of oxygen transport from the blood to the tissues. Tissue oxygen tension may be decreased directly through a reduction in oxygen content by a lowered arterial oxygen tension, as well as through the presence of COHb. The oxygen dissociation curve is shifted to the left. The clinical effects of CO are usually attributed to tissue hypoxia, but they do not always correlate with COHb levels. Because CO combines with extravascular proteins such as myoglobin, its combination with cytochrome C-oxidase and cytochrome P-450 has been considered possibly to cause cellular hypoxia by inhibiting the mitochondrial respiratory chain.

Effects of CO on Various Systems of the Body

CO involves most parts of the body, but the areas most affected are those with high blood flow and high oxygen

---

Table 12.4
Effect of CO on Various Systems of the Body

Cardiovascular system
- Precipitation of myocardial ischemia in patients with angina
- ECG abnormalities
- Cardiomyopathy as an acute effect and cardiomegaly as a chronic effect
- Hypertension and atherosclerosis as chronic effects

Elements of the blood and hemorrheology
- Increased platelet aggregation
- Lower RBC deformability
- Increased plasma viscosity and hematocrit
- Erythrocytosis as a chronic effect

Nervous system
- Brain: cerebral edema, focal necrosis
- Peripheral nerves: neuropathy and delayed motor conduction velocity

Special senses
- Visual system: retinopathy and visual impairment
- Auditory system: hearing loss due to hypoxia of the cochlear nerve

Lungs
- Pulmonary edema

Muscles
- Myonecrosis, compartment syndrome

Exercise physiology
- Decrease of physical work capacity and $V_{2\,max}$

Liver
- Impaired function due to inhibition of cytochrome P-450

Kidneys
- Impairment of renal function, renal shutdown

Endocrines
- Impairment of hypophysis, hypothalamus and suprarenals

Bone and joints
- Degenerative changes, hypertrophy of bone marrow

Skin
- Erythema and blisters

Reproductive system
- Impaired menstruation and fertility in women
- Impotence in men
- Fetal toxicity with low conceptus weight and growth retardation

---

requirement, such as the brain and the heart. The effects of CO on various systems are shown in Table 12.4.

Acute Effects on the Heart

The heart is particularly vulnerable to CO poisoning, because CO binds to cardiac muscle three times as much as to skeletal muscle. Studies on isolated animal hearts have shown that CO may have a direct toxic effect on the heart regardless of the formation of COHb. At levels of 1 to 4% COHb, myocardial blood flow is higher, but no adverse effects are demonstrated. If the perfusion medium of an isolated rat heart muscle is gassed with 10% CO, there is a 40% increase in coronary blood flow, which is likely to be due

Table 12.5
ECG Abnormalities Due to CO Poisoning

1. Arrhythmias, extrasystoles, atrial fibrillation
2. Low voltage
3. Depression of S-T segment
4. Prolongation of ventricular complex, particularly the Q-T interval
5. Conduction defects
   – Increased P-R interval
   – A-V block
   – Branch bundle block

to vasodilatation secondary to anoxia. Increase in myocardial blood flow occurs mostly without an increase in COHb levels.

Angina patients are particularly susceptible to CO exposure. The onset of angina during physical exertion can be accelerated by elevating COHb levels to the 5 to 9% range. CO precipitates ischemia by reducing oxygen delivery to the myocardium. Changes in ECG have been shown to occur in workers chronically exposed to CO when COHb levels reach 20 to 30%. These changes are reversible after withdrawal from exposure to CO. Various abnormalities in the ECG reported in CO poisoning are summarized in Table 12.5. Depression of the S-T segment is the most common ECG finding in these cases and may precede myocardial infarction resulting from exposure to CO. Conduction abnormalities may be the result of anoxia or a direct toxic effect of CO on hemorrhages into the conducting system of the heart. Abnormalities of the motion of the left ventricular wall, as shown by echocardiography, are frequently seen in CO poisoning, and these correlate with a high incidence of papillary muscle lesions in fatal cases.

Hemorrheological Effects of CO

Viscosity of the whole blood as well as of the plasma increases after inhalation of 400 ppm of CO. An increase in COHb levels also decreases the deformability of erythrocytes, thus impairing the microcirculation.

Effect of CO on Blood Lactate

Levels of COHb over 5% have been shown to raise blood lactate levels. This is presumed to be an effect of hypoxia. Severity of CO poisoning depends on the duration of exposure rather than on COHb levels alone. Severe poisoning associated with long exposure is accompanied by high blood lactate and pyruvate levels.

Effect of CO on the Lungs

Pulmonary edema is present in 36% of patients with CO poisoning and is considered to be caused by hypoxia. X-rays of the lungs show a characteristic ground-glass ap-

pearance. Perihaler haze and intraalveolar edema may also be present. Vomiting in an unconscious patient may lead to aspiration pneumonia.

Exercise Capacity

Endurance and $VO_{2\,max}$ decrease as the COHb levels rise. Fatigue and reduced exercise capacity may also be caused by the accumulation of lactate resulting from exposure to CO. Lactate levels over 4 mmol hinder physical training.

Sleep

Sleep is severely disturbed by CO, without a detectable effect on the respiratory frequency and pulmonary ventilation. The aortic body receptors mediating circulatory reflexes are more sensitive to CO than the carotid body receptors mediating respiratory reflexes. Disruption of sleep could result from afferent discharges from aortic receptors in response to CO or low oxygen content. Anoxia is known to abolish REM sleep.

Effect on Pregnancy

Studies of the effects of CO inhalation on the conceptus weight in gravid rats leads to the following conclusions:

- Continuous CO inhalation lowered the conceptus weight on days 14 and 20 of pregnancy.
- The effect was more pronounced in the group exposed to cigarette smoke (CO plus nicotine) than the group exposed to CO alone.
- CO affects the fetus more adversely during the last trimester of pregnancy, which is the phase of rapid growth.

Experimental studies in neonatal animals have shown that acute exposure to CO can alter neurotransmitter function in the brain and that some of the effects persist for several weeks. Exposure of neonatal rats to CO has also been shown to produce hyperactivity that persisted for up to 3 months of age.

Musculoskeletal System

Compartment syndromes of the lower extremities may be caused by necrosis and swelling of the muscles.

Skin

Cutaneous blisters occur in CO poisoning. It seems possible that necrobiosis in eccrine glands starts early, but that the epidermal basal cells, notably at the papillary apices, suffer the same change only after temporary pressure anoxia and reactive hyperemia.

Gastrointestinal System

Extensive bowel ischemia with infarction has been reported in a patient who died following CO poisoning (Balzan *et al* 1993).

Effects on the Peripheral Nervous System

Peripheral neuropathy can be caused by CO poisoning. Possible causes include anoxia, the toxic effect of CO on the nerves, and positional compression of the nerves during the comatose stage.

Effects on the Visual System

Measurable decreases in sensitivity to light and adaptation to darkness have been shown to result from low levels of CO exposure. These alterations persist even after elimination of COHb from the blood, indicating that a significant amount of CO may be retained in the tissues. Retinal hemorrhages have been observed on ophthalmoscopy of patients with acute CO poisoning. Retinal venous engorgement and peripupillary hemorrhages resemble those seen in hypoxia. CO retinopathy has been recorded as an acute effect of CO poisoning leading to visual impairment.

Effect on the Auditory System

Hearing loss of a central type caused by anoxia from CO poisoning is only partially reversible. The loss of auditory threshold activity is pronounced at the level of the auditory cortex; the relative vulnerability of the central auditory pathway has been demonstrated. Vestibular function is more frequently involved than the auditory function. Recovery from hearing loss is uncommon; this is the result of hypoxia of the cochlear nerve and the brain stem nuclei.

Effect on the Central Nervous System

The most important lesions of CO poisoning are in the central nervous system (CNS). This subject has been discussed in detail elsewhere (Jain 2003c).

Neuropathology. Of the cells of the CNS, the astrocytes are more sensitive than neurons to the effects of CO. The critical lesions in CO poisoning are in the brain. There are three stages in the evolution of the brain lesions:

- In immediate death after CO poisoning, there are petechial hemorrhages throughout the brain, but no cerebral edema
- In patients who die within hours or days after poisoning, cerebral edema is present. There is necrosis of the globus pallidus and substantia nigra.
- In patients who die days or weeks later from delayed sequelae of CO poisoning, edema has usually disappeared.

Degenerative and demyelinative changes are usually seen.

Necrosis of the globus pallidus in a patient is revealed by CT scan as a low-density area. The corpus callosum, hippocampus, and substantia nigra may also be affected. In the late stages, there is cerebral atrophy, which is also demonstrated by CT scan; this usually correlates with poor neurological recovery. White matter damage is considered to be significant in the pathogenesis of parkinsonism in patients with carbon monoxide poisoning (Sohn *et al* 2000).

Pathophysiology. The tendency for effects on certain areas of the brain such as the globus pallidus and substantia nigra has been considered to be caused by a hypoxic effect of CO. Clinical instances of "pure hypoxia" are rare, and many investigators consider CO intoxication to represent cerebral hypoxia aggravated by relative ischemia, as the lesions are similar to those induced by other forms of hypoxia and/or ischemia. Putnam *et al* (1931) showed that CO damages the blood-brain barrier, particularly in the cerebral white matter, where the venous drainage pattern predisposes to focal edema. This may lead to hypoxia and set up the cycle of hypoxia-edema-hypoxia. Delayed neurological deterioration can occur following anoxia from other causes and can explain similar deterioration after CO poisoning, in the absence of elevated levels of COHb

The mechanism of delayed neurological toxicity is based on several reactions triggered by increased calcium concentrations in the cell, which persist long enough to produce alterations in cell function and delayed neurological damage. White matter demyelination is believed to be responsible for delayed neuropsychiatric syndrome.

Harmful effects of an acute nonlethal CO exposure do not cease with a decrease in COHb concentration. The decreased cytochrome oxidase activity may later on be mediated by a loss of mitochondria because of lipid peroxidation, rather than by specific inhibitory effects of CO. A similar mechanism would explain the acid proteinase activity in the glial cell fraction within 24 h of reoxygenation.

CO may alter the oxidative metabolism of the brain independently of a COHb-related decrease in oxygen delivery. Binding of CO to cytochrome oxidase in rat brain cortex has been observed by reflectance spectroscopy, and this is a possible explanation of a non-hypoxic mechanism of CO toxicity (Brown & Piantadosi 1990). Zhang and Piantadosi (1992) have studied the generation of partially reduced oxygen species (PROS) in the brains of rats subjected to 1% CO for 30 min and then reoxygenated on air for 0 to 180 min. They propose that PROS generated in the brain after CO hypoxia originate primarily from mitochondria and contribute to CO-mediated neuronal damage during reoxygenation after severe CO intoxication. CO-mediated brain injury is a type of postischemic reperfusion phenomenon and xanthine-oxidase-derived reactive oxygen species are responsible for lipid peroxidation (Thom 1992). These observations may provide an explanation for a number of poorly understood clinical observations regarding CO poisoning, particularly the neuropsychological effects at concentrations below 5%. Nabeshima *et al* (1991) have shown that delayed amnesia induced by CO exposure in mice may result from delayed neuronal death in the hippocampal CA1 subfield and dysfunction of the acetylcholinergic neurons in the frontal cortex, the striatum, and/or the hippocampus. In studies on mice it has been shown that N-methyl-D-aspartate (NMDA) receptor/ion channel complex is involved in the mechanism of CO-induced neurodegeneration, and that glycine binding site antagonists and NMDA-antagonists may have neuroprotective properties.

In spite of various explanations that have been offered, nothing is known with certainty about the pathomechanism of CO poisoning. A recent finding that CO may act as a putative neural messenger by interacting with the enzyme guanylyl cyclase (Verma *et al* 1993), may provide an important clue to the pathomechanism of CO toxicity. Endogenously formed carbon monoxide arises from the enzymatic degradation of heme oxygenase to release a molecule of CO, which acts as a neuromodulator. In addition to its physiological role, CO that arises subsequent to the appearance of heme oxygenase-1 may underlie various pathological states (Johnson & Johnson 2000).

Relative cerebral hyperperfusion has been observed during CO-hypoxia and is considered to be due to a fall in the P_{50} (PO_2 at 50% saturation of non-CO bound sites on hemoglobin) rather than a direct tissue effect of CO. Cerebral blood flow has been shown to increase more than two-fold in anesthetized rabbits exposed to 1% CO, despite a 28% fall of mean arterial blood pressure (Meyer-Witting *et al* 1991). In the presence of tissue hypoxia with undiminished plasma PO_2, the brain vasculature allows greater flow of blood while the microvasculature adjusts to reduce the diffusion distance for O_2 (Sinha *et al* 1991).

Clinical Features of CO Poisoning

Signs and symptoms of CO poisoning are nonspecific and involve most of the body systems. They vary according to the COHb levels, as shown in Table 12.6. The clinical signs and symptoms depend on both the dose of CO and the duration of exposure. COHb levels do not necessarily correlate with the severity of clinical effects.

Neuropsychological Sequelae of CO Poisoning

The neurological sequelae of CO poisoning as reported in the literature are summarized in Table 12.7. There is some disparity in the results of the studies summarized here. However, psychological impairment can be detected at COHb levels between 2.5 and 5% by appropriate tests.

Table 12.6
Degree of Severity of CO Poisoning, COHb Levels, and Clinical Features

Severity	COHb level	Clinical features
Occult	> 5%	No apparent symptoms Psychological deficits on testing
	5%–10%	Decreased exercise tolerance in patients with chronic obstructive pulmonary disease Decreased threshold for angina and claudication in patients with atherosclerosis Increased threshold for visual stimuli
Mild	10%–20%	Dyspnea on vigorous exertion Headaches, dizziness Impairment of higher cerebral function Decreased visual acuity
Moderate	20%–30%	Severe headache, irritability, impaired judgment Visual disturbances, nausea, dizziness, increased respiratory rate
	30%–40%	Cardiac disturbances, muscle weakness Vomiting, reduced awareness
Severe	40%–50%	Fainting on exertion Mental confusion
	50%–60%	Collapse convulsions Paralysis
Very severe	60%–70%	Coma, frequently fatal within a few minutes
	Over 70%	Immediately fatal Respiratory and cardiac arrest

Higher levels of COHb during acute exposure may lead to impairment of consciousness, coma, and convulsions. Most of the neurological manifestations of CO poisoning are late sequelae (listed in Table 12.8); these late sequelae are also referred to as "secondary syndromes." The complications may develop a few days to 3 weeks after exposure to CO, and as late as 2 years after apparently complete recovery from acute CO poisoning. Neuropsychiatric symptoms are prominent in the late sequelae. The incidence of secondary syndromes varies from 10 to 40%. Patients poisoned by CO and treated by oxygen still developed late sequelae but such sequelae are rare in patients treated by HBO therapy.

Choi (1983) reported that of 2360 victims of CO poisoning, delayed neurological sequelae were diagnosed in 11.8% of those admitted to hospital and 2.75% of the total group. The lucid interval before appearance of neurological symptoms was 2 to 40 days (mean, 22.4 days). The most frequent symptoms were mental deterioration, urinary incontinence, gait disturbance, and mutism. The most frequent signs were masked face, glabellar sign, grasp reflex, increased muscle tone, short-step gait, and retropulsion. Most of these signs indicate parkinsonism. There were no

Table 12.7
Neuropsychological Sequelae of CO Poisoning

Authors and year	Subjects	COHb level or CO/ppm	Effects
Lilienthal and Fugitt (1946)	Humans	5%–10% COHb	Impairment in the FFT test
Trouton and Eysenck (1961)	Humans	5%–10% COHb	Impairment of the precision of control Multiple limb incoordination
Schulte (1963)	Humans	2%-5% COHb	Decrease in cognition and psychomotor ability Increase in the number of errors and the completion time in arithmetic tests, t-crossing test, and visual discrimination tests
Beard and Wertheim (1967)	Humans	90 min at 50 ppm shorter time at 250 ppm (= COHb of 4%–5%)	Impaired ability to discriminate short
	Rats	100 ppm for 11 min	Disruption of ability to judge time (assessed by differential reinforcement at a low rate of response
Mikulka et al (1973)	Humans	125–250 ppm briefly (COHb 6.6%)	No effect on time estimation No disruption of tracking
Gliner et al (1983)	Humans	100 ppm for 2.5 h Controls (room air)	Decreased arousal and interest with fatigue resulting in decrease in performance
Schrot et al (1984)	Rats	500 ppm – 90 min (40% COHb) 850 ppm – 90 min (50% COHb) 1200 ppm – 90 min (60% COHb)	Disruption of the rate at which the rats acquired a chain of response
Schaad et al (1983)	Humans	COHb 20%	No impairment on a tracking simulator device
Yastrebov et al (1987)	Humans	900 ± 20 mg/m^3 for 10 min (COHb of 10% – +0.5%)	Impairment in a two-dimensional compensatory tracking task combined with mental arithmetic. Symptoms of mild CO intoxication at COHb levels of 10%

Table 12.8
Delayed Neuropsychological Sequelae of CO Poisoning

- Akinetic mutism
- Apallic syndrome
- Apraxia, ideomotor as well as constructional
- Ataxia
- Convulsive disorders
- Cortical blindness
- Deafness (neural)
- Delerium
- Dementia
- Depression
- Diminished IQ
- Dysgraphia
- Gilles de la Tourette syndrome
- Headaches
- Memory disturbances
- Movement disorders, parkinsonism, choreoathetosis
- Optic neuritis
- Peripheral neuropathy
- Personality change
- Psychoses
- Symptoms resembling those of multiple sclerosis
- Temporospatial disorientation
- Urinary incontinence
- Visual agnosia

important contributing factors except anoxia and age. Previous associated disease did not hasten the development of sequelae. Of the 36 patients followed for 2 years, 75% recovered within 1 year.

Clinical Diagnosis of CO Poisoning

Few symptoms of CO poisoning occur at COHb concentrations of less than 10%. The presence of symptoms and history of exposure to CO and the circumstances in which the patient is found should lead to strong suspicion of CO poisoning. Therapy may be started before the laboratory investigations are completed.

Pitfalls in the Clinical Diagnosis of CO Poisoning

The following points should be taken into consideration in making a diagnosis of CO poisoning:

1. Clinical signs and symptoms of CO poisoning do not always correspond to COHb levels.
2. The cherry red color of the skin and the lips, usually considered to be a classical sign, is not present when the COHb levels are below 40% and there is cyanosis caused by respiratory depression. In practice this sign is rarely seen.
3. Some of the symptoms are aggravated by preexisting disease, such as intermittent claudication.
4. Tachypnea is frequently absent, because the carotid body is presumably responsive to the oxygen partial pressures rather than the oxygen content.
5. Examples of frequent misdiagnosis of CO poisoning are: psychiatric illness, migraine headaches, stroke, acute alcohol intoxication or delirium tremens, heart disease, and food poisoning.

6. CO poisoning in infants is a frequently missed diagnosis. When unexplained neurological symptoms occur in an infant who has been a passenger in a car, COHb determinations should be made and CO poisoning should be considered in the differential diagnosis.

7. A bit of detective work may be required to locate the source of carbon monoxide poisoning. A simple tool based on the CH2OPD2 mnemonic (Community, Home, Hobbies, Occupation, Personal habits, Diet and Drugs) is helpful in obtaining an environmental exposure history (Abelsohn *et al* 2002).

Occult CO Poisoning

This is a syndrome of headache, fatigue, dizziness, paresthesias, chest pains, palpitation, and visual disturbances associated with chronic CO exposure. Headache and dizziness are early symptoms of CO poisoning and occur at COHb concentrations of 10% or more. Among patients taken to an emergency department during the winter heating season with complaints of headache or dizziness, 3 to 5% have COHb levels in excess of 10%. They are usually unaware of exposure to toxic levels of CO in their home prior to the visit to the emergency department.

In patients who present with ill-defined symptoms and no history of CO exposure, CO poisoning must be considered when two or more patients are similarly or simultaneously sick.

Laboratory Diagnosis of CO Poisoning

Various laboratory procedures that may be used in the diagnosis of CO poisoning are as follows:

1. Determination of CO in the blood
   Direct measurement of the COHb levels
   Measurement of CO released from the blood
   Measurement of CO content of the exhaled air
2. Arterial blood gases and lactic acid levels
3. Screening tests for drug intoxication and alcohol intoxication
4. Biochemistry
   Enzymes: creatine kinase, lactate dehydrogenase, SGOT, SGPT
   Serum glucose
5. Complete blood count
6. Electroencephalogram
7. Electrocardiogram
8. Brain imaging: CT scan, MRI, SPECT
9. Magnetic resonance spectroscopy
10. Neuropsychological testing

COHb measurement. This is the most commonly used investigation. Measurement is done spectrophotometrically,

offering an accurate and rapid determination of the patient's COHb levels. An instrument like the CIBA Corning 2500-CO oximeter determines various selected wavelengths from 520 to 640 nm, and the following hemoglobin derivatives are measured: oxyhemoglobin (O_2Hb), deoxyhemoglobin (HHb), carboxyhemoglobin (COHb), and methemoglobin (MetHb).

Determination of CO Released from the Blood. Several methods are available for releasing CO from samples of blood. CO is then measured by gas chromatography. The amount of CO in the blood sample is calculated from the ratio of the CO content to the full CO capacity of the same sample.

CO Measurement in Exhaled Air. This can be measured by gas chromatography. A bag can be used to collect exhaled air and CO is determined by a flame ionization detector after catalytic hydration with tomethane. The values are given as parts per million (ppm) in the range of 0 to 500.

Clinical Significance of Monitoring Blood COHb. Fang *et al* (1986) monitored COHb in 192 Patients with acute CO poisoning:

1. Blood COHb greater than 10% has diagnostic significance and, COHb greater than 30% should be considered serious.
2. Clinical manifestations should be primary and COHb secondary when judging the degree of CO poisoning.
3. Treatment should be continued even when COHb levels have returned to normal, if the clinical symptoms are still present.
4. COHb sampling need not be continued when the patient has been away from the toxic environment for more than 8 h.
5. Monitoring of COHb is useful in making a differential diagnosis and in the event of death, a definitive diagnosis.

Pitfalls in the Diagnosis of CO Poisoning from COHb Level Determinations. COHb levels may be normal when first obtained and not reflect the true insult. This is likely to happen when:

- There is delay in obtaining samples following cessation of exposure to CO.
- Oxygen is administered before blood samples are withdrawn.
- COHb is calculated from oxygen partial pressures using a sliderule nomogram. Arterial pO_2 may be normal in the presence of CO if the patient is not dyspneic. The calculated oxyhemoglobin saturation may be grossly wrong in this case.

Changes in Blood Chemistry. Increased levels of lactate, pyruvate, and glucose are influenced by the duration of exposure to CO, and are more pronounced after prolonged acute exposure than after a short exposure. Hyperglycemia may occur as a result of hormonal stress response.

Electroencephalographic Changes. Various EEG abnormalities noticed in CO poisoning are diffuse abnormalities (continuous theta or delta activity) and low voltage activity accompanied by intervals of spiking or silence, as well as rhythmic bursts of slow waves.

Topographic quantitative EEG methods may have promise in the study of acute and long-term effects of CO poisoning. Longitudinal and quantitative EEG recording after acute CO poisoning may show the following:

1. Elevated Absolute Power of all EEG frequencies with the most marked voltage increases occurring in the alpha-theta range.
2. Sharply defined regional increases in the absolute power of delta activity over the posterior temporal-parietal-occipital cortex bilaterally.
3. Increased relative power of the alpha wave that is most marked over the prefrontal cortex.
4. Decreased relative power of the alpha wave that is most marked over the prefrontal cortex.
5. Pronounced decreases in interhemispheric coherence for most frequency bands.

The multimodality evoked potentials have proved to be sensitive indicators in the evaluation of brain dysfunction and in the prognosis of acute CO poisoning and development of delayed encephalopathy. Pattern shift visual evoked potential (PSVEP) N75 and P100 latencies were evaluated as an objective, widely available and rapid test of brain dysfunction in a group of 11 patients in the acute phase (first 6 h) of mild-to-moderate CO poisoning (Emerson & Keilor 1998). N75 and P100 latency results were compared to nearly simultaneously obtained standard CO Neuropsychological Screening Battery (CONSB). Patients were sought in whom treatment decisions concerning HBO vs. normobaric oxygen (NBO) might be difficult, and were excluded from the study if confounding variables existed for CONSB or PSVEP. N75 and P100 latencies were also obtained after completion of NBO2 or HBO2 therapies. Only one patient, judged clinically to have the mildest poisoning in the series, had significantly abnormal initial PSVEP latencies. This patient's simultaneous CONSB was normal and the abnormal PSVEP latencies failed to normalize post treatment with NBO2. PSVEP latencies were not found to be a sensitive screening tool for treatment decision making in a group of acutely CO poisoned patients where treatment decisions might be difficult.

Neuropsychological Testing

It has long been known that CO poisoning has a spectrum of effects on cognitive functioning. Neuropsychological impairments in carbon monoxide-poisoned subjects include memory, intellectual, executive, and visuospatial defects (Rahmani *et al* 2006). Various psychological tests have been designed for patients with CO poisoning. One neuropsychological screening battery for use in assessment of such patients consists of 6 tests: general orientation, digit span, trail making, digit symbols, aphasia, and block design (Messier & Myers 1991). These tests can be administered in an emergency by a non-psychologist in 20 min. There is a strong correlation between abnormalities detected on psychometric testing and COHb levels. The former measures actual neurological disability and is a better index of severity of CO poisoning.

McNulty *et al* (1997) have investigated the effects of CO poisoning on short-term verbal memory, both rote and context aided. Impairment was measured before and after HBO treatment. Twenty-six patients who had been admitted for emergency treatment after exposure to significant CO poisoning were tested using a measure of short-term recall for word lists with no or varying degrees of internal context-aided structure. Impairment of context-aided memory (but not rote memory) has been previously reported to be associated with low relative frontal volume in psychiatric patients. Carbon monoxide poisoning was significantly associated with impairment of context-aided memory, with the degree of pretreatment impairment predicting the number HBO treatments judged to be necessary on the basis of clinical monitoring of the patient. In patients with poisoning of moderate severity, pretreatment performance in context-aided memory improved after the first HBO treatment. The memory measure used in this study appears to have considerable potential usefulness in the clinical assessment of the severity of CO poisoning in patients treated in an emergency setting.

Brain Imaging Studies

Various brain imaging studies have been found to be useful in assessing the brain involvement in CO poisoning, The are described in the following pages and a comparison of the value of various techniques is shown in Table 12.9

CT Scan. The CT scan is the most widely used neuroimaging method for patients with CO poisoning. Common CT findings are symmetrical low-density abnormalities of the basal ganglia and diffuse low-density lesions of the white matter. The globus pallidus lucencies may be unilateral and white matter involvement may show marked asymmetry. Post-contrast CT offers an advantage when non-contrast CT is normal in CO poisoning. Acute transient hydrocephalus has been observed in acute CO poisoning in one case and this resolved

Table 12.9
Comparative Value of Brain Imaging Studies in CO Poisoning

	CT	MRI	SPECT
Basal ganglia lesions	+	++	
White matter lesions	+	+++	
Both white and gray matter	+	++	+++
Cerebral edema	+	++	
Cerebral perfusion			+++
Predicting late sequelae	+	++	++
Assessing response to HBO	+	++	+++

6 weeks later (Prabhu *et al* 1993). In the interval form of CO poisoning, low-density lesions bilaterally in the frontal regions, centrum semiovale, and pallidum have been correlated with demyelination of white matter of the corresponding parts at autopsy. An initial normal CT scan in a comatose patient does not rule out CO poisoning. Serial CT scanning showed no low-density lesions of the frontal lobes and basal ganglia until three days after exposure to CO).

Magnetic Resonance Imaging (MRI). In patients with CO poisoning, MRI can demonstrate bilateral edematous lesions in the globus pallidus and it is considered to be a more sensitive examination than serial CT in acute CO poisoning. Although the severity of white matter lesions correlates with the prognosis in acute CO poisoning, it does not always correspond to the neurological outcome in the subacute stage.

MRI has been used less often in cases of delayed encephalopathy after CO poisoning. The main finding in such cases is a reversible demyelinating process of the cerebral white matter. Lesions of the anterior thalami, which may be missed on CT scan, can be demonstrated by MRI. A spectrum of MRI changes has been seen even years after relatively mild CO poisoning. Patients with severe CO intoxication may develop persistent cerebral changes independently of their neuropsychiatric findings in the chronic stage, which may present with characteristic MRI findings.

Positron Emission Tomography (PET). PET studies in acute CO poisoning show a severe decrease in rCBF, rOER, and rCMRO in the striatum and the thalamus, even in patients treated with HBO. These changes are temporary and the values return to normal in patients without clinical sequelae or only transient neurological disturbances. PET findings remain abnormal in patients with severe and permanent sequelae. In one case with persistent impaired responsiveness for one year after CO poisoning, PET showed a 20% decrease of rCBF and rCMRG in the frontal cortex, whereas MRI and CT scans had shown only lesions of basal ganglia (Shimosegawa *et al* 1992). Diffusion tensor MRI is a promising technique to characterize and track delayed encephalopathy after acute carbon monoxide poisoning (Villa *et al* 2005).

Most of the knowledge of MRI findings in carbon monoxide poisoning is based on case studies of patients in the subacute or chronic phase following exposure. MRI studies in the acute phase of carbon monoxide poisoning show that, although the globus pallidus is the commonest site of abnormality in the brain, the effects are widespread. The white matter hyperintensities seen on MRI do not correlate with carbon monoxide poisoning severity. In one study white matter hyperintensities occurred in both the periventricular and the centrum semiovale regions but only those in the centrum semiovale were significantly associated with cognitive impairments (Parkinson 2002).

Single Photon Emission Computed Tomography (SPECT). This can provide imaging of cerebral perfusion. Diffuse hypoperfusion has been shown in both the gray and the white matter of the cerebral cortex in CO poisoning. SPECT is helpful in documenting the increase in cerebral perfusion along with clinical improvement as a result of HBO treatment. Cerebral vascular changes may be the possible cause of hypoperfusion in patients with CO poisoning and there is a good correlation between the clinical outcome and the findings of SPECT. SPECT can be used for predicting and evaluating the outcome of delayed neurological sequelae after CO poisoning. SPECT performed on a patient 10 days after CO poisoning showed hypoperfusion which preceded the onset of neurological sequelae by 20 days (Choi & Lee 1993). In comparison to traditional brain imaging techniques, 99 mTc-HMPAO brain imaging with fanbeam SPECT in combination with surface 3-dimensional display is a better tool for early detection of regional cerebral anomalies in acute CO poisoning. HMPAO-SPECT has been used in the management of patients with acute and delayed neurological sequelae of CO poisoning and found to be helpful in identifying potentially recoverable brain tissue and the response to HBO (see Chapter 19). The case history and SPECT scans of one of the patients are reproduced in Chapter 19.

Magnetic Resonance Spectroscopy (MRS). MRS is a non-invasive method that provides information about brain metabolites such as N-acetyl aspartate, choline and creatine. MRS can reflect the severity of delayed sequeale of CO poisoning precisely. Increase in choline in the frontal lobes indicates progressive demyelination. Appearance of lactate and decrease in N-acetylaspartate reflect the point at which neuron injury becomes irreversible. These findings have been correlated with those of MRI and SPECT. It may be a useful method to determine neuron viability and prognosis in CO poisoning. The combination of proton MRS and diffusion tensor imaging is useful for monitoring the changes in brain damage and the clinical symptoms of patients with delayed encephalopathy after CO poisoning and response to HBO treatment (Terajima *et al* 2008).

Table 12.10
Guidelines for the Management of CO Poisoning

1. Remove patient from the site of exposure.
2. Immediately administer oxygen, if possible after taking a blood sample for COHb.
3. Endotracheal intubation in comatose patients to facilitate ventilation.
4. Removal of patient to HBO facility when indicated.
5. General supportive treatment: for cerebral edema, acid-base imbalance, etc.
6. Keep patient calm and avoid physical exertion by the patient.

Table 12.11
Half-life of COHb

	Pressure	Time
Air	1 ATA	5 h 20 min
100% oxygen	1 ATA	1 h 20 min
100% oxygen	3 ATA	23 min

General Management of CO Poisoning

General guidelines for the management of CO poisoning are shown in Table 12.10. Once the patient is removed from CO environments, CO slowly dissociates from the Hb and is eliminated. The half-life of the COHb is shown in Table 12.11. At atmospheric pressure in fresh air, the circulating half-life of CO is 5 h 20 min. This time decreases to 23 min with HBO at 3 ATA using 100% oxygen. These half-lives are not constant, as they depend on a number of variable factors. They are particularly inaccurate when COHb levels are high. The objectives of treatment in CO poisoning are as follows:

- To hasten elimination of CO
- To counteract hypoxia
- To counteract direct tissue toxicity.

A triage chart for handling patients with CO poisoning is shown in Figure 12.3. HBO therapy is the most important factor in treatment, but the following adjunctive measures should be considered:

- Treatment of cerebral edema. HBO therapy itself is effective against cerebral edema, but the use of steroids and mannitol may be helpful.
- Cellular protection. Mg^{2+} can be used; the usual dose is 20 to 30 mmol/day.
- Fluid and electrolyte balance should be carefully maintained and overhydration, which may aggravate cerebral edema and pulmonary complications, should be avoided. Acidosis should not be corrected pharmacologically,

Table 12.12
Experimental Studies on the Effect of HBO on Carbon Monoxide Poisoning

Authors and year	Experimental subjects	Mode of oxygen therapy	Results
End and Long (1942)	Dogs and guinea pigs	HBO 3 ATA, 100% oxygen	HBO more effective than normobaric oxygen in eliminating CO from the body
Pace *et al* (1950)	Human volunteers	HBO 2 ATA	Rate of diminution of CO accelerated
Ogawa *et al* (1974)	Dogs	HBO	Hemoconcentration (20% decrease of blood volume reversed by HBO
Koyama (1976)	Dogs	Half of the animals treated by conventional methods and the other half by HBO 2 ATA	COHb determination and biochemical studies showed that HBO was more effective than the conventional methods
Sasaki (1975)	Dogs	HBO	Acceleration of the half-clearance time of COHb. Proposed procedure for HBO therapy based on it: 1. For severe CO poisoning, HBO at 2.8 ATA for 20 min followed by 1.9 ATA for 57 min 2. For moderate CO poisoning, 2.8 ATA oxygen for 20 min followed by 1.9 ATA for 46 min 3. For light CO poisoning, 2.8 ATA oxygen for 20 min followed by 1.9 ATA for 30 min
Jiang and Tyssebotn (1997)	Rats with occluded left carotid artery	NBO in one group vs HBO in the other, Normoxic animals as controls.	1. Compared to the normoxic treatments, the HBO, but not the NBO, significantly reduced the mortality and the neurologic morbidity. 2. HBO was also significantly better than NBO in increasing surviving time and survival rate. 3. The results support the value of HBO in improving short-term outcome of acute CO poisoning in this rat model.

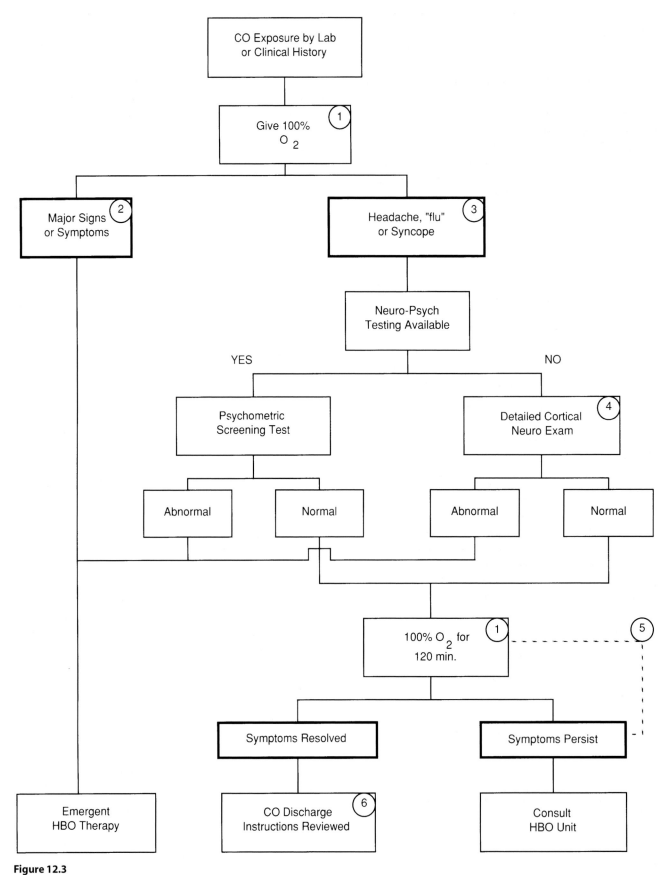

Figure 12.3
Carbon monoxide triage decision chart (Reproduced from Kindwall & Goldmann 1988, *Hyperbaric Medical Procedures*, Milwaukee, St. Luke's Hospital, by permission).

Notes for Figure 12.3 (see opposite)

1. O_2 should be delivered by tight-fitting system such as Scott mask, anesthesia mask, endotracheal tube, or CPAP mask.
2. Major signs and symptoms include: abnormal EKG, metabolic acidosis, lab or clinical findings of pregnancy, chest pain, confusion, disorientation, personality change, lethargy, or drug overdose with mental status change.
3. Headache may be severe and mimic intracranial hemorrhage in severity. Any suggestion of postsyncopal neurological dysfunction is a major sympton.
4. Detailed cortical neurological examination should include: general orientation, phone number, address, date of birth, serial 7s, digit span, forward and backward spelling of three and four-letter words, and short-term memory.
5. OPTION: One repeat 2 h O_2 cycle (4 h of surface O_2 total) is permissible. If symptoms persist beyond this point, con-sultation and possible referrals is indicated.
6. Follow-up of CO exposed patients is critical. Recurrent or indolent symptoms or family observation of abnormalities should be reevaluated as they appear.

as slight acidosis aids in the delivery of oxygen to the tissues by shifting the oxygen dissociation curve to the right. HBO usually limits the metabolic acidosis associated with CO poisoning.

- Management of cardiac arrhythmias. Cardiac arrhythmias are a common complication of CO poisoning. They may subside with reversal of tissue hypoxia but may require pharmacological management.

Rationale for Oxygen Therapy (Normobaric and Hyperbaric) for CO Poisoning

Hyperoxygenation enhances oxygen transfer into the anoxic tissues. At normal concentrations of tissue oxygen it should physically dilute the CO and possibly halt the movement of CO from Hb to Mb and cytochrome enzymes. Hyperoxygenation may be achieved by breathing 100% oxygen either at atmospheric pressure (normobaric) or under hyperbaric conditions. HBO is more effective. HBO accomplishes the following therapeutic goals in CO poisoning:

- Immediate saturation of plasma with enough oxygen to sustain life and to counteract tissue hypoxia in spite of high levels of COHb.
- It causes a rapid reduction of CO in the blood by mass action of O_2. In the equation $HbO_2 + CO = HbCO + O_2$, an increase in either oxygen or CO results in a comparable increase in the corresponding compound with hemoglobin.

- It assists in driving CO away from cytochrome oxidase and in restoration of function. The increase in oxygen tension in plasma and not simply an increase in dissolved oxygen is responsible for the efficacy of HBO.
- HBO reduces cerebral edema.
- Brain lipid peroxidation caused by CO is prevented by 100% oxygen at 3 ATA.
- HBO prevents immune-mediated delayed neurologic dysfunction following exposure (Thom *et al* 2006).

Experimental Evidence

The results of some experimental studies of the use of HBO in CO poisoning are shown in Table 12.12.

Clinical Use of HBO in CO Poisoning

Guidelines for the use of HBO versus normobaric oxygen are given in Table 12.13. Some open clinical studies of CO poisoning treated by HBO are shown in Table 12.14.

Hyperbaric oxygen, if available, should be used at COHb levels of 25% or above, but the clinical picture of the patient with a history of CO exposure is the deciding factor for the initiation of HBO therapy, and the COHb levels should be a secondary consideration. Because of the cost and limited availability of hyperbaric chambers, a decision regarding transfer of the patient to a hyperbaric facility is not always easy, particularly when the patient is critically ill. If possi-

Table 12.13
Hyperbaric Oxygen (HBO) versus Normobaric Oxygen

Hyperbaric facilities available	COHb > 25%	HBO
	COHb < 25%	HBO if symptoms, NBO if none
No hyperbaric facilities	COHb > 40%	Immediate referral to HBO center
	COHb < 40% no symptoms	NBO
	COHb < 40% with symptoms	Referral to HBO center

Table 12.14
Open Clinical Studies of HBO in CO Poisoning

Authors and year	No. of patients	Pressure	Results
Smith *et al* (1962)	22	2 ATA	All recovered
Sluitjer (1963)	40	3 ATA	Group I: conscious or drowsy. 21 patients. Excellent results. Group II: comatose with neurological abnormalities. 10 patients. Two died, 7 recovered fully and one had severe neurological sequelae. Group III: Attempted suicide with combination of CO and barbiturates. 9 patients. Cardiorespiratory depression mainly with little localizing neurological signs. All recovered completely.
Goulon *et al* (1969)	302	2 ATA	Mortality when treatment started before 6 h was 13.5%, and when after 6 h 30.1%
Heyndrickx *et al* (1970)	11	3 ATA	Clinical improvement more than in another 11 patients treated by NBO.
Kienlen *et al* (1974)	370	2–3 ATA	93.7% of the patients recovered.
Adamiec *et al* (1975)	44	2.5 ATA	80% showed good recovery
Yun and Cho (1983)	2242	?	98.2 recovered
Mathieu *et al* (1985)	203	?	Mortality 1.7%; Incidence of secondary syndromes, 4%: rest recovered.
Norkool & Kirkpatrick (1985)	115	?	88% recovered fully
Colignon and Lamy (1986)	111	83 ATA	0.5% died in emergency room; 3.3% admitted to ICU; rest 96.2% had minor symptoms and recovered completely.
Tirpitz & Baykara (1988)	276	2–2.5 ATA	4 deaths. Rest recovered. Many treated and released to home the same day
Sloan *et al* (1989)	297	3 ATA	Extremely ill patients with mortality of 6%. Rest recovered.
Abramovich *et al* (1997)	24	2.8 ATA	20 (84%) recovered recovered consciousness during one treatment, 3 required a second treatment, and one who arrived in deep coma died.

ble, the patient should be transferred to a multiplace chamber with facilities for critical care and suitably qualified personnel. During transport to such a facility, the patient should receive 100% oxygen, using a mask, and care should be taken that the patient does not rebreathe the exhaled air. The argument that normobaric oxygen is always satisfactory for severe CO poisoning can no longer be sustained. A pO_2 of 1800 mmHg achieved by HBO is definitely more effective than the maximal pO_2 of 760 mmHg attainable by normobaric 100% oxygen. In practice, it is much lower than this, since few oxygen masks exist that are suitable for administering oxygen to achieve a pO_2 above 600 mmHg.

Clinical Trials of HBO in CO Poisoning

Clinical trials of HBO in CO poisoning are listed in Table 12.15. These are discussed in more detail below.

Raphael *et al* (1989) carried out a trial of normobaric and hyperbaric oxygen for acute CO intoxication in 629 adults who had been poisoned at home in the 13 h preceding admission to hospital. It was a randomized study with grouping based on whether or not there was initial loss of consciousness. In those without any loss of consciousness HBO was compared with normobaric oxygen (NBO) treatments, with no difference being noticed in the recovery rate. Those who had an episode of loss of consciousness were treated either by a single session of 2 h of HBO at 2 ATA followed by 4 h of NBO, or by 4 h of NBO with 2 sessions of HBO 6 to 12 h apart. Two sessions of HBO were shown to have no advantage over a single session. The authors concluded that those who do not sustain initial loss of consciousness should be treated by NBO regardless of the COHb levels. The authors did not deny the usefulness of HBO in those with loss of consciousness, but stated that two sessions of HBO had no advantage over a single session. The methodology in the study is questionable.

Ducassé *et al* (1995) carried out a randomized study to compare the effects of normobaric oxygen versus HBO therapy in patients with moderate CO poisoning. In conscious patients without neurological impairment, one HBO treatment at 2.5 ATA for 0.5 h, within the first 2 h after admission, had the following advantages:

- Faster recuperation from symptoms such as headache and nausea.
- Quicker elimination of CO during the first 2 h. After 12 h, there was no difference in blood COHb levels between the two groups.
- Fewer EEG abnormalities after 3 weeks in the group treated with HBO.
- Recovery of the cerebral vasomotor response in the group treated with HBO, as shown using the acetazolamide test.

In a longitudinal study of 100 consecutive patients, the frequency of neuropsychiatric sequelae among patients who received oxygen at atmospheric pressure was 63%, among those who received one HBO treatment it was 46%, and in those who received two or more HBO treatments it was 13%

Table 12.15
Clinical Trials of HBO in CO Poisoning

Authors and year	Study design	HBO pressure	Results
Weaver et al (2002)	Double-blind, randomized trial to study the effect of HBO on cognitive sequelae of acute CO poisoning. Control with normobaric oxygen + air.	HBO (2–3 ATA)	3 HBO treatments within a 24-hour period reduced the risk of cognitive sequelae 6 weeks and 12 months after acute carbon monoxide poisoning.
Scheinkestel et al (1999)	Randomized controlled double-blind trial and sham treatments in a multiplace hyperbaric chamber. Neuro-psychological assessments.	HBO (2.8 ATA/1 H) or 100% oxygen	Both groups received high doses of oxygen but HBO therapy did not benefit.
Thom et al (1995)	Prospective, randomized study in patients with mild to moderate CO poisoning who presented within 6 H. Incidence of delayed neurological sequelae (DNS) compared between groups treated with oxygen or HBO.	Normobaric 100% oxygen or HBO (2.8 ATA for 30 min + 2 ATA for 90 min)	HBO treatment decreased the incidence of DNS after CO poisoning.
Ducassé et al (1995)	Randomized study in acute CO poisoning: normobaric oxygen (NBO) versus hyperbaric oxygen.	2 h treatment with normobaric oxygen or HBO (2.5 ATA)	Patients treated with HBO had a significant clinical improvement compared with patients treated with NBO.
Raphael et al (1989)	Randomization of patients with acute CO intoxication to normobaric or hyperbaric oxygen. Grouping based on whether or not there was initial loss of consciousness.	Single session of HBO (2 ATA/2 h) followed by 4 h of NBO, or by 4 h of NBO with 2 sessions of HBO, 6 to 12 h apart	Better recovery with HBO treatment in those with initial loss of consciousness. There was no advantage of 2 sessions of HBO over a single session.

(Gorman et al 1992). The frequency of sequelae was greater if HBO treatment was delayed. In a prospective randomized clinical study, delayed neuropsychiatric sequelae were found to be less frequent with HBO treatment as compared with normobaric oxygen administration (Thom et al 1992).

These authors recommend that HBO should be used in the initial treatment of all patients with CO poisoning, regardless of the severity of their initial clinical manifestations. It is difficult to compare the results of different reported studies, because the patient conditions differed widely and the HBO technique used also varied. The overall results of HBO therapy, however, were favorable. Some patients in critically ill condition died from other complications, and in some other cases the HBO therapy was instituted too late to be life-saving.

The treatments may be carried out in a monoplace or a multiplace hyperbaric chamber. A large chamber with intensive care facilities is preferable in case of a critically ill patient. Various regimens have been used for the treatment of CO poisoning. The pressures used vary between 2 and 3 ATA. The most commonly used protocol is an initial 45 minutes of 100% oxygen at 3 ATA followed by further treatment at 2 ATA for 2 hours or until the COHb is less than 10%. HBO is the treatment of choice in patients who lost consciousness during toxic exposure, who are comatose on admission to hospital and who have persisting neurological abnormalities (Wattel et al 1996). Complications of HBO in comatose patients include rupture of the eardrum in about 10% of the patients. Seizures may occur in patients with brain injury who are subjected to high HBO pressures. In a series of 300 consecutive CO-poisoned patients, there was one seizure at 2.45 ATA (0.3%), nine seizures at 2.80 ATA (2%) and six seizures at 3 ATA (Hampson et al 1996). This difference is statistically significant and

should be considered when selecting the HBO treatment pressure for CO poisoning. Concern has been expressed that patients with severe CO poisoning, who are intubated and mechanically ventilated, may not achieve adequate hyperbaric oxygenation in a multiplace chamber. In a review of 85 such patients, pO_2 greater than 760 mmHg was documented in 95% of the patients (Hampson 1998). Such patients should not be excluded from HBO treatment for fear that adequate oxygenation cannot be achieved.

North American HBO facilities were surveyed to assess selection criteria applied for treatment of acute CO poisoning (Hampson et al 1995). Responses were received from 85% of the 208 facilities in the United States and Canada which treated a total of 2,636 patients in 1992. A majority of facilities treat CO-exposed patients in coma (98%), transient loss of consciousness (77%), focal neurologic deficits (94%), or abnormal psychometric testing (91%), regardless of carboxyhemoglobin (COHb) level. Although 92% would use HBO for a patient presenting with headache, nausea and a COHb value of 40%, only 62% of facilities utilized a specified minimum COHb level as the sole criterion for HBO therapy of an asymptomatic patient. It was concluded that when COHb is used as an independent criterion to determine HBO treatment, the level utilized varies widely between institutions.

HBO for CO Intoxication Secondary to Methylene Chloride Poisoning

Methylene chloride is converted to CO by cytochrome P-450 after it enters the human body. Rioux and Myers (1989) treated two cases of CO poisoning secondary to exposure to methylene chloride. Both recovered following treatment with HBO. Youn et al (1989) reported 12 cases of methylene chloride poisoning from a single exposure. Nine of these required HBO treatment and made a good recovery. The authors observed that CO derived from methylene chloride has an effective half-life 2.5 times that of exogenously inhaled CO.

Rudge (1990c) reported a case of CO poisoning from exposure to methylene chloride that was successfully treated by use of HBO. He pointed out that in the case of methylene chloride poisoning, tissue levels of CO continue to rise after exposure, whereas in CO poisoning, the CO levels begin to fall after the exposure is terminated. The practical implication of this observation is that patients with methylene chloride poisoning should be observed for 12 to 24 h after exposure and should be treated adequately with HBO.

Treatment of CO Poisoning in Pregnancy

In the past, pregnancy was considered to be a relative contraindication for the use of HBO, because of the possible toxic effects of oxygen on the fetus. Dangers of hyperoxic exposure to the fetus have been demonstrated in animals. However, these experimental exposures exceeded the time and pressures routinely used in clinical therapy. If 100% oxygen given to pregnant women with CO intoxication, it should be prolonged to five times what the mother needs, because of the slow elimination of CO by the fetus. Van Hoesen et al (1989) treated CO intoxication (COHb 47.2%) in a 17-year-old pregnant woman at 37 weeks of gestation using HBO at 2.4 ATA for a 90-min treatment. The patient recovered and produced a healthy baby at full-term normal delivery. If the mother had been left untreated, considerable morbidity would have been anticipated for the mother as well as for the fetus. These authors reviewed the literature on the subject and made the following recommendations:

- Administer HBO therapy if the maternal COHb level is above 20% at any time during the exposure.
- Administer HBO therapy if the patient has suffered or demonstrated any neurological signs, regardless of the COHb level.
- Administer HBO therapy if signs of fetal distress are present, that is, fetal tachycardia, decreased beat-to-beat variability on the fetal monitor, or late decelerations, consistent with the COHb levels and exposure history.
- If the patient continues to demonstrate neurological signs or signs of fetal distress 12 h after initial treatment, additional HBO treatments may be indicated.

In a prospective uncontrolled study on 44 pregnant women, HBO treatment for acute CO poisoning was well tolerated without any hazards to the fetus or the mother (Elkharrat et al 1991). Results of the first prospective, multicenter study of acute CO poisoning in pregnancy showed that severe maternal CO toxicity was associated with signifi-

cantly more adverse fetal cases when compared to mild maternal toxicity (Koren et al 1991). Because fetal accumulation of CO is higher and its elimination slower than in the maternal circulation, HBO may decrease fetal hypoxia and improve outcome. Careful documentation of the experience with this treatment is necessary to determine the long-term sequelae and effectiveness of treatment with HBO during pregnancy.

Treatment of Smoke Inhalation

Smoke inhalation involves multiple toxicities and pulmonary insufficiency, as well as thermal and chemical injury. CO intoxication is the most immediate life-threatening disorder in such cases As a practice guideline, the following patient groups in smoke inhalation injury should be directed by rescue personnel to an emergency service with a hyperbaric facility:

- Those who are unconscious
- Those who are responsive but combative
- Those not responding to verbal instructions or painful stimuli.

If the patient meets these criteria, 100% oxygen is administered initially during transport to a hyperbaric emergency medical center. If the COHb is over 20% and the surface burns are cover less than 20% of the patient's body, the patient should be treated initially with HBO and then transferred to a burn center, unless the burn service is located in the hyperbaric facility itself. HBO is given at 2.8 ATA for 46 min using 100% oxygen. Patients with surface burns more extensive than 10% should be treated initially at a burn center.

Experimental pulmonary edema caused by smoke inhalation is lessened by HBO. This may be the explanation of benefit of HBO on respiratory insufficiency associated with smoke inhalation and CO poisoning. Administration of HBO 2.8 ATA for 45 min inhibits adhesion of circulating neutrophils subsequent to smoke inhalation in rats whether used in a prophylactic manner before smoke inhalation, or as treatment immediately after the smoke insult (Thom et al 2001). However, the beneficial effect appears related to inhibition of neutrophil adhesion to the vasculature rather than prevention of CO poisoning.

Prevention and Treatment of Late Sequelae of CO Poisoning

Several reports indicate that the incidence of secondary syndromes is reduced by adequate treatment with HBO in the acute stage of CO poisoning. Empirical overtreatment has been used in the belief that it would prevent late sequelae. The half-life of CO bound with cytochrome a_3 oxidase, which is the determining factor for late sequelae, is not known. Further research is required to evaluate the CO bound to cytochrome a$_3$ oxidase, so that the necessary duration of HBO treatment can be determined more realistically.

HBO has been used for the treatment of late sequelae of CO poisoning (Gibson *et al* 1991;. Patients with severe CO poisoning who have abnormalities on CT scan, which persist after HBO treatment still develop neuropsychiatric sequelae (Fife *et al* 1989). Samuels *et al* (1992) reported a case of CO poisoning which was misdiagnosed as conversion disorder. Cognitive deficits demonstrated at time of assessment were successfully reversed by HBO, despite the delay of one week between the exposure and treatment.

Thom *et al* (1995) measured the incidence of delayed neurologic sequelae (DNS) in a group of patients acutely poisoned with CO and tested the null hypothesis that the incidence would not be affected by treatment with HBO. They conducted a prospective, randomized study in patients with mild to moderate CO poisoning who presented within 6 hours. Patients had no history of loss of consciousness or cardiac instability. The incidence of DNS was compared between groups treated with ambient pressure 100% oxygen or HBO (2.8 ATA for 30 min followed by 2 ATA oxygen for 90 minutes). DNS were defined as development of new symptoms after oxygen treatment plus deterioration on one or more subtests of a standardized neuropsychologic screening battery. In 7 of 30 patients (23%), DNS developed after treatment with ambient-pressure oxygen, whereas no sequelae developed in 30 patients after HBO treatment (P < .05). DNS occurred 6 ($\pm$ 1) days after poisoning and persisted 41 ($\pm$ 8) days. At follow-up 4 weeks after poisoning, patients who had been treated with ambient pressure oxygen and had not sustained DNS exhibited a worse mean score on one subtest, Trail Making, compared with the group treated with HBO and with a control group matched according to age and education level. The authors concluded that HBO treatment decreased the incidence of DNS after CO poisoning.

Controversies in the Use of HBO for CO Poisoning

Even those who recognize the value of HBO question its role in CO poisoning, because there are no definite correlations of clinical manifestations with COHb levels, and COHb levels are not a definite guide for therapy. There is a particularly poor correlation between carboxyhemoglobin levels and neurological presentation. Neurological effects are due to unmeasured tissue uptake of CO, which increases during hypoxia because of competition between CO and oxygen at the oxygen-binding sites on hemopro-

teins. The efficacy of HBO therapy cannot be ascribed to hastened dissociation of carboxyhemoglobin. Additional mechanisms of action of HBO found in studies in animals include:

- Improved mitochondrial oxidative metabolism
- Inhibition of lipid per oxidation
- Impairment of adherence of neutrophils to cerebral vasculature.

Among the clinical trials reviewed, Weaver *et al* (2002) report on the latest and most carefully controlled investigation of HBO for acute CO poisoning. Among the strengths of this trial are its large size, its use of a sham-treatment control group with blinding of both patients and investigators to the treatment-group assignment, its selection of seriously poisoned patients representative of those encountered in emergency departments, its employment of treatment regimens similar to those in common use, its very high rates of follow-up evaluation, and its explicit definitions of cognitive sequelae. This trial showed that HBO treatment significantly reduces the incidence of CO-induced delayed neurologic sequelae. The assessment of the primary end point (identification of patients in whom cognitive sequelae developed) took place 6 weeks after poisoning, but evaluations at 6 and 12 months also showed a large benefit of HBO. These findings lend further support to the use of HBO, particularly because neurologic manifestations may persist for variable intervals after CO poisoning. Randomized controlled trials have shown that HBO is the only effective therapy for acute CO poisoning if delayed neurologic sequelae are to be minimized (Stoller 2007). Normobaric oxygen should not be used between multiple hyperbaric oxygen treatments, as this can contribute to oxygen toxicity.

Review of all the available evidence indicates that HBO has a definite place in the management of CO poisoning. COHb levels cannot be used as a guide for treatment as they do not correlate with with the clinical severity of CO poisoning. The following approach is recommended for HBO treatment for CO poisoning (Prockop & Chichkova 2007):

- Patients with severe poisoning must receive HBO regardless of their COHb levels.
- Pregnant patients must be treated with HBO regardless of signs and symptoms.
- Administration of more than one course of HBO treatment to those who remain in coma remains controversial.

It would be helpful to have an objective biochemical serum marker that could help in the evaluation of CO poisoning and indication for HBO therapy. In two case reports, where the established criteria for the CO poisoning were not optimum for the decision regarding HBO therapy, S-100B protein could be used as a biochemical marker of CO-induced brain injury (Brvar *et al* 2003).

There is some controversy regarding the pressure of HBO. Use of pressures between 2.5 and 3 ATA seems appropriate for CO poisoning (Thom 2002).

Mg^{2+}, a physiological calcium antagonist, helps in the prevention of late sequelae of CO poisoning by blocking cellular calcium influx.

Cyanide Poisoning

Cyanide is one of the most rapidly acting and lethal poisons known. Cyanide exists as either a gas or as the liquid hydrogen cyanide (HCN), also known as prussic acid. It is one of the smallest organic molecules that can be detected: inhalation of as little as 100 mg of gas can cause instantaneous death. An oral dose of the sodium or potassium salt (lethal dose 300 mg) acts more slowly; symptoms may not appear for several minutes and death may not occur for 1 h. Cyanide poisoning is mostly suicidal, but exposure can occur in the electroplating industry, in laboratory procedures, and in fumigation. Propronitrile, a substituted aliphatic nitrile commonly used in manufacturing industry, is capable of generating cyanide. Cyanogenic glycosides are found in several plant species, including apricot kernels and bitter almonds. The iatrogenic source is sodium nitroprusside, which is used as a vasodilator and as a hypotensive agent. Cyanide is a metabolite of nitroprusside, and toxicity results from rapid infusion, prolonged use, or renal failure.

Pathophysiology

Cyanide combines with cytochrome-a_3-oxidase, and exhibits a great affinity for oxidized iron (Fe^{3+}). This complex inhibits the final step of oxidative phosphorylation and halts aerobic metabolism. The patient essentially suffocates from an inability to use oxygen.

Rationale for Use of HBO in Cyanide Poisoning

Theoretically it appears unlikely that HBO would exert its effect in cyanide poisoning by competing with cyanide at a receptor site in cytochrome-a_3-oxidase. Possible mechanisms for the positive effect of HBO are:

- The equation

  cytochrome oxidase + cyanide = cytochrome oxidase cyanide

  is pushed to the left by high pO_2 levels.

- Increased detoxification of cyanide by elevated oxygen pressures.
- Sufficient cellular respiration may continue via cyanide-

Table 12.16
Experimental Evidence for the Effectiveness of HBO in Cyanide Poisoning

Authors and year	Evidence
Ivanov (1959)	HBO restored normal activity of the brain in mice poisoned with cyanide
Skene *et al* (1966)	Drop in mortality from 96% to 20% in a group of mice treated with HBO at 2 ATA compared with those treated at 1 ATA
Takano *et al* (1980)	HBO at 2 ATA was shown to reduce the pyridine nuclide fluorescence (which represents the degree of blockage of respiratory chain) in the renal cortices of rabbits poisoned with cyanide
Isom *et al* (1982)	Showed that recovery of brain cytochrome oxidase was more rapid in rats poisoned with cyanide and treated by oxygen breathing, compared with those breathing air

insensitive pathways under hyperbaric conditions to counteract effects of hypoxia.

The value of high tensions of oxygen in the management of cyanide poisoning in experimental animals was shown by Cope (1961). However, HBO at 4 ATA was not shown to be more effective than NBO as an adjunct to conventional antidotes in cyanide poisoning in mice (Way *et al* 1972). Other experimental studies showed HBO to be effective in cyanide poisoning; these are listed in Table 12.16.

Clinical Features of Cyanide Poisoning

Signs and symptoms of acute cyanide poisoning reflect cellular hypoxia and are often nonspecific. The central nervous system is the most sensitive target organ with initial stimulation followed by depression.

Laboratory Diagnosis

Blood cyanide levels are useful in confirming toxicity, but treatment has to be initiated before the results of this test are available. Changes in ECG and EEG are nonspecific.

Treatment

The basic treatment of cyanide poisoning is chemical (Cyanide Antidote Kit, Eli Lilly). The object is to bind the cyanide in its harmless form as a stable cyanmethemoglobin by giving sodium nitrite. Cyanide is later liberated by dissociation of cyanmethemoglobin. To convert this to thiocyanate, a harmless substance, intravenous sodium thiosulfate is given. Litovitz *et al* (1983) reported the unsuccessful use of HBO in a case of cyanide poisoning. Later Trapp and Lepowski (1983) reported five cases of cyanide poisoning

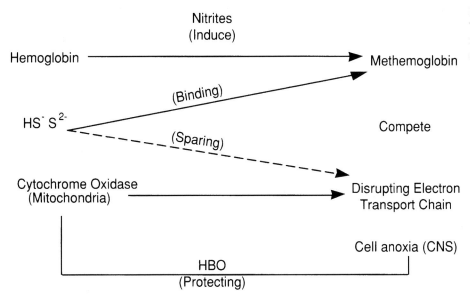

Figure 12.4
The role of hyperbaric oxygenation and nitrites in acute hydrogen sulfide poisoning (reproduced from Hsu *et al* 1987).

treated successfully by means of HBO. There are several anecdotal reports of cases of cyanide poisoning in which HBO was useful for treatment. Scolnick *et al* (1993) treated one patient with cyanide poisoning resulting from exposure to substituted nitrile using HBO for residual symptoms after initial treatment with sodium nitrite and sodium thiosulfate. A man who deliberately drank a potassium-gold cyanide solution survived after treatment with the Lilly Cyanide Antidote kit and hyperbaric oxygen (Goodhart 1994).

Hydrogen Sulfide Poisoning

Hydrogen sulfide (H_2S) is a highly toxic, inflammable, colorless gas, readily recognized by its characteristic odor of "rotten eggs." The mechanism of toxicity is similar to that of cyanide and CO poisoning. Hydrogen sulfide is a mitochondrial toxin and inhibits cellular aerobic metabolism. Therapies for toxic exposures include removal from the contaminated environment, ventilation with 100% oxygen, and nitrite therapy if administered immediately after exposure. The rationale for the use of HBO in H_2S poisoning is shown in Figure 12.4. Nitrates aid the conversion of hemoglobin to methemoglobin. The latter, by binding free sulfide ions, spares intracellular cytochrome oxidase.

Bitterman *et al* (1986) studied the effect of oxygen at 3 ATA, both alone and in combination with intraperitoneal sodium nitrite in rats poisoned with LD_{75} hydrogen sulfide. They found that pure oxygen at 1 ATA was effective in preventing death, but oxygen at 3 ATA was more effective. The best therapy was the combination of oxygen at 3 ATA with sodium nitrite. The clinical usefulness of HBO in H_2S poisoning is based on the relief of cerebral edema and protec-

tion of the vital organs from hypoxia. Single case reports have shown that HBO treatment was successful in treating H_2S poisoning (Smilkstein *et al* 1985; Whitecraft *et al* 1985). Hsu *et al* (1987) reported five patients with severe H_2S poisoning who were treated successfully with HBO in combination with the use of nitrates. Pontani *et al* (1998) reported a patient in whom delayed neurologic toxicity from hydrogen sulfide was treated successfully with HBO. The pressure used was 3 ATA for 90 min during the initial treatment and this resulted in significant improvement. Daily treatments at 2.4 ATA were continued and neurological deficits resolved completely in three days. HBO therapy was used succeessfully in the management of two cases of hydrogen sulfide toxicity, who had not responded to normobaric oxygen (Belley *et al* 2005).

Carbon Tetrachloride Poisoning

Carbon tetrachloride (CCl_4) poisoning is not an uncommon occurrence in clinical practice. In moderate cases, the clinical course is benign. When severe hepatorenal injury occurs, the prognosis is grave because of hepatic insufficiency.

Although ischemic anoxia can damage the sinusoidal capillaries, the popular theory of CCl_4-induced hepatic injury is based on free radicals. CCl_4 exerts its toxicity through its metabolites, including the free radicals CCl_3 and CCl_3OO. Oxygen strongly inhibits the hepatic cytochrome P-450 mediated formation of CCl_3 from CCl_4 and promotes the conversion of CCl_3 to CCl_3OO. Both of these free radicals can injure the hepatocyte by lipoperoxidation and by binding covalently to the cell structures. Under conditions of hypoxia most of the free radicals are CCl_3, whereas under hyperoxia most are CCl_3OO. A reduced glutathione (GSH)-dependent mechanism can protect against CCl_3OO but not against CCl_3, so there is an advantage in using HBO in CCl_4 poisoning. Burk *et al* (1986) showed that oxygen at 2 ATA given 6 h after administration of CCl_4 to rats improved the survival rate from 36% to 50%. HBO inhibited the in vivo conversion of CCl_4 to its volatile metabolites $CHCl_3$ and CO_2 by 52%. The predominant effect was on CO_2, which is quantitatively the more significant metabolite.

Animal experimental studies of the effect of HBO on CCl_4 poisoning have been reviewed by Burkhardt *et al* (1991). Most of these studies show that the mortality of the HBO-treated animals is lowered and there is less impairment of the liver function tests (Bernacchi *et al* 1984). Troop *et al* (1986) conducted a carefully controlled study of the effects of HBO on rats poisoned with CCl_4 and concluded:

- HBO improves survival from CCl_4 poisoning.
- The response rate is time-related. There was a better survival rate in animals treated within 1 h of poisoning compared with those treated after 4 h.
- The improved survival with HBO is the result of decreased hepatotoxicity.

Although the mechanism of the protective effect of HBO on the liver is not well understood, it has been used in patients with CCl_4 poisoning. Larcan *et al* (1973) described a case of CCl_4 poisoning treated by HBO. The treatment was begun 24 h after ingestion of 150 ml CCl_4, when severe hepatic necrosis was already present. The patient recovered, and a liver biopsy on the twelfth day showed only minimal hepatic centrilobular necrosis. Other cases of CCl_4 poisoning successfully treated by HBO have been reported (Montani & Perret 1967; Saltzman 1981; Truss & Killenberg 1982).

CCl_4 poisoning is rare these days as this toxic solvent is no longer used industrially. However, when a case occurs there is no satisfactory conventional treatment. HBO has been shown to be useful, and free radical scavengers such as vitamin E seem to be effective only if given before or with HBO.

Methemoglobinemias

The reversible oxygenation and deoxygenation of Hb at physiological partial pressures of oxygen require that the heme iron of deoxyhemoglobin remain in the Fe^{2+} form. In methemoglobinemias iron is already oxidized to the Fe^{3+} form, rendering the molecule incapable of binding oxygen. When Hb is oxygenated during the process of respiration, an electron is transferred from the Fe^+ atom to the bound oxygen molecule. Thus, in oxyhemoglobin, the iron pos-

sesses some of the characteristics of the Fe^{3+} state, whereas the oxygen takes on the characteristic of the superoxide (O_2^-) anion, which is a free radical.

Many drugs and chemicals have toxic effects on the Hb molecule and produce methemoglobinemia. Nitrobenzene and nitrites provide examples. The methemoglobinemia is usually asymptomatic. As methemoglobin levels increase, patients show evidence of cellular hypoxia in all tissues. Death usually occurs when methemoglobin fractions approach 70% of total hemoglobin. The diagnosis depends upon the demonstration of methemoglobin and the causative agent.

Treatment

Methylene blue remains an effective treatment for methemoglobinemias but HBO can be a useful adjunct. Comparison of antagonism to the lethal effects of sodium nitrite displayed by various combinations of methylene blue, oxygen, and HBO shows that HBO is the most effective agent, with or without methylene blue. Timchuk *et al* (1981) treated three patients with drug-induced methemoglobinemia (methemoglobin levels 50–70%) who were admitted in a comatose state. HBO at 2.2 ATA was given. Methemoglobin decreased at a rate of 5 to 8% per hour of exposure to HBO, and the patients recovered. In another patient, who was accidentally intoxicated with isobutyl nitrite by a threefold lethal dose, a blood exchange transfusion was performed under HBO and the patient recovered (Jansen *et al* 2003). In a patient with severe life-threatening isobutyl nitrite-induced methemoglobinemia of 75% of total hemoglobin, toluidine-blue was administered as first-line antidotal therapy immediately, followed by HBO and the patient recovered uneventfully (Lindenmann *et al* 2006)

Miscellaneous Poisons

Quinine

Toxic effects of quinine and related antimalarial drugs includes cardiotoxicity with vascular collapse. Neurotoxicity and visual loss may also occur. Good recovery of visual activity and visual field defects resulting from quinine intoxication and treated with HBO at 2 ATA, has been reported.

Organophosphorus Compounds

Organophosphorus compounds have been used as pesticides and as chemical warfare nerve agents such as soman and sarin. The mechanism of toxicity of organophosphorus compounds is the inhibition of acetylcholinesterase, resulting in accumulation of acetylcholine and the continued stimulation of acetylcholine receptors. The management of poisoning with organophosphorous compounds consists of atropine sulfate and blood alkalinization with sodium bicarbonate and also magnesium sulfate as an adjunctive treatment. Neurotoxicity is a serious concern. Experiments on rabbits have shown that accumulated poisoning with paraoxon leads to development of hypoxia with a rapid fall in oxygen tension in the muscles and the venous blood, and a shift of the acid-base balance toward the uncompensated metabolic acidosis. HBO at 3 ATA for 2 to 4 h considerably prolongs the survival of the poisoned animals. The role of HBO in potential management of organophosphorus poisoning with neurotoxicity requires further investigation.

Amanita Phalloides

Cases of *Amanita phalloides* (mushroom) poisoning have been treated by using HBO with good results.

Ethacrynic Acid

Ototoxicity of ethacrynic acid on the inner ear can be reduced by HBO, with improvement of hearing.

Conclusions: Poisoning Other than with CO

There are only anecdotal reports of the use of HBO in cases of cyanide, hydrogen sulfide, and CCl_4 poisoning and methemoglobinemias; in situations like this one cannot have controlled studies. In a critical case HBO should be considered as a supplement to conventional methods. The liver is the target organ for injury caused by toxins that are activated by drug-metabolizing enzymes to reactive molecular intermediates. These intermediates cause cell injury by forming chemical bonds with cell proteins, nucleic acid, and lipids, and by altering the biological function of these molecules. The hepatocyte, in particular, is affected by toxic drug injury because it is the main site in the body where these toxins are activated. HBO has a marked effect on toxic liver damage by blocking the injury caused by toxins activated by oxidative biotransformation. HBO has no effect on damage caused by toxins that do not require biotransformation to induce liver damage. HBO may increase the hepatic necrosis induced by compounds which undergo oxidative biotransformation (e.g. thioacetamide, aflatoxin, dimethylnitrosamine), but this can be overcome and inhibited by prolonged hyperoxia.

13

HBO Therapy in Infections

K.K. Jain

HBO has been shown to be a valuable adjunct to the medical and surgical treatment of various infections. The topics covered in this chapter are:

Host Defense Mechanisms Against Infection

Phagocytic leukocytes present the first and the most important line of defense against microorganisms introduced into the body. The capacity of the leukocytes to kill depends largely on the amount of oxygen available to them. Bacterial killing usually consists of two phases. The first phase involves degranulation, in which ingested bacteria are exposed to various antimicrobial substances derived from the leukocyte granules. The second phase is the oxidative phase (see Figure 13.1), which depends on the molecular oxygen captured by the leukocytes and converted to high energy radicals such as superoxide, hydroxy radicals, peroxides, aldehyde hypochlorite, and hypochlorites. The rate of production of free radicals and hence of the oxidative bacteria killing depends on the local oxygen tension. The killing sequence can be replicated to some extent *in vitro* by incubating bacteria in the presence of halide ions, hydrogen peroxide, and myeloperoxidases, a mixture that generates hypohalite free radicals.

Impairment by Anoxia

The oxidative killing mechanism is also related to the nonoxidative pathway. The energy for this pathway is provided by the hexose-mono-phosphate shunt. Absence of the enzyme primary oxidase (NADPH) means absence of the substrate on which it acts – oxygen – and is equal to anoxia. Therefore, lack of oxygen leads to loss of killing power of the leukocytes. The major loss of killing capacity occurs when tissue pO_2 levels fall below 30 mmHg.

Oxygen as an Antibiotic

The characteristics of oxygen as an antibiotic are shown in Table 13.1. The effect of hyperbaric oxygenation (HBO) in anaerobic infections is well recognized. The high levels of oxygen in the tissues are detrimental to organisms that thrive in the absence of oxygen. The aerobic bacteria, however, show a biphasic response on exposure to HBO. At pressures of 0.6–1.3 ATA the growth is enhanced, but above 1.3 ATA it is inhibited. The toxicity of oxygen to the microbes is time-dependent. The aim is to have an exploitable difference in specificity to the drug between the host and the parasite. The greater the specificity of the drug for the parasite, the safer the drug is for clinical use. As a drug, oxygen acts indiscriminately, however; the quantities of oxygen required to raise tissue pO_2 to a level that would adversely affect the growth or metabolism (including toxin production) of the microorganisms is in the same range that produces symptoms of pulmonary and central nervous system toxicity. There are, therefore, two goals:

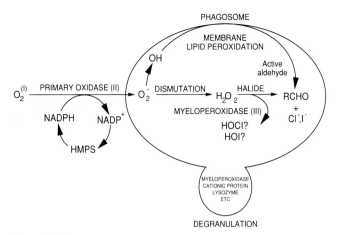

Figure 13.1

Schema of oxidative killing mechanism and its relation to nonoxidative pathway (Reproduced by permission from Rabkin and Hunt, (1988). Infection and Oxygen. In Davis JC, Hunt TK (Eds.): Problem Wounds – Role of oxygen. Elsevier, New York, by permission). HOCl, hypochlorite; HOI, hypoiodite; HMPS, hexose-monophosphate shunt.

Table 13.1
Oxygen as an Antibiotic and Rationale for HBO Therapy in Infections

1. Oxygen acts as an antibiotic by impairing the bacterial metabolism. The effect of HBO is not selective but covers a broad spectrum of grampositive as well as gram negative organisms. It is most effective in anaerobic infections.
2. HBO improves the phagocytosis, which is impaired by hypoxia.
3. Hypoxia impairs the immune mechanism of the body, whereas HBO improves it.
4. HBO produces free radicals which are toxic to the microorganisms.
5. HBO has a synergistic effect when combined with sulfonamides and increases the effect five to ten fold.
6. HBO is effective in drug resistant infections.
7. Adequate tissue oxygen tension is required for achieving an optimal effect of the antibiotics. The effect of aminoglycosides is reduced in anoxic conditions as oxygen is needed for transporting the drug into bacteria.
8. Oxygen has a direct bactericidal or bacteriostatic effect equal to that of some antibiotics.
9. HBO inhibits the exotoxin production, e.g., alpha-toxin of *C. perfringans* or detoxifies the oxygen-labile exotoxins, e.g., theta-toxin of *C. perfringans*

- To expose the microorganisms to a given pO_2 for a time long enough to affect the microbial physiology adversely and give the host defense mechanisms an opportunity to prevail. The exposure should not be so long as to produce tissue toxicity.
- To raise tissue pO_2 sufficiently to bolster the body's defense mechanisms without altering the physiology of the microbe simultaneously.

Bacteria in culture are exposed to intermittent HBO to simulate clinical situations and to determine the time-dose relationships. The growth of *Myobacterium tuberculosis* is greatly retarded after twice-daily 3-h exposures to 2.87 ATA oxygen for 5 days, while twice-daily 2-h exposures to 1.87 ATA are less effective. There are species differences in response to increased pO$_2$.

Oxygen may enhance the effects of other antimicrobial agents, particularly para-aminobenzoic acid (PABA) antagonists such as sulfonamides. Hyperbaric oxygen at 2.87 ATA increases the effectiveness of sulfisoxazole five to tenfold. There is no oxygen enhancement of PABA analogs on *Corynebacterium diphtheriae*. The only drug-resistant organism that is susceptible to oxygen-induced synergy is *M. tuberculosis*.

Improving tissue oxygen by administration of normobaric oxygen decreases infectious necrosis as effectively as prophylactic antibiotics, and has an additive effect. In several animals models of peritonitis due to pathogenic organisms, HBO reduces mortality and has a synergistic effect with antibiotics which further reduce the mortality.

In a murine model of group A streptococcal myositis, HBO treatment alone does not decrease mortality significantly *in vivo* whereas penicillin therapy alone improves outcome significantly but the combined treatment of penicillin and HBO exerts synergistic effects in both decreasing bacterial counts *in vivo* and increasing survival in this model (Oztas *et al* 2001).

HBO in the Treatment of Infections

For oxygen to be effective as a bactericidal agent, it has to be delivered to the infected areas. Normobaric oxygen may not reach the affected area, but HBO is more effective. The presence of normal blood flow and normal oxygen content of the blood does not exclude the possibility of hypoxia of the infected tissues, such as ulcers in the lower extremities.

For most infections 100% oxygen is used at 2.5 ATA for 1 h sessions, which can be given once a day or preferably twice a day. The treatment is continued until the infection subsides. There are two reasons for choosing 2.5 ATA:

- It is a safe pressure well below the upper limit of 3 ATA. This is an important consideration because of the debilitated state of some patients and the lengthy treatment required.
- The immune system is stimulated by oxygen pressures up to 2.5 ATA (see Chapter 25), whereas higher pressures have an immunosuppressive effect.

HBO exposures should be intermittent, as continual exposure of experimental animals to high oxygen pressures has been found to be detrimental to phagocytosis. Finally, it must be pointed out that HBO therapy is used as an adjunct to other well-recognized methods of treatment of infection, and it should not replace the antibiotics used in accordance with the results of the culture and sensitivity studies on the organisms.

Not all doses of HBO have an antibacterial effect. The use of HBO at pressures lower than 1.3 ATA promotes the growth of aerobic bacteria *in vivo* by enhancing oxygen delivery to bacteria in the injured tissues. Pressures have to be increased to sufficient levels for oxygen to be bacteriostatic or bactericidal.

Microbes with adequate antioxidant defenses are resistant to the toxic effect of oxygen-free radicals. Some bacteria even use free radical production to injure host cells. Two virulent strains of *Listeria monocytogenes* exhibit maximal production of H_2O_2 and O^{2-}. Virulence can be correlated with survival of *L. monocytogenes* in macrophage monolayers. A virulent strain of *L. monocytogenes* and an isolate of *Staphylococcus aureus* do not release O_2 in significant amounts. Addition of exogenous H_2O_2 results in a significant loss of macrophage viability.

Bacterial antioxidant enzymes are important in resisting x-dependent microbicidal activity in human polymorphonuclear neutrophils (PMN). Surface-associated SOD and high levels of catalase act together to protect strains of *Nocardia asteroides* from the bactericidal effect of PMN. Interaction between oxygen-derived free radicals and antioxidant defense mechanisms may be a crucial factor in the establishment of bacterial infections. The outcome of *in vitro* or *in vivo* HBO treatment of aerobic bacteria depends on the particular organism and the experimental conditions.

HBO has been shown to be beneficial in septicemia. Although hyperoxia may lead to increased lipid peroxidation and free radical damage, it is also possible that lesser degrees of hyperoxygenation such as 2–3 ATA may antagonize lipid peroxidation, which has been implicated in tissue damage in septicemia.

Infections for which HBO has been studied and is recommended by the Undersea and Hyperbaric Medicine Society include necrotizing fasciitis, gas gangrene, chronic refractory osteomyelitis (including malignant otitis externa), mucormycosis, intracranial abscesses, and diabetic foot ulcers that have concomitant infections (Kaide & Khandelwal 2008). In all of these processes, HBO is used adjunctively along with antimicrobial agents and aggressive surgical debridement.

HBO in the Treatment of Soft Tissue Infections

These infections are usually necrotizing and occur in traumatic or surgical wounds, around foreign bodies; they affect patients who are compromised by either diabetes mellitus, vascular insufficiency, or both. Anaerobic soft tissue infections are still life threatening infections. Although their frequency is actually moderate; they remain severe because physicians are often insufficiently aware of them. Their origin is often traumatic or surgical but may also be secondary to an ulcer or a small wound in a high-risk patient with arteriosclerosis or diabetes mellitus. Hypoxia, traumatic muscle crush, heavy bacterial contamination as well as incorrect antibiotic prophylaxis are the major reasons for their occurrence. Management consists of antibiotics adapted to both anaerobic and associated aerobic bacteria, large and early surgical debridement, but with conservative excision, and intensive hyperbaric oxygen therapy. Strict prevention measures must be applied to avoid their occurrence.

Various factors influence outcome in a large group of patients presenting with necrotizing soft tissue infections, and analyses of risk factors for mortality have been performed, producing conflicting conclusions regarding optimal care. In particular, debate exists regarding the impact of concurrent physiologic derangements, type and extent of infection, and the role of HBO in treatment. A retrospective chart review of 198 consecutive patients with documented necrotizing soft tissue infections, treated at a single institution during an 8-year period, was conducted. Using a model for logistic regression analysis, characteristics of each patient and his/her clinical course were tested for impact on outcome. The mortality rate among these patients was 25.3%. The most common sites of origin of infection were the perineum (Fournier's disease; 36% of cases) and the foot (in diabetics; 15.2%). By logistic regression analysis, risk factors for death included age, female gender, extent of infection, delay in first debridement, elevated serum creatinine level, elevated blood lactate level, and degree of organ system dysfunction at admission. Diabetes mellitus did not predispose patients to death, except in conjunction with renal dysfunction or peripheral vascular disease. Myonecrosis, noted in 41.4% of the patients who underwent surgery, did not influence mortality. The authors concluded that necrotizing soft tissue infections represent a group of highly lethal infections best treated by early and repeated extensive debridement and broad-spectrum antibiotics. Hyperbaric oxygen appears to offer the advantage of early wound closure. Certain markers predict those individuals at increased risk for multiple-organ failure and death and therefore assist in deciding allocation of intensive care resources.

Common necrotizing soft tissue infections are described below.

Crepitant Anaerobic Cellulitis

This includes clostridial as well as nonclostridial cellulitis. It manifests itself as a necrotic soft tissue infection with abundant soft tissue gas. This condition usually occurs with local trauma and vascular insufficiency in the lower extremities. Multiple organisms isolated from these infections include bacteroides species, peptostreptococcus species, clostridium species, and enterobacteriaceae.

Progressive Bacterial Gangrene

This is a subacute to chronic ulcer formation on the abdominal or the thoracic wall with a zone of gangrene surrounding it. The major symptom is pain. Microorganisms found in the gangrenous margin are microaerophilic or anaerobic streptococci, and the central part of the lesion contains *Staphylococcus aureus* and enterobacteriaceae. This synergistic bacterial combination is necessary to produce gangrenous lesions.

Necrotizing Fasciitis

This is a rare infection of soft tissues considered to be due to streptococcal infection and first described as a generalized condition by Meleney (1924). Fournier's gangrene (described in this chapter) is considered to be a localized variant of it. Several hundred cases have been reported in the literature. Patients usually complain of pain which is disproportionate to minor skin changes in early phases. Deeper changes are more widespread than the skin changes. Shock with multiorgan failure can occur later in the course of the disease. Microscopic examination of tissue aspirates shows the infective organisms and imaging techniques show the infection spreading along tissue planes.

Primary, aggressive but tissue-saving debridements together with antibiotics are the cornerstones of therapy of necrotizing fasciitis. HBO therapy can oxygenate infected hypoxic tissues to help marginally viable tissues survive, reduce the inflammatory response, improve leukocyte bacterial oxidative killing capacity, and achieve infection control and healing (Flam *et al* 2008).

Nonclostridial Myonecrosis

This is also a synergistic necrotizing cellulitis and is similar to clostridial myonecrosis because of extensive muscle and fascia involvement. It occurs most commonly in the perineal area and Fournier's gangrene is a variant of it. Multiple organisms that have been isolated include peptostreptococcus species, bacteroides species, and enterobacteriaceae.

Differential diagnosis and treatment of these infections is listed in Table 13.2. The treatment of these infections is a combination of aggressive surgery, debridement, appropriate antibiotics, good nutritional support, and optimal oxygenation of the infected tissues. HBO treatment has

Table 13.2
Differentiation and Treatment of the Common Necrotizing Bacterial Soft Tissue Infections

	Crepitant Anaerobic Cellulitis	Progressive bacterial synergistic gangrene	Necrotizing fasciitis	Nonclostridial myonecrosis
Incubation	More than 3 days	2 weeks	1–4 days	Variable, 3–14 days
Onset	Gradual	Gradual	Acute	Acute
Toxemia	None or slight	Minimal	Moderate to marked	Marked
Pain	Absent	Moderate	Moderate to severe	Severe
Exudate	None or slight	None or slight	Serosanguinous profuse	Dishwater pus
Odor to exudate	+Foul	+Foul	Foul	+Foul
Gas	Abundant	May be present	Usually not present	Not pronounced
Muscle	No change	No change	Viable	Marked change
Skin	Little change	Shaggy ulcer, gangrenous margin	Pale red cellulitis	Minimal change
Mortality	5%–10%	10%–25%	30%	75%
Treatment				
· Antibiotics	Yes	Yes	Yes	Yes
· Surgery	I & D	I & D	I & D	Muscle removal
· Adjunctive HBO	No	Yes (severe cases)	Yes (compromised host)	Yes

I & D = incision and drainage
(from Mader 1988, reproduced by permission)

been used successfully as adjunctive therapy in mixed soft tissue infections. An objective evaluation of the use of HBO in these infections is difficult because of the multitude of variable factors in patients and other treatment methods used.

Fournier's gangrene. Many controversial issues exist surrounding the disease pathogenesis and optimal management of Fournier's gangrene. In Fournier's original descriptions in 1883, the disease arose in healthy subjects without an obvious cause. Most contemporary studies, however, are able to identify definite urologic or colorectal etiologies in a majority of cases. Intercurrent diseases include diabetes mellitus, ethanol abuse, and use of systemic immunosuppressants. Management involves prompt surgical debridement with initiation of broad-spectrum antibiotics. Multiple debridements, orchiectomy, urinary diversion, and fecal diversion are performed as clinically indicated. HBO is used as adjuvant therapy, with considerable reduction in overall mortality. Although a grim prognosis usually accompanies the diagnosis, significant improvement is reported by combining traditional surgical and antibiotic regimens with HBO therapy.

Successful use of HBO in Fournier's gangrene has been reported in several studies. In some cases, the infection was progressive in spite of surgery and antibiotics, and was arrested only with the use of HBO treatment. It is concluded that HBO is very effective in the treatment of Fournier's gangrene (Ayan *et al* 2005).

Gas Gangrene

Gas gangrene is an acute painful necrotic condition of the soft tissues usually associated with trauma of surgery, but it may occur spontaneously. It is due to infection with various species of gas-forming anaerobic organisms and is also referred to as clostridial myonecrosis, and as *Gasödem* or *Gasbrand* in German. Although one-third of all wounds of violence are contaminated with such organisms, only 3% develop the clinical disease. The annual incidence in the USA is about 1000 cases.

Bacteriology and Pathogenesis

Clostridia are putrefactive, gram-positive, anaerobic, spore-forming, and encapsulated bacilli comprising more than 150 species. They are mostly soil contaminants but have also been isolated from the human gastrointestinal tract and the skin. *Clostridium welchii* was first recognized as a cause of gas gangrene by Welch in 1892. Subsequently renamed *C. perfringans*, this organism is implicated in 50%–100% of all cases of gas gangrene. Clostridia thrive in tissues that have low oxygen tensions as a result of trauma or ischemia. They release exotoxins that set a vicious circle in motion: there is tissue edema around the area of necrosis, which further diminishes the blood supply and oxygen tension and diminishes the numbers of leukocytes, leading to rapid spread of the necrotizing process. The patient may become moribund within 12 h and die.

Alpha-toxin, a C-lecithinase, is the major lethal toxin of *C. perfringans*; it precedes hemolysis and necrosis. It is stable under oxygen pressures of 2–3 ATA, although there is experimental evidence that further production of toxin is halted. Other toxins assist in destroying, liquefying, and dissecting the adjacent tissues with resulting rapid spread of the process. Some toxins affect vascular permeability and cause edema. The proteolytic and saccharolytic enzymes are responsible for the production of hydrogen sulfide. The toxins produce dysfunction of the brain, heart, and kidneys.

The local condition of the wound is far more important than the presence of clostridia and can be considered a deciding factor in the evolution of the infection and its clinical sequelae. Gas gangrene has been recorded after:

1. Soft tissue trauma
2. Foreign bodies, hemorrhage, or necrotic tissue in the wound
3. High velocity missile wounds
4. Compound fractures
5. Deep contamination of wounds
6. Prolonged delay in surgery
7. Traumatic or surgical interruption of blood supply
8. Careless abortion procedure
9. Too-tight plaster casts or dressings
10. Any kind of surgery
11. Other (often minor) injuries in the immune-compromised host.

Diagnosis

The clinical picture of gas gangrene is quite typical. There is a swollen wound with bronze, gray, or purple discoloration, bullae, and watery discharge (Figure 13.2). Pain is an early symptom. Crepitation is a late sign. Signs of systemic toxicity may be fever, tachycardia, and mental impairment. A gram stain of the wound is the most rapid method of

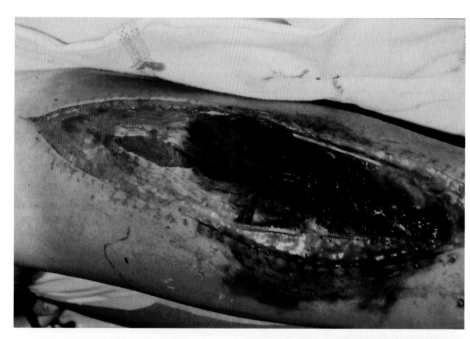

Figure 13.2
Photograph showing the appearance of gas gangrene (courtesy of Prof. D. Bakker, Amsterdam).

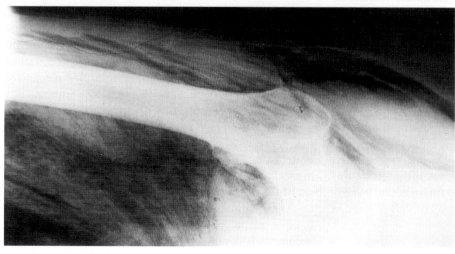

Figure 13.3
X-ray of the affected limb in gas gangrene showing the typical pattern of distribution of gas in the tissues.

Table 13.3
Classification of Clostridial Infections

Category	Type	Subtype	Examples
I	Clostridial myonecrosis (gas gangrene)	(a) Spreading (b) Diffuse	Crepitant: edematous Noncrepitant
II	Primary organ involvement		Uterus, gallbladder
III	Clostridial cellulitis	(a) Anaerobic toxemia (b) Localized	
IV	Clostridial contamination		

Table 13.4
Differential Diagnosis of Soft Tissue Gas

Bacterial		Nonbacterial
I	Aerobic aerogenic infections	Mechanical effect of trauma
	a) Hemolytic staphylococcal fascitis	Air hose injury, injection
	b) Hemolytic streptococcal gangrene	Hydrogen peroxide irrigation
	c) Coliform	Injection of benzine
II	Anaerobic streptococcal infections	Barotrauma; dysbarism
III	*Bacteroides* infections	Postoperative
IV	Clostridia	Aberrant sexual activity
V	Mixed aerobic and anaerobic infections	

diagnosis. Presence of gram-positive bacteria with the typical symptoms and signs should be considered a case of gas gangrene unless proven otherwise. Treatment should be initiated before confirmation by culture can be obtained, as this requires 48–72 h. A rapid method of diagnosis involves measurement of sialidase activity in the serum or the muscle tissue of the patient.

X-rays will not reveal gas consistently, and when present, gas is not pathognomonic of gas gangrene. Gas distribution in a feathery pattern indicating spread along muscle fasciculi, however, is pathognomonic (Figure 13.3). Large gas bubbles are usually associated with open wounds or necrotizing fasciitis. The classification of clostridial infections is presented in Table 13.3. This classification is used as a guide for initiating treatment: categories I and II require surgical treatment, whereas categories III and IV may be managed medically. Category III may progress to category II or I if not managed properly. The combination of gas in tissues and necrotizing myositis does not always mean gas gangrene. Differential diagnosis of soft tissue gas is given in Table 13.4.

The history and the findings on physical examination assist in diagnosis. Extensive gas in the tissues in the absence of systemic toxicity suggests gas-forming fasciitis.

Treatment of Gas Gangrene

The essentials of treatment of gas gangrene are:

- General supportive measures for seriously ill patients. The patients usually require intensive care. Tissue perfusion, oxygenation, and fluid as well as electrolyte balance have to be maintained. Blood transfusions may be necessary because of hemolysis caused by clostridia. HBO may be used at this stage for a patient who is too ill to undergo surgery. A few treatment sessions may stabilize the condition of the patient so surgery may be carried out.
- High doses of antibiotics. Penicillin is preferred but other antibiotics may be combined depending on the nature of the superimposed infections.
- Surgery. This has an important place in the management of gas gangrene. The main object is the removal of necrotic tissue and blood, because the erythrocytes containing catalase counteract the effect of HBO treatment.
- Hyperbaric oxygenation. This is a useful adjunct to surgery and antibiotics.

HBO in the Treatment of Gas Gangrene: Clinical Results

The action of HBO in clostridial and other anaerobic infections is based on the formation of free radicals and the lack of free radical degrading enzymes such as superoxide dismutase, catalase, and peroxidases.

Brummelkamp *et al* (1961) were the first to report the successful use of HBO at 3 ATA in the management of gas gangrene. The major benefit of HBO treatment in gas gangrene is the inhibition of toxin production, which stops at tissue oxygen tensions of 60 mmHg and above. HBO counteracts the hypoxic environments in which the clostridia thrive. Peroxidase develops within the organisms to inactivate or kill them, but the presence of catalase in muscle or blood inactivates the peroxidase. Hence the removal of necrotic tissue by surgery is essential for the proper effect of HBO. Tissue pO_2 levels of 250 mmHg are required for inhibition of clostridia.

It is doubtful whether the toxins already formed by the bacteria can be eliminated any faster with the help of HBO. The use of HBO can be a guide to the demarcation of the necrotic and the viable tissue after initial debridement. A more definite excision can be performed after HBO treatments. HBO has no effect on the necrotic tissue itself. Neither oxygen nor antibiotics can penetrate such tissue, which should be surgically removed. HBO treatment results in a marked increase in tissue oxygenation in both healthy tissue and in the vicinity of infected tissue. The hyperoxygenated tissue zone surrounding the infected area may be of significance in preventing the extension of invading microorganisms (Korhonen 2000).

For the initial management of gas gangrene the "Amsterdam therapeutic regimen." (Bakker 1988) is as follows. Before a patient suspected of gas gangrene is transferred to the hyperbaric unit, doctors from the referring hospital are advised to refrain from surgical intervention and to treat the patient with 1–2 million units of penicillin-G intravenously. Thereafter, the following protocol is carried out:

1. Wound inspection to evaluate the clinical picture, discoloration of skin, muscle necrosis, swelling of the infected area, discharge and smell from the wound, in order to ascertain whether gas gangrene is involved.
2. Removal of sutures and opening of the wound is performed in sutured postoperative or posttraumatic wounds. In cases of gas gangrene after injections or minor injuries, wounds are not surgically handled (i.e. no incision or excision).
3. Bacteriology, including a direct smear for gram stain, aerobic and anaerobic blood and wound cultures, and tissue specimens for histology. A gram stain with gram-positive clostridial rods supports the clinical diagnosis of gas gangrene, and HBO treatment is indicated. However, before the results of cultures are known, treatment is started because the alpha toxin production has to be stopped as quickly as possible.
4. Demarcation of the boundaries of discoloration and crepitance.
5. Blood sampling for laboratory investigation, including hemoglobin, hematocrit, leukocytes, electrolytes, kidney and liver function tests, arterial blood gases, etc.
6. Infusion therapy and treatment for shock as soon as the patient arrives in the hospital.
7. X-rays for signs of clostridial myositis.
8. Antibiotics (6 × 1 million units penicillin-G/day).
9. Chloral hydrate as a sedative (1 g rectally) has proved useful. Interaction of other sedatives, and their use under hyperbaric conditions has been outlined in Chapter 9.
10. Myringotomy performed in patients (small children, very old, and seriously ill patients) who are not capable of "clearing the ears," to equalize the pressure on both sides of the eardrum during treatment. Myringotomy is easily and quickly performed under local anesthesia and is virtually without complications. The opening in the eardrum remains competent during the 3 days of treatment. If, for other reasons, HBO treatment has to be continued, tympanotomy tubes are inserted.

The HBO pressures recommended for gas gangrene vary from 2.5 ATA to 3 ATA while breathing oxygen and the treatment sessions should last about 90 min. This usually leads to an oxygen partial pressure of 200 mmHg in the infected tissues. Frequency of the treatments should vary from three to four per 24 h during the first 48 h and then two treatment sessions daily until the infection is controlled. More than seven sessions in 3 days are seldom required.

The reported number of cases of gas gangrene where HBO treatment was used exceeds 2500. The true number is greater as HBO is an accepted mode of treatment for gas gangrene and many surgeons do not report such cases. With few exceptions, the reported results of HBO were favorable; details for some of the larger reported series are given in Table 13.5. Although there are no randomized trials of HBO in these infections, *in vitro* data and meta-analysis of clinical cases strongly support the use of HBO.

The emphasis should be on prophylaxis and prevention of gas gangrene by proper wound management. The use of gas gangrene antitoxins is obsolete. Patients with trauma and overwhelming infection should be transferred to a major trauma center with hyperbaric facilities (Hitchcock 1987). HBO should be used early, but it is worth a try even at a later stage before any ablative surgery of the limbs is undertaken.

Fungal Infection

Actinomycosis

Actinomycosis is an anaerobic infection with four clinical forms: cervicofacial, thoracic, abdominal-pelvic, and disseminated. The cervicofacial form responds well to antibiotic treatment; the other forms often require surgical procedures. Due to low tissue oxygen levels, the prognosis for

Table 13.5
Results in Some Large Series of Cases of Gas Gangrene Where HBO Was Used as an Adjunctive Therapy

Authors and year	Cases	Survival	Remarks
Hart *et al* (1983)	139	70	Limb salvage rate 80%
Tirpitz (1986)	480		Survival rate increased to 90% with use of IgG therapy
Bakker (1988)	409	79.5	Amputation rate only 8.7% after
Hirn and Niinikoski (1988)	32	72.9	All patients who died had been transferred from other hospitals in moribund condition
De Sola (1990)	85	80	Multicenter study. Outcome was satisfactory in 67.1% of survivors
Korhonen et al (1999)	53	77.4%	Conclusion was that patient survival can be improved if the disease is recognized early and appropriate therapy applied promptly

cure is low. An increase in the oxygen tension with subsequent oxygen radical formation is lethal for the actinomycosis organisms. HBO is recommended as an adjunct to surgical care and antimicrobial therapy.

Mucormycosis

Mucormycosis is a devastating fungal disease that occurs most commonly in immune-suppressed patients who have burns, who are on long-term corticosteroid therapy, or who present with diabetic acidosis. The major location of the infection is the rhinocerebral area, lungs, and intestine. The mortality rate prior to the advent of amphotericin B (AMB) was 70%, but this decreased to 40% with the use of AMB. Mucormycosis has been reported in patients who undergo multiple bone marrow transplant for thalassemia and are in advanced phase of disease with severe acquired hemochromatosis. HBO is used in fulminating mucormycosis on the following theoretical basis:

- To provide oxygen to the tissues distal to the occluded vessels in order to achieve local tissue survival
- To reduce acidosis
- To exercise a fungicidal effect

Rhinocerebral mucormycosis. The disease is fatal when cerebral extension occurs. The mainstay of the treatment is surgery, AMB, and eradication of the underlying cause. Several cases of rhinocerebral mucormycosis in immunocmpromised states and patients with diabetes mellitus as a predisposing cause. Progressive loss of vision may occur in rhino-orbital-cerebral mucormycosis and CT-imaging reveals bony defects in sinus borders to orbits or endocranium. Immediate diagnosis and therapy are essential. Radical procedures like orbital exenteration must be considered in all cases Therapeutic success can be achieved due to advances in antimicrobial therapy, HBO and treatment of the underlying disease (Arndt *et al* 2008).

HBO treatment has been used for patients with brain abscesses, secondary to mucormycosis where the disease progresses despite aggressive debridement, surgery, and AMB therapy.

Candida Albicans

Effect of HBO treatment and antifungal agents on *Candida albicans* has been examined *in vitro*. There was no response to increased atmospheric pressure alone, but addition of 100% oxygen under pressure led to growth inhibition of pO_2 of 900 mmHg and killing of organisms at a pO_2 value of 1800 mmHg. Clinical use of HBO for this infection and a study of the interaction of HBO with antifungal agents has been suggested by but not tested clinically.

Nocardia Asteroides

This opportunistic infection occurs in patients receiving chemotherapy. Patients with *Nocardia asteroides* abscesses respond dramatically to HBO therapy.

Phycomycotic Fungal Infections

Necrotizing fasciitis can occur in the extremities due to invasive phycomycotic fungal infection. A standard HBO gas gangrene protocol can be used to stop the progression of the fungal infection.

HBO in the Management of AIDS

Currently this viral infection is receiving much attention and no cure for it has been found, although combination chemotherapy can keep the infection under control for long periods. In 1987, I suggested the use of HBO as a supplement to chemotherapy for the following reasons:

- Free radicals generated by HBO and accelerated by mild hyperthermia (38.5° C) can penetrate the lipid covering of the virus, particularly before its entry into the monocytes (free form) and after its entry into the brain after crossing the blood-brain barrier, whence it may be released from the monocytes and attack the neurons. The toxic effects of free radicals on the normal cells of the body can be blocked by the use of Mg^{2+}, a cell membrane protector (see Chapter 6).
- HBO increases the production of reactive oxygen intermediates (ROIs), responsible for producing cellular oxidative stress (and their enhancement or diminution of viral replication). ROIs are virucidal against enveloped-viruses such as HIV (Baugh 2000).
- HBO treatment has been shown to be effective against opportunistic infections found in AIDS (Holmes & Gargas 1987).
- HBO pressures up to 2.5 ATA have an immune-stimulating effect and bring about an increase in the number of lymphocytes.

The limitation of this therapy is that very little of the virus is found in a free form in the body, where it would be susceptible to the effect of free radicals. It is difficult to eradicate the virus entrenched in tissue cells without killing the cells. However, it is conceivable that HBO treatment in conjunction with drug therapy may reduce AIDS encephalopathy.

Reillo and Altieri (1996) have reported on results of *ex vivo* and *in vivo* quantitative assays on HIV-infected plasma and peripheral blood mononuclear cells (PBMCs) at baseline and after treatment. The authors also HBO-treated uninfected PBMCs and then exposed them to HIV at ambient pressure. HIV viral load was decreased in the infected cells, and few viruses entered uninfected PBMCs exposed to HBO. The results of this study were used to support the theory that HBO has an antiviral effect but these observations have not been reproduced by other authors.

During the past few years, over 300 hundred AIDS patients have been treated with HBO (Reillo 1997).

Concluding remarks. There is no doubt that HBO helps the secondary infections in AIDS patients and thus improves their condition and reduces the mortality. However, the direct effect in eradicating AIDS remains to be proven. At present, very many potent and effective chemotherapeutic agents are available for treating these patients and molecular diagnostics can enable viral loads to be estimated. Any HBO claims have to tested against other drug regimens as controls. The problem may be denying effective drugs to AIDS patients. HBO has a definite place as an adjunct to antimicrobial drugs for treatment of secondary infections in AIDS patients but claims of a direct anti-HIV effect will have to be verified by researchers in this field.

Miscellaneous Infections

Leprosy (Hansen's Disease)

Leprosy is a chronic infectious disease caused by *Mycobacterium leprae*. It principally affects the peripheral nerves and skin. The spinal cord and brain are not involved.

Leprosy is prevalent in tropical countries and the total number of leprosy patients in the world is estimated to be 12 million. Effective chemotherapy was introduced only in the 1950s and the number of patients currently under treatment remains less than 33%. Endemic foci of the disease are found in the USA, where the number of leprosy sufferers is estimated to be about 5000; they are mainly refugees from the Far East and South America.

The pathology, clinical features, and treatment of leprosy have been reviewed by Yawalkar (2002). Effective chemotherapy is available in the form of dapsone, rifampicin, and clofazamine. Leprosy can be definitely controlled by the judicious use of these drugs, individually or in combination to overcome drug resistance. Duration of therapy ranges from 6 months to 2 years or until negative skin smears are obtained. Cell-mediated immunity to *Mycobacterium leprae* is impaired in patients with leprosy, but there is no generalized immune deficiency. The procedures for immune therapy with significant long-term effects are still under development. A vaccine may prevent new cases; however, eradication of leprosy and rehabilitation of the patients is still a tremendous problem.

Role of HBO in Leprosy

Ozorio de Almeida and Costa (1938) of Brazil were the first to report the use of HBO therapy in conjunction with methylene blue in the treatment of leprosy. They treated nine patients using a variety of oxygen regimens for a total treatment duration of 10 h (in several sessions), using pressures from 3 ATA to 3.5 ATA. Posttreatment changes consisted of a marked decrease of skin infiltration, disappearance of tubercles, and generalized improvement in the condition of the patients. In six of the nine cases, the bacilli disappeared completely from the lesions. This report is of interest for several reasons:

- Hyperbaric air had been used previously for the treatment of tuberculosis, but this is the first recorded use of HBO for an infectious disease.
- No effective chemotherapy for leprosy was available in 1938. The rationale for using methylene blue was that, since this substance stains the tissues, it must fix the organisms for exposure to oxygen.
- The object of the treatment was to expose the organisms to oxygen. This was in line with the thinking of the time when tuberculosis patients were exposed to fresh air and oxygen inhalation.

Gottlieb (1963), in the USA, unaware of the work in Brazil, also suggested the use of HBO in leprosy. Wilkinson *et al* (1970) treated 50 patients suffering from leprosy, each with four sessions of HBO at 3 ATA for 30 min. The interval between the first and the second treatment was 24 h; that between the second and third was 30 days. All the 45 patients available for evaluation improved; definite improvement was observed in 51.11%, moderate improvement in 40%, and slight improvement in 8.88%. Wilkinson's colleague Rosasco (1974) reported the results of 200 cases of leprosy treated with HBO at 3 ATA for 60 min twice daily for 3 consecutive days. Chemotherapy was stopped during this period and not resumed. Ten patients were available for follow-up examination 5 years later and showed no sign of recurrence of the disease. This is a very small percentage of the original number of patients and therefore has no statistical significance. It is difficult to explain why there was no further work on this subject for 30 years, following the original observation of the effectiveness of HBO treatment in leprosy in 1938.

Mokashi *et al* (1979, personal communication), of Bombay, reported on a controlled study of the effect of HBO in drug-resistant intractable leprosy. Twenty such patients were divided into two groups of ten each. Drug therapy was stopped and one group was treated with HBO at 2.5 ATA (1 h twice daily) for 3 days while the other group served as a control. These patients were followed for one year by periodic biopsy and smear examinations. The biopsy specimens of the patients treated with HBO became negative after 8 months, whereas there were no changes in the lesions of the patients not exposed to HBO.

Youngblood (1984) devised a protocol for investigation of the effect of HBO on leprosy that included the following:

- Pretreatment biopsy of the lesion and inoculation into the mouse footpad model.
- Repetition of (1) after 5 days of HBO treatment at 3 ATA (1-h session twice daily).
- Microscopic examination of the pre- and post-HBO inoculated footpads and comparison of the viability, morphology, and the relative number of bacteria in the treated group with those in the untreated controls. Only one patient was reported to have been treated according to this protocol and was shown to have improved clinically; no further information was published on this project.

In conclusion it can be stated that no definitive study of the effect of HBO on leprosy has been carried out. There is need for such a study. The adjunctive role of HBO in the drug treatment of leprosy should be considered in the following situations:

- Patients who are severely anemic and have to wait until their blood hemoglobin levels improve before chemotherapy is started
- In drug-resistant cases with drug toxicity
- In patients with ulcers and those who require surgery.

There is good evidence that HBO helps in wound-healing and shortens the recovery period after plastic surgery (see Chapters 15 and 28).

It is doubtful whether enough HBO facilities can be provided on a scale large enough to deal with this problem for millions of patients in underdeveloped countries.

Nosocomial Infections

These are infections acquired in hospital. About 80% of nosocomial infections are caused by aerobic bacteria. The *Pseudomonas aeruginosa* is a Gram-negative bacterium pertaining to the Pseudomonadaceae family. *P. aeruginosa* is responsible for 6–22% of all hospital infections. Marmo *et al* (1986) have evaluated the efficacy of HBO alone at 2 ATA for 35 min/day alone for 8 days as well as in combination with antibiotic therapy (amikacine 15 mg/kg/day for 8 days intraperitoneal), in rats infected via pulmonary and subcutaneous routes. In rats affected by *P. aeruginosa*, HBO induces a significant reduction in mortality and morbidity with eradication of bacteria in blood cultures, bronchial aspirate and skin biopsies. These effects were enhanced by the use of amikacine – an antibiotic used for the treatment of Gram-negative bacteria. HBO is worth a clinical trial for nosocomial infections.

Tuberculosis

It has been shown experimentally that HBO inhibits the growth of *Mycobacterium tuberculosis* and has a synergistic action with the antitubercular drugs isoniazid, P-aminosalicylic acid, and streptomycin (Gottlieb 1970). There is not much interest in clinical uses of HBO in tuberculosis, perhaps because the current drug therapy is adequate. HBO may, however, be considered for drug-resistant organisms.

Osteomyelitis

Osteomyelitis is an inflammatory process with bacterial infection involving the bone. Additionally, ischemia as well as hypoxia are present in the infected bone tissue. The condition may be acute, subacute, or chronic. Chronic osteomyelitis is defined as bone infection that persists beyond 6 months with exposed bone and drainage, histological or radiological evidence of infection, or a positive bone culture. The term "refractory osteomyelitis" refers to those cases that fail to heal in spite of surgical and antibiotic therapy. The basic principles of management of osteomyelitis are as follows:

- Surgery:
  (a) drainage of abscess;
  (b) removal of foreign bodies;
  (c) debridement of sequestrum;
  (d) removal of barrier to normal vascularization; and
  (e) obliteration of dead spaces as a result of debridement.

- Antibiotics:
  appropriate antibiotics at optimal dosage to be administered for an adequate length of time.

The optimal surgical objectives are not always achievable, and this is one of the common causes of refractory osteomyelitis. Surgical treatment is effective in 70%–80% of chronic osteomyelitis cases. (This does not include cases that are denied surgery because of poor prognosis.) One does not know how many of the remaining 20%–30% would benefit from HBO therapy. The role of HBO in the management of refractory osteomyelitis is shown in Figure 13.4.

HBO Treatment of Osteomyelitis

Osteomyelitis is a hypoxic condition as shown by intramedullary pO_2 measurements, which usually give values below 30 mmHg. There are three possible causes of the hypoxia:

- Oxygen consumption by the microorganisms
- Oxygen consumption by inflammatory cells
- Interference with local perfusion due to tissue edema.

REFRACTORY OSTEOMYELITIS

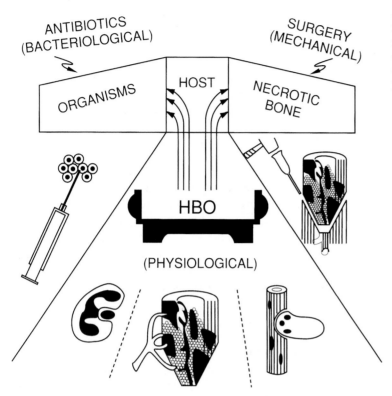

Figure 13.4
Although antibiotics will help kill microorganisms in the nonossified tissues around the focus of infection and surgery will remove the macroscopic portions of dead, infected bone, HBO improves host responsiveness by making the environments more favorable to WBC oxidative killing, neovascularization, and resorption of dead, infected bone (reproduced from Strauss 1987, by permission).

The possible mechanisms of action of HBO in osteomyelitis are:

1. HBO can raise the tissue oxygen tension in partially ischemic, hypoxic tissues.
2. HBO, by providing adequate oxygen, enhances the leukocyte killing mechanisms that are oxygen-dependent through hydrogen peroxide and superoxide production. HBO, by itself, has been shown to be as effective as cephalosporins in controlling staphylococcal osteomyelitis in the animal model.
3. Optimal wound pO_2 can enhance osteogenesis or neovascularization to fill the dead space with vascular or structurally sound bony tissue. Improved vascularity facilitates entry of leukocytes, antibodies, and antibiotics to the infective focus.
4. HBO enhances osteoclastic activity to remove bony debris.
5. The effectiveness of HBO in osteomyelitis may be due to the enhancement of host factors rather than to a direct effect on microorganisms causing the disease. Oxygen tensions in the infected tissues cannot always be raised to levels considered high enough to be directly toxic to the microorganisms.

The direct effect of HBO on bacteria is not important in osteomyelitis. The optimal pO_2 for these effects should be maintained at 100 mmHg. Hamblin (1968) determined the effect of intermittent HBO on experimental staphylococcal osteomyelitis in rats. Osteomyelitis was established (21 days) with discharging sinuses or abscesses and confirmed radiologically. This was a controlled study and no animal received antibiotics or surgery. The treatment was given for 21 days and the treated animals were divided into groups according to the pressures of oxygen used. The best results were obtained in the group treated with HBO at 2 ATA for 2 h 3 times a day. Since HBO given prophylactically did not prevent the development of infections, it was concluded that the effectiveness of HBO on established osteomyelitis is due to the enhancement of host defenses and not to a direct effect on the organisms.

Esterhai *et al* (1986) studied the effect on the intramedullary tension of 100% oxygen exposure at 1, 2, 3, and 4 atm pressure in rabbits with chronic right tibial osteomyelitis. The oxygen tensions were measured polarographically through implanted electrodes. The tension in the left tibia (normal, control) was low (below 30 mmHg), and the infected side still lower. It rose in response to HBO on both sides but returned to baseline in 15 min after cessation of therapy.

Mendel *et al* (1999) studied staphylococcal osteomyelitis using a rat tibia model to compare the effect of the following three modalities of treatment:

- HBO alone
- Antibiotic cefazolin
- HBO and cefazolin.

The infection rate in this model was 96% and mortality was 0%. HBO was found to be effective in that the number of colony forming bacteria (CFB) per gram decreased from 106 to 105. Animals receiving cefazolin had a mean CFB count of 104. The best results were obtained in animals treated by a combination of HBO and cefazolin but bone sterilization was never recorded.

Clinical Results of HBO Treatment in Osteomyelitis

Clinical results of the treatment of chronic osteomyelitis are shown in Table 13.6.

There are many other reports of improvement of chronic osteomyelitis with HBO therapy, but there are no controlled studies. All the studies emphasize the important role of good surgical and antibiotic management and point out that HBO is not a substitute but a supplement to these treatments. The overall success rate in various studies ranges from 60% to 85%. These are good results if one considers the severe nature of the cases treated with HBO. In some cases the alternative to HBO was amputation of the involved extremity.

HBO plays a vital role in treatment of osteomyelitis of the skull and the spine. In the latter the involved bone cannot be removed entirely.

In two identical publications, Esterhai *et al* (1987 1988) have reported no benefit of HBO treatment in their patients with chronic refractory osteomyelitis. This is the only reported study with negative effects of HBO in osteomyelitis.

Osteomyelitis of the Jaw

Osteomyelitis of the mandible is usually due to untreated odontogenic infections, postextraction complications, and untreated or poorly managed mandibular fractures. Because the mandible receives less blood than the maxilla it is more susceptible to infections. Nevertheless, the prognosis for osteomyelitis of the jaw is better than for osteomyelitis of the long bones. The reasons for this are the jaw's easy accessibility for debridement and its proximity to a richly vascular area with collateral circulatory pathways. The usual organisms found are:

- *Actinomyces israelii*, an obligatory anaerobe
- *Eikenella corrodens*
- *Bacteroides fragilis*
- *Staphylococcus aureus*.

Treatment of osteomyelitis of the jaw should include the following measures:

1. Removal of the source of infection; tooth extraction or root canal therapy
2. Debridement of necrotic tissue
3. Staining and culture of the infected tissue
4. Insertion of drains and irrigation with Dakin's solution
5. Immobilization; use of fixation pins if necessary
6. Antibiotic therapy.

Most cases of osteomyelitis of the jaw respond to appropriate debridement and antibiotic therapy, but some are refractory to all the measures outlined above. HBO treatment is indicated in these cases. There are few published reports of large series of patients of this type treated by HBO. Although successful treatment of patients with suppurative osteomyelitis of the jaw by surgery and antibiotics without HBO has been reported, it is difficult to eradicate diffuse sclerosing osteomyelitis, which is characterized by recur-

Table 13.6
Clinical Results of Treatment of Chronic Osteomyelitis with HBO

Authors and year	Cases	Pressure	Results and comments
Slack *et al* (1966)	5	2 ATA	Successful. Organisms included Staphylococcus pyogenes and Proteus vulgaris
Davis (1977)	98	2 ATA	Disease process arrested in 50% and remained so at 5-year follow-up
Eltorai *et al* (1984)	40[1]	2 ATA[2]	30 patients (68%) were cured
Sheftel *et al* (1985)	5		Methicillin resistant staphylococcal osteomyelitis. 5 of 7 episodes were arrested in these patients by a combination of surgery, antibiotics and HBO
Moorey *et al* (1979)	40		Cure rate at 2-year follow-up was 85%. HBO used as an adjunct to surgery and antibiotics
Davis *et al* (1986)	38	2 ATA[3]	34 (89.5%) of these patients became free from clinical signs of osteomyelitis for 34 months. HBO plus wound debridement plus antibiotics

[1]spine, ischia, hips sacrum and calcaneus, [2]average 50 sessions, [3]48 daily HBO sessions

rent episodes of swelling, pain, and trismus, without abscess formation or discharge. Clinical trial of conventional therapy and of additional HBO treatments have shown that patients for whom additional HBO was used were fully relieved of symptoms, whereas those treated without HBO continued to have further minor recurrences. Adjuvant HBO is successful in the treatment of patients with chronic recurrent osteomyelitis of the mandiblend is an treatment option which can avoid ablative surgery in some cases (Handschel *et al* 2007).

Osteomyelitis of the Sternum

HBO has been used with good results in the treatment of chronic sternal osteomyelitis. Infectious sternal dehiscence is a serious complication after open heart surgery. Stassano *et al* (1989) treated 7 patients with infected sternal wounds by a combination of surgical debridement, antiseptic irrigation, antibiotics and HBO (2.8 ATA). All the infected sternal dehiscences resolved.

Malignant Otitis Externa

This syndrome was first described by Chandler (1968) and consists of an antibiotic resistant *Pseudomonas aeruginosa* infection of the external auditory meatus with osteomyelitis of the temporal bone. It usually affects patients with long-standing diabetes mellitus and a weakened immune system. Over 120 cases have been described in the literature. The overall mortality is 35%.

Spread of infection beyond the external auditory meatus can produce lethal invasive osteomyelitis. Such patients should be investigated by using radiological procedures such as tomography of the temporal bone and intensive management with antibiotics, surgery, and HBO is recommended. The multimodal treatment approach of malignant otitis externa by surgical debridement, combinations of antibiotics, specific immunoglobulins, and adjunctive HBO has proved to be highly effective in improving the survival and quality of life of the patients s justifies the high costs that this therapy may involve (Tisch & Maier 2006).

14 HBO Therapy in Chronic Lyme Disease

William P. Fife and Caroline E. Fife

Some Lyme disease patients fail to respond to antibiotic therapy. The possible role of HBO and its rationale in chronic Lyme disease are discussed in the following sections:

Introduction

Lyme disease and its longer-term sequitur, chronic Lyme disease, is one of the most challenging arthropod-borne infectious diseases to diagnose, study, and treat. Although named after the town in Southwest Connecticut in the United States where epidemiological cluster investigations were performed in the mid 1970s, the European medical literature predating this period suggests there was considerable knowledge of this disease prior to this date.

In Europe and the United States, the disease is caused by the spirochete *Borrelia burgdorferi*, although several other *Borrelia* species have been identified as causative organisms in various parts of the world (Krupka *et al* 2007). The spirochete is primarily tick-borne, the most common vector being the *Ixodes* genus, although its presence in mosquito genera has also been reported (Halouzka *et al* 1999; Zakovská *et al* 2002). In the United States, 23,000 individuals were bitten by *Borrelia*-infected *Ixodes* ticks in 2005, which makes Lyme disease the most common arthropod-borne infectious disease in that country (Centers for Disease Control and Prevention [CDC], 2007).

Following the tick bite, an erythema migrans or "bull's-eye" rash typically develops several days or weeks later, which is capable of expanding until it can measure 30 cm across. An array of flu-like symptoms appears weeks to months thereafter, the most common of which are joint swellings akin to arthritis. Unfortunately, as many as half of bitten individuals do not notice the bite, and the rash itself may not appear bull's-eye-shaped, nor appear at all in many cases (Edlow 2002; Stricker & Phillips 2003).

Although diagnostic tests are very specific (99%–100%), and thus good for surveillance, they have relatively poor sensitivity (50%–75%) (Stricker 2007); thus, diagnosis is made clinically. CDC recommends a 2-tiered approach of ELISA or immunofluorescence as a screening test, followed by Western blotting for confirmation if the test is positive.

Prompt treatment with 14 to 30-day courses of antibiotics cures the infection in 80%-90% of infected individuals (Marques 2008; Smith *et al* 2002). The most appropriate choices are doxycycline or ceftriaxone for adults and amoxicillin for children, although it should be stressed that other antibiotics may be better suited to different *Borrelia* species. Our knowledge of the efficacy of antibiotic treatment is far from adequate (Dinser *et al* 2005; Smith *et al* 2002).

Chronic Lyme Disease

Despite antibiotic therapy, a minority of patients do not respond or continue to report ongoing symptoms, such as fatigue, myalgia, arthralgias, sleep disturbances, cognitive disorders, and depression (Marques 2008), and herein lies a controversy. One school of thought, endorsed by the Infectious Diseases Society of America (IDSA) (Wormser *et al* 2006), maintains that in patients properly treated with antibiotics, such symptoms are not caused by the persistence of the organism, but are due to the presence of pre-existing conditions, such as fibromyalgia or chronic fatigue syndrome, or the presence of chronic inflammatory states induced by the *Borrelia* species. On the other hand, other researchers and clinicians believe that the problems stemming from chronic Lyme disease are caused by *Borrelia* species that continue to evade the immune system by a variety of mechanisms (Stricker 2007). This view is endorsed by the International Lyme and Associated Diseases Society. The controversy is fueled in part by the extraordinary defensive capabilities of the *Borrelia* species, which include immunosuppression factors, genetic, phase, and antigenic variation, physical seclusion in various intracellular and extracellular sites, and secreted factors whose actions range from damaging cartilage (Behera *et al* 2006) to autoresuscitation, a faculty similar to the tubercle bacillus (Chan & Flynn 2004; Von Lackum *et al* 2006). Given that *B burgdorferi* has some 1500 genes sequences, at least 132 functioning genes, and 21 plasmids (the record-holder for bacteria) (Stricker 2007), that complications should arise from infection should be no surprise.

As a result of the Connecticut Attorney General's recent antitrust investigation of chronic Lyme disease, the ISDA has agreed to review its disease-specific guidelines (Associated Press 2008). At the heart of this controversy are two issues: (a) acknowledgment that persistent or "silent" infection is possible, and (b) a determination whether longer-term antibiotic treatment is appropriate in such cases. While there is certainly some evidence that the former is true (Stricker 2007), the latter issue is more problematic. To date, there have been 4 double-blinded, placebo-controlled randomized controlled trials (RCTs) of antibiotic therapy in individuals with chronic Lyme disease (Fallon *et al* 2007; Klempner *et al* 2001; Krupp *et al* 2003). Unfortunately, no trial has demonstrated a sustained improved benefit; moreover, potentially serious adverse events have occurred (Marques 2008). The real issue here is determining whether these represent true treatment failures. Some researchers have argued that the treatment regimen of the three earlier trials (the report of the Klempner *et al* trial actually contained the results of two RCTs) (Klempner *et al* 2001; Krupp *et al* 2003) was too short (1 month of intravenous ceftriaxone, and 1 month of intravenous ceftriaxone followed by 2 months of oral doxycycline) for patients who have had the condition for an average of 4–5 years (Bransfield *et al* 2001; Cameron 2006). In addition, Cameron (2006) persuasively argued that the exclusion criteria in these trials precluded results that could be generalized to the population with chronic Lyme disease. The most recent RCT, which employed 10 weeks of intravenous ceftriaxone in the treatment arm, also showed no sustained improvement in cognitive impairment.

Although one can certainly make the case that there might have been design flaws in all of these trials, at the same time, the strong possibility must be faced that long-term antibiotic treatment may not provide any benefit. Since chronic Lyme disease patients constitute the group in which delayed treatment occurs or initial treatment fails, they must represent patients in which the spirochete becomes more entrenched, there is more severe immunosuppression, or imbalances in cytokine signaling leading to chronic inflammation are more pronounced. Furthermore, the organisms in these cases could have become antibiotic-resistant or simply inaccessible to the antibiotic. All of these unsolved issues demand a different approach to treating chronic Lyme disease, whether one believes the organism is capable of persistent infection or not.

Rationale for Using Hyperbaric Oxygen Therapy

The effects of oxygen on *B Burgdoferi* were demonstrated by the work of Austin (1993), who showed that *in vitro* cultures in which oxygen and carbon dioxide were ambient (PO_2 = 160 mm Hg), there was a loss of infectivity. Conversely, if the organism was cultured in 4% O_2/5% CO_2, (PO_2 = 30 mm Hg), the infectivity remained viable. Since under normal conditions the partial pressure of oxygen at the tissue level is only approximately 30 mm Hg, it would appear doubtful that the organism could be suppressed while the host was breathing air. These findings suggest that the organism may be sensitive to elevated tissue oxygen levels, which can be achieved by hyperbaric oxygen therapy. Furthermore, it is well known that neutrophil function is inhibited at low tissue oxygen levels, due to the suppression of the oxidative burst phenomenon, the rapid production of reactive oxygen species in response to a pathogenic invasion (Allen *et al* 1997). Thus, elevating tissue oxygen levels has been shown to enhance neutrophil killing in osteomyelitic bone (Mader *et al* 1978).

Breathing pure oxygen at a barometric pressure of 2.36 ATA, the inspired PO_2 will be 1,794 mm Hg, and the tissue oxygen approximately 300 mm Hg. This increase in tissue PO_2, which may be inhibitory to the spirochete, together with a possible increase in leukocyte effectiveness, suggests the possibility that therapy may either destroy *B burgdorferi* or enhance its response to antimicrobials.

Pilot Program at Texas A&M University

A pilot program to assess the possible benefit of HBO in mitigating chronic Lyme symptoms was carried out at Texas A&M University and was approved by the Institutional Review Board. It was initiated in the 1990s and lasted 6 years. Potential subjects were referred by physicians who were experienced in the treatment of Lyme disease. All subjects presented with a positive diagnosis of Lyme according to the CDC criteria. All had failed intravenous antibiotics and many were continuing to deteriorate even though still on various antibiotics. Some patients were wheelchair-bound due to arthritis, one was semicomatose, and several were children. Those already on antibiotics (67%) continued with their pre-HBO regimen while treatments were in progress.

Subjects were educated regarding the risks of HBO and signed an informed consent. All were treated at 2.36 ATA in a multiplace hyperbaric chamber compressed with air, and provided with 100% oxygen via a standard plastic "head tent." Treatments were 60 minutes in duration and were administered twice a day for five consecutive days, followed by a two day period of rest. From 10 to 30 treatments were delivered followed by a re-assessment. One subject received 145 treatments over 3 months.

Ninety-one subjects completed a total of 1,995 HBO (average 21.9 treatments per patient). Subject evaluation was carried out by an abbreviated questionnaire derived from an evaluation used by several Lyme specialists. This questionnaire was designed so that zero reflected no symptoms and ten reflected severe symptoms. Using the questionnaire, 84.8% of treated patients showed significant improvement based on a decrease or elimination of symptoms. Eleven subjects (12%) claimed no benefit. Prior to treatment, subjects had an average score of 114.12 (of a possible 270), and following treatment, an average of 49.27 (p = 0.000). The standard deviation of scores was 56.00 prior to treatment and 44.14 after treatment (p = 0.057 by Fisher's F-test). Further, 58% of subjects reduced their score b y 41.86 points or more.

All but one of 91 subjects developed severe Jarisch-Herxheimer (JH) reaction, similar to the effect of aggressive and extensive antibiotic treatment, within approximately 3 days of HBO initiation (Pound & May 2005). This was manifested by myalgias, chills, and a low-grade temperature. Typically the reaction abated after 2–3 weeks, although in many cases the reaction continued throughout the series of treatments. After discontinuation of HBO, many subjects continued to show improvement for up to 8 months.

Follow-up (from 6 years to 6 weeks) showed that the benefit was sustained in approximately 70% of patients. Many patients claimed improved cognitive abilities including improved concentration; others who had depression reported much improvement or disappearance of this symptom. No adverse events were reported. The details of three cases are reported below as typical examples.

Case Examples

Case 1

A female, age 40, married with 2 children: At age 19, she began to have constant pain in the right hip and knee that gradually expanded to other areas. She lived in a Lyme disease-infested area but denied any tick bite or bull's-eye rash. At age 26 she was diagnosed with "non-convulsive epilepsy and migraine headaches," and was placed on Tegretol without benefit. At age 35 she was diagnosed with Lyme disease and treated initially with clarithromycin, followed by cefixime without improvement. Later she was placed on intravenous ceftriaxone for 45 days, also without benefit. In 1996, amoxicillin and probenicid were started, followed by sodium divalproex, clonazepam, cefotaxime, and imipenem-cilastatin. Except for intravenous imipenem-cilastatin, all other drugs were terminated due to lack of benefit. Her IGM demonstrated three positive bands for Lyme disease. At presentation she was chronically fatigued, unable to walk more than a few feet, described constant joint pain, and had serious cognitive difficulties as well as suicidal ideation.

This subject underwent 32 HBO over a 3-week period, during which she experienced a severe JH reaction. At the end of the treatment series she still suffered from considerable joint pain and felt there had been little benefit from the treatments. However, 2 months after finishing HBO she noted improved walking distance and improved cognitive function. She discontinued all antibiotics and noted continued improvement such that five months post-HBO she was able to do family shopping and resume many normal social activities.

Case 2

A 39-year-old female, who suffered from Lyme disease for 6 years, presented with neurological symptoms including partial loss of vision in her left eye, paresthesia on the left side, generalize fatigue, and reduced mental alertness. Additional symptoms included joint stiffness, muscle pain, and weakness of the left leg. Her serum, tested by Western blot, was equivocal for IgM.

No change was noticed after the first two HBO treatments. After the third treatment she felt extremely fatigued, likening it to her previous JH reaction to antibiotics. After the 4th and 5th HBO treatments she noticed a tingling in her left foot. After subsequent treatments she noted improved energy and decreased pain in the left foot as well as resolution of leg weakness. Four months after completing HBO she terminated antibiotic use. Five months after HBO she felt well with only occasional "down days."

Case 3

A 16-year-old female had been diagnosed with Lyme disease 3 years prior to start of HBO therapy, although her medical records suggested recurring symptoms for 10 years or more. While there was no history of a bull's-eye rash or tick bite, she lived in a Lyme disease-endemic area, and received aggressive long-term antibiotic treatment with some short-term cessation of symptoms, which included fatigue, joint and muscle pain, mood swings, weight gain and loss, insomnia, encephalopathy, short-term memory problems, and headaches. These symptoms were aggravated by stress and she had been removed from high school. Her Western blot was equivocal. She was due to enter college but did not feel that her memory and physical health would allow her to compete academically. At the time of evaluation, all antibiotics had been discontinued due to severe adverse reactions.

After the third HBO treatment she complained of fever and headache akin to the JH reaction she had once experienced with antibiotics. After 4–5 treatments, her ability to read and comprehend without losing concentration increased from 30 minutes to 3 hours. Five months after cessation of treatment she continued to improve and became an honors student in college.

Implications for Treatment

One of the challenging aspects of treating Lyme disease is to know if the organism has been truly eradicated. There are instances in which Western blot positive bands appear and disappear as the disease progresses, and bands may persist for a year or more after the signs and symptoms of the disease appear to have resolved. The paradox of a positive clinical diagnosis of Lyme in the presence of negative serology has been studied by Schutzer and his associates (1990), who found that in some instances the sequestration of antibodies in immune complexes prevented their appearance in the Western blot bands. They showed that although the patient was seronegative, Lyme antibodies actually were present and could be dissociated by a modified polyethylene glycol precipitation from their immune complex into components that then could be demonstrated by Western blot. For these reasons, objective serological tests must be considered unreliable, and we may have to depend more upon clinical symptomology as an endpoint.

Although the appearance of the JH reaction in virtually all patients may indicate that a competent immunological assault against the *Borralia* spirochete did occur, this in itself is not diagnostic of eradication, since several patients had experienced such reactions during previous antibiotic treatment that evidently failed to effect a cure. Nevertheless, two patients who were retested 2 months after completing the HBO treatment, were both serologically negative for Lyme disease and one had been free of symptoms or need for medication for 6 years. On the other hand, a few subjects still had some symptoms persisting after 5 months, although the symptoms appeared to be much diminished, by both verbal report and questionnaire results. In some instances, little benefit was subjectively noted until 1–3 weeks after the treatments ended. While we do not completely understand the reasons for such a delay, it could be that such a time is required to reduce chronic inflammation and cytokine hyperactivity to more normal levels.

The question concerning the presence of confusing clinical depression with Lyme disease needs to be considered. Some of Lyme disease patients manifested depression, but it usually appeared after they failed to respond to all of the treatment modalities in the armamentarium of current medical practice, raising the possibility that depression was a response to prior failed treatments rather than part of the neurological problems caused by chronic Lyme disease. Depression, along with the other symptoms, resolved after conclusion of HBO therapy.

Can the spirochete be transferred to the fetus if the mother is infected during pregnancy? MacDonald (1989) demonstrated that even if the mother is seronegative, the fetus can still be infected with *Borrelia* spirochetes, sometimes with severe consequences. Although more recent literature reviews suggest this is an uncommon event (Walsh *et al* 2007), as five of the children we treated appeared to have been infected *in utero*, this problem may be underestimated. The issue of HBO in pregnancy is a complex one. Oxygen causes uterine artery vasoconstriction which affects the PO2 achieved in the fetus during HBO (Jackson *et al* 1987), but we can assume that there is still a significant increase in tissue PO2.

We do not know the optimal HBO treatment regimen. The above study was open and HBO was administered in conjunction with varying antibiotic protocols. For other infections such as necrotizing fasciitis and osteomyelitis, HBO is considered adjunctive to be an adjunctive treatment, in part for its ability to enhance antibiotic efficacy. Prospective trials are needed to evaluate the optimal use of HBO in conjunction with standard treatment. Questions regarding twice daily vs. once daily treatments, and the advantages or disadvantages of a "weekend off" must be assessed. Twice daily treatments are fatiguing for subjects but were generally well tolerated. The 2-day weekend interruption in the HBO sequences appeared to be beneficial because it often allowed time for the JH reaction to subside.

Ethical Considerations in Using HBO for Unproven Indications

At this time, Lyme disease remains an unproven use of HBO. Ethical "off-label" use of HBO has been discussed in an article, which is recommended for study by physicians using off-label HBO (Chan & Brody 2001). The important ethical considerations regarding the use of HBO in Lyme disease (and all unproven indications) are those of beneficence and non-maleficence. The principle of beneficence refers the moral obligation to act for the benefit of others, whereas non-maleficence can be condensed to the phrase, "Do no harm." Physicians must not do anything that would purposely harm patients. However, providing an ineffective treatment to patients with no possibility of benefit, particularly if there is any chance of harm, could constitute maleficence. The assessment of whether to provide an unproven therapy is a balance between beneficence and non-maleficence. In fact, virtually every medical decision involves weighing the risks versus the benefits of treatment. By providing informed consent, physicians give patients the information necessary to understand the scope and nature of the potential risks and benefits in order to make a decision. The informed consent process allows patient autonomy. The potential benefits of any intervention must outweigh the risks in order for the action to be ethical.

Is It Research?

The first question that must be determined is whether the physician is performing research. Case-by-case decisions to treat a patient constitute practicing medicine, but repeated off-label use with the intention to apply any information obtained to other patients is research. Research requires a protocol approved by an institutional review board (IRB). If they are participating in a research protocol, patients must be informed that they are research subjects and must consent to participate in the study.

Informed Consent

Even in routine medical practice, physicians must obtain informed consent for all procedures, whether considered off-label use or not. However, off-label use of HBO requires that certain types of information be included in the informed consent that are not otherwise required. HBO involves the use of a drug (oxygen) and a device (the hyperbaric chamber). While informed consent can be written or oral, since one must document in the chart that it was performed, consent is usually obtained in writing. For off-label use, informed consent must cover 5 specific areas of information:

1. Are there alternative medical treatments?
2. What is the level and type of scientific data to support the use of HBOT for this condition?
3. Are the risks of HBOT acceptable?
4. Does the patient understand that they are responsible for the cost?
5. Physician disclosure of any financial issues which might affect the physician-patient relationship

It is imperative that patients undergoing HBOT for off-label use are aware of alternatives to HBO for their illness. "Level of scientific evidence" refers to whether the rationale is supported only by animal data, or by human data, and if by the latter, from what sort of trials. In the case of Lyme disease, we have only unblinded, uncontrolled data from small case series. This represents the lowest level of human scientific evidence with the exception of expert opinion. However, we note that the patients included in the Texas A&M series were quite ill and had failed other therapies, and their disease represented a category likely to have been rejected for participation in the randomized, controlled trials performed to assess antibiotic efficacy.

Many patients interested in HBO therapy fall into a similar category of illness. Risk assessment requires an attempt to weigh the risk of HBO against the potential chance of benefit. The risks of HBO treatment are low but are not zero. Between 0.5% and 10% of patients have otic barotrauma, and the risk of more serious oxygen toxicity seizures is 1:3,000 to 1:50,000. In the case of Lyme disease, HBO risk may also include the JH reaction, which, ironically, may be a sign of subsequent benefit. In the context of HBO and chronic Lyme, it must be remembered that the value of long term antibiotic therapy is yet to be proven and has been demonstrated to have some risk.

It is not ethical to disguise the reason for treatment as some other medical problem for the purpose of obtaining coverage by a third party payer. It is possible for a physician to charge for providing HBO under off-label use but charges must be reasonable and similar to those for other indications. In the US, patients do sometimes pay to participate in research, or for unproven treatments. However, it is not usual for patients to pay to participate in trials if they receive only placebo treatment. Normally patients who pay to participate in trials do have access to active therapy at some point in the protocol; also, the treatment/research protocol must conform to ethical standards. If the physician is in a position to realize substantial financial gain from the patient's course of treatment (perhaps because he or she is owns the facility and is thus the beneficiary of payments beyond the usual professional fees), this information is considered to have a potential effect on the physician-patient relationship and should be disclosed.

Regulatory Aspects of HBO in Relation to Lyme Disease

In the United States, according to the Food and Drug Administration (FDA) which regulates drugs as well as medical devices, hyperbaric chambers are "Class II devices"; i.e., they do not support or sustain human life as is the definition of Class III, but they are not as innocuous as tongue depressors ("Class I devices"). Devices developed after 1976 are split into two groups: those that are substantially equivalent to pre-1976 devices, and those that are genuinely new products.

Manufacturers of new chambers must notify the FDA with a pre-market notification system, referred to as the 510(k). Devices that are determined to be equivalent to a pre-1976 device must be marketed with the same restrictions as their pre-1976 predecessors. Since 1978, the Undersea and Hyperbaric Medical Society (UHMS) Committee report has been recognized by the FDA as a guide in establishing the "indications of use" for hyperbaric chambers in a manufacturer's claim of substantial equivalency for the 510(k) pre-market notification requirements. This means that, in the US, all hyperbaric chambers are cleared for marketing for *only* those conditions that are listed as approved in the UHMS Hyperbaric Oxygen Therapy Committee Report. A chamber could be approved to treat an indication that is not on the list, but this would require data to support the use of HBO in that condition be submitted to the FDA for review. Although the US Federal Food, Drug, and Cosmetic (FDC) Act does not authorize FDA to regulate the practice of medicine, it specifically directs FDA to regulate the promotion of drugs and devices. Promotional materials are unlawful if they promote an unapproved use for the product. US facilities with web sites advertising the use of HBO for Lyme disease (or any other off-label use) are in violation of FDA regulations, *even if treatment is being given as part of an IRB-approved research protocol.*

Since the majority of randomized controlled trials are undertaken by pharmaceutical companies, the likelihood of a large RCT focused on the efficacy of HBO in Lyme disease seems low. Chan and Brody (2001) suggested that registries could be employed as a tool to assess the potential benefit of HBOT for certain relatively rare diseases. Registry data cannot substitute for RCT data when it comes to proving efficacy, but can assist in defining treatment protocols, and can certainly define a subset of patients who are *not* likely to benefit and who might need to be excluded from a future RCT. A registry does require that a defined treatment protocol be established and approved by the sponsoring IRB. Individual facilities must have this protocol approved by their individual IRBs, and patients must sign a consent to participate. Patients all receive the active therapy, but undergo standardized treatment and assessments, and outcome data are complied in a central repository for analysis. Lyme disease would seem an ideal candidate for such a registry.

Conclusions

In summary, it cannot be stated that HBO cures or permanently suppresses chronic Lyme disease, although it can be said that the HBO protocol used in the preliminary study at Texas A&M reduced the symptoms and greatly improved the quality of life among this series of very ill patients. It remains to be seen if HBO can be considered to be an adjunctive treatment to a rigorous regimen of antibiotic therapy. It does seem clear that HBO improves or eliminates the symptoms in patients who have been treated with antibiotics for several years and have shown no further mitigation of disease symptomology. Moreover, the results described here suggest that the further improvement observed is due to HBO, which is the only factor that changed in the long-standing treatment regimen. Lyme disease is an unproven indication for HBO and specific ethical practices should be followed whenever physicians engage in the off-label use of HBO.

15 HBO Therapy in Wound Healing, Plastic Surgery, and Dermatology

K.K. Jain

HBO promotes wound healing by counteracting tissue hypoxia and is a valuable adjunct in management of ischemic, infected, and nonhealing wounds. HBO also improves the survival of skin flaps. It reduces the mortality and morbidity in burns. This chapter contains the following sections:

Introduction

These three topics are lumped together in this chapter because nonhealing wounds frequently come under the care of plastic surgeons and disorders of the skin form a common bond between plastic surgery and dermatology.

A wound is a disturbance in the continuity of intact tissue structures, mostly associated with loss of substance. The damage may be the result of mechanical, thermal, physical, surgical, or chemical influences. An ulcer is a local defect, or excavation of the surface of an organ or tissue, which is produced by sloughing of inflammatory necrotic tissue. The cutaneous wound is described as an ulcer if there is focal loss of dermis and epidermis.

The rapidly aging population and patients with multiple concomitant pathologies present an increasing population of patients with nonhealing and problem wounds causing an unwelcome challenge for all health care providers. Methods that may be used to heal soft tissue wounds are shown in Table 15.1.

Traditional surgical procedures have not solved the problem of non-healing wounds. Many of the patients are not surgical candidates and there are problems with healing of donor sites of the skin graft. Wound closure alone does not suffice as there is a high rate of wound dehiscence. Several non-surgical methods are in development. A revolution in the wound care has been the introduction of Apligraf® to cover the skin ulcer. It will be described further in the management of venous ulcers for which it has been approved and is in clinical trials for the management of diabetic and pressure ulcers. Keratinocyte growth factor

(repifermin) is in phase II studies. It stimulates the growth of epithelial cells and might attract fibroblasts to the site of the wound, thereby stimulating the production of new connective tissue.

Hyperbaric medicine is only an adjunctive and rather slow method of promoting wound healing. Undue emphasis has been placed on this approach with some hyperbaric centers specializing only in wound healing. Application of HBO to wound healing has been recommended by the Undersea and Hyperbaric Medicine Society and approved by the health care providers on the basis of economic studies carried out prior to the introduction of new methods. HBO will remain an important adjunct to wound healing but its role needs to be redefined. Because the focus of this textbook is on HBO, wound healing and the role of oxygen in this process will be described as a prelude to the discussion of the use of HBO in wound care.

Wound Healing

Wound healing is a complex process involving multiple interacting cell types and biochemical mediators. Following tissue injury, platelets and fibrin are attracted to the wound site. Macrophages, fibroblasts, smooth muscle cells, and endothelial cells follow. These cells become organized, interact, and produce cytokines that stimulate cell growth. Angiogenesis and collagen production follows. Macrophages phagocytize dead tissue and contaminants and the wound becomes filled with granulation tissue. Finally the wound site is populated by cells normally present at that location and the wound is considered to have healed.

Role of Oxygen in Wound Healing

Oxygen is a critical nutrient of the wound and plays an important role in wound repair. Fluctuations of oxygen tension within the physiological range control the proliferation of fibroblasts by altering the activity of a stable intermediate substance that regulates the cellular response to growth factors. Oxygen is required for hydroxylation of proline and lysine, a step that is necessary for the release of collagen from the fibroblasts and its incorporation into the healing wound matrix.

Some local hypoxia is an inevitable result of tissue injury and may act as a stimulus to repair. Wound perfusion also depends on angiogenesis. An angiogenic factor is produced by macrophages under hypoxic conditions or exposure to high lactate levels. This process is not inhibited by oxygen administration as tissue levels are maintained constantly at high oxygen tension to inhibit this process.

Table 15.1
Methods of Treatment of Ulcers

A. Surgical
- Surgical debridement and closure
- Conventional skin grafting

B. Non-surgical
- Wound dressings with application of various chemicals
- Exogenous application of growth factors: Keratinocyte growth factor, platelet-derived growth factor
- Application of bioengineered skin implant, e.g., Apligraf®)
- Electrical stimulation
- Hyperbaric oxygen
- Vacuum-assisted closure system

C. Correction of underlying cause
- Stripping of varicose veins for venous ulcers
- Management of chronic venous insufficiency by drugs, e.g., Venoruton®
- Control of diabetes in case of diabetic ulcers
- Treatment of infections
- Eradication of underlying osteomyelitis
- Correction of malnutrition
- Counteracting vasoconstriction: idiopathic or drug-induced
- Reduction of steroid use

Pathophysiology of Non-healing Wounds

A chronic (non-healing) wound or the so called "problem wound" is defined as any wound which fails to heal within a reasonable period by the use of conventional medical and surgical methods. Conditions associated with nonhealing of wounds include arterial insufficiency, diabetes, cancer, infections, stress and use of corticosteroids. Nonhealing in a wound is mostly related to hypoxia and ischemia. The metabolic requirements of the dividing fibroblasts are increased. Since the energy needs for repair are the greatest at the time the local circulation is impaired, there is an energy crisis in the wound. Hypoxia thus impairs collagen synthesis and the collagen fibers that are formed have low tensile strength. When the environmental oxygen tension is less than 10 mmHg, fibroblasts do not migrate properly.

Anoxia leads to accumulation of metabolites such as ammonia that cause swelling of cells and impair healing. Hypoxia can activate enzymes that synthesize collagen. This paradox is partially explained by the observation that synthesis of collagen is doubled by elevation of lactate (5–15 mmol) induced by hypoxia. If the tissue pO_2 is raised to 40 mmHg, collagen production rises sevenfold.

Wounds in ischemic areas are highly susceptible to infection which is known to interfere with wound healing.

Regardless of etiology, a common denominator of nonhealing wounds is tissue hypoxia. This has been confirmed by tissue oxygen studies. The extent of the "problem" is a clinical definition that is partially proportional to the degree of hypoxia. Ischemia is a common cause of nonhealing wounds, but ischemia and hypoxia are not the same. Ischemic wounds are usually hypoxic, but not all hypoxic wounds are ischemic. A wound with adequate perfusion may be relatively hypoxic as infection in the wound can raise the oxygen requirements.

Some common causes of cutaneous ulceration with examples are listed in Table 15.2.

Table 15.2
Some Common Causes of Cutaneous Ulcers

1. Vascular: arterial or venous insufficiency
2. Metabolic: diabetes
3. Physical trauma: decubitus ulcers, burns, radiation, frostbite
4. Infections: bacterial, fungal, etc.
5. Neuropathic: tabes dorsalis and syringomyelia
6. Neoplastic: squamous cell carcinoma
7. Toxic: drug-induced

Wound Healing Enhancement by Oxygen

Rationale of Use of Oxygen

The rationale of using oxygen in wound healing can be summarized as follows:

1. Hypoxia in the wounds can be corrected by oxygen therapy, which varies from inhalation of 40% oxygen at ambient pressure to 100% oxygen at 2.5 ATA. High pressures are needed to oxygenate the hypoxic center of chronic nonhealing wounds.
2. Hypoxia can arise in a normally perfused tissue when it is the site of an inflammatory reaction, and HBO at 2 ATA has been shown to improve the tissue oxygenation in this situation.
3. Intermittent correction of wound hypoxia by oxygen therapy increases fibroblast replication and collagen production.
4. Improvement of oxygen supply raises the RNA/DNA ratio in the tissues, indicating increased formation of rough endoplasmic reticulum by the cells of the wounded area, and a higher degree of cellular differentiation.
5. Raising the wound oxygen tension increases the capability of the leukocytes to kill pathogenic bacteria (see Chapter 13).
6. The increased oxygen supply meets the increased oxygen needs of the healing wound.
7. Oxygen administered at 1–2 ATA promotes the rate of epithelialization in ischemic wounds.
8. HBO promotes neoangiogenesis in wounds.

The benefit of HBO in hypoxic wounds is depicted schematically in Figure 15.1.

New tissues striving to fill the dead space of a wound need to be supplied by a new vasculature, which follows the formation of collagen. Capillaries grow into the hypoxic area, and collagen synthesis is carried further into the wound in this manner. Obliteration of the dead space proceeds in cyclical fashion. Increasing the capillary pO_2 ten-

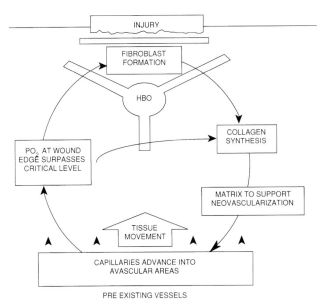

Figure 15.1
Benefits of HBO to ischemic and hypoxic wounds. Note that HBO acts at the same points where hypoxia interferes with wound healing.

sion by HBO increases the amount of oxygen reaching the advancing cells. These cells are able to migrate further and retain the ability to synthesize. This enables the vascular supply to advance more quickly, which ensures faster closure of the wound.

Experimental Studies

In controlled experiments, HBO (2.5 ATA for 2 h) used three times has been shown to increase the bursting strength and stimulate angiogenesis in the early stages of healing of incisions in rats. HBO-induced Ang2 expression may occur through transcriptional stimulation, and requires the nitric oxide signaling pathway, which may play an important role in HBO-induced angiogenesis (Lin *et al* 2002). Wounds exposed to oxygen at 2.5 ATA show linear strength increase in the first week. Prolonged hyperoxygenation beyond the optimal needs can retard healing. HBO has been shown to reduce the severity of damage in cryobiologic wounds in rats and to stimulate faster and better tissue repair.

The complex cell interaction involved in wound healing and the effect of HBO on this is not fully understood. The healing effect of O_2 in chronic wounds is not explained by increased phagocytosis or increased adhesions of macrophages.

Results of a study in a rat model of ischemic wound indicate that HBO improves wound healing by downregulation of HIF-1a and subsequent target gene expression with attenuation of cell apoptosis and reduction of inflammation (Zhang *et al* 2008).

HBO for Impairment of Wound Healing by Stress

Psychological stress has been shown to dysregulate healing in both humans and animals. Stress launches a sequence of events that constrict blood vessels and deprive the tissues of oxygen, which is an important mediator of wound healing. Decreased oxygen supply combined with increased oxygen demand in the wounds of the stressed animals can impair healing rate by as much as 45%. The hypothesis that HBO would ameliorate the effect of stress on dermal wound healing was tested in a mouse model of impaired healing due to stress induced by confinement (Gajendrareddy *et al* 2005). HBO therapy twice a day during early wound healing significantly ameliorated the effects of stress, bringing healing to near-control levels. There was no significant effect of HBO on the wounds of control animals. Gene expression of inducible nitric oxide synthase (iNOS) in the wound, modulated by psychological stress and oxygen balance, was studied by real-time PCR. Expression of iNOS increased in stressed mice on days 1, 3, and 5, post-wounding. HBO treatment of the stressed animals decreased iNOS expression by 62.6% on day 1 post-wounding. There was no significant effect of HBO on wound healing and iNOS expression in the control animals. Nitric oxide is critically involved in wound healing, by increasing blood flow and the delivery of oxygen. Thus, methods aimed at increasing tissue oxygenation, such as HBO, have a high therapeutic potential.

Tissue Oxygen Tension Measurement

The rational approach to treatment of nonhealing wounds by HBO should include tissue oxygen tension monitoring. Tissue oxygen tensions during normobaric as well as hyperbaric oxygen breathing are shown in Figure 15.2 and Table 15.3.

The ideal method of wound oxygen tension measurement is tissue tonometry. Oxygen tension of 30 mmHg is required for normal cell division and wound healing. The oxidative phosphorylation process in the mitochondria requires a minimum oxygen tension of 0.5 to 3 mmHg in the

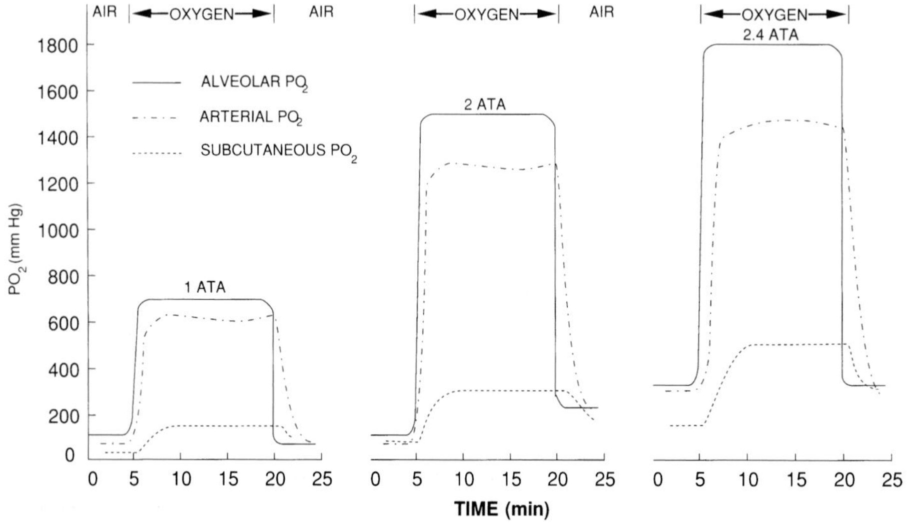

Figure 15.2
Tissue oxygen tension during normobaric and hyperbaric oxygen breathing (from Sheffield & Heimbach (1985): Respiratory Physiology, in Dehart RL (Ed.): Fundamentals of Aerospace Medicine, Philadelphia, Lea & Febiger, p. 87, by permission).

Table 15.3
Range of Tissue Oxygen Tensions (mmHg) with HBO Therapy

	1 ATA (air)	1 ATA (O_2)	2 ATA (O_2)	2.5 ATA (O_2)
Arterial pO_2	100	600	1400	1800
Transcutaneous pO_2	70–75	450–550	1200–1300	1400–1500
Muscle pO_2	30–35	60–75	220–300	No data available
Subcutaneous pO_2	30–50	90–150	200–300	300–500
Wound pO_2	5–20	200–400	600–800	800–1100

mitochondria. Cytochrome c activity is reduced progressively as tissue pO_2 falls and is markedly reduced below 30 mmHg. These changes are reversible when the oxygen tension is elevated again. These basic metabolic functions should be present for the tissues to heal.

Transcutaneous oxygen pressure ($tcpO_2$) is a noninvasive method and its measurements have been shown to correlate with wound healing. These measurements are taken on the area surrounding the wound and not directly on the wound surface. It is generally considered that $tcpO_2$ greater than 20 mmHg in room air predicts a positive response to HBO. The value should double on 100% oxygen and increase to 100 mmHg at 2 ATA. $TcpO_2$ has been measured in edematous wounds before and after a regimen of HBO therapy, in patients breathing normobaric air (AIR), 100% normobaric oxygen (O_2), and 100% O_2 at 2.36 ATA (Dooley et al 1996). Wounds also were scored for severity, including three ratings for periwound edema. Only during AIR was pre $tcpO_2$ of markedly edematous wounds significantly lower than that of moderately edematous and non-edematous wounds ($P < 0.001$). After HBO therapy, wound severity score and periwound edema rating decreased significantly ($P < 0.001$), and periwound edema ratings could no longer be distinguished by $tcpO_2$. Although pre periwound $TcpO_2$ measured during both O_2 and HBO evaluations was significantly greater than that measured during AIR ($P < 0.0001$) and was positively correlated with subsequent change in wound severity ($P < 0.05$), regression analyses failed to yield a significant prediction equation. The authors concluded that: a) dramatically marked increases in $tcpO_2$ of normally hypoxic (< 30 Torr O_2) edematous wounds during O_2 and HBO challenges demonstrate that periwound edema is an O_2 diffusion barrier during normal conditions; b) HBO therapy significantly reduces periwound edema in markedly edematous wounds; c) despite significant correlations between pretherapy periwound $tcpO_2$ measured during O_2 and HBO challenges and changes in wound severity, single $tcpO_2$ measurements are not predictive of changes in periwound edema or overall wound severity.

A retrospective analysis of 1,144 patients with diabetic lower extremity ulcers treated by HBO shows that the reliability of in-chamber $TcPO_2$ as an isolated measure was 74% with a positive predictive value of 58% (Fife et al 2002). Better results may be obtained by combining information about sea-level air and in-chamber oxygen. A sea-level air $TcP O_2 < 15$ mmHg combined with an in-chamber $TcP O_2 < 400$ mmHg predicts failure of hyperbaric oxygen therapy with a reliability of 75.8% and a positive predictive value of 73.3%.

Clinical Applications

LaVan and Hunt (1990) recommend the use of supplemental oxygen for all patients considered to be at high risk of infection who are either undergoing or recovering from surgery.

A critical review of hyperbaric oxygen for wound healing includes 57 studies, 7 randomized clinical trials, 16 nonrandomized studies, and 34 case series involving more than 2000 patients (Wang et al 2003). None of the studies selected used wound tissue hypoxia as a patient inclusion criterion. Results of the studies suggest that HBO is helpful for some wounds. The main criticism by the reviewer was that there were inadequate or no controls in most studies. Given the clinical nature of the problem, it is not possible to design optimal controlled studies. It is now established that HBO treatments in selected patients can facilitate healing by increasing tissue oxygen tension, thus providing the wound with a more favorable environment for repair (Zamboni et al 2003). Therefore, HBO has become an important component of any comprehensive wound care program.

The optimal dose of oxygen for a nonhealing wound is not yet determined. The optimal pO_2 for the wound is about 50–100 mmHg. Oxygen is only an adjuvant treatment; the primary care of the wound by debridement and meticulous dressing is necessary. The primary cause of the ulcer should be eliminated where possible. Three methods of oxygen administration are usually available:

1. Normobaric oxygen (100%) inhalation
2. Topical hyperbaric oxygen
3. Hyperbaric oxygenation by inhalation in a chamber

Normobaric Oxygen

Normobaric oxygen (100%) inhalation is the most commonly used method and is usually adequate in acute wounds where the wound pO_2 is over 30 mmHg. Methods of oxygen inhalation have been described by Jain (1989b).

Topical Hyperbaric Oxygen

Topical application by a small hyperbaric chamber (TOPOX) which encloses the affected limb has been described in Chapter 7. This technique has been used for treatment of leg ulcers. Treatment with topical oxygen is associated with an induction of vascular endothelial growth factor (VEGF) expression in wound edge tissue and an improvement in wound size (Gordillo *et al* 2008).

Fischer (1969) was the first to describe healing of leg ulcers under topically applied HBO in 52 patients. Fischer (1975) described another 30 patients with leg ulcers due to different causes. HBO was administered by a topical chamber applied to the affected extremity. Pressure of 1.03 ATA was not exceeded to avoid obstruction of capillary blood flow. The oxygen delivery was maintained at 4 l/min, and treatment was performed twice daily, each session lasting 2–3 h. Wound debridement was done as necessary. The patients served as their own controls, as they had been treated by other methods before with no success. Most of the ulcers healed well, but HBO failed to heal those associated with severe ischemia. There was absorption of oxygen through the ulcer as evidenced by the rise of capillary pO_2 in the area of the ulcer, without an increase of systemic capillary pO_2. In some cases the stimulation of the granulation tissue was so effective that it rose above the skin surface. Fischer felt that HBO is a simple, safe, and inexpensive treatment to reduce the time required for healing of ulcers, and in some cases served as a good preparation for surgical intervention.

Ignacio *et al* (1984) conducted a prospective study of 36 patients with extensive skin ulcers treated with HBO at 16–20 mmHg above atmospheric pressure. A healing rate of 77% was reported. Ravina *et al* (1983) described a simple disposable polyethylene bag device for application of HBO to leg ulcers and treated 18 patients with ulcers of various types with good results.

A recent review of the published data on the oxygen diffusion properties of skin indicates that the upper skin layers to a depth of 0.25–0.40 mm are almost exclusively supplied by external oxygen, whereas the oxygen transport of the blood has only a minor influence (Stucker *et al* 2002). This is almost 10 times deeper than previous estimates. This zone includes the entire outermost layer of living cells – the epidermis – and some of the dermis below, which contains sweat glands and hair roots. As a consequence, a malfunction in capillary oxygen transport cannot be the initiator of the development of superficial skin defects such as those observed in chronic venous incompetence and peripheral arterial occlusive disease. Peripheral vascular disease contributes to ulceration by poor blood supply, which starves tissues of nutrients. These concepts indicate that ulcer management should not involve bandaging but atmospheric exposure. Although environmental oxygen may suffice in superficial ulcers, nonhealing deep ulcers with hypoxic wounds would require supplemental exposure to oxygen, which may be more effective by topical application than systemic exposure to HBO. The advantages of topical application of HBO are:

1. The ischemic areas are separated from the oxygen by a thin layer of tissue only a few microns thick whereas systemic oxygen must traverse a much larger distance to reach the ischemic tissue at the base of the ulcer.
2. This method avoids the toxicity of hyperbaric oxygen.
3. No special equipment is required. Only a disposable polyethylene bag is used.
4. Low cost.

The limitations of this method are:

1. It is effective in open wounds. Encrustation of ulcers prevents the oxygen from diffusing to the base of the ulcer.
2. Pressure applied to the limb may impair the circulation of the limb.
3. Ulcers penetrating into deep tissues do not respond well to this method.

Electrical stimulation has been combined with hyperbaric oxygen for promotion of wound healing. In an open study, no significant differences in healing were observed between patients receiving topical hyperbaric oxygen alone and those receiving topical hyperbaric oxygen/electrical stimulation (Edsberg *et al* 2002). Preliminary data indicate that topical hyperbaric oxygen facilitates wound healing and full closure for pressure ulcers in patients with and without diabetes mellitus. A multicenter, prospective, randomized, double-blind controlled study is currently underway.

Adjuncts to HBO for Wound Healing

alpha-Lipoic acid (LA) has been shown to accelerate wound repair in patients with chronic wounds undergoing HBO therapy. In a study, patients undergoing HBO therapy were randomized into two groups in a double-blind manner: The LA group and the placebo group (Alleva *et al* 2008). Gene expression profiles for matrix metalloproteinases (MMPs) and for angiogenesis mediators were evaluated in biopsies collected at the first HBO session, at the seventh HBO session, and after 14 days of HBO treatment. ELISA tests were used to validate microarray expression of selected genes. LA supplementation in combination with HBO therapy downregulated the inflammatory cytokines and the growth factors which, in turn, affect expression of MMPs. LA regulates MMP expression in cells that are involved in wound repair The disruption of the positive autocrine feedback loops that maintain the chronic wound state promotes progression of the healing process.

Role of HBO in Nonhealing Wounds and Ulcers

If the wound pO_2 cannot be raised to above 30 mmHg by normobaric 100% oxygen inhalation, HBO should be tried at pressures of 2 to 2.5 ATA. The treatments should last for 1–2 h and should be repeated every 24 h. Such a schedule correlates with the cell cycle of human fibroblasts, which lasts about 24 h, and the duration of mitosis, which takes about 1 h. Lack of rise of wound pO_2 in response to HBO therapy is usually an indicator that further treatments may be ineffective.

HBO therapy is used in the following types of wounds and ulcers:

1. Ulcers due to arterial insufficiency
2. Diabetic ulcers
3. Venous stasis ulcers
4. Decubitus ulcers
5. Infected wounds
6. Frostbite
7. Intractable wounds associated with spider bite
8. Refractory perineal Crohn's disease

Ulcers Due to Arterial Insufficiency

Many of the peripheral vascular diseases reviewed in Chapter 24 are accompanied by ulceration of skin on the legs or even gangrene. Local rather than regional blood flow insufficiency is the cause of skin lesions in peripheral vascular disease. Satisfactory results are obtained with HBO (2 ATA) in ulcers typical of thromboangiitis obliterans. In arteriosclerosis the response is less satisfactory unless prolonged courses of treatment are instituted.

Kidokoro et al (1969) treated 22 patients with leg ulcers and pain due to chronic vascular insufficiency by means of HBO at 2–2.5 ATA for up to 70 sessions. Fifteen patients obtained relief of rest pain and 12 had healing of ulcers. Hart and Strauss (1979) used HBO (2 ATA) to treat 16 patients with arteriosclerotic ulcers that were refractory to conventional treatments. In 75% of cases the ulcers healed completely

Perrins and Barr (1986) described their results in 50 patients with arteriosclerotic ulcers treated with HBO alone (1.5–3.0 ATA). Healing was achieved in 52% and improvement in 20%. These were all geriatric patients, and amputation was avoided in 65% of them. The same authors treated eight further patients with split skin grafts and HBO. Seven of them healed and no effect was observed on the remaining patient. The conclusions reached by these authors were:

- Many patients with ulcers associated with peripheral vascular disease that have resisted treatment by other means can be healed by prolonged courses of HBO.
- The response is dose-dependent. Some ulcers respond to 1.5 ATA, while others require up to 3 ATA. Some fail to respond to treatment for a total of 2 h per day, others heal with less than 1 h a day.
- The period required for healing can be reduced consid-

erably if the ulcer bas is prepared with a course of HBO before split skin grafting.
- Of all the different types of ulcers, those due to rheumatoid vasculitis showed the best results. Of the 15 patients, 73% healed with HBO alone, and all of the three that had split skin grafts healed.

Wattel et al (1991) reported complete healing of arterial insufficiency ulcers in all patients where the distal transcutaneous pO_2 could be raised above 100 mmHg by HBO treatments at 2.5 ATA (100% oxygen) with daily sessions of 90 min each. An average of 46 sessions per patient were required. HBO was ineffective in those patients where the distal transcutaneous pO_2 could not be raised above 100 mmHg.

Diabetic Ulcers

Introduction and epidemiology. Diabetic ulcers usually involve the foot and hence the term "diabetic foot." The United States' incidence of diabetic ulcers is about 80,000 per year of which 25–30% are not healed by standard therapy. Approximately 20% of all diabetics who enter hospital are admitted because of foot problems with ulcers. Even when hyperglycemia is controlled by insulin, the vascular pathology of diabetes continues to progress. It may result in large vessel occlusive disease or pathology of the microvasculature. An additional pathology is diabetic neuropathy and the secondary infections in the wound leading to the term "diabetic foot syndrome." The whole lower extremity may become gangrenous and require amputation which carries a high mortality in the elderly diabetic patients. A diabetic has 15–20 higher chance of having an amputation of the lower extremity as a non-diabetic individual. According to the American Diabetic Association, 42 out of 10,000 diabetics in the United States have an amputation yearly because of diabetic foot syndrome. HBO has been shown to reduce the leg amputation rate in diabetic gangrene.

General management. Standard care for diabetic ulcers includes good wound care, control of diabetes and treatment of infections. Recent advances in the treatment of diabetic ulcers include the introduction of skin substitutes such as Apligraf (Organogenesis Inc) to close the skin ulcer. A platelet-derived growth factor, Regranex (Janssen Pharmaceutica), has also been approved for the treatment of diabetic ulcers of the lower extremities in the United States. The growth factor stimulates the migration of cells to the ulcer site, encouraging the patient's body to grow new tissue to heal the ulcers. If gangrene sets in, the lower extremity is amputated below the knee.

Role of HBO in the management of diabetic foot. HBO reduces insulin requirements in diabetics (see Chapter 27)

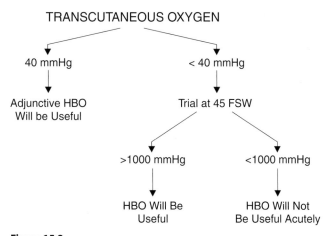

Figure 15.3

Algorithm for decision-making in offering HBO as an adjunct to the diabetic patients (Reproduced by permission from Emhoff and Myers (1987): Transcutaneous oxygen measurements in wound healing in the diabetic patient. In Kindwall EP ed) Proceedings of the Eighth International Congress on Hyperbaric Medicine, Best, San Pedro, pp. 309–313).

but no effect on diabetic neuropathy has been demonstrated. HBO may have an important role in preventing gangrene by counteracting the vascular insufficiency and this issue needs to be examined further. The rationale of HBO in diabetic wound is based on the known effect of HBO in counteracting hypoxia, edema and infection. Before considering HBO treatment one has to consider whether tissue oxygen in the ulcer can be augmented by HBO.

Whether or not the oxygen tension can be raised in the diabetic wound by HBO depends upon the patency of the vasculature around the ulcer. The decision regarding use of HBO is made after vascular evaluation of the extremity involved and the transcutaneous pO_2 determination. A decision tree based on this is shown in Figure 15.3. Emhoff and Myers studied 10 diabetic patients and measured oxygen tensions transcutaneously to assess the adequacy of microcirculation in the affected areas. The normal range of pO_2 measured transcutaneously over the leg is 45–95 mmHg. Only two of these patients had pO_2 above this value, eight had a lower value. The authors believe that in diabetics, the pO_2 value has to be raised much higher for optimal healing. If pO_2 cannot be raised to 1000 mmHg when the patient breathes 100% oxygen at 2.36 ATA, it can be stated that the patient's microcirculation is defective and would not allow adequate supply and flow of oxygen to the wound, and HBO may not be useful (Emhoff & Myers 1987).

Adjuncts to HBO in the management of diabetic ulcers. Endothelial progenitor cells (EPCs) are the key cellular effectors of neovascularization and play a central role in wound healing, but their circulating and wound-level numbers are decreased in diabetes, implicating an abnormality in EPC mobilization and homing mechanisms. The deficiency in EPC mobilization is presumably due to im-

pairment of endothelial nitric oxide synthase-nitric oxide cascade in bone marrow. Hyperoxia, induced by a clinically relevant HBO protocol, can significantly enhance the mobilization of EPCs from the bone marrow into peripheral blood. However, increased circulating EPCs failed to reach the wound tissues, partly as a result of downregulated production of SDF-1α in local wound lesions with diabetes. Administration of exogenous SDF-1α into wounds reverses the EPC homing impairment and, with HBO, synergistically enhances EPC mobilization, homing, neovascularization, and wound healing (Liu & Velazquez 2008).

Clinical use of HBO in diabetic foot. Various studies of the use of HBO in treating diabetic foot are summarized in Table 15.4. Most of the studies used HBO at 2–3 ATA and the number of sessions varied from 4 to 79. A standard problem wound protocol is 100% oxygen at 2 ATA/2 hour daily/5 days a week.

The study of Stone et al (1995) can be criticized for a low proportion of the patients who completed the study. The study of Faglia et al (1996) is considered to be a good example. This study was done on 70 diabetic subjects were consecutively admitted to a diabetology unit for foot ulcers. Only two subjects, one in the arm of the treated group and one in the arm of nontreated group, did not complete the protocol and were therefore excluded from the analysis of the results. Finally, 35 subjects received HBO and another 33 did not. Of the treated group (mean session = 38.8 ± 8), three subjects (8.6%) underwent major amputation: two below the knee and one above the knee. In the nontreated group, 11 subjects (33.3%) underwent major amputation: 7 below the knee and 4 above the knee. The difference is statistically significant ($p = 0.016$). The relative risk for the treated group was 0.26 (95% CI 0.08–0.84). The transcutaneous oxygen tension measured on the dorsum of the foot significantly increased in subjects treated with HBO therapy: 14.0 ± 11.8 mmHg in the treated group, 5.0 ± 5.4 mmHg in the nontreated group ($p = 0.0002$). Multivariate analysis of major amputation on all the considered variables confirmed the protective role of s-HBOT (odds ratio 0.084, $p = 0.033$, 95% CI 0.008–0.821) and indicated as negative prognostic determinants low ankle-brachial index values (odds ratio 1.715, $p = 0.013$, 95% CI 1.121–2.626) and high Wagner grade (odds ratio 11.199, $p = 0.022$, 95% CI 1.406–89.146). It was concluded that HBO, in conjunction with an aggressive multidisciplinary therapeutic protocol, is effective in decreasing major amputations in diabetic patients with severe prevalently ischemic foot ulcers.

The decision on using HBO may be correlated with following classification of the diabetic foot:

- Grade I: Superficial lesions. No need for hyperbaric treatment
- Grade II: Deep ulceration reaching tendons and bone. HBO is indicated as cost effective treatment.

Table 15.4
Studies of Use of HBO for Diabetic Foot

Authors and year	No. of patients	Success rate	Comments
Hart and Strauss (1979)	11	18%	All of the patients improved but ulcer healed completely only in 2.
Perrins and Barr (1986)	24	67%	Amputation was avoided in 18% of the cases
Baroni *et al* (1987)	26	83%	
Davis (1987)	168	70%	
Wattel *et al* (1991)	20	75%	Mixed pathology: 9 patients with arterial insufficiency and 11 with diabetic ulcers.
Doctor *et al* (1992)	30	?	Prospective study. Thirty patients were randomized to a study group (HBO plus conventional treatment) and a control group (conventional treatment only). The treatment group showed better results in that the number of positive bacterial cultures decreased from 19 to 3 (in the control group from 16 to 12). Only two patients in the treatment group required amputations as compared to 7 patients in the control group.
Oriani *et al* (1992)	80	96%	Prospective study. Sixteen of the patients in this study either refused HBO or had contraindications for the use of HBO and were identified as controls. Of the 62 who received HBO, 59 (96%) recovered versus 12 (67%) in the control group. Only three patients in the HBO group required amputation as compared to six in the control group.
Stone *et al* (1995)	87	72%	Of the 501 patients in the study, 382 received conservative treatment. The endpoint was salvage of both lower extremities. Of the 119 treated patients, only 87 were available for follow-up.
Faglia *et al* (1996)	68	92.4%	The endpoint was amputation. The amputation rate was 8.6% in the HBO-treated patients and 33.3% in the control group.
Zamboni *et al* (1997)	5	100%*	Prospective with 5 controls for duration of 7 weeks.
Landau and Schattner (2001)	100	81%	Open study of topical hyperbaric oxygen and low energy laser radiation of the ulcer.
Kalani et al (2002)	38	76%	Success rate in patients treated conventionally was 48%. Seven patients (33%) in this group compared to two patients (12%) in HBO-treated group went to amputation.
Ong (2008)	45	71%	77% of successful cases were at risk of amputation proior to treatment

*Reduction of wound size and not complete healing

• Grade III: Involvement of deep tissues with infection: HBO is indicated as an adjunct to debridement.
• Grade IV: Gangrene of a portion of the foot. HBO treatments may reduce the size of the gangrenous portion which needs to be excised.
• Grade V: Gangrene of the whole foot. Usually amputation is required.

Economic analysis. Estimation of the cost of hospitalization and rehabilitation associated with amputation has shown that use of HBO as an adjunct in cases of problem wounds of the limbs has resulted in a high rate of salvage of the limbs, which would be expected to lower the cost of medical care. Experience with use of HBO in non-healing wounds both diabetic and those due to arterial insufficiency has been rather disappointing (Ciaravino *et al* 1996) From 1989 to 1994, fifty-four patients with nonhealing lower extremity wounds resulting from underlying peripheral vascular disease and/or diabetes mellitus were treated with HBO at Orlando Regional Medical Center, Florida. Wounds were grouped into the following five categories: (1) diabetic ulcers (n = 17 [31%]); (2) arterial insufficiency (n = 8 [15%]); (3) gangrenous lesions (n = 6 [11%]); (4)

nonhealing amputation stumps (n = 13 [24%]); and (5) nonhealing operative wounds (n = 10 [19%]). Each patient received an average of 30 treatments. Outcomes for all 54 patients treated with HBO in this study were dismal. None of the patients experienced complete healing, six (11%) showed some improvement, 43 (80%) showed no improvement, and in five cases (9%) results were inconclusive because these patients underwent concomitant revascularization or amputation. Thirty-eight of the 43 patients who showed no improvement (88%) ultimately required at least one surgical procedure to treat their wounds. Thirty-four patients (63%) developed complications, most commonly barotrauma to the ears, which occurred in 23 patients (43%). The average cost of 30 HBO treatments was $14,000 excluding daily inpatient charges. The authors found it is difficult to justify such an expensive, ineffective and complication-prone treatment modality for problem extremity wounds.

Concluding remarks. No definitive studies on the usefulness of HBO in limb salvage have been carried out as yet. The Orlando study quoted above may also have been done poorly as the technique of HBO treatment may not have been proper as indicated by the high barotrauma rate. Hospitalization is not required for HBO treatment and inpatient charges should not be included in any economic analysis as part of HBO therapy costs. Nevertheless, this study indicates a controversy surrounding the use of HBO for diabetic foot. Because most published studies suffer from methodological problems, there is an urgent need for a collaborative, international, randomized prospective clinical trial for the application of HBO in diabetic foot lesions, as part of a multidisciplinary treatment approach, before HBO can be recommended as standard therapy in patients with foot ulcers (Bakker 2000).

The problem of management of a diabetic foot should be divided into two parts: healing of ulcer and the limb salvage. For treatment of ulcer, the definitive primary treatment should be application of a skin substitute. One product, Apligraf® (Organogenesis Inc), which is a living skin equivalent engineered from human skin cells, is already approved for the treatment of venous ulcers and is commercially available. It is in clinical trials for diabetic and pressure ulcers. It is a one-time application as an outpatient at a wound center or similar facility. Another similar product which is in clinical trials is Dermagraft (Advanced Tissue Sciences). More promising than skin substitutes are the cell and gene therapies in development for wound healing (Jain 2004e). If the foot is threatened with gangrene, the role of HBO should be investigated in controlled and well designed studies. Current economic analyses favor HBO as it is less expensive than amputation in some countries. If prolonged HBO expenses exceed the one time expense of amputation, the quality of life may be the only justification for the use of HBO which may help limb salvage.

Venous Ulcers

Pathophysiology. A review of various studies suggests that 1% of the general population will suffer from a chronic venous ulcers at some point in their lives. A venous ulcer (also referred to as stasis ulcers) is one of the manifestations of chronic venous insufficiency (CVI), which is defined as hypertension involving either the superficial or both the superficial and the deep venous systems. The term CVI is also used to describe the stigmata of this disease: pigmentation, atrophy blanche, induration, varicose eczema and ulceration. CVI is a common condition if one includes a related condition, varicose veins, which arises from the same underlying cause, i.e., incompetence of valves in the perforator veins.

Chronic venous hypertension and repeated pressure peaks, provoked by calf muscle contractions, which are transmitted to the skin microvasculature lead to microangiopathy which is characterized by enlarged blood capillaries, reduced capillary numbers, microvascular thrombosis and increased permeability of microlymphatics. These changes have been documented by using fluorescent videomicroscopy and microlymphography. Transcutaneous oxygen measurements and laser Doppler fluxometry have shown that transcutaneous oxygen tension is decreased whereas Doppler reflux is enhanced. These findings indicate hypoperfusion of the superficial skin layers with paradoxical hyperperfusion of the deeper layers. Transcutaneous (tc) measurements show a decrease of $tcpO_2$ and this correlates with the degree of alterations of skin capillaries. Trophic changes leading to venous ulcerations are caused by microvascular ischemia and edema is due to increased capillary permeability and deficient lymphatic drainage. Edema further hinders tissue nutrition and transdermal diffusion of oxygen. This mechanism is supported by the demonstration of decreased transcutaneous pO_2 (measured as postischemic response) in patients with severe venous disease. Pericapillary deposition of fibrin in response to venous hypertension acts as a diffusion barrier to oxygen and thus impairs the nutrition of the skin. However, it is not certain that venous ulceration is attributable to failure of diffusion of oxygen and other small nutritional molecules to the tissues of the skin. It is likely that neutrophils attach themselves to the cutaneous microcirculation, become activated and produce endothelial injury by release of cytokines, oxygen free radicals, proteolytic enzymes and platelet activating factors. Repeated over many months or years, this process leads to chronic inflammation. The microvascular changes in the skin are characterized by activated endothelium and perivascular inflammatory cells. In conclusion, the exact pathomechanisms of venous ulcers remain to be resolved.

Treatment of venous ulcers. It appears that ulcers associated with CVI have a different pathomechanism and the management of the ulcer should be based on treatment of the CVI. The venous ulcers need to be differentiated from several other types including those due to arterial insufficiency because the management strategies are different. General measures for all leg ulcer patients should include the following (Jain 1998c):

- Elevation of the leg at night. This diminishes the exudate from the ulcer and reduces edema.
- Compression: by special stockings or intermittent pneumatic compression. The compliance rate of compression stockings or bandage is quite poor.
- Ulcer dressing and topical treatment
- Surgical treatment is directed at debridement of the ulcer and correction of the underlying cause. This may involve procedures to correct venous hypertension or stripping of varicose veins
- Pharmacotherapy. Oxyrutins (Venoruton, Novartis) is an established treatment for chronic venous insufficiency
- Growth factors. Several growth factors are being evalu-

ated for this purpose. One of these in clinical trials is keratinocyte growth factor.

- Apligraf® (Organogenesis Inc) is approved for treatment of venous ulcers. Like human skin, Apligraf is composed of two layers. The outer epidermal layer is made of living keratinocytes and the dermal layer consists of fibroblasts, both derived from human donor tissue that is thoroughly screened to exclude pathogens. It is applied by a physician in an outpatient facility or a wound care center. Apligraf heals more ulcers faster than compression therapy alone and is expected to become the treatment of choice for this condition.

HBO for treatment of venous ulcers. Rationale of HBO for venous ulcers is based on the hypoxia theory which has not been proven to be the sole pathomechanism. HBO promotes healing of venous ulcers but is not necessary for the healing. Oxygen tension measurements show low pO_2 values with microcirculatory disturbance of the ulcer tissue. After a compression bandage had been applied to the legs, the tissue oxygen tension of the ulcers increases markedly, probably as the result of diminished venous stasis. These ulcers heal without any special HBO treatment.

An example of a venous stasis ulcer treated by HBO and the results are shown in Figure 15.4. Slack *et al* (1966) reported on HBO treatment of 17 patients with varicose ulcers of the legs. They used HBO at 2.5 ATA once a day in a monoplace chamber until maximum benefit was achieved. Five of their patients healed completely, six showed had marked improvement, and another four had slight improvement. Fischer (1969) treated 16 cases of ulcers due to venous stasis with HBO via topical application. Improvement was noted within 8 h of beginning treatment in all cases. Bass (1970) obtained complete relief in 17 of 19 cases of venous stasis ulcers by use of HBO at 2 ATA after conventional treatment had failed.

Combination of HBO with skin grafting is more effective than HBO alone. Skin grafting is carried out for large ulcers and HBO is also used as an adjunct to promote healing of skin grafts. Perrins and Barr (1986) treated 12 patients with HBO (1.5–3 ATA) and there was healing in 50%. In another six patients with split skin grafts treated by HBO there was 100% healing. Saphenectomy wounds may not heal properly and HBO therapy is useful in the management of these (Horowitz *et al* 1992).

Recommendations for management of non-healing venous ulcers are as follows. The only one of these established by clinical trials is Apligraf®. Further clinical studies need to be carried out to support the supplementary use of HBO and venoruton.

- Primary treatment by application of Apligraf® which is a substitute for skin graft.
- Supplementary treatment with HBO until the ulcer has healed.

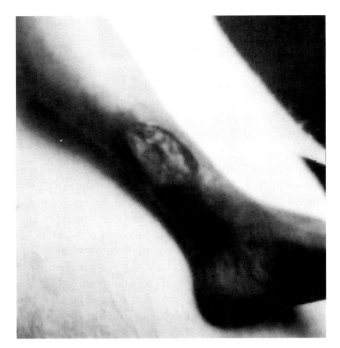

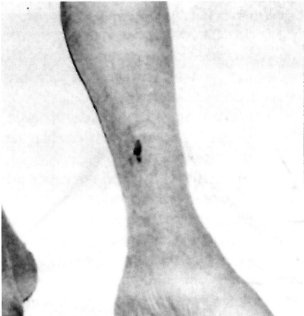

Figure 15.4
Example of an arterial insufficiency ulcer of the leg treated by HBO. (top) before treatment; (bottom) after treatment.

- Prophylactic treatment of CVI with Venoruton to prevent recurrence of venous ulcer.

Decubitus Ulcers

Pathophysiology. The cause of decubitus ulcers is pressure on the skin, which interferes with circulation at the point of contact. Prolonged rest or immobilization in one position, as with hemiplegics and paraplegics, may lead to this within a few hours. Poor skin hygiene, malnutrition, and debility are contributing factors. These ulcers are usually located over bony prominences such as the sacrum and the heel. The ulcer results from breakdown of the ischemic skin and subsequent bacterial invasion and inflammatory reaction. Persistence of the latter leads to microvascular thrombosis, which further aggravates ischemia.

Role of HBO. Seiler *et al* (1984) measured the oxygen tension of the tissues under pressure transcutaneously. Pressure of 15 kPa on a point leads to anoxia and a pressure sore in 2 h. Fischer (1969) treated 26 patients with pressure sores on the hips and the sacral areas using topical HBO at 1.03 ATA. He noticed improvement in almost all cases with 6 h of treatment. A pinkish color developed and the inflammatory reaction subsided. This was followed by granulation and epithelialization. Lesions less than 6 cm in diameter eventually healed, but in three patients where the lesions were larger than this, HBO suppressed bacterial growth and stimulated granulation tissue before plastic surgical repair.

Eltorai (1981) reported 28 cases of pressure sores treated conservatively because of anaerobic infections, osteomyelitis, and septic arthritis, which contraindicated surgical intervention. Eighteen of these patients (65%) healed completely. Another 27 patients with ulcers covered by inadequately vascularized flaps were given HBO shortly after surgery. In 20 (74%) of them the flaps healed completely. He recommended HBO for consideration when a skin flap is in danger of ischemia during surgery for pressure sores.

Future status of HBO for pressure ulcers. Introduction of skin substitutes such as Apligraf® may obviate the need for HBO treatments alone or as an adjunct to surgery for pressure ulcers. However, HBO may be useful for preparation of patients with infected pressure ulcers before a skin substitute is applied. In some cases it may be used as an adjunct to accelerate healing after application of the skin substitute. In any case, the role of HBO in the treatment of pressure ulcers needs to be redefined. Prevention of such ulcers will remain the most important part of medical management.

Infected Wounds

The role of HBO in the treatment of infections is described in Chapter 13. Use of HBO should be considered if an infected space cannot be sufficiently vascularized with debridement and flap construction. Yagi (1987) reported that 62 out of 95 (65%) infected ischemic ulcers healed in response to HBO therapy.

Frostbite

Pathogenesis. Frostbite usually results from exposure to temperatures below −2°C. The extent of injury is determined by the duration of exposure, humidity, high altitude (decrease of oxygen tension), and the rapidity of cooling. Predisposing factors such as peripheral vascular disease may influence the extent of tissue damage in frostbite.

Damage to the tissues is caused by freezing or by ischemic changes that occur during rewarming. Intracellular ice formation leads to indirect damage from dehydration. The vascular complications are vasoconstriction, thrombosis, and ischemic swelling of soft tissues such as muscles, which can cause a compartment syndrome. The ischemic lesions may take several weeks to evolve.

Research into the pathophysiology of frostbite has revealed marked similarities in inflammatory processes to those seen in thermal burns and ischemia/reperfusion injury (Murphy *et al* 2000). Evidence of the role of thromboxanes and prostaglandins has resulted in more active approaches to the medical treatment of frostbite wounds.

Clinical features. Most of the clinical experience has been in the two world wars and the Korean conflict, representing over 1 million cases. Clinically, frostbite can be classified into three stages:

- Erythema; only superficial redness
- Blistering of the skin
- Necrosis of the skin and soft tissues.

Laboratory studies. The following laboratory studies have been found to be helpful in the assessment of such cases:

- Noninvasive vascular studies; Doppler and digital plethysmography.
- X-rays. Tissue edema is seen in early cases. Osteoporosis is noted in 50% of the cases, 4–10 weeks following the injury. Damage to the epiphyseal plates can occur in children.
- EMG and nerve conduction studies may be useful in assessing the lesions of the peripheral nerves.

Management. This consists of the following measures:

1. Emergency management; rewarming
2. Chemical sympathectomy (reversible blocking by intra-arterial injection)
3. Vasodilators
4. Heparin and infusion of low molecular weight dextran to reduce the sludging in microcirculation
5. Wound care
6. Delayed debridement 1 to 3 months after demarcation
7. Hyperbaric oxygenation.

HBO has been found to be useful in limiting tissue loss and enhancing healing after frostbite. The successful use of HBO has been reported in several cases. HBO is capable of improving nutritive skin blood flow in frostbitten areas more than 2 weeks after the injury (Finderle & Cankar 2002). In a case where HBO was started three days after frostbite and amputation of the affected fingers had been considered, complete recovery occurred following two weeks of daily HBO treatments (von Heimburg *et al* 2001). A case is reported of frostbite to all fingers of a mountain climber, who was treated by HBO, resulting in healing of all fingers to full function, except some cosmetic deformity of the tip of the most severely affected finger (Folio *et al* 2007). There are no controlled clinical studies and the results of controlled animal studies are conflicting.

HBO counteracts tissue hypoxia and reduces tissue edema. It promotes wound healing and prevents infection. Eventually it helps to demarcate the necrotic area from the viable area so that a greater part of the involved tissue can be salvaged and restored to function. HBO is indicated when there is evidence of ischemia that is refractory to other measures, and where surgery is considered to cover soft tissue defects.

Spider Bite

Introduction. A significant number of persons are bitten by the brown recluse spider *(Loxosceles reclusa)* each year. It is widely distributed in the central and southern United States. The bite is accompanied by pain, pruritus, and erythema at the site of skin puncture. This is followed by a vesicle formation a few hours later that ruptures, leading to the formation of an ulcer. The bite may go unnoticed, which delays treatment until tissue necrosis occurs. The underlying tissue, including the muscle, is involved with enlargement of the ulcer and plastic surgery may be required for repair. The cause of tissue necrosis may be hypoxia or vasospastic and thrombotic action of the venom. The necrotizing component of the brown spider venom is considered to be the enzyme lipase sphingomyelinase D, which contains sulfhydryl groups that are susceptible to HBO. Systemic symptoms that may be present in 25% of patients usually occur within 24 to 72 hours. These include fever, chills, malaise, nausea, vomiting, myalgia, rash, jaundice, hemolytic anemia, renal failure, shock and disseminated intravascular coagulation. Death has been reported in children.

Animal experimental studies. Brown recluse spider venom has been injected intradermally in albino rabbits and the effect of HBO has been studied on the resulting ulcers (Strain *et al* 1991). Although there was no difference in lesion healing as assessed by measuring the lesion area, animals receiving HBO had complete re-epithelialization while those not receiving any HBO developed necrotic cavities extending into the dermis with myonecrosis. Maynor *et al* (1997) performed a prospective controlled study on New Zealand rabbits to delineate the effects of HBO therapy on these lesions. The animals were divided into 5 groups: 1) venom and no HBO; 2) venom and one immediate HBO treatment (100% O_2); 3) venom and immediate HBO with 10 treatments (100% O_2); 4) venom and then delayed (48 h) HBO therapy with 10 treatments (100% O_2); and 5) venom and immediate hyperbaric treatment with normal inspired PO_2 for 10 treatments (8.4% O_2). Three animals in group 2 also received a control sodium citrate buffer injection. HBO treatments were at 2.5 ATA for 90 min twice daily. Daily measurements were made of the lesion diameter and skin blood flow using a laser Doppler probe. There was no significant effect of HBO on blood flow at the wound center or 1–2 cm from the wound center. Standard HBO significantly decreased wound diameter at 10 days, whereas hyperbaric treatment with normoxic gas had no effect. Histologic preparations from two animals in each group revealed that there were more polymorphonuclear leukocytes in the dermis of all the HBO-treated animals when compared with the venom-alone and sodium-citrate controls. It was concluded that HBO treatment within 48 h of a simulated bite from *L. reclusa* reduces skin necrosis and results in a significantly smaller wound in this model. The mechanism appears unrelated to augmented local blood flow between treatments.

Treatment with HBO in humans. Svendsen (1986) has described six cases of brown recluse spider *(L. reclusa)* bite where HBO treatment (2 ATA, 90 min, twice daily for 1–3 days) was started 2–6 days postbite. All the patients recovered without any surgery or hospitalization. Broughton (1997) has reported the case of soldier who was bitten on the glans penis by a brown recluse spider and received HBO treatment within 24 hours of the bite and twice daily for 5 days. He recovered in a week without any sequelae. A patient with brown recluse spider bite to the left lower eyelid was treated by HBO in addition to canthotomy as well as administration of dapsone, antibiotics, and steroids (Jarvis *et al* 2000). Complete recovery with occurred with cicatrization at the site of the bite. Another case of brown recluse spider bit with necrotic wound and hemolysis was managed successfully with dapsone and HBO (Wilson *et al* 2005). Results of HBO treatment in the reported cases shows that it is possible to avoid surgery and other sequelae of this spider bite.

Refractory Perineal Crohn's Disease

Perineal Crohn's disease (CD) is an extremely difficult condition to treat medically or surgically. Current surgical methods include procedures such as incision and drainage, debridement, fistulotomy, muscle flaps, colostomy, etc. Medical treatments involve use of sulfasalazine, metronidazole, broad spectrum antibiotics, and immunosuppressive agents. Brady *et al* (1989) reported a patient who responded dramatically to HBO treatment after failure of multiple medical and surgical treatments. Nelson *et al* (1990) reported another case of intractable perineal Crohn's disease where integration of HBO in a comprehensive management program including debridement and metronidazole therapy resulted in a complete and sustained closure of the lesion.

Weisz *et al* (1997) have recently reported a good clinical effect of HBO treatment in perineal CD. Seven patients with perineal CD were subjected to daily sessions of HBO in a multiplace hyperbaric chamber. Each patient received a total of 20 sessions during a time period of 1 month, and IL-1, IL-6, and TNF-a measurements were done several times during the initial sessions and after completing therapy. Pretreatment cytokine levels were elevated in patients compared to age-matched normal controls. During the first 7 days of treatment, IL-1, IL-6, and TNF-α levels in supernatants of LPS-stimulated monocytes derived from patients' peripheral blood were decreased compared to pretreatment levels. Parallel measurements of serum IL-1 levels revealed an initial elevation and thereafter decreased levels, which remained low throughout the first week of HBO treatment. After completion of therapy, cytokine levels increased to pretreatment values. The authors concluded that alterations in secretion of IL-1, IL-6, and TNF-α may be related to the good clinical effect of HBO treatment in CD patients with perianal disease.

The role of HBO in larger groups or less severely affected patients with perinal CD has not yet been studied, nor has the minimum number of treatments required for initial or complete healing of perineal disease in this population been described (Noyer & Brandt 1999).

HBO as an Aid to the Survival of Skin Flaps and Free Skin Grafts

Basic Considerations

Skin coverage for open wounds is obtained by transposition of skin as a flap or a pedicle graft or by application of grafts of split or full-thickness skin. Naturally, there is some risk, as ischemia is an unavoidable consequence of these procedures. The tissue damage incurred may result in failure of 21% of replants and 11% of free flaps. The raising and transfer of a pedicle flap takes 2–3 months, and if even one stage fails, this period may be doubled.

The problem of closing large open wounds was partially solved by the introduction of split skin grafting. After excision, the vessels of the graft collapse, and the fibrinogen-free fluid they contain bathes the graft to meet its metabolic requirements for some days. During this period, there is low oxygen tension in the wound area. Remarkably, this healing skin can survive with a flow of only 1–2 ml of blood per 100 g tissue per min, contrasting markedly with the flow to normal skin of 90 ml per 100 g per min.

Ischemic injury to the skin flaps plays a role in the evolution of skin necrosis. Free radicals contribute to ischemic damage; superoxide dismutase, given immediately after the injury, exerts a protective effect in the viable zones in the microvasculature, where free radicals are generated by neutrophils contained in the gaps between the endothelium and the vessel wall.

The chemical changes that occur in the skin, fat, and blood vessels of the skin flap, as well as the muscles in the myocutaneous flap, include a breakdown of the Na/K pump and inflammation of the perivascular tissue, with a concomitant increase in the number of free radicals. The edema resulting from these changes may cause constriction of the lumen, particularly in the microvasculature. Tissue levels of energy in the form of ATP and oxygen are usually depleted, leading to sequential necrosis of myocytes, smooth muscle cells, fat cells, and endothelial cells lining the vasculature. Endothelial damage may result in the exposure of subendothelial collagen, leading to platelet aggregation and thrombus formation after revascularization. Plasma levels of creatine kinase in the first 24 h postischemia are significantly higher in the ischemic flaps that fail, compared with those that survive. This parameter has been proposed as a means of predicting potential failure of the flap after an ischemic insult and an indication to take appropriate measures to remedy the situation.

Tissue hypoxia is the common denominator in the pathogenesis of ischemia and infection that can lead to skin flap necrosis. The effectiveness of HBO is based on relief of tissue hypoxia. Boerema (1963) noticed an apparent beneficial effect of HBO on a compromised skin graft, and his observation has been confirmed by many other surgeons in the past quarter of a century.

Animal Experimental Studies

HBO has been shown to be of definite value in preventing necrosis in the pedicle flaps, and also limits the extent of necrosis in the free composite grafts.

Champion *et al* (1967) achieved survival of all experimental flaps in rabbits exposed to HBO at 2 ATA for 2 h twice daily. None of the flaps in the controls treated with hyperbaric air survived. Gruber *et al* (1970a,b) found that the tissue oxygen tension of pedicle flaps, skin grafts, and third-degree burns in experimental rats was significantly lower at 24 h than in normal skin. There was no significant increase in tissue oxygen tension after exposure to 100%

oxygen at ambient pressure. The response of these tissues to HBO at 2 ATA, however, was rapid and large in most cases. The high oxygen tensions returned to preexposure levels after discontinuation of HBO.

Winter and Perrins (1970) conducted studies in pigs with shallow wounds and found that treatment with HBO at 2 ATA for 16 h of a 48-h period resulted in 80% epidermal coverage, as against 49% in controls. This has relevance for the healing of sites of skin graft removal in human patients, which epithelialize faster under HBO.

Jurrel and Kaisjer (1973) found that immediate postoperative HBO increased the flap survival area to twice that in nontreated control rats. Better results were obtained with HBO at 2 ATA than at 3 ATA. If the start of HBO was delayed by more than 24 h after surgery, the beneficial effect was diminished considerably.

In a controlled study by Kivisaari and Niinikoski (1975), HBO at 2 ATA for 2 h twice daily for 30 days had no effect on the healing of full thickness wounds in rats if the circulation was intact. When the circulation was interrupted locally, the control group had impaired healing, whereas healing in the HBO-treated group approached normal parameters. The results of their experiments indicate that HBO is not effective in improving the flap survival unless ischemia is a factor for non-healing.

Tan et al (1984) studied the effect of HBO and air under pressure on skin survival in acute 8 × 8 cm neurovascular island flaps in rats. Skin flaps treated with 8% oxygen at 2.5 ATA (equivalent to room air at standard pressure) exhibited no improvement in skin survival. Skin flaps treated with hyperbaric air (21% oxygen) and hyperbaric 100% oxygen exhibited significant increase in survival.

The controversy in the literature between survival of flaps in rats and nonsurvival in pigs with HBO can be explained. The flap in a pig is a true random flap, while the one in a rat is a myocutaneous flap incorporating the panniculus cavernosum and has a different blood supply than the flap in the pig.

Preoperative or postoperative HBO treatment has been shown to improve the survival rate of free flaps in rats to 66% as compared to 20% without the use of HBO (Kaelin et al 1990). This beneficial effect was explained by the increase of superoxide dismutase activity induced by intermittent exposure to HBO and is an important factor in protection from reperfusion injury.

The number and size of blood vessels in the microvasculature is significantly greater in animals skin flaps treated with HBO as compared with controls ($p > 0.01$) and HBO enhances flap survival by this mechanism. HBO treatment of ischemic rat skin flaps in the acute phase improves distal microvascular skin perfusion as measured by Laser Doppler flowmetry and this correlates with improvement of skin flap survival (Zamboni et al 1992).

Kerwin et al (1992) tested the effect of HBO on pedi-cled skin flap in the cat based on the caudal superficial artery which was ligated. There was no significant difference in the total flap survival between treated and non-treated control animals. The limitation of this study was that HBO at 2 ATA was used for 90 min once a day instead of the usual twice daily treatments. However, HBO did improve the color and decrease the exudate produced by the skin flap in the early postoperative period, factors that may be important in skin flap survival in less controlled conditions. The authors suggested the use of larger samples and a more sensitive model for future studies.

Intensive and tapering HBO therapy has been shown to demonstrate a mean 35% less necrosis as compared with controls in random skin flaps in swine (Pellitteri et al 1992).

Survival of free flaps of rats stored under HBO conditions increased from 10% (in room air) to 60% ($p > 0.05$) after 18 hours of preservation. Inhibition of xanthine oxidase system was postulated to be one of the mechanisms of improved success of skin flap transplantation with HBO (Tai et al 1992).

HBO treatment significantly increases flap survival in rat axial skin flap model and reduces deleterious effects of ischemia reperfusion injury (Agir et al 2003).

Comparison of HBO with Other Methods for Enhancing Flap Survival

Corticosteroids. Esclamado et al (1990) showed that in the rat dorsal skin flap model, perioperative corticosteroids improved the skin viability and that this therapy alone was as efficacious as HBO or HBO combined with corticosteroids.

Nicotinamide. Nicotinamide, which is considered to be angiogenetic, can provide benefit equal to that of HBO in improving survival rate of skin flaps in rats. No additive effect between nicotinamide and HBO has been observed.

Clinical Applications

Perrins and Barr (1986) described their experience of using HBO as an adjunct to flaps in a plastic surgery unit where the usual failure rate for such operations was 10%. With the use of HBO this incidence was reduced significantly to 4.5%. The authors recommended starting HBO treatment as soon as there is any doubt about the viability of the flap, rather than as a last resort. The pressure should be raised until the flap is pink and held at that level for 60–90 min. During this time the edema usually resolves, although it reappears between treatments, and additional treatments are required. Perrins (1979) carried out a controlled study that revealed contrasting effects on patients undergoing split skin grafting. After surgery, these patients were treated either conventionally or by exposure to 100% oxygen at 2 ATA for 2 h twice daily for 3 days. The better results were obtained in the HBO-treated group of 24 patients, where 92% of the surface area of the graft survived compared with 63% in the controls. A complete and successful graft occurred in 65% of the treated patients but only 17% of the controls.

In certain situations pedicle skin grafts can be replaced by full-thickness grafts with intensive HBO.

Complete survival of full-thickness grafts has been achieved in patients in whom free skin transfer would not normally have been contemplated.

With interruption of blood supply, the mechanism by which free skin grafts are revascularized is not fully understood. They either connect to the existing vessels of the host, or atrophy and are replaced by vessels invading the graft. In any case the graft is hypoxic in the initial stages and may not survive. HBO applied in this situation can penetrate the skin to a depth of up to $70\,\mu m$ by direct diffusion. Oxygen permeability of the skin is a function of the richness and pressure of the oxygen: 100% oxygen at ambient pressure applied topically does not elevate the tissue oxygen tension of the dermis, while HBO can elevate the tissue oxygen tension of the superficial layers of the dermis only. Skin color changes under HBO can be noted even in dead animals, indicating transdermal diffusion of the oxygen.

Under HBO treatment, the donor site from which the grafts are taken heals remarkably quickly. Perrins and Barr (1986) continue to hold the view that HBO improves the success rate of skin grafting. They did not recommend use of HBO routinely, but stated that it is valuable in treating cases of severe burns in children by making it possible to obtain further grafts from donor sites sooner than is normally practicable.

It is generally accepted that composite grafts of full-thickness skin and cartilage are unreliable for tissues farther than 0.75 cm from a viable source of blood. However, Nichter et al (1991) have reported a case of successful reimplantation of nose using HBO as an adjunct therapy. Prewitt et al (1989) described a case of successful reattachment, by microvascular anastomosis, of an avulsed ear using HBO as an adjunct therapy. HBO has been found to be a useful adjunct to microvascular transfer of free osteocutaneous flaps, pedicled on deep circumflex iliac vessels, for mandibular reconstruction.

Conclusion

There is considerable disparity in the results of animal experiments carried out to evaluate the effect of HBO on the survival of graft flaps. Apart from the controversy regard-ing the rat versus the pig experimental model, there are other variations in the experiment designs that make comparison of various studies impossible. Various studies indicate that when ischemia threatens the viability of a graft, HBO improves the chances of survival mainly by one or more of the following mechanisms:

- Relief of hypoxia/ischemia of the tissues
- Diminished metabolic disturbances in the ischemic/hypoxic tissues.
- Improvement of the microcirculation and reduction of platelet aggregation
- Increase in the number and size of blood vessels within the microvasculature
- By counteracting free radical-mediated reperfusion injury
- By accelerating the formation of healthy granulation tissue over bone

HBO is not recommended for routine use as an adjunct to flaps and grafts. Indications for its use are:

1. Significant local ischemia/hypoxia
2. Graft in an irradiated field
3. Previous graft failure

HBO appears to be most effective when given within the first 24 h following surgery. Usually pressure of 2–2.4 ATA are used for 90 minutes twice a day and the treatment duration varies from 3–10 days depending on the flap type and its condition of viability (Kindwall et al 1991a). It would be difficult to carry out double-blind, prospective studies in the circumstances in which HBO is used in these highly variable wounds.

HBO as an Adjunct in the Treatment of Thermal Burns

Basic Considerations

Thermal injury results in coagulation necrosis of the cellular elements of the epidermis and dermis; the depth of injury is determined by the intensity and duration of heat exposure. With tissue injury, vessels are disrupted or thrombosed and cells destroyed; interstitial fluid, cellular elements, and connective tissues interact. Adjacent intact vessels soon dilate and platelets and leukocytes begin to adhere to the vascular endothelium as an early event in the inflammatory response. Increased capillary permeability is then observed as plasma leaks from the microvasculature into the area of damage. Wound edema is followed by influx of numerous polymorphonuclear neutrophilic leukocytes and monocytes that accumulate at the site of injury.

Following these initial inflammatory events, new capillaries, immature fibroblasts, and newly formed collagen fibrils appear within the wound. The neovasculature and other components of wound repair support the rapidly regenerating epithelium that covers a partial-thickness injury. With full-thickness burns, these elements form a luxurious bed of granulation tissue that readily accepts a split-thickness skin graft.

Normal repair processes do not proceed smoothly in third-degree burns. Ischemic process in the tissues can increase threefold during the 48 h following injury. Burns are at risk for infection for the following reasons:

- There is loss of integrity of the skin, which is a barrier against invading micro-organisms.
- There is impairment of the immune system.
- The presence of necrotic tissue predisposes to infection.

Due to increased vascular permeability, there is extravasation of plasma in burns. This response is not limited to the burned area, as there may be systemically released vasoactive mediators (prostaglandins). It has been suggested that oxygen-induced vasoconstriction may limit the perfusion of the tissues having increased vascular permeability. There is animal experimental evidence that plasma extravasation decreases after HBO exposure.

Most of the recent research on burn wound pathophysiology has been directed toward the third-degree component of the burn wound. The accepted clinical approach is excision of the third-degree burn and coverage of the debrided area.

In partial thickness (second-degree) burns, not covered by stratum corneum, there is massive fluid loss. The resulting dehydration deepens the wound and may convert it into a full-thickness loss. Efforts have been directed at salvaging the viable tissue. Desiccation can be prevented by keeping the wound covered. Epithelialization of a burn wound depends upon: (a) the total cell population surviving the injury, (b) migration, and (c) mitosis. HBO appears to affect the burn wound by allowing earlier reversal of capillary stasis. There is lessening of desiccation and increased oxygen supply to the hypoxic, thermally damaged cells, which might not survive otherwise. There is, therefore, a larger surviving mass of epithelial cells to resurface the wound. The major effect of HBO is facilitation of normal healing, whether by stimulation of mitosis or by migration remains to be seen.

Experimental Studies

Healing takes 30% less time in burned rabbits treated with HBO than in controls. They also reported more rapid revascularization of full-thickness burn wounds in rats (Ketchum *et al* 1967).

There is faster epithelialization of blister-removed second-degree burn wounds in guinea pigs treated by HBO (2 ATA) with early return of capillary patency. Investigations of the effect of HBO on burns of different depths in guinea pigs show spontaneous healing, as well as good integration of the graft, regardless of the depth of the burn (second or third degree). Immediate and consistent application of HBO to burn wounds in guinea pigs infected with *Pseudomonas aeruginosa* resulted in better healing than in those animals not treated by HBO.

The following effects of HBO have been demonstrated in a rat scald burn model:

- Reduction of tissue edema
- Repletion of depleted ADP and PCr stores
- Decrease of elevated lactate levels
- Prevention of reduction of phosphorylase activity, a sensitive marker for muscle cell damage.

In standardized third-degree burns in guinea pigs, untreated animals show a considerable increase in the wound area as compared to the initial lesions whereas the wound area is reduced in animals treated with HBO.

Hammarlund *et al* (1991) used a model of skin blister with ultraviolet radiation in human volunteers. HBO was shown to have a beneficial effect on this superficial dermal lesion. Edema, exudation, and hyperemia decreased but rate of epithelialization was not accelerated. Niezgoda *et al* (1997) designed a protocol to either confirm or challenge these previous findings in a randomized, blinded format. Twelve healthy, nonsmoking volunteers were screened for contraindications to HBO therapy and given a single test hyperbaric exposure. A standardized wound model was employed for the painless creation of a volar forearm lesion on volunteers by applying a suction device to form a blister, excising its epidermal roof, and irradiating the exposed dermis with ultraviolet light. Subjects were randomized into either a hyperbaric oxygen group (100% oxygen at 2.4 ATA, n = 6) or the sea-level air-breathing equivalent control group (8.75% oxygen at 2.4 ATA, n = 6). Both groups then underwent standard hyperbaric therapy. The wounds were studied noninvasively prior to treatment and once per day over 6 days for size, hyperemia, and exudation, with epithelialization as the endpoint. The averages for each measurement of the hyperbaric oxygen group versus the control group were computed by means of a one-tail t test; p was considered significant at less than 0.05. Daily wound size, hyperemia, and exudation measurements were significantly different on day 2. The hyperbaric oxygen group showed a 42% reduction in wound hyperemia, a 35% reduction in the size of the lesion, and a 22% reduction in wound exudation (p values of 0.05, 0.03, and 0.04, respectively). No significant difference was noted for epithelialization. Observed differences in wound size, hyperemia, and exudation were attributable to hyperbaric oxygen therapy. This study further supports earlier conclusions that hyperbaric oxygen therapy is beneficial in a superficial dermal wound.

Clinical Applications

Wada *et al* (1965) were the first to observe that burned coal miners with CO poisoning who were treated with HBO appeared to do better than those treated conventionally. Their wounds dried earlier, had fewer infections, and healed faster.

Hart *et al* (1974) presented a randomized double-blind study of 191 burn patients. They concluded that application of HBO within the first 24 h decreases the healing time, morbidity, and mortality significantly. The healing time is related directly to the percentage of burns. Hart *et al* recommended the monoplace chamber as a safe, economical, and convenient means of HBO treatment for burns patients. They stated that HBO therapy in burns is an adjunctive measure: it does not replace resuscitative, topical, or surgical care, and is not a panacea.

Grossman (1978) presented his experience with HBO treatment of burns in 800 patients during 6 years at Sherman Oaks Community Hospital in California. His treatment schedule was as follows:

- Treatment was given within 4 h of admission of the patient to the burn unit.
- Treatment was given in a monoplace chamber at 2–2.5 ATA (100% oxygen) for varying periods of time.
- Tissue pO_2 was monitored. In second-degree burns the tissue pO_2 achieved at 2 ATA was 1200 mmHg, compared with 25 mmHg at 1 ATA. This value dropped to 40 mmHg 2 h after treatment. In third-degree burns, the tension achieved at 2 ATA was 1500 mmHg, dropping to 400 mmHg 2 h after treatment.

The results were reductions in (1) patients' fluid requirements; (2) second-degree burn healing time; (3) eschar separation time; (4) donor graft harvesting time; (5) length of hospital stay; (6) complications such as Curling's ulcer, infections, pulmonary emboli etc.; and (7) mortality (by 10% compared with the non-HBO-treated patients).

Grossman and Grossman (1982) presented their accumulated experience with 1,130 burn patients and continued to have the good results reported by Grossman in 1978.

Niu *et al* (1987) presented a comparative study of human patients with burns treated by adjunctive HBO therapy. They used HBO at 2.5 ATA, for a 90- to 120-min session, which was repeated two to three times daily in the first 24 h and then one to two times per day. The overall mortality in the HBO-treated and non-HBO-treated patients was not different, but in a high risk group of patients the mortality was reduced considerably. There was less fluid loss and earlier reepithelialization in the HBO-treated patients.

Cianci *et al* (1989) carried out a historically controlled study of HBO in burns patients and their conclusions were:

- In patients with burns involving 18%–39% of total body surface, there was a 37% reduction in the length of hospital stay.
- In patients with partial to full-thickness burns involving 40%–80% of total body surface, there was a reduction of the number of surgical procedures for debridement and grafting.
- HBO-treated patients showed a reduction of fluid requirements. The authors recommended HBO in a carefully controlled setting and in combination with a recognized burns care program.

Hart and Grossman (1988) have the following protocol for the treatment of burns patients:

- General supportive care: care of the airway, intravenous buffered Ringer's lactate solution for rehydration, avoidance of morphine and narcotics prior to HBO session.
- Silver sulfazine is applied to the burn wound every 8 h. Mafenide (Sulfamylon) cream should be carefully removed before placing the patient in the hyperbaric chamber (see Chapter 9).
- HBO is applied in a monoplace chamber at 2 ATA for 90-min sessions that are repeated every 8 h during the first 24 h postburn, and then twice a day until all the wounds are epithelialized.
- Debridement and grafting procedures are performed when eschars start to separate. This occurs characteristically from the 10th to the 14th day. HBO is applied again after recovery from the anesthetic.

Conclusions

There are adequate experimental studies to support the beneficial effect of HBO in thermal burns. The rationale for HBO therapy in thermal burns is summarized in Table 15.5.

The Undersea and Hyperbaric Medical Society approves the treatment of patients with burns by HBO provided the treatment is carried out in an approved facility for care of burns according to a strict protocol which involves use of HBO at 2 ATA for 90 minutes twice daily. HBO as an adjunct to comprehensive management of patients with burns has resulted in a statistically significant 25% reduction in the length of hospital stay (p < 0.012), and 19% reduction in overall cost of care (Cianci *et al* 1989, 1990).

Table 15.5
Summary of Rationale for HBO Therapy in Thermal Burns

During the first 24 h:	After the first 24
1. HBO counteracts vasodilatation and exudation of plasma by its vasoconstricting effect, and prevent burns shock.	1. It relieves paralytic ileus (see Chapter 25).
2. It inhibits wound infection.	2. It has a beneficial effect on stress ulceration of the stomach (Curling's ulcers).
3. It promotes epithelialization of the wound.	3. It reduces hypertrophic scarring and ulcerations.
4. It is a useful adjunct to survival of skin grafts and flaps.	4. It counteracts burns encephalopathy/cerebral edema (see Chapter 17).
5. It is effective against other serious problems accompanying serious burns, such as smoke inhalation injury and CO poisoning.	5. It reduces the length of hospitalization.
6. It reduces fluid requirements.	6. It reduces the need for surgical procedures.
7. It counteracts ischemia of the tissues.	
8. It helps to maintain the integrity of the wound by minimizing RBC aggregation and platelet thrombi and their propagation from the zone of heat coagulation.	

Applications of HBO in Dermatology

Necrobiosis Lipoidica Diabeticorum

This is chronic cutaneous complication of diabetes mellitus but similar lesions may appear in non-diabetics as well. The characteristic typical plaques with indurated periphery and central atrophy, are prone to ulceration which may be refractory to medical and surgical treatment. Corticosteroids have been used but this therapy may not be tolerated by some diabetic patients.

Diabetic microangiopathy is an important factor in the pathophysiology of this disease and there is significant hypoxia in the wound. Weisz *et al* (1993) used HBO in a diabetic patient with necrobiosis lipoidica of 7 year's duration that had remained refractory to medical treatment. The lesions healed after 98 daily sessions of HBO at 2.5 ATA for 90 min. Bouhanick *et al* (1998) reported the case of a 28-year-old insulin-dependent diabetic woman with a disease duration of 23 years who spontaneously developed ulcerated necrobiosis lipoidica on pretibial skin. The disease progressively improved during 113 sessions of HBO therapy and local corticosteroids.

Pyoderma Gangrenosum

This disease is characterized by the appearance of one or more bluish-black, boggy, undermined ulcers, which appear most frequently on the legs. The pathogenesis of pyoderma gangrenosum is obscure. Present conventional management of this disease consists of local treatment of the wound, systemic corticosteroid therapy, and treatment of any underlying disease. Vasculitis, wound ischemia, and infections are common in this disease.

The rationale for the use of HBO in pyoderma gangrenosum is based on the effectiveness of HBO in skin wound healing and as an adjunct to antibiotics. Several successful cases have been reported in the literature. Skin grafting can fail in this condition because of the rejection of the autograft. Davis *et al* (1987a) used HBO in four patients with pyoderma gangrenosum to prepare the wound for skin grafting, which was successful in all the cases.

Purpura Fulminans

Purpura fulminans is an acute and often fatal disease of children characterized by the sudden occurrence of ecchymotic lesions on the lower extremities that rapidly progress to necrotic gangrene. Disseminated intravascular coagulation is a major component of the disease. Waddell *et al* (1965) and Kuzemko and Loder (1970) described one case treated successfully with HBO. Dudgeon *et al* (1971) treated two patients with HBO, along with other standard treatments, and found it useful.

Toxic Epidermal Necrolysis

Ruocco *et al* (1986) have used HBO (2 ATA, 1–2 h sessions once a day) in three patients with drug-induced epidermal necrolysis. Reepithelialization occurred in all the patients with approximately ten treatments. The reasons stated for the beneficial effect of HBO in this condition are:

- Activation of dermal metabolism
- Antibacterial action
- Possibly an immunosuppressive effect.

Psoriasis

Shakhtmeister and Savrasov (1987) have used HBO as an adjunct to phototherapy in the treatment of 45 patients. The treatment was well tolerated and the course of the disease was shortened as compared with the results of conventional treatment. The average duration of remission of the disease was 1.5 years.

Maulana and Djonhar (1987) treated five patients with psoriasis using HBO. Good results were obtained in two patients with lessening of desquamation and erythema after 2 weeks, and disappearance of the lesions after 4 weeks. Treatment failed in one patient and two patients were lost to follow-up. No conclusions can be drawn from this report.

Leprosy

The possibly important role of HBO in leprosy is described in Chapter 13 (infections).

Scleroderma

Diffuse and progressive scleroderma is one of the connective tissue disorders. Ninety percent of these patients suffer from Raynaud's phenomenon. Zhou (1986) treated five patients with scleroderma using HBO. In all cases there was improvement in the symptoms of peripheral vascular disturbances. Further investigations of the long-term effect are required.

Delektorsky et al (1987) studied the electron-microscopic changes in patients with scleroderma treated by HBO. Some of the abnormalities of mitochondria improved and a larger number of "energy" mitochondria appeared after the HBO treatments.

16 HBO Therapy in the Management of Radionecrosis

K.K. Jain

HBO has been used with good results in the management of radionecrosis. This chapter reports on the applications after discussing important background topics, following this outline:

Introduction

Radiation therapy has proven to be effective in the treatment of malignancies. The goal is to irradiate tumors with minimal adverse effects on the surrounding normal tissue. This is difficult to achieve, and in practice there is usually some degree of residual damage to the tissues after radiotherapy. Theoretically it is possible to destroy all malignancies if the dosage of radiation is raised to high levels. With the limitations of the human body's tissue tolerance to radiation, optimal dosage schedules are followed that provide an acceptable benefit/damage ratio for the patient. Radiation-induced tissue necrosis is a complication even when accepted dosage schedules are followed. A basic knowledge of radiation physics and radiation biology is essential for understanding the pathology of radio-necrosis.

Radiation Physics

There are two types of ionizing radiations with significant biological effects.

- Electromagnetic radiation: a combination of electric and magnetic fields, consisting of bundles of energy called photons. This form of radiation is termed gamma rays if it originates from the atomic nucleus, and x-rays if it originates from the shell around the nucleus.
- Particulate radiation. Examples of this are the heavy radiation particles such as protons and neutrons.

Unit of Radiation

A rad is the amount of radiation of any type that results in deposition of 100 ergs of energy/g of tissue. Directly ionizing radiation transfers energy to the tissue by direct disruption of the atomic structure of the tissue. Indirectly ionizing radiations such as neutrons transfer energy by being absorbed by the tissue atom nuclei, which, in turn, give off directly ionizing charged particles as well as gamma rays and x-rays.

X-rays scatter in tissues whereas heavy radiation particles like proton beams can be focused on targets at depths with peak effect. The tissues in the path of the beam receive minimal radiation.

Radiation Biology

In the initial stages of radiation tissue interaction there are several metastable states and energy transfer processes that precede chemical changes in the tissues. The indirect effects of radiation are due to reactive species (free radicals derived from water molecules). The chemical changes resulting from radiation are:

- Damage to the protein structure
- Lipid peroxidation
- DNA damage

The cell DNA is a critical target. There is breakage of hydrogen bonds between the strands of DNA and formation of cross links with other DNA molecules and chromosomal proteins. There is some correlation between DNA molecules and chromosomal proteins, and between DNA damage and cellular radiosensitivity. The radiosensitivity of a cell depends upon the stage of the cell cycle at the time of radiation and is greatest just prior to mitosis. The radiosensitivity of the cells is directly proportional to their mitotic activity and inversely proportional to their level of specialization.

The effect of ionizing radiation on the tissues is the sum of the damage to cells in the tissues: damage to the critical cell components of a certain tissue can cause death of the whole tissue or even the whole organ.

Connective tissue (including vascular epithelium) has a radiosensitivity that is intermediate between differentiating intermitotic cells and reverting postmitotic cells. Damage to vascular epithelium with obliteration of the vessels may be responsible for the delayed necrosis following radiation.

Radiation Pathology

Clinicopathological Correlations

The clinicopathological correlation of the sequence of events following radiation is divided into four periods:

- Acute period. First 6 months. During this period there is accumulation of acute organ damage, which may be clinically silent.
- Subacute period. Second 6 months. This is the end of the recovery from the acute period. Persistence and progression of permanent tissue damage is evident during this period.
- Chronic period. Second to fifth year. There is further progression of chronic progressive residual damage. There is deterioration of microvasculature with resulting hypoperfusion, parenchymal damage, and reduced resistance to infections.
- Late clinical period. After the fifth postirradiation year. Further progression of changes in the chronic period with additional effects of aging (premature), and radiation carcinogenesis may manifest during this period.

Whole body irradiation may cause acute radiation sickness, but the localized radiation-induced damage that manifests during the subacute and the chronic periods is relevant to our discussion in this chapter.

Radiation damage progresses slowly and continues long after the radiotherapy has been discontinued. Damaged cells do not reproduce and otherwise normal cells may fail to reproduce because of loss of vascularity. There is loss of collagen and increased fibrosis in the radiated tissues due to low oxygen gradient. Oxygen tension at the center of an uncomplicated radiated area is 5–10 mmHg (Marx & Johnson 1988).

Effect of Radiation on Blood Vessels

Radiation has been shown to produce swelling, degeneration, and necrosis of the endothelium with resulting thickening of the vessel wall. These vascular changes progress slowly after radiation and have been referred to as proliferative endarteritis and necrotizing vasculitis. The arterioles and the capillaries suffer the most damage, whereas the larger vessels are spared.

Effect on Soft Tissues

Skin is the tissue that has been most extensively studied for the effects of radiation in the acute, subacute, and chronic periods. Skin atrophy occurs in the chronic stages and the skin is prone to ulceration with minor trauma. Skin incisions made through previously irradiated areas heal poorly. The underlying soft tissues undergo necrosis due to microvascular occlusion. Radiation may directly affect the mucosal cells of the gastrointestinal and genitourinary tracts producing gastroenteritis and cystitis respectively. A case of laryngeal radionecrosis was treated successfully with HBO (Hsu et al 2005).

Radiation Effects on the Nervous System

The effects of radiation on the nervous system are reviewed elsewhere (New 2001). The normal neurons are fairly resistant to the usual doses of radiation. Radiation necrosis is thought to result from complex dynamic interactions between parenchymal and vascular endothelial cells within the CNS.

Radiation Effects on Bone

Bone is 1.8 times as dense as soft tissues and absorbs a larger portion of the incident radiation than do soft tissues.

Radiation affects both the vascular and the cellular components of bone. High doses of radiation damage the blood vessels passing between the periosteum and the surface of the bone, leading to bone death. Radiation upsets the balance between the constantly occurring osteoclastic destruction and osteoblastic construction of adult bone. This leads to osteoporosis and finally osteonecrosis, which usually takes place 4 months to several years following radiation. The usual sites of necrosis are:

- The mandible, generally following radiotherapy of soft tissue tumors of the head and the neck. The mandible absorbs more radiation than the maxilla because of its greater density and shows more necrosis due to its lesser vascularity.
- The ribs, clavicle, and the sternum, usually following radiotherapy of breast cancer.
- The skull, usually following radiotherapy of brain tumors and soft tissue tumors of the scalp.
- Vertebral column, usually following radiation of spinal cord tumors.
- Pelvis and femoral head following radiation of pelvic tumors.

HBO Therapy for Radionecrosis

Rationale

There is no satisfactory treatment of radiation necrosis using the available conventional methods. It is difficult to provide adequate nutrients and oxygen to the devascularized tissues. Radiation ulcers are painful and use of narcotic analgesics can lead to addiction. Reconstructive surgery in the radiated areas has a high failure rate due to healing problems. Frustration with the use of conventional methods has led to the trial use of HBO in the management of radiation necrosis.

HBO raises the tissue pO_2 to within the normal range and stimulates collagen formation at wound edges. This, in turn, enhances the formation of new microvasculature. This provides reepithelialization of small ulcers and provides a better nutritive bed to support grafts and pedicle flaps. Tissue oxygen studies have shown that angiogenesis becomes measurable after 8 treatments with HBO, reaches a plateau at 80%–85% of non-radiated tissue vascularization after 20 treatments, and remains at this level whether or not HBO is continued (Marx et al 1985).

The rationale of the use of HBO for nonhealing wounds also applies to radiation necrosis. Osseous implants are sometimes required for reconstruction of bone in radionecrosis. Larsen et al (1993) have exposed rabbit tibias to tumoricidal doses of radiation. Adjuvant HBO therapy was shown to improve the amount of histologic integration of the implants in this compromised situation as compared with contralateral control implants.

HBO is not used in the early postradiation period as it may potentiate the effects of radiation. HBO may have no effect as a prophylactic for radionecrosis because a certain amount of vascular damage should be evident before HBO effect can be observed. In some situations HBO, by resolution of the swelling of the involved tissues, permits a better definition of the tumor tissue, which can be resected surgically. The presence of residual tumor in an ulcer bed, on the other hand, would lead to failure of a skin graft, even if HBO is used.

The benefit of treating radiation injuries with HBO was first reported in 1973 (Mainous et al 1973; Greenwood & Gilchrist 1973). Hart & Strauss (1986) reported their treatment of 378 patients with this diagnosis. After deaths and drop-outs for various reasons, 336 patients completed the treatment course of HBO. The reasons for discontinuance of the therapy (contraindications) were recurrence of the tumor, viral infections, and smoking by patients. HBO was considered as an adjunct to surgery and other appropriate medical regimens. Each patient was treated at 2 ATA for 2 h daily in the case of outpatients, or 1.5 h twice daily in the case of inpatients for a total of 120 h or less. If healing is not adequate, the treatment is repeated after a rest period of 3–6 months. As HBO immediately following radiation may have deleterious effects, the authors do not start HBO therapy until 2 months after the last radiotherapy treatment. They concluded that HBO combined with other appropriate treatments reduces the morbidity of radiation injury.

After a review of the literature and his own experience, Davis (1981) concluded:

The clear physiological basis, supported by experimental data, upon which hyperbaric oxygen is useful in radiation necrosis, confirmed by almost identical beneficial results in multiple centers, makes the use of adjunctive hyperbaric oxygen in both soft tissues and osteoradionecrosis compelling indications.

This conclusion still holds good. Review of a cumulative 14-year experience with 124 patients has shown that HBO therapy led to significant improvement in 94% of the cases (Slade & Cianci 1998). The average number of treatments for these patients was 33.1 and the average HBO treatment costs were $15,800. The patient material covered a wide range of soft tissues affected by radiation necrosis and the treatment protocol was HBO at 2 ATA for 90–120 min daily and occasionally twice daily. The authors feel that a minimum of 30 treatments are necessary and there is need to develop more definite outcome predictors and treatment protocols for soft tissue radiation damage indicators.

The role of HBO in radiation necrosis in the adults is well established now. In order to evaluate this approach in the pediatric population, Ashamalla et al (1996) reviewed the experience at the University of Pennsylvania, Philadelphia. Between 1989 and 1994, ten patients who underwent radiation therapy for cancer as children were referred for HBO therapy. Six patients underwent HBO therapy as a prophylactic measure prior to maxillofacial procedures; dental extractions and/or root canals (four patients), bilateral coronoidectomies for mandibular ankylosis (one patient), and wound dehiscence (one patient). Therapeutic HBO was administered to four other patients; one patient for vasculitis resulting in acute seventh cranial nerve palsy and the other three after sequestrectomy for osteoradionecrosis (mastoid bone, temporal bone, and sacrum, respectively). Osteoradionecrosis was diagnosed both radiologically and histologically after exclusion of tumor recurrence. The number of treatments ranged between 9–40 (median, 30). Treatments were given once daily at 2 ATA for 2 hours each. Adjunctive therapy in the form of debridement, antibiotics, and placement of tympanotomy tubes was administered to two patients. Ages at HBO treatment ranged from 3.5 to 26 years (median, 14 years). The most commonly irradiated site was the head and neck region. The interval between the end of radiation therapy and HBO treatment ranged between 2 months and 11 years (median, 15 years). The median follow-up interval after HBO therapy was 2.5 years (range, 2 months–4 years). Except for two patients who had initial anxiety, nausea, and vomiting, HBO treatments were well tolerated. In all but one patient, the outcome was excellent. In the six patients who had prophylactic HBO, all continued to demonstrate complete healing of their orthodontal scars at last follow-up. In the four patients who received HBO as a therapeutic modality, all 4 had documented disappearance of signs and symptoms of radionecrosis and two patients demonstrated new bone growth on follow-up CT scan. One patient with vasculitis and seventh cranial nerve palsy had transient improvement of hearing; however, subsequent audiograms returned to baseline. It was concluded that the use of HBO for children with radiation-induced bone and soft tissue complications is safe and results in few significant adverse effects. It is a potentially valuable tool both in the prevention and treatment of radiation-related complications.

Management of Osteoradionecrosis

Basic Studies

Several studies have been carried out to demonstrate the protective effect of HBO on osteoradionecrosis. Wang et al (1998) carried out experiments to test for a protective effect of HBO and basic fibroblast growth factor (bFGF) on bone growth. Control C3H mice received hind leg irradiation at 0, 10, 20, or 30 Gy. HBO-treated groups received radiation 1, 5, or 9 weeks before beginning HBO. The remaining groups began bFGF ± HBO 1 or 5 weeks after 30 Gy. HBO treatments were given 5 days per week for 4 weeks at 2 ATA for 3 h/day. At 18 weeks control tibia length discrepancy was 0.0, 4.2, 8.2, and 10.7% after 0, 10, 20, and 30 Gy, respectively. HBO beginning in week 1, 5, or 9 following 10 Gy decreased these discrepancies to 2.0% ($p < 0.05$), 1.8% ($p < 0.05$), and 2.4% ($p < 0.05$), respectively. After 20 Gy, HBO decreased these discrepancies to 7.0% ($p = $ ns), 4.9% ($p < 0.05$), and 3.6% ($p < 0.05$), respectively. At 30 Gy, HBO alone had no effect on bone shortening. bFGF improved tibia length discrepancy with or without HBO. At 18 weeks length discrepancies were 6.5% ($p < 0.05$) and 7.3 ($p < 0.05$), and after bFGF alone were 6.8% ($p < 0.05$) and 7.3% ($p < 0.05$) for treatment beginning in week 1 or 5, respectively. Tibial growth at 18 and 33 weeks following radiation were similar. This study showed that radiation effects on bone growth can be significant reduced by HBO after 10 or 20 Gy, but not after 30 Gy. At 30 Gy bFGF still significantly reduced the degree of bone shortening, but HBO provided no added benefit to bFGF therapy.

HBO therapy was found to be effective in the treatment of complications of irradiation for cancer in head and neck area (Narozny et al 2005). Impact of perioperative HBO therapy on the quality of life of maxillofacial patients who undergo surgery in irradiated fields has been assessed in 66 patients (Harding et al 2008). The Head and Neck submodule identified significant improvements in teeth, dry mouth and social contact. It was recommended that adjunctive HBO should be considered for the treatment and prevention of some of the long-term complications of radiotherapy.

Osteoradionecrosis of the Mandible

Mandibular osteoradionecrosis is a late complication of radiotherapy for cancers of the head and neck, particularly of the oral cavity. Mandibular osteoradionecrosis is also the most frequently reported radiation injury – 235 of 378 patients (62.2%) in the series of Hart and Strauss (1986). This high frequency is because of the singularity of the blood supply running through the matrix of the bone and the proximity of the tumor to the mandible. Radiation decreases the number of osteoclasts and osteoblasts in the irradiated mandible, and if the mandible is fractured, the healing is delayed. In a normal mandible, after fracture, the alveolar processes remodel, and tooth sockets will heal in 9–12 months.

X-rays of the mandible in osteonecrosis show a variety of lesions including osteolysis and pathological fracture. In some cases, x-rays do not show any abnormalities and when present, the abnormalities do not necessarily correlate with the clinical severity of the disease. In the past, infection was considered to play a role in the pathogenesis of osteoradionecrosis, although it is now considered essentially a nonbacterial process. The following conventional treatments have been used during the past 30 years on the assumption that osteoradionecrosis is an infection:

- Irrigation of the wound with a variety of solutions ranging from saline to hydrogen peroxide and other disinfectants
- Antibiotic therapy
- Superficial sequestrectomy

These treatments are obsolete now and HBO has an important role in the management of osteoradionecrosis of the mandible (Guernsey & Clark 1981, Patel et al 1989, Fattore & Strauss 1987). Of the 206 patients of Hart and Strauss (1986) who underwent treatment with HBO as an adjunct, 72% had an excellent result, 10% a good result, and 15% a fair response. The remaining 3% were failures.

There are some variations in the technique of combination of HBO with surgery. The Marx/University of Miami protocol (Marx & Johnson 1988) consists of three stages:

Stage I

This includes all patients having osteoradionecrosis of the jaw with three exceptions: cutaneous fistulae, pathological fractures, and radiological evidence of bone absorption at the inferior border of the mandible. Patients with these exceptions are allocated to stage III. Treatment of stage I includes daily HBO treatments at 2.4 ATA (90 min), wound care by saline rinses, no bone removal, and discontinuance of antibiotics. If improvement continues, ten further sessions of HBO are given. If there is no improvement, the patient is considered a nonresponder in stage I and moved to stage II.

Stage II

A local wound debridement is attempted to identify patients with only cortical bone involvement who do not require jaw resection. A transoral alveolar sequestrectomy is performed. If healing continues satisfactorily, ten further HBO treatments are given. If the wound dehisces, the patient is considered to be a nonresponder in stage II and is moved to stage III.

Stage III

The patient is given 30 HBO treatments followed by transoral partial jaw resection and a stabilization procedure (extraskeletal or mandibulo-maxillary fixation). A further ten HBO treatments are given and the patient is advanced to stage III-R (reconstruction).

Stage III-R

The emphasis in this stage is on early reconstruction and rehabilitation. Ten HBO sessions are given in the postoperative period and jaw fixation is maintained for 8 weeks.

Marx treated 268 patients over a period of 8 years using this protocol. Resolution of the lesions was achieved in 38 patients in stage I (14%), 48 patients in stage II (18%), and 182 patients in stage III (68%). Marx et al (1985) carried out a randomized clinical trial of HBO vs penicillin for prevention of radiation-induced osteoradionecrosis after tooth extraction in a high-risk population. One group received only penicillin before and after extraction; the other group received no antibiotics, but did receive HBO at 2.4 ATA for 20 daily sessions of 90 min each. One-half of the sessions were given before the extractions and the other half afterwards. The incidence of osteoradionecrosis was 29.9% in the antibiotic group and only 5.4% in the HBO group. The conclusion was that HBO should be considered as a prophylactic measure when postradiation dental care (e.g., tooth extraction) involving trauma to the tissues is necessary.

Mounsey et al (1993) carried out a retrospective analysis of 41 patients with osteoradionecrosis of the mandible treated at the Hyperbaric Chamber Unit of the Toronto Hospital and reported that 83% of these patients had a significant improvement. These authors concluded that HBO is of benefit in the management of these cases and that mild cases will heal with HBO alone but in severe cases surgery is necessary to remove the dead tissue. The authors recommended that such patients should receive dental evaluation, local wound care, and a strict oral hygiene. Diseased teeth should be removed prior to radiotherapy and any teeth that develop abscesses subsequently should be extracted in conjunction with prophylactic HBO.

Epstein et al (1997) carried out a study was to assess the long-term progress of 26 patients who experienced postradiation osteonecrosis of the jaw between 1975 and 1989. Of 26 patients who had been previously managed with HBO therapy as a part of their treatment for postradiation osteonecrosis of the jaw, 20 were evaluated to determine their current status of the condition: resolved, chronic persisting (unresolved), or active progressive (symptomatic). Two of 20 patients experienced recurrences of the condition. In one of these patients, surgical treatment was identified as the stimulus of postradiation osteonecrosis. In the other patient, the recurrence appeared to be related to periodontal disease activity. In 60% (12 of 20) of the patients, the condition remained resolved, improvement in clinical staging occurred in 10% (2 of 20) (from symptomatic to unresolved or resolved), and 20% (5 of 20) of the patients continued to demonstrate chronic persisting postradiation osteonecrosis at the end of the long-term follow-up period. This study supports the contention that postradiation osteonecrosis can occur at any time after radiation therapy, and that patients remain at risk up to 231 months after treatment of the cancer and probably indefinitely after radiation therapy. These findings also suggest that risk of second episodes of the condition after management of an ini-

tial episode is low. In addition, the follow-up study revealed that chronic nonprogressive postradiation osteonecrosis can remain stable without extensive intervention including combined HBO therapy and surgery.

Osteonecrosis of the Temporal Bone

Temporal bone is susceptible to the development of osteoradionecrosis because it is covered by a thin layer of skin, has a limited blood supply, and is composed mainly of compact bone. The latent period for the development of clinically manifest osteoradionecrosis of the temporal bone is 8 months to 23 years with an average of 8 years (Ramsden et al 1975). Surgical treatment involves removal of all necrotic bone.

Rudge (1993) treated a patient with osteoradionecrosis of the temporal bone using HBO as an adjunct and the result was complete resolution.

Osteoradionecrosis of the Chest Wall

There were 20 cases of osteonecrosis of the chest wall in the series of Hart and Strauss (1986). The osteonecrosis developed following radiation therapy for cancer of the breast, lung or mediastinum and involved the sternum and/or ribs. All the patients recovered.

Kaufman et al (1979) presented three cases of postradiation osteomyelitis of the chest wall that were treated successfully by a combination of HBO and surgery.

Osteoradionecrosis of the Vertebrae

Four cases of necrosis of the vertebrae in the series of Hart and Strauss (1986) were treated by HBO and minor debridements. All four patients recovered, and three had spontaneous fusions.

Management of Radionecrosis of CNS

Radiation Myelitis

Radiation myelitis of the cervical spinal cord was first reported more than 60 years ago following radiation therapy for pharyngeal cancer (Ahlbom 1941). The pathology of radiation injury usually involves interstitial tissue damage and microvascular endothelial injury causing thrombosis with secondary regional ischemia. Provision of HBO during the period of ischemia should, theoretically, minimize the effect of radiation injury. However, HBO has also been shown to potentiate the effects of radiation. One of the practical problems is that adverse neurological effects of radiation may not manifest clinically for several months following exposure.

Poulton and Witcofski (1985) investigated the use of HBO in rats with radiation-induced myelitis. The animals were randomized into HBO-treatment and control groups. Eight weeks following radiation therapy, the animals in the treatment group were given HBO at 2.5 ATA for 30 min 5 times a week for 4 weeks. Serial neurological examinations did not shown any benefit or harm as a result of HBO therapy.

Feldmeier et al (1993c) carried out an animal experimental study to investigate HBO as a treatment or prophylaxis for radiation myelitis. All animals received identical amounts of radiation. Group I received no HBO, group II began HBO at onset of myelitis, group III received HBO as prophylactic beginning 6 weeks after radiation, and group IV received HBO and radiation on the same day but following it after no less than 4 h. HBO consisted of 90 min sessions at 2.4 ATA for 20 daily treatments. All animals progressed to myelitis but it was least severe in group III and most severe in group IV.

Glassburn et al (1977) investigated the efficiency of HBO for established radiation myelitis. They reported 9 patients in whom radiation myelitis had appeared 5–21 months after receiving 400–6300 rads for a variety of tumors in or overlying the spinal cord. Patients were treated 2–5 times weekly for 2–30 min at 2.5–3.0 ATA. The total number of treatments ranged from 21 to 61. They concluded that 6 of the 9 patients improved as a result of therapy. Torubarov et al (1983) studied the cerebral hemodynamic changes under HBO in 23 patients with brain vascular pathology in the late period of radiation-induced disease. Clinical improvement was observed in all patients.

Hart and Strauss (1986) reported 10 patients (8 males and 2 females, average age 46 ± 8 years) who had radiation myelitis. The patients were given HBO at 2 ATA for 90 min twice daily for 2 weeks. Three patients with established neurological deficit did not show any response. Three patients who were treated within 1 year of onset showed cessation of progression of disease and slight improvement. Four patients who had symptoms for less than 6 months showed marked improvement in function. The authors concluded that HBO is useful in radiation myelopathy; however, patients should not be given treatment immediately following the radiation, but at least 2 months after the last radiation treatment.

In a retrospective analysis of 9 patients with radiation myelopathy treated with HBO, 6 (66%) were been stabilized or improved by HBO (Angibaud et al 1995). There are few case reports of use of HBO for radiation myelitis in recent years. One report describes a case of radiation myelitis with a progressive improvement in the clinico-radiologic picture following HBO that was documented by MRI (Calabro & Jinkins 2000). Controlled studies are required to prove the value of HBO in this disease.

Radiation Encephalopathy

Radiation encephalopathy has been reported following radiation therapy for brain tumors and is sometimes difficult to differentiate from the recurrence or extension of the brain tumor. Hart and Strauss (1986) reported two patients with radiation-induced encephalopathy who were treated with a combination of vasodilators and HBO and showed marked improvement in cerebral function. Radiation-induced necrosis (RIN) of the brain is a complication associated with the use of aggressive focal treatments such as radioactive implants and stereotactic radiosurgery. Ten patients who presented with new or increasing neurologic deficits associated with imaging changes after radiotherapy received HBO treatments (Chuba et al 1997). Necrosis was proven by biopsy in eight cases. HBO was comprised of 20–30 sessions at 2–2.4 ATA, for 90–120 minutes. Initial improvement or stabilization of symptoms and/or imaging findings were documented in all ten patients studied and no severe HBO toxicity was observed. Four patients died, with the cause of death attributed to tumor progression. Five of six surviving patients were improved by clinical and imaging criteria; one patient was alive with tumor present at last follow-up. The authors concluded that HBO is an important adjunct to surgery and steroid therapy for RIN of the brain.

Two patients with arteriovenous malformations, who developed radiation encephalopathy following treatment with Gamma Knife, were treated by HBO at 2.5 ATA in sessions of 60 minutes per day (Leber et al 1998). This treatment was repeated 40 times in cycles of ten sessions. Both patients responded well to HBO, one lesion disappeared and the other was reduced significantly in size. No adjuvant steroids were given. Although these results provide evidence for the potential value of HBO in treating radiation encephalopathy, further experience will be needed to confirm its definite benefit.

Kohshi et al (2003) described the use of HBO therapy to manage radiation necrosis of the brain, which developed after two treatments with stereotactic radiosurgery to the same lesion. Treatment was continued with steroids alone for 2 months, but the patient started to deteriorate clinically and radiographically. Improvement started again following the resumption of HBO therapy.

Radiation-Induced Optic Neuropathy

Radiation-induced optic neuropathy (RION) is a devastating complication of radiotherapy to the head and neck. Cumulative doses of radiation that exceed 50 Gy or single doses to the anterior visual pathway or greater than 10 Gy are usually required for RION to develop. RION has been reported years after external beam radiation therapy. Patients commonly presents with unexplained, painless visual loss in one or both eyes, visual field defects, pupillary abnormalities, and defective color vision. Various theories of pathomechanism implicate vascular occlusion, demyelination, free radical injury, direct damage to cellular DNA, and damage to the blood-brain barrier. MRI with or without contrast is an important diagnostic tool. Visual outcome is poor and there is no established treatment. Corticosteroids and free-radical scavengers showsome efficiency in treatment, especially in acute phases. Guy and Schatz (1986) suggested HBO treatment of RION. Roden et al (1990) treated 13 patients with RION using a combination of corticosteroids and HBO. Recurrence of tumor and other causes of loss of vision were ruled out by appropriate studies. There was no improvement of vision in any of these patients. Borruat et al (1993) and Liu (1992), however, have presented cases RION where visual recovery occurred after HBO therapy. Partial visual recovery from RION after HBO has been reported in a patient with Cushing disease treated with stereotactic radiosurgery of the pituitary galnd (Boschetti et al 2006).

Management of Radionecrosis of Soft Tissues

Delayed Radiation Injuries of the Extremities

Radiation injuries of the extremities usually present as nonhealing wounds within the radiation fields of previously treated skin cancer. Feldmeier et al (1998) have presented their experience with 17 such patients. They were treated in a multiplace chamber at 2.4 ATA daily and wound care was maintained. Eleven of these patients had complete resolution of the wounds, one had improvement but not complete healing while 4 failed to heal and went on to have amputations. The success rate of HBO in this setting was 65% and non-responders to HBO had a 80% rate of going on to amputations. It is thus important that these patients should have an adequate trial with HBO as the first line treatment.

Soft Tissue Necrosis of the Head and Neck

Radiotherapy, which is often used for cancer in the head and neck, leads to damage of tissue cells and vasculature. Surgery in such tissues has an increased complication rate, because wound healing requires angiogenesis and fibropla-

sia as well as white blood cell activity, all of which are jeopardized. HBO raises oxygen levels in hypoxic tissue, stimulates angiogenesis and fibroplasia, and has antibacterial effects. There were 48 patients with soft tissue necrosis of the head and neck in the series of Hart and Strauss (1986). All of these presented after operative procedures with breakdown. With the exception of one lethal aspiration, all the patients improved.

In a consecutive retrospective study, 15 patients with soft-tissue wounds without signs of healing after surgery in full-dose (64 Gy) irradiated head and neck regions were treated with HBO and adjuvant therapy (Neovius et al 1997). The patients in this study were also compared with patients examined in an earlier study, with corresponding wounds treated without HBO. The healing processes seemed to be initiated and accelerated by HBO. In the HBO group, 12 of 15 patients healed completely, 2 patients healed partially, and only 1 patient did not heal at all. There were no life-threatening complications. In the reference group, only 7 of 15 patients with corresponding wounds without signs of healing eventually healed without surgical intervention, and 2 patients had severe postoperative hemorrhage, which in one case was fatal. Evaluation of results supports the hypothesis that HBO therapy has a clinically significant effect on initiation and acceleration of healing processes in irradiated soft tissues.

Radionecrosis of the Larynx

Radiation therapy is the treatment of choice for early stages of laryngeal cancer and larynx is often included in the field of radiation of head and neck cancer. Postradiation edema of the larynx usually resolves spontaneously but occasionally persists as long as 6 months. Laryngeal radionecrosis is an uncommon complication of radiotherapy for carcinoma of the head and neck. The interval between conclusion of radiation therapy and development of radionecrosis ranges from 3 to 12 months. Neither computed tomography nor magnetic resonance imaging differentiate between necrotic tissue and recurrent tumor. Tissue ischemia and hypoxia play an important role in its pathogenesis. This is a debilitating disease with pain, dysphagia, and respiratory obstruction. Biopsy is required to differentiate it from recurrent cancer. The pathological changes are fibrosis, endarteritis, and chondroradionecrosis. Tracheostomy and laryngectomy is required in some cases.

Chandler's grading system (Feldmeier et al 1993b) is a useful guide to the evaluation of the therapy of laryngeal necrosis. It is summarized as follows:

• Grade 1: Slight hoarseness. Laryngeal edema and telangectesia.

- Grade II: Moderate hoarseness. Slight impairment of vocal cord mobility and moderate edema.
- Grade III:Severe hoarseness with dyspnea and dysphagia. Severe impairment of cord mobility.
- Grade IV: Respiratory distress. Fistula, fixation of the skin to the larynx, laryngeal obstruction

Humidification, broad spectrum antibiotics, steroids, and hyperbaric oxygen, with or without surgery, are successful in many cases. Ferguson *et al* (1987) presented 8 patients with advanced radionecrosis of the larynx who were treated with adjuvant HBO therapy. Four of these patients were Chandler's grade IV laryngeal necrosis. Signs and symptoms of radionecrosis were markedly ameliorated in 7 of the 8 patients. Only one patient required laryngectomy. As compared with a previous series of cases where HBO was not used, there was a definite improvement of the outcome in these cases treated by HBO therapy as an adjunct.

Feldmeier *et al* (1993a) treated 9 patients with laryngeal necrosis using HBO. Eight of these patients were Chandler's grade IV and the ninth was grade III. All the nine patients were able to maintain their voice until death or last follow up. All patients with tracheostomies could be decannulated and the fistulae were closed. The authors recommended HBO as a therapeutic option whenever laryngeal necrosis occurs and there is a chance to save the larynx.

Delayed Radiation Injuries of the Abdomen and Pelvis

Radiation therapy is less commonly applied for malignancies of the abdomen but is still used for some cancers of the pancreas, biliary tree, stomach and colon. Radiation doses are limited due to poor tolerance of normal organs located in the abdomen. Whole abdomen radiation for ovarian cancer with local spread can have about 20% risk of complications. The most serious complications usually occur after a period of 6 months or longer and result from vascular compromise and hypoxia secondary to reactive fibrosis in the irradiated tissue. Some of these complications require surgical interventions. Feldmeier *et al* (1996) have reviewed 44 patients with radiation injury involving abdomen and pelvis and 41 of these were available for follow-up examination. Twenty-six of these patients healed, six failed to heal and nine patients had inadequate HBO therapy (less than 20 treatments). Overall, the success rate in patients receiving at least 20 treatments was 81%.

Clinical improvement of malabsorption due to radiation enteritis has been reported following HBO therapy (Neurath *et al* 1996). Hamour and Denning (1996) reported a patient who developed severe diarrhea with blood and pain in the rectum following post-operative radiation therapy for uterine cancer. She was advised to have a colostomy but declined. After 98 hours of HBO treatments (2.5 ATA) over a period of four weeks, she improved and the rectal ulceration decreased in size until it healed completely two months later. The patient did not have any recurrence of these symptoms.

Radiation-Induced Hemorrhagic Cystitis

This is an adverse effect of therapeutic radiation administered for a variety of pelvic malignancies. Clinical features are:

1. Recurrent hemorrhage (hematuria)
2. Urinary urgency
3. Pain

Bladder biopsy in these cases shows the following:

1. Mucosal edema
2. Vascular telangiectasis
3. Submucosal hemorrhages
4. Obliterative endarteritis
5. Smooth muscle fibrosis

It is a progressive disease and does not resolve spontaneously. Conventional treatment of this complication has included the following modes of treatment:

- Intravascular instillation of formalin, alum, and silver nitrate
- Systemic use of steroids and aminocaproic acid (inhibitor of fibrinolysis)
- Antibiotics
- Cauterization of bleeding vessels
- Bilateral ligation of the hypogastric arteries

Most of these approaches treat symptoms but none of these promote healing and may even have undesirable side effects. Because these complications are partially due to endothelial damage as well as to decreased vascularity and oxygenation to pelvic tissues, HBO may be able to improve oxygenation and induce angiogenesis in damaged organs, resulting in recovery from radiation injury. Rijkmans *et al* (1989) treated 10 patients with radiation-induced cystitis with HBO at 3 ATA (90-min sessions/day, 5 days/week) for an average of 20 sessions. In 6 patients hematuria stopped after 12 sessions of HBO. In another 4 patients where there was only partial resolution of hematuria, residual tumor was found in the bladder mucosa and was better defined after resolution of the edema of the surrounding tissue. The tumor was resected in these patients.

Hart and Strauss (1986) presented 15 patients with radiation cystitis, 11 of whom were relieved of symptoms of tenesmus and hematuria by a combination of HBO and surgery.

Weiss and Neville (1989) treated each of their 8 patients suffering from radiation-induced cystitis with a series of 60 HBO sessions (2 h at 2 ATA daily). They were able to document the improvement in 7 of these patients by cystoscopy. The hypervascularity of the bladder wall was diminished. The authors stated that the symptomatic relief was accompanied by a significant reversal of tissue injury. Clinical remissions were an average of 24 months (range 6 to 43 months). Only one patient failed to respond. The authors recommended HBO as the primary treatment for patients with symptomatic radiation-induced hemorrhagic cystitis.

Other cases of radiation-induced cystitis treated successfully by use of HBO have been reported by other authors (Shoenrock & Cianci 1986, Velu & Myers 1992, Kindwall 1993, Nakada et al 1992, Shameem et al 1992, Morita et al 1994). The largest series is that of Norkool et al (1993) who treated 14 patients with radiation-induced cystitis using HBO at 2.4 ATA for 90 min daily sessions for an average of 28 treatments per patient. There was complete resolution or marked improvement in 10 of these (74%). Of the 4 patients with poor outcome, 3 had recurrence of malignancy that was not present before HBO treatment. The cost of HBO therapy compared favorably with that of conservative treatment.

In conclusion, HBO has been shown to have a favorable effect on the course of radiation-induced cystitis as observed in 50 of the 63 published cases and several other cases which have not been reported. There is a difference in pressure used. It appears that use of 2.4 ATA instead of 2 ATA reduces the number of treatments from about 60 to about 30. aA prospective (but not controlled) study has shown beneficial effect of HBO on radiation cystitis (Bevers et al 1995). There is a lack of randomized trials to definitively demonstrate the effectiveness of HBO for cystitis. Concern still exists regarding the durability of the beneficial effects.

Radiation Proctitis

Chronic proctitis is a well-known complication of therapeutic irradiation. Most patients had previously been treated with radiotherapy for prostate carcinoma. Radiation-induced proctitis is a difficult clinical problem to treat and will probably become more significant with the rising incidence of diagnosis of prostate cancer. Patients with proctitis mainly suffer from bleeding, diarrhea, incontinence, and pain.

Charneau et al (1991) reported a case of a male patient

suffering from severe radiation-induced hemorrhagic proctitis which healed after HBO therapy. Williams et al (1992) carried out a prospective observational study on 14 patients with radiation-induced soft tissue necrosis following treatment of pelvic malignancy and after the wounds had failed to heal after 3 months of conservative therapy. All of the patients received 15 courses of HBO. All those with radiation necrosis of vagina or rectovaginal fistula healed. There was only one treatment failure.

Warren et al (1997) treated 14 patients with chronic radiation-induced proctitis with HBO. Nine patients were treated in a monoplace chamber at 2 ATA, and five patients were treated at 2.36 ATA. Eight patients experienced complete resolution of symptoms and one patient had substantial improvement for a total response rate of 64%. Follow-up ranged from 5 to 35 months. Five patients (36%) were classified as non-responders.

Three experienced significant improvement during treatment but relapsed soon after therapy was discontinued, whereas two had no symptomatic improvement. Responders who had sigmoidoscopy after therapy showed documented improvement whereas no non-responders showed improvement. The authors concluded that HBO therapy should be considered in patients with chronic radiation proctitis.

In more than half of the patients with radiation proctitis, symptoms partially or completely resolved after HBO treatment (Woo et al 1997). HBO should be considered in the treatment of radiation-induced proctitis. Further prospective trials with strict protocol guidelines are warranted to definitively demonstrate the effectiveness of HBO for proctitis.

Effect of HBO on Cancer Recurrence

Because there may be residual cancer in some of the patients treated for radiation necrosis, there is some concern that HBO may promote cancer growth or recurrence. Eltorai et al (1987) presented a historical review of the effects of HBO on malignancy. They reported 3 cases of occult carcinoma that manifested clinically after HBO was started and presumably led to the proliferation of the tumor in all 3 cases. The authors considered HBO therapy to be contraindicated in malignancy. There is no evidence to substantiate this view.

Squamous cell carcinoma transplanted in mice neither progresses or regresses when the animals are exposed to HBO (Sklizovic et al 1993). Other studies suggest that HBO may even have an inhibitory effect on cancer growth (Ehler et al 1991, Headley et al 1991, Mestrovic et al 1990). McMillan et al (1989) studied the effect of HBO on dimethylbenzathracene-induced oral carcinogenesis in an animal model. The group that received simultaneous HBO had fewer tumors but these were larger than those in the non-HBO group. They concluded that HBO has a tumor-suppressive effect during the induction phase of oral carcinoma and appears to have a stimulatory effect during the proliferative phase. In a survey of this topic, majority of the hyperbaric practitioners who responded, did not did not consider HBO to have cancer-promoting or cancer-accelerating properties (Feldmeier *et al* 1993b).

Feldmeier *et al* (1994) reviewed the pertinent literature to answer the question: Does hyperbaric oxygen have a cancer-causing or -promoting effect? Several of the studies showed a positive effect of HBO in suppressing tumor growth whereas other studies failed to demonstrate this effect. One explanation of this difference is that generation of free radicals by HBO may diminish superoxide dismutase and affect the susceptibility of tumor cells to HBO (Mestrovic 1996).

Conclusions

Radiation wounds are difficult to treat and in the past there have been few non-surgical options. Now, there is considerable evidence of the beneficial effect of HBO on radiation necrosis and it has become a useful adjunct to surgery. Among the bony structures, the effect on osteoradionecro-

sis of the mandible is most striking. Among the soft tissues, the effect on laryngeal necrosis is impressive. The effect on the radionecrosis of the neural tissues other than the brain is not striking.

There are no controlled studies to prove the efficacy of HBO in radionecrosis. Apart from the variations in clinical presentation, there is difficulty in controlling other methods of treatment.

Feldmeier and Hampson (2002) reviewed 74 publications reporting results of applying HBO in the treatment or prevention of radiation injuries and appraised these in an evidence-based fashion. All but seven of these publications report a positive result when HBO is delivered as treatment for or prevention of delayed radiation injury. These results are particularly impressive in the context of alternative interventions. Without HBO, treatment often requires radical surgical intervention, which is likely to result in complications. Other alternatives including drug therapies are rarely reported, and for the most part have not been the subject of randomized controlled trials. Based on this review, HBO is recommended for delayed radiation injuries for soft tissue and bony injuries of most sites.

Growth factors show promise in the management of chronic irradiated tissues and it would be worthwhile to investigate the effect of combination of HBO with growth factors.

17 The Use of HBO in Treating Neurological Disorders

K.K. Jain

HBO appears to have a number of interesting effects regarding neurological problems. Many such applications remain in their infancy. This chapter reviews evidence concerning the following implications:

Introduction

Since hypoxia and ischemia are involved in the pathophysiology of many disorders of the nervous system, hyperbaric oxygen (HBO) therapy has an important role in their management. To understand the role of HBO in neurological disorders, a basic knowledge of cerebral metabolism, cerebral blood flow, and the neurophysiology of the brain is essential.

Effect of HBO on Cerebral Metabolism

The effect of HBO on cerebral metabolism in the healthy state has been described in Chapter 2. The response of the injured brain to HBO is quite different.

There is evidence for a Pasteur effect (inhibition of glycolysis by oxygen) with hyperoxia in the case of carbohydrate metabolism in cerebrovascular disease. Inhalation of 100% oxygen significantly decreased cerebral metabolic rate (CMR) for lactate and pyruvate. Since cerebral blood flow (CBF) decreased and cerebral pO_2 increased slightly, total glycolysis was decreased. Cerebral pO_2 plotted against CMR lactate showed evidence of the Pasteur effect.

Holbach *et al* (1977) studied the effect of HBO on cerebral metabolism in cases of brain injury. They noted that normally there is aerobic glycolysis with phosphofructokinase as the regulating enzyme. The activity of this enzyme and the glycolysis are inhibited when, through the oxidation of glucose, citrate concentration and adenosine triphosphate rises (the Pasteur effect). Conversely, glycolysis is stimulated when ATP and citrate levels fall from high energy use, as in hypoxia (reverse Pasteur effect).

Since 1 ml of oxygen oxidizes 1.34 mg of glucose, the glucose oxidation quotient (GOQ) is:

$$\text{AVD of glucose} - \text{AVD of lactate} = 1.34 \text{ AVD of oxygen,}$$

where AVD is the arteriovenous difference.

The normal GOQ is 1.34 because the brain consumes oxygen almost exclusively from the oxidative metabolism of glucose. GOQ increases in anaerobic glycolysis as there is too high an amount of glucose still available for oxidation, even after subtracting the considerably increased AVD lactate.

In patients treated with 100% oxygen at 1.5 ATA (measurements made 10–15 min after the exposure) there was a moderate increase in AVD glucose and AVD lactate. The AVD oxygen remained constant. This resulted in a balancing of the cerebral glucose metabolism as reflected in the normal or near normal GOQ values.

When Holbach *et al* (1977) tried HBO at 2 ATA in similar situations, there was an increase of AVD glucose and a decrease of AVD oxygen compared with the values measured prior to the treatment. The GOQ increased. They concluded that in the injured brain, HBO at 1.5 ATA has beneficial effects, whereas raising the pressure to 2 ATA has deleterious effects.

Contreras *et al* (1988) measured cerebral glucose utilization using the autoradiographic 2-deoxyglucose technique in rats injured by focal cortical freeze lesions. They treated these animals with HBO at 2 ATA (90-min sessions) for 4 consecutive days. There was an overall increase of cerebral glucose utilization measured 5 days after injury when compared with the lesioned control animals exposed only to air (Figure 17.1). The data indicate that the changes in cerebral glucose metabolism persisted beyond the period of exposure to HBO. This observation is important as it explains the persistence of clinical improvement in patients after exposure to HBO.

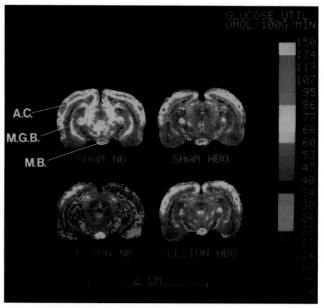

Figure 17.1
Color-coded transformation of autoradiographs of brain sections at the level of the auditory cortex into a quantitative map of glucose utilization. Three of these areas that demonstrate a statistically significant interaction between the lesion and the HBO therapy are the auditory cortex (A.C.), the medial geniculate body (M.G.B.), and the mammillary body (M.B.). The lesion was performed on the right side of the brain and is shown on the right side of these photographs (From Contreras *et al* 1988).

Effect of HBO on Cerebral Blood Flow

Various studies of the effect of HBO on cerebral blood flow (CBF) are shown in Table 17.1 It is generally recognized that oxygen has a vasoconstrictive action and reduces CBF, though the mechanism is unknown. Extracellular superoxide dismutase plays a critical role in the physiological response to oxygen in the brain by regulating nitric oxide (NO) availability. Cerebral blood flow responses in geneti-

Table 17.1
Summary of Cerebral Blood Flow under HBO as Reported by Various Authors

Authors and year	Method	Material	Inhalant	Pressure	Change
Kety and Smith (1948)	Nitrous oxide	Man	O$_2$ 85%–100%	1 ATA	Decrease 13%
Lambertson et al (1973)	Nitrous oxide	Man	O$_2$ 100%	3.5 ATA	Decrease 25%
Jacobson and Lawson (1963)	Krypton-85 clearance	Dog	O$_2$ 100%	1 ATA 2 ATA	Decrease 12% Decrease 21%
Tindall et al (1965)	Electromagnetic flow-meter	Baboon, internal carotid (5 min.)	O$_2$ 90%	1 ATA 3 ATA 3 ATA	Decrease 9% Decrease 13% Decrease 18% (10 min.)
Harper et al (1965)	Krypton-85 clearance	Dogs made hypotensive by bleeding	O$_2$ 100%	2 ATA	No change
Di Pretoro et al (1968)	Rheography	Man	O$_2$ 100% Air	2 ATA 2 ATA	Reduced No change
Wuellenweber et al (1969)	Thermal probes	Patients with brain injuries	O$_2$ 100%	2.5 ATA	Increase
Miler et al (1970)	rCBF	Dogs, cryogenic sprobe lesions	O$_2$ 100%	2 ATA	
Hayakawa (1974)	Ultrasonic rheography	Man, internal carotid	O$_2$ 100%	1 ATA 2 ATA	Decrease 1% Decrease 8%
Artru et al (1987)	133 Xe clearance	Patients with brain injury	O$_2$ 100%	2.5 ATA	Increase (in patients with cerebral edema)
Ohta et al (1987a)	133 Xe	Healthy volunteers	O$_2$ 100%	1 ATA 1.5 ATA 2 ATA 3 ATA	Decrease 9% Decrease 23% Decrease 29% Decrease 14%
Omae et al (1998)	Transcranial Doppler to	Human volunteers	O$_2$ 100%	HBO 2 ATA, control with hyperbaric air	Velocity of blood flow in the middle cerebral artery decreased with HBO as compared to hyperbaric air
Demchenko et al (1998)	Hydrogen (H$_2$) clearance method	Rats	O$_2$ 100%	HBO 3 ATA	Decrease 26–39%
Di Piero et al (2002)	SPECT	Divers Healthy non-diver controls	O$_2$ 100%	HBO 2.8 ATA	Normobaric O$_2$ (NBO) No difference in CBF distribution between controls and divers in both NBO and HBO
Demchenko et al (2005)	Platinum electrodes in globus pallidum Rats	Air	100% O$_2$	2 to 6 ATA	Doubling of CBF with HBO led to 13-64 fold increase in pallidum in a linear manner.
Meirovithz et al (2007)	Fiber optic probe	Awake restrained rats	100% O$_2$	1.75 to 6 ATA	The maximal level of microcirculatory Hb O$_2$ at 2.5 ATA is double the normoxic level

cally altered mice to changes in PO$_2$ demonstrate that SOD3 regulates equilibrium between superoxide (O$_2$-) and NO, thereby controlling vascular tone and reactivity in the brain. That SOD3 opposes inactivation of NO is shown by absence of vasoconstriction in response to PO$_2$ in the hyperbaric range in SOD3+/+mice, whereas NO-dependent relaxation is attenuated in SOD3–/–mutants (Demchenko et al 2002). Thus, extracellular SOD promotes NO vasodilation by scavenging O$_2$-, while hyperoxia opposes NO and promotes constriction by enhancing endogenous O$_2$- generation and decreasing basal vasodilator effects of NO. The explanation of increase of CBF in some reports is as follows:

- If the probe was measuring flow in the area of the damaged brain, the increase in flow could be an "inverse steal phenomenon" (Lassen & Palvölgyi 1986) due to vasoconstriction elsewhere.
- The area of brain under the probe might have lost its

power of autoregulation, and the increase of blood flow could be due to an increase of perfusion pressure owing to a decrease of intracranial pressure (ICP) consequent upon vasoconstriction elsewhere in the brain.

The conflict among the reports in the literature on this subject arises from the variable effect of HBO on the normal versus the injured brain. If CBF is impaired by cerebral edema or raised ICP it can be improved by HBO. Leniger-Follert and Hossman (1977) made observations on the microcirculation and cortical oxygen pressure, during and after prolonged cerebral ischemia, that are relevant to the effect of HBO. According to these authors, complete cerebral ischemia of 1 h in cats followed by reactive hyperemia, and recirculation as well as reoxygenation of the brain can occur. However, there is a critical phase of a few hours after the recommencement of circulation as soon as reactive hyperemia ceases. If brain swelling occurs during this period, cerebral hypoxia may develop. If brain swelling can be prevented, however, the distribution of oxygen pressure in the cortex can be restored to normal. HBO has a beneficial effect on cerebral edema.

Bean *et al* (1971) suggested that HBO had a dual influence on the central vasculature initial vasoconstriction followed by vasodilatation – and that prolonged exposure to HBO – results in the loss of oxygen vascular constrictive controls. Based on the evidence available, it may be concluded that HBO generally causes vasoconstriction and results in a reduction of CBF. The detailed response of cerebral vessels to HBO, however, varies according to the degree of compression, exposure time, region of the brain, and pathological process in the brain and blood vessels. Ohta *et al* (1987a) believe that too much oxygen disturbs the regulatory oxygen response of CBF and may explain the pathogenesis of oxygen toxicity. These investigators state that reduced CBF under HBO is a protective response against oxygen toxicity.

Bergö *et al* (1993) measured the changes in CBF distribution during HBO (5 ATA for 5 and 35 min) exposure in rats with unilateral frontal decortication lesions. CBF was reduced in most cerebral regions on the lesioned side. Brainstem showed reduction of CBF below the increased oxygen content after 35 min of HBO. The hypoxia as well as the disturbed balance between glutaminergic and GABAergic neurotransmitter systems was considered to have contributed to the increased frequency of convulsions in these animals. Cerebral blood flow decreases during HBO treatment at a constant $PaCO_2$. Hypercapnia prevents this decline and elevated $PaCO_2$ augmented oxygen delivery to the brain, but increases the susceptibility to oxygen toxicity (Bergö & Tyssebotn 1999).

Omae *et al* (1998) have conducted a study to clarify the relationship between HBO and CBF in humans. Middle cerebral arterial blood flow velocity (MCV) was measured using transcranial Doppler (TCD) technique in a multiplace hyperbaric chamber. The Doppler probe was fixed on the temporal region by a head belt, and the transcutaneous gas measurement apparatus ($tcPO_2$ and $tcPCO_2$) was fixed on the chest wall. MCV and transcutaneous gas were measured continuously in eight healthy volunteers under four various conditions: 1 ATA air, 1 ATA O_2, 2 ATA air, and 2 ATA O_2. Next, the effect of environmental pressure was studied in another eight healthy volunteers, in whom the $tcPO_2$ was kept at almost the same level under conditions of both 1 ATA and 4 ATA by inhaling oxygen at 1 ATA. MCV of 1 ATA O_2, 2 ATA air, and 2 ATA O_2 decreased, and $tcPO_2$ increased significantly in comparison with that of 1 ATA air. A significant difference in MCV was observed between the O_2 group and the air group under the same pressure circumstance. On the other hand, there were no differences in MCV or $tcPO_2$ between 4 ATA air and 1 ATA plus O_2, and the influence for the MCV of the environmental pressure was not observed. The authors concluded that hyperoxemia caused by HBO reduces the CBF, but the high atmospheric pressure per se does not influence the CBF in humans.

A decrease in nitric oxide (NO)availability in the brain tissue due to the inhibition of nitric oxide synthase (NOS) activity during the early phases of HBO exposure is involved in hyperoxic vasoconstriction leading to reduced rCBF. Increased levels of asymmetric dimethylarginine , an endogenous inhibitor of NOS, have been demonstrated in rat brains exposed to HBO (Akgül *et al* 2007).

Effect of HBO on the Blood-Brain Barrier

Some earlier animal experimental studies indicated that HBO increases the permeability of the cerebral vessel walls in normal animals. These findings were not substantiated in later studies. Blood brain barrier (BBB) is disturbed in certain disorders such as cerebrovascular ischemia, and HBO may serve to decrease the permeability of BBB. Intraischemic HBO therapy reduces early and delayed postischemic BBB damage and edema after focal ischemia in rats and mice (Veltkamp *et al* 2005).

Effect of HBO on Oxygen Tension in the Cerebrospinal Fluid

Hollin *et al* (1968) studied the effect of HBO on the oxygen tension of cerebrospinal fluid (CSF). They found that CSF levels usually reflect the arterial pO_2 tensions. Katsurada *et al* (1973) studied ventricular fluid oxygen tension in head injury patients and concluded that in severe brain injury, intracranial arteriovenous shunts or capillary blocks may prevent the rise of CSF oxygen tension with a rise of respiratory oxygen, and that this difference may be an index of the degree of injury to the brain. This may also mean that in a brain with multiple injuries, HBO may not affect the damaged part.

Rationale for the Use of HBO in Neurological Disorders

The following are the main mechanisms of the effectiveness of HBO in neurological disorders:

- Relief of hypoxia
- Improvement of microcirculation
- Relief of cerebral edema by vasoconstrictive effect
- Preservation of partially damaged tissue and prevention of further progression of secondary effects of cerebral lesions
- Improvement of cerebral metabolism

Relief of hypoxia is the most significant effect of HBO. Hypoxia has been described in Chapter 5. Hypoxemia can be corrected by normobaric 100% oxygen inhalation, but hypoxia of some lesions of the CNS requires HBO for correction.

The beneficial effect of HBO on cerebral hypoxia has been shown by biochemical studies. It is well known that there is an increase of lactate in brain and CSF in cerebral injury and anoxia. Mogami *et al* (1969) showed that there was a decrease

in the CSF lactate:pyruvate ratio under HBO, suggesting reduction of anaerobic in favor of aerobic metabolism.

The rational basis of the use of HBO in some neurological disorders is understandable in view of one concept of the pathogenesis of multiple sclerosis. According to James (1982, 1987), the following phenomena may occur in multiple sclerosis:

- Failure of pulmonary filtration of fat microemboli.
- Blood-brain barrier dysfunction that allows access of fat emboli to the brain parenchyma.
- Focal areas of perivenous edema preceding demyelination.

Vascular disturbances in the pathogenesis of multiple sclerosis may provide the rational basis for HBO therapy in this disease.

Cerebral Hypoxia

Oxygen is vital for the brain, and oxygen deficiency, regardless of the cause, starts a vicious circle of pathological changes in brain tissue:

$$\text{Primary brain damage} \rightarrow \text{hypoxia} \rightarrow \text{edema} \rightarrow$$
$$\text{aggravation of hypoxia} \rightarrow \text{secondary brain damage}$$

The object of HBO therapy in brain injuries is to supply the brain tissue with adequate oxygen and to interrupt this process.

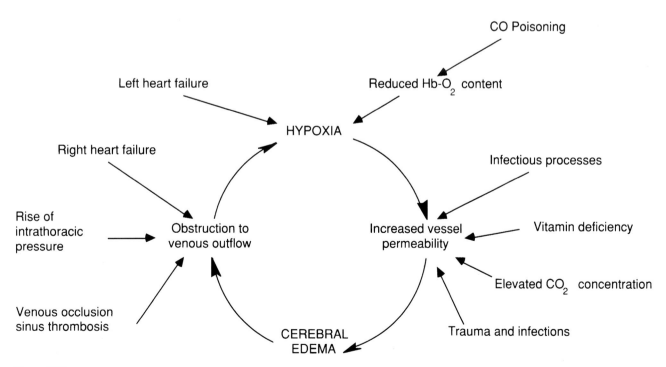

Figure 17.2
Pathophysiology of cerebral edema.

Cerebral Edema

Brain edema is divided into three types:

- *Vasogenic*. There is cerebral vasomotor paresis with transudation of plasma proteins into the extracellular space of the brain, e.g., brain injury, abscess, tumor, or infarction.
- *Cytotoxic*. Swelling in the intracellular space, e.g., CO poisoning, hypoosmolarity.

- *Interstitial*. Fluid escapes from the ventricle to enter the extracellular space of the periventricular white matter. This is unique to hydrocephalus.

Cerebral edema is a frequent finding in many disorders of the CNS. Its pathogenesis is depicted in Figure 17.2.

Generalized edema is a life-threatening process due to the rise of intracranial pressure (ICP) associated with it. The role of localized edema in aggravating the neurological deficits resulting from focal vascular and demyelinating le-

---

Table 17.2
Experimental Studies of the Effect of HBO on Cerebral Edema

Authors and year	Experimental animals and methods	Results and comments
Jamieson and Van Den Brenk (1963)	Rats. Oxygen tension measured in the brain under HBO (2 ATA).	Decrease of edema. Increase of brain oxygen tension in spite of vasoconstriction.
Coe and Hayes (1966a,b)	Rats. 2 groups with brain injury by liquid nitrogen. One group treated by HBO at 3 ATA.	Treated group survived longer and had less cerebral edema and less neuronal damage than the untreated group.
Dunn and Connolly (1966)	Dogs. One group treated by HBO, the other by normobaric 100%. Single 2 h treatment.	Reduction in mortality in both groups equal. Authors concluded that any any additional benefits from HBO was not manifest because of vasoconstriction.
Jinnai *et al* (1967)	Cats and rabbits.	Extradural balloons and intracarotid injections. Group tested by HBO at 3 ATA for 1 h.
Sukoff *et al* (1967)	Dogs. Psyllium seed injections in brain.	HBO at 3 ATA given at every 8 h starting 25 h after injury. Decreased mortality and morbidity in treated animals as compared with untreated ones.
Moody *et al* (1970)	Dogs. Injuries simulating extradural hematomal. Assisted respiration with 100% oxygen (1 ATA) in one group and 100% oxygen at 1 ATA or 2 ATA in other groups with spontaneous respiration.	Best reduction in mortality was in animals breathing spontaneously with 100% oxygen at 2ATA for 4 h.,
Hayakawa *et al* (1971)	Dogs with and without brain injury at HBO 3 ATA. CSF pressure measurements.	In dogs without brain damage CSF pressure decreased initially but rose later due to CBF disturbances. There was more consistent decrease in brain injured animals.
Dunn (1974)	Freeze lesions to produce cerebral edema. Four groups 1. control 2. ventilated for 2–3 h with air 3. 3 h of 97% oxygen + 3% CO_2 hyperventilation 4. 3 h of HBO at 3 ATA (97% oxygen + 3% CO) + hyperventilation	The lowest mortality (29%) was in group 4 (mean survival 5.3d). The highest mortality was in group 3 (mean survival 2d). HBO with hyperventilation was shown to reduce ICP definitely.
Nagao *et al* (1975)	25 dogs. Anesthetized and ventilated.	ICP raised by extradural balloons. HBO reduced ICP only when cerebral circulation was responsive to CO_2. In animals treated by HBO, CO_2 reactivity was maintained until high levels of ICP.
Miller (1979)	Dogs. Cerebral edema by liquid nitrogen. Effect of HBO on CBF and ICP.	HBO caused a 30% reduction of ICP and 19% reduction of CBF so long as the cerebral vessels remained responsive to CO_2.
Gu (1985)	Rabbits. Experimental edema. Treated by various mixtures of nitrogen and oxygen as well as 100% O2 at 1 and 4 ATA.	No effect of mixtures of oxygen and nitrogen 100% caused a drop of ICP at both 1 and 4 ATA.
Isakov *et al* (1985)	30 rabbits. Head injury 15 treated by HBO. The rest were controls.	Ten sessions of HBO led to significant reduction of tissue water in the brain of animals treated by HBO.
Nida *et al* (1995)	Fluid percussion (FP) injury or cortical injury (CI) in rats. Treated with HBO (1.5 ATA for 60 min), starting 4 h after head trauma.	HBO reduced edema produced by FP but not by CI although both were equally severe.

sions is generally not well recognized. With modern neuroimaging techniques, it has become possible to demonstrate focal brain edema *in vivo*.

The ICP represents the sum of three components: the volume of the brain substance, the CSF, and the blood present in the cranial cavity at any time. Reduction of any of these components can lower ICP. The conventional treatments for brain edema and raised ICP include corticosteroids, osmotic diuretics, hyperventilation, barbiturate coma, and ventricular drainage.

Experimental Studies

Most of the research regarding the effect of HBO on cerebral edema and raised ICP has been done on experimental animals. These studies are shown in Table 17.2.

Clinical Studies

Clinical studies of the effect of HBO on cerebral edema are shown in Table 17.3. Pierce and Jacobson (1977) reviewed the role of HBO in cerebral edema. Their classical conclusion, which is still valid is as follows:

"this therapy directly decreases vasogenic brain edema and due to improvement of O_2 delivery to anoxic tissue acts on cytotoxic brain edema as well. The mechanism underlying the potentially beneficial action of HBO appears clear and is well supported by animal and clinical studies. HBO should be considered an adjunct for patients who are not sufficiently responsive to standard methods. Treatment levels should not exceed 2 ATA and an effort should be made to prevent the rebound phenomenon by titrating pO_2 downwards, preferably by varying O_2 concentrations while maintaining hyperbaric pressure levels."

Table 17.3
Clinical Studies of the Effect of HBO on Cerebral Edema

Authors and year	Diagnosis and no. of patients	Results and comments
Jinnai *et al* (1967)	Head injuries, 7; Post-operative neurosurgery, 8	Neurological and EEC improvement but not long lasting
Hayakawa *et al* (1971)	Brain trauma or neurosurgery, 15 continuous monitoring of ICP and CBF before, during and after HBO at 2 ATA	Three types of responses: I CSF pressure decreased initially and then rose (n = 9) II ICP was lowered and remained so (n = 2) III Little or no response of ICP to HBO (n = 4)
Miller (1973)	Head injury patients 30% reduction of ICP at 2 ATA (PAO2 1227 mmHg)	No further education when pressure raised to 3 ATA
Sukoff and Ragatz (1982)	Head injury patients, 50	Considerable reduction of cerebral edema as shown by CT scan and clinical evaluation

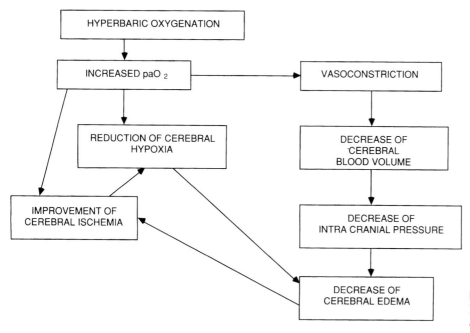

Figure 17.3
Mechanism of effectiveness of HBO in cerebral edema.

The favorable results of HBO on cerebral edema in experimental animals have been confirmed by the clinical use of HBO for the relief of traumatic cerebral edema (Sukoff & Ragatz 1982). HBO (1.5 ATA) treatment of patients with severe brain injury reduces raised intracranial pressure and improves aerobic metabolism (Rockswold *et al* 2001; Sukoff 2001).

Application of HBO during the early phase of severe fluid percussion brain injury in rats significantly diminished ICP elevation rate and decreased mortality level (Rogatsky *et al* 2005). In conclusion, it can be stated that HBO relieves cerebral edema by the following mechanisms (Figure 17.3):

- Reduction of CBF but maintenance of cerebral oxygenation.
- HBO counteracts the effects of ischemia and hypoxia associated with cerebral edema and interrupts the cycle of hypoxia/edema.

HBO lowers raised ICP in traumatic cerebral edema as long as the cerebral arteries are reactive to CO_2. It is ineffective in the presence of vasomotor paralysis and is contraindicated in terminal patients with this condition. The effects of HBO can persist after the conclusion of a session and there is no rebound phenomenon, as is the case with the use of osmotic diuretics. If the ICP is elevated due to obstruction in the CSF pathways, as is the case in intraventricular hemorrhage, HBO and dehydrating agents have only a temporary effect in lowering ICP. Ventricular drainage is important in these patients, not only to lower the ICP but also to improve the CBF that decreases as an effect of raised ICP. Persistence of raised ICP can cause further cerebral damage. Studies of the effect of HBO on raised ICP in patients with brain tumors and cerebrovascular disease indicate that reduced ICP is initially due to direct vasoconstriction caused by hyperoxia but tends to rise again. However, the secondary rise can be prevented by induced hypocapnia.

The injured brain is susceptible to oxygen toxicity if high pressures are used. This is usually not a problem as the pressures seldom exceed 2.5 ATA; 1.5 ATA is used for most neurological indications.

Indications for the Use of HBO in Neurological Disorders

Various neurological conditions where HBO has been reported to be useful are listed in Table 17.4. Most of these are based on a review of the literature. There are few controlled clinical studies. The Undersea and Hyperbaric Medical Society USA does not list any of these conditions (with the exception of cerebral air embolism) as approved for payment by third-party insurance carriers.

Table 17.4
Neurological Indications for the Use of HBO Therapy

1. Cerebrovascular disease
   Acute cerebrovascular occlusive disease
   Chronic poststroke stage
   Treatment of spasticity
   Aid to rehabilitation
   Adjunct to cerebrovascular surgery
   Selection of patients for IC/EC bypass operation on the basis of response to HBO
   Postoperative complications of intracranial aneurysm surgery: cerebral edema and ischemia
   Carotid endarterectomy under HBO as a cerebral protective measure

2. Cerebral air embolism

3. Head injuries: cerebral edema and raised intracranial pressure

4. Spinal cord lesions
   Acute traumatic paraplegia within 4 h of injury
   Spinal cord decompression sickness (spinal cord "hit")
   Ischemic disease of the spinal cord
   Aid to the rehabilitation of paraplegia and quadriplegia
   Residual neurological deficits after surgery of compressive spinal lesion

5. Cranial nerve lesions
   Occlusion of the central artery of the retina
   Facial palsy
   Sudden deafness
   Vestibular disorders

6. Peripheral neuropathies

7. Multiple sclerosis

8. Cerebral insufficiency (decline of mental function): multi-infarct dementia

9. Infections of the CNS and its coverings: brain abscess, meningitis

10. Radiation-induced necrosis of the CNS: radiation myelopathy and encephalopathy

11. CO poisoning

12. Migraine headaches

13. Cerebral palsy

There are several good reviews of the use of HBO in neurological disorders (Hayakawa 1974; Kapp 1982; Sukoff 1984). The role of HBO in cerebrovascular disease is described in Chapter 18. HBO for the management of anoxic encephalopathies is dealt with in Chapter 19, neurosurgical disorders in Chapter 20, HBO as an adjunct to the management of multiple sclerosis is discussed in Chapter 21, cerebral palsy in Chapter 22, and migraine headaches in Chapter 23. The rationale for the use of HBO is discussed, along with the indications.

Diagnostic Procedures Used for Assessing the Effect of HBO

Routine neurological procedures are not necessarily useful in assessing the effects of HBO therapy but the following are worthy of consideration.

Clinical Neurological Assessment of Response to HBO

Neurological examination in the hyperbaric chamber is important in determining the effect of hyperbaric oxygen. Some of the effects are transient and may not been seen after removal of the patient from the chamber. It is not necessary to have a specialist provide a simple brief neurological examination, because any physician should be able to carry out such an investigation. Due to constraints of space and time, the examination should be limited to less than 5 min and repeated as often as possible, but at least three times during a hyperbaric session – once during the compression phase, once during the oxygenation phase, and once during decompression. A simple procedure such as measurement of the handgrip by a hand dynamometer can be done more often. The following are some examples as guidelines. Each hyperbaric center should develop its own protocol for the minimum neurological testing acceptable to the attending neurologist.

Comatose Patients

For comatose patients, the following should be included in the testing:

1. Reaction to painful stimuli by movement of limbs
2. Presence or absence of decerebrate rigidity
3. Pupil size and reaction to light
4. Fundoscopic examination – look for any vasoconstriction
5. Glasgow coma scale in case of patients with head injury

Paraplegics

1. Mark the level below which the sensory loss begins and chart the sensory loss, if partial
2. Grading of the major muscle group power if incomplete lesion
3. In subacute or chronic cases with spasticity, clinical grading of spasticity by passive range of motion

Hemiplegics (Stroke Patients)

1. Fundoscopic examination, visual acuity and visual fields by confrontation
2. Motor power testing, proximal muscles of the arm and the leg; test the time it takes for the stretched out (in sitting position) and the raised leg (in supine position) to drift; measurement of the hand grip by a hand-held dynamometer
3. Testing for spasticity; clinical grading of spasticity (see Chapter 18); measurement of spasticity of fingers by a handy muscle tonometer

A patient's response to a single HBO treatment is sometimes used for determining the response to HBO therapy and to make a decision regarding continuation of the therapy but this may not be adequate. In some patients, the

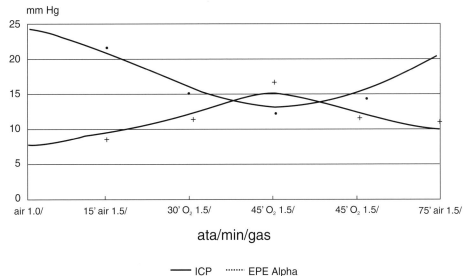

Figure 17.4
HBO therapy of a patient with severe cerebral edema and raised intracranial pressure (ICP). Continuous recording of arterial pO_2, pCO_2, ICP, and electrical power equivalents (EPEs) of alpha EEG activity. (From Wassman and Holbach 1988).

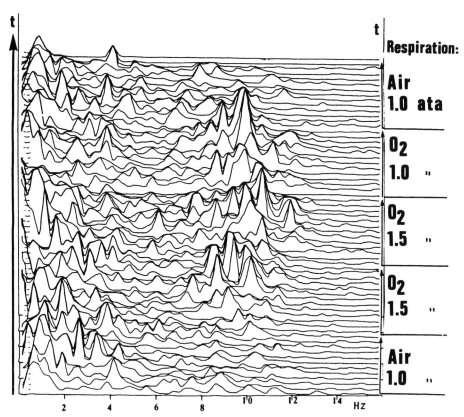

Figure 17.5
Illustration of EEG power spectrum during HBO treatment of a patient suffering from cerebral hypoxia. A definite increase of alpha activity is seen during the rise of oxygen partial pressure. (From Wassmann and Holbach 1988).

improvement resulting from HBO therapy is noticeable only after several treatments.

Electrophysiological Studies

The EEG has been found to be useful in assessing the response of patients to HBO treatment. Wassmann (1980) described the technique of interval amplitude EEG analysis (power spectrum) of patients during HBO therapy sessions. Two examples of the use of EEG in evaluating the response to HBO are shown in Figures 17.4 and 17.5. Matsuoka and Tokuda (1983) observed that slow waves tended to decrease and alpha activity tended to increase on the side of the lesion in patients undergoing HBO at 2 ATA. Topographic EEG mapping is an acceptable objective parameter of the effect of HBO on the brain (Tsuru *et al* 1983). In normal subjects somatosensory evoked potentials (SSEP) are reproducible under hyperbaric conditions and can be used to assess the response of spinal cord injury patients to HBO therapy. EEG is used little now for the evaluation of HBO treatment effects. The emphasis is now on brain imaging methods.

Cerebral Blood Flow (CBF)

This is most relevant to stroke and its management using HBO. Brain dysfunction after stroke closely relates to the site

and extension of lesions and thus correlates with the degree of reduction of CBF and metabolism. The most commonly used method in the past few years has been the ^{133}Xenon (Xe) inhalation method. The technique is based on gamma scintillation counting on NaI crystals after inhalation of ^{133}Xenon. This gives the values for regional CBF (rCBF). More recently positron emission tomography (PET) has been used for measuring rCBF. Relations between rCBF. Glucose metabolism, oxygen consumption and the structural lesions have been studied in the acute stroke to assess the impact of various treatments on the evolution of stroke during the first few ours after the onset. rCBF is also useful in the subacute and chronic phases of stroke. The severity of hemiparesis correlates with degree of asymmetry of CBF. Bilateral reductions of CBF are more likely to be associated with cognitive impairment. Quantitative CBF in acute ischemic stroke can be determined by XeCT and these measurements correlate with early CT findings (Firlik *et al* 1997). This system is commercially available as the XeCT System + (Diversified Diagnostic Products, Houston, Tx) and the advantages of this method are that CBF can be determined by the CT-staff along with routine CT without waiting for the CBF-staff. Results are available within 20 minutes.

Computerized Tomography (CT)

Principles. Computerized tomography (CT) permits the examination of tissue by the same principle as conventional x-ray imaging, except that the radiation passes successively through tissue from multiple different directions, detectors measure the degree of attenuation of the exiting radiation relative to the incident radiation, computers integrate the information and construct the image in cross section. Administration of a contrast agent increases x-ray attenuation owing to the high atomic number and electron density of the iodinated compounds used. Use of intravenous contrast agent enables the assessment of the integrity of the BBB. CT angiography (CTA) can also be performed after intravenous infusion of a nonionic contrast agent. Recent experimental studies indicate that contrast CT can detect cytotoxic edema (Von Kummer & Weber 1997).

Advantages and disadvantages. Advantages of CT are the widespread availability, short study time, sensitivity for detection of calcification and acute hemorrhage. It can be used in situations where MRI cannot be used in persons with intracranial metallic clips, pacemakers and other metal prostheses. It is preferred in rapidly evolving neurologic disorders where direct observation of the patient and life support systems is essential during scanning procedure. CT usually costs about half as much the MRI scan. Main disadvantages of CT scan are that it involves radiation and is less sensitive than MRI. More than 90% of the hospitals in the USA with 200 or more beds has this equipment. The distribution of this diagnostic facility is much lower in Europe and rare is confined mostly to large medical centers in developing countries.

Uses. This is the most widely used diagnostic procedure in neurological disorders. CT scan is the method of choice for assessment of ischemic injury to the brain. It is done without contrast to determine whether the stroke is hemorrhagic or ischemic. It is absolutely essential because all subsequent therapeutic decisions depend on the results of this examination. It can detect almost all of intracranial hematomas more than 1 cm in diameter and more than 95% of subarachnoid hemorrhages. Definite changes of infarction are usually not seen for 24 to 48 hours after onset but subtle signs of ischemia may appear before 3 h.

CT scan is used for detecting traumatic hematomas, brain tumors, abscesses and other infectious granulomas such as tuberculomas. Edema surrounding intracranial lesions such as those due to brain tumor and injury can be detected. Changes from cerebral edema include a local mass effect with distortion of the ventricular system.

Magnetic Resonance Imaging (MRI)

Principle of MRI. A tissue, when placed in a strong magnetic field, causes certain naturally occurring isotopes (atoms) within the tissue to line up within the field, orienting the net tissue magnetization in the longitudinal direction.

Current MRI uses signals derived from ^{1}H, the most plentiful endogenous isotope. Within a magnetic field, these atoms do not orient precisely with the axis of the field, but wobble a few degrees off center. Application of a radio-frequency pulse perpendicular to the applied magnetic field reorients the net tissue magnetization from the longitudinal to the transverse plane. When the radio-frequency pulse is turned off, the net tissue magnetization returns to its previous orientation, resulting in a magnetic resonance signal that can be detected by receiver coils. Application of different-gradient magnetic fields to the tissue under study permits reconstruction of the signal from individual volume units in space. The result is a clear image of the tissue in space.

Sequences such as T_1 and T_2, proton-density, and spin-echo weighted images enhance the utility of the MRI. Use of intravascular contrast material gandolinium-diethyleneamine pentaacetic acid with MRI enhances the magnetic susceptibility of the adjacent tissue, thereby providing information about the integrity of the BBB. Diffusion-weighted imaging can detect cytotoxic edema and is sensitive to early ischemic changes in the brain. Magnetic resonance angiography (MRA) enables noninvasive visualization of the cerebral and extracerebral vessels. Magnetic resonance spectroscopy provides a noninvasive method of studying brain metabolites, brain pH, and some neurotransmitter without the use of ionizing radiation. Functional MRI is a method of imaging the oxygen status of hemoglobin in order to visualize local changes in cerebral blood flow that reflect changes in neuronal activity in response to a specific sensory stimulus or motor task.

Advantages and disadvantages. The advantages of MRI are the absence of ionizing radiation, sensitivity to blood flow, high soft tissue contrast resolution and capacity to produce images in any plane. MRI is superior to CT for detecting most CNS lesions including cerebral infarction but is not as effective as CT for detecting subarachnoid hemorrhage. MRI may show evidence of ischemic stroke sooner than CT. Drawbacks of MRI include the lack of general availability and difficulty in monitoring seriously ill patients during the examination, and the time needed to perform it which is longer than that for unenhanced CT scan. SAH can be missed by MRI scan.

Uses. With newer MRI techniques such as diffusion-weighted and perfusion-weighted imaging, immediate identification of ischemic injury is possible and reversible ischemia can be estimated (Lutsep *et al* 1997). MRI is superior to CT in detecting cerebral edema and for detecting small lacunar lesions, particularly those located deep within the cerebral hemispheres and in the brain stem.

MRI is also used for evaluating the progression or regression of lesions of multiple sclerosis.

Positron Emission Tomography (PET)

This is a method of radionuclide scanning which requires the intravenous radioligand with a positron-emitting isotope, accumulation of the ligand in the brain and subsequent emission of the positrons from the ligand into the adjacent tissue during radioactive decay. Positrons are the antimatter equivalent of electrons. The collision of an electron and a positron annihilates both particles, converting their masses to energy in the form of two photons (gamma rays) that leave the brain at an angle of 180 degrees to each other and can be decayed. The radioligands that are most frequently used are ^{18}F-fluorodeoxyglucose and ^{15}O-water for determining cerebral blood flow. The use of PET is limited by a high cost, the need for a nearby cyclotron to produce radioisotopes with short half-lives, and its restricted spatial and temporal resolution. Routine use for neurodiagnostics is not currently practical. PET is referred to as functional imaging because, by using appropriate tracers, one can determine CBF and regional cerebral metabolic rate for oxygen (CMR O$_2$) and CMR for glucose (CMR glu). These techniques are extremely sensitive in the early detection of a cerebrovascular disturbance and can delineate the natural course of an episode that can lead to cerebral infarction. Evidence of ischemia is clearly demonstrated by substantial reduction in CBF and elevated CMR O$_2$ and CMR glu. The effect of a therapeutic intervention can be assessed by demonstrating the complete or partial reversal of these physiological and biochemical parameters.

Permanently and irreversibly damaged cortex in acute stroke can be detected by flumzenil PET. Evidence of tissue damage might be of relevance in selection of individualized therapeutic strategies. PET can be utilized in pilot trials for selection of patients who might benefit from particular therapeutic strategies and can be used to evaluate therapeutic effects in an experimental setting which then might form the basis for large clinical trials (Heiss *et al* 1998).

Kitani *et al* (1987) presented the use of PET with radioactive ^{15}O to compare CBF and regional cerebral oxygen consumption in a group of patients with CO poisoning and patients with acute cerebral ischemia treated by HBO. The findings proved to be a useful guide to the prognosis of HBO as well as to HBO treatment. The results suggested that HBO confers protection against ischemic brain damage. PET is expensive, not easily available, and its use is limited.

SPECT (Single Photon Emission Computed Tomography)

This is a useful tool for assessing the effect of HBO in neurological disorders. SPECT uses principles similar to those of PET but the radioligands decay to emit only a single photon. Conventional brain scanning uses highly polar radiopharmaceuticals such as ^{99m}Tc-pertechnitate. These tracers do not penetrate the normal brain but can cross a damaged BBB and appear as focal areas of increased activity in the region of the brain pathology. The long half-life of these tracers is a disadvantage. A radiolabeled lipid-soluble amine, Iofetamine (^{123}I-IMP) is an indirectly agonistic amphetamine derivative that readily crosses the BBB, is taken up by the functioning neurons, and its distribution in the brain mirrors that of the CBF. Brain activity is observed 30 s after injection (Holman *et al* 1983) and can be detected for up to 4–5 h. The areas of the brain affected by stroke show a reduced uptake of the tracer material and can be used to document the pathophysiology in stroke patients (Raynaud *et al* 1987). This test has been used in many of the studies to monitor the natural recovery and effect of therapy on stroke patients. The ^{123}I SPECT scan is ideal for evaluating the effect of HBO on stroke patients for the following reasons:

1. It is more widely available and less costly than PET scan. Any nuclear medicine facility with a gamma camera has the capability for this procedure.
2. There is a short waiting period for uptake of the isotope. The procedure can be integrated with HBO sessions and a post-HBO scan can be done with the same injection as for the pre-HBO scan.
3. This scan documents the area of cerebral infarction as diminished uptake, and any improvement is easy to document by noting the increased uptake of the tracer.
4. Improvement in the scan can be correlated with clinical improvement, which is not always the case when CT scan is used.
5. Recent work by Raynaud *et al* (1989) has indicated that two areas, the central area representing the infarct core and the peripheral area or the peri-infarct zone, may be differentiated during the subacute period of the stroke. The pathophysiology and outcome are different in these two areas, and studies of subacute infarction should refer to the area involved. The central area is the site of wide variations of rCBF and IMP uptake during the development of necrosis. The peripheral area, with its slight decrease in rCBF and IMP uptake without morphological changes, appears stable because it is present early after stroke and may persist for years. Knowledge of the spontaneous changes in rCBF and IMP uptake in these two areas during the subacute period will facilitate the evaluation of new treatment for cerebral infarction.
6. SPECT performed within 24 hours may be helpful in predicting outcome in clinical practice and in appropriately categorizing patients into subgroups for clinical trials (Laloux *et al* 1995).

IMP is no longer available commercially and its use has been replaced by ^{99m}Tc in hexamethylpropyleneamine oxime (HM-PAO). In HM-PAO scans half of the dose of the tracer is given initially and the brain is imaged. The patient is then exposed to HBO for 60 to 90 min and the other half of the dose is given following by brain imaging. Alternatively, the second scan using full dose HM-PAO can be done at a later time, 24 to 48 h after the initial scan (also using full dose) followed by the HBO session. The difference between the two scans helps to determine whether there is potentially recoverable brain tissue present (Neubauer & Gottlieb 1993). Hypometabolic but potentially viable areas in the brain can be identified using HM-PAO SPECT in conjunction with HBO. Data from Neubauer et al (1992) supports the hypothesis that idling neurons are capable of reactivation when given sufficient oxygen. Changes in tracer distribution after HBO may be a good prognostic indicator of viable neurons. Recoverable brain tissue can be identified and improved with cerebral oxygenation using HBO and the results can be documented with SPECT (Neubauer & James 1998).

One study has used archival data to compare 25 older and 25 younger subjects who were investigated with SPECT scans for evaluation of HBO for chronic neurological disorders: pretherapy, midtherapy, and posttherapy (Golden et al 2002). ANOVAs using the SPECT scans as a within subjects variable and age as a between subjects variable confirmed the hypothesis that the cerebral measures all changed but that the cerebellar and pons measures did not. Post-hoc t-tests confirmed that there was improvement in blood flow from the beginning to the end of the study. An age effect was found on only two of the five measures; however, there were no interactions. Analysis by post-hoc t-tests showed that the younger group had higher blood flows, but not more improvement than the older group. The results provided the first statistical research data to show the effectiveness of HBO in improving blood flow in chronic neurological disorders.

Use of HBO in Miscellaneous Neurological Disorders

The use of HBO in significant neurological disorders is described in separate chapters that follow. A few miscellaneous indications, particularly benign intracranial hypertension and peripheral neuropathy, that do not fit into these are described here.

HBO in the Treatment of Benign Intracranial Hypertension (BIH)

This syndrome is characterized by prolonged raised intracranial pressure without ventricular enlargement, focal neurological signs, or disturbances of consciousness and intellect. The most frequent symptoms are headaches, diplopia, and impairment of visual acuity. It occurs most frequently in obese women in the child-bearing period. The cause is not known, but the following explanations have been considered for the pathophysiology of BIH:

1. An increased rate of CSF formation
2. Sustained increase in intracranial venous pressure.
3. A decreased rate of CSF absorption by arachnoid villi apart from venous occlusive disease.
4. Increase in brain volume because of an increase in cerebral blood volume or interstitial fluid. There is histological evidence for cerebral edema

Diagnostic criteria of BIH are as follows:

1. Signs and symptoms of raised intracranial pressure.
2. No localizing neurological signs in an awake and alert patient except for abducent palsy.
3. Documented elevation of intracranial pressure (250 mm H_2O).
4. Normal CSF composition.
5. Normal neuroimaging studies except for small ventricles and empty sella turcica.

Various methods are used for lowering the intracranial pressure, including lumbar punctures, dehydrating agents such as mannitol, diuretics, and corticosteroids. Ventriculo-peritoneal shunts have been performed frequently and afford good relief from headaches, but the small ventricles present a technical difficulty in inserting catheters into this space. The main concern is preservation of vision and the preferred operation is fenestration of the sheath of the optic nerve.

Luongo et al (1992) treated various groups among 53 patients with BIH by several methods. Eight of the patients were treated only by HBO at 2 ATA, daily for 15 days. In all patients a gradual disappearance of signs and symptoms of elevated intracranial pressure was observed. However, the intracranial pressure was elevated again after discontinuation of HBO. The mechanism of this effect is not clear, but reduction of CSF production and an anti-edema effect of HBO are possible explanations. Further studies are required to assess this therapy for BIH but to date there have been no further publications on this topic.

Peripheral Neuropathy

Clioquinol-induced damage to the peripheral nerves has been shown to be decreased in animals treated using HBO as compared with controls (Mukoyama et al 1975). The authors speculated that oxygenation might prevent the death of intoxicated neurons in the spinal root ganglia and resuscitate them, as well as accelerate the sprouting and regeneration of nerve fibers in the peripheral part. They indicated that HBO may be useful in the treatment of peripheral nerve lesions.

Peripheral neuropathy in streptozotin-induced diabetic rats has been shown to be partially reversed by HBO treatment (2 ATA, 2 h, 5 days/week) for 4 weeks (Low *et al* 1988). There was enhancement of nerve energy metabolism in the HBO-treated animals as compared with the control animals with similar lesions, not treated by HBO.

Neretin *et al* (1988), after a review of their experience in treating polyradiculoneuritis with HBO have concluded that: "The results of clinico-electromyographic examinations point to a sufficiently high effectiveness of hyperbaric oxygenation in polyradiculoneuritis and permit its inclusion into the multimodality treatment of the latter. Hyperbaric oxygenation (HBO) accelerates regression of neurological disorders, with the predominant effect on the severity of motor and autonomic-trophic disturbances. HBO makes it possible to reduce the doses of glucocorticoids and the period of treatment and hospitalization of patients."

HBO in Susac's Syndrome

The Susac syndrome consists of a clinical triad of encephalopathy, loss of vision, and hearing defects (Jain 2003f). It is caused by microangiopathy of unknown origin affecting the small arteries of the brain, retina, and cochlea. This rare disorder, with 75 cases documented in the literature, affects mainly young women. The course of the illness is self-limiting. The deficit of visual acuity is caused by occlusion of tributaries of the retinal artery. The auditory defect is bilateral and symmetrical, and particularly affects medium and low frequencies. NMR is of great diagnostic value, showing multiple lesions in the gray and white matter. Li *et al* (1996) were the first to report HBO treatment with favorable outcome in a young woman with Susac syndrome who presented on two separate occasions with visual acuity loss from a recurrent branch retinal artery occlusion. Meca-Lallana *et al* (1999) reported the case of a young woman who presented with psychiatric symptoms and migraine followed by clinical encephalopathy and acute/subacute coma. There were also visual and auditory deficits. The patient responded to systemic treatment with cortico-steroids and HBO. The encephalopathy resolved in a few days and 2 months later she had resumed her former daily activities. Treatment with HBO was considered to have definitely reduced visual sequelae in this case. In another similar case, combination of intravenous steroids and HBO reduced the ischemic lesions (Cubillana Herrero *et al* 2002).

Cerebral Malaria

Cerebral malaria (CM) is a syndrome characterized by neurological signs, seizures, and coma. Despite the fact that CM presents similarities with cerebral stroke, few studies have focused on new supportive therapies for the disease. An experimental study has explored the use of HBO for CM. Mice infected with *Plasmodium berghei* ANKA (PbA) were exposed to daily doses of HBO (100% oxygen at 3 ATA for 1–2 h per day) before or after parasite establishment (Blanco *et al* 2008). Cumulative survival analyses demonstrated that HBO therapy protected 50% of PbA-infected mice and delayed CM-specific neurological signs when administered after patent parasitemia. HBO reduced peripheral parasitemia, expression of TNF-α, IFN-γ and IL-10 mRNA levels and percentage of gammadelta and alphabeta $CD4^+$ and $CD8^+$ T lymphocytes sequestered in mice brains, thus resulting in a reduction of BBB dysfunction and hypothermia. These data indicate that HBO treatment could be used as supportive therapy, perhaps in association with neuroprotective drugs, to prevent CM clinical outcomes, including death.

Neurological Disorders in Which HBO Has Not Been Found to Be Useful

This section presents historical information on several diseases where HBO has been used. Dementia and neuromuscular diseases are two examples. There have been no further studies done to prove the efficacy of HBO in these areas, and at present HBO cannot be recommended for these conditions except in the few cases noted.

Dementia

Dementia is defined as "a global impairment of higher cortical function, including memory, the capacity to solve problems of everyday living, the performance of learned motor skills, the correct use of social skills and the control of emotional reactions, in the absence of gross clouding of consciousness."

The causes of dementia are varied, and no single mode of treatment is applicable uniformly to the varied causes. HBO has been used as a treatment for dementia. Interest in the use of hyperbaric environments for central nervous system pathology has existed since the report by Corning (1891). McFarland (1963) theorized that sensory and mental impairment in the elderly are due to diminished availability or utilization of oxygen in the nervous system.

Various clinical trials of HBO in dementia are shown in Table 17.5.

Table 17.5
Clinical Trials of HBO in Dementia

Authors and year	Indication	Patients (n)	Technique	Results and comments
Jacobs et al (1969)	Cognitive deficits of the elderly	80	HBO sessions of 390 min each daily using 100% oxygen at 2.5 ATA. 5 patients were used as controls, breathing 10% oxygen + 90% nitrogen so that their pO2 did not rise above prepressurization levels	Psychological improvement in all patients which persisted beyond the of oxygen tension
Jacobs et al (1972)	Cognitive deficits in the elderly	52 incl. the previously reported 8	as above Psychological testing EEG. Cerebral blood flow. Blood and CSF pO2 pCO2 and lactate and pyruvate	Patients divided into 4 groups of 13 each. Group I, above study of 1969; Group II, Psychological evaluation performed 72 h after the last HBO treatment; Group III, evaluation performed 1 week after the last treatment; Group IV, evaluation performed 10 days after the last treatment. Improvement in mental function in all groups but was the in Group IV
Ben-Yishai and Diller (1973)	Cognitive deficits in the elderly	?	Same technique as that of Jacobs et al (1969) but combined with cognitive training	Cognitive improvement in patients persisted 3 months after treatment
Edwards and Hart (1974)	Decline of mental function	20	HBO at 2 ATA (100% oxygen) 15 daily sessions of 2 h each	Maximum improvement in those patients whose memory quotient was 70–100 before the treatment. Little or no improvement above and below those values
Harel et al (1974)	Senile dementia	8	?	No significant effect of HBO on CBF or cerebral metabolism which was already reduced
Imai (1974)	Memory disturbance of presenile dementia, chronic alcoholism, cerebrovascular disease and CO poisoning	?	HBO at 1.5 ATA (100% oxygen) 15 daily sessions of 2 h each	Improved performance on psychological testing
Thompson et al (1976)	Cerebrovascular disease and cerebral atrophy	21	100% oxygen at 2.5 ATA for 90 min twice daily for 15 days	Double-blind study. No effect of HBO on psychological function, EEG or CFF
Ben-Yishai et al (1978)	Cognitive deficits in the elderly	?	Same as in 1973 study by the author except that the control group received only cognitive training	No difference between the combined HBO treatment and the cognitive treatment alone. The latter was considered to be responsible for improvement in 1973 study

Considerable criticism followed publication of the study by Jacobs et al (1972), some of which can be summarized as follows:

1. Lack of oxygen supply to the brain was the main reason for using hyperoxygenation therapy. According to Sokoloff (1966), however, the proportional relationship between oxygen supply and oxygen consumption is near normal in patients with chronic brain syndrome.
2. The study failed to sort out the various reversible psychotic states that need to be differentiated from senility.
3. The validity of some of the psychological tests used was questioned by discussants of the paper. There was paucity of measurement.
4. There was no randomization regarding inclusion in the study or division into groups.
5. A wide variety of symptoms and signs were manifested by the patients and they belonged to a large number of diagnostic categories. Such a heterogeneous group would make the interpretation of the most precise and the most concrete results difficult.
6. The treatment is time-consuming and expensive. Elderly patients may dislike it or refuse it. The results are short-lived.
7. The placebo treatment of five patients with 10% O2 + 90% N2 is dangerous in elderly patients. Thomas et al (1976) studied the interaction of hyperbaric nitrogen and oxygen mixtures on behavior in rats. Raised oxygen

pressure modulated and interacted with the narcotic effect of nitrogen on behavior – an initial increase in response rate was followed by decline.

Raskin et al (1978) assigned 82 elderly subjects with significant cognitive impairment to treatment with HBO, hyperbaric air, normobaric air, or normobaric oxygen. Treatment consisted of two 90-min sessions per day for 15 days. Psychological evaluation immediately after treatment and 1, 2, 3, and 8 weeks later did not reveal any enhanced cognitive function in experimental subjects (who received normobaric or hyperbaric oxygen) as compared with controls (who received normobaric or hyperbaric air). Kron et al (1981) reviewed the published literature on the application of HBO in senile dementia and their own experience. They made a number of observations about the difficulties encountered in evaluating this therapy's usefulness in treating mental dysfunction, and came to the following conclusions:

1. The definitive study on the efficacy of HBO in the treatment of senile dementia has yet to be performed.
2. The gross discrepancies in the published reports may be attributed to inadequate design of experiments, poor research methodologies, and great variability in the clinical research populations. They noted that many of the psychological test instruments used in these studies lack the precision and reliability necessary to demonstrate small changes in mental capacity in response to therapeutic intervention. Further, because of logistical and safety considerations, the administration of HBO does not lend itself to well-controlled double-blind studies. Also, there is lack of agreement on the etiology and diagnosis of mental dysfunction in the aged, contributing to the difficulty in determining which patients may benefit from HBO therapy.

Schmitz (1977, 1981) evaluated HBO therapy for senility and concluded:

"At the present time, there is no basis for claiming that HBO is beneficial in reversing senility or any other central nervous system deficit that occurs in the aged . . . the only indication for HBO therapy in senility would be as a part of research study . . . Subjecting older people to hyperbaric environments, even if the risks are minimal, is contraindicated."

HBO in the Management of Neuromuscular Disorders

Muscular Dystrophy. The muscular dystrophies are hereditary degenerative disorders of the muscles. Most of the theories of the etiology of muscular dystrophy relate to the neuromuscular system. According to other theories, however, the primary disturbance is in the vascular supply to the skeletal muscles; blood flow is reduced to the exercising muscles. Biochemical abnormalities in the muscles may either be the cause or the effect of muscle degeneration.

Hirotani and Kuyama (1974) treated ten patients with muscular dystrophy using HBO. Five were of the Duchenne type and five of the limb-girdle type; 100% oxygen was used at 2 ATA daily and 19 sessions were completed in 3 weeks. Along with this an intravenous infusion of fructose + adenosine triphosphate (cytidine phosphatase choline), reduced glutathione, and sodium carbazochrome sulfanate was given. As controls, three patients with muscular dystrophy of the Duchenne type were subjected to HBO without the intravenous medications. There was improvement in muscle strength in the group given HBO plus medications but none in the group given HBO alone. The effect, however, was transient, and 5 years later there was no difference in condition between the controls and the treated group. The authors concluded that HBO in combination with ATP and CDP-choline may be effective in the symptomatic relief of muscular dystrophy.

Badalian et al (1975) summarized their experience in treating 306 patients with muscular dystrophy during different phases of the disease. The treatment was carried out keeping in mind the disturbance of protein metabolism and decreased permeability of the cell membranes. The treatment consisted of HBO with anabolic hormones, amino acids, vitamins, muscle electrostimulation, and so forth. There was no clinical progression of symptoms in 3 years of follow-up.

There has been no further progress in this area during the past 20 years and there appears to be no rational basis for the use of HBO for this indication. Considerable advances are taking place in molecular genetics and gene therapy for muscular dystrophy is a reasonable possibility.

Myasthenia gravis. Myasthenia gravis is an autoimmune disease. A specific antibody against the acetylcholine receptor is found in 85% of the patients, and the major component of this antibody is IgG.

Li et al (1987) carried out a controlled trial of HBO in 40 patients with myasthenia gravis; one group was treated with HBO alone and the other with HBO plus steroids. The rate of improvement with HBO alone was 88.9%, with HBO plus steroids it was 86.5%, and in the control group treated by steroids alone, it was 45%. IgA and IgM were reduced in the HBO group, indicating an immunosuppressive effect.

There has been no further work done in this area during the past decade. The immunosuppressive effect of HBO has not been demonstrated conclusively. There appears to be no justification for using HBO in myasthenia gravis at present.

18 The Role of Hyperbaric Oxygenation in the Management of Stroke

K.K. Jain

HBO, by counteracting the hypoxia of ischemic brain tissue, aids the recovery of stroke patients. The use of HBO in stroke patients is dealt with here in the following sections:

Introduction

"Stroke" is the term commonly used to describe the sudden onset of a neurological deficit such as weakness or paralysis due to disturbance of the blood flow to the brain. The term is applied loosely to cover ischemic and hemorrhagic episodes. The preferred terms are "ischemic stroke" or "cerebral infarction." A completed (established) stroke is an acute, nonconvulsive episode of neurologic dysfunction that lasts longer than 24 h. A transient ischemic attack is a focal, nonconvulsive episode of neurologic dysfunction that lasts less than 24 h, and often lasts less than 30 minutes. An ischemic stroke occurs when a thrombus or an embolus blocks an artery to the brain, blocking or reducing the blood flow to the brain and consequently the transport of oxygen and glucose which are critical elements for brain function. Ischemic strokes may also occur due to spasm of the cerebral arteries without any obstruction of the lumen such as in patients with migraine. Cerebral infarction can also occur as a result of obstruction to the venous outflow from the brain. Two distinct types of hemorrhage are intracerebral hemorrhage due to hypertension and subarachnoid hemorrhage due to rupture of an aneurysm (ballooning of the intracranial artery).

The World Health Organization (WHO) defines stroke as "rapidly developing clinical signs of focal (or global) disturbance of cerebral function with symptoms lasting 24 h or longer or leading to death, with no apparent cause other than of vascular origin" (WHO MONICA Project, 1990). This definition includes subarachnoid hemorrhage but excludes transient ischemic attacks and brain hemorrhages or infarctions due to non-vascular causes.

Fundamentals of epidemiology, pathophysiology, diagnosis and current management of stroke are described briefly in this chapter as a background to discuss the role of HBO.

Epidemiology of Stroke

Stroke is the third leading cause of death and an important cause of hospital admissions in most industrialized countries. Stroke accounts for 10% of deaths in all industrialized countries. It is the most common cause of disability worldwide. There are over 2 million stroke survivors in the United States and about 500,000 patients are discharged annually from acute care hospitals. It has been estimated that only 10% of the stroke survivors return to work without disability, 40% have mild disability, 40% are severely disabled, and 10% require institutionalization (Figure 18.1).

The incidence of stroke in the US is was approximately 800,000 cases per year. More than 4 million Americans are living with the consequences of stroke currently. In the year

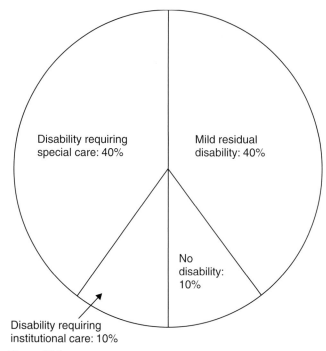

Figure 18.1
Functional results for stroke survivors.

2008, over 2 million new stroke patients are expected in USA, Europe, and Japan. About half of these will be in the US. Stroke is less common in developing countries, though accurate statistics are not available. Despite the improvement in the care of stroke, the incidence is rising by 2% per year. The incidence of stroke in western Europe was 635,700 during the year 1996 and is expected to increase to 663,001 in the year 2000. The incidence in Japan was 271,900 in 1996 and is expected to increase to 298,900 in the year 2000. The largest epidemiological study of stroke within the past decade has been conducted in China involving investigation of 5,800,000 persons out of a total population of nearly one billion (Guang-Bo *et al* 1991). The incidence of stroke was 109.95 per 100,000 in 1986. The age-standardized mortality was 80.94 per 100,000. The incidence, prevalence and mortality increased with age.

Risk Factors for Stroke

Various risk factors for stroke are:

- Aging
- Alcohol
- Atherosclerosis involving major vessels
  Atherosclerosis of aortic arch
  Carotid stenosis
- Cardiovascular
  Heart disease
  Atrial fibrillation
  Endocarditis

Left ventricular hypertrophy
Mitral valve prolapse
Myocardial infarction
Patent foramen ovale
- Coagulation disorders
- Cold
- Endocrine disorders
  Diabetes mellitus
  Hypothyroidism
- Female sex
- Genetic
  Angiotensin-converting enzyme gene deletion polymorphism
  Genetically determined cardiovascular, hematological and metabolic disorders causing stroke
- Hemorrheological disturbances
  Increased blood viscosity
  Elevated hematocrit
  Red blood cell disorders
  Leukocytosis
- Heredity: parental history of stroke is associated with increased stroke risk in the offspring
- Hyperlipidemia
- Hypertension
- Hypotension
- Lack of physical activity
- Metabolic disorders
  Hyperuricemia
  Hyperhomocysteinemia
- Migraine
- Nutritional disorders
  High salt intake
  Malnutrition
  Vitamin deficiency
- Obesity
- Psychosocial factors: anger, aggression, stress
- Pregnancy
- Race: Strokes more common in black Americans than whites.
- Raised serum fibrinogen levels
- Sex: Strokes more common in men than in women
- Sleep related disorders: snoring and sleep apnea
- Smoking
- Transient ischemic attacks

Pathophysiology of Stroke

The term "cerebrovascular disease" is used to mean any abnormality of the brain resulting from pathological processes of the blood vessels. The "pathological processes" are defined as lesions of the vessel wall, occlusion of the vessel lumen by an embolus or a thrombus, rupture of the vessel, altered permeability of the vessel wall, and increased viscosity or other changes in the quality of blood.

Causes of Stroke

The causes and risk factors for ischemic stroke overlap. Causal relationship is more definite than a risk factor which implies an increase in the chance of stroke in the presence of that factor. The interaction between risk factors and causes of stroke is shown in Figure 18.2. Various causes of stroke are:

- Atherosclerosis of arterial wall
  Atherosclerotic occlusion of cerebral arteries
  Carotid stenosis
- Arterial occlusion secondary to infections
  Bacterial meningitis: *H. influenzae* and tuberculosis
  Meningovascular syphilis
  Cysticercosis
  Cerebral malaria
  Herpes zoster
  Viral infections: AIDS
- Arterial occlusion secondary to head and neck trauma
  Closed head injury
  Blunt trauma to neck
  Fractures and dislocations of the cervical spine
  Chiropractic manipulations of the neck
  Beauty parlor stroke syndrome
- Cervical spondylosis with compression of vertebral arteries
- Congenital abnormalities of the cerebral vessels: hypoplasia of arteries
- Coagulation disorders
- Drug-induced stroke
  Therapeutic drugs
  Drug abuse
- Embolism
  Cardiogenic embolism: atrial fibrillation
  Embolism from peripheral arteries
  Tumor emboli
- Hematological disorders: e.g., sickle cell anemia
- Genetic
- Iatrogenic as complications of:
  Anesthesia
  Cerebral angiography
  Cardiovascular surgery
  Neurosurgical procedures
- Infections
  AIDS
  Bacterial meningitis
  Chickenpox
  Cysticercosis
  Subacute bacterial endocarditis
  Syphilis

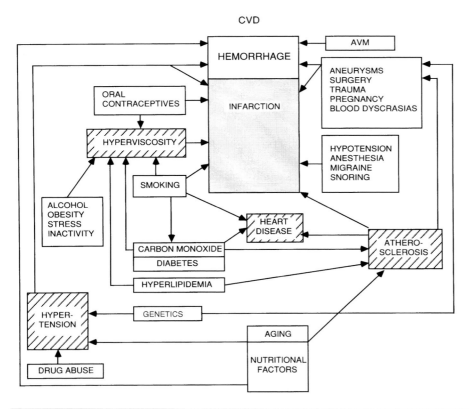

Figure 18.2
Interaction of risk factors for stroke.

Table 18.1
Factors that Influence the Extent of Infarction

Factors that increase infarction	Factors that decrease infarction
Hypotension; reduction of cardiac output	Increase of pressure
Lack of collaterals	Adequate collaterals
Hypoxia	Oxygenation
Sudden occlusion of the vessel	Gradual occlusion of the vessel
Increased viscosity of blood	Decreased viscosity of blood
Increased metabolism; hyperthermia	Decreased metabolism; hypothermia; sedation
Cerebral edema	Absence of cerebral edema

- Inflammatory diseases
  Systemic: e.g., rheumatoid arthritis and systemic lupus erythematosus
  Of the cranial arteries:
  – temporal arteritis
  – aortic branch arteritis (Takayasu's disease)
  – granulomatous intracranial arteritis
- Myocardial infarction
- Nonatherosclerotic vasculopathies
  Moyamoya disease
  Thrombangitis obliterans (Buerger's disease)
  Radiation vasculopathy
  Spontaneous cervical artery dissection
  Fibromuscular dysplasia
  Cerebral amyloid angiopathy

Among the different causes of stroke, 70% are due to an ischemic infarct, of which 9% are due to large-artery occlusion, 5% are due to tandem arterial pathology, 26% are lacunar, 19% are from a cardiac source, and 40% are of uncertain cause. The three disease processes responsible for most ischemic strokes are:

1. Large vessel atherothrombotic disease, which accounts for about 14% of the cases.
2. Small vessel atherothrombotic disease (lacunar stroke), accounting for about 27% of the cases.
3. Embolic disease, accounting for about 59% of the cases.

Changes in the Brain During Ischemic Stroke

Changes that occur in the brain during a stroke are both histological and biochemical (metabolic). The brain re-

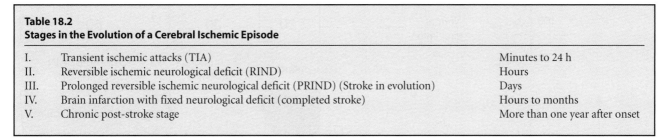

Table 18.2
Stages in the Evolution of a Cerebral Ischemic Episode

I.	Transient ischemic attacks (TIA)	Minutes to 24 h
II.	Reversible ischemic neurological deficit (RIND)	Hours
III.	Prolonged reversible ischemic neurological deficit (PRIND) (Stroke in evolution)	Days
IV.	Brain infarction with fixed neurological deficit (completed stroke)	Hours to months
V.	Chronic post-stroke stage	More than one year after onset

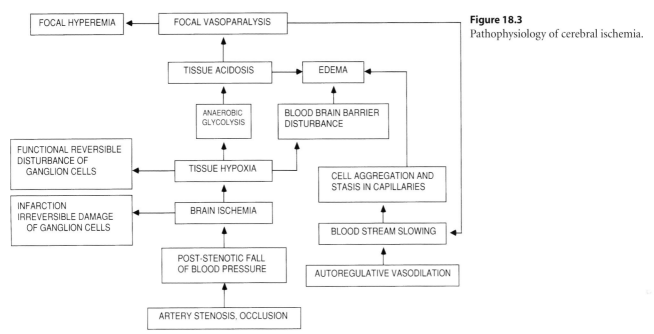

Figure 18.3
Pathophysiology of cerebral ischemia.

quires 500–600 ml oxygen/min (25% of the total body consumption). One liter of blood circulates to the brain each minute. If this flow is interrupted completely, neuron metabolism is disturbed after 6 s, brain activity ceases after 2 min, and brain damage begins in 5 min. Brain tissue deprived of its oxygen supply undergoes necrosis or infarction (also called "zone of softening" or encephalomalacia). The infarct may be pale if devoid of blood, or hemorrhagic if blood extravasates from small vessels in the area of infarction. Depending on the degree of ischemia, the changes are reversible up to a few hours and some recovery of function can take place after days, weeks, months or even years. The first 3 h after acute stroke are usually considered to be the therapeutic window during which therapeutic interventions can stop the progression of stroke and reverse the biochemical disturbances to some extent.

Two major types of strokes are ischemic and hemorrhagic. Most ischemic lesions (infarcts) are due to occlusion of cerebral vessels, although they may occur in the absence of demonstrable occlusion of the vessels. The pathophysiology of cerebral ischemia is shown in Figure 18.3 and various factors influencing the size of a cerebral infarct are shown in Table 18.1.

Clinicopathological Correlations

Various stages in the evolution of stroke are shown in Table 18.2.

The symptoms of a stroke vary according to the arterial system or the branch involved. Most stroke syndromes are designated by the name of the artery supplying the area of the brain that is infarcted. Neurological deficits due to stroke depend upon the type and location of the disease process. A common presentation is hemiplegia due to occlusion of the carotid artery or the middle cerebral artery, with aphasia if the dominant hemisphere is involved. In vertebral-basilar territory strokes, the neurological picture is more varied with involvement of cranial nerves and the sensory pathways. In the most severe form, the patient becomes comatose.

There are variations in the arterial supply and collateral circulation, and sometimes an artery may be occluded without any infarction, or infarction may not be clinically manifest. The major cause of cerebrovascular disease is atherosclerosis, a noninflammatory degenerative disease that can affect segments of almost any artery in the body. Atherosclerosis is the commonest vascular disorder, although other diseases also affect the cerebral circulation. Some of these are embolic occlusion of the cerebral arteries by detached thrombi from

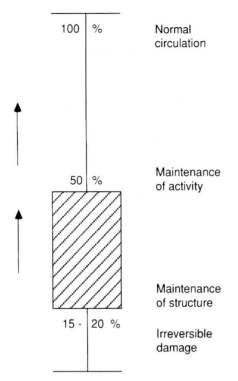

Figure 18.4
Critical levels of cerebral blood flow required for maintenance of structure and function.

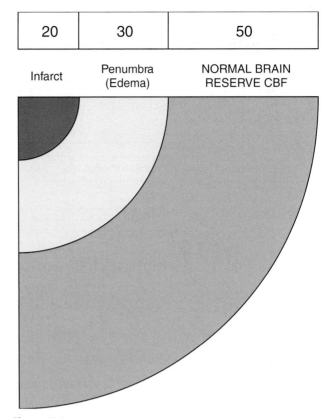

Figure 18.5
Penumbra zone in cerebral infarction. Numbers indicate the percentage of cerebral blood flow in this model to correlate with that in Figure 18.4.

the heart or major vessels, intracranial vascular malformations, and microvascular disorders.

Structure of a Cerebral Infarct

There are three phases of evolution of morphological changes with infarction: coagulation necrosis, liquification necrosis, and cavitation. The three zones of histological alterations within an infarct are:

- A central zone with variable neuronal necrosis ranging from pale ghost cells to shrunken neurons with pyknotic nuclei.
- A reactive zone at the periphery of the central zone within which there is neuronal necrosis and leukocytic infiltration and neovascularization.
- A marginal zone peripheral to the reactive zone within which there are shrunken neurons and swollen astrocytes in various stages of hyperplasia and hypertrophy.

The traditional concept of infarction, that the brain tissue dies from a shortage of blood and oxygen lasting more than a few minutes, is no longer valid. The interruption of blood flow is seldom total and a drop of CBF to as low as 50% can maintain function. The neuronal structure can be preserved with CBF as little as 15%–20% of the normal (Figure 18.4). Between the zones of infarction and normal

brain is a third zone referred to as the "penumbra" (Figure 18.5) containing the so-called dormant or idling neurons (Symon 1976). These neurons are nonfunctional but anatomically intact and can be revived. The presence of viable brain tissue in the penumbra explains why the acute clinical presentation of a stroke is a rather poor predictor of the outcome (Astrup *et al* 1981). A trickle of blood flow is maintained to the penumbra zone, which is hypoxic. It can be presumed that the critical parameter for cellular function is oxygen availability rather than blood flow.

Cerebral Metabolism in Ischemia

The cascade of biochemical events following cerebral ischemia is shown in Figure 18.6. The outcome of cerebral ischemia depends on cerebral metabolic reactions to the failing circulation. Although ischemia is a circulatory disorder, its impact on the brain is determined by neurochemical events at the subcellular level. Several investigative therapies for stroke are based on an attempt to prevent detrimental biochemical events. The correlation between the metabolic changes and hemodynamic changes in an ischemic focus is shown in Table 18.3.

Table 18.3
Hemodynamic and Metabolic Changes in an Ischemic Focus

Area	Cerebral blood flow	Characteristics
Central zone	< 0.10 ml/g/min	Rise of extracellular K; fall of ATP; increase of lactate and intracellular acidosis
Boundary	0.10–0.15 ml/g/min	Extinction of neuronal electrical activity; limited rise of extracellular K
Collateral	> 0.15 ml/g/min	Undisturbed metabolism, hyperemia

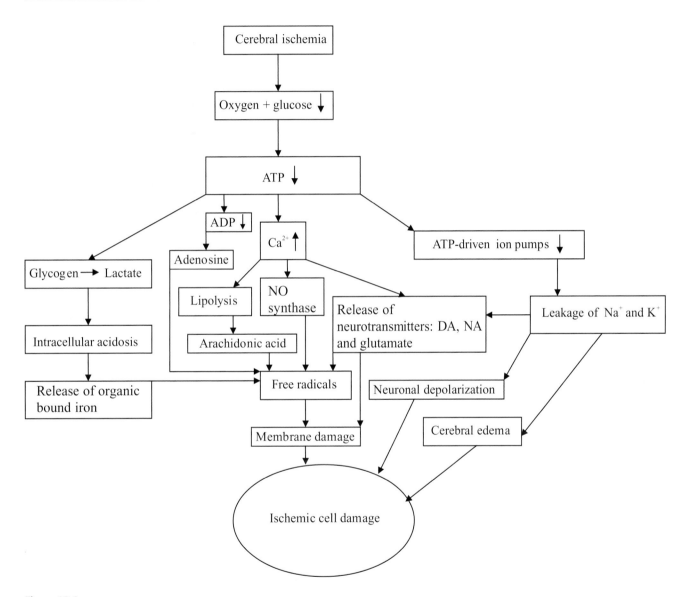

Figure 18.6
Sequence of biochemical events following cerebral ischemia. CBF, cerebral blood flow; FFA, free fatty acids; K_e, extracellular potassium ion; Ca_i, intracellular calcium ion; Na_i, intracellular sodium ion; GABA, gamma-aminobutyric acid (Welch & Barkley 1986).

Glutamate as a Marker of Stroke

Excitotoxic injury, triggered by inappropriately high levels of extracellular glutamate and possibly other excitatory amino acids, has been identified as the dominant mechanism underlying calcium-mediated injury of gray matter in a number of experimental models. Glutamate levels are elevated in the CSF of patients with progressive cerebral infarcts. Glutamate levels in patients with cortical infarcts have been found to be higher than in patients with deep infarcts. The explanation of this may be that underlying molecular mechanisms of anoxic/ischemic injury are different in the white and the gray matter. These results also suggest that there may be different molecular signatures of different types of stroke.

Role of Oxygen Free Radicals in Cerebral Ischemia

Free radicals are formed during normal respiration and oxidation. Oxidation is a chemical reaction in which a molecule transfers one or more electrons to another. Stable molecules usually have matched pairs of protons and electrons whereas free radical have unpaired electrons and tend to be highly reactive, oxidizing agents. Damage to cells caused by free radicals includes protein oxidation, DNA strand destruction, increase of intracellular calcium, activation of damaging proteases and nucleases, and peroxidation of cellular membrane lipids. Furthermore, such intracellular damage can lead to the formation of prostaglandins, interferons, TNF-α, and other tissue damaging mediators, each of which can lead to disease if overproduced in response to the oxidative stress. Free radicals can be measured *in vivo* and some of the antioxidant mechanisms have been studied in transgenic mice. Free radicals has been linked to numerous human diseases including ischemia/reperfusion injury resulting from stroke. Reoxygenation provides oxygen to sustain neuronal viability and also provides oxygen as a substrate for numerous enzymatic oxidation reactions that produce reactive oxidants. In addition reflow following oxidation also increases oxygen to a level that cannot be utilized by mitochondria under normal physiological conditions.

Damaging effect of free radicals is controlled to some extent by the antioxidant defense systems and cellular repair mechanisms of the body but at times it is overwhelmed.. Enzymes such as superoxide dismutase, catalase and glutathione peroxidase, and vitamins such as tocopherol, ascorbate and beta carotene act to quench radical chain reactions. Many of these agents have been investigated as potential therapeutic agents. Unfortunately, most studies testing naturally occurring antioxidants have resulted in disappointing results. Generally, natural antioxidants must be produced on site within the cell to be effective in disease prevention. Free radicals are normally scavenged by superoxide dismutases (SODs) and glutathione peroxidases. Vitamin E and ascorbic acid are also likely to be involved in the detoxification of free radicals but these mechanisms may be overwhelmed during reperfusion and damage may occur to the brain parenchyma.

Free radicals have been a topic of discussion in relation to HBO therapy because oxygen administration is considered to increase oxidative stress. This issue remains unresolved. There is no convincing evidence that HBO induces any oxidative stress that is harmful to the patient with stroke.

Reperfusion Injury

Reperfusion implies resumption of the blood flow either spontaneously or as a result of thrombolysis or surgical procedures, there is resumption of the principal functions of tissue perfusion: oxygen delivery, provision of substrates for metabolism and clearance of metabolic wastes. This has beneficial effects as well as a dark side-reperfusion injury. Interactions between blood and the damaged tissues can lead to further tissue injury. Major mechanism postulated to participate in this injury are loss of calcium homeostasis, free radical generation, leukocyte-mediated injury, and acute hypercholesterolemia.

Molecular Mechanism in the Pathogenesis of Stroke

Various molecular mechanism are involved in the pathophysiology of ischemic stroke and form the basis of experimental interventions. It is beyond the scope of this textbook to describe these in detail but some important ones are as follows.

Gene expression in response to cerebral ischemia. During the early postischemic stages, protein synthesis in the brain is generally suppressed, but specific genes are expressed and their corresponding proteins may be synthesized. There is expression of a range of genes in cerebral ischemia which may have either a beneficial or a detrimental effect on the evolution of neuronal injury. The first set of genes to be activated following neuronal injury in focal cerebral ischemia are the c-fos/c-jun complex which are involved in the induction of target genes that regulate cell growth and differentiation. According to the excitotoxic hypothesis, ischemic neuronal death is induced by the release of excitatory amino acid glutamate. Activation of the NMDA receptor operated and voltage-sensitive calcium channels cause calcium influx which activates degrading enzymes leading to disintegration of nuclear and cell membranes and generation of oxygen free radicals. Calcium influx also induces expression of c-fos. The induction of neurotrophin genes by c-fos/c-jun has been demonstrated although the role of these induced proteins in the overall adaptive response is not certain. Gene regulation, including immediate early genes is required for programmed neural death after trophic factor deprivation and is predicted to be involved in apoptosis triggered by cerebral ischemia. Novel therapies following cerebral ischemia may be directed at genes mediating either recovery or apoptosis.

Induction of heat shock proteins (HSP). Heat shock protein concentrations increase in the brain after experimentally induced strokes. Induction of HSP 70 does not occur until reperfusion for 24 h following cerebral ischemia and occurs only in areas with earlier induction of c-fos/c-jun, suggesting that induction of HSP occurs in neurons that survive to that point. HSP does not participate in early response for neuronal survival after global cerebral ischemia. Although the proteins are known to protect cells against damage caused by various stresses, it was not known that they were doing anything useful. It is now realized that HSPs may be factors in ischemia tolerance and neuroprotection against ischemia. Insertion of gene for HSP 72 into the brain of rats, using a viral vector, has been shown to protect against ischemia and this forms the basis of a potential gene therapy approach.

Role of cytokines and adhesion molecules in stroke. Inflammatory-immunologic reactions are involved in the pathogenesis of cerebral ischemia. In addition to this cells such as astrocytes, microglia or endothelial cells have been found to be activated by cerebral injuries including stroke. These cells then become immunologically reactive and interact with each other by producing substances including cytokines and adhesion molecules. Three major cytokines, tumor necrosis factor (TNF)-α, interleukin (IL)-1 and IL-6, are produced by cultured brain cells after various stimuli.

Increased expression of adhesion molecules such as ICAM-1 and VCAM are observed in cultured microglial cells after treatment with TNF-α. ELAM and P-selectin were also found to be expressed. The induction of these adhesion molecules in the ischemic brain is time-locked and appears to be controlled in a highly regulated manner during the process of ischemic cascade. An understanding of the cytokine-adhesion molecule cascades in the ischemic brain may allow us to develop new strategies for the treatment of stroke. Further work is required to define the role of these cytokines and other signaling molecules in cerebral ischemic infarcts. This may open the way for gene therapy of cerebral infarction: antisense methods and use of genetically engineered overexpressors.

DNA damage and repair in cerebral ischemia. There is evidence of DNA damage in experimental stroke and this is an important factor in the pathophysiology of stroke. DNA repair may be an important mechanism for the maintenance of normal physiological function. Research in the science of DNA injury and repair will likely provide new and important information on mechanisms of cell damage and provide opportunities for the development of novel and effective therapies to reduce CNS injury in stroke. Techniques for measuring DNA damage are available that are applicable to *in vitro* and *in vivo* models of cerebral ischemia.

Role of neurotrophic factors. Neurotrophic Factors (NTFs) are polypeptides which regulate the proliferation, survival, migration and differentiation of cells in the nervous system. By definition, a neurotrophic factor is synthesized by and released from target cells of the neurons, bound to specific receptors, internalized and retrogradely transported by the axon to the cell soma where multiple survival-promoting effects are initiated. The major hypotheses for the functional effects of cerebral insult-induced neurotrophin changes are protection against neuronal damage and stimulation of neuronal sprouting as well as synaptic reorganization. Basic fibroblast growth factor (bFGF) is one of of the NTF's that has been studied extensively in relation to stroke and is in clinical trials.

Role of Poly(ADP-ribose) polymerase (PARP) gene. DNA damage can lead to activation of the nuclear enzyme PARP, which catalyzes the attachment of ADP ribose units from NAD to nuclear proteins following DNA damage. Excessive activation PARP can deplete NAD and ATP, which is consumed in regeneration of NAD, leading to cell death by energy depletion. Genetic disruption of PARP provides profound protection against glutamate-NO-mediated ischemic insults *in vitro* and major decreases in infarct volume after reversible middle cerebral artery occlusion. This provides evidence for a primary involvement of PARP activation in neuronal damage following focal cerebral ischemia and suggest that therapies designed toward inhibiting PARP may provide benefit in the treatment of cerebrovascular disease.

Classification of Ischemic Cerebrovascular Disease

A practical comprehensive classification of stroke is needed for evaluation of new therapies. With many variations in the initial presentations, pathology, brain imaging, and the clinical course, it is essential that a patient with stroke be labeled with these variables. This status would change in the natural course of the disease as well as by modifications with treatment. A proposed classification of ischemic cerebrovascular disease is shown in Table 18.4.

The case summary of a patient should include information on these essential points which can be coded under the letters and numerals for sorting out categories from a large series.

The patient presented with right hemiplegia (I1), showed an infarct on CT (II2), severe atherosclerotic narrowing of left internal carotid artery (III–A1, B1, C3), recovered partially over a period of 3 weeks, and was found to have hypertension (V1).

Recovery from Stroke

It is well recognized that spontaneous, often dramatic improvement occurs in patients with acute ischemic stroke.

Table 18.4
A Practical Classification of Ischemic Cerebrovascular Disease for Evaluating Therapy

I.   Initial clinical features
         1. Asymptomatic
         2. TIA
         3. Neurological deficits: hemiplegia, aphasia

II.   Brain imaging studies
         1. Normal
         2. Infarction
         3. None carried out

III.   Vascular pathology
         A. Location
             1. Cerebral arteries (including neck arteries)
             2. Heart and the great vessels
             3. Blood elements (coagulation disorders)
         B. Type
             1. Atherosclerotic occlusive disease
             2. Thromboembolic
             3. Other
         C. Severity
             1. Minimal
             2. Moderate
             3. Severe

IV.   Clinical course
         (state time period)
         1. Single event. No recurrence
         2. Partial recovery
         3. Complete recovery
         4. Fixed neurological deficits

V.   Major risk factors
         1. Hypertension
         2. Heart disease
         3. Atherosclerosis
         4. Old age
         5. Diabetes
         6. Smoking
         7. Other risk factors
         8. None identified

- Presence of collateral blood supply. The degree of motor improvement has been shown to correlate significantly (positively) with CBF values in the undamaged motor cortex of the opposite cerebral hemisphere.
- Regression of cerebral edema
- Volume of penumbra that escapes infarction offers opportunities for secondary perifocal neuronal reorganization. Mapping of the extent of penumbra enables prediction for potential of recovery and select the most appropriate candidates for therapeutic trials.
- There is considerable scope for functional plasticity in the adult human cerebral cortex. Cortical reorganization is associated with functional recovery in stroke. Retraining after stroke can extend cortical representation of the infarcted area and improve skilled motor performance.

Recovery of cerebral energy metabolism is a prerequisite for the recovery of brain function and depends, to some extent, on the restoration of blood flow following ischemia. Postischemic resynthesis of ATP is limited. The recovery process is far more complex than the simple process of reversal of ischemia by revascularization.

The size of the penumbra zone is an important factor in the recovery of brain function. In the patient with an acute stroke, it is difficult to distinguish between the deficits due to areas of infarction and those due to the penumbra zone with potential for recovery. The duration of survival of neurons in the penumbra zone is not known but can extend to years, as evidenced by the recovery following HBO (Neubauer 1981).

The time course of clinical recovery from stroke is variable and controversial. Most of the motor recovery usually occurs in the first 3 months and functional recovery can continue for 6 months to 1 year after stroke. the possible. The following are important neurophysiological mechanisms underlying recovery from stroke:

- Unmasking or release from inhibition of previously ineffective pathways
- Synaptic sprouting and formation of new dendritic connections for pathways for transmission of neural messages.

About one-fourth of patients with acute ischemic stroke show some degree of spontaneous improvement by 1 h and nearly half of the patients show some improvement by 6 h. Few of these patients, however, show complete motor recovery. Ninety percent of these patients remain improved on long-term follow-up indicating that improvement during the first 48 h after acute ischemic stroke is a predictor of favorable long-term outcome. This is correlated with absence of early hypodensity seen on CT. This improvement should be taken into consideration in design of any clinical trial of acute treatment of stroke. Mechanisms of recovery following acute ischemic stroke are:

Table 18.5
Factors that Influence the Recovery from Stroke

1. Neurological status of the patient:
    (a) prior to stroke
    (b) immediately following stroke
2. Age
3. Type of Stroke
4. Location of lesion in the cerebral arteries
5. Risk factors of stroke
6. Treatment of stroke

These mechanisms are the basis of the concept of neuro-plasticity, which is the term used for the ability of the central nervous system (CNS) to modify its own structural organization and function.

Recovery from stroke depends upon several factors, listed in Table 18.5.

Complications of Stroke

Various complications of stroke have been reported in the literature. These can be divided into neurological and medical or systemic complications. They have an adverse effect on the outcome of stroke and many are preventable. Deterioration of the neurological status, including a decrease in consciousness or progression of neurological deficits, occurs during the first week in 26–43% of the patients with acute stroke. In some the causes are extension or hemorrhagic transformation of the infarct. Other causes are metabolic disturbances such as hypoglycemia and hyponatremia and adverse effects of drugs. Early deterioration is associated with a poor prognosis. Determinants of neurological worsening may include causative aspects rather than just the evolution of the ischemic or hemorrhagic process itself. Acute neurological complications of ischemic stroke are:

- Progressive neurological deficits
- Cerebral edema with transtentorial herniations
- Extension of infarction or appearance of a new infarct
- Hemorrhagic transformation of infarct
- Seizures

Stroke may be aggravated by treatment. Examples of this are complications of surgery on the cerebral blood vessels. Adverse effect s of several drugs used in stroke patients may aggravate the condition. One example of this cerebral hemorrhage resulting from anticoagulant or thrombolytic therapy in patients with ischemic infarction.

Sequelae of Stroke

The chronic poststroke stage may manifest some neuropsychological sequelae, as shown in Table 18.6. These are an extension of the neurological deficits seen in the acute phase of stroke. These are important but not always detected or emphasized. Two of them – spasticity and dementia – are important and will be considered here as they are amenable to treatment with hyperbaric oxygen.

Spasticity. This is the most troublesome complication of stroke and interferes with the physical rehabilitation of the

Table 18.6
Neuropsychological Sequelae of Stroke
• Persistence of neurological deficits
• Epilepsy
• Spasticity
• Central pain syndrome
• Neuropsychological disturbances
Memory disturbances
Intellectual and cognitive impairment
Dementia
Depression
Pseudodepressive manifestations
Anxiety
Apathy
Pathological laughing and crying
Mania

patients. Spasticity is defined as a velocity-dependent response of a muscle to passive stretching, increased resistance to passive manipulation of the paretic limb, and is most marked in the antigravity muscles. Spasticity does not bear any definite relation to the degree of paralysis or the time of onset of the stroke; usually it becomes noticeable a few weeks after the onset of stroke. The underlying mechanism is controversial. The final common pathway for the expression of muscle tone is the anterior horn cells and myoneural junction. Spasticity may be viewed as alpha-overactivity. A slight amount of spasticity of the paretic leg may be helpful in ambulation, but spasticity in the hand interferes with fine movements. Persistent spasticity can lead to contractures of muscles, tendons, and joint capsules.

Vascular dementia. Dementia is defined as deterioration in intellectual function which is sufficient to interfere with customary affairs of life, which is not isolated to a single category of intellectual performance and is independent of level of consciousness. Vascular dementia may be the leading cause of cognitive impairment in the world but there is no general agreement as to its definition. The term "vascular" may be obsolete and "dementia" implies that a patient has reached a state from which recovery is unlikely. The alternative term of vascular cognitive impairment has been used. Another term used in the literature is multi-infarct dementia but vascular dementia has a broader connotation and is the most widely used to describe cognitive impairment after stroke. Post-stroke dementia is another term used to describe this condition. The only catch to this is that a patient with vascular disease may develop dementia without any manifest stroke.

Stroke patients are at risk for dementia. The prevalence of dementia 3 months after an ischemic stroke in patients over the age of 60 years is over 25% and about 10 times that in controls. Poststroke dementia is the second most common cause of dementia after Alzheimer's disease in Europe and the US. In Asia and many other countries it is more common than the dementia of Alzheimer's disease. Vascular risk factors are dominant in this form of dementia although there may be some genetic factors and some overlap with Alzheimer's disease. Treatable vascular risk factors occur more frequently in patients with vascular cognitive impairment than in patients with Alzheimer's disease. The importance of this distinction is that the vascular risk factors are more amenable to treatment. A single explanation for poststroke dementia is not adequate; rather, multiple factors including stroke features (dysphasia, major dominant stroke syndrome), host characteristics (level of education), and prior cerebrovascular disease each independently contribute to the risk. Dementia is relatively frequent after a clinical first stroke in persons younger than 80 years and aphasia is very often associated with poststroke dementia.

Two main causes of infarction in vascular dementia are hypoperfusion and vessel obstruction resulting in different types of lesions. Hypoperfusion is due to blood pressure fall in combination with vascular stenosis. Most of these infarcts are of an incomplete nature, i.e., an attenuation of the tissue leaving some axons with axon sheaths or intact neurons with scarring. Vascular obstruction may involve both the large extracerebral arteries as well as the small intracerebral vessels. Small vessel disease is usually due to hypertensive angiopathy, amyloid angiopathy or microembolism.

Diagnosis

The diagnosis of stroke is basically clinical but confirmation requires laboratory procedures. In the case of acute stroke, the primary diagnosis at site of occurrence is important as it effects the treatment decisions. With the availability of treatment for acute stroke, the reliability of prehospital diagnosis has been examined. In a study in Ohio, emergency medical dispatchers correctly identified 52% and paramedics 72% of patients with stroke (Kothari *et al* 1995). At the physician's level, neurologist's obviously make a more accurate diagnosis than primary care physicians. False positive rate without supplementary laboratory investigations varies from 1 to 5%. This increases if the patient is unable to give a history because of impairment of consciousness or loss of speech. Diagnostic errors are most likely to arise in patients with atypical presentations and those with other diseases associated with cerebrovascular complications. Diagnosis of stroke depends on the clinical stage. Clinical diagnosis is important for classification of stroke which is an important part of clinical research for testing new therapies.

The diagnosis of stroke should be confirmed by laboratory investigations. Various laboratory diagnostic procedures used for stroke patients are:

- General laboratory examination
  Hematology: full blood count, thrombophilia screen, erythrocyte sedimentation rate, etc
  Biochemistry: blood glucose, electrolytes, etc
- Lumbar puncture and CSF examination
- Biomarkers of stroke in blood and CSF
- Doppler ultrasound
- Radioisotope imaging of atherosclerotic plaques
- Electroencephalography (EEG)
- Magnetoencephalography
- Neuro-ophthalmic examination: fundoscopy and ophthalmodynamometry
- Cerebral blood flow
- Cerebral angiography
- Brain imaging studies
  Computerized tomography (CT)
  Magnetic resonance imaging (MRI)
  Positron emission tomography (PET)
  Single photon emission computerized tomography (SPECT)
- Cardiac investigations
  Electrocardiography (ECG)
  Transthoracic echocardiography
  Transesophageal echocardiography

The most important of the imaging methods in relation to acute ischemic stroke are the brain imaging methods. These are discussed in Chapter 23. Currently CT scans are done routinely and MRI or SPECT are still limited to certain centers. The last two are the most relevant to evaluation of the effect of HBO on acute ischemic stroke.

Stroke Scales

The most commonly used functional scales in stroke patients, which measure only basic activities of daily living, are the Barthel Index and the Rankin scale. Two global scales frequently used in clinical trials are the Unified Neurological Scale and the NIH Stroke scale. These will be described in the following pages.

Barthel Index. The Barthel Index scores the patient's performance in 10 basic activities of daily life, chosen and weighted as to reflect the amount of help required. For example 15 points are given for walking and transfers; 10 points for feeding, bowel, bladder, toileting and dressing; and 5 points are given for bathing and grooming. The maximum score is 100, which corresponds to full independence, and the lowest score is 0, which corresponds to bed-ridden state with full dependence. Most of the patients being discharged home have a score of 60 or above at that time. At a score of 85, most patients can dress themselves and transfer from bed to chair without help. The scores are not arbitrary but represent a definite average level of autonomy. The advantage of the thresholds of the Barthel Index is that they can be used in different types of statistical analyses. The reliability of the Barthel Index is high as reflected by an interobserver agreement of more than 85%. It is a more reliable and less subjective scale for assessing disability, from which a Rankin Handicap score can then be derived to enable those managing the stroke patients to assess aspects of handicap as well as disability.

Rankin Scale. This scale has the following scoring system:

0 No symptoms at all.
1 No significant disability despite symptoms, able to carry out all usual duties and activities.
2 Slight disability, unable to carry out all previous activities but able to look after own affairs without assistance.
3 Moderate disability, requiring some help, but able to walk without assistance and attend to own body needs without assistance.
4 Moderately severe disability, unable to walk without assistance and unable to attend to body needs without assistance.
5 Severe disability, bedridden, incontinent and requiring constant nursing care and attention.
6 Dead.

National Institutes of Health Stroke Scale. National Institutes of Health (NIH) Stroke Scale is a standardized measure of neurological function to assess outcome after investigative therapy for acute stroke (Brott *et al* 1989, Wityk *et al* 1994). It has 15 items which cover level of consciousness, pupillary response, best motor, limb ataxia, sensory, visual, neglect and dysathria items. This scale was used for the earlier tPA studies.

Unified Neurological Stroke Scale. The Unified Neurological Stroke Scale (UNSS) is composed of the Neurological Scale for Middle Cerebral Artery Infarction (MCANS) and Scandinavian Neurological Stroke Scale (SNSS). This scale is constructed specifically to assess patients with hemiparesis due to MCA infarction (Orgogozo & Dartigues 1991). Most of the items deal with testing the motor function. Consciousness and verbal communication are rated but it excludes sensory and cognitive dysfunction items which are known to be less reliable and difficult to assess in evaluation of stroke in general. Disability evaluation items are omitted as they are included in scales for functional evaluation. The Unified Neurological Stroke Scale demonstrates good reliability and high construct and predictive validity and its use is supported in ischemic and hemorrhagic stroke. Structural equation modeling is

an appropriate technique for use with scales of this type (Edwards *et al* 1995).

Canadian Neurological Scale. The Canadian Neurological Scale (CNS) is a highly reliable and validated stroke scoring system (Goldstein & Chilukuri 1998). Long-term outcome can be predicted soon after acute stroke with a simple mathematical model based on the patient's age and initial CNS score. In contrast to other scales, which include assessment of neglect, coordination, sensation and gait, the CNS focuses on level of consciousness, speech and strength. Because impairment of these modalities is basic to the evaluation of any stroke patients, the data required for retrospective application of the CNS is more likely to be available in hospital records. Retrospective scoring of initial stroke severity using an algorithm based on the CNS is valid and can be reliably performed using hospital discharge summaries.

Evaluation of various scales. Stroke scales were originally devised to quantify disturbances in neurological function explained by a stroke induced brain lesions. In the course of evolution of these scales disagreements have arisen as to the weighting of certain elements in these scales. For example, coma is considered more serious than sensory disturbances of a limb. Considerable controversy still exists regarding the utility of these scales. The main finding of these analyses supports that the scales in popular use share many items but emphasize different features of the standard clinical examination. The scales most closely approximate one another for assessment of sensorimotor function. They vary widely when it comes to assessment of higher cerebral function.

De Haan *et al* (1993) compared five classic stroke impairment scales (NIH, SNSS, UNSS, CNS, Mathew Scale) with scales measuring disability, handicap and quality of life (Barthel Index and Rankin Scale). They concluded that stroke scales only partially explain functional health and that the impact of impairment on functional outcome seems to be underestimated by stroke scale weights. In a reappraisal of reliability and validity of 9 stroke scales, the following were found to be the most reliable, based on interobserver agreement: NIH Scale, CNS Scale and the European Stroke Scale (D'Olhaberriague *et al* 1996). The Barthel Index was found to be the most reliable disability scale. In the NIH tissue plasminogen activator (tPA) stroke trial, no measure of disability was found to describe all dimensions of recovery for stroke patients at 90 days. To compare treatments, the NINDS tPA Stroke Trial Coordinating Center proposed the use of a global statistical test. This test allowed an overall assessment of treatment efficacy for a combination of correlated outcomes (Tilley *et al* 1997).

An Overview of the Conventional Management of Stroke

The management of stroke will be discussed according to whether it is the acute phase or chronic post-stroke stage. Treatment of acute ischemic stroke is more critical because there is a chance to prevent or limit irreversible damage to the brain. This is a challenge because of the limitations of feasible methods and of the short time window, which is considered to be no more than 3 h. The management of post-stroke stage is more rehabilitation-oriented and is aimed at recovery of the lost function.

Acute Ischemic Stroke

Until the approval of thrombolytic therapy by tissue plasminogen activator (tPA) 1996, there was no definite treatment of acute stroke. The availability of thrombolytic therapy has opened the door for improved and more definitive care for acute stroke patients. It is now considered important to bring the acute stroke patients to a medical center within the first few hours following stroke. The ideal place for a patient is a stroke center, and if this is not available, a major general hospital with neurological service would be adequate. Objectives of acute stroke therapy are:

- To reduce the mortality rate in those who survive stroke to below 20%
- Restoration of normal cerebral blood flow
  Thrombolysis of blood clot obstructing cerebral arteries
  Surgical procedures such as carotid endarterectomy
- Cerebral protection against the effects of cerebral ischemia
  Hyperbaric oxygen
  Neuroprotectives
- Supportive medical care
  Maintenance of airway and oxygenation
  Management of concomitant diseases such as heart disease and hypertension
  Maintenance of fluid and electrolyte balance
  Prevention of complications such as aspiration pneumonia
- Preservation of life and management of systemic effects of stroke
- Neurologic intensive care
  Monitoring for increased intracranial pressure
  Management of neurological complications, e.g., cerebral edema and seizures
- Prevention disease extension and recurrence
  Anticoagulation/antiplatelet therapy
  Risk factor management
- Rehabilitation: To enable 70% of the stroke survivors to live independently 3 months after stroke

Table 18.7
Current Management of Acute Stroke
• Medical Therapies
Thrombolytic therapy
Anticoagulant therapy
Antiplatelet agents
Hemorrheological agents: Trental
Drugs for reduction of cerebral edema
Management of hypotension
Complementary medical therapies: herbs and acupuncture
Hyperbaric oxygen
• Management of concomitant disorders
Antihypertensive medications
Drugs for cardiac disorders
• Surgical therapies
Evacuation of intracerebral hematomas
Decompressive craniotomy
Carotid endarterectomy
Embolectomy
Transluminal angioplasty
Surgical procedures for revascularization
• Start of rehabilitation

These goals are ideal but extremely difficult to attain. To achieve these objectives, all patients with acute ischemic stroke should be treated on an emergency basis within 1 h of occurrence. The current management of acute stroke is summarized in Table 18.7.

The acute stroke is a medical emergency and most of these patients are transported by ambulance to a hospital. Trained and experienced ambulance attendants are able to recognize stroke in fair percentage of patients. In some countries a physician accompanies the ambulance. Care during transport varies according to the type of medical attendants in the ambulance. Most of the patients receive basic medical care according to the condition. Unconscious patients are observed and airway is maintained if necessary with intubation. Supplementary oxygen is usually given and an intravenous line is established. Monitoring of cardiovascular function varies in different countries. Blood pressure is checked regularly and ECG monitoring is done in some countries. The emergency medical facility is notified to have necessary personnel and equipment ready on arrival, including the readiness of emergency CT scan and alerting the emergency physician for the possibility of the patient as a candidate for tPA therapy. On arrival in the emergency department, the level of care varies according to the facility, e.g., a stroke center or a small general hospital. Airway and circulation are checked. Supplemental oxygen and intravenous saline or lactate Ringer solution is started. An eyewitness history of the onset is obtained as the patient's account may not be reliable. Establishing the time and mode of onset is important. A careful clinical neurovascular examination is done. Neurological dysfunction is recorded and examination repeated to see if it is recovering, stable or increasing. Most of the acute care in the US is done by emergency room physicians who also administer tPA.

Major questions that remain unanswered and are under investigation for treatment of acute stroke are:

- Redefinition of indications and modifications of thrombolytic therapy).
- Value of early intravenous heparin following acute ischemic stroke
- Value of antiplatelet therapy given during the first 6 h after stroke onset
- Neuroprotective therapy for acute stroke
- Value of hyperbaric oxygenation in acute ischemic stroke
- Value of hypothermia in acute ischemic stroke
- Combination of various therapies

Over 150 compounds are in various stages of development for acute stroke by the pharmaceutical industry. These fall into the following categories and are discussed in detail elsewhere (Jain 2009d).

- Thrombolytics
- Anticoagulants
- Defibrogenating agents
- Agents to improve hemorheology
- Neuroprotectives
  Adenosine analogs
  Anti-inflammatory agents
  Apoptosis inhibitors
  – Calpain inhibitors
  – Cycloheximide
- Ion Channel modulators
  – Ca^+ channel blockers
  – Na^+ channel blockers
- NMDA antagonists
  NMDA receptor antagonists – competitive and non-competitive
  AMPA antagonists
  Glycine site antagonists
- Non-NMDA excitatory amino acid antagonists
  5-HT agonist
  GABA agonists
  Opioid receptor antagonists
- Nitric oxide scavengers
- Free radical scavengers
- Drugs counteracting lactate neurotoxicity
- Agents for regeneration and repair
  Neurotrophic factors
  Nootropic agents
  Phosphotidylcholine synthesis
- Hormonal modulators of cerebral ischemia
- Anti-edema agents
- Antihypoxic agents

- Miscellaneous agents
- Oxygen carriers
- Cell therapy
- Gene therapy

Neuroprotectives. A neuroprotective agent is one that aims to prevent neuronal death by inhibiting one or more of the pathophysiological steps in the processes that follow occlusion (or rupture) of a cerebral artery. Neuroprotection is an important part of acute therapy of stroke to protect the neural tissues from the ischemic cascade that increases the damage. Even if the ischemia is reversed by thrombolytic therapy, reperfusion injury may be responsible for further tissue damage.

The time window during which initiation of treatment with neuroprotective agents may rescue brain tissue is limited. The ideal time window for thrombolytic therapy is considered to be < 3 h and most of the neuroprotectives in clinical trials are used in a time window of > 3 h. Ideally a neuroprotective should be given as soon as possible after the ischemic insult, i.e., within the first 3 h. It should precede the use of thrombolytic therapy and at least overlap it.

Oxygen carriers. Two main categories of pharmaceutical agents have been used for delivery of oxygen to the tissues: perfluorocarbons (PFCs) and hemoglobin-based oxygen carriers. Both are primarily blood substitutes. Here we are interested in the use of these substances as oxygen carriers to the ischemic brain in stroke. Theoretically, cell-free carriers should transfer oxygen to the tissues more efficiently than red cells but so far, this has not been readily demonstrable. A third category is liposome encapsulated Hb where Hb is entrapped in a bilayer of phospholipid. A modifier of heme function is also enclosed to adjust the oxygen-carrying capacity of HB. The half life of this product can be increased by coating the liposome surface with sugar. Various oxygen carriers have been discussed in detail elsewhere (Jain 2009d). Some of them are:

- Hemoglobin-based oxygen carriers (HBOCs). Preparation of HBOCs involves the removal of the cellular capsule of Hb and modifying the structure of Hb to prevent it from degradation, to enable it to function in simple electrolyte solutions and avoid toxic effects in the body.
- Diaspirin cross-linked hemoglobin. Purified diaspirin cross-linked hemoglobin (DCLHb) is a cell-free hemoglobin that is intramolecularly cross-linked between the two alpha subunits, resulting in enhanced oxygen offloading to tissues and increased half-life. It is prepared from outdated human red cells. Because Hb molecules are minute compared with red cells, free Hb may perfuse into capillaries that have been shut down and thus prevent secondary damage.
- Perfluorocarbons (PFCs). PFCs are inert organic substances produced by substituting fluorine for hydrogen

in specific positions within highly stable carbon chains. They are not metabolized by the body and are excreted via the lungs, urine and feces although a small amount may be stored in the reticuloendothelial system. The two major mechanisms underlying the efficacy of PFCs for oxygen transport and delivery are: (1) a high solubility coefficient for oxygen and CO_2 and (2) PFCs release O_2 to the tissues more effectively because their O_2 binding constant is negligible. They have been investigated intensively over the past 30 years. PFC-based oxygen carriers, while more recent than HBOCs, have some advantages over HBOCs. They are synthetic, chemically inert and inexpensive. PFCs have a high affinity for oxygen and carbon dioxide. PFCs can substitute for red blood cells transport oxygen as a dissolved gas rather than as chemically bound as in the case of HBOCs. This makes a difference to the way the oxygen is presented to the tissues. It is not yet certain if PFCs can provide more oxygen to the tissues than simple oxygen inhalation. Other drawbacks are adverse characteristics such as instability, short intravascular half-life and uncertainty concerning toxic effects.

Cell therapy. Cell therapy is the prevention or treatment of human disease by the administration of cells that have been selected, multiplied and pharmacologically treated or altered outside the body (ex vivo). Cells may repair the damage or release therapeutic molecules. The scope of cell therapy can be broadened to include methods, pharmacological as well as non-pharmacological, to modify the function of intrinsic cells of the body for therapeutic purposes. Various types of cells have been used for this purpose but most of the current interest in cell therapy centers on stem cells. Cell therapy can be combined with HBO. HBO can promote the mobilization and multiplication of stem cells. This topic is dealt with in detail in a special report on this topic (Jain 2009e). Examples of some of the strategies are:

- Implantation of genetically programmed embryonic stem cells.
- Intravenous infusion of marrow stromal cells.
- Intravenous infusion of umbilical cord blood stem cells.
- Intracerebral administration of multipotent adult progenitor cells.
- Neural stem cell therapy for stroke.

Gene therapy. Gene therapy can be broadly defined as the transfer of defined genetic material to specific target cells of a patient for the ultimate purpose of preventing or altering a particular disease state. Carriers or delivery vehicles for therapeutic genetic material are called vectors which are usually viral but several non-viral techniques are being used as well. The broad scope of gene therapy covers implantation of genetically engineered cells, repair of defective gene in situ, excision or replacement of the defective

gene by a normal gene and inhibition of gene expression by antisense oligodeoxynucleotides. Gene therapy has been described in detail in a textbook as well as a report on this topic (Jain 1998b; Jain 2008). Examples of some of the strategies that are under investigation to reduce cerebral infarction are:

- Transfer of glucose transporter gene to neurons/HSV vector.
- Adenovirus vector coding for $bFGF_{1–154}$ may be used to induce angiogenesis in vivo.
- Intracerebroventricular injection of antisense c-fos oligonucleotides.
- Intracerebro-ventricular injection of oligonucleotide antisense to NMDA-Ra receptor
- Intracerebro-ventricular injection of adenovirus vector carrying a human IL-2 receptor antagonist protein.
- Intraparenchymal injection of HSV-packaged amplicon vector expressing bcl-2.

Combination of approaches to management of stroke. In view of the multiple choices available for experimental therapies of stroke, some thought has been given to combination therapies. This has been done within the same category and also between compounds from different categories. Some examples of potential combinations are:

- Thrombolytics and neuroprotectives. The two therapies address different problems. Can be used simultaneously. Neuroprotectives may counteract reperfusion injury as a sequelae of thrombolysis.
- Thrombolytics and HBO. HBO may protect the brain against ischemia/hypoxia during the first hour until the patient can be transported and investigated to have thrombolytic therapy. Should improve the results in survivors. Also counteracts edema associated with stroke.

Management of the Chronic Post-Stroke Stage

In contrast to the tremendous efforts being made for the management of acute stroke, little is done for the patients in the chronic post-stroke stage. Most of the patients have been discharged to home at this stage and very few receive regular physical therapy. Physicians are seldom interested in these patients who are considered to have fixed neurological deficits due to irreversible brain damage. They come to the attention of physicians only because of neurological and systemic complications which sometimes require hospitalization and surgery. However, conventional and sometimes innovative efforts have been made in patients in the chronic post-stroke stage for the management of spasticity, for improvement of motor deficits and treatment of dementia.

Table 18.8
Currently Used Methods for the Management of Spasticity

1. Physical medicine:
   Physical modalities: heat, cold, vibration, electrical stimulation
   Physical therapy: use of proper splints, proper positioning of patient, spasm inhibiting exercises, slow and prolonged stretch
2. Drugs: dantrolene, baclofen, diazepam, phenytoin plus chlorpromazine
3. Surgery:
   Orthopedic: lengthening, sectioning, release and transposition oftendons
   Neurosurgical: intramuscular neurolysis and rhizotomy, spinal cord stimulation, intrathecal baclofen, tizanidine

Management of spasticity. Current methods for the management of spasticity are shown in Table 18.8. None of these methods is satisfactory in the long term: all the drugs have toxic effects. Physical therapy helps, but the effects are of short duration.

Strategies to facilitate motor recovery in the chronic post-stroke stage. The following measures have been used in an attempt to improve motor deficits:

- Drugs that may improve motor function
  ACH chlorohydrate
  Amphetamine
  Apomorphine
  Caffeine
  Carbaminol choline
  Fluoxetine
  GM$_1$ gangliosides
  Levodopa
  Neostigmine
  Norepinephrine
  Phenylpropanolamine
  Yohimbine
- Promotion of neural regeneration and enhancement of synaptic plasticity
- Surgical procedures
  Cerebral revascularization
  Neural transplantation

It is generally believed that there is a significant interaction between acetylcholine (ACh) and norepinephrine (NE) in the CNS. NE modulates the direct release of ACh from the cerebral cortex by way of alpha-1 receptors. This release is also mediated by gamma amino butyric acid (GABA). There are anatomical connections between the locus coeruleus (LC) located in the floor of the fourth ventricle and the cholinergic cells in the septum, hippocampus and cerebral cortex. The current hypothesis is that release of NE from LC is the integral factor in recovery of motor function after stroke.

Of all the drugs studied in animal models, amphetamine was most consistently reported to accelerate recovery of function. Amphetamine has a variety of effects primarily on the brain neurons releasing NE. Intraventricular infusions NE of mimic the effect of amphetamine whereas similar infusions of dopamine have no effect. In a rat model of cerebral infarction, amphetamine appears to promote alternate circuit activation – a pharmacological property that may be advantageous for recovery after stroke (Dietrich *et al* 1990). Evidence that amphetamine combined with physical therapy promotes recovery of motor function was provided by Crisostomo *et al* (1987) in a double-blind pilot study. Amphetamine has been reported to promote recovery of motor function in stroke patients but the objections to this approach are:

- Amphetamine aggravates rather than improves spasticity.
- Amphetamine is contraindicated in several conditions including hypertension, which is frequent in stroke patients.
- Amphetamine is habit-forming and has other undesirable side effects

The role of surgical procedures in the chronic post-stroke stage is described in Chapter 20.

Treatment of vascular dementia. It is important to establish the pathogenetic type of dementia before starting the treatment. Vascular dementia is potentially preventable and more responsive to treatment than degenerative dementias such as Alzheimer's disease. Effective and early treatment of risk factors for stroke is likely to prevent recurrent cerebral infarctions and progression of dementia. The main form of therapy is prevention, but several pharmacotherapeutic approaches are:

- Antiplatelet therapy
- Agents for improving hemorrheology
- Cerebral blood flow enhancers
- Nootropics (cerebral metabolic enhancers)
- Neuroprotectives
- Ergot derivatives

There is no hard evidence that any of these drugs can improve dementia significantly.

Role of HBO in the Management of Acute Stroke

Scientific Basis

The role of HBO in relieving ischemia and hypoxia has already been described in Chapter 17. These are the most important reasons for using HBO in cerebral ischemia. HBO also has an important role in improving the microcirculatory disturbances. Logistic problems in the use of HBO in the management of stroke have been reviewed (Jain & Toole 1998a).

The resistance to blood flow is greater in vessels in which the diameter is less than 1.5 mm, e.g., the capillaries. The viscous effect is less, because the red blood cells (RBC) are aligned in a column as they pass through the lumen (Fahraeus Lindqvist effect) instead of moving randomly. In microcirculatory disturbances, such as occur with clumping of RBC and slowing of circulation, the viscosity of the blood increases tremendously. RBC can get stuck where the endothelial cells protrude into the lumen of the capillary. The blood flow can become totally blocked for a fraction of a second or a longer period. Some plasma may, however, seep across the obstruction.

HBO has a beneficial effect in cerebral ischemia through the following mechanisms:

1. Oxygen dissolved in plasma under pressure raises pAO_2 and can nourish the tissues even in the absence of RBC (Boerema *et al* 1959).
2. Oxygen can diffuse extravascularly. Diffusion is facilitated by the gradient between the high oxygen tension in the patent capillaries and the low tension in the occluded ones. The effectiveness of this mechanism depends upon the abundance of capillaries in the tissues. Because the brain is a very vascular tissue, this mechanism can provide for the oxygenation of the tissues after vascular occlusion.
3. The supply of oxygen to the tissues can be facilitated by decreasing the viscosity of the blood and reducing platelet aggregation and increasing RBC deformability.
4. HBO relieves brain edema. By its vasoconstricting action, HBO counteracts the vasodilatation of the capillaries in the hypoxic tissues and reduces the extravasation of fluid.
5. HBO also reduces the swelling of the neurons by improving their metabolism.
6. HBO, by improving oxygenation of the penumbra that surrounds the area of total ischemia, prevents glycolysis and subsequent intracellular lactic acidosis and maintains cerebral metabolism in an otherwise compromised area.

HBO in Relation to Cerebral Ischemia and Free Radicals

Free radical generation and possible relation to hyperbaric oxygen has been discussed in Chapter 2. The role of free radicals in mediating oxygen toxicity has been discussed in Chapter 6. Free radical generation is increased during reperfusion following ischemia. This may result in damage to the myelin although neurons and axons are preserved by hyperoxic perfusion. Various free radical scavengers may be useful adjuncts to HBO therapy in acute stroke. In experimental studies, administration of HBO to rabbits after global ischemia showed no evidence of aggravation of the brain injury even though free radical production was increased.

Animal Experiments

Animal models of stroke. Investigation of pathophysiology and therapy of cerebral ischemia requires animal experimental models where effects of ischemia can be produced under controlled conditions. This goal is not easy to achieve because of the diversity of the scientific issues related to brain ischemia research that are relevant to therapy. Although larger animals (cats, dogs, and subhuman primates) have been used to study brain ischemia, rats are the most popular and desirable animals for this purpose. The important features are low cost, resemblance to the human brain vasculature, small brain size that is suited to whole brain fixation procedures, and their greater acceptability (for example, in comparison with subhuman primates). The last is an important point with the current trends in animal rights movement. Transgenic models of stroke are also available. One example is of nitric oxide synthase knockout mice that are more resistant to ischemic stroke. These models may be helpful for understanding the pathophysiology of ischemic stroke but are not relevant to HBO.

Models of focal ischemia are most relevant to human stroke and involve the occlusion of a selected artery. The methods used for occlusion vary. Middle cerebral artery occlusion in the rat is a standard model of experimental focal vascular ischemia and has gained increasing acceptance because of its predictive validity. It is used for studying the pathophysiology of stroke as well as for efficacy of neuroprotective agents. A convenient method to evaluate the therapeutic effect is the measurement of infarct volume by brain sectioning. Magnetic resonance imaging (MRI) has also been used in animal stroke models for *in vivo* evaluation of neuroprotective effects of various compounds in cerebral ischemia. Traditional T_2– weighted MRI has a very limited use in identifying ischemic issue destined for infarction because accurate measurements can only be made at time points of > 4 h. Diffusion-weighted (DW) MRI has enabled accurate assessment of early ischemic changes occurring within 30–40 minutes of temporary or permanent MCA occlusion in animals.

No animal model can mimic the human stroke and there are fallacies of testing neuroprotective compounds in animal models. Some of these results are difficult to translate into human clinical trials. One advantage, however, of these models is that a standard model can be used to compare various therapies. Stroke models may be quite appropriate for evaluating the effects of HBO in acute cerebral infarction.

Animal experimental evidence for the effect of HBO in ischemia/hypoxia is summarized in Table 18.9. These are mostly studies of focal cerebral ischemia. Experimental studies of global ischemia/hypoxia are described in Chapter 19. Smith *et al* (1961) carried out one of the earlier studies showing the protective effect of HBO against cerebral ischemia. In dogs made hypoxic by CO_2, inhalation of HBO at 2 ATA facilitated recovery. In another series of animals, the same authors observed the diameter of cortical vessels through burr holes. They noted no changes in arterial diameter whether the animals breathed room air or oxygen at 2 ATA, as long as the arterial pCO_2 was kept at 40 mmHg. Of the eight studies, only one failed to find any beneficial effect of HBO. Another seven studies, done on different animals and different time periods (1961 to 1987), have shown the beneficial effect of HBO in cerebral ischemia.

Breathing 100% oxygen at ambient pressures does not appear to have the same effect. In one study it has been shown to lead to a threefold increase in mortality in gerbils when administered 3 to 6 h after 15 min of ischemia induced by vascular occlusion (Mickel *et al* 1987). The explanation given was that oxygen-free radical toxicity aggravates the lipid peroxidation following ischemia. Apparently this aggravation does not occur with oxygen at 1.5 ATA. Oxygen toxicity may, however, occur at higher pressures and after prolonged application. Survival rates were 30% in control group vs. 70% in the group treated with HBO. Neurological recovery with slight disability was in 1 of 10 control animals vs. 6 out of 9 animals in the HBO-treated group.

Review of Clinical Studies

Most of the studies of HBO in acute stroke are uncontrolled. Only a few controlled studies have been done in recent years and further studies are planned. Considerable background information can be extracted from the uncontrolled studies reported in the literature.

Uncontrolled studies. Various studies on the clinical applications of HBO in cerebrovascular disease, as reported in the literature, are summarized in Table 18.10. The total number of cases reported in the literature is over 1000. The reported rate of improvement is 40% to 100% and is much higher than the natural rate of recovery, particularly because many of the reported cases were in a chronic post-stroke stage with stable neurological deficits. A major criticism of these studies is that none of them was a randomized controlled study. The report of Lebedev was labeled a controlled study but it did not meet the usual criteria of such studies; therefore, it is included among the uncontrolled studies.

Illingworth *et al* (1961) were the first to suggest that HBO could be beneficial in cerebrovascular disease. Ingvar and Lassen (1965) were the first to use HBO for treatment of patients with cerebral ischemia and proposed the following rationale:

a. An acute ischemic lesion implies a rapid fall to zero of the oxygen tension within the central part of the lesion.
b. There is little chance of reaching this anoxic part by any form of currently available therapy.
c. With HBO at 2–2.5 ATA, diffusion of oxygen into the nonvascularized part of the brain is enhanced.

The authors treated four patients, and three improved. The fourth, who died with extensive thrombotic lesions of the brain stem, showed dramatic initial improvement with recovery from coma. Although the authors obtained good results, the argument about the extravascular diffusion of oxygen is questionable. The maximum distance that oxygen may have to diffuse in the extravascular tissue from the capillary to the neuron is 0.1 mm. Even at 3 ATA of oxygen, this diffusion distance extends to only 0.075 mm.

Neubauer and End (1980) used HBO in 122 patients with strokes due to thrombosis in both the acute and the chronic stages. The patients were investigated thoroughly with EEG, CT scan, and CSF examination, as indicated. Generally, the patients with completed stroke had previously been given the conventional medical and physical therapy. HBO was given at 1.5–2 ATA, and the duration and frequency of treatments were adjusted according to current signs after improvement with initial HBO sessions. The duration of the sessions was as long as 1 h and the sessions were as frequent as every 12 h. Of 79 patients who received treatment, 5 months to 9 years after onset of stroke 65% reported improvement in the quality of life. It was also shown that patients treated with HBO spent fewer days in the hospital (standard treatment 287 days, versus HBO 177 days). The authors noted that using HBO in this way as a supplement to other methods of treatment makes appraisal of the role of HBO difficult. They could not identify the type of patient that would benefit most from HBO, but stated that a significant number of patients would benefit to some extent. They suggested randomized controlled studies. Neubauer has continued to treat stroke patients with HBO since his 1980 report; he has documented the effects using rCBF measurements (Neubauer 1983) and MRI, as well as SPECT (Neubauer 1988). HBO is used for stroke in clinical practice at the discretion of the treating physician. Prompt use of HBO in some situations can save considerable disability. An example is a case reported by Bohlega and McLean (1997) from Saudi Arabia. HBO was used in a young women who developed hemiplegia and seizures after accidental catheterization of the right common carotid artery and infusion of parenteral nutrition. Carotid angiography and

Table 18.9
Animal Experimental Studies Regarding the Effect of HBO in Cerebral Ischemia/Anoxia

Authors and year	Animal model	Technique of ischemia/anoxia	Treatment protocol	Measurements and results
Smith et al (1961)	Dogs	CO inhalation	HBO 2 ATA, 100% oxygen controls, no treatment	Neurological recovery facilitated; cortical vessel diameter, no change if CO_2 is 40 mmHg
Jacobson and Lawson (1963)	Dogs anesthetized	Middle cerebral artery clipping, transcranial	1. HBO 2 ATA 2. Controls, no clipping 3. Hypothermia + air 4. Hypothermia + HBO	Decreased CBF; less protection than hypothermia Decreased CBF with vasoconstriction Protective effect Protective effect same as in 3 (breathing air)
Moore et al (1966)	Dogs	Total circulatory arrest with hypothermia	HBO 3 ATA, 100% oxygen; controls room air	Extension of safe period of occlusion from 1–2 min under normothermia to 2–3 min with hypothermia
Whalen et al (1966)	Dogs	Induced cardiac fibrillation	HBO 3 ATA, 100% oxygen Controls, no treatment	Prolonged the period from fibrillation to cessation of EEG activity; cerebral protection
Corkill et al (1985)	Gerbils	Carotid ligation	HBO 1.5 to 2 ATA with 100% oxygen; controls air	Calorimetric videodensimetric estimation of cerebral ischemia through intact cranium; best results obtained in HBO groups
Shiokawa et al (1986)	Rats-spontaneous hypersensitive	Bilateral caratoid ligation	HBO 2 ATA, 100% oxygen; controls, room air	HBO prevented increase in cerebral lactate and prolonged survival time if started 3 h after ligation but no effect if started 1 h post ligation
Weinstein et al (1986)	Cats (awake)	Temporary occlusion of middle cerebral artery for 6 or 24 h (from previously implanted vessel occluder via transorbital approach)	HBO 1.5 ATA 100% oxygen for 40 min during or after 6 h occlusion and before, during, or after 24 h occlusion; controls room air	Neurological assessment, grade 0–10. Brain examined after cats killed on day 10 1. HBO during first 3 h of 6 h occlusion results in a 4 grade improvement which persisted during rest of the occlusion period. 2. Average grade of neurological deficit 94% less with HBO than in controls 3. Infarct size in HBO group was 58% less than in controls in 6 h group and 40% less in 24 h group
Burt et al (1987)	Gerbils	Right carotid ligation	HBO 1.5 ATA, 100% oxygen 1. 36 h with 5-min air breaks/hr treatment 2. 36 h with 1-h air break/h treatment 3. 18 h with 5-min air breaks/h treatment 4. controls; room air Unligated controls	Neurologic; brain staining with tetrazolium 1. Infarcts in 26% but all animals died within 24–36 h from oxygen toxicity 2. 44% had cerebral infarcts 3. 11% had infarcts during the first 18 h; no infarcts during the next 18 h 4. 72% had cerebral infarcts; no mortality when subjected to protocol 1
Kawamura et al (1990)	Rats	Middle cerebral artery occlusion for 4 h.	HBO at 2 ATA 100% oxygen for 30 min. Treatment given between 2.5–3.5 h following ischemic insult	HBO reduced ischemic neuronal injury and brain edema
Reitan et al (1990)	Gerbils	Unilateral carotid artery interruption	HBO at 2.5 ATA 100% oxygen for 2–4 h after occlusion. Controls: pentobarbital and superoxide dismutase	Increased survival in HBO-treated group
Yatsuzuka (1991)	dogs	Complete cerebral ischemia for 18 min.	HBO at 2 ATA for 170 min	CBF, EEG and indicators of oxidative stress. HBO reduced brain damage without increasing oxidative stress
Takahashi et al (1992)	Cats	Global ischemia induced by occlusion of ascending aorta and caval veins for 15 min.	HBO at 3 ATA 100% oxygen for 1 h at 3, 24, and 29 h after ischemia. Controls: room air	Survival rates were 30% in control group vs. 70% in group treated with HBO. Neurological recovery with slight disability was in 1 of 10 control animals vs. 6 out of 9 animals in the HBO-treated group.

Table 18.9 continued

Authors and year	Animal model	Technique of ischemia/anoxia	Treatment protocol	Measurements and results
Wada et al (1996)	Gerbils	Occlusion of both common carotid arteries under anesthesia	1 h to male Mongolian gerbils either for a single session or every other day for five sessions. Two days after HBO pretreatment, the gerbils were subjected to 5 min of forebrain ischemia.	Seven days after recirculation, neuronal density per 1-mm length of the CA1 sector in the hippocampus was significantly better preserved in the five-session HBO pretreatment group. Tolerance against ischemic neuronal damage was induced by repeated HBO pretreatment, which is thought to occur through the induction of HSP-72 synthesis.
Atochin et al (1998)	Rats	Reversible occlusion of one carotid artery. Cerebral reperfusion model.	Pretreatment with HBO at 2.8 ATA for 45 min and estimation of cerebral myeloperoxidase (MPO)	Cerebral MPO was elevated in both hemispheres of rats subjected to ischemia/reperfusion and this was prevented by pretreatment with HBO, indicating that HBO may be useful for ameliorating reperfusion injury.
Krakovsky et al (1998)	Rats	Acute global ischemia by four-vessel occlusion.	Two groups: (1) control animals that breathed air at atmospheric pressure and (2) rats exposed to oxygen at 3 ATA	Survival rate was significantly higher (45%) in the HBO group than in the control group (0%). Even among the animals that did not survive the 14-day period, those exposed to HBO survived longer than the control animals.
Roos et al (1998)	Rats	Middle cerebral artery occlusion	Group I received a single 30-minute HBO treatment at 2 ATA Group II received 30-minute HBO treatments at 2 ATA daily for 4 consecutive days.	Daily neurologic examinations and computerized quantal bioassay was used to determine the ET50 – the occlusion time required to cause a neurologic abnormality in half of the animals. HBO therapy showed no apparent benefit in a rat model as a treatment modality for acute cerebral ischemia with reperfusion.
Atochin et al (2000)	Rats	Reversible occlusion of the middle cerebral artery	HBO (2.8 ATA 100% oxygen for 45 m)	HBO reduced functional neurologic deficits and cerebral infarct volume by inhibiting neutrophil accumulation
Chang et al (2000)	Rats	Occlusion of the middle cerebral artery	HBO (3 ATA) 2 × 90 min at a 24-h intervals.	Also hyperbaric air at similar schedule.
Prass et al (2000)	SV129 or C57BL/6 mice	Focal cerebral ischemia induced 1 day after the 5th HBO session	HBO (3 ATA, 1 h daily/5 days), 100% oxygen	HBO can induce tolerance to focal cerebral ischemia, but this effect is strain dependent
Sunami et al 2000	Rats	Ligation of the right middle cerebral and right common carotid arteries	HBO (3 ATA) 2 h initiated 10 min after onset of ischemia	Reduced infarct volume by increasing oxygen supply to the ischemic periphery without aggravating lipid peroxidation
Veltkamp et al (2000)	Rats	Reversible occlusion of middle cerebral artery	HBO 1.5 or 2.5 ATA	Controls with 100% normobaric oxygen
Badr et al (2001a)	Freely moving rats	Middle cerebral artery occlusion. After 2 h of occlusion the suture was removed and reperfusion was allowed	HBO (3 ATA, 1 h), 100% oxygen	Neuroprotective effect as HBO normalized brain energy metabolites and excitatory amino acids disturbances that occur during cerebral ischemia
Yang et al (2002)	Rats	Focal cerebral ischemia was by occlusion of the middle cerebral artery	HBO (2.8 ATA 100% oxygen) during ischemia. Room air for control animals.	HBO offered significant neuroprotection. The mechanism seems to partly imply reduced level of dopamine
Hjelde et al (2002)	Wistar rats	Right middle cerebral occluded for 4 h	HBO (2 ATA, 100% oxygen for 230 min)	HBO did not reduce tissue damage
Yin et al (2002)	Rata	Transient middle cerebral artery occlusion with focal ischemia	HBO (3 ATA, 100% oxygen for 1 h) given 6 h after reperfusion	HBO within 6 h reduced infarction. There was inhibition of COX-2 over-expression in cerebral cortex accompanying the neuroprotective effect.

Table 18.9 continued

Authors and year	Animal model	Technique of ischemia/anoxia	Treatment protocol	Measurements and results
Qin et al (2007)	Rat	Middle cerebral artery occlusion	3 ATA for 1 h 30 min after	Reduction of hemorrhagic transformation
Hou et al (2007)	Rat	Middle cerebral artery occlusion with ischemia/reperfusion	NBO control HBO at 2 ATA	The infarct size after HBO was smaller than for NBO
Eschenfelder et al (2008)	Rat	Middle cerebral artery occlusion with ischemia/reperfusion	HBO at 1.5, 2,2.5 or 3 ATA for 1 h.	Reduction in infarct volume with HBO 2.5 and 3.0 ATA over 1 week
Sun et al (2008)	Rat	Filament-induced middle cerebral artery occlusion for 2 h.	HBO at 3 ATA for 95 min.	HBO improves penumbral oxygenation in focal ischemia. by modification of the hypoxia-inducible factor-1α

Table 18.10
Uncontrolled Studies of the Application of HBO in Cerebrovascular Disease

Authors and year	Diagnosis	No. of patients	HBO protocol	Method of evaluation and results
Ingevar and Lassen (1965)	Focal cerebral ischemia	4 single treatment	2 2.5 ATA 1.5 to 2.5 h	Improvement in 3 patients; clinical and EEG
Saltzman et al (1966)	Acute cerebrovascular insufficiency	25	2–3 ATA, 1 h; single session	8 improved dramatically; 5 improved during but regressed later; 12 did not improve
Hart and Thompson (1971)	Occlusion of right middle cerebral A.	1	2.5 ATA, 2 h/day; 15 treatments	Patient improved during 15 treatments but regressed during the following month; improvement recurred following resumption of HBO treatments
Sarno et al (1972)	Cerebrovascular disease, most of patients were aphasics; at least 3 months poststroke	32	2 ATA, 90 min; single session	Patients served as their own controls while breathing 10.5% oxygen (instead of 100%in the treated group); no improvement in aphasia
Charcornac et al (1975)	Cerebrovascular insufficiency	26	2.5 ATA, 1 h; single session	Clinical assessment and EEG; improvement in 20 patients
Larcan et al (1977)	Acute cerebral artery occlusion; both acute and chronic cases	36	2 ATA + urokinase	17 recovered and 18 died (52% compared with 77% deaths in those treated by intensive care alone)
Holbach and Wassman (1979)	Internal carotid and MCA occlusion; both acute and chronic cases	131	1. 5 ATA, 1 h/day	Clinical, neurological, and EEG power spectrum; improvement in 80% of acute and 43% of chronic cases
Knapp (1980)	Cerebral infarction	22	1.5 ATA, 40 min/day; 14 days	Clinical assessment, 10 patients improved during HBO, 9 had surgical revascularization, 6 of these maintained improvement; neurological deficits recurred in 3 patients with unsuccessful operations
Neubauer and End (1980)	Stroke; acute and chronic cases	122	1.5–2 ATA, 1 h/day 10 sessions acute, 20 sessions chronic	Total hospitalization stay of treated patients was 177 days (287 days in untreated patients); 65% of chronic patients (5 months to 9 years) improved
Newman and Manning (1980)	Vertebrobasilar occlusion (?air embolism); locked in syndrome	1	6 ATA for 1 h within 1 h of onset of stroke	Full recovery
Gismondi et al (1981)	Acute stroke	4	2 ATA	All patients improved
Isakov et al (1981a)	Ischemic stroke	140	1.6–2 ATA, 1 h/day; 6–15 sessions	Clinical, neurological, and cardiovascular assessment; rheoencephalography; 80% improved; in 52% improvement coincided with HBO treatment

Table 18.10 continued

Authors and year	Diagnosis	No. of patients	HBO protocol	Method of evaluation and results
Nagakawa et al (1982)	Occlusive CVD	22	2 ATA, 1 h/day; 12 treatments	Excellent recovery in 6, moderate in 7, slight in 6, and 3 patients were unchanged
Shalkevich (1982)	Vertebrobasilar insufficiency	54	2–3 ATA, 1 h/day; 10–15 sessions	Clinical, EEG, and vestibular testing; 47 patients improved
Lebedov et al (1983)	Acute occlusive CVD	124	2 ATA; duration?	Improved level of consciousness and alpha activity in HBO-treated patients as compared with controls
Akimov et al (1985)	Cerebrovascular disease	104	2 ATA 6 to 15 sessions	Clinical, electrophysiological, psychological, and biochemical assessment; 74 patients showed good results, 22 satisfactory, and in 8 the results were doubtful; 3–5 year follow-up
Ohta et al (1985)	CVD including infarction and hemorrhage	134	2 ATA	Overall improvement in 72% of patients; CBF decreased with decrease in intracranial pressure; EEG and SSEP improved
Jia et al (1986)	Cerebral thrombosis 1 month – 3 years after onset	104	2.5 ATA, two 40-min sessions per day, with 10 min air breaks per day; 30–50 treatments	Recovery in 33 patients (31.7%), marked improvement in 32 cases (30.8%), improvement in 35 cases (33.7%) and ineffective in 4 cases (3.8%); recovery coincided with HBO treatment
Kazantseva (1986)	Acute ischemic stroke	60	1.6–2 ATA; variable schedule	Clinico-polygraphic study: EEG, ECG, rheoencephalograpy, sphygmography of the temporal arteries, phlebography
Hao and Yu (1987)	Cerebral thrombosis (782) Cerebral embolism (16) TIA (31) Cerebral arteriosclerosis (149)	978	pressure and duration? 20–30 sessions	Improvement in 82.3% of cases
Sugiyama et al (1987)	Cerebral infarction 1–3 months after onset	142	2 ATA for 75 min; 20 daily sessions	Very good results in 15%, moderate improvement in 33%, and 20% showed no effect
Jain and Fischer (1988)	Hemiplegia; chronic post stroke	21	1.5 ATA, 45 min/day; 6 weeks	Neurological assessment during HBO treatments; measurement of handgrip with dynamometer; improvement of handgrip and spasticity in all patients during HBO and maintained by use of physical therapy and repeated treatments
Gusev et al (1990)	Acute stroke	220	1.2–1.3 ATA	Normalization of EEG, acid-base balance and decrease of raised free radicals by activation of lipid peroxidation

MRI showed evidence of arterial occlusion and ischemic infarction. HBO treatment at 2.5 ATA was instituted 6 h after this episode and the patient showed improved considerably within a few hours of the treatment. This was followed by daily HBO treatments for one week and she recovered with minimal residual neurological deficit. MRI showed considerable regression of the infarct.

Controlled clinical trials. Such trials are considered necessary because the value of HBO therapy in acute stroke remains controversial. Controlled trials will be required for proving the efficacy of HBO in acute stroke because it is difficult to prove that the recovery is due to treatment and not natural recovery. The other issue is demonstrating the safety of HBO in acute stroke patients. For a number of

logistical problems, it has not been easy to carry out clinical trials of HBO in acute stroke. There have been only three controlled trials reported at the time of writing (see Table 18.11) and others are in progress.

Anderson et al (1991) administered HBO in a double-blind prospective protocol to 39 patients with acute ischemic cerebral infarction. They aborted the study when no dramatic improvement was noted in the HBO treated patients. Rather, there was a trend favoring the control patients (treated with air only) who has less severe neurological deficits and smaller infarcts. This trend was considered to be an artifact of randomization process. The treatment protocol was broken in 19 of the 39 patients and 8 patients refused to continue treatment. The results of this trial neither prove or disprove the usefulness of HBO in acute

Table 18.11
Controlled Clinical Trials of the Application of HBO in Acute Ischemic Cerebral Infarction

Authors and year	No. of patients	Study design	HBO protocol	Results
Anderson *et al* (1991)	39	Double-blind prospective study. Patients treated within 2 w of onset.	HBO 1 h at 1.5 ATA repeated every 8 h for total of 15 treatments.	Same schedule of hyperbaric air in sham group. Study aborted as no dramatic improvement was noted in the HBO treated patients
Nighogossian *et al* (1995) reported the results of a air	34	Randomized: half of the patients received HBO, the other half were treated in hyperbaric air. Patients treated within 24 h of onset.	HBO 40 m at 1.5 ATA, daily for 10 treatments.	Control group received hyperbaric air. HBO was safe in these patients and there was an outcome trend favoring HBO therapy
Rusyniak *et al* 2003	33	Randomized, prospective, double-blind, sham-controlled study.	HBO 1 h at 2.5 ATA (100% O_2) or 1.14 ATA in the sham group.	No differences between the groups at 24 h. At 3 months sham patients had a better outcome as defined by their stroke scores
Vila *et al* (2005)	26	Randomized but not blinded	Daily 45 min exposures of HBO for 10 d or hyperbaric air in controls	Improvement of function in HBO treated patients
Imai *et al* (2006)	38	Randomized, prospective	HBO combined with intravenous edaravone (free radical scavenger)	6/19 patients in the HBO group, but 1/19 in the control group, had favorable outcomes

stroke and can be disregarded. They merely point out the difficulties in carrying out such trials.

Nighogossian *et al* (1995) reported the results of a randomized trial on 34 patients. These were enrolled over a period of three years. Half of these received HBO whereas the other half were treated in hyperbaric air. There was no significant difference at inclusion between the two groups regarding age, time from stroke onset to randomization, and Orgogozo scale. The mean score of the HBO group was better at one year but no statistically significant improvement was observed in the HBO group on the Rankin score. There authors concluded that HBO was safe in these patients and there was an outcome trend favoring HBO therapy. They recommended large scale controlled trials. In a recent review these authors suggested a large double-blind trial of HBO, possibly in combination with thrombolytic therapy (Nighogossian & Trouillas 1997).

Rusyniak *et al* (2003) conducted a randomized, prospective, double-blind, sham-controlled pilot study of 33 patients presenting with acute ischemic stroke who did not receive thrombolytics over a 24-month period. Patients were randomized to treatment for 60 min in a monoplace hyperbaric chamber pressurized with 100% O_2 to 2.5 ATA in the HBO group or 1.14 ATA in the sham group. Primary outcomes measured included percentage of patients with improvement at 24 h using NIHSS scale and 90 days (NIHSS, Barthel Index, modified Rankin Scale, Glasgow Outcome Scale). Secondary measurements included complications of treatment and mortality at 90 days. Results revealed no differences between the groups at 24 h. At 3 months, however, a larger percentage of the sham patients had a good outcome defined by their stroke scores compared with the HBO group (NIHSS, 80%

versus 31.3%; P = 0.04; Barthel Index, 81.8% versus 50%; P = 0.12; modified Rankin Scale, 81.8% versus 31.3%; P = 0.02; Glasgow Outcome Scale, 90.9% versus 37.5%; P = 0.01) with loss of statistical significance in a intent-to-treat analysis. It was concluded that HBO does not appear to be beneficial and in fact may be harmful in patients with acute ischemic stroke. The design of this study, however, invalidates any conclusions because HBO at 1.5 ATA has been established to be a safe pressure to treat patients with acute stroke. The control group was closer to this parameter. This study should have included a group treated with HBO at 1.5 ATA (Jain 2003h).

HBO dose is adjusted either by changing the pressure or the duration of exposure and number of treatments. was found on the dose/effect of HBOT in patients with AIS. Rogatsky *et al* (2003) have analyzed retrospectively the published data of clinical studies performed in different hyperbaric centers (a total of 265 patients). The total dose of HBO therapy (D_{HBOT}) was calculated as follows:

$$D_{HBOT} = pO_2 \times Ts \times Nt,$$

where pO_2 is measured as ATA, Ts is the duration of a single treatment and Nt is the number of treatments.

This method was used to analyze the HBO dose-effect relationship in patients with acute ischemic stroke. D_{HBOT} can be easily understood and analyzed when measured within a limit of 50 units defined as unit medical dose (UMD) of HBO therapy. Efficacy of HBO (Ef_{HBOT}) represents the percentage of the total number of patients who showed significant clinical improvement of their neurologic status in the course of the treatment. The level of Ef_{HBOT} in each study was compared with a corresponding value of D_{HBOT}. A comparison of the data shows a pronounced tendency for higher values of Ef_{HBOT} as the level of the average values of the total D_{HBOT} increases. The coefficient of correlation between these parameters appears to be fairly high ($r = 0.92$). The maximum possible value of Ef_{HBOT} is 100%, which corresponded to the average values of D_{HBOT} at a level of no less than 30 agreed units. The examined data suggest that applying optimal total D_{HBOT} may provide a maximum possible Ef_{HBOT} in treating patients with acute ischemic stroke.

HBO as a Supplement to Rehabilitation of Stroke Patients

The objective neurological improvement in chronic poststroke patients undergoing HBO therapy was first documented by Jain in 1987 (Jain & Fisher 1988) and a long-term follow-up was presented (Jain 1989a). This was also the first documentation of relief of spasticity due to stroke by HBO. Wassmann (1980) has reported the power spectrum of the EEG recording during an HBO session and the improvement of this parameter in responders. The neurological assessment of his patients was not done until after the HBO session. The transient neurological improvement of these patients, which might have occurred in the chamber and reversed afterwards, may have been overlooked. Under these circumstances the allocation of a patient to the "nonresponder" group may not be justified.

The study conducted by Jain at the Fachklinik Klausenbach in Germany was aimed at assessing the effect of HBO on motor deficits in strokes objectively, using a simple repeatable method that could be applied in the hyperbaric chamber. The protocol was such that it did not interfere with the application of two other methods – mental training and physical exercise – used in the hyperbaric chambers, which have been found to be useful adjuncts in previous studies.

Fifty patients with occlusive cerebrovascular and residual hemiparesis or hemiplegia were investigated during the period December 1987–May 1989. There was no selection of patients as the HBO therapy has become a standard procedure in the rehabilitation of stroke patients in the Fachklinik Klausenbach. Only those patients were included in this study who were available to the author for examination prior to HBO treatment, during the sessions in the chamber, and subsequently. Data on other patients treated during the author's absence were available but not included in this study. Neurological and functional assessment was done on admission and at discharge, but the most constantly measured parameter was the handgrip, using a handheld dynamometer, which recorded pressures up to 1 kg or more. Motor power and spas-

Table 18.12
Grading of Motor Power of Hemiplegic Hand

Grade 0: No movement
1: Flicker of finger movement
2: Measurable handgrip: 1 to 5 kg
3: Measurable handgrip: 5 to 15 kg
4: Handgrip 15 kg but less than that of the healthy hand
5: Full strength with normal movements

Table 18.13
Grading of Spasticity in the Hemiplegic Hand

Grade 0: Normal tone and movements
1: Stiffness of fingers, slow finger tapping
2: Partially closed fist, minimal force required to open it
3: Partially closed fist, moderate force required to open it
4: Fully closed fist, can be partially opened with moderate force
5: Clenched fist, can be partially opened with extreme force

ticity of the hand were graded clinically according to the scales shown in Tables 18.12 and 18.13. The duration of stay of the patients was limited to 6 weeks by hospital rules. During the first week following admission, the patient underwent investigative procedures and assessment, and received the standard medical treatment and physical therapy. The visit to the hyperbaric chamber was limited to familiarization and a session of breathing 100% normobaric oxygen. Dynamometer readings during this week and during a visit to the hyperbaric chamber were used as baseline values. Repeated measurements made with a handheld dynamometer on the paralyzed side are considered to be reliable.

Daily HBO sessions were started during the second week. Each session lasted 45 min (10 min compression plus 30 min at 1.5 ATA plus 5 min decompression). Handgrip and spasticity were measured every 5 min during the stay in the chamber. In the first eight patients, physical therapy was initially given immediately following the HBO session. When it was observed that a trial session of physical therapy in the chamber prolonged the relief from spasticity, physical therapy was routinely given in the chamber during the HBO session.

Most of the patients were transferred to the Fachklinik Klausenbach from acute care facilities for stroke, including university hospitals. Those where surgery was indicated had been operated on. The shortest period of time from the stroke episode to the admission was 3 weeks and the longest 5 years. Most of the patients were in a chronic poststroke stable condition with no day-to-day neurological changes during the first week of admission to the hospital.

Results

The overall results of this study are summarized in Table 18.14, and the effect on spasticity is shown in Table 18.15. The course of one patient at various phases before, during, and after HBO treatments is shown with regard to motor power and spasticity (Figure 18.7). An example of the effect of HBO on spasticity of the hand is shown in Figure 18.8. The near normal posture of the hand after HBO demonstrates the effectiveness of HBO in spasticity. The overall improvement of mobility and gait was shown by videotapes before and after HBO.

At one-year follow-up, patients continued to maintain the improvement noted at the time of discharge without any further HBO treatments. There were no complications resulting from this treatment. Other patients treated by a similar protocol by other clinic staff members during this period showed a response to HBO by an increase of handgrip power in all cases. Those with aphasia and cognitive deficits also improved during this period.

Discussion

All of the fifty patients in this series showed response to HBO by improvement of neurological status. The degree of improvement varied according to the extent of neurological deficit at onset and the interval between the onset of stroke and the institution of HBO therapy. The most marked improvement was in those patients where the treatment was started earlier, the neurological deficits were less severe, and the spasticity was minimal. Twenty-one of the patients had significant spasticity between grades 2–5 (on a scale of 1–5). In all these, the spasticity was reduced during HBO sessions by 1 to 2 grades. This improvement was transient initially and started to regress during 1 to 8 h following HBO treatment. However, the beneficial effect of HBO on spasticity was prolonged by conducting physical therapy exercises against spasticity in the chamber during HBO.

The treatment has a cumulative effect, as shown in Figure 18.9. However, as the "ceiling" of improvement is reached, the peaks of improvement with each session become smaller. After a patient has reached the peak, further HBO treatments are superfluous.

Conclusions

1. All patients with neurological deficits due to occlusive cerebrovascular disease showed a response to HBO at 1.5 ATA by measurable increases of power of handgrip on the paralyzed side.
2. The response to HBO was initially transient but reproducible with sessions repeated daily. After 6 weeks, the improvement was maintained in most of the patients.
3. The peaks of response to HBO got smaller as the plateau of maximum improvement was reached. When there was no further measurable response to HBO, the treatments were terminated.
4. The benefit from HBO was limited by the size of the penumbra and the total neuronal damage done during the insult.
5. The spasticity was reduced during the HBO session and improvement maintained for longer periods if physical therapy was carried out simultaneously.
6. Some of the improvement in motor power was due to relief of spasticity, but considerable improvement was also noted in patients without spasticity.
7. Patients who respond to HBO therapy and are considered candidates for the EC/IC bypass operation may improve with long-term HBO therapy and may not require surgery. HBO, by improving oxygenation, may be more effective than an EC/IC bypass operation.
8. HBO therapy should be instituted early in the management of stroke. In our series, those treated within 3 months of the initial episode did not develop spasticity. Since the number of these patients is small, a larger number of patients should be treated with HBO in the first week following stroke, to test the hypothesis that early HBO therapy may prevent the development of spasticity.

Table 18.14
Long Term Results of Treatment of Stroke Patients with Combined HBO & Physical Therapy

Neurological dysfunction	No. with dysfunction	No. improved
Impairment of mental function	35	30 (86%)
Impairment of gait	24	10 (41%)
Motor power impairment (paralysis)	50	50 (100%)
Spasticity	21	21 (100%)
Speech impairment	8	2 (25%)

Total number of patients 50. Some had more than one deficit.

Table 18.15
Effect of HBO on Grades of Hand Spasticity in Stroke in 21 Patients

Pre-HBO	No.	During HBO	After 6 weeks of HBO	At 6 months to 1 year
5	1	4	4	4
	1	2	3	3
4	4	2	3	3
	2	3	3	3
3	6	1	1	1
	3	2	2	2
2	4	1	1	1

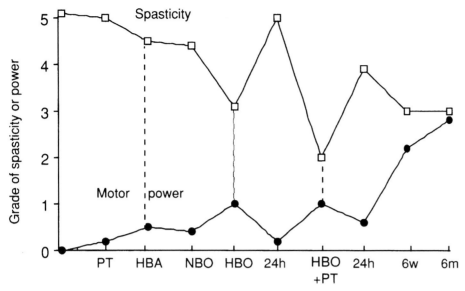

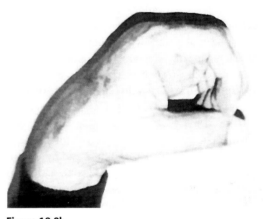

Figure 18.7
Course of spasticity and motor power of the paralyzed left hand of a patient with right middle cerebral artery occlusion. Initial spasticity was grade 5 and motor power 0. At 6 mo follow-up, the spasticity was reduced to grade 3 and the motor power rose to grade 3. **Broken lines** indicate measurements made in the hyperbaric chamber. **PT,** physical therapy; **HBA,** hyperbaric air at 1.5 ATA for 45 min; **NBO,** 100% normobaric oxygen by face mask for 45 min; **HBO,** hyperbaric oxygen (100%) at 1.5 ATA for 45 min. (From Jain KK (1989) Effect of hyperbaric oxygenation on spasticity in stroke patients. *J Hyperbaric Med* 4: 55–61).

Figure 18.8a
Posture of the left hand before HBO (grade 5).

Figure 18.8b
Posture of the hand after HBO therapy alone (grade 3).

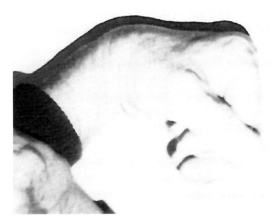

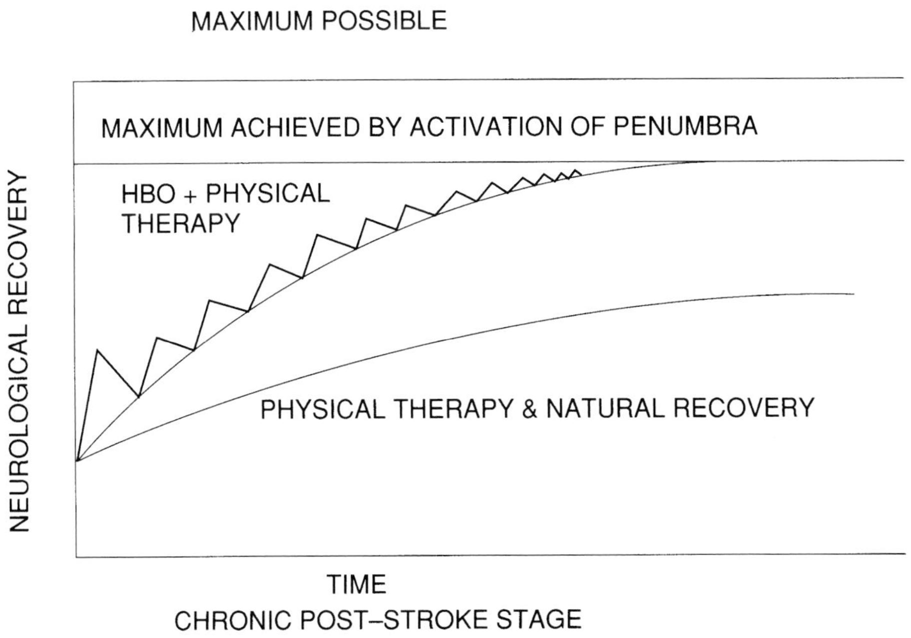

Figure 18.9
Pattern of recovery of stroke patients treated by combination of HBO therapy and physical therapy.

9. Hyperbaric oxygen therapy at 1.5 ATA is safe and well tolerated by stroke patients. So far we have no evidence that higher pressures would extend the improvement in patients who have reached a "ceiling" effect with 1.5 ATA.

10. In view of the 100% response rate and the limitation of length of stay of our patients, we cannot justify a randomized controlled study where one-half of the patients would not receive HBO. Longitudinal studies, however, are in progress, to compare simultaneous HBO and physical therapy with the two treatments given separately.

11. Response to HBO is not necessarily seen during the first session. A few treatments may be required for the initial improvement to be demonstrated.

12. Fixed neurological deficits persisting for years after stroke are no contraindication of HBO therapy. Neubauer and End (1980) and Holbach et al (1977) have shown response to HBO in these cases. We have shown response in a case 5 years after stroke and fixed neurological deficits.

13. If a patient is seen at a stage where there are no potentially viable neurons or if the maximum possible recovery has taken place through other methods of treatment, no response to HBO would be expected. Since the start of the present study, we have not yet encountered such a patient.

14. Effort was made to control the risk factors for stroke in these patients, such as obesity, smoking, and hyperlipidemia. Those with high hematocrit had venesection for lowering the hematocrit. All these measures were already in effect at the time of admission or were instituted during the first week. These measures may contribute to the overall improvement of the patients and the lack of any recurrence of stroke during the period of observation. The role of HBO only in the prevention of stroke recurrence remains to be determined by properly designed studies and longer follow-up.

15. Although natural recovery may still occur in the chronic poststroke stage, in no case treated by any other method did the recovery of motor function take place so dramatically as it did during HBO therapy.

16. HBO is superior to the currently used methods for the control of spasticity, the duration of the effect is longer, and no side effects have been encountered.

17. A hyperbaric chamber with 100% oxygen at 1.5 ATA is the ideal place to combine physical therapy with mental training and should be included in the routine management of stroke patients. Under HBO conditions, physical exercise improves cerebral blood perfusion and oxygenation. This leads to improved mental performance.

Conclusions

Modern concepts of the pathophysiology of stroke provide a rational basis for using HBO in stroke management. Conventional methods of stroke management are not satisfactory and the role of many surgical procedures for stroke remains controversial. Animal experimental studies and uncontrolled human trials have shown the effectiveness and safety of HBO therapy after stroke. At the Fachklinik Klausenbach (FRG) simultaneous HBO and physical therapies were used in the rehabilitation of stroke patients. Objective evaluation of patients during the HBO session showed a 100% response rate (improvement of spasticity or motor power or both). The improvement was initially transient but could be maintained, following a course of daily treatments (1.5 ATA for 45 min) for 6 weeks, in most of the cases. The most significant finding was the striking reduction of spasticity under HBO conditions and the prolongation of this benefit if physical therapy was combined with HBO therapy and repeated daily. The mechanism of relief of spasticity has not been demonstrated conclusively. At present the most likely explanation is that it is related to improvement of function of the neurons in the affected areas of the brain. Rise of tissue pO_2 in the spastic, inactive, and hypoxic muscles affected by spasticity seems to play a secondary role.

The response to HBO has been considered a criterion for selecting patients for the EC/IC bypass operation (see Chapter 20). There are some patients in the chronic poststroke stage who can be managed by the long-term combination of physical therapy and HBO without the need for an operation. HBO does not change the vascular pathology, but improves the cerebral function by activation of the partially affected neurons in the penumbra zone that survive the insult due to a trickle of blood supply by collaterals. The hypothesis that long-term alterations of hypoxia/ischemia with hyperoxia may promote collateral circulation remains to be proven.

Objective measurement of spasticity and motor power as well as the SPECT scan have provided the evidence for the improvement following HBO therapy in post-stroke patients with fixed neurological deficits. With the evidence available, it may not be necessary to carry out randomized double-blind studies in such patients to evaluate the effect of HBO therapy.

However, the role of HBO in acute stroke is not well-defined. Because recovery spontaneously takes place in this stage, controlled studies should be done to assess the effect of HBO. The three controlled clinical trials completed to date have not been encouraging, and the methodology needs to be improved. Two important issues are the time window and pressure at which the treatments should be conducted. As HBO is used for neuroprotective effect in acute stroke, it should be ideally used within the 3-h window and not over 6 h following the initial insult. Use of

HBO as an aid to rehabilitation in the subacute and chronic phase is safe because some of the initial biochemical disturbances following initial insult are stabilized by that time. There is animal experimental evidence that use of HBO in the acute stage after the 6 h time window may be harmful. In one study of use of HBO in rat middle cerebral artery occlusion model, the percentage of infarcted area increased significantly in animals treated 12 h and 23 h following arterial occlusion as compared to the beneficial effect of HBO within 6 h after the occlusion (Badr *et al* 2001b). The results of this study suggest that applying HBO within 6 h of ischemia-reperfusion injury could benefit the patient but that applying HBO 12 h or more after injury could harm the patient.

HBO at or below a pressure of 2 ATA was used in the majority of over 2000 stroke patients that have been treated in published studies. Pressure of 1.5 ATA is optimal for recovery of the cerebral ischemic injury. Higher pressures used in animal studies cannot be transposed into humans.

Rehabilitation of stroke patients should also be planned during the first few months following stroke. Long-term follow-up studies are required to determine whether such measures would reduce the chronic disability from stroke and reduce the incidence of severe spasticity in stroke patients. The use of HBO may also reduce the need for some surgical procedures.

There has been an ongoing study of HBO for cerebral ischemia, and a review of the current publications supports further investigation of this therapy for stroke (Al-Waili *et al* 2005). The failure of some clinical trials of HBO in stroke is probably attributable to factors such as delayed time to therapy, inadequate sample size, and use of excessive chamber pressures (Singhal 2007). Previous trials did not assess long-term benefit in patients with tissue reperfusion. In this modern era of stroke thrombolysis and advanced neuroimaging, HBO may have renewed significance. If applied within the first few hours after stroke onset or in patients with imaging evidence of salvageable brain tissue, HBO could be used to lengthen the window for the administration of thrombolytic or neuroprotective drugs.

19 HBO Therapy in Global Cerebral Ischemia/Anoxia and Coma

Paul G. Harch and Richard A. Neubauer[†]

Hyperbaric oxygen therapy has been used in a number of conditions characterized by global ischemia (as opposed to focal ischemia of stroke), and anoxia, and leading to impairment of consciousness. Conditions such as coma due to brain injury and anoxia associated with drowning and hanging are discussed under the following headings:

Introduction

For a discussion of the effectiveness of hyperbaric oxygen (HBO) therapy in global cerebral ischemia/anoxia and coma, we define HBO as a medical treatment that uses high pressure oxygen as a drug by fully enclosing a person or animal in a pressure vessel and then adjusting the dose of the drug to treat pathophysiologic processes of the diseases. Like all drugs, the dose of HBO is crucial and should be customized to each patient's response. It is dictated by the pathological target and is determined by the pressure of oxygen, duration of exposure, frequency, total number of treatments, and timing of the dose in the course of the disease. As diseases and their pathologies evolve, different doses of HBO are required at different times. In addition, patients have individual susceptibility to drugs, manifest side-effects and toxicity. Unfortunately, the ideal dose of HBO in acute or chronic global ischemia/anoxia and coma is unknown. The studies reviewed below suggest higher pressures (2 ATA or higher) and lesser numbers of treatments very early in the disease process whereas lower pressures (2 ATA or lower) and a greater number of treatments have been used as the brain injury matures. While this general trend seems justified, the absolute or effective pressures delivered to the patients in these reports may be slightly less than what is stated since many studies do not specify the HBO delivery system that was employed. For example, an oxygen pressurized chamber has an effective HBO pressure equal to the plateau pressure administered during the treatment, whereas an air pressurized chamber in which oxygen is administered by aviators mask can achieve a far lower effective HBO pressure, depending on the fit of the mask and the amount of its air/oxygen leak. In the later cases, the dose of oxygen is less. This concept is particularly important when analyzing the studies in this chapter performed prior to the late 1980s when the aviator mask dominated delivery systems in multiplace chambers.

In reviewing the data in this chapter, it is surprising that HBO has not enjoyed widespread use for neurological diseases in the United States. This has been partly due to institutional reservations and overt therapeutic nihilism for neurological injuries, both of which are presently waning. To assume that HBO could have efficacy and benefit when liberally applied to various "accepted" indications, yet have none in the great majority of neurological conditions is perplexing. After all, the brain is enclosed within the same body in the same pressure vessel and is exposed to the same elevated oxygen pressure. To justify this distinction, one would have to postulate that an entire set of pathophysiological processes of brain that are insensitive to HBO and distinct from those in the rest of the body's organ systems which are sensitive to HBO and to which we routinely apply HBO. This is illogical and unlikely. Such reasoning is indefensible when one considers the "accepted" neurolog-

ical indications include carbon monoxide poisoning, brain decompression sickness, cerebral air embolism, brain abscess, and cyanide poisoning. We conclude that HBO should benefit other hypoxic/ischemic conditions of the brain, provided the dose is correct, i.e., target specific.

Other reasons for nonrecognition of HBO in neurological conditions concern methodologies. The standard for proof in scientific medicine has been the randomized prospective controlled double-blinded clinical trial. While some of the studies in this chapter meet this rigor (except for double-blinding), many do not. Some are randomized, prospective, and controlled and thus exceed the quality of studies used to sanction reimbursement for some HBO indications. Other studies are uncontrolled series, case-controlled, or individual cases. All of this clinical data, in conjunction with the animal data, makes a strong case for at least attempting HBO in what are otherwise untreatable conditions with debilitating, tragic, and expensive outcomes, especially when the visual medium is used to prove single-case causality (Kiene & von Schön-Angerer 1998; Harch 1996). In addition, case-controlled series with chronic neurological maladies make powerful statements of efficacy from the statistical (Glantz 1992) and logical perspectives where the counterargument of placebo effect is minimized (Kienle & Kiene 1996). If these considerations are kept in mind when analyzing this chapter, it appears that the bulk of data is solidly in favor of a beneficial effect of HBO in global ischemia/anoxia and coma.

Pathophysiology

The effect of global ischemia/hypoxia on the brain has been discussed in Chapter 5. Oxidation of glucose is the primary energy source for the brain. Deprivation of oxygen causes deep psychological unresponsiveness in 8 s while glucose and energy stores take a few minutes to exhaust (Plum & Pulsinelli 1992). Global deprivation of oxygen delivery can be achieved by reduction in blood flow (ischemia), oxygen (hypoxia/anoxia), or both (hypoxic or anoxic ischemia). Unfortunately, clinical syndromes and animal models are rarely pure and often result from combinations or sequences and varying degrees and durations of hypoxia/anoxia and ischemia. Since the insult, oxygen deprivation, is similar whether by lowered blood flow or oxygen content the two are often considered as a single type of insult and this concept will be followed in this chapter.

Global ischemia/anoxia is a severe transient insult to the brain that causes a stereotypic pathophysiology characterized by reperfusion hyperemia followed by progressive ischemia which is often heterogeneous (Safar 1986; Dirnagl 1993). The extent of injury is governed by a complex interplay of patterns of systemic and local respiratory and circulatory function and selective vulnerability of cells (Meyers 1979). The result is both immediate and delayed cell death (Cormio *et al* 1997). The deterioration of blood flow and late cell death occur in the absence of microvascular disruption by formed blood elements unless the global ischemia is prolonged (Dirnagl 1993) in which case both cellular and noncellular mechanisms may be responsible. The mechanisms of eventual neuronal energy failure are poorly understood (Siesjö *et al* 1995, Katsura *et al* 1995).

Coma, on the other hand, is a neurological state resulting from a wide variety of cerebral insults that is caused by diffuse disruption (functional or anatomical) of the bilateral cerebral cortices, proximal brainstem (reticular activating system), or both (Rossor 1993). Coma is characterized by an alteration in the level of awakeness, ranges from mild somnolence to deep coma, and is graded on a number of scales, the best known of which is the Glasgow Coma Scale (Teasdale & Jennett 1974). In the studies reviewed below, coma usually refers to the more severe end of the continuum: unresponsiveness, posturing, and neurovegetative signs, however, a number of studies are unclear about the exact level of coma.

Rational Basis of HBO Therapy

HBO in acute global ischemia/anoxia is complicated by a lack of knowledge of the exact pathological targets and their oxygen sensitivity. It has been postulated that postischemic hypoperfusion may be a neurogenic reflex (Dirnagl 1993) and/or characterized by a block in the transduction of physiologic stimuli and hence protein synthesis (Siesjö 1981). Assuming short-lived (minutes) global ischemia/anoxia and cell death independent of the microcirculation (Dirnagl 1993), positive effects of HBO under these conditions must be due to effects on hypoxia, cellular energy metabolism, ion homeostasis, membrane integrity, gene induction, and/or a plethora of as yet unidentified targets. The dramatic effect of even one HBO exposure on recovery of brain function, as indicated in many of the studies below, implies a powerful on/off drug effect that simultaneously quenches a degradative process and energizes the cell. It is easy to envision HBO acting at some or multiple points of blockade in the above mentioned reflex or at a physiologic impasse. However, in the past 5 years the site of action of HBO is increasingly pointing to genes and gene products (see below). In the chronic state, a similar action of a single HBO on some of these targets may be responsible for the awakening of idling neurons (Neubauer *et al* 1990), and when delivered repetitively considered a signal transducer (Siddiqui 1995). The signal transduction mechanism is inferred in multiple noncerebral HBO wound models where trophic tissue changes result from repetitive HBO (HBO Committee Report 2003), measured molecularly in two studies (Wu *et al* 1995, Buras *et al* 2000),

suggested in a replicated chronic traumatic brain injury rat model (Harch & Kriedt 2007), and reaffirmed in a controlled human trial of HBO in chronic traumatic brain injury directed by Harch in Texas (Barrett *et al* 1998). In the rat model repetitive 1.5 ATA/90 min HBOT induced increased blood vessel density and cognitive function in injured hippocampus. This finding likely underpins much of the trophic effect of HBOT in chronic brain injury and represents the first ever improvement of chronic brain injury in animals. Future studies should be focused on elucidating the molecular effects of HBO in this model and in global cerebral ischemia/anoxia.

With prolongation of global ischemia/anoxia or the recovery phase of reperfusion pre-therapeutic intervention the microcirculation is disturbed (Dirnagl 1993) and the pathophysiology begins to resemble that in acute traumatic brain injury (Cormio *et al* 1997): lipid peroxidation, edema, arterial spasm, cellular reperfusion injury, and anaerobic metabolism in the setting of penumbral lesions (Cormio *et al* 1997). HBO has been shown to have positive effects on all of these: ischemic penumbra (Neubauer *et al* 1990; Neubauer *et al* 1998; Barrett *et al* 1998), cerebral edema (Sukoff *et al* 1982), arterial spasm (Kohshi *et al* 1993, Kawamura 1988), anaerobic metabolism (Holbach 1977d), and peroxidation/cellular reperfusion injury (Thom 1993a). This last HBO sensitive pathophysiological target is most exciting since it seems to be a generic ischemic model-, species-, and organ-independent HBO effect (Harch 2000). In a carbon monoxide rat model Thom (1993b) showed a powerful inhibitory action of HBO on white blood cell mediated brain lipid peroxidation when delivered 24 hours before the poisoning or 45 min after removal from carbon monoxide. Zamboni *et al* (1993) demonstrated a similar finding in a four hour global ischemic rat gracilis muscle model, using intravital microscopy. Follow-up work by Khiabani *et al* (2001) identified a plasma mediator(s) of this phenomenon. This HBO inhibition of WBCs is inferred in brain decompression sickness and cerebral air embolism (Harch 1996) when one combines the Dutka *et al* (1989), Helps & Gorman (1991) and Martin (2001) data, which implicates WBCs in the pathogenesis of these disorders, with Thalmann's (1990) review which shows a 90% single treatment cure rate in decompression sickness when hyperbaric recompression is delivered within the first 1–2 h of injury. Similarly, the data of Bulkley & Hutchins (1977) and Engler *et al* (1986) that document a WBC-mediated pathogenesis in cardiac reperfusion injury, in conjunction with the Thomas *et al* (1990) tissue plasminogen activator/HBO/acute myocardial infarction dog model and the congruent human study of Shandling *et al* (1997) strongly suggest an HBO directed action on cellular reperfusion injury, among other effects. Lastly, the recent Rosenthal paper (2003) demonstrates a positive effect on the microcirculation similar to the findings of Zamboni *et al* (1993). All of the above actions of HBO on the pathophysiology in acute traumatic brain injury should sum to provide a beneficial effect. In fact, such is the case as a review of the studies in Table 19.2 shows a convincing argument for the use of HBO in acute severe traumatic brain injury. Similarly, if global ischemia/anoxia is prolonged or incomplete, e.g., unsuccessful hanging, microcirculatory disturbances are incomplete. Under these circumstances, HBO-induced inhibition of cellular reperfusion injury may partly explain the very positive results of the studies listed in Tables 19.1 and 19.2.

For HBO to be effective in coma it must be directed at diffuse targets in the bilateral hemispheric gray and white matter, the brainstem, or both. Acutely, regardless of the nature of the targets, e.g., microcirculatory, nonvascular, cellular, or other, HBO can conceivably act equally effectively on the hemispheres, brainstem, or both. As the pathology progresses to anatomic damage and eventually to penumbral lesions, a significant HBO effect on hemispheric coma is very unlikely because of the large tissue volumes and low ratios of umbra to penumbra. Smaller tissue volumes are favored such that brainstem coma would be expected to have better results. This is suggested by the positive HBO data in the large traumatic mid-brain report of Holbach (1974b), the brainstem contusion subgroup of Artru (1976), the GCS 4-6 group of Rockswold (1992), and the coma patients of Heyman et al (1966) and Neubauer (1985a). In all of these clinical trials, a recovery of just a few millimeters of reticular activating system can translate into far-reaching effects in the hemispheres, e.g., awakening. Additional work will be necessary to confirm this hypothesis.

In chronic global ischemia/anoxia and coma the pathological targets become more speculative. The ischemic penumbra (Astrup et al 1981) argument of Neubauer and Gottlieb (1990) and sympathetic hibernating myocardium concept of Swift et al (1992) remain, but given the numbers of treatments reported below the element of time enters the equation and implies a trophic effect. This effect, which could include stimulation of axon sprouting, or possibly an alteration or redirection of blood flow as suggested above (Harch 2007), or both, may be indiscriminately effective on the final common pathway of a variety of brain injuries similar to HBOT's generic effect on reperfusion injury (Harch 2000). Given the diversity of reports (Neubauer et al 1998; Harch 1994a,b,c; Harch 1996; Keim et al 1997; Myers 1995a) and the multitude of studies listed below this maybe so. Regardless of the nature of this generic effect, in the past 22 years (PGH) and 38 years (RAN) these authors have noted a upward sawtooth response (Chapter 18 Stroke, Figures 18.7 and 18.9) during HBOT in sub-acute and chronic brain injury with a partial regression once each round of HBOT ends. This implies permanent and transient components to the treatment (see Chapter 44 Neuroimaging). While the net HBO result appears uniform, the biochemical, molecular, cellular, and anatomic complexities of the transient, permanent, and final effects will need to be developed in the future.

Review of Animal Experimental Studies

A review of the studies listed in Table 19.1 leads to the conclusion that HBO is unequivocally beneficial in acute global ischemia/anoxia regardless of treating pressure, frequency, duration, or number of treatments, but may be sensitive to time to onset of HBO post insult. Since the first publication of this chapter in the third edition of the Textbook in 1999, the data has been fortified with each successive edition of the text. Thirty-one of thirty-three studies gave positive results, one study did not show any benefit, and the last study used normobaric oxygen. In the complete ischemia models, Moody et al (1970) showed a nearly 50% reduction in mortality without the benefit of artificial ventilation using a prolonged 2 ATA exposure (four hours). Mrsic-Pelcic (2004a) performed two metabolic studies assessing delay to HBOT as long as 168 h and found that HBOT at 2 ATA could prevent decline of ATPase and increase SOD in hippocampus if initiated as late as 24 h and 168 h, respectively. When they looked at the optic nerve (Mrsic-Pelcic (2004b), however, HBO was effective with ATPase only if begun within 6h of ischemia and had no effect on SOD regardless of time of initiation. Clinical parameters were not measured in either study, but it appears that optic nerve is more sensitive to complete global ischemia. Kapp (1982) measured EEG recovery time and CSF lactate change, demonstrating significant improvement with a lower pressure, 1.5 ATA, for a prolonged 2.5 hours. Ruiz et al (1986) was the sole insignificant result with a 2 ATA/1 hour exposure, but this lack of efficacy may be partially explained by hemodilution with hetastarch prior to HBO. Yatsuzuka (1991) generated a significant decrease in ICP and oxidative stress metabolites with a 2 ATA/170 min staged protocol.

Using higher pressures, Takahashi et al (1992), Iwatsuki et al (1994), Krakovsky et al (1998), and Zhou (2003) at 3 ATA, Mink and Dutka (1995a,b) at 2.8 ATA, and Rosenthal et al (2003) at 2.7 ATA obtained statistically significant positive results on survival, neurological recovery, and various physiological or metabolic measures. In the Rosenthal experiment survival improved with increased oxygen extraction ratio but without a change in oxygen delivery or cerebral metabolic rate for oxygen, suggesting an improvement of the microcirculation similar to the Zamboni et al (1993) HBO/peripheral global ischemia reperfusion model in rats. The Zhou experiment underscored the more permanent trophic effects of early HBO by showing a persistent elevation of Ng-R and RhoA, which are both associated with the inhibition of growth cone collapse, i.e., improvement of growth. Despite the tissue slice model of the

Table 19.1
Hyperbaric Oxygen Therapy in Global Ischemia, Anoxia, and Coma – Animal Studies

Authors and year	Model	Animal species	Length of ischemia/ anoxia	Initiation of HBO	HBO protocol	Results and conclusions
Moody et al 1970	Temporary complete global ischemia/anoxia using bilateral extradural balloons	50 dogs (20 controls)	Flattening of EEG for 3 min plus spontaneously rising intracranial pressure to equal systolic blood pressure. Evaluation after 10 days.	Immediately after balloon deflation	Group 1: Controls 1 ATA air, spontaneous respiration Group 2: 1 ATA O_2/4 h on a ventilator Group 3: 1 ATA O_2/4 h, spontaneous respiration, no ventilator Group 4: 2 ATA O_2/4 h, spontaneous respiration, no vent.	Group 1: 95% mortality within 30 h after ischemia Group 2: 30% mortality Group 3: 70% mortality within 72–96 h after ischemia Group 4: 50% mortality within 72–96 h after ischemia Quality of survivors was poor in Group 2 and good in Groups 3 and 4.
Kapp 1982	Temporary complete global ischemia/anoxia. Total circulatory arrest with occlusion of aorta, superior vena cava, and inferior vena cava	10 cats	5 min	3–5 min after ischemia release	Group 1: 5 controls, 1 ATA O_2/2.5 h Group 2: 5 HBO, 1.5 ATA O_2/2.5 h	Beneficial effect of HBOT with significant reduction in EEG recovery time and CSF lactate change.
Ruiz 1986	Temporary complete global ischemia/anoxia. Ventricular fibrillation and no ventilation for 12 min then cardiac resuscitation. Evaluate survival times, cardiac function, and neurological scoring 7 days post arrest.	16 dogs	12 min	Approximately 13 min after end of arrest (resuscitation within 6 min + 7 min of hemodilution)	Group 1: Controls No treatment Group 2: Normovolemic hemodilution with hetastarch/$MgSO_4$ to hematocrit of 20–30% Group 3: Group 2: plus 2 ATA O_2/1 h	No significant difference in survival, cardiac function, or neurological scoring between control and HBO. Decreased hematocrit due to hemodilution felt to possibly be detrimental.
Shiokawa et al 1986	Permanent incomplete global ischemia/anoxia. Bilateral carotid artery ligation. Measure survival times and lactate/ATP.	60 Spontaneously hypertensive rats	1.5 or 3.5 h for survival experiment, 2.5 or 4.5 h for metabolic studies	At 1 h or 3 h post ligation	Group 1: (Survival) a. 1 ATA air/1.5 h b. 1 ATA air/3.5 h c. 2 ATA O_2/30 min at 1 h post ligation d. 2 ATA O_2/30 min at 3 h post ligation Group 2: (Metabolic) Same as for survival experiment but assays at 2.5 (a. and c.) and 4.5 h (b. and d.) of ligation	All HBOT animals survived at least 1.5 or 3.5 h. Control animals that died in less than these times were excluded from analysis. Animals with HBOT at 3 h survived significantly longer than controls with significantly less lactate accumulation. Trend toward more ATP accumulation in HBO Group D.
Weinstein et al 1986	Temporary incomplete global ischemia/anoxia. Permanent unilateral carotid occlusion. Temporary opposite carotid artery occlusion for 2, 5, 10, 20, or 60 min. Autopsy studies. Separate DMSO experiment.	30 gerbils	2, 5, 10, 20, or 60 min	After 20 min of temporary occlusion.	Group 1: Controls at 2, 5, 10, 20, or 60 min with bilateral carotid artery occlusion. Group 2: HBO 1.5 ATA/15 min after 20 min of occlusion. Group 3: Intra-peritoneal DMSO at 5 or 10 min of bilateral occlusion. Group 4: Controls-surgery without carotid occlusion	Mortality: Group 1: 2 min 0%, 5 min 33%, 10 min 33%, 20 min 100%, 60 min 100% Group 2: HBO 16% (p < .001) Extent of damage much less in HBO survivors. Group 3: DMSO 86% mortality each.
Van Meter et al 1988	Temporary complete global ischemia/cardiac arrest. Measured return of cardiac function by EKG and thermodilution cardiac output.	Guinea pig	15 min	Immediately after 15-min arrest period	Group 1: Control. 1, 2.8 or 6 ATA air/maximum 30 min Group 2: HBOT at 1, 2.8, or 6 ATA oxygen/30 min maximum	Maximum initial post resuscitation survival at 2.8 ATA O_2 > 6 ATA air or 6 ATA O_2, maximum mean post resuscitation survival time with 6 ATA O_2 > 2.8 ATA O_2 > 1 ATA O_2 > 6 ATA air.
Mickel 1990	Temporary incomplete global ischemia. Bilateral carotid artery occlusion. Histological evaluation at death or up to 28 day limit.	60 gerbils	15 min	None	Group 1: 1 ATA O_2/first 3 h of reperfusion. Group 2: 1 ATA air for 3 h of reperfusion	In the oxygen group: (1) Increased myelin damage, but better preservation of axons. (2) Better preservation of neurons in the deeper laminae of the cerebral cortex (3) Increased mortality.

Table 19.1 continued

Authors and year	Model	Animal species	Length of ischemia/ anoxia	Initiation of HBO	HBO protocol	Results and conclusions
Yatsuzuka 1991	Temporary complete global ischemia. Cross clamp of ascending aorta. Measure intracranial pressure, cerebral blood flow, EEG, and oxidative stress (metabolites) before, during, and after HBO	34 dogs	18 min	60 min post ischemic release	Group 1: Ischemic controls Group 2: HBOT without global ischemia Group 3: HBO 2 ATA/170 min	Significant decrease in intracranial pressure and oxidative stress metabolites in HBOT
Grigoryeva et al 1992	Permanent incomplete global ischemia. Bilateral carotid artery occlusion. Survival and histology measurements of cortical neurons	Approximately 60 rats	24 h	2 h after occlusion	Group 1: HBOT 2 ATA/1 h Group 2: Air 2 ATA/1 h Group 3: HBOT 1.2 ATA/30 min Group 4: Controls, sham, operation, sacrifice at 2.5 h Group 5: Controls, operation, air treatment, sacrifice at 2.5 h	At 24 h: Group 1: 30% survival with 25–30% sparing of neurons Group 2: 50% spared neurons (did not mark mortality) Group 3: 50% survival with 50–60% sparing of neurons Group 4: Used for baseline histologic studies Group 5: 100% mortality, when allowed to proceed to 24 h Pronounced protective effect in HBO groups with preservation of transcription and increased survival; 1.2 ATA was superior to 2 ATA.
Takahashi et al 1992	Temporary complete global ischemia/anoxia. Occlusion of the ascending aorta and caval veins. EEG and neurological recovery scores measured over a period of 14 days post ischemia	19 dogs	15 min	3, 24, and 29 h after release of ischemia	Group 1: 3 ATA O_2/1 h at 3, 24, and 29 h Group 2: Controls air 1 ATA	Survival: 30% in control group 78% in hyperbaric group with significantly greater EEG and neurological recovery scores.
Iwatsuki et al 1994	Temporary complete global ischemia. Same model as Takahashi's study.	19 dogs	15 min	3, 24, and 29 h after release of ischemia	Group 1: nicardipine bolus immediately at the end of ischemia then nicardipine drip × 3 days plus HBOT – 3 ATA/1 h at 3, 24, and 29 h after ischemia Group 2: no nicardipine or HBOT	Survival rate and time, neurological recovery, and EEG scores all significantly better in HBOT/nicardipine group.
Mink 1995a	Temporary complete global ischemia. CSF infusions to subarachnoid space to increase intracranial pressure to mean arterial pressure. Measure cortical somatosensory evoked potentials and oxyradical brain damage.	18 rabbits	10 min	Immediately on reperfusion.	Group 1: 1 ATA air for 75 min Group 2: 2.8 ATA O_2/75 min with air breaks	HBOT significantly increased evoked potentials and free radical generation but lipid peroxidation was unchanged.
Mink 1995b	Same model as above	22 rabbits	10 min	30 min after the end of ischemia. On room air during the 30 min	Group 1: 2.8 ATA O_2/125 min with air breaks then 1 ATA O_2/90 min Group 2: Control 1 ATA O_2/215 min	HBO significantly reduced brain vascular permeability and blood flow while somatosensory evoked potentials were unchanged.
Yaxi et al 1995	Temporary incomplete global ischemia. Temporary clamping of bilateral common carotid arteries (CCA) plus (?) internal jugular veins. Histochemical analysis of LDH, isocitratedehydrogenase:(ICDH), cytochrome a_3, ATPase, and cAMP. Also pathological study of tissue.	52 rabbits	20 min	(?) Immediately after release of clamp	Group 1: Control. Room air × 20, 40, or 120 min Group 2: (HBA- hyperbaric air): 8.4% O_2 at 2.5 ATA/20, 40, or 120 min Group 3: HBOT at 2.5 ATA (by "mask")/20, 40, or 120 min. Tissue analysis immediately post hyperbaric treatment.	Improvement in LDH, ICDH, cytochrome a_3, and ATPase levels in 40 and 120-min HBO groups with concomitant reduced tissue injury on pathological examination.

Table 19.1 continued

Authors and year	Model	Animal species	Length of ischemia/ anoxia	Initiation of HBO	HBO protocol	Results and conclusions
Yiqun *et al* 1995	Temporary incomplete global cerebral ischemia. Bilateral common carotid artery (CCA) clamping. Measured Na, K-ATPase activity in groups 1, 2, 3, 4, and 5 and histologic and electron microscope analysis in groups 1, 2, and 4.	98 gerbils	60 min	(?) Immediately after treatment	Group 1: Control. Skin incision only. Group 2: Control CCA clamping plus 80-min. room air exposure. Group 3: CCA clamping plus 1 ATA O_2/80 min Group 4: CCA clamping plus 2.5 ATA O_2/80 min Group 5: CCA clamping plus 2.5 ATA air/80 min Group 6: CCA clamping plus immediate sacrifice.	Significant decrease ATPase activity in all groups except group 4 HBO. Least pathological changes in same group.
Kondo *et al* 1996	Temporary incomplete global ischemia/anoxia. Bilateral common carotid artery ligation. Histological exam of hippocampal neurons 3 weeks post op and histochemical examination of heat shock proteins 36 h post op	47 gerbils	10 min	2, 6, or 24 h post op.	Group 1: 6 h post ischemia: 2 ATA O_2/60 min tid × 7 days, then qd × 14. Group 2: 24 h post ischemia: 2 ATA O_2/60 min 1 × day/14 days. Group 3: surgery, no HBO Group 4: 2 ATA O_2/60 min 1 × day for 14 days. No surgery Group 5: No HBO, no surgery. Sacrifice at 36 h: Group 6: Surgery, single HBO 2 ATA/60 at 2 h post op Group 7: Surgery, single HBO at 2 ATA/60 min 24 h post op Group 8: Surgery, no HBO	Preservation of hippocampal neurons in HBO animals (6 h animals > than 24 h animals) with less heat shock protein induction in HBO animals than controls. Increase in lysozomes and myelinoid structures in hippocampal neurons in HBO group. HBO prevented delayed neuronal death without oxygen toxity.
Wada *et al* 1996	Temporary incomplete global ischemia/anoxia, bilateral common carotid artery occlusion. Evaluate neuronal density 7 days post ischemia and heat shock protein production in the hippocampus	49 gerbils	5 min (2 days after last HBOT)	Pre ischemia	Group 1: 2 ATA O_2/1 h × 1 treatment Group 2: 2 ATA O_2/1 h every other day × 5 treatments Group 3: Sham operation, no HBO Group 4: Surgery, no HBO Group 5: Groups 1, 2, and 3 without ischemia; measurement of heat shock proteins	Significant preservation of neurons in the 5 HBO pre treatment group with significant increase in heat shock protein production. Repetitive HBOT protects against ischemia neuronal damage possibly through heat shock protein induction.
Krakovsky *et al* 1998	Temporary complete global ischemia (cauterization of bilateral vertebral arteries then temporary occlusion of the bilateral common carotid arteries). Measure brain blood flow by direct laser/Doppler flowmetry and 14-day survival.	18 rats	60 min	"Brief delay to transfer to HBO chamber".	Group 1: Control. Room air Group 2: HBOT: 3 ATA/1 h	Significantly increased survival in HBO (45%) versus controls (0%). In < 14-day survival, significant increase in survival time with HBO (59.8 h) versus controls (17.9 h).
Van Meter *et al* 1999	Temporary complete global ischemia/cardiac arrest. Measure initial return of circulation with BP > 90/50 and sustained circulation for 2 h.	36 swine	25 min	Immediately after the 25-min arrest period	Group 1: Control. 1 ATA O_2/maximum 30 min Group 2: 2 ATA O_2/maximum 30 min Group 3: 4 ATA O_2/maximum 30 min	Initial return of circulation and sustained returnf circulation at 2 h only present in group 3; 4 ATA HBOT groups at 80% and 67%, respectively. All animals in all other groups failed to be resuscitated.

Table 19.1 continued

Authors and year	Model	Animal species	Length of ischemia/ anoxia	Initiation of HBO	HBO protocol	Results and conclusions
Hai 2002	Temporary incomplete global ischemia/hypoxia. (?) Right common carotid artery, internal carotid artery, and external carotid artery ligation (?) then 5.5% oxygen environment (same model as Calvert 2002 study). Measure brain fibroblastic growth factor (bFGF) and bFGF mRNA after ten-day treatment period.	44 rats (< 7 days old)	2 h	7 days	Group 1: Control Room air for 10 days Group 2: HBOT 2.5 ATA/90 min qd × 10 Group 3: HBA (hyperbaric air) 2.5 ATA/90 min qd × 10 ("concentrations oxygen controlled under 25%") Group 4: "Untreated". "Free growing × 10 days" Group 5: Sham operation	Increased bFGF levels in HBA and HBO groups, especially in precortex and hippocampus. Increased bFGF mRNA only in HBO group.
Van Meter *et al* 2001a	Temporary complete global ischemia/cardiac arrest. Measure initial return of circulation with BP > 90/50 and sustained circulation for 2 h. Measure malondialdehyde.	36 swine	25 min	Immediately after the 25-min arrest period	Group 1: Control. 1 ATA O_2/maximum 30 min Group 2: 2 ATA O_2/maximum 30 min Group 3: 4 ATA O_2/maximum 30 min	Significant reduction in brain lipid peroxidation in 4 ATA HBOT group only.
Van Meter *et al* 2001b	Temporary complete global ischemia/cardiac arrest. Measure initial return of circulation with BP > 90/50 and sustained circulation for 2 h. Measure myeloperoxidase content.	36 swine	25 min	Immediately after the 25-min arrest period	Group 1: Control. 1 ATA O_2/maximum 30 min Group 2: 2 ATA O_2/maximum 30 min Group 3: 4 ATA O_2/maximum 30 min	No effect of any treatment group on myeloperoxidase content. Implies the target of ischemia reperfusion injury reduction with HBOT in this model is not leukocytes.
Calvert *et al* 2002	Temporary incomplete global ischemia. Right common carotid artery ligation then 8% oxygen exposure. Measure brain weights and examine with light microscopy and electron microscopy at 24, 48, and 72 h., and 1, 2, and 6 weeks, and perform sensory motor functional test 5 weeks post hypoxia.	229 rats (7 days old)	2½ h of hypoxia post 2 h carotid ligation	1 h after hypoxia	Group 1: Control Group 2: Ischemia/ hypoxia plus room air recovery Group 3: HBOT 3 ATA/60 min	Significant preservation of brain weight in the right hemisphere of HBO rats at 2 and 6 weeks with less atrophy and apoptosis on light and electron microscopy. Sensory motor function also significantly improved at 5 weeks in HBO group.
Rosenthal *et al* 2003	Temporary complete global ischemia (cardiac arrest/resuscitation). Measure neurological deficit score 23 h after resuscitation, sacrifice at 24 h and measure apoptosis in hippocampus and cerebral neocortex, arterial and sagittal sinus oxygenation and cerebral blood flow(CBF), cerebral oxygen extraction ratio(ERc), oxygen delivery(DO_2c), and metabolic rate for oxygen($CMRO_2$) at baseline, 2, 30, 60, 120, 180, 240, 300, and 360 min after restoration of spontaneous circulation.	20 dogs	1 h	1 h	Group 1: Control Room air resuscitation Group 2: HBO 2.7 ATA/60 min	Improvement in neurological deficit score in HBO group with significantly fewer dying neurons. Magnitude of neuronal injury correlated with the neuro deficit score. HBO decreased the oxygen extraction ratio without a change in oxygen delivery or $CMRO_2$.
Zhou *et al* 2003	Temporary complete global ischemia. Bilateral carotid occlusion. Measure Nogo-A, Ng-R, and RhoA proteins at 6, 12, 24, 48, 96 h, and 7 d.	78 rats	10 min	1 h after ischemia	3ATA/2 h. Thirteen groups: 1 sham, 6 global ischemia, 6 global ischemia + HBO	HBO significantly reduced neurological injury (neuronal loss) and the levels of Nogo-A, Ng-R, and RhoA in injured cortex

Table 19.1 continued

Authors and year	Model	Animal species	Length of ischemia/ anoxia	Initiation of HBO	HBO protocol	Results and conclusions
Mrsic-Pelcic et al 2004a	Temporary complete global ischemia (vertebral cautery + transient bilateral carotid occlusion). Measure hippocampal SOD or Na,K ATPase.	84 rats	20 min	2, 24, 48, or 168 h after ischemia (for SOD), or .5, 1, 2, 6, 24, 48, 72, or 168 h after ischemia (for ATPase)	2 ATA/1 h daily for 7d.	HBO significantly increased hippocampal SOD only when delayed 168 h and prevented ATPase decline only if begun during 1st 24 h of reperfusion.
Mrsic-Pelcic et al 2004b	Temporary complete global ischemia (vertebral cautery + transient bilateral carotid occlusion). Measure optic nerve SOD or Na,K ATPase	84 rats	20 min	2, 24, 48, or 168 h after ischemia (for SOD), or .5, 1, 2, 6, 24, 48, 72, or 168 h after ischemia (for ATPase)	2 ATA/1 h daily for 7 d.	HBO prevented ATPase decline in the optic nerve only if begun during 1st 6 h of reperfusion and no effect on SOD regardless of time of initiation.
Gunther 2004	Complete global ischemia (brain slices post decapitation). Measure purine nucleotide content and morphological changes	Rat(s)	5 or 30 min	After 5 or 30 min of anoxia	2.5 ATA/1 h, 1ATA/1 h, 2.5 ATA air/1 h, or 1 ATA air/1 h	HBO and NBO equally effective at 5 min Less so after 30 mins hypoxia while only HBO lessened morphological cell injury.
Li Y et al 2005	Temporary incomplete global ischemia (bilateral common carotid occlusion + hypotension to 30–35 mm Hg). Measure HIF-1 alpha, p53, caspase-9, 3, & 8, bcl-2 and cell death at 6, 12, 24, 48, 96 h, and 7d.	78 rats	10 min	1 h after ischemia	3 ATA/2 h Thirteen groups: 1 sham, 6 global ischemia, 6 global ischemia + HBO	HBO reduced HIF-1 alpha, p53, caspase 9 and 3, and apoptosis, yet increased proapoptotic caspase 8 and decreased antiapoptotic bcl-2.
Calvert 2005	Temporary incomplete global ischemia (unilateral carotid ligation + 8% oxygen exposure). Measure ATP, creatine, phosphocreatine, glucose at 4 and 24 h. Brain weight at 2 weeks.	7 d old rat pups	2h	1 h after ischemia	3 ATA/2 h or 1 ATA/2 h	Significant reduction of brain injury and increase in ATP, cr, Pcr over controls with HBO and NBO.
Yu 2006	Temporary incomplete global ischemia (unilateral carotid ligation + 8% oxygen exposure). Measure neural stem cells and myelin in hippocampus at 3 weeks.	7d old rat pups	2 h	1 h after ischemia	2 ATA/? Oxygen or air daily x 7 d	HBO increased hippocampal stem cells and nestin expression. Both HBO and hyperbaric air mitigated myelin damage.
Liu, X-h (2006)	"Hypoxic-ischemic brain damage". Article in Chinese, model not described in English abstract. Measure hippocampal and cortical cell density at 48 h and neurobehavioral testing at 5 and 6 weeks.	7 d old rat pups (n = 84)	1 h	1, 3, 6, 12, or 24 h after ischemia	2.5 ATA/1.5 h at 1, 3, 6, 12, or 24 h	Neuronal density, sensorimotor, grip test, and treadmill were significantly increased over controls when HBO was delivered up to 6 h after ischemia.
Liu, M-N (2006)	Temporary incomplete global ischemia (unilateral common carotid ligation + hypoxia). Measure spatial learning/memory 37 and 41d and morphology 42d after ischemia.	7 d old rat pups (n = 52)	2 h	.5–1 h after ischemia, daily x 2 d	2 ATA/?	HBO significantly improved spatial learning/memory and alleviated morphological and histological damage

Table 19.1 continued

Authors and year	Model	Animal species	Length of ischemia/ anoxia	Initiation of HBO	HBO protocol	Results and conclusions
Calvert (2006)	Temporary incomplete global ischemia (unilateral carotid ligation + 8% oxygen exposure). Measure HIF-1 alpha, glucose transporter, LDH, aldolase, and p53	7 d old rat pups	2 h	1 h after ischemia	2.5 ATA or 1 ATA oxygen	HBOT > NBOT significantly reduced elevated HIF-1 alpha, promoted a transient increase in glucose transporter, LDH, Ald, and decreased HIF-1 alpha-p53 interaction and expression of p53.
Yang (2008)	Temporary incomplete global ischemia (unilateral carotid ligation + 8% oxygen exposure). Measure hippocampal stem cells at 7 and 14 d and nestin 6h-14d, myelin basic protein and pathological changes at 28d.	7 d old rat pups	2 h	Within 3 after ischemia	2 ATA/? daily x 7 d	HBOT caused proliferation of stem cells which peaked at 7 d and migrated to the cerebral cortex at 14 d. New neurons, oligodendrocytes, and myelin basic protein was seen in the HBO group at 28 d.

Table 19.2
Hyperbaric Oxygen Therapy in Global Ischemia, Anoxia, and Coma – Human Studies

Authors and year	Diagnosis	No. of patients	Length of coma/ neuro insult pre-hyperbaric oxygen therapy (HBOT)	Timing of HBOT	HBOT protocol	Results and conclusions
Category I: Hyper Acute Period (0–3 h post cerebral injury)						
Hutchison et al 1963	Global ischemia/anoxia. Asphyxiated neonates (apnea). No in chamber ventilator support available.	65	3–38 min	3–38 min	2–4 ATA/30 × 1, 14 patients treated more than 1	79% resuscitation rate (25% died later of other causes). Overall, 55% discharged from hospital as well. Most deaths due to Hyaline membrane disease or stillborn.
Ingvar & Lassen 1965	Coma: Progressive thrombotic CVA of the brainstem. Patient was pre-terminal.	1	Not mentioned	At signs of failing circulation	2.0– 2.5 ATA ... for 1.5– 2.5 h	Rapid awakening in chamber with increase in blood pressure and decrease in heart rate. Death shortly after the end of 1 HBOT.
Saltzman et al 1965	Various forms of cerebral ischemia. Some in coma but only 5 of 25 is level of consciousness specifically identified.	25 (2 patients in coma in hyperacute or acute coma, 23 patients a few hours to 30 days after CVA)	1. 5 hours 61-year-old patient with stupor and hemiplegia, suspected embolic clot. 2. 2.5 hours 58-year-old with deep coma and hemoplegia, suspected air embolism	1. 5 hours 2. 2.5 hours	1. 2.02 ATA/> 1 hour, 1 treatment 2. 2.36 ATA/5 hours, 1 treatment	First patient dramatic awakening 5 min into HBO with improvement of hemiplegia. Discharged from hospital with mild residual deficit. Second patient dramatic awakening 10 min into HBO with improvement of hemiplegia. Discharged from hospital with only partial paralysis of the right leg. Remainder of patients probably described in Heyman study: 3 patients dramatic temporary improvement, 8 patients less dramatic temporary improvement, 12 patients no change during HBOT. 24 of 25 patients with only 1 treatment. One patient with 3 treatments.

Table 19.2 continued

Authors and year	Diagnosis	No. of patients	Length of coma/ neuro insult pre-hyperbaric oxygen therapy (HBOT)	Timing of HBOT	HBOT protocol	Results and conclusions
Viart *et al* 1969	Hepatic coma infants (2 viral, 1 toxic); HBOT plus exchange transfusions.	3	Not mentioned	Not mentioned	Not mentioned, but extreme profile implied	One died of pulmonary oxygen toxicity with 36 h of HBOT, two survived. All three with normalization of consciousness, EEG, and neurological examination, (One transient, two permanent). Cardiac conduction abnormalities during HBO in the two survivors? difficult to assess the effect of HBO; authors feel high complication rate of HBOT makes exchange transfusion standard of care.
Hayakawa *et al* 1971	Acute coma: 9 TBI, 4 post-op brain tumor. 7 patients ventilator dependent. Measure CSF pressure pre, during, and post-one HBOT.	13	Acute post-trauma and immediately post-op. Exact time not mentioned	Acute post-trauma and immediately post-op. Exact time not mentioned.	2 ATA/1 h × 1	Three patterns of response: (1) 9 patients: CSF pressure decreased at beginning of HBOT and rose at end of HBOT. (2) 2 patients: CSF pressure decreased with HBO and remained significantly lower at end of HBOT. (3) 2 patients: no change in CSF pressure. Conclusion: HBOT has two actions, decreases edema in injured brain and produces edema in normal brain. If HBOT produced significant change in CSF pressure, clinical improvement was remarkable and neurological deficit was mild. If no change CSF pressure with HBOT, severe brain damage and little clinical improvement.
Voisin 1973	Global ischemia/anoxia/coma: Near-hanging	35 (33 by suicide attempt)	14 controls with normobaric oxygen (NBO) prior to installation of HBO chamber in 1968	(2/3 of cases: < 3 h from discovery to hospitalization	Exact timing not stated	(1) HBO 2 ATA/1 h × 1 or more Rxs. Total 51 Rxs in 35 patients (2) Control: NBO
Larcan *et al* 1977	Coma: Thrombotic CVA (HBOT + Urokinase)	77 (36 in varying degrees of coma, 10/36 in severe coma)	Only reported for urokinase/HBO group 16 patients < 24 h 20 patients > 24 h Only 1 patient treated in less than 3 h	Only reported for urokinase/HBO group 16 patients < 24 h 20 patients > 24 h	2.0 ATA/60–90 BID: 5 groups: (1) standard medical treatment (2) HBOT (3) HBOT + urokinase + heparin (4) HBOT + urokinase + plasma or heparin (5) HBOT + heparin	1 patient (< 2 hrs) had excellent outcome. All 10 patients with profound coma (Grades III and IV) died. HBO treatment alone ineffective. Very complicated article – difficult to assess group assignment, time to initiation of treatment, etc. Incomplete data. Conclusion: Urokinase plus HBO did the best, especially coma Grades I, II, and III, and the best results were in those patients treated in less than 6h.
Baiborodov 1981	(1) Newborns with birth asphyxia (2) Syndrome of respiratory disturbance (3) Aspiratory syndrome	1555 2165 3110	> 15 min or > 1030 min	1–5 min after artificial pulmonary ventilation (APV) or 1030 min after APV	HBOT 23 ATA/1.52 h for 10–15 min and 1.41.5 ATA/1.5–2.5 h	HBOT decreased cerebral circulatory disorders by 4 times and/or mortality by 8 times.

Table 19.2 continued

Authors and year	Diagnosis	No. of patients	Length of coma/ neuro insult pre-hyperbaric oxygen therapy (HBOT)	Timing of HBOT	HBOT protocol	Results and conclusions
Mathieu *et al* 1987	Global ischemia/anoxia: Post-hanging suicide attempt. 88% in coma or brain dead.	170 (136 HBO 34 NBO) HBO only for patients with impaired consciousness. NBO patients with minor neurological problems.	81% < 3 h 19% > 3 h	81% < 3 h 19% > 3 h	(1) 2.5 ATA/90 Q6H with NBO intervening until normal. (2) Controls NBO	Worse coma requires more HBO. Recovery without neurological sequelae significantly better when HBO initiated < 3 h post-hanging (85 vs. 56%).
Kohshi *et al* 1993	Subarachnoid hemorrhage, status post aneurysm surgery. Grade III and IV coma. Measure infarct incidence and Glasgow Outcome Scale on all, SPECT and EEG on some.	43	Soon after onset of symptomatic	vasospasm; exact time not	mentioned	Soon after onset of symptomatic vasospasm; exact time not mentioned. (1) Control: mild hypertensive hypervolemia (2) HBOT 2.5 ATA/70 QD to BID, 2–21 treatments, avg. 10.
Shn-Rong 1995	Coma (95 cerebral ischemia/hypoxia: 23 near drownings, 44 near hangings, 2 electrocution, 14 narco-operation accidents, 1 Stokes-Adams, 4 barbital poisoning, 2 asphyxia, 5 Cover-Bedding syndrome; 56 of 95 with cardiac arrest). Moderate acute CO poisoning 156; serious acute CO 70 (up to 3 months coma); 12 hydrogen sulfide (2 h–20 days), 3 TBI (10, 20, and 30 days post).	336	Variable: Implied early treatment – first day	Variable: Implied early treatment – first day.	(1) Ischemia/hypoxia: 2–2.5 ATA/120 × 2–3 days BID. Then 2 ATA/variable time × up to 40 to 60 treatments (average 2–7) (2) Carbon monoxide: 2 ATA/120 BID × 1–2 days then 2 ATA/2 hrs QD (Avg 1–3 treatments moderate cases, 2–5 serious up to 40 total). One case, 3 months of coma treated 30, 60, and 60 treatments for a total of 150.	Ischemia/hypoxia: 75% recovery of consciousness (62.5% of those with cardiac arrest, 92% without cardiac arrest). Carbon monoxide: 100% recovery in moderate poisoning, 93% in serious poisoning. Eleven of 12 recovery. TBI: 3 of 3 recovery
Sanchez *et al* 1999	Intestinal ischemia, necrotizing enterocolitis or anoxic encephalopathy	7 neonates (3 with anoxic brain injury) over 34 weeks of age and 1200 grams. All ventilator dependent	< 6 h to > 24 h	< 6 h to > 24 h	HBOT 2.0 ATA/45 min b.i.d.	All patients treated within 6 h of delivery resolved with only one treatment. Those treated after 24 h required more than one treatment, two of whom developed pulmonary oxygen toxicity which was easily treated. Sepsis, DIC, and cerebral edema resolved after one treatment. 3-month follow-up was performed.
Van Meter 1999	Cardiac arrest with massive decompression illness and (?) near drowning	1	< 22 min	22 min	U. S. Navy Treatment Table 6A with 100% oxygen at 6 ATA. Converted to U. S. Navy Treatment Table 7 air saturation decompression with intermittent 3 ATA oxygen-breathing periods.	Returned to functional life. 20-year follow-up: patient married with children and works as a custom furniture carpenter.
Mathieu *et al* 2000	Near-hanging	305 (136 in Mathieu 1987 study)	All patients irrespective of delay to treatment	All patients irrespective of delay	HBOT 2.5 ATA/90 min t.i.d. in the 1st 24 h then b.i.d. to total of 5 treatments	76% total recovery with 16% death rate, persistent neurological sequelae in 8%. Best results of HBO < 3 h post rescue.
Liu Z (2006)	Hypoxicischemic encephalopathy	Review of Chinese literature	Hours to 24 days	Hours to 24 days	?1.2–2.0 ATA/60–100 min, daily, 5–50 treatments	Significant reduction in mortality and neurological sequelae

Table 19.2 continued

Authors and year	Diagnosis	No. of patients	Length of coma/ neuro insult pre-hyperbaric oxygen therapy (HBOT)	Timing of HBOT	HBOT protocol	Results and conclusions
Category II: Acute (> 3–48 h post cerebral insult)						
Illingworth *et al* 1961	Coma: Barbiturate overdose	1	13 h	13 h	2 ATA/95 min	Immediate benefit . . . later course uncomplicated
Koch 1962	Global ischemia/anoxia after 3 min cardiac arrest	1	6 h	6 h	3 ATA/103 min (includes 60 min at 3 ATA)	Rapid recovery. Minimal visual field defect at discharge.
Sharp *et al* 1962	Pentobarbital overdose	1	> 12 h. Patient brought to emergency room in coma; 12 h later, significant deterioration with low blood pressure, cyanosis, and assisted ventilation for 25 min. Resuscitative efforts failing.	> 12 h	2 ATA/65 min at depth	Rapid improvement within a few min in chamber. Discharged from hospital four days later well.
Saltzman *et al* 1965	See above hyper acute period					
Heyman *et al* 1966	Coma: Various forms of cerebral ischemia	22 (2 in coma with quadriplegia, 2 stuporous or semi-comatose)	(1) 4 h (2) 7 h (3) 7 days (4) 11 days	(1) 4 h (2) 7 h (3) 7 days (4) 11 days	(1) 2.36 ATA/79 × 1 (2) 2.36 ATA/45 × 1 (3) 2.0 2 ATA/26 min (4) 2.02 ATA/32 min	(1) Partial transient improvement during HBO (2) No significant change during HBO (3) No mention of immediate effect of HBOT; patient died 3 months later (4) No mention of immediate effect of HBOT; patient died 2 days later
Holbach 1967–1971	Coma: Neurosurgical cases (43 traumatic brain injury (TBI), 47 CVA, 7 tumor, 3 infection, 2 ischemia); life threatening TBI, acute CVA, severe post-op and post-TBI brain edema	102	Questionably in first 48 h	Questionably in first 48 h	(1) 52 patients: 2–3 ATA/not mentioned (2) 50 patients: 1.5 ATA/not mentioned. Overall average 2.6 HBOTs per patient	1.5 ATA group showed a significant 92% increase in number of markedly improved patients over the 2–3 ATA group
Dordain 1968	Hepatic coma due to viral hepatitis	1	12 h	12 h	2.4 ATA/not mentioned × 3 in 24 h	Patient became normal
Mogami 1969	Coma: Severe acute cerebral damage Measure EEG in 24 patients, CSF pressure, lactate and pyruvate in 13	66 (51 severe acute trauma, 10 tumor, 2 CVA, 3 cerebral ischemia). Most in coma, 26 on vent.	Acute cases, but length of coma not mentioned.	Acute cases, but time of initiation of HBOT not mentioned.	2 ATA/1 hr QD or BID; 6 treatments at 3 ATA/30. Average 2 treatments per patient.	Neurological improvement in 50% of cases, EEG in 33%, mostly during HBO with regression post treatment. Best response in least injured; least response in coma patients. High variation in CSF fluid pressure, but mostly decreased during treatment with rebound post-treatment. Mixed carbon dioxide/oxygen inhalation treatment gas dangerous. Slight decrease in lactate: pyruvant in CSF.
Viart 1969	See above hyper acute period					
Hayakawa *et al* 1971	See above hyper acute period. TBI patients most likely in acute period.					
Voisin 1973	See above hyper acute period					
Holbach 1975	Acute mid-brain syndrome with coma (traumatic brain injury)	99	Between 2nd and 10th day of intensive care	Between 2nd and 10th day of intensive care	(1) Controls-standard intensive care (2) HBOT: 1.5 ATA/45 × 1–7	Survival rate and time increased in HBO group, especially less than or equal to 30 years old. 21% decrease in mortality and apallic state with HBO with 450% increase in complete recovery.

Table 19.2 continued

Authors and year	Diagnosis	No. of patients	Length of coma/ neuro insult pre- hyperbaric oxygen therapy (HBOT)	Timing of HBOT	HBOT protocol	Results and conclusions
Sheffield & Davis 1976	Prolonged cerebral hypoxia: Blind, disoriented, combative, severe thrashing disoriented with severe visual impairment at time of HBO	1	6–8 min	6.5 h	2.8 ATA (US Navy TT 6) ® US Navy TT 6A	Clearing of symptoms at 1.9 ATA, mild cognitive residual at end of 6 h treatment. Patient normal after 1.5 days.
Holbach 1977d	Coma: 7 CVA, 23 TBI, all somnolent to stuporous	30		few days	few days post-accident	(1) Room air ® 1 ATA O_2 ® 1.5 ATA O_2 × 35–40 min ® 1 ATA O_2 room air. 10 min each stop (2) Room air ® 1 ATA O_2 ® 1.5 ATA O_2 ® 2.0 ATA O_2 ® 1.5 ATA O_2 ® 1.0 ATA O_2 ® room air
Holbach 1977e	Coma: TBI patients. High severity and acuity implied by ICP monitor and reference to comparable severe TBI patients in Holbach (D) study above who were evaluated a few days post-accident. Measure CBF, blood pressure, temperature, EKG, arterial blood gases, pyruvate, and lactate. 5% CO_2 test used to verify CO_2 reactivity of cerebral blood vessels.	14	Exact time not mentioned.	Exact time not mentioned	(1) 6 patients: room air ® 1 ATA O_2 ® 1.5 ATA O_2 ® 2 ATA O_2/30 min ® 1.5 ATA O_2 ® 1.0 ATA ® Room air. 15 min stops at each pressure except highest pressure. (2) 8 patients: room air ® 1 ATA O_2 ® 1.5 ATA O_2 ® 2 ATA O_2 ® 2.5 ATA O_2/30 min ® 2.0 ATA O_2 ® 1.5 ATA O_2 ® 1.0 ATA O_2 ® Room air. 15 min stops at each pressure except highest pressure.	Oxygen causes vasoconstriction up to 2 ATA. After about 15 min at 2 ATA and 2.5 ATA vasoconstriction is lost and 11 of 17 show marked increase in CBF with 4 of 11 having persistent increase after HBOT. This effect is nearly reversible on return to room air, but is a function of pressure and duration of oxygen exposure. CO2 levels were stable. Simultaneously lactate decreased as proceeded to 2–2.5 ATA, but after 30 min at these pressures, no further change in lactate.
Holbach (Companion to above article Holbach 1977e) 1977f	Same as Holbach 1977e. Measure EEG.	14	Same as Holbach 1977e	Same as Holbach 1977e	Same as Holbach 1977e	Correlation between CBF and EEG up to 1.5 ATA with decrease in CBF and improvement in EEG. At 2.0 and 2.5 ATA there is a dissociation of vasoconstriction and EEG with severe alterations in EEG while CBF generally increases, due to oxygen toxicity. Upon return to room air, the changes are mostly reversible.
Larcan et al	See above hyper acute period					
Isakov 1982a	Coma: Acute ischemic stroke (some status post surgery for sub-arachnoid hemorrhage). Includes 11 internal carotid artery and 10 vertebral-basilar artery strokes. 30 patients in coma of varying degree. Authors measured a variety of pulmonary function parameters.	53	< 6 days post-stroke	or two days post-surgery	< 6 days post-stroke or two day post-surgery	Based on patients age, severity, and associated diseases. 1.6–2.0 ATA/55–90 min (exact total bottom time unclear by description) × 6–10 treatments Groups and data assignment unclear at times, but improved neurological condition in all groups and normalization of initial abnormal external respiration by eliminating pathological rhythms and decreasing hyperventilation. This effect occurred with a variable number of HBOT sessions. In the vertebral basilar artery group, significant decrease in respiratory volume and minute respiratory volume. (In 50 % stabilization of external respiration by the middle of the HBO course.)

Table 19.2 continued

Authors and year	Diagnosis	No. of patients	Length of coma/ neuro insult pre- hyperbaric oxygen therapy (HBOT)	Timing of HBOT	HBOT protocol	Results and conclusions
Sukoff & Ragatz 1982	Coma: Acute severe traumatic cerebral edema	50	Approximately 6 h	Less than 6 h	after admission	Group 1: 40 patients, 2 ATA/45 Q8h × 48–96 hrs Group 2: 10 patients, 2 ATA/45 Q8h × 48 if ICP > 15 after Osmitrol Group 1: 22/40 improved. Better and more sustained results in lesser injured patients. Group 2: significant reduction in ICP
Smilkstein et al 1985	Hydrogen sulfide coma	1	10 h	10 h	2.5 ATA /45 initially then 2.0/75 × 1, then 2.0/90–120 TID initially to QD. Total 12 treatments.	Asymptomatic at discharge, but bilateral Babinski and slight difficulty with complex tasks
Hsu et al 1987	Hydrogen sulfide coma	1	6 h	6 h	2.5 ATA/80 TID in first 24 h, then QD for a total of 15 treatments	Normal neurologically
Mathieu et al 1987	See above hyper acute period					
Belokurov et al 1988	Coma. Pediatrics (13 TBI, 2 subarachnoid hemorrhage, 7 hypoxia, 1 diabetic coma), measured coma score	23		4 h–17 days, when exclude 3 cases greater than 1 week old each, average = 21.6 h	21.6 h	1.7–2.0 ATA/60 × 1/day 1–11 treatments
Rockswald 1992	Coma: Acute TBI (Glasgow Coma Scale 9 for 6 h)	168 (Randomized prospective controlled)	Average 26 h post injury	Average 26 h post injury	(1) 1.5 ATA/60 Q8h × 2 weeks until brain dead or awake (avg. 21 treatments) (2) Control group: no HBO	Nearly 60% reduction in mortality in HBO group, especially for those with ICP > 20 or GCS of 4–6
Thomson et al 1992	CO poisoning with persistent coma after 1st HBO treatment and normal carboxyhemoglobin	1	5.5 h	5.5 h	3 ATA × 1 2 ATA/90 BID × 3 days, QD × 10 days with one day break. Total 17 treatments.	Normal at 5 weeks with maintenance of recovery measured by neuropsychometric testing
Dean et al 1993	Coma: Carbon monoxide poisoning	1	Day of poisoning	Day of poisoning	2.4 ATA/90 BID × 3 days, total 6 treatments	Awakening after 6 HBO. No evidence of significant neurological sequelae at one month.
Kohshi 1993	See above hyper acute period					
Shn-Rong 1995	See above hyper acute period					
Snyder 1995	Hydrogen sulfide poisoning coma, GCS = 3	1	11–12 h post exposure	11–12 h post exposure	3 ATA/60 then 2.5 ATA/90 BID × 1 day, 2.0 ATA//90 BID × 5, 2.0 ATA/90 QD × 10 23 total	Stepwise neurological improvement with HBOT. Significant cognitive residual.

Table 19.2 continued

Authors and year	Diagnosis	No. of patients	Length of coma/ neuro insult pre- hyperbaric oxygen therapy (HBOT)	Timing of HBOT	HBOT protocol	Results and conclusions
Yangsheng *et al* 1995	Respiratory and heart sudden stopping	27 (13 hanging, 7 electric shock, 2 cardiomyo-pathy, 1 overdose, 1 encephali-tis-B, 1 se-vere CO, 1 acute an-oxia, 1 se-vere crush injury. (Part of group of 324 pa-tients which in-cluded CO/H2S/ CN and se-vere TBI	Cardiac and/or respira-tory arrest, 211 min, 7 patients unknown.	(?)	HBOT 2.5 ATA/60 min q.d. × 10 = 1 course. Repeat course as needed. Average 29 treatments (range, 4-50).	59% cured, 37% died, 4% im-proved.
Liu Z (2006)	Hypoxicischemic en-cephalopathy	Review of Chinese lit-erature	Hours to 24 days	Hours to 24 days	1.2–2.0 ATA/60–100 min, daily, 5–50 treatments	Significant reduction in mor-tality and neurological seque-lae
Category III: Sub-Acute (49 h – 1 month post cerebral insult)						
Heyman *et al* 1966	See above acute period and Saltzman study					
Holbach 1967–1971	See above acute period					
Holbach 1975	See above acute period					
Artru *et al* 1976a	Coma (TBI). Measure cortical blood flow, cere-bral metabolic rate for oxygen, cerebral meta-bolic rate glucose and lactate, glucose, lactate, and CSF parameters, (PO2, glucose, lactate), pre and 2 1/3 h after HBO2 133Xenon tech-nique	6 (3 post-op, plus 3 brainstem contusion) 12 normals plus con-trols with multiple sclerosis, and medi-cal litera-ture nor-mal con-trols, all for cortical blood flow measure-ment	5–47 days post injury	5–47 days post in-jury	2.5 ATA/90 × 1; 1 patient 2.2 ATA. 1 patient 3 studies, 1 patient 2 studies, 4 patients 1 study.	Arterial PO2 decrease in 8 of 9 patients, cortical blood flow variable due to differential ef-fects on normal and injured brain
Artru *et al* 1976b	Coma (TBI)	60 (57 intubat-ed or with tracheos-tomy) 9 subgroups	4.5 days	4.5 days	(1) 2.5 ATA/90 min QD × 10, 4 day break, repeat se-quence until recovery of consciousness or die. (2) No HBO	One sub-group (brainstem contusion) significantly high-er rate of recovery of con-sciousness at one month with HBO and lower rate of persis-tent coma.
Holbach 1977e	See above acute period					
Holbach 1977f	See above acute period					

Table 19.2 continued

Authors and year	Diagnosis	No. of patients	Length of coma/ neuro insult pre-hyperbaric oxygen therapy (HBOT)	Timing of HBOT	HBOT protocol	Results and conclusions
Larcan et al 1977	See above hyper acute period					
Isakov 1982a	See above acute period					
Belokurov et al 1988	See above acute period					
Kawamura et al 1988	Subarachnoid hemorrhage after operative intervention: 81% with vasospasm on angiography. Measure SSEPs pre, during, and after HBO. The during and post measurements were done on different HBOTs.	26 patients (some in coma)	2–62 days after the last subarachnoid hemorrhage	2–62 days after last subarachnoid hemorrhage	HBOT 2 ATA/70 min ? 1.3 ATA/10 min (loosely fitted mask during HBO treatment)	Significantly improved SSEPs during HBO in 57% of cases between 2 and 14 days post hemorrhage. Retention of effect highest in those treated within first 5 days of SAH and those with mild neurological deficits or mild brain swelling. Minimal effect in moderate to severe cases.
Satoh et al 1989	Global ischemia/anoxia: post-hanging patient in coma	1	5th hospital day	5th hospital day	Not mentioned in English abstract of Japanese author	Gradual progress
Shn-Rong 1995	See above hyper acute period					
Neubauer et al 1998	Global ischemia/anoxia. 1 Status epilepticus/hypoglycemia, 1 patient near drowning, SPECT brain imaging performed.	2	Patient 1: over 1 week post insult ambulatory, poor speech, agitated, combative Patient 2: 1.5 months post-near drowning	Patient 1: over 1 week post insult ambulatory, poor speech, agitated, combative Patient 2: 1.5 months post-near drowning	(1) 1.5 ATA/60 QD to BID total 88 (2) 154 treatments	Improved SPECT and neurological outcome in both patients
Rockswold 2001	Acute severe TBIs. GCS < 8. Measure CBF, AVDO2, CMRO2, CSF lactate, ICP pre-, during, and post HBOT.	37	Average 23 h (9–49 h)	Delayed HBOT averaged 23 h (9–49 h)	HBO 1.5 ATA/60 min at depth q 24 h × 7 maximum, average 5/patient. 2nd Rx began > 8 h after 1st treatment.	Improved CMRO2 and CSF lactate, especially in patients with decreased CBF or ischemia, recoupling of flow and metabolism, persistent effect lasting > 6 h, reduction elevated ICP and CBF. Rec: shorter, more frequent sessions.
Ren (2001)	Acute severe TBI. Average GCS = 5.3 (controls), 5.1 (HBOT)	55 (20 control, 35 HBOT), randomized	"On the third day"	"On the third day"	2.5 ATA/40–60 min, x10/4days (1 course), x 3–4 courses	Significant improvement of: GCS and BEAM (with successive courses of HBOT), Glasgow Outcome Scale at 6 months, and morbidity and mortality.
Liu Z (2006)	Hypoxicischemic encephalopathy	Review of Chinese literature	Hours to 24 days	Hours to 24 days	1.2–2.0 ATA/60–100 min, daily, 5–50 treatments	Significant reduction in mortality and neurological sequelae
Category IV: Chronic (> one month post cerebral injury)						
Neubauer 1985a	TBI. Prolonged coma, random selection.	17	7.5 months	7.5 months	HBO 1.5 ATA/60 min, × 40–120 treatments	Average 88% improvement on Glasgow Coma Scale. Twelve of 17 substantial improvement on GCS, five of 17 qualitatively improved.
Kawamura et al 1988	See above subacute period					
Eltorai & Montroy 1989	Coma: TBI plus anoxia	1	48 days	48 days	2 ATA/90 daily × 24	Recovery of consciousness; cognitive deficits. Extubated at day treatment center.

Table 19.2 continued

Authors and year	Diagnosis	No. of patients	Length of coma/ neuro insult pre-hyperbaric oxygen therapy (HBOT)	Timing of HBOT	HBOT protocol	Results and conclusions
Neubauer 1989b	Global ischemia/anoxia/carbon monoxide and natural gas	1	2 years post insult	2 years post	insult	1.5 ATA/60 × 21 treatments. Dramatic cognitive improvement and decrease in spasticity.
Neubauer 1992c	Global ischemia/anoxia: 12 years previously	1	12 years	12 years	1.5 ATA/60 QD, 61 treatments in 5 months	Marked neurological and cognitive improvement
Harch 1994	Global ischemia/anoxia	4	(Average age 3.25 years)	Average age 3.25 years	1.5 ATA/90 QD × 80	All patients improved, some substantially. SPECT brain imaging improved
Neubauer 1995	TBI: Coma, semi-apallic	1	12 months	12 months	1.5 ATA/60 × 188	Improved from coma to ambulation and self-sufficiency
Shn-Rong 1995	See above hyper acute period					
Neubauer et al 1998	Severe anoxic/ischemic encephalopathy: Abruptio placenta (1), near-drowning (4), choke-hold (1), natural gas + CO (1), and CO (1). Measured clinical outcomes and performed SPECT brain imaging before and after at least one hyperbaric treatment. SPECT and clinical outcomes measured.	8	Unknown	3 months to 12 years post event	HBOT 1.5 ATA, occasional 1.75 ATA/1 h q.d. to b.i.d. × 1, 27, 122, 181, 27, 200, 19, and > 200 treatments	Clinical improvement in all patients and on SPECT
Neubauer 1998	See above sub-acute period					
Montgomery 1999	Cerebral palsy. Measure gross motor functional measures (GMFM), Jebsen hand test, Ashworth spasticity scale, and video exams pre and post treatment.	25	Unknown	Average age 5.6 years	Control each patient served as his own control	HBOT: 1.75 ATA 95% oxygen/60 min at depth q.d., 5 days per week × 20 treatments or 1.75 ATA 95% oxygen/60 min at depth b.i.d., 5 days per week × 20 treatments
Collet et al 2001	Cerebral palsy measure GMFM, psychometric test, and PEDI questionnaire pre, post, and 3 months after treatment.	111	History of perinatal hypoxia	Average age = 7.2 years	Control 1.3 ATA air/60 min at depth q.d., 5 days per week × 40 HBOT 1.75 ATA 100% oxygen/60 min at depth q.d., 5 days per week × 40	Improvement in GMFM in both groups which persisted at three months. Greatest changes in children with lowest scores which were independent of age. Improvement in language production, attention, memory, and PEDI in both groups. Caregiver scores for PEDI favored the air group. Improvement in oral facial structure and functional speech and language test in the air group.

Table 19.2 continued

Authors and year	Diagnosis	No. of patients	Length of coma/ neuro insult pre-hyperbaric oxygen therapy (HBOT)	Timing of HBOT	HBOT protocol	Results and conclusions
2nd International Symposium on Hyperbaric Oxygenation and the Brain Injured Child (authors: Neubauer, Harch, Chavdarov, Lobov, Zerbini) 2001	Chronic brain injury: Great majority of patients were cerebral palsy or global ischemia, anoxia and coma. Variety of tests performed including physical exam, laboratory testing and functional brain imaging with SPECT.	361	(?)	Vast majority < 10 years of age	1.5–2 ATA oxygen/60–90 min q.d. to b.i.d., × 1 to > 500 treatments (rare case)	Average 50% of patients with noticeable improvements in different tests
Golden et al 2002	Chronic neurological disorders: CP 30%, TBI 26%, anoxic/ischemic encephalopathy 16%, CVA 12%, lyme disease 6%, other 10%. Measure SPECT pre, after at least 15 HBOTs, and after a course of at least 50 HBOTs.	50 (25 under 18 years old and 25 over 18 years old)	Unknown	Average 5–1/3 years postinsult	HBOT 1.25–2.5 ATA/60 min b.i.d. (12 × per week)	Improvement in SPECT from first to last scan for both hemispheres and cortex with the 3rd SPECT showing more improvement than the 2nd SPECT, which was improved over the 1st. Main increase in blood flow didn't occur until after 2nd SPECT scan and a substantial number of treatments (> 15). No change in blood flow to the pons and cerebellum.
Hardy et al (E) 2002	Cerebral palsy. Psychometric testing pre and post treatment.	75	(?)	3–12 years of age. No average age given.	Control 1.3 ATA air/60 min at depth q.d., 5 days per week × 40. HBOT 1.75 ATA oxygen/60 min at depth q.d., 5 days per week × 40.	Better self-control and significant improvements in auditory attention, and visual working memory both groups. No difference between groups. Sham group significantly improved on 8 dimensions of parent rating scale vs. 1 dimension in HBO. No change in verbal span, visual attention, and processing speed in either group.
Muira et al (E) 2002	Overdose with loss of consciousness and cyanosis x unknown amount of time. Secondary deterioration fifteen days later with akinetic mutism. Measure EEG, MRI, MRS, and SPECT.	1	(?)	50 days	HBO 2.0 ATA/90 min, 5 days a week × 71	Progressive improvement through 33 Rxs. Deterioration with strange behavior by 47th Rx. 52nd Rx disoriented, restless, and agitated with decreased memory. Excitability by 71st Rx requiring Valium, Tegretol, and Haldol. Behavior improved post HBOT but disorientation and amnesia worsened. Nine months later patient better than pre-HBO. MRI, MRS, and EEG tracked patients course.
Waalkes et al (E) 2002	Cerebral anoxia: 8 with CP, 1 near-drowning. Measured GMFM, spasticity, WEEFIM, video exams, parent questionnaire, and time spent in any 24-hr. period by caregivers.	9	(?)	6.4 years average age	1.7 ATA oxygen/60 min q.d., five days a week × 80	58% average improvement in GMFM, minimal improvement WEEFIM, no change spasticity. Significant reduction in time spent with caregiver in 24-h period. Patients still improving at end of study.

Table 19.2 continued

Authors and year	Diagnosis	No. of patients	Length of coma/ neuro insult pre-hyperbaric oxygen therapy (HBOT)	Timing of HBOT	HBOT protocol	Results and conclusions
Golden (2006)	Chronic brain injury (Children: CP 29%, TBI 26%, HIE 17%, Stroke 12%, Lyme 7%, other 9%; adults: TBI 26%, stroke 26%, anoxia 21%, hypoxia 7%, other 20%.	21 children, 21 adults, each compared to 42 untreated brain injured and normal children or adults. Prospective, non-randomized.	Not stated.	Static level of function for at least 1 year, but many patients were years post insult. Adults were at least 2y post insult.	Not stated, but HBOT protocol well known at this clinic: 1.15–(<)2.0 ATA/60 qd-bid. Children: avg. 28 Rx's in 28 days. Adults: avg. 35 Rx's in 35d.	Children: significant improvement in measures of daily living, socialization, communication, and motor skills. Adults: significant improvements on all neuropsychological measures, including attention, motor, tactile, receptive & expressive language, word fluency, and immediate and delayed memory
Senechal (2007)	Cerebral palsy	Review of literature	Not mentioned	Years post insult	All published HBOT studies. Compared HBOT studies using the Gross Motor Functional Measures (GMFM) outcome to standard therapies using the GMFM	Significantly greater rate of GMFM improvement compared to all but one study which used dorsal rhizotomy. HBOT was the only therapy that also improved cognition.

Gunther (2004) experiment the results were interesting because they suggested equal sensitivity of pathological targets to both HBO and NBO very early after ischemia (5 minutes), but only HBO had a positive effect after 30 minutes of ischemia. In addition, only the HBO dosage had any effect on morphology regardless of early or later initiation. These results reinforce the points made in the introduction to this chapter about hyperbaric dosage differences with evolving pathology and the possible difference in efficacy of HBO depending on the route of delivery. The dose by aviator mask is lower than by oxygen hood or in a pure oxygen environment. Similarly, the dose of HBO in tissue slices is markedly different when 1 ATA and 3 ATA oxygen are used. Lastly, the study by Mink and Dutka (1995b) had conflicting results with a simultaneous decrease in brain vascular permeability and blood flow while somatosensory evoked potentials were unchanged. This implies concomitant beneficial and detrimental effects which are difficult to explain without more data.

The five Van Meter et al studies (1988, 1999, 2001a, 2001b, and 2008) are unique in that they showed resuscitation of animals using HBO, rather than delivering HBO after resuscitation as in the Rosenthal article. These combined experiments were dose-response evaluations of HBO at 1.0, 2.0, 2.8, 4.0, and 6.0 ATA. The swine study proved the ability of 4 ATA HBO to resuscitate animals after 25 min of cardiac arrest, simultaneously truncating white blood cell-independent brain lipid peroxidation. This is the longest successful arrest/resuscitation reported in the medical literature and has profound implications for application to human cardiac arrest (see Chapter 39, HBO in Emergency Medicine). In 12 of the 16 studies the benefit

of HBO was generated with one treatment, in 2 studies with 3 treatments, and in the remaining two studies with 7 treatments. No consensus emerges for the ideal dose of HBO after complete global ischemia, but the Van Meter dose-response study suggests that HBO at 4 to 6 ATA was effective in resuscitating animals with cardiac arrest. More importantly, in the sixteen studies, a beneficial effect on global ischemia, anoxia, and coma was demonstrated even when the ischemic insult was as long as one hour (two studies) and the delay to treatment as long as six hours after the ischemic insult. When metabolic parameters only are considered the delay to treatment can be as long as 24 h (Zhou 2003).

The results are similarly impressive and uniformly positive in the group of incomplete global ischemia/anoxia experiments. As in the complete models no consensus emerges as to best HBO pressure, duration, frequency, or number of treatments, but there maybe an intervention time limit of 6h for improvement in behavioral/neurological outcomes. Shiokawa et al (1986) demonstrated an improvement in survival with 2 ATA HBO for only 30 min, with best results at three hours post-insult as opposed to one hour. Weinstein et al (1986) achieved an 84% reduction in mortality with a 15 min 1.5 ATA treatment and Grigoryeva (1992) demonstrated a superior effect of 1.2 ATA/30 min over 2 ATA/60 min on survival and preservation of neuronal transcription. Yaxi et al (1995) and Yiqun et al (1995) both showed improvements in brain enzymatic function from a single HBO treatment at 2.5 ATA with the Yaxi article suggesting a minimum 20–40 min duration of HBO exposure for efficacy. Kondo et al (1996), meanwhile, showed that repetitive HBO at 2 ATA/60 preserves hippocampal neurons and decreases heat shock proteins; there was a greater effect when the HBO was started at six h instead of 24 h. Essentially, HBO prevented delayed cell death (apoptosis) without oxygen toxicity. This anti-apoptotic effect was also proven by Calvert *et al* (2002 and 2005), Li (2005) and indirectly by Liu X-h (2006) and Liu M-N (2006) who measured neuronal density and morphological changes, respectively. The Li article varied the time to initiation of HBO and reinforced a 6 h window similar to Kondo and Liu. It also underscored the complexity of the microscopic brain injury milieu and the myriad of possible targets by its beneficial effect on apoptosis while increasing pro-apoptotic Caspase 8 and decreasing antiapoptotic bcl-2. In Calvert's 2005 article the antiapoptotic effect occurred with both 3ATA and 1ATA oxygen, while Liu X-H (2006) and Liu M-N (2006) used 2.5 and 2.0 ATA (2 treatments), respectively, suggesting that the intermittency of dosing pioneered in HBO therapy maybe more important than the actual dose of oxygen. In other words, early after incomplete or complete global ischemia pathological targets may be sensitive to a wide range of oxygen doses as long as they are short.

The clinical importance of these three studies is that, along with the Hai *et al* (2002) study, they used similar animal models to simulate human neonatal ischemia/hypoxia, a research and clinical subject of intense interest that has been heightened by review of the important neonatal resuscitation paper by Hutchison *et al* (1963) in the 1999 edition of this textbook. In the Hai study repetitive 2.5 ATA HBO delivered 7d post insult had a signal induction effect on brain fibroblastic growth factor (bFGF) while also increasing the amount of bFGF; bFGF increase also occurred in the hyperbaric air group. Most importantly, Calvert (2002), Liu X-h (2006), and Liu M-N (2006) all showed that the short-term effect on apoptosis, neuronal density, and improved morphology/histology with either one or two early HBO treatments translated to improved behavioral/neurological outcomes at 5–6 weeks. This underscores the Hutchison clinical findings and strongly argues for additional human application of these animal findings.

The remaining two studies by Yu (2006) and Yang (2008) are important for the demonstration of increased hippocampal stem cells with 7 HBO' treatments at 2 ATA. In the Yang study these stem cells migrated to cerebral cortex by 14d and new tissue growth was seen at 28d. These findings underscore the known trophic effects of HBOT in noncentral nervous system models and suggests a similar process in the chronic brain injury study of HBO (Harch 2007). The underlying mechanism in the acute phase of injury may be due to HBO effects on HIF-1α, which was demonstrated at both 2.5 and 1 ATA (Calvert 2006).

The only equivocal study, Mickel *et al* (1990), showed that normobaric oxygen (NBO) gave mixed results: increased production of white matter lesions while sparing cortical neurons. Lastly, the Wada *et al* (1996) study, the only model with pre-ischemic HBO, proved an anti-apo-ptotic effect of HBO. This is somewhat similar to the protective effect of pre-carbon monoxide exposure HBO in the Thom (1993a) model. Despite the inability to establish clear guidelines regarding HBO parameters in incomplete global ischemia/anoxia, the results of HBO treatment have been uniformly positive across the range of ischemic exposures (up to 3.5 h), with delays in starting HBO treatments up to 7d, treatment pressures as low as 1.2 ATA and HBO durations as short as 15 min.

Most of the above studies initiated HBO within three hours of insult and showed positive results with a maximum of seven treatments and in most cases only one. The four exceptions to this were the Kondo *et al* (1996) experiment which began HBO at either 6 or 24 h (a 2-h group was used for a separate histological oxygen toxicity examination) after insult and continued treatment to a total of 14 or 35 treatments, the Wada *et al* (1996) experiment which used pre-ischemia/anoxia HBO a maximum of 5 times, the Hai *et al* (2002) study which delayed 10 daily HBO's for 7d, and the Liu X-h (2006) study which used a single HBO up to 24 h after ischemia. All of these four studies except Liu were biochemical or pathological, not outcome/survival experiments. Interestingly, despite the prolonged course of HBO exposure in Kondo's study, no overt oxygen toxicity was delineated. The near uniform success of all of the above animal experiments suggests that pre-ischemic HBO or single HBO soon after ischemia, possibly as late as 6h, is highly beneficial and probably the most important factor in positive outcomes while the absolute HBO pressure is less important. Even NBO appears to have a positive effect. The consistency of data reinforces the earlier discussion (vide supra) where global ischemia may activate the microcirculation and when this occurs, provides a convenient HBO target, white blood cells. The only exceptions to this conclusion are the Van Meter studies which strongly suggest that HBO pressures of at least 2.8 ATA and ideally 4–6 ATA are necessary for resuscitation from cardiac arrest. Interestingly, this model showed no effect on a derivative pathology of WBC involvement, myeloproxidase.

Review of Human Clinical Studies

The human HBO experience in cerebral ischemia/anoxia and coma is extensive, complicated, incomplete at times, and spread across multiple medical conditions. Despite the heterogeneous group of studies, the data shows a beneficial effect of HBO, especially in the large series and particularly in traumatic brain injury (TBI).

Since the last edition of this chapter a number of important reviews have been published that support HBO across the time spectrum in pediatric neurologic injury. This data is consistent with previous reports and the above-mentioned animal studies.

To facilitate review of the literature all reports have been categorized somewhat arbitrarily by amount of time delay to initiation of HBO. Some reports span multiple categories and are unclear about exact times of HBO intervention. In these a rough estimate was attempted based on the implications and inferences in the study, and references to companion articles. The four categories are hyperacute ($\leq$ 3 h post insult), acute (4–48 h post), subacute (49 h to 1 month post), and chronic (greater than 1 month after insult).

The studies of Mathieu *et al* (1987, 2000), Voisin (1973), Hutchison *et al* (1963), Kohshi *et al* (1993), Shn-Rong (1995), Larcan *et al* (1977), Viart *et al* (1969), Hayakawa *et al* (1971), Saltzman *et al* (1966), Ingvar and Lassen (1965), Baiborodov (1981), Sanchez *et al* (1999), and Van Meter *et al* (1999) address the hyperacute period of global ischemia/anoxia and coma. The most clearcut of these are the studies reported by Mathieu *et al* (1987) and Hutchison *et al* (1963). Mathieu used HBO in 170 cases of unsuccessful hanging, 34 of whom received NBO and 136 HBO, and found statistically significant greater recovery without sequelae if HBO was delivered < 3 hours post hanging (85 vs. 56%). Worse coma required more treatment, but even the worst only averaged 3.9 HBO's. The 34 NBO patients were those with minor neurological problems; only patients with impaired consciousness received HBO. The pressure used in this study was 2.5 ATA/90 min. HBO for near-hanging had become the standard of care at Mathieu's facility in northern France following installation of the HBO chamber in 1968 and the results of their historically controlled study of 1973 (Voisin). The study compared 14 patients with standard treatment (normobaric oxygen) pre-1968 to 35 patients with HBO after 1968. HBO reduced mortality by 39% and neurological sequelae by 59%. The authors stated that HBO provided "a recovery both quicker and of better quality". This series of 170 patients has been extended to 305 patients (Mathieu *et al* 2000) with nearly identical results, again strongly arguing for HBO-responsive pathology within the first few hours of rescue from near-hanging. These are similar to the initial results (79%) reported by Hutchison *et al* (1963) in resuscitation from neonatal asphyxia, but one-third of those patients regressed after the first treatment. Overall, 54% were discharged from the hospital as "well". HBO was used at 2–4 ATA in this study and treatment was initiated 2–38 min after birth. These findings were replicated by Baiborodov (1981) at 2–3 ATA and 1.4–1.5 ATA in 555 infants. Although the HBO protocol is confusing and the details of the paper are limited due to publication of only the abstracts [the manuscripts were too numerous (350) and subsequently lost in a fire at one of the editors' homes] the eightfold reduction in mortality is compelling and consistent with Hutchison's data. More recently Sanchez *et al*

(1999) has reported the same positive findings at 2 ATA in a small number of infants. Altogether these experiences with HBO in neonatal ischemia/hypoxia/"asphyxia" are remarkable and significantly supported by the animal data, particularly the Calvert *et al* (2002) model.

Most of the other papers in this group imply hyperacute and acute treatment or do not state the time of HBO intervention. Kohshi *et al* (1993) initiated HBO soon after onset of symptomatic vasospasm in subarachnoid hemorrhage post-neurosurgical comatose patients using 2.5 ATA and an average 10 treatments which decreased subsequent progression to infarcts. Shn-Rong (1995) applied HBO in 336 cases of cardiac arrest, near-drowning, unsuccessful hanging, electrocution, carbon monoxide, TBI, and other toxic and asphyxial coma patients, implying at least some treatment hyperacutely, with 75–100% recovery rates at 2–2.5 ATA. Best results were with earlier treatment; delays to treatment required greater numbers of HBO's. In the Larcan *et al* (1977) paper it appears that only one patient was treated in the hyperacute period with both urokinase and HBO. The result was excellent and the best in their study, but the effect can't be necessarily attributed to HBO alone. The Viart *et al* (1969) paper does not mention time to HBO in the three cases of infant hepatic coma, but the profile of HBO seemed extreme since one patient died of pulmonary oxygen toxicity with 36 h of HBO and the other two experienced cardiac conduction abnormalities during HBO, an extremely rare complication of HBO. Despite the apparent complications, all three patients had normalization of consciousness, EEG, and neurological exam with HBO, two permanently and one transiently. Hayakawa *et al* (1971) performed a single 2ATA/1 h HBO immediately after surgery on four comatose brain tumor patients and nine acute TBI patients. The time to initiation of HBO was not stated but was probably < 3 hours in the post-operative patients. The authors found three patterns of CSF pressure and clinical response that corresponded to differential effects on normal and injured brain; HBO decreases edema in injured brain and produces edema in normal brain. Most patients had an initial decrease of CSF pressure with HBO and then return to pre-HBO level at the end of HBO. The patients with a major decrease in CSF pressure during HBO had remarkable clinical improvement and a mild neurological deficit If there was no change in CSF pressure the reverse was true. The duration of the HBO neurological improvement was not mentioned.

The coma case reported by Ingvar and Lassen (1965) showed a transient rapid awakening of a patient with "failing circulation" but died at the conclusion of a 2–2.5 ATA/1.5– 2.5 h HBO. This could be the natural history of the patient's disease and/or an oxygen toxicity effect. The other single case reports are of a "dramatic" near-complete cure of a suspected air embolism patient treated with a 2.36 ATA/5 h session of HBO (Saltzman *et al* 1966) and the Van Meter *et al* (1999) example of AGE, massive DCS, and cardiac arrest. The Saltzman treatment was similar to the United States Navy Treatment Table VI for air embolism and serious decompression sickness and may explain the near-complete cure without oxygen toxicity after a higher pressure very prolonged oxygen exposure (5 h). The Van Meter case also used a very prolonged deep oxygen exposure, 6 ATA pure oxygen on a modified US Navy TT6A extended to a US Navy TT7 with oxygen breathing periods at 3 ATA. This case spawned the guinea pig and swine resuscitation experiments of 1988 (Van Meter *et al*) and 1999/2001a,b/2008 (Van Meter *et al*), respectively. The success of the Saltzman and Van Meter cases are likely due to the large proportion of the pathology caused by intravascular gas. Overall, the preponderance of data in these 14 HBO studies and 1,388 global ischemia/anoxia and coma patients is strongly positive with pressures greater than or equal to 2 ATA and a minimum of 1–7 treatments.

The publication of Liu Z (2006) deserves particular attention since it is a review of 20 randomized or "quasi-randomized" controlled Chinese studies. While there are many methodological criticisms of the studies, there is an overwhelming consistency of the results between the 20 studies and with the above 14 studies in this category, which show a reduction in mortality and neurological sequelae with HBO in term neonates (> 36 weeks gestation) with hypoxic-ischemic encephalopathy. It appears likely that most of the patients treated were beyond the 3 h time limit of this category, falling into the acute category. The pressures used were 1.5–1.7 MPa or 1.5–1.7 ATA, which is supportive more of the pressures used in the acute category, particularly for TBI. These lower pressures are similar to the pressure (< 2 ATA) used by Baiborodov in his pediatric study.

Thirty-two studies fall into the second or acute category. Once again the preponderance of data is positive, either transiently or permanently, regardless of the etiology of coma. Kohshi *et al* (1993), Mathieu *et al* (1987), Voisin (1973), Shn-Rong (1995), Viart *et al* (1969), and Liu Z (2006) papers span this and the hyperacute period and were already reviewed. The Larcan *et al* (1977) study had one patient in the hyperacute period mentioned above and 35 coma patients in the acute period. HBO appeared to have no effect and, in fact, was no different from the medical treatment group, but the data is incomplete, lacking a pure urokinase group and exact times to initiation of treatment. All ten severe coma patients died with lesser coma grades I–III showing the best response to combined urokinase plus HBO, and minimization of time to treatment the best predictor of success. The Saltzman *et al* (1966) report also had one patient in both the hyperacute and acute periods. The acute patient had an embolic clot CVA and was treated 5 h post CVA at 2.02 ATA/>1 h with near total permanent improvement. Lastly, nine TBI pa-

tients of Hayakawa's *et al* (1971) 13 patients were most likely in the acute period, but the results have already been summed above.

Of the remaining 24 studies, 15 were at pressures greater than or equal to 2 ATA: Sharp *et al* (1962), Heyman *et al* (1966), Mogami *et al* (1969), Sukoff (1982), Thomson *et al* (1992), Dean *et al* (1993), Snyder *et al* (1995), Yang-cheng (1995), Dordain (1968), Illingworth *et al* (1961), Koch *et al* (1952), Hsu *et al* (1987), Smilkstein *et al* (1985), Sheffield *et al* (1976); 7 used 1.5 ATA:(Holbach a, b, d, e, f), Rockswald (1992), and Rockswold *et al* (2001); and two used 1.6–2 ATA: Belokurov *et al* (1988), Isakov *et al* (1982); with near uniform transient or permanent positive results. Four of the seven 1.5 ATA reports (Holbach *et al* 1974a, 1977d, e, f) compared 1.5 ATA to either 2, 2.5, or 2–3 ATA and demonstrated better results at 1.5 ATA, using a variety of clinical, biochemical, and physiological outcome measures. Four of the seven studies (Holbach *et al* 1974b, 1977d; Rockswald 1992, Rockswold *et al* 2001) initiated treatment > 24 h after injury and the fourth (Holbach *et al* 1974a) does not mention time to treatment, but implies treatment in the acute period since the patients are neurosurgical cases and they are reported incidentally in a paper on cerebral glucose metabolism in acute brain-injured patients which is a preliminary version of patients who were a "few days" post injury (Holbach 1977d). The fourth and fifth 1.5 ATA papers (Holbach 1977e, 1977f) span the acute and subacute periods and are similar patients to those in the other Holbach papers. In (Holbach 1974a) 1.5 ATA had significantly better clinical results than 2–3 ATA. This is confirmed with CBF measurements (Holbach 1977e), EEG (Holbach 1977f), and cerebral glucose metabolism (Holbach 1977d) where 15–30 min excursions to 2 and 2.5 ATA caused deterioration in the measured parameters. While the Holbach (1977d) experiment did not explore pressures between 1.5 and 2 ATA, the Belokurov study affirmed the efficacy of 1.7–2 ATA pressures in 23 comatose children with 100% recovery of consciousness. Their results were maximal in TBI and if initiated < 24 h post coma. Similarly, Isakov *et al* (1982) experienced good results between 1.6 and 2 ATA in patients with cerebrovascular accidents. The final study (Rockswold *et al* 2001) deserves special comment. This was an elegant follow-up study to Rockswald (1992) to evaluate the cerebral and biochemical physiological effects of 1.5 ATA HBO on acute severe TBI. The authors demonstrated that 30 min total dive time had achieved the maximum reduction of elevated ICP in chamber, one HBO recoupled flow/metabolism in injured brain and reduced lactate levels, and the HBO changes persisted at least six h after HBOT. The importance of the study is its duplication of the Holbach studies' elucidation of HBO effects on pathophysiology in acute severe TBI and the underpinning of all of the clinical studies, most notably the Rockswald 1992 study with its HBO induced 47–59%

reduction in mortality. The study emphatically argues for HBO in acute severe TBI. 518 of the 705 patients reviewed in this category (excluding Kohshi, Mathieu, Voisin, Shn-rong, and Viart) had TBI; the data strongly argues for the routine use of HBO in TBI at 1.5 ATA. Overall, treatment courses tended to be longer in the acute category than the hyperacute, using higher HBO pressures earlier (less than or equal to 24 h) and lower pressures later, with overall positive effects regardless of coma etiology: chemical/toxic gas, trauma, CVA, surgery, etc.

In the third category, subacute (49 h–1 month) sixteen studies are presented. The papers of Holbach (1974a,b, 1977e,f), Larcan et al (1977), Shn-Rong (1995), Isakov et al (1982), Belokurov (1988), and Liu Z (2006) were discussed above, but to reiterate, many of the TBI cases of Holbach started HBO 2–10 days post injury. Results were positive and favored treatment at 1.5 ATA for 1–7 times. Lareng et al (1973) reported two additional late TBI coma cases and had excellent outcomes with prolonged treatment at 2.0 ATA. In the Shn-Rong series a number of carbon monoxide cases presented with > 6 days of coma. In general they required more treatment, and one case of 90 day coma was cured finally with normal EEG after 150 treatments in three stages. Three patients with TBI coma of 10, 20, and 30 days regained consciousness after 7–20 treatments. Almost all except the initial few treatments were at 2 ATA. Two additional TBI studies by Artru et al (1976a, 1976b) had mixed results. The first involved 60 TBI patients 4.5 days post injury, HBO at 2.5 ATA, and an average 10 treatments with multiple breaks in protocol, and few receiving much treatment in the first week. Only one of nine sub-groups (brainstem contusion) achieved significant improvement with HBO (see above discussion on penumbra/umbra size considerations in brainstem vs. cortical coma). The second study with 6 patients, 5–47 days post insult, examined blood flow, metabolism, and CSF biochemistry before and after 2.5 ATA HBO. Results were inconclusive, but arterial partial pressure of oxygen declined in 8 of 9 patients, CSF oxygen remained elevated above baseline for 2 h after HBO, and the authors concluded that HBO has different effects on normal and injured brain circulation. Both of these studies featured high pressure, 2.5 ATA, later in the course of illness and are consistent with an oxygen toxicity effect as Holbach demonstrated in multiple reports above.

In contrast, the randomized, prospective-controlled Ren study (2001) reported significant positive results in acute severe TBI using a high pressure protocol and intensive dosing of HBOT. The treatment regimen was ten 2.5 ATA/60 minutes HBO treatments in 4 days, repeated in blocks up to a total of 40 HBO treatments. The patients experienced improvement in BEAM, GCS, and Glasgow Outcome Scale. The results are hard to reconcile with the Holbach and Artru data, and questions are raised about the uneven numbers of patients in the control (20) and

HBO (35) groups for a randomized study. Despite this intensive high dose of HBO, there was no report of complications in the study.

The final five studies deal with subacute CVA (Holbach 1976c), (Heyman et al 1966), subarachnoid hemorrhage with postoperative vasospasm (Kawamura et al 1988), post-hanging (Satoh et al 1989), and status epilepticus/hypoglycemia (Neubauer et al 1998). Holbach reported excellent results at 1.5 ATA, Heyman did not mention immediate effects at 2.02 ATA, Kawamura noted sustained improvement in SSEP's at 2 ATA, Satoh noted "gradual progress" of his unsuccessful hanging patient and Neubauer found significant progress at 1.5 ATA. In summary, with delay to treatment of 2–30 days generally positive results are achieved with HBO with a tendency to lower pressures and longer treatment courses.

The final category, chronic (> 1 month), now has 18 studies, most of which address pediatric brain injury. Six of these are single cases and the remainder are prospective and retrospective case series, prospective controlled trials, and a review article. All of the reports used 1.5– 2.0 ATA oxygen with most < 1.75 ATA, except for Golden et al (2002 and 2006) and Miura et al (2002), which used 1.25–2.5 ATA (2002) or < 2.0 ATA (2006) and 2.0 ATA, respectively. Treatment times were mostly < 60 min at depth and extended from 1 to over 500 treatments; most involved 20 to 40 treatments. The 2nd International Symposium studies were grouped together due to their heterogeneity of subjects, protocols, and hypotheses. For example, the Harch (2001) article addressed and identified oxygen toxicity and/or negative side effects of lower pressure HBO in chronic brain-injured patients with prolonged treatment courses at 1.5 ATA (average 119 treatments) and 1.75 ATA (91 treatments) or early in treatment at 1.75 ATA or greater. In addition, a withdrawal syndrome (4 patients) was described in brain-injured individuals habituated to 1.75 ATA HBO. In two of these four cases the author intervened and truncated the neurological deterioration with additional HBO at a lower pressure. These toxicity findings were reaffirmed by Miura et al (2002) in a case of delayed neuropsychiatric sequelae from drug overdose complicated by hypoxia. The patient recovered acutely then deteriorated to akinetic mutism. The authors initiated HBO at 2.0 ATA/ 90 min and the patient improved then worsened during prolonged HBO, identical to cases in Harch (2001). The behavioral problems slowly abated upon cessation of HBO, but his cognitive decline continued. The case suggests over-treatment with HBO resulting in transient and permanent negative side-effects against a background of permanent clinical improvement. MRI FLAIR, MRS, and EEG tracked the clinical course in a manner that was almost identically to the SPECT findings in the cases of Harch (2001).

One of the most important additions to this category is the Senechal report (2007). This study is described in detail in the chapter on cerebral palsy. In short, improvements in gross motor functional measures were the highest, fastest, and most durable in HBOT studies compared to studies using the GMFM for other types of therapies with the exception of two dorsal rhizotomy studies. The second important addition is the Golden study (2006), a controlled nonrandomized study of HBOT in a group of children and adults with chronic stable brain injury. Both groups showed significant improvements in nearly all measures after 28–35 HBO treatments at low pressure.

In conclusion, additional experience with HBO in chronic global ischemia, anoxia and coma that was supported by SPECT, standardized motor, and psychometric testing has accumulated in the past five years, strongly suggesting a positive trophic effect of HBO. These results are underpinned by the addition of the sole animal study in the literature that demonstrated a highly correlated improvement in vascular density and cognition using an HBO protocol originally designed for humans and used in many of the human studies above (Harch 2007). This animal study strongly reinforces the human studies, especially in TBI, and argues for further application of HBO to other chronic forms of brain injury.

Case Studies

To illustrate the effect of HBO in both acute and chronic global cerebral ischemia/anoxia and coma several cases treated by these authors are presented below. In each case the visual medium of SPECT brain blood flow imaging on a high resolution scanner (7 mm; Picker Prism 3000) registers in a global fashion the neurocognitive clinical improvement experienced by the patients and witnessed by the authors. The SPECT brain scans presented below are CT technology with the patient's left brain on the reader's right and vice versa, with the 30 frame images registering transverse slices from the top of the brain in the left upper corner to the base of the brain in the lower right corner. Images are approximately 4 mm thick. Brain blood flow is color coded from white-yellow to yellow to orange to purple, blue and black from highest brain blood flow to lowest. Normal human brain shows predominantly yellows and oranges, but, more importantly, has a fairly smooth, homogeneous appearance. The companion image (B) to the 30 slice transverse set of images is a three-dimensional surface reconstruction of the transverse images. Abnormalities in perfusion are registered as defects and as coarseness of the brain's surface.

Patient 1: HBO Treatment for Coma Due to Traumatic Brain Injury

A 19-year-old male was inadvertently ejected from a motor vehicle at 65 mph with impact on the left frontal/parietal region of the skull. Within one-half hour Glasgow coma scale was 6–7 and the patient was ventilator dependent. CT of the brain revealed diffuse edema, midline shift, petechial hemorrhages, subarachnoid hemorrhage, small subdural hematoma, and basilar skull fracture. HBO was given 19 h post injury at 1.75 ATA/90 bid. On the first treatment the patient began to fight the ventilator. Initial SPECT brain imaging obtained five days post injury on a single-head low-resolution scanner was "normal." Repeat SPECT imaging on a triple-head high-resolution scanner occurred 30 days post injury (Figure 19.1, A and B) and now clearly demonstrated the significant injury to the left frontal area as well as the contra coup injury to the right parietal/occipital area characterized by luxury perfusion. Nine days later and two hours after a fifth additional HBO, SPECT was repeated (Figure 19.2, A and B) and showed a dramatic "filling in" of the injured areas thus giving functional neurophysiological support to the clinical decision to continue HBO. The patient, meanwhile, progressed rapidly on twice daily HBO for four weeks with often new neurological or cognitive findings occurring in the chamber and then continued on HBO 4 times a day for seven weeks, at which time he was conversant and independently ambulatory with slight spasticity. At 11 weeks the patient was transferred to a rehabilitation center and his HBO discontinued by the new medical team. SPECT imaging at this time (Figure 19.3, A, B, and C) registers the patient's clinical progress with a persistent increase in flow to the left frontal region while some deterioration occurs to the area of previous luxury perfusion on the posterior right. The patient made transient limited initial progress at the rehabilitation center then quickly leveled off cognitively while his spasticity and balance worsened. Three months after discontinuance of HBO the patient's father requested further HBO and repeat SPECT brain scan (Figure 19.4, A and B), psychometric, and motor testing were obtained. SPECT now demonstrates a significant deterioration in the right frontal and posterior areas, while the left frontal normalization persists. The right posterior area has infarcted on simultaneous MRI. To assess recoverable brain tissue the patient underwent a single 1.75 ATA/90 min HBO followed by SPECT imaging (Figure 19.5, A and B); SPECT showed improvement in the right frontal and parietal/occipital lesions along the ischemic penumbral margins. HBO was resumed for an additional 80 treatments, once/day at 1.75 ATA/90 min. The patient made a noticeable improvement in cognition (40 percentile gain in written computational mathematics), insight (the patient now verbalized for the first time the understanding that he had sustained a brain injury and could no longer aspire to be a surgeon), and balance (improvement in gait and progression from a 3-wheel tricycle to a 2-wheel bicycle). HBO (188 treatments total) was discontinued when the patient desired enrollment in remedial courses at a community college. SPECT imaging at this time (Figure 19.6, A and B) shows improve-

balance (improvement in gait and progression from a 3-wheel tricycle to a 2-wheel bicycle). HBO (188 treatments total) was discontinued when the patient desired enrollment in remedial courses at a community college. SPECT imaging at this time (Figure 19.6, A and B) shows improvement in perfusion in the ischemic penumbral areas of the right-sided lesions. The left hemisphere remains intact. In summary, HBO, when reinstituted following SPECT and

relapse after discontinuation of HBO, prevented further deterioration and improved SPECT image as well as neurocognitive function in TBI, demonstrating the benefit of HBO in the chronic stage of TBI

Patient 2: Near Drowning, Chronic Phase

The patient is a 4-year-old male who was found at the bottom of a swimming pool after an estimated 5 min of sub-

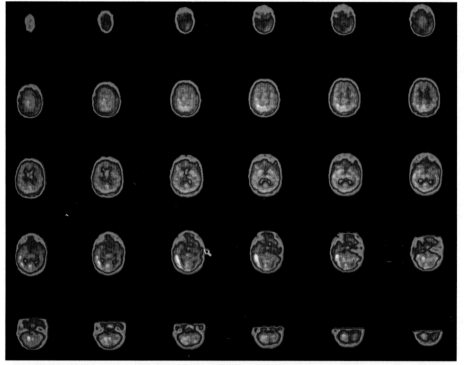

Figure 19.1A
HMPAO SPECT brain imaging, transverse slices, one month post injury. Note severe reduction in left frontal, parietal, and temporal brain blood flow with luxury perfusion in the right occipital parietal region.

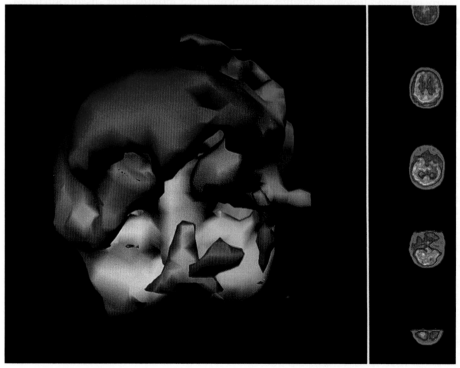

Figure 19.1B
Frontal projection three-dimensional surface reconstruction of Figure 19.1A. Non cerebral uptake is shown in scalp and neck soft tissues.

mersion. Resuscitation measures were instituted and a pulse was regained 45 min after removal from the pool. Two years after the injury, the patient was wheelchair bound with significant motor disabilities, inability to speak and communicate, and problems with drooling, attention span, and swallowing. SPECT brain imaging was performed on a high resolution scanner before (Figure 19.7, A and B) and two hours after (Figure 19.8, A and B) a

1.5 ATA/60 min HBO. The baseline scan in Figure 19.7A shows a severe reduction in blood flow to the frontal lobes, while Figure 19.8A shows a generalized improvement in brain blood flow, particularly to the frontal lobes, and denotes recoverable brain tissue after the single hyperbaric treatment. The patient embarked on a course of 80 hyperbaric treatments at 1.5 ATA/60 min four times a day, 5 days per week with a 3 week break at the 40 treatment point. At

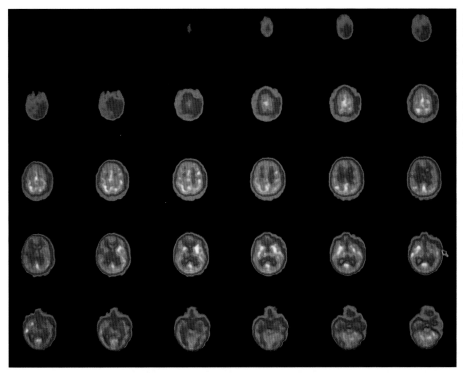

Figure 19.2A
HMPAO SPECT brain imaging, transverse slices, 9 days after Figure 19.1A and 19.1B and 2 hours post 5th additional hyperbaric treatment. Note improvement in flow to the left frontal, parietal, and temporal regions while defects begin to appear in the right frontal and parietal area. Luxury perfusion is no longer evident.

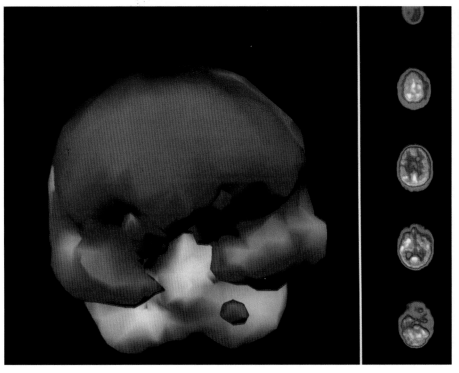

Figure 19.2B
Frontal projection three-dimensional surface reconstruction of Figure 19.2A.

the end of 80 treatments, he returned for evaluation and was noted to have a generalized improvement in spasticity, movement of all 4 extremities, increase in trunk and head control as well as improvements in swallowing, awareness, non-verbal communication, and attention span. There was a global increase in blood flow on SPECT brain imaging performed at that time (Figure 19.9, A and B).

Patient 3: Near Drowning, Chronic Phase

Case 3: The patient is a 4-year-old boy who is 2 years status post 30 min submersion in a pond. Resuscitation regained a pulse 45 min after removal from the water. Two years later, the child is severely disabled with almost no cognition, frequent posturing, inconsistent tracking, extreme difficulty swallowing fluids, choking, and 10 petit

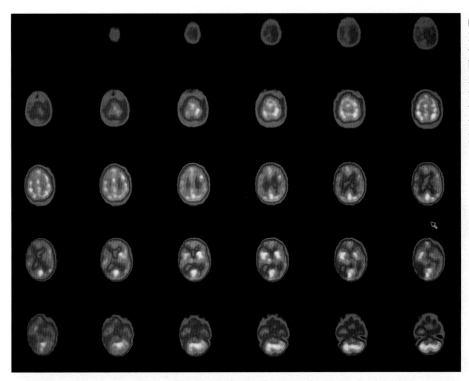

Figure 19.3A
HMPAO SPECT brain imaging, transverse slices, 11 weeks and 108 hyperbaric treatments post injury. Note maintenance of perfusion in the left frontal, parietal, and temporal regions with further progression of defects in the right frontal-parietal and posterior parietal-occipital areas.

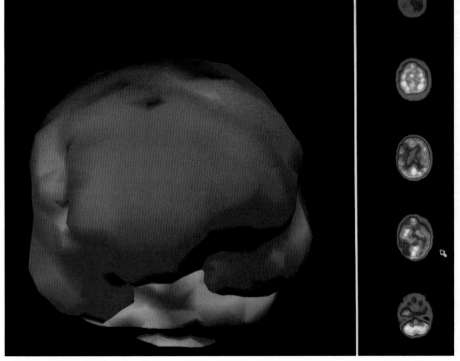

Figure 19.3B
Frontal projection three-dimensional surface reconstruction of Figure 19.3A.

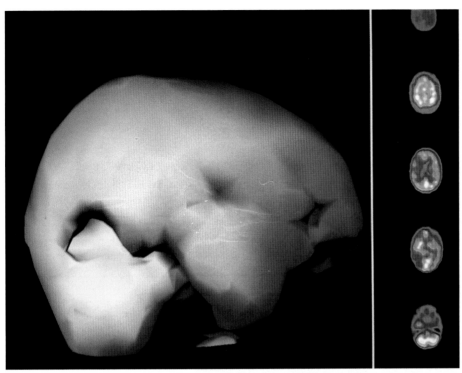

Figure 19.3C
Right lateral projection three-dimensional surface reconstruction of Figure 19.3A.

mal seizures a day. Baseline SPECT brain imaging is shown in Figure 19.10 with prominent abnormalities in the inferior frontal lobes. The patient underwent a single HBO at 1.5 ATA/60 min with repeat SPECT imaging 2 h after chamber exit (Figure 19.11). A generalized improvement in flow is noted, particularly to the frontal lobes, identifying potentially recoverable brain tissue. The patient underwent a course of 80 hyperbaric oxygen treatments at 1.5 ATA/ 60 min QD, 5 days per week with approximately one month break after 40 treatments. On return evaluation, SPECT brain imaging was repeated (Figure 19.12). Improvement in frontal lobe blood flow is noted over the baseline scan. The child exhibited greater awareness, control of his head, eye tracking, alertness, nonverbal communication, performance of some simple commands, improvement in swallowing and decrease in seizure frequency.

Patient 4: Battered Child Syndrome

Case 4: The patient is a 6-month-old girl who was slammed against the mattress of her crib by her father on multiple occasions over a four day period at two months of age. One of the first episodes was characterized by a short period of apnea; paramedics arrived at the house and found the child to be apparently normal. Three days later another episode of shaking ended with deliberate suffocation and cardiac arrest. Resuscitation was complicated by multiple recurrent arrests en route to and at the hospital. CT of the brain revealed bilateral subdural hematomas and subarachnoid hemorrhage and CT of the cord, L1 to L4 subdural hemato-

ma. The child was ventilator dependent for 12 days. Seizures developed. Repeat CT 18 days after arrest showed severe diffuse encephalomalacia, bilateral infarcts, and bilateral hemorrhages with sparing of the basal ganglia, posterior fossa, and brainstem. EEG showed seizure activity on a background of minimal electrical activity. The mother unsuccessfully sought HBO therapy. Four months after the injury the child was stable enough to travel to New Orleans where she was found to be paraplegic with rectal prolapse secondary to loss of sphincter tone. She was unable to suck and was dependent on a feeding tube. She had 5–8 seizures/day and was unable to interact socially. The patient received 38 HBO sessions at 1.5 ATA/60 min TDT, 5d/wk with progressive neurological improvement. She was more awake and aware, starting to interact with her mother, had better head control, use of her arms, and no seizures. SPECT brain imaging reflects this improvement in Figure 19.13; baseline scan is on the right and one after 38 HBO's is on the left. There is a remarkable diffuse increase in cortical blood flow after HBO with a relative absence of flow on the baseline scan, consistent with the EEG.

The day after her 38th HBO treatment the patient began a four week phenobarbital taper. HBO was re-instituted at 1.5ATA/60 qd, six treatments in 5d/week for 42 more treatments (total of 80 HBO treatments) 2 weeks into the taper. By the 80th HBO treatment, the patient had begun a phenytoin taper, was eating baby food, had been weaned off Propulsid for her reflux disorder, was much more alert, had increased motor activity, truncal balance, improved social interaction/early smile, much less irritability, a return of rectal tone, and resolution of rectal prolapse, but was still paraplegic. Repeat SPECT brain imaging after 80 HBO treatments again captures this increased clinical activity with increased cortical blood flow in Figure 19.14 (baseline scan is again on the right and after 80 HBO treatments on the left). Three dimensional surface reconstructions of the three scans are shown in chronological order in Figures 19.15, 19.16, and 19.17. Repeat EEGs after 65 HBO treatments (patient off phenobarbital, now only on phenytoin) and one month after her 80th HBO treatment (off all anticonvulsants) showed no seizure activity. EEG also showed new background rhythm and bursts of frontal activity.

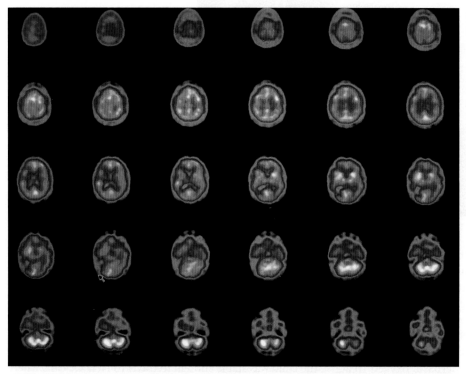

Figure 19.4A
HMPAO SPECT brain imaging, transverse slices, 3 months after Figures 19.3A, 19.3B, and 19.3C. Left frontal, parietal, and temporal perfusion is maintained with further deterioration of the right frontal and posterior defects.

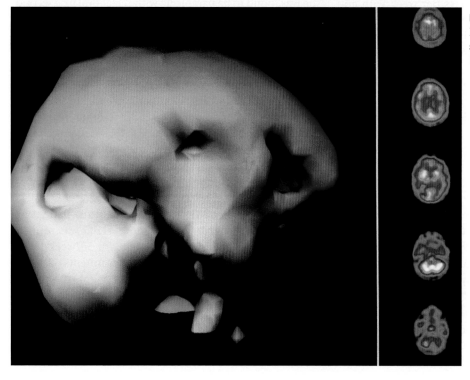

Figure 19.4B
Right lateral projection three-dimensional surface reconstruction of Figure 19.4A.

Conclusions

There are several causes of coma and global cerebral ischemia/anoxia. HBO has been used in a variety of animal models and in over 2500 patients with these conditions worldwide. Although HBO protocols have varied, the results have been remarkably consistently positive with improvement in a variety of physiological and biochemical measures and outcomes, the most important of which was improvement in overall clinical condition and consciousness. This consistent success rate suggests a generic effect of HBO on common brain pathophysiological processes at different stages in global ischemia/anoxia and coma. Importantly, this review excluded thousands of cases of acute carbon monoxide (CO) coma in the medical literature treated with HBO because of the confusion over HBO ef-

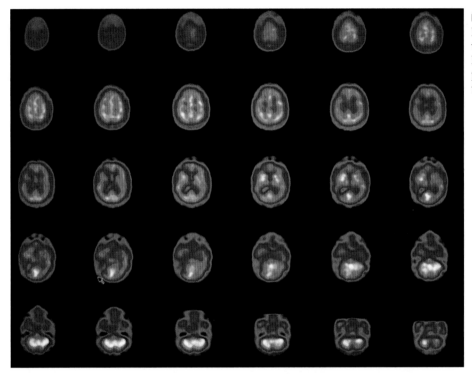

Figure 19.5A
HMPAO SPECT brain imaging, transverse slices, 2 hours following single HBO at 1.75 ATA/90min. Note improvement in the right frontal and posterior defects.

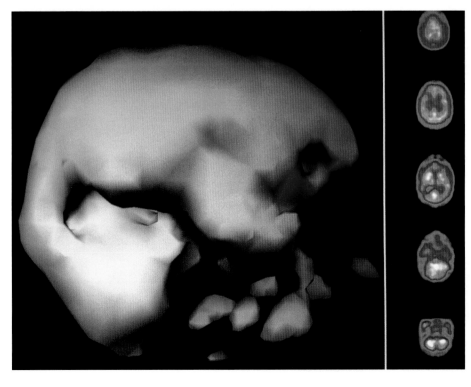

Figure 19.5B
Right lateral projection three dimensional surface reconstruction of Figure 19.5A.

fects on the metabolic poison and COHb dissociation vs. hypoxia and other pathophysiology. No doubt hypoxia is a major contributing insult to the patient's overall condition in CO and reperfusion injury a significant component of the pathophysiology, and both of these are treated definitively by HBO early after extrication, but many patients arrive for HBO hours after extrication (Thom 1992; Goulon *et al* 1969; Raphael *et al* 1993), adequately oxygenated, with low or normal COHb levels, and outside the 45 min HBO window identified in Thom's rat model of CO reperfusion injury. Clearly, HBO is effective treatment for CO coma, irrespective of COHb and hypoxia, and it is acting on yet unidentified pathological targets (see Chapter 12). Cerebral arterial gas embolism (CAGE) of diving and non-diving etiology (thousands of cases) similarly was excluded because of the argument that bubbles are the primary

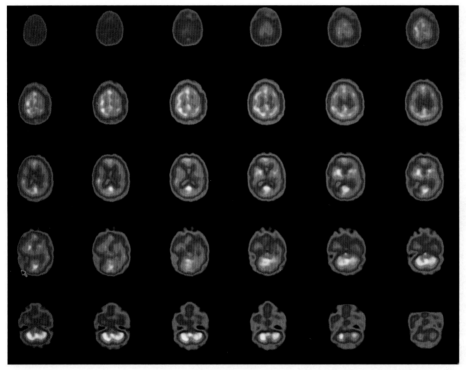

Figure 19.6A
HMPAO SPECT brain imaging, transverse slices, 5 months and 80 HBO's after Figure 19.4A. Note improvement in flow to the ischemic margins of the right frontal and posterior defects.

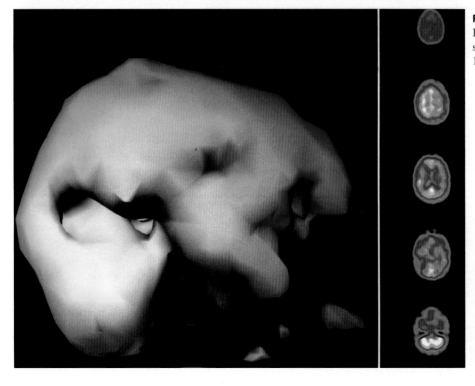

Figure 19.6B
Right lateral projection three dimensional surface reconstruction of Figure 19.6A.

pathophysiological target and not ischemia/hypoxia (for discussion see Chapter 11). It has been proposed that most bubbles in CAGE/cerebral decompression sickness have passed the cerebral circulation by the time of HBO and the primary pathological target of treatment is reperfusion injury which is responsive to HBO (Harch 1996). In conclusion, the collective experience of HBO in many of the cases of coma due to CO (especially with delayed treatment 6 h or so) and CAGE is strongly positive and further bolsters the above conclusion on usefulness of HBO in coma and global ischemia/anoxia.

Another conclusion drawn from this review is that the earlier the HBO intervention the more impressive the results. In particular, if HBO is instituted within about 3 h of cerebral insult, over 75% of patients will be noticeably improved or cured. This finding very strongly suggests targets

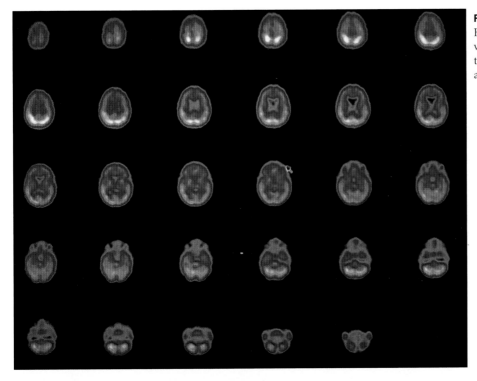

Figure 19.7A
HMPAO SPECT brain imaging transverse slices, baseline study two years status post near drowning. Note considerable reduction in frontal blood flow.

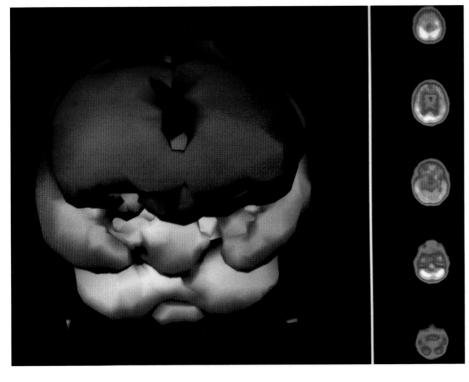

Figure 19.7B
Frontal projection three dimensional surface reconstruction of Figure 19.7A.

that are both inhibited and stimulated by oxygen. A single hyperacute HBO greater than or equal to 2 ATA is possibly quenching an on-going injurious cascade, re-energizing stunned neurons similar to the hibernating myocardium reactivation by HBO (Swift *et al* 1992), and simultaneously reversing any hypoxia or anoxia. The best examples of this are the resuscitation experiments of Van Meter *et al* (1988, 1999, 2001a, 2001b) and Calvert *et al* (2002). The Van Me-

ter experiments resuscitated arrested animals 25 min after arrest and truncated brain lipid peroxidation, but had no effect on any white blood cell mediated pathology. The Calvert experiment was a neonatal asphyxia model which inhibited apoptosis. When ischemia is incomplete, prolonged, or treatment is delayed > 45 min HBOT likely inhibits reperfusion injury as demonstrated by the animal data of Thom, Zamboni, and other models (Harch 2000).

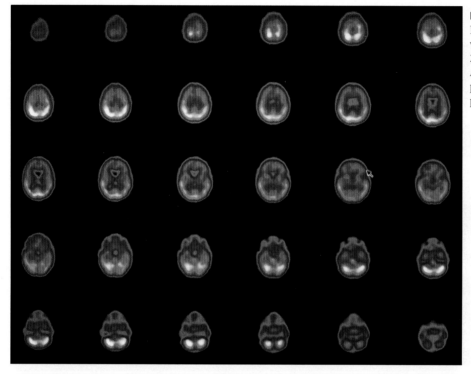

Figure 19.8A
HMPAO SPECT brain imaging, transverse slices, 1 day after Figure 19.8A and 2 hours following single HBO at 1.5 ATA/60 min. Note diffuse increase in perfusion to the frontal lobes and improvement in overall brain blood flow.

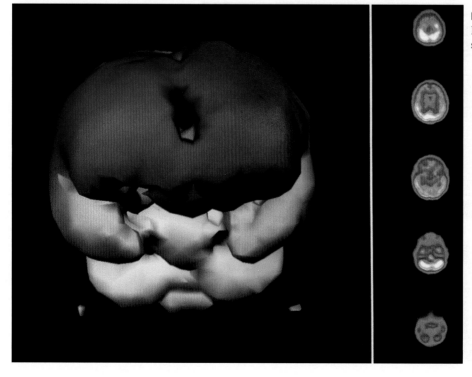

Figure 19.8B
Frontal projection three dimensional surface reconstruction of Figure 19.8A.

As treatment is delayed to 6 h, pressures above 2 ATA are still very effective, but they lose their effectiveness as delays approach 24 h. At this time lower pressures and more treatment are required and suggests treatment of different pathology. Most of the data in this time period derives from TBI studies performed at 1.5 ATA; the results show a dramatic reduction in mortality. With delays longer than one month, HBO assumes a trophic role stimulating brain repair and possibly manipulating brain blood flow and metabolism as demonstrated in the Harch (1996) animal study, which was replicated in Harch (2001). In both of these experiments (same model, larger numbers in the 2001 experiment) a human low pressure (1.5 ATA) protocol successfully employed from 1990 to 1994 was applied to rats with chronic traumatic brain injury. A series of 80 HBO treatment improved cognition and increased blood

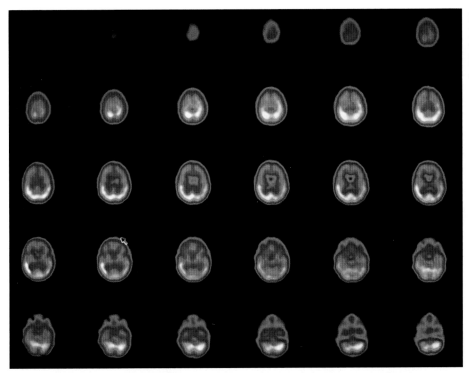

Figure 19.9A
HMPAO SPECT brain imaging, transverse slices, 4 months and 80 HBO's following Figure 19.9A. Note persistent increase in perfusion to the frontal lobes.

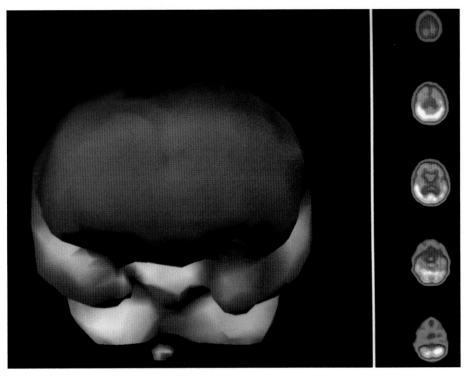

Figure 19.9B
Frontal projection three dimensional surface reconstruction of Figure 19.9A.

vessel density in the injured hippocampus. This study duplicates the known trophic effect of HBO in chronic shallow perfusion gradient radionecrosis head wounds (Marx 1990) and likely underpins the mechanism of action of HBO in the multiple subacute and chronic neurological conditions reported in this chapter.

A more obscure point from this chapter that merits attention is the suggestion of an upper limit to HBO dosing in chronic brain injury (Harch 2001). Acute oxygen toxicity (overdose) is well known in HBO such that proper dosing requires a balance of therapeutic benefit with a minimum of negative side effects. Oxygen toxicity in chronic brain injury at pressures < 2 ATA has been considered nonexistent in clinical HBO. The 35 examples in the Harch (2001) article and the case of Miura *et al* (2002) suggest the opposite in a dose-response fashion. In general this is consistent

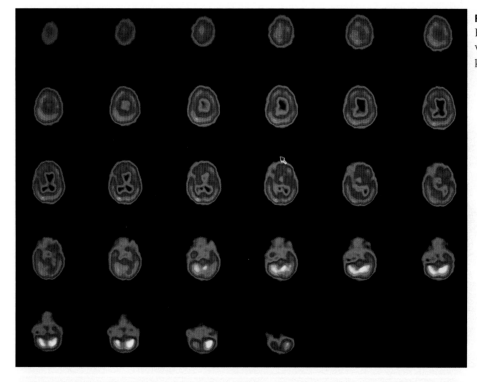

Figure 19.10
HMPAO SPECT brain imaging, transverse slices, baseline study two years post near drowning.

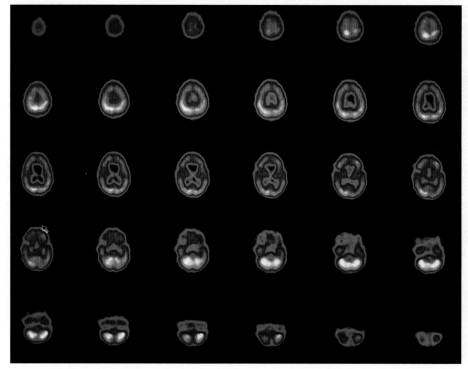

Figure 19.11
HMPAO SPECT brain imaging transverse slices one day after Figure 19.10 and two hours after a single HBO treatment at 1.5 ATA/60min. Note generalized improvement to frontal lobe brain blood flow.

with the known oxygen toxicity inverse relationship of pressure and duration at pressure, but this finding requires further confirmation by other authors.

HBO in acute cerebral ischemia/anoxia and coma appears to satisfy the cardinal rule of medicine, primum non nocere. In the multitude of cases above and those not reviewed (CO and CAGE) the incidence of serious side-effects of HBO is surprisingly small. In one review of nearly 1,000 CO poisoned patients (Hampson *et al* 1994), the maximum seizure frequency was 3% and only occurred at the highest pressures, 2.8–3 ATA, which is greater than the pressure in 49 of the 58 human studies in Table 19.2. The rate dropped ten-fold to 0.3% with pressures of 2.4 ATA. These facts alone argue overwhelmingly for a reasonable attempt, without endangering patients in transport, to perform HBO in acute cerebral ischemia/anoxia and coma, es-

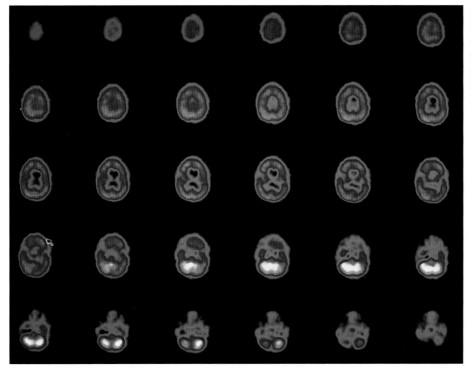

Figure 19.12
HMPAO SPECT brain imaging transverse slices four months and 80 HBO treatments after Figure 19.10. Note persistent improvement to blood flow to the frontal lobes over baseline scan of Figure 19.10A.

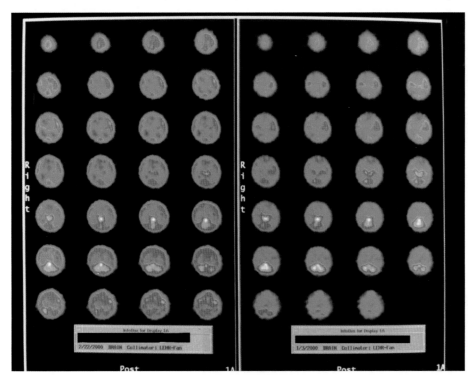

Figure 19.13
ECD SPECT brain imaging transverse slices. Baseline study is on the right and after 38 HBO treatments on the left. Note the predominant thalamic, midbrain, brainstem, and posterior fossa flow and lack of cortical flow on the first study which is augmented by cortical flow on the after HBO study.

pecially where no other treatment modality exists or has shown clearcut superiority. In essence, HBO is a simple treatment with potentially profound impact after a single hyperacute administration on devastating incurable neurological conditions that generate monumental long-term tolls of material and human capital and suffering. An increasing number of animal and human experiments/articles are drawing attention to this potential.

HBO in acute cerebral ischemia/anoxia and coma satisfies the second cardinal rule of medicine – treat until the patient no longer benefits from treatment. In many of the hyperacute and acute studies HBO benefit was observed on the first or second treatment and was a prelude to further improvement with 1–2 weeks of treatment. The advance in care levels of such patients makes a powerful cost/effectiveness argument from human and financial perspectives. Unfortunately, the

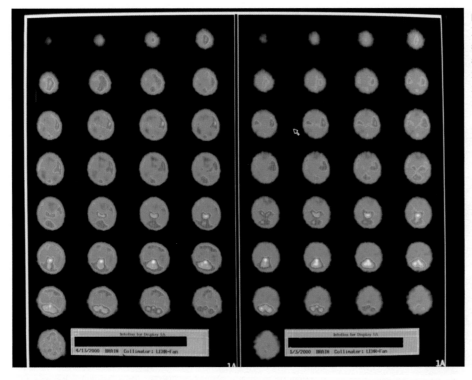

Figure 19.14
ECD SPECT brain imaging transverse slices. Baseline study is on the right again and study after 80 HBO treatments is on the left. Note the improvement in cortical blood flow after HBO.

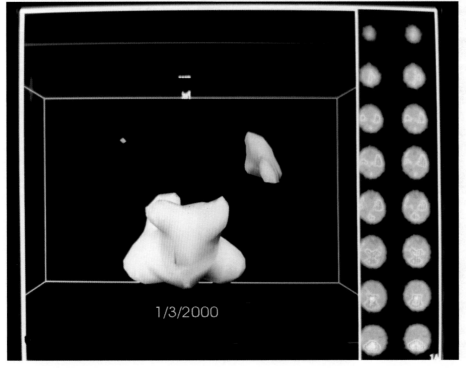

Figure 19.15
Frontal projection three-dimensional surface reconstruction of baseline study in Figure 19.13. Note the relative absence of cortical and striatal flow.

tradition in hyperbaric medicine has been to treat once or twice based on the U. S. Navy's miraculous early results with hyperacute treatment of decompression sickness and air embolism, results not attained equally in the sport scuba diving arena. This stereotyped thinking has subsequently governed the approach to treatment of carbon monoxide poisoning, stroke, and other neurological maladies, ignoring the fact that HBO initiated at different times after a neurological in-

sult is treating different neuropathology as has been discussed in this chapter. Such an approach may explain the limited positive results of Saltzman (11 of 25 patients with temporary improvement after single HBO) and Rockswold (47–59% reduction in mortality with 21 treatments, but no long term effect on functional outcome) among others. The greater consideration of the fixed HBO approach to neurologic injury and the finite, predetermined endpoint of the

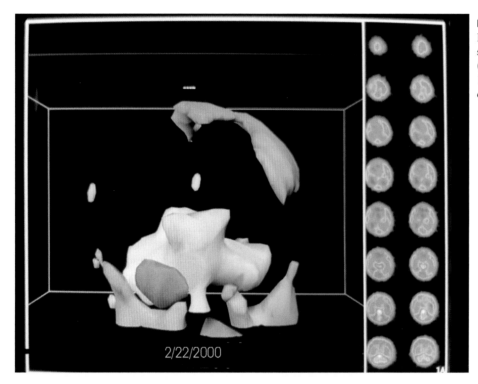

Figure 19.16
Frontal projection three-dimensional surface reconstruction of second study (after 38 HBO treatments) in Figure 19.13. The patient has developed some cortical blood flow.

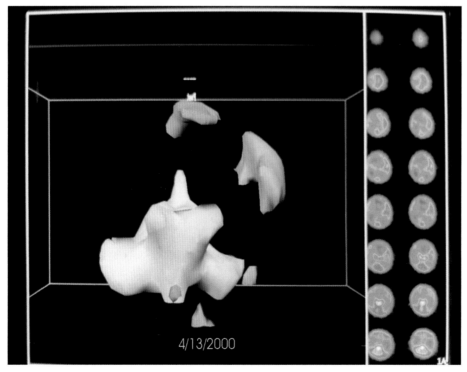

Figure 19.17
Frontal projection three-dimensional surface reconstruction of third study (after 80 HBO treatments) in Figure 19.14. Note persistence of cortical blood flow.

prospective controlled clinical trial is raised by asking the question of why stop HBO when the patient is continuing to benefit from treatment or showing neurological gains in the chamber at depth (See Patient 1). New neurological activity at depth strongly suggests ischemic neurological tissue, e.g., ischemic penumbra that would benefit from further HBO. This arbitrariness is most evident in DCI and CO poisoning where after 5–10 treatments a treating physician is asked how he knows that the patient would not continue to improve on his own. No one knows for sure with each individual case. However, we ask why this factor is not considered at the outset, or after the 2nd, 4th, 7th, 11th, or any other subsequent HBO treatment when the patient is making stepwise improvement with each or a few HBO treatments, it is known that it takes one year for a human tissue injury to mature (e.g., wound healing tensile strength and time for neurological injury to be considered chronic), smoldering inflammatory cascades are the underlying pathology, and the analogy of a single HBO "jump starting a failed engine with a dead battery" is grossly inadequate. In fact, the deciding factor in determining the number of HBO treatments may be the point in the injury process at which HBO is initiated, not financial considerations, a factor increasingly dominating medical decision-making in the United States today.

In our accumulating extensive experience, repetitive HBO appears to be trophic, stimulatory to brain repair, and may not be complete in some cases until 200–300 treatments (see Patient 1). Perhaps the best and most expedient method to assess the HBO potential and endpoint of treatment at any time after injury for any brain pathology is SPECT brain imaging on a high resolution camera (see Figures 19.1 to 19.6). SPECT before and after any single HBO at any point in the treatment process may help identify the injured brain's potential for any or further HBO. HBO can then be initiated or continued and combined with multiple other treatment modalities. This approach may help document cost-effectiveness of prolonged HBO by choosing endpoints. Currently, there are over 600 hyperbaric centers in the United States but less than 12 of these routinely treat the neurological conditions addressed in this chapter with the exception of decompression sickness and CO poisoning. In the last edition of this chapter, we wrote that "As hyperbaric medicine continues to experience a resurgence in use and expansion of applications and research, the proliferation of chambers and increasing ease of access will facilitate use of HBO in acute cerebral ischemia/anoxia and coma and will be driven by ever greater lay public and physician knowledge of the above data through widespread computer-assisted dissemination." These words were prophetic as we are now seeing an Internet driven explosion in HBO application to chronic neurological conditions. Efforts are currently underway to collect this massive amount of accruing data, publicize the results, leverage scientific proof of efficacy, and achieve reimbursement. The ultimate result will be a retrospective look and application of HBO to the highest impact targets, acute ischemic/hypoxic brain injury and resuscitation. The outcome will be a large scale dramatic improvement in mortality, morbidity, and quality of life. We predict that this will revolutionize the treatment of brain injury.

20 HBO Therapy in Neurosurgery

M. Sukoff and K.K. Jain

Introduction

Investigations of applications of hyperbaric oxygenation (HBO) in neurosurgery continue to evolve. A number of new publications have confirmed the efficacy of HBO in cerebral edema, which was initially reported over 40 years ago. Uncertainty amongst clinicians about using HBO in the therapy of cerebral pathology because definitive established mechanisms of action are still lacking has been addressed (Calvert *et al* 2007).

The use of hyperbaric oxygenation (HBO) for diseases of the central nervous system is based on the ability of HBO to increase oxygenation and reduce cerebral blood flow. The pathophysiological sequelae of both head and spinal cord trauma include hypoxia and hyperemia. However, the complexity of central nervous system trauma involves events at multiple levels: cellular integrity and metabolism, blood flow, enzymatic disruption, and all their implications. Consequently, not only is multimodality therapy essential in central nervous system trauma, but also the specific effects must be carefully monitored inasmuch as the treatment of the brain and spinal cord with HBO is somewhat paradoxical, and carries with it the potential for therapeutic success as well as aggravation.

Role of HBO in the Management of Traumatic Brain Injury

Therapy for traumatic brain injury (TBI) must address the cascade of events that occurs subsequent to brain injury. The rationale for success must first be based on the potential of the damaged brain for recovery. This must be followed by the use of agents to prevent the cyclical events of ischemia, edema, elevated intracranial pressure (ICP), cellular disruption, and the metabolic and enzymatic derangements that occur subsequent to brain injury. The enclosure of the brain in the rigid and compartmentalized skull adds an additional challenge. HBO along with other non-operative care must be considered as an adjuvant to surgery or as the primary therapy in nonsurgical cases.

Osmotic and renal diuretics continue to be used for control of cerebral edema but their use is not quite satisfactory The current emphasis on treatment of TBI involves investigation of pharmacological methods and control of intracranial pressure in an effort to produce an environment that will either allow the injured brain to heal, and/or prevent the development of progressive damage. Use of various neuroprotective agents in TBI has been reviewed (Jain 2008). There has been experimental and clinical experience with various cerebral protective agents such as calcium channel blockers, barbiturates, glutamine antagonists, free radical scavengers, steroids, receptor antagonists, and volatile anesthetics..

On a practical and accepted level, we now have very adequate monitoring facilities for TBI patients. To support our clinical judgment, we have neuro-imaging and improved methods of measuring ICP, cerebral blood flow (CBF) and cerebral metabolism. These would facilitate the development of comprehensive approaches to deal with the complexity of brain injury. Because the traumatized brain can respond to the therapeutic effects of HBO, continued efforts to develop appropriate regimes utilizing this modality are mandatory. Virtually any trauma to the central nervous system (CNS) includes the vicious cycle of interacting ischemia, hypoxia, edema, and metabolic-enzymatic disturbances. The metabolic disturbances include the production of free radicals capable of causing vasodilatation and vascular wall damage. Hypoxia causes a shift in glycolysis with the production of lactic acid and lowering of the pH. An imbalance of energy demand and availability results in the consequent ischemia-like state with loss of ATP available to the neurons and glia. In addition to the oxygen free radicals, excitatory amino acids are released as a consequence of vascular injury. The initial or subsequent loss of cellular integrity, combined with the ionic derangements and vascular dilatation effects of free radicals, and compounded by fluid and electrolyte shifts both into the interstitial spaces and extracellular components, will result in cerebral edema and increased ICP. Thus, the main therapeutic efforts of treating the head injured patient are directed toward the above noted pathophysiological changes. Agents must be used to reduce increased ICP, ischemia, and metabolic and enzymatic derangements.

The properties of HBO that have enabled both clinical and investigational advances in the management of TBI are well known. As we have seen in previous chapters, vasoconstriction reduces cerebral blood flow, and the increased oxygenation of the blood mitigates against ischemia. The decrease in blood flow reduces a major element of ICP. However, there are additional mechanisms involved in the therapeutic effects of HBO. Studies of CBF and damaged cerebral tissue in humans demonstrates that variations of CBF are minimized by HBO. The hypothesis is that if the reduction of ICP by HBO is the result of decreased cerebral edema, then hyperoxia causes a reduction in CBF and the damaged areas manifest an increased flow after HBO. This statement does contradict the fact that hyperoxia reduces blood flow. Rather, it supports the multimechanisms that are present when using hyperoxia and are necessary in the treatment of cerebral trauma, a complex and multidimensional pathological entity. Variations in CBF, cerebral autoregulation have been well investigated (Jaeger *et al* 2006)

HBO alone has been demonstrated to reduce ICP. Even normobaric hyperoxia has been shown to improve brain oxidative metabolism and reduce intracranial pressure in TBI (Tolias *et al* 2004). This nonrandomized study suggests further verification and defines hyperoxia as treatment with 100% oxygen, FIO2 = 100% for 24 hours. The importance of cerebral metabolism was emphasized in this study.

Brain tissue O_2 was monitored, but there is no notation that blood O_2 was measured. ICP fell after institution of the normobaric oxygen treatment and continued to decrease post therapy. During baseline periods there was no difference between the control patients and those receiving 100% oxygen. Their findings including elevated brain oxygen and improved metabolism and patient outcome and provides a strong impetus for the use of oxygen in TBI. Other authors have also suggested the therapeutic benefits from normobaric oxygen (Alves *et al* 2004). The essence of oxygen therapy, as we have indicated, is that O_2 should be treated as a drug. Therefore dosimetry and monitoring are necessary. The correct utilization of HBO involves documentation of the patient's neurological status, measurement of ICP, and cerebral metabolism; particularly the lactate/pyruvate ratio effects an increase in the pH by decreasing the lactate level. This facilitates the decision as to when to treat, how often to treat and at what atmosphere of oxygen. Clearly, if the same results can be obtained with normbaric O_2 than the clinician must reserve HBO for those patients that respond better to this treatment than to normobaric "hyperoxia" as assessed by multimodality monitoring and neurological status. Avoidance of oxygen toxicity is paramount. The use of continuous 100% oxygen must be accompanied by evidence of the absence of oxygen toxicity. Because HBO is dosimetry controlled the patient's clinical status is monitored (ICP, cerebral metabolism), and if it is used intermittently, the patient has time to recover from potential O_2 toxicity with the normal indigenous anti-oxidant mechanisms. If confirmation of ICP reduction and improved metabolism aid is obtained, a combination of HBO and "hyperoxia" should be considered for TBI. Alternate sessions of HBO and normobaric oxygen can be considered. Differences in response reflect the differences and complexity of TBI. In any event, there is more than ample evidence of the need to adequately use oxygen in TBI and measure partial pressure of brain 02 in TBI. Similarly, safety and understanding the issues of ischemia and altered metabolism continue to be stressed (Verweij *et al* 2007).

The use of hyperventilation to diminish cerebral blood volume (secondary to hypocarbia causing increased pH and vasoconstriction) can be enhanced by hyperbaric oxygenation. The complexities of the use of HBO for TBI, however, must not be understated. Vasoconstriction secondary to hyperventilation can cause areas of cerebral ischemia. In addition, after 30 h of hyperventilation, the cerebral spinal fluid (CSF) pH returns to normal. Vessel diameter becomes greater than that at baseline during this time frame. It is unlikely that under hyperoxic conditions vasoconstriction itself could be deleterious. However, it has been shown that under excessive hyperoxic conditions, cerebral metabolism can be adversely affected. Thus, as in any treatment, both dosimetry and appropriate indications are essential. CBF measurements, before and after HBO, will assist in determining the efficacy of the treatment and in deciding upon dosimetry and schedules

of HBO treatments. HBO is contraindicated when a stage of vasomotor paralysis has developed. In that condition, the vasoconstrictive effects of oxygen are absent and toxic hyperoxia can result. Patients receiving hyperoxygenation, therefore, must show a response to hyperventilation by reduction in ICP. They must not have fixed and dilated pupils. Continuous monitoring of the neurological status when using HBO for the acute brain damaged patient is necessary. It must include jugular venous lactate and pH determinations, and periodic evaluation of cerebral blood flow. This, along with measurement of ICP and periodic neuro-imaging and clinical evaluation, will allow the appropriate application of HBO therapy. Each individual patient will require a specific dose with a specific frequency of administration during well defined times if HBO is to be appropriately and successfully utilized.

Toxic effects of hyperoxia should be avoided (see Chapter 6). Oxygen toxicity involves metabolic production of partially reduced reactive oxygen species. These oxygen free radicals include superoxide, peroxide, and hydroxyl radicals. They are produced by a univalent reduction of oxygen during aerobic metabolism. Thus, the use of HBO to reduce edema and oxygenate ischemic tissue may pose a dilemma because the original cerebral injury itself may alter cerebral metabolism, resulting in anaerobic metabolism and the production of oxygen free radicals. Free radical production in experimentally injured animals, however, has been shown to be reduced by HBO application (Wan & Sukoff 1992). In spite of this observation, caution should be exercised in the use of HBO in brain injury and free radical scavengers may be used as adjuncts to HBO.

Oxygen toxicity is a dose-related phenomena because oxygen is a drug. Dosimetry, therefore, must be appropriate. Monitoring must be continuous and accurate. HBO is administered intermittently to allow the anti-oxidant defenses to recover. Concomitant drugs that may potentiate oxygen toxicity must be avoided. These include adrenal cortical steroids which have been used in acute head injury patients. Untoward results from the use of HBO in head trauma is seen at pressures over 2 ATA. Usually HBO at 1.5–2 ATA is used in CNS disorders and is considered to be quite safe. Modifications of this will depend upon the metabolic monitoring factors and ICP measurements.

Experimental studies confirm some of the findings observed in earlier studies of TBI patients with HBO. In a rat model of chronic TBI, a 40-day series of 80 HBO treatments at 1.5 ATA produced an increase in contused hippocampus vascular density and an associated improvement in cognitive function as compared to controls and sham-treated animals (Harch *et al* 2008). These findings reaffirm the favorable clinical experience of HBO-treated patients with chronic TBI.

In our experience, when HBO is utilized as an adjunct to the treatment of TBI, the following regime should be followed:

Table 20.1
Clinical and Investigative Work on HBO in Traumatic Brain Injury – Classical Studies

CEREBRAL METABOLISM

Experimental

Meyer *et al* (1968): Pasteur effect (inhibition of glycolysis by oxygen) produced by hyperoxia in cerebrovascular injury.

Miller *et al* (1970): Increase in CSF lactate with hyperventilation but not HBO.

Contreras *et al* (1988): HBO increased the overall cerebral glucose utilization measured five days after injury and had a persistent positive effect.

Wan, Sukoff (1992): Demonstrated reduction in free radical and water content in experimental brain injury treated with HBO.

Clinical

Fasano *et al* (1964): HBO improved metabolic abnormalities in cerebral trauma patients.

Mogami *et al* (1969): HBO resulted in decrease CSF lactate-pyruvate ratio suggesting cerebral repair potential of HBO on metabolic basis.

Artru *et al* (1976): HBO assisted impaired cerebral metabolism by improved CSF lactate content and acid base balance.

Holbach *et al* (1977): HBO had favorable effect on cerebral glucose metabolism at 1.5 ATA but at 2 ATA increased cerebral glycolysis and resulted in decreased cerebral glucose uptake. HBO maintained aerobic glucose metabolism.

Kaasik (1988): HBO diminished the metabolic acidosis in patients with acute stroke.

CEREBRAL TRAUMA

Experimental

Coe (1966): Increased life span in experimentally injured rats treated with HBO.

Sukoff (1968): Psyllium seed induced cerebral edema and acute epidural balloon inflation successfully treated with HBO.

Wan J, Sukoff MH (1992): Demonstrated improved neurological status and mortality in experimentally produced brain injury when HBO utilized.

Clinical

Fasano *et al* (1964): HBO in traumatic brain injury demonstrated to be therapeutic.

Holbach (1969, 1974): Acute and subacute brain injuries were demonstrated to have better results when treated with HBO. ICP and cerebral metabolism improvement documented.

Mogami *et al* (1969): Traumatic brain injuries and post operative edema after brain tumor surgery successfully treated with HBO. ICP, EEG and clinical improvement most favorable in the lesser injured patients.

Artru (1976): The neurological status, ICP and metabolism of certain patients with traumatic encephalopathies improved when treated with HBO. Patients under 30 without mass lesions fared better than similar control group.

Orszagh, Simacek (1980) and Isaacov (1981): Positive results in patients treated with HBO for traumatic encephalopathies.

Sukoff (1982): Clinical and ICP improvement seen in those patients with mid level coma scales undergoing HBO therapy for acute head trauma.

Rockswold (1992): Increased survival in acute head injury with HBO.

Barrett *et al* (1998): Cognitive and cerebral blood flow improvement in chronic stable traumatic brain injury by use of HBO at 1.5 ATA.

ICP

Experimental

Miller, Ledingham (1970, 1971) and Miller (1973): HBO demonstrated to reduce ICP in experimental cerebral edema. Vasomotor changes in response to CO_2 are necessary for the vasoconstrictor effects of HBO to lower ICP. HBO and hyperventilation causes a greater reduction in ICP than hyperventilation alone. Additionally, cerebral vasoconstriction does not occur when arterial PO_2 is above 1800 mmHg. Cerebral nervous pH at 2 ATA were also shown to increase.

Clinical

Mogami *et al* (1969): Patients with the least severe symptoms had the greatest ICP reduction (traumatic encephalopathy).

Artru *et al* (1976): Improvement in patients treated with HBO for traumatic head injuries.

Sukoff (1982): Statistically significant reduction in ICP in all patients monitored (traumatic encephalopathy).

- A neurosurgeon is involved with the patient care.
- Treatments must be initiated within 12 h of the trauma, unless there has been a recent deterioration of the patient's condition.
- An ICP monitor must be in place.
- Concurrent methods to reduce ICP include hyperventilation for the first 48 h and consideration for barbiturate coma.
- An experienced hyperbaric team.
- The protocol must consist of exposure to HBO at between 1.5 and 2 ATA on an intermittent basis.
- Treatments can be given every 4, 6, 8, or 12 h depending upon the clinical status, ICP, and results of measurement of cerebral metabolism, neuro-imaging, and CBF measurements.
- Jugular venous glucose, pH and lactic acid determinations are necessary. The goal is to achieve a diminished lactic acid concentration and an increased pH.
- Cerebral perfusion pressure must be adequate (70 mmHg or above).
- The patient must have therapeutic levels of an anticonvulsant.

Table 20.1 gives a brief summary of the literature dealing with the clinical and investigative work on this topic, which indicates that HBO has an important place in the management of the severely injured but therapeutically responsive patient with TBI. A study on the effect of HBO in TBI evaluated CBF and cognitive improvement (Barrett *et al* 1998). In this study five patients with TBI, at least three years after injury, underwent 120 HBO treatments each at 1.5 ATA for 60 min. There was a rest period of five months before the first set of 80 treatments and the second set of 40 treatments. Sequential studies of SPECT scanning, CBF, speech, neurological and cognitive function were carried out. Six patients with TBI, who were not treated with HBO, served as controls. Results of SPECT scanning showed that there was no significant change over time whereas HBO-treated patients had permanent increases in penumbra area CBF. Speech fluency improved in the HBO group as well as memory and attention. The improved peaked at 80 HBO treatments. The authors concluded that HBO therapy can improve cognitive function as CBF in the penumbra in chronic stable TBI patients where no improvement would ordinarily be expected three years after the injury.

Increased cerebral metabolic rate of oxygen and decreased level of lactate in CSF found in TBI patients treated with HBO indicate that HBO can improve cerebral metabolism. The correlation between CBF and cerebral metabolic rate and HBO is important in understanding why HBO may be useful in the treatment of severe TBI. Intracranial pressure is the sum total of brain blood volume, brain tissue volume, and water, and may be lowered by reducing blood volume. HBO can reduce blood volume. ICP responds better to HBO when the rate of CBF is lowered.

There is no correlation between the response of ICP to HBO therapy and the level of CBF. In patients with elevated ICP, HBO tends to decrease it.

It must be noted that HBO is a drug, so that dosimetry is necessary. Complete monitoring is essential including frequent neurological examinations, ICP measurements as well as analysis of CSF, blood pH, and lactic acid. Each patient must be treated according to an individual schedule, and the dose should be based on response and results. The authors are correct in stating that HBO is not established in the treatment of severe head injury. However, they have demonstrated that therapeutic effectiveness may be determined when full analysis including total monitoring of another randomized clinical trial is accomplished. One would hope that therapeutic sensitivity will be apparent, and that the subgroup of appropriate patients for treatment can be identified. For these patients the ideal pressure, duration and frequency of HBO sessions can be determined.

Summary and Conclusions

Hyperbaric oxygenation has been shown both experimentally and clinically to improve the outcome of TBI. Its therapeutic effects are based on the ability of the hyperoxic environment to reduce CBF by vasoconstriction, reduce ICP, and increase oxygenation. There is supportive evidence for increasing tissue pO_2 as a consequence (tissue and microcirculation). Cerebral trauma results in a cascade of events characterized by ischemia, hypoxia, edema, increased ICP, increased CBF, and metabolic and enzymatic alterations. This results in a lowering of the pH and increase in lactic acid production, and free radical release resulting in vasodilatation, impaired carbon dioxide reactivity, and damage to the cerebral vascular endothelium. The ability of HBO to modify these pathophysiological changes is postulated, and there is sufficient experimental and clinical evidence to support this.

The toxic effects of oxygen itself is explained by the free radical theory of molecular oxygen toxicity and parallels the metabolic effects initiated subsequent to head injury; the release of toxic oxygen free radicals. However, when utilized appropriately as regards dosage, patient selection, CBF, and cerebral metabolic monitoring, the vasoconstrictive effect of HBO, while enabling increased tissue oxygenation, will maintain the tissue pO_2 at a level that allows the cellular anti-oxidant defense mechanisms to overcome the potential of hyperoxia to induce oxygen toxicity. It appears that the most favorable patients to treat are those with mid-level Glasgow coma scales using HBO pressure between 1.5 and 2 ATA, on an intermittent short-term basis. Intriguing issues in the use of HBO to manage cerebral injury include the fact that HBO has persistent effects. Additionally, the use of HBO with pharmacological agents such as oxygen radical scavengers may potentiate their therapeutic effects.

The hemodynamic phases following TBI are well defined. Autoregulation impairment after even minor brain trauma, and the importance and manner of CBF in cerebral trauma, have been well studied and are well defined. This, along with experimental and clinical success, support the use of HBO for TBI.

Historically, cerebral vasoconstriction and increased oxygen availability were seen as the primary mechanisms of HBO in TBI. HBO now appears to improve cerebral aerobic metabolism at a cellular level, i.e., by enhancing damaged mitochondrial recovery. HBO given at the ideal treatment paradigm, 1.5 ATA for 60 minutes, does not appear to produce oxygen toxicity and is relatively safe (Rockswold et al 2007).

The authors believe that, by virtue of over 40 years of experimental and clinical evidence, supported by their own experience, HBO has stood the test of time and can be considered a valuable therapeutic modality in the treatment of TBI. The importance of monitoring, clinically, analysis of the ICP and metabolism; and realization that HBO is a drug, remains important. Multicenter prospective randomized clinical trial are still needed to resolve some of the controversies and to definitively define the role of HBO in severe TBI. Such clinical trials are in progress.

Role of HBO in the Management of Spinal Cord Injury

The concept of using HBO for spinal cord injury (SCI) parallels the application of this therapy for brain injuries. The ability of HBO to reduce both edema and ischemia are the key factors. Traumatic myelopathies are characterized by ischemia and edema, which may be a consequence of vasoparalysis and direct injury to the spinal cord and its vasculature. There is compromise of spinal cord microvasculature, resulting in decreased blood flow and oxygen supply to the gray matter with surrounding hyperemia. Anatomical or physiological cellular disruption may occur as a result of the initial injury, or consequent to the pathophysiological changes that occur over a period of 2–4 h. The evolution of SCI entails gray matter ischemia and increased spinal cord blood flow with subsequent white matter edema. There are numerous publications reporting experimental work supporting the effectiveness of HBO in TBI. Clinical studies, including our own, have suggested but not substantiated the potentially beneficial effects of HBO for the TBI. Encouraging reports have been anecdotal at best. However, none of the clinical studies but ours deals with patients treated within 2–4 h post-injury. This time period represents the window of opportunity that relates to the progression of pathophysiological sequelae of SCI resulting in permanent anatomical disruption of an originally physiologically functional cord. Initially, they may be indistin-

guishable. In our experience, patients without definite evidence of anatomical disruption of the spinal cord treated within 2–4 h of their trauma may respond to HBO treatment. Clinical monitoring of the patient must be accompanied by somatosensory evoked potentials (SSEPs). Magnetic resonance imaging (MRI) must not show evidence of anatomical disruption of the spinal cord. Computerized tomography (CT) and plain x-ray films similarly must not show evidence of anatomical disruption. Our protocol includes the necessity for beginning HBO no greater than 4 h post-injury. Treatment sessions are either at 1.5 or 2 ATA, depending upon the initial and subsequent clinical evaluation and pre- and post-treatment SSEPs. If there is evidence of either clinical or electrodiagnostic improvement, a justification for continuing HBO is present. The patient's spine must be maintained in proper alignment with traction at all times in cervical injuries. A portable traction-gurney, compatible with HBO therapy as well as ground and air ambulance transfer, initial emergency hospital care, neuro-diagnostic procedures, surgery, and initial nursing care, including prone and supine positioning, is used.

Spinal Cord Injury

There are two major effects of trauma to the spinal cord:

- Anatomical disruption and secondary vascular compromise following venous stasis, edema, and hypoxia. If uncorrected, it leads to tissue necrosis.
- Functional loss and paralysis below the level of the lesion.

Various surgical and drug treatments have been advanced for SCI, with little or no cure. The role of conventional surgery is confined to removal of compressive lesions and stabilization of the bony spine. Currently, research is in progress for stem cell transplantation and regeneration of the spinal cord. Major advances in SCI research during the past quarter of a century. include use of SSEP, rCBF, methods to detail the morphology and content of the spinal cord tissues, and use of HBO.

The rationale of the use of HBO in SCI is as follows:

- Some neuronal damage, due to bruising rather than laceration, is reversible by HBO.
- HBO relieves ischemia of the gray matter of the spinal cord.
- HBO reduces edema of the white matter.
- HBO corrects biochemical disturbances at the site of injury in the spinal cord substance; lactic acidosis is an example.

Below is a summary of the literature dealing with the clinical and investigative work on this topic. This leads to the

Animal Experimental Studies

The initial experimental studies suggesting the use of HBO in SCI were published by Maeda (1965). He demonstrated tissue hypoxia resulting from injury to the spinal cords of dogs induced by clamp crushing. When the animals were subjected to HBO at 2 ATA, significant elevations in spinal cord pO_2 were observed as long as 72 h after the injury. Hartzog et al (1969) demonstrated reversibility of the neurological deficit in cord-traumatized baboons by administration of 100% oxygen at 3 ATA during the first 24 h after trauma.

Locke et al (1971) found that lactic acid accumulates in the injured spinal cord. This supports the concept that ischemia plays a role early in the traumatic process following SCI. The lactic acid levels remain elevated up to 18 h.

Kelly et al (1972) studied the tissue pO_2 of the normal and the traumatized spinal cord in dogs. The tissue pO_2 of the normal spinal cord rose on breathing 100% oxygen. After trauma the tissue pO_2 dropped to near zero and did not respond to 100% oxygen at ambient pressure. However, at 2 ATA the tissue pO_2 rose to high levels during the period of mechanical compression of the cord. The animals rendered paraplegic and then given HBO recovered to a greater degree than the untreated animals in the control group. The beneficial effects were similar to those of glucocorticosteroids and hypothermia. The authors suggested a clinical trial of HBO in patients with acute spinal cord injury.

Yeo (1976) reported the results of use of HBO therapy (3 ATA) to control the onset of paraplegia after SCI induced in sheep. Institution of HBO within 2 h of injury resulted in improved motor recovery over the following 8 weeks. Yeo's further research into the effect of HBO on experimental paraplegia in sheep (1977) confirmed his earlier findings. The degree of central cord cystic necrosis and degeneration of surrounding white matter was compared in the controls and the treated animals. Not only was there motor improvement in the HBO-treated group, there was also less cord degeneration.

Yeo et al (1977) compared the recovery of motor power and histopathology at the level of lesion after controlled contusion to the spinal cords of sheep. The treatments used were prednisolone, α-methyl-para-tyrosine (AMT, an inhibitor of norepinephrine synthesis that produces some recovery of motor activity in SCI), mannitol, or HBO. There was significant motor recovery in the untreated (control) animals, but none regained the ability to stand or walk. There was no significant recovery with methylprednisolone. In AMT-treated as well as HBO-treated groups there was significant motor recovery. Examination at 8 weeks showed cystic necrosis of the central portion of the spinal cord at the level of the lesion in all animals, but it was least marked in those treated by HBO.

Higgins et al (1981) studied the spinal cord evoked potentials in cats subjected to transdural impact injuries and treated with HBO, and demonstrated beneficial effects on the long tract neuronal function. The authors suggested that HBO may afford protection against the progression of intrinsic post-traumatic spinal cord processes destructive to long tract function if this treatment is applied early.

Sukoff (1982) reported the effects of HBO on experimental SCI. Seventeen cats were treated immediately after graded SCI by intermittent exposure to 100% oxygen at ambient pressure. No animals treated with HBO were paralyzed, whereas six of the 13 controls were. Five treated animals recovered fully and all but one could walk. Only one of the control cats could do so.

Gelderd et al (1983) performed spinal cord transection in rats and tested the therapeutic effects of dimethylsulfoxide (DMSO) and/or HBO at various pressures in different groups of animals. The animals were killed 60–200 days after the treatment and the spinal cord was examined with light microscopy, scanning electron microscopy, and transmission electron microscopy. Normally, the growth of axons is aborted within a few days following transection. In animals treated with DMSO and HBO, Gelderd et al found naked axons 90–100 days post-lesion. These findings suggest that both DMSO and HBO can prolong the regeneration process for extended periods following injury. There was less cavitation in the spinal cords of animals treated with DMSO and HBO than in the controls which did not receive any treatment.

An additional study using 20 gerbils with controlled and graded spinal cord trauma caused by aneurysm clip has confirmed the therapeutic effect of HBO, and the decrease in pathological changes has been verified histologically (Sukoff 1986b).

The effects of HBO have been compared with that of methylprednisolone regarding the oxidative status in experimental SCI (Kahraman et al 2007). Clip compression method was used to produce acute SCI in rats. HBO was administered twice daily for a total of eight 90 min sessions at 2.8 ATA. Tissue levels of superoxide dismutase and glutathione peroxidase were evaluated as a measure of oxidant antioxidant status and were elevated in nontreated animals. Methylprednisolone was not able to lower these levels, but HBO administration diminished all measured parameters significantly. Thus, HBO, but not methylprednisolone, seems to prevent oxidative stress associated with SCI.

Clinical Studies

Jones et al (1978) treated seven SCI patients with HBO within 12 h of injury. Two of these patients had functional recovery, and three patients' complete lesions became incomplete (partial recovery). One of the patients had enough motor and sensory recovery after two treatments to allow the functional use of calipers.

Gamache *et al* (1981) presented the results of HBO therapy in 25 of 50 patients treated during the preceding years. HBO was generally initiated 7.5 h after injury. The patients continued to receive conventional therapy for SCI, and their pretreatment and post-treatment motor scores were compared with those of patients not receiving HBO. Patients paralyzed for more than 24 h failed to make any significant recovery with or without HBO. The authors concluded:

The fact that HBO patients, at 4–6 months, were closer to the one year results of the patients treated conventionally is a reflection of the alterations in the rate of recovery rather than a difference in the overall outcome. Ideally the HBO therapy should be initiated within 4 h of the injury.

Sukoff (1983) treated 15 patients with traumatic myelopathy according to the following protocol:

1. Initial evaluation, including complete neurological and systemic examination, took place in the shock-trauma unit.
2. Respiratory function was assisted as necessary to maintain pO$_2$ above 90 mmHg. Problems outside the nervous system were treated and BP was maintained at 100–130 mmHg systolic.
3. X-rays of the spine were obtained and skeletal traction was applied to maintain the alignment in cases of fracture-dislocation.
4. IV mannitol was given as long as BP was above 110 mmHg systolic.
5. Cisternal myelography or metrizide-assisted CT scan was promptly obtained.
6. HBO treatment was performed in a Sechrist monoplace chamber. A special traction device was used in the chamber and nursing attention was maintained.
7. Treatment consisted of 100% oxygen at 2 ATA for 45 min repeated every 4–6 h for 4 days. If no response had occurred by that time, treatment was discontinued.

Motor improvement was seen in those patients who were treated within 6 h of injury. Two patients with sensory problems obtained relief. Two patients showed significant reduction of myelographic block, although neither improved clinically. In three patients there was dramatic recovery. Sukoff felt that his clinical success with HBO therapy, as well as that reported by others to date, was anecdotal. He suggested that clinical trials using double-blind techniques should be initiated on patients within 4 h of SCI. Kondrashenko *et al* (1981) treated patients with incomplete spinal cord injury with HBO at 2 ATA for 8–10 sessions and showed that this led to earlier return of sphincter function as compared with the controls. Yeo and Lowrey (1984) reviewed their experience with the use of HBO therapy in 45 patients with SCI over the period 1978–1982. Patients were given one, two, or three treatments, usually 90 min in duration at 2.5 ATA. Thirty-five of the patients had upper motion neuron lesions. Twenty-seven of these could tolerate two or three treatments, and 15 (56%) of them recovered functionally. During the same period of time, 29 (46%) of the 63 patients who did not receive HBO also recovered. The difference in the recovery rate is significant, considering that the average delay from the time of injury to the commencement of treatment was 9 h. All patients who showed recovery had incomplete lesions with some preservation of function below the level of the lesion.

Role of HBO in Rehabilitation of SCI Patients

Rehabilitation is the most important part of the management of SCI patients. The role of HBO in physical therapy and rehabilitation is discussed in Chapter 35. HBO can be a useful aid in the rehabilitation of paraplegics in the following ways:

Capacity for physical exercise can be increased in neurologically disabled persons by using HBO at 1.5 ATA (see Chapter 4). Metabolic complications associated with fatigue are reduced. Quadriplegics have a reduced vital capacity. Hart and Strauss (1984) tested the effect of HBO on 22 quadriplegics with an average vital capacity of 2.38 liters, as compared with the expected normal of 5.10 liters for that age group. HBO at 2 ATA for 2 h per day for 3 weeks did not impair pulmonary function, vital capacity, or inspiratory and expiratory forces. The vital capacity of 41% of the patients was improved by more than 10%.

Spasticity is a major hindrance in rehabilitation, but it can be reduced by HBO, particularly when combined with physical therapy (Kieper 1987).

Treatment should be instituted in the first 4 h following injury, but in practice this is difficult to achieve. Perhaps the treatment of acute spinal cord injuries in a mobile hyperbaric chamber could resolve the time factor. Such a mobile facility should have all the standard emergency equipment and a physician competent to deal with spinal injuries. Sensory evoked potentials should be used to monitor the progress of the patient, and eventually the patient should be transferred to an SCI center where further treatment should be given, along with any surgery and rehabilitation measures deemed necessary. In the first few hours of SCI, it may be difficult to sort out the serious damage to the spinal cord from spinal cord concussion and contusions. Because time is such an important factor, we suggest that all SCI patients with any degree of neurological involvement (minor or major) be treated with HBO prophylactically during the first few hours following injury. This may possibly prevent edema at the site of contusion with spinal cord compression.

Role of HBO in Compressive and Ischemic Lesions of the Spinal Cord

Compressive lesions of the spinal cord. Holbach *et al* (1978) reported three patients with compressive lesions of the spinal cord: one with a protruded cervical disc, one due to arachnoidal adhesions of the spinal cord, and one due to an arachnoid cyst of the lower thoracic cord. There was no improvement of the neurological deficits of these patients in spite of surgical correction of the lesions. HBO therapy was given in the hope of correcting the ischemic process associated with the compressive lesions. The first patient improved after the first HBO session but regressed afterwards. Fifteen sessions at 1.5 ATA, each lasting 35–40 min, were then given on a daily basis to all three patients, who all improved. CSF oxygen was monitored and showed a significant increase during HBO. Linke *et al* (1974) used the EMG technique to obtain an insight into the mode of action of HBO on the spinal cord lesions treated by Holbach *et al* (1978). Recordings were taken from many muscles corresponding to the level of the lesion in the spinal cord. In all three cases there was a marked increase in the density of the muscular reaction potentials after each course of HBO. The improvement reverted to some extent in the new few hours but never dropped to the pretreatment level. The cumulative result of a series of treatments was progressively increased action potentials, and the record had the appearance of an ascending steplike curve.

Holbach *et al* (1977) reported use of HBO in the treatment of 13 patients with compressive spinal cord lesions. The therapy was administered postoperatively when neurological deficit persisted. Six of the 13 patients improved markedly, particularly in motor function, while the others showed slight changes. There were no adverse effects. Neretin *et al* (1985a) used HBO for treatment of 43 patients with dyscirculatory myelopathy in developmental anomalies and spondylosis. Regression of neurological deficits was observed in patients with spastic tetraparesis within 5–6 days, in contrast to the control group, which was given only vasodilators. There was little improvement in patients with syringomyelia.

Cervical myelopathy. The effectiveness of HBO in predicting the recovery after surgery in patients with cervical compression myelopathy was evaluated by Ishihara et al (1997). This is the first paper to utilize HBO as a diagnostic tool to evaluate the functional integrity of the spinal cord. The study group consisted of 41 cervical myelopathy patients aged 32–78 years. Before surgery, the effect of HBO was evaluated and was graded. The severity of the myelopathy and the recovery after surgery were evaluated by the score proposed by the Japanese Orthopedic Association (JOA score). The correlation between many clinical parameters including the HBO effect and the recovery rate of JOA score was evaluated. The recovery rate of JOA score was found to be $75.2 \pm 20.8\%$ in

the excellent group, $78.1 \pm 17.0\%$ in the good group, $66.7 \pm 21.9\%$ in the fair group and $31.7 \pm 16.4\%$ in the poor group. There was a statistically significant correlation between the HBO effect and the recovery rate of the JOA score after surgery ($r = 0.641$, $p < 0.0001$). The effect of HBO showed a high correlation with the recovery rate after surgery as compared to the other investigated parameters. HBO can be employed to assess the chance of recovery of spinal cord function after surgical decompression.

Spinal epidural abscess. Ravicovitch and Spalline (1982) obtained good results with HBO as an adjunct to laminectomy for drainage of epidural spinal abscesses and to antibiotic therapy. Some of these cases are associated with osteomyelitis of the vertebrae, for which HBO has proven to be very useful.

Conclusion

From the available evidence in the literature, it appears that HBO has beneficial effects in some patients with spinal cord injury. Inasmuch as it is difficult to distinguish between anatomical and physiological disruption during the initial stages of spinal cord trauma, we believe that unless otherwise contraindicated (MRI, CT, or plain films), all patients should be treated in a hyperbaric chamber if seen within 4 h after a spinal cord injury. Pressures of 1.5–2 ATA are utilized. Monitoring of these patients must include SSEPs and neuro-imaging studies. Determination of spinal fluid glucose metabolism utilizing ventricular CSF samples may significantly advance the treatment of traumatic myelopathies with HBO. As in brain injury, dosimetry and periodicity of treatment will depend upon the results of clinical, electrodiagnostic and metabolic monitoring.

Experimental studies showing positive effect of HBO on SCI continue to be published (Kahraman *et al*, Hillard *et al*). These combined with ours support the role of HBO in acute SCI and we advocate its use.

HBO as an Adjunct to Radiotherapy of Brain Tumors

HBO has been used as an adjunct to radiotherapy (Chapter 36) of brain tumors. Chang (1977) carried out a clinical trial on the radiotherapy of glioblastomas with and without HBO. Eighty previously untreated patients with histologically proven glioblastoma were evaluated. Thirty-eight were irradiated under HBO and 42 (controls) in atmospheric air. At the end of 18 months the survival rate appeared considerably higher in the HBO group (28%) than in the controls (10%). After 36 months no patients in the control group survived, whereas two patients in the HBO group were alive beyond 45 and 48 months respectively. The median survival time was 38 weeks for the HBO group and 31 weeks for the controls. Owing to the small population samples and the pilot nature of the study, the difference in the survival rate between the two groups was not statistically significant. The quality of survival in the HBO group was equal to or slightly better than that of the control group.

A study of preconditioned experimental TBI under 3 ATA HBO found a protective effect of the HBO and suggested it may be a method of limiting brain injury during invasive neurosurgery. (Zhiyong *et al* 2007). We had previously observed that experimental extradural hematoma produced in a hyperbaric chamber caused no adverse effects. When the same mass lesion was produced under normobaric conditions, the animal suffered a seizure and did not survive.

The results of radiotherapy combined with HBO in 9 patients with malignant glioma were compared with those of radiotherapy without HBO in 12 patients (Kohshi *et al* 1996). This is the first report of a pilot study of irradiation immediately after exposure to HBO in humans. All patients receiving this treatment showed more than 50% regression of the tumor, and in 4 of them, the tumors disappeared completely. Only 4 out of 12 patients without HBO showed decreases in tumor size, and all 12 patients died within 36 months. So far, this new regimen seems to be a useful form of radiotherapy for malignant gliomas.

Role of HBO in the Management of CNS Infections

Two types of infections are of particular concern to the neurosurgeon: postoperative infections and brain abscess. HBO has a proven value in the management of infections (Chapter 13). Role of HBO in the management of these will be discussed in this section.

HBO for Postoperative Infections

A study was conducted to evaluate the clinical usefulness of HBO therapy for neurosurgical infections after craniotomy or laminectomy (Larsson *et al* 2002). The study involved the review of medical records, office visits, and telephone contacts for 39 consecutive patients who were referred to a neurosurgical department in 1996 to 2000. Infection control and healing without removal of bone flaps or foreign material, with a minimum of 6 months of follow-up monitoring, were considered to represent success. Successful results were achieved for 27 of 36 patients; one patient discontinued HBO therapy because of claustrophobia, and two could not be evaluated because of death

resulting from tumor recurrence. In Group 1 (uncomplicated cranial wound infections), 12 of 15 patients achieved healing with retention of bone flaps. In Group 2 (complicated cranial wound infections, with risk factors such as malignancy, radiation injury, repeated surgery, or implants), all except one infection resolved; three of four bone flaps and three of six acrylic cranioplasties could be retained. In Group 3 (spinal wound infections), all infections resolved, five of seven without removal of fixation systems. There were no major side effects of HBO treatment. The study concluded that HBO treatment is an alternative to standard surgical removal of infected bone flaps and is particularly useful in complex situations. It can improve outcomes, reduce the need for reoperations, and enable infection control without mandatory removal of foreign material such as that used for the reconstruction of cranial operative defects. HBO therapy is a safe, powerful treatment for postoperative cranial and spinal wound infections, it seems cost-effective, and it should be included in the neurosurgical armamentarium.

HBO for Brain Abscess

Brain abscesses may stem from a variety of infective organisms, but anaerobic organisms predominate, which make the abscess difficult to treat by antibiotics, normally the first mode of treatment. Surgical drainage is reserved for encapsulated abscesses that do not resolve and situations where increased intracranial pressure occurs. Brain abscesses are associated with a high mortality and the survivors have severe neurological sequelae. Lampl *et al* (1989) treated a series of 10 unselected consecutive patients with brain abscess using HBO as an adjunct. All the patients recovered and only one had residual neurological disability. HBO therapy in children with brain abscesses seems to be safe and effective, even when they are associated with subdural or epidural empyemas (Kurschel *et al* 2006). It provides a helpful adjuvant tool in the usual multimodal treatment of cerebral infections and may reduce the intravenous course of antibiotics and, consequently, the duration of hospitalization. The rationale of the use of HBO for treatment of brain abscesses is based on the following:

- HBO has a bactericidal effect on predominantly anaerobic organisms.
- HBO has a synergistic effect with the antibiotics used for the treatment of the brain abscess.
- Intermittent opening of the blood-brain barrier (BBB) as an effect of HBO facilitates entry of the antibiotics into the abscess cavity.
- HBO reduces cerebral edema surrounding the abscess and reduces the intracranial pressure.

Experimental studies in the rat have shown that BBB is

damaged in staphylococcal cerebritis and that there is surrounding edema in the early stage of the formation of the brain abscess (Lo *et al* 1994). This would provide an additional rationale for the use of HBO in the early stages of human brain abscesses, because oxygen entry into the area of cerebritis would be facilitated and brain edema would also be reduced.

Role of HBO in Cerebrovascular Surgery

HBO has a role as an adjunct in the following situations in cerebrovascular surgery:

- As a measure for cerebral protection during cerebral vascular procedures requiring vascular occlusion. Complicated neurosurgical procedures requiring lasers and electrocoagulation cannot be performed in a hyperbaric operating room; simpler procedures such as endarterectomy of the cervical portion of the carotid artery can be carried out.

- HBO should be particularly considered in the high risk carotid endarterectomy patients to afford cerebral protection from stroke during preoperative waiting period.
- Postoperative complications of cerebrovascular surgery; particularly those associated with surgery of intracranial aneurysms.
- As a decision-making measure to select patients for carotid endarterectomy and extracranial/intracranial (EC/IC) bypass operation.
- For cerebral protection during the preoperative waiting period for patients with cerebrovascular occlusive disease.

Use of HBO in Relation to Carotid Endarterectomy

Early attempts to employ HBO as an adjunct to cerebrovascular surgery were made by Illingworth (1962) and Jacobson *et al* (1963a). Oxygen at 2 ATA was used during carotid endarterectomy, but it did not afford protection against temporary carotid occlusion, and an intraluminal bypass had to be used. There was, however, an increase in

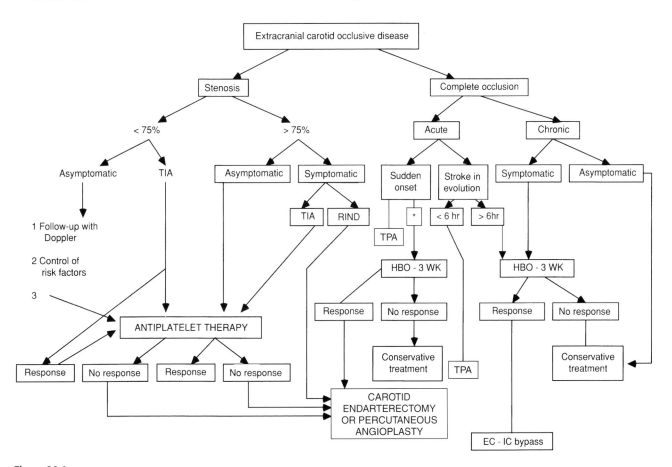

Figure 20.1

Decision-making for conservative versus surgical management of extracranial carotid occlusive disease. HBO, hyperbaric oxygen; EC/IC, extracranial-intracranial bypass. TIA = transient ischemic attack; RIND = reversible ischemic neurological deficit; TPA = tissue plasminogen activator; * = not eligible for TPA.

cerebral oxygenation. McDowall *et al* (1966) believed that Jacobson's failure was due to cerebral vasoconstriction from HBO and halothane anesthesia, and they subsequently performed a carotid endarterectomy under HBO using chloroform anesthesia, which had a vasodilating effect on cerebral vessels. The procedure was successful. Fitch (1976) has reviewed the role of HBO in carotid artery surgery.

Lepoire *et al* (1972) described the beneficial effect of HBO in six cases of post-traumatic thrombosis of the terminal part of the internal carotid artery. Those lesions are amenable to surgical procedures – direct or bypass – but it is important to give supportive treatment to prevent brain damage from infarction and edema in the acute stage before the surgery can be performed.

Carotid endarterectomy is the most commonly performed surgical procedure for stroke. HBO can be included in the decision tree for the management of a patient with carotid occlusion, as shown in Figure 20.1. Reversibility of neurological deficit can be determined by response to HBO and improvement seen on SPECT scan (Neubauer & Gottlieb 1992).

As an alternative to carotid endarterectomy, a less invasive procedure – percutaneous angioplasty with stenting – is being carried out. An incidence of 5% of minor strokes and 1% major strokes has been reported to be associated with this procedure (Jordan *et al* 1997). Yadav *et al* (1997) described a combined 7.9% complication rate for death in the initial 30 days following the procedure of percutaneous angioplasty and carotid stenting. It is feasible to reduce this complication rate by the use of HBO which has a beneficial effect in cerebral ischemia (see Chapter 18).

Use of HBO for Postoperative Complications of Surgery for Intracranial Aneurysms

Neurological deficits after aneurysm surgery stem from a number of causes, including vasospasm, vascular occlusion, and cerebral edema. Holbach and Gött (1969b) used HBO in a patient with a large middle cerebral artery aneurysm who developed hemiplegia and seizures after surgical repair of the aneurysm. The patient recovered. Ugrimov *et al* (1980) used HBO in managing the postoperative complications of intracranial aneurysm surgery. The authors found that HBO prevented the development of severe and fixed neurological deficits in many cases.

Kitaoka *et al* (1983) tried HBO treatment in 25 patients with postoperative mental signs after direct operations on anterior communicating aneurysms. Ischemia and edema of the frontal lobes occurred due to spasm of the anterior cerebral arteries. The HBO treatments were started in the "chronic phase" after cerebral edema had subsided. The effects of HBO were marked in three cases, moderate in six cases, slight in eleven cases, and insignificant in four cases.

Generally the results were favorable. The degree of efficacy of HBO was closely related to the previous condition of the patient. HBO was distinctly effective in patients who did not have marked spasm of the anterior cerebral arteries or infarction of the frontal lobes before or after the operation. In contrast, the treatment was ineffective in patients who were in a poor condition (grade) before surgery, e.g., coma. Many patients improved mentally, although EEG, rCBF, and CT scan showed no changes. The authors recommended the use of HBO therapy for postoperative mental signs as soon as cerebral edema disappears.

Isakov *et al* (1985) also used HBO in the postoperative care of patients with complications of aneurysm surgery. They used oxygen at 1.6–2.0 ATA. The course of 47 patients treated with HBO was compared with that of 30 patients not subjected to HBO (control group). The conclusions were that in patients with HBO therapy:

1. The serious phase was less prolonged
2. The duration of meningeal syndrome (fever, headache) was shorter by 6 days
3. The number of patients with good results from surgery increased by 18%
4. Mental disorders were prevented in patients who had no frontal lobe hematoma
5. There was a decrease of postoperative wound infections

Kawamura *et al* (1988) found HBO to be useful in the management of patients with neurological deficits resulting from vasospasm associated with subarachnoid hemorrhage. HBO is a useful adjunct in moderate cerebral edema, but it is not as effective in severe edema with midline shifts seen on CT scan.

Kohshi *et al* (1993) evaluated the usefulness of HBO in 43 patients who developed vasospasm following surgery in the acute stage following rupture of intracranial aneurysms. They found that HBO was a useful adjunct to mild hypertensive hypervolumia for the treatment of mild symptomatic vasospasm.

HBO has been shown to ameliorate disturbances following experimental subarachnoid hemorrhage in rats: decreased Na^+, K^+, and ATPase activity and impaired function of cerebrocortical cell membrane proteins (Yufu *et al* 1993). This may be one basis of useful effect of HBO in patients with subarachnoid hemorrhage.

HBO as an Adjunct to Surgery for Intracerebral Hematoma

Holbach and Gött (1969b) reported the use of HBO in a patient with a massive intracerebral hematoma (caused by an angioma) who was comatose and did not regain consciousness after surgery. HBO at 2 ATA was started on the

7th postoperative day, and the patient showed improvement in EEG and in level of consciousness. Sugawa *et al* (1988) used HBO therapy on a patient who did not recover from coma after evacuation of an intracerebellar hematoma. The patient regained consciousness but motor recovery was incomplete in spite of continuation of HBO treatments.

Kanno *et al* (1993) have used a favorable response to HBO in deciding on surgery in patients with hypertensive putaminal hemorrhage. These patients are more likely to continue to improve with the use of HBO following surgery. Patients who do not respond to HBO show a poor outcome regardless of subsequent surgery. Kanno and Nonomura (1996) reviewed 81 patients with hypertensive putaminal hemorrhage treated with HBO after an initial CT scan. The surgical technique used was mostly stereotactic aspiration of the clot. Open craniotomy was used only in 3 cases. The patients were divided into four groups: (1) patients who showed improvement with HBO and underwent surgery (n = 21); (2) patients who showed improvement with HBO but did not undergo surgery; (3) patients who showed no improvement with HBO but underwent surgery; and (4) patients who showed no improvement with HBO and did not undergo surgery. Of all the groups, patients who had shown clinical improvement with HBO had significantly better outcomes that those who did not respond to HBO. The number of surgical procedures for intracerebral hemorrhage have declined considerably at the authors' institution following the adoption of the policy that only responders to HBO are operated on. The authors have not tried to maintain the patients only on HBO stating that the effects of HBO are not durable. It is conceivable that HBO alone may be able to sustain clinical improvement in these patients in the acute phase and it may not be necessary to operate on these patients at all. This approach has not been tested in any clinical study.

Role of HBO in Extracranial/Intracranial (EC/IC) Bypass Surgery

The EC/IC bypass operation was devised to bypass the obstruction in a major cranial artery by anastomosis of an extracranial branch with an intracranial branch, using microsurgical techniques. The most common type of operation was an anastomosis between the superficial temporal and the middle artery branches. The usual indications for this procedure in the past were:

- TIA or RIND (reversible ischemic neurological deficit) or a slowly evolving stroke
- Bilateral carotid occlusion
- Unilateral carotid occlusion with contralateral carotid stenosis (prior to endarterectomy of the stenosed artery)

- Occlusive disease of the intracranial arteries: internal carotid, middle cerebral, or basilar
- Generalized cerebrovascular insufficiency
- Moyamoya disease
- Generalized (primary orthostatic) cerebral insufficiency usually associated with multiple occlusions of intracranial vessels
- As a preoperative adjunctive measure for the treatment of giant intracranial aneurysms requiring carotid occlusion, or vertebral artery aneurysms requiring vertebral artery occlusion.

The Cooperative Study of IC/EC bypass (1985) conducted a multicenter review of more than 1400 patients, and compared the medical versus the surgical treatment. The study concluded that the operation had no advantage over medical management, and that it was useless in preventing TIA and stroke. The 30-day mortality of the surgically treated patients was 0.6% and the morbidity 2.5%. A decrease of TIA was noted in 77% of the surgically treated patients, as compared with a decrease in 80% of the medically treated patients.

The shortcomings of the EC/IC bypass operation are as follows:

- The operation aims at increasing blood flow to the brain, but this alone may not be effective in preventing stroke and limiting the size of the infarct. Large vessel occlusion is not the only cause of stroke, and the problem may lie at the microcirculatory level (e.g., capillary endothelium) or in the blood perfusing the brain. McDowell and Flamm (1986) stated that EC/IC bypass may have applications, but not in preventing stroke due to atherosclerosis.
- EC/IC bypass does not prevent embolization from the stump of the occluded extracranial carotid artery, which may be the cause of the TIA. A patent bypass may even increase the possibility of passage of emboli through it.
- Many studies have reported the short-term benefits of EC/IC bypass on rCBF, neurological, and psychological function, but the long-term effects are debatable. Di Piero *et al* (1987) monitored the rCBF using SPECT (single photon emission computed tomography) in 14 patients before and after EC/IC bypass operation performed because of carotid occlusion. Preoperatively, all patients showed hypoperfusion in the affected cerebral hemisphere. Shortly after surgery rCBF was shown to improve in six of the patients, but studies repeated at the 6- and 12-month postoperative follow-ups did not show any difference from the preoperative status.

The health technology assessment report of the United States Department of Health and Human Services (Holohan 1990) admits the shortcomings of the cooperative study of 1985, but maintains that no objective evidence has come up since this study to alter its conclusions. The burden of the proof rests on those who advocate the prophylactic value of this surgery for stroke.

Selection of Patients for EC/IC Bypass Operation

Most of the bypass operations reviewed in the cooperative study were carried out on the basis of angiographic studies. CT scan was not available in some of the centers during the earlier part of the study. Many methods of investigation have evolved during the past decade. They are shown in Table 20.2. Of all the methods used for evaluation of patients who are considered for an EC/IC bypass operation,

---

Table 20.2
Investigation of Patients for EC/IC Bypass Operation

Preoperative
1. Methods for detection of cerebral infarction CT scan and MRI
2. Assessment of vasodilatory capacity of the intracranial arteries
   - Acetazolamide response with rCBF
   - CO_2 response by transcranial Doppler
3. rCBF measurement
   - Xenon 133
   - PET
   - Xenon and CT blood flow mapping
   - SPECT (single photon emission computerized tomography
4. Cerebral blood volume
   - C11 carboxyhemoglobin and PET
5. Cerebral metabolism
   - radioactive markers for glucose and oxygen
   - PET
6. Electrophysiological
   - SSEP
   - EEG analysis
   - power spectrum
7. Neuropsychological testing
8. Methods to show reversibility of the cerebral ischemic effects
   - HBO therapy
   - HBO and EEG analysis
   - HBO + EEG + rCBF
   - SPECT

Intraoperative
1. Measurement of blood flow through bypass using Doppler and electromagnetic flowmeter
2. Fluorescein angiography
3. pO_2 measurement over the cerebral cortex

Postoperative
1. Angiography
2. rCBF
3. EEG analysis
4. Psychometric tests
5. PET response to HBO may be of use in selecting patients with neurological deficits who could benefit from surgical revascularization

---

EEG analysis and the SPECT scan are the most practical and most useful when combined with response to HBO.

Holbach et al (1977) treated 35 patients in the chronic poststroke stage with HBO. These patients had had internal carotid occlusion for an average of 10 weeks, and their neurological deficits were fixed. The treatments were given at 1.5 ATA for 40 min daily and continued for 10–15 days. Fifteen of these patients improved neurologically; when subsequent EC/IC arterial bypass was carried out, with the improvement was maintained. Fifteen patients who did not improve were not operated on. A small group of five patients who did not improve with HBO nevertheless underwent EC/IC bypass, but still did not improve. The authors therefore suggested that the response to HBO be used as a guideline to selection of patients for EC/IC bypass. Response of the patients to HBO was considered a sign of reversibility of the brain lesion, and hence an indicator of a good chance of continuing improvement after a cerebral revascularization procedure. Holbach et al (1977) believe that EC/IC bypass is useful not only for transient ischemic attacks but also for completed strokes if there is a response to HBO and thus neuronal viability in the penumbra zone.

Kapp (1979) reported two cases to illustrate the use of HBO as an adjunct to revascularization of the brain. In both these patients – one with embolism of the middle cerebral artery and the other with occlusion of the left internal carotid artery – circulation was restored to the ischemic areas by surgical means. Both of these patients recovered. In the first case, HBO was used to reverse the patient's neurological deficits while the operating room was being prepared for surgery. A successful embolectomy then restored the patency of the middle cerebral artery. In the second case, HBO treatment stabilized the patient during occlusion of the blood supply to the left hemisphere while the operation was developing enough flow to nourish this hemisphere.

Ohta et al (1985) elaborated on Holbach's technique and described a method of choosing EC/IC bypass candidates by topographic evaluation of EEG and SSEP with concomitant rCBF studies under HBO.

In 1980, Kapp reported on the treatment by HBO at 1.5 ATA of 22 patients with cerebral infarction secondary to occlusion of the carotid or the middle cerebral arteries. Ten patients demonstrated motor improvement during HBO. Seven of these had successful surgical revascularization and no recurrence of neurological deficits. In three patients who were not successfully revascularized, the neurological deficits recurred. It was concluded that the response to HBO may be of use in selecting patients with neurological deficits who could benefit from surgical revascularization. The author confirmed the views of Holbach, and agreed that HBO is useful in about 40% of patients in the chronic stroke stage. Sukoff (1984) also found the response to HBO and improvement of EEG to be good selection criteria for EC/IC bypass operation.

Rossi *et al* (1987) performed the EC/IC bypass operation on 50 patients using the response to HBO and EEG analysis. Neurological improvement was observed in 43 patients, and in 40 of these the improvement persisted.

The EC/IC bypass study failed to take into consideration any subgroups such as those patients selected by response to HBO (Holbach *et al* 1977). The lack of a favorable response to HBO in a stroke patient can help to exclude those who are unlikely to benefit from surgery, who are then spared the expense and risk of unnecessary surgery.

This operation should now be reevaluated critically. It is known that the clinical improvement of the patient may be independent of the improvement of CBF. An increase in CBF is not necessarily accompanied by improved oxygenation of the brain tissue. A response to HBO means that the "idling" cerebral neurons show improved function when their hypoxic environments are corrected by raising the tissue oxygen tension. This does not mean that restoring the blood flow to the infarcted area will provide an equivalent effect by carrying only normal amounts of oxygen dissolved in the blood. Although the HBO response test can show the viability of the neurons affected by stroke, its effects cannot be compared quantitatively with those of cerebral revascularization.

In an effort to better define the indications for cerebral revascularization in patients with carotid artery occlusion or middle cerebral artery stenosis, a group of 29 patients was examined. Exposure to HBO (1.5 and 2 ATA) for 30 min each with computer analysis of the EEG was utilized. It proved to be confirmatory for denying surgery in patients with large infarctions or diffused intracranial vascular disease. In clinically stable or transient ischemic episode patients, an improved EEG (increase in alpha activity) supported the indications for EC/IC bypass.

The EC/IC bypass operation is contraindicated in the following situations:

1. Stroke patients who show no response to HBO therapy: They are unlikely to benefit from EC/IC bypass.
2. Patients with completed cerebral infarcts who have shown no neurological recovery and have no further ischemic episodes.
3. Patients with single TIA and recovery: Even though these patients may have carotid occlusion, the risk of stroke is not high enough to justify an operation.
4. TIA with marginal circulation and no fixed neurological deficit (EC/IC Bypass Study 1985).
5. Stroke due to thromboembolism.
6. In the acute phase of a stroke in the presence of edema and hemorrhagic infarct: The operation should not be performed within 3 weeks of the onset of infarction.
7. Patients with infarcts located in a strategic location, such as internal capsule with dense hemiplegia are not candidates for EC/IC bypass.
8. Elderly patients with cerebral atrophy and mental impairment associated with chronic cerebrovascular ischemia are not candidates for this operation.

Redefinition of the Indications for EC/IC Bypass Operation in Cerebral Ischemia

The EC/IC bypass is a useful and safe operation. It has been technically refined using sutureless laser microvascular anastomosis (Jain 1984). Its use as a planned supplement to permanent occlusion of the internal carotid artery for the treatment of a giant intracranial aneurysm is justified in some circumstances. HBO may be useful for identifying patients with viable yet nonfunctional ischemic brain, who may benefit from cerebral revascularization (Andrews & Weinstein 1990). There is need for a controlled study to compare the effect of the EC/IC bypass operation in responders to HBO, where the control group would be maintained on long-term HBO treatments. The objective of such a study would be to determine if long-term HBO treatment may make the use of an EC/IC bypass operations unnecessary. Redefinition of the indications of the EC/IC bypass operation would involve further separation of the HBO responders into those who should be maintained on long-term HBO therapy and those who should have the operation. Stroke patients who do not respond to HBO therapy are unlikely to benefit from an EC/IC bypass operation.

Cerebral Ischemia

The use of HBO for primary cerebral ischemia remains controversial in spite of many clinical and experimental demonstrations of its effectiveness. The rationale for increased tissue and microcirculatory oxygenation has been presented in previous chapters.

Role of HBO for acute ischemic stroke is described in Chapter 18. Potential of combination of HBO with thrombolysis by tPA has been discussed. Direct thrombolysis of the clot by intraarterial administration of streptokinase and urokinase is also under clinical investigation. This involves manipulation of the clot and has the advantage of a lesser dose of the thrombolytic and less risk of intracerebral hemorrhage. HBO may be used as an adjunct during the preparation of the patient for the procedure which may be performed by a neuroradiologist/neurosurgeon and also in the postoperative period to reduce cerebral edema and possible reperfusion injury.

Conclusions

The most important application of HBO appears to be in the management of acute TBI. The bulk of the evidence available indicates the effectiveness of HBO in reducing cerebral edema and intracranial pressure. Sufficient experimental and clinical studies have demonstrated the effectiveness of HBO as a part of comprehensive multimodality management of survivors of head injury to improve the outcome. Dosimetry and monitoring are the essence of success with HBO in TBI.

Post-operative cerebral edema is still a problem in neurosurgery, and the use of HBO in reducing this is well documented and should be utilized. There is still no satisfactory treatment for acute spinal cord injury. Experimentally and anecdotally HBO has proven more effective in the acute stages than any pharmacological method. Its potential is high.

A decision regarding the removal of intracerebral hematomas can be facilitated by response to HBO. Additionally, it will afford protection to the patient during the period that the decision to operate or not to operate is being deliberated. Parallel to the potential of HBO in redefining the indications for extracranial/intracranial bypass operation based on favorable response to HBO is the usefulness of this therapy in the treatment of acute vascular occlusive disease. TBI had received the most support and investigation and has arrived at a stage, in our opinion, of acceptance.

21 HBO Therapy in Multiple Sclerosis

P.B. James

Multiple sclerosis is a progressively disabling disease associated with multiple demyelinating lesions of the central nervous system. The exact cause is not known, but there is evidence for failure of oxygen delivery. The role of hyperbaric oxygen in the management of multiple sclerosis is described under the following headings:

Introduction

Multiple sclerosis (MS) has generally been considered to be a progressively disabling disease associated with multiple demyelinating lesions of the central nervous system. The exact cause is not known, but there is evidence for failure of oxygen delivery. A MS lesion is classically described as "demyelination with relative preservation of axons." The axon loss in typical lesions in the spinal cord has been shown to be about 20% (Putnam & Alexander 1947). There are between 100 and 150 patients per 100,000 of the population of Western countries, but MRI has demonstrated asymptomatic lesions in up to 40% of the population (James 1997). The disease runs an intermittent course and the initial diagnosis conventionally requires a minimum period of a month between attacks. Single attacks of the same disease process can occur, as in optic neuritis, and may result in permanent disability.

In such patients the disease may remain monosymptomatic, but about three quarters of them when imaged at the time of presentation have other lesions in the brain. There is poor correlation between the patient's disability and the pathology found in the brain at post-mortem, but small lesions in the brainstem and spinal cord are usually associated with clinical signs and symptoms. The clinical course is extremely unpredictable. Patients who satisfy the criteria for multiple sclerosis are described, after several attacks and often with increasing disability, as having "relapsing remitting disease". In a much smaller number the disease may be "chronic progressive" from the onset. Sometimes the patient stabilizes but with disability and is then described as having "chronic static" disease.

New evidence indicates that MS is far from being a progressively disabling disease for the majority of patients, as only 25% of patients so labeled become wheelchair dependent. It is also not just a demyelinating disease – the myth that has been used to support autoimmunity. About 20% of fibers are lost in typical spinal cord lesions. Also retinal periphlebitis illustrates that BBB breakdown is not dependent on myelin destruction as there is no myelin in the retina (McDonald 1986).

Pathogenesis

MS is a disease of the nervous system caused by intermittent breakdown of the BBB, inflammation, and hypoxia. Involvement of sensory or motor tracts may cause disability, though silent lesions are common in the general population. Increasing plasma oxygen tension under hyperbaric conditions reduces inflammation and may resolve the barrier dysfunction, which otherwise may lead to permanent scarring.

Damage to the BBB, as has been shown in vivo by imaging with enhancement, allows release of plasma proteins into the nervous system tissue is associated with activation of the complement cascade. Although autoimmunity has been a popular etiological concept, all the immune markers investigated in MS have also been found in stroke patients and at the same levels (Wang et al 1992). The abrupt onset of symptoms, dissemination in time, the affected sites, and the blood-brain barrier dysfunction all point to a vascular mechanism. There is strong circumstantial evidence that the common cause of the disease is microembolism due to failure of the pulmonary filtration of circulating debris, including fat (James 1982). Neuropathologists have observed that the late lesion of acute fat embolism is indistinguishable from the acute lesions of MS (Scheinker 1943; Courville 1959; Sevitt 1962; Lumsden 1970). The same focal lesion results from microbubble damage to the blood-brain barrier in decompression sickness (Hills & James 1991). However, other mechanisms may also cause focal breakdown of the barrier which is associated with edema, and inflammatory cell invasion. Magnetic resonance spectroscopy has shown a lactate peak in acute new lesions, indicating a failure of oxygen delivery (Miller et al 1991).

Rationale for HBO Therapy

The focal edema that characterizes lesions typical of MS inevitably increases the diffusion distance for oxygen and provides a sound rationale for increasing the oxygen concentration of the plasma under hyperbaric conditions. This increases the gradient for transfer into the tissue. The caliber of the cerebral vasculature is related to the oxygen tension of the perfusing blood and the blood-brain barrier is oxygen dependent. The effectiveness of HBO in the reduction of global cerebral edema has been demonstrated by direct measurement in man (Sukoff & Ragatz 1982) and Rockswold et al (1992) have shown that HBO reduces the mortality of severe head injury by 50%. In 1986 Neubauer et al showed the effect of HBO on the edema associated with MS (Figure 21.1). They found that one or more lesions shown on MRI disappeared in 11 of 35 patients (31.4%) after 1 hour of treatment, which suggests that it is the resolution of focal edema that accounts for the improvement.

Administering oxygen under hyperbaric conditions allows a substantial increase of plasma oxygen tension despite paradoxically reducing blood flow and this improves the gradient for oxygen transport to tissue enabling the relief of severe tissue hypoxia and resumption of normal aerobic metabolism in acute areas affected by the disease process. However, it also reduces inflammation by downregulating the transcriptional protein hypoxia-inducible factor 1α (HIF 1α). This protein, which is continually produced by every cell is normally destroyed by the action of the Von Hippel Landau protein (VHL). Falling oxygen levels reduces the production of VHL leading to an increase in the level

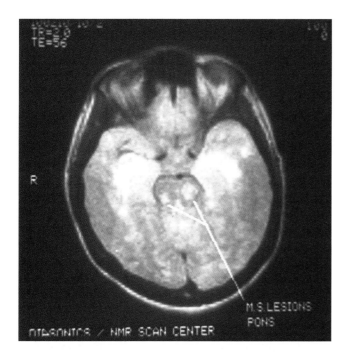

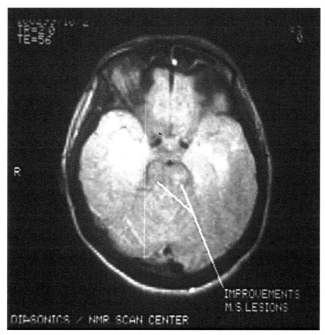

Figure 21.1a (above)
Magnetic resonance image of a patient with MS showing two large lesions in the pons.

Figure 21.1b (below)
Image after oxygen treatment showing improvement of the lesions (Illustrations courtesy of Dr. Robert Kagan, MRI Scan Center, Fort Lauderdale, Florida).

of HIF α, which in turn upregulates the inflammatory response. This is valuable as a short-term response when tissue is infected as it ensures neutrophil attraction to the area, but is misdirected in the aseptic inflammation which results from the localized BBB breakdown in MS.

A second, recently described, mechanism likely to contribute to the repair of focal areas of damage in the nervous system is the release of stem cells by HBO treatment. A course of 20 sessions at 2 ATA 5 days a week for a month in patients undergoing HBOT for complications of treatment for head and neck cancer increases circulating stem cells eight-fold (Thom *et al*, 2006).

When natural remission occurs in MS, the critical factor in barrier and tissue repair in the CNS is the availability of tissue oxygen. The driving force to increase the delivery to the tissue is the plasma oxygen tension. A mild disturbance of the barrier may simply increase the water content of the nervous tissue, but more severe failure is associated with the extravasation of plasma constituents, including proteins into the extracellular space and thence to neural tissue. This degree of barrier failure primarily causes damage to myelin. The most severe form of BBB failure is associated with perivascular extravasation of red blood cells and tissue necrosis.

Using the animal model *experimental allergic encephalomyelitis* (EAE), Warren *et al* (1978) showed that daily HBO completely suppresses the development of paralytic disease in rodents for at least 34 days. Prockop and Grasso (1978) also found amelioration of EAE in guinea pigs. Hansbrough *et al* (1980) demonstrated that HBO is immunosuppressive in mice. Abbot *et al* (1994) showed that the inflammation produced by the tuberculin reaction in man can be associated with a developing tissue hypoxia that results from edema limiting the rate of oxygen flux at a time when the area is being invaded by highly metabolically active cells.

Clinical Trials of HBO in Multiple Sclerosis

Boschetty and Cernoch (1970) were the first to report the use of HBO in MS patients. In 26 patients they used two 30 min sessions at 2 ATA daily for 10–20 days. Symptomatic improvement occurred in 15 but was of limited duration. Baixe (1978) compared the symptoms of MS to those of decompression sickness and reported favorable results in 11 patients. Neubauer (1978) independently confirmed the effect when, in 1975, he used HBO for a patient with osteomyelitis who was also suffering from MS. The course of HBO markedly improved the patient's neurological symptoms. Italian reports (Pallotta *et al* 1980a; Formai *et al* 1980) also described a beneficial effect and some longer term studies were undertaken.

These uncontrolled studies influenced the design and execution of the first randomized, placebo-controlled, double-blind study by Fischer *et al* (1983). They studied only patients with a low Kurtzke disability score – KDS

(Kurtzke 1961) and matched patients in the experimental and control groups according to age, sex, age at onset of the disease, duration and type of disease, and disability before randomization. It was shown that at 2 ATA once a day for 90 min, 5 days a week to a total of 20 treatments, objective improvement in mobility, fatigue, balance and bladder function occurred in 12 of 17 patients ($p < 0.0001$). Those patients having a less severe form of the disease had a more favorable and long lasting response. In contrast, only 1 out of 20 placebo-treated patients showed a positive change. After one year, with no further treatment the treated patients had deteriorated less than the controls ($p < 0.0008$). The authors appreciated the necessity for further studies, particularly in the treatment of acute attacks and the effect of long-term treatment.

This was the first double-blind controlled study and has provided a standard against which other studies should be compared and indeed no other trial has been undertaken in this way. It also set several unfortunate precedents. It used a fixed pressure (2 ATA), limited the number of sessions to 20, and did not employ continuation therapy. The blood-gas measurements indicated that oxygen breathed from a mask gave an effective average alveolar paO_2 of 998 mmHg or 1.3 ATA with a range of 1.1 to 1.5 ATA. Most other studies have been undertaken at 2.0 ATA or more with arterial oxygen tensions in the range equal or greater than 1.8. to 1.9 ATA. There is good evidence that the reduction in vessel caliber in the lesions of chronic MS will make patients more sensitive to the vasoconstriction induced by oxygen. Holbach *et al* (1972) have produced evidence that the optimal inspired partial pressure of oxygen in the injured brain of stroke patients is about 1.75 ATA.

Subsequent trials have been of variable quality and have used patients with very long disease duration and often with stable disabilities. They have been extensively reviewed by Gottlieb and Neubauer (1988). Barnes *et al* (1985), after dismissing HBO therapy on the basis of preliminary findings, despite overall significance ($p < 0.01$), called for further studies in their final report (Barnes *et al* 1987). Their follow-up of patients who received HBO showed that the bladder improvement present after one month of treatment ($p < 0.03$) was maintained for 6 months without additional treatment. After a year there was less deterioration in cerebellar function compared to controls ($p < 0.05$). Wiles *et al* (1986), in the second UK study, recorded objective improvement in bladder function in their most severely affected patients under controlled conditions ($p < 0.03$) using cystometry.

Two controlled studies have reported sustained benefit with follow-on treatment. Oriani *et al* (1990) used patients with a low KDS disability score and compared 22 controls with 22 patients treated each week for a year. They detected an appreciable difference in outcome ($p < 0.01$). Pallotta *et al* (1986) followed 22 patients for 8 years. All received an initial course of 20 HBO treatments, and 11 were treated

thereafter with 2 exposures every 20 days. The frequency of relapses decreased dramatically in the prolonged treatment group whereas they gradually increased in the group which received only an initial course of treatment (Figure 21.2).

Following these reports, patients established a charity now known as *The Federation of Multiple Sclerosis Treatment Centers*, and they have installed multiplace HBO facilities throughout the United Kingdom (Figure 21.3).

The problems associated with the evaluation of any treatment for MS are widely appreciated. Dr. George Schumacher (1974), a former chairman of the International Federation of Multiple Sclerosis Societies, considered that MS does not readily lend itself to double-blind studies because of the unpredictable fluctuation of signs and symptoms. He believed that the best experimental design for investigating the effectiveness of a therapeutic regime is a longitudinal one involving large numbers of patients who serve as their own controls. He suggested that the sole criterion of efficacy should be the arrest of further downhill progression in an overwhelming majority of patients over a two year period, a view now supported by the fact that only long term studies have shown persistent benefits from HBO.

Since 1982 the Federation have treated over 14,000 patients and more than 1,500,000 individual exposures have been administered without significant incident. They are therefore in a unique position to evaluate the effectiveness of prolonged courses of HBO in a considerable number of patients over 10 or more years.

Seven hundred and three patients were followed in detail since first receiving treatment (Table 21.1).

They breathed oxygen from a face mask in a chamber compressed with air. Five daily treatments of one hour were given at 1.25 ATA. If two or more symptoms improved, a course of twenty treatments in 4 weeks was completed at this pressure. Otherwise the pressure was raised in weekly increments of 0.25 ATA until a response was obtained or five treatments at 2.0 ATA had no effect. Thereafter the patients were invited to return for a "follow-on" treatment on a weekly basis, or failing that, as often as they felt the need or found it possible.

Table 21.1
Patients Recruited to the Study

	Females	Males	Total
	464 = 66%	239 = 34%	703
Mean age years (range)	47 (20–70)	47 (19–73)	
Average duration of MS	14 (0–54)	15 (0–50)	
Diagnosis confirmed by a neurologist.		670 = 95%	
MS Type			
Relapsing/Remitting	126 = 18%	41 = 6%	167
Chronic Progressive	262 = 37%	155 = 22%	417
Relapsing/Remitting	76 = 11%	43 = 6%	119

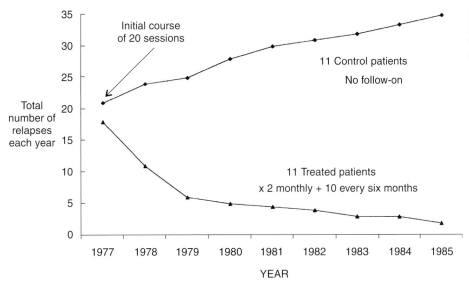

Figure 21.2
Incidence of relapses in 22 patients with and without regular HBO treatment, followed for 8 years. From Pallotta *et al* (1986), with permission.

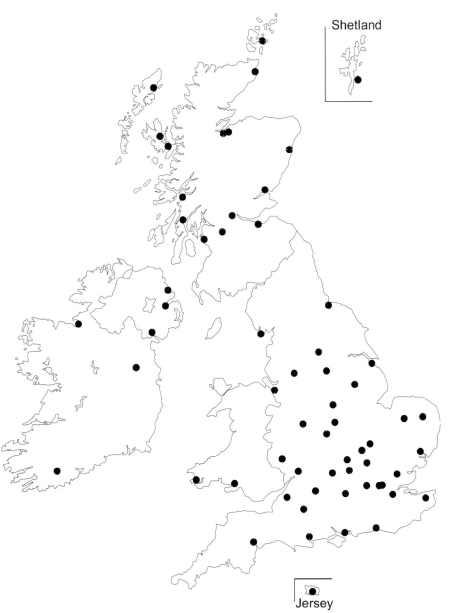

Figure 21.3
The location of the Centers.

Table 21.2
The Patients Assessment of Symptomatic Response to the Initial Course

	n	Improved %	No change %	Worse %
Fatigue	567	70	22	8
Speech	187	64	34	1
Balance	562	59	37	4
Bladder	523	68	30	0
Walking	638	77	19	4

Table 21.3
Urinary Frequency of 523 Patients – Before and After the Initial Course

	Before initial course $\bar{x}$		After initial course $\bar{x}$		Improvement
Frequency					
– at night	1232	2.4	651	1.2	47%
– during the day	3873	7.4	2960	5.7	24%

Patients were interviewed and assessed immediately before the initial course when the MS Type and the KDS were determined. A further assessment was made immediately after the initial course of 20 daily treatments. About 70% of patients obtained relief of two or more symptoms (Table 21.2)

The bladder improvements observed in other studies were confirmed (Tables 21.2 and 21.3).

In general, the response was better in patients with less advanced disease. Lower pressures than those used by others were found to be effective, while the initial response was found to be an unreliable guide to the outcome of prolonged treatment.

Further assessments were made between two and four years, and again between six and eight years after the initial course (Perrins & James 1994). They suggested that the initial improvements were being maintained by regular treatment (Table 21.4).

A third survey was conducted between ten and fourteen years. By now 126 patients had died (8% were over 60 years old when first treated), 99 had become "lost to follow up," 29 had suffered injuries that affected their Kurtzke value and 2 had had their original diagnosis revised; 447 patients therefore remained for an assessment (Table 21.5). This shows that 103 (23%) were no worse after regular treatment for 10–14 years. Even more remarkable are the 30 patients (7%) who have actually improved.

An analysis reveals that about 300 treatments in 10 + years (about one treatment a fortnight) are required to retard the progression of Relapsing/Remitting patients, while more than 500 treatments (say, once a week) are more effective (Figure 21.4).

Very long-term double-blind controlled studies are not possible as patients do not comply with their allocation. However it is possible to compare groups of patients who have received different treatment regimes (Figure 21.5). The importance of regular treatment is shown at all points examined.

Although there is wide variation in the rate and pattern of decline, the majority of MS patients deteriorate over a two year period of observation (Schumacher 1974). In this study the five Relapsing/Remitting patients who had less than 10 follow-on treatments had deteriorated by 2.0 on the KDS after 10 + years, while the 31 who received more than 400 had only deteriorated by 1.1 ($p \leq 0.001$). This represents a difference of being able to walk without assistance and the need to use two sticks, or the ability to walk 200 m and being confined to a wheelchair.

A search of the records has revealed 1384 patients who

Table 21.4
Specific Abilities Regained After Initial Course and Maintained 2 or 4 Years Later

n = 703	After the initial course %	With 0–27 treatments in 2 years after the initial course %	With 1–104 treatments in 4th year %
Brushing teeth	39	26	20
Doing up buttons	81	54	40
Threading a needle	50	34	29
Holding a cup	54	46	23
Brushing hair	48	33	26
Fastening brassiere	25	22	11
Cutting up food	36	11	18
Shaving	30	11	18

Abilities
Regained 67% of 410   Maintained 73% of 276

Table 21.5
Patients Who Were No Worse After Regular Treatment for 10–14 Years

447 patients	112 Relapsing/ Remitting	259 Chronic Progressive	76 Chronic Static	Total
Improved	14 (13%)	12 (5%)	4 (5%)	30 (7%)
Unchanged	23 (21%)	31 (12%)	19 (25%)	73 (16%)
No worse	37 = 33%	43 = 17%	23 = 30%	103 = 23%
Mean no. of treatments	*338*	*257*	*266*	

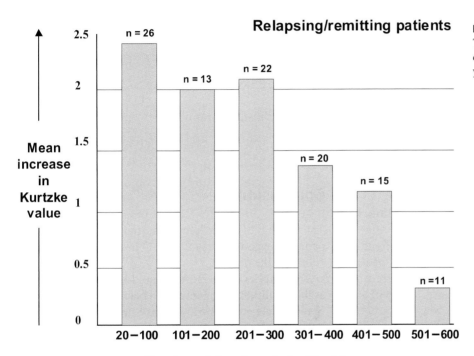

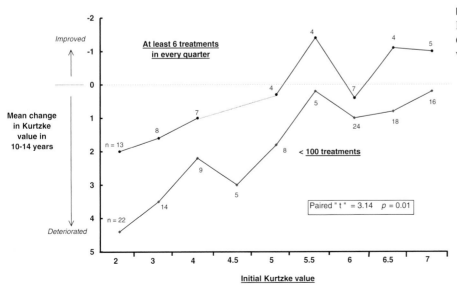

Figure 21.4
The mean change in Kurtzke value related to the number of treatments in 10–14 years.

Figure 21.5
Patients, of all types, who received at least 6 treatments in every quarter versus those with less than 100 in 10–14 years.

Table 21.6
117 Patients Who Have Attended Regularly for 5–17 Years

Years attended	No. of patients	MS type	Average difference in Kurtzke value	Average no. of treatments
5–10	13	Relapsing/Remitting	.6	351
	19	Chronic Progressive	1	323
	2	Chronic Static	.75	248
10–15	17	Relapsing/Remitting	1	464
	24	Chronic Progressive	.8	523
	8	Chronic Static	.5	488
> 14	12	Relapsing/Remitting	0	466
	16	Chronic Progressive	1	494
	6	Chronic Static	2	664
Total	117			

were first treated 17 or more years ago and 104 (11%) are still attending for regular treatment. The fate of 117 patients who have been attending regularly without interruption for 5 to 17 years are shown in Table 21.6. It is noteworthy that between and 15 years the Kurtzke value has not increased by more than 1 point.

The treatment, as administered by the Federation, has been shown to be practicable and cost-effective. After 10 or more years 38% of the 447 patients were still attending regularly. There were no side effects. The cost of each HBO treatment is about the same as for a haircut, so that relief may be obtained for less than £300 (US$ 450) a year.

Many patients continue to attend as their symptoms, particularly frequency of micturition, are only controlled by regular attendance. Some arrange their holidays so as to be near a Center. Some patients have difficulty in reaching a Center and are so dependent on regular treatment that they have installed monoplace chambers in their own homes.

Conclusions

The findings of all the long-term studies of established MS patients suggest that regular HBO favorably influences the course of the disease.

This implies that treatment should be instigated as soon as the condition is diagnosed and before irreversible lesions have become established (Perrins & James 2005). As might be expected, the response has been shown to be better in patients with less advanced disease and is related to the frequency and continuity of treatment. The social and economic advantages to be gained from regular and prolonged treatment are obvious. There are no side effects.

22 HBO in the Management of Cerebral Palsy

Paul Harch, Richard A. Neubauer[†], and Virginia Neubauer

Cerebral palsy is a chronic neurological disorder that can be due to several causes of brain damage in utero, in the perinatal period, or postnatally. Hyperbaric oxygen has been shown to be useful in treating children with cerebral palsy. This topic is discussed under following headings:

Causes of Cerebral Palsy

The term *cerebral palsy* (CP) covers a group of nonprogressive, but often changing, motor impairment syndromes secondary to lesions or anomalies of the brain arising in the early stages of development. Between 20 to 25 of every 10,000 live-born children in the Western world have the condition (Stanley *et al* 2000). Problems may occur in utero, perinatal, and postnatal. Infections, traumatic brain injury, near-drowning and strokes in children suffering from neurological problems come under the heading of cerebral palsy. Diagnosis of cerebral palsy resulting from in utero or early perinatal causes may be made immediately after birth, but more commonly occurs between 15 and 24 months. It is possible that CP may be misdiagnosed for years because specific symptoms may show up very late in childhood. Some of the possible causes of CP and are listed in Table 22.1.

Although several antepartum causes have been described for CP, the role of intrapartum asphyxia in neonatal encephalopathy and seizures in term infants is not clear. There is no evidence that brain damage occurs before birth. A study using brain MRI or post-mortem examination was conducted in 351 full-term infants with neonatal encephalopathy, early seizures, or both to distinguish between lesions acquired antenatally and those that developed in the intrapartum and early postpartum period (Cowan *et al* 2003). Infants with major congenital malformations or obvious chromosomal disorders were excluded. Brain images showed evidence of an acute insult without established injury or atrophy in (80%) of infants with neonatal encephalopathy and evidence of perinatal asphyxia. Although the results cannot exclude the possibility that antenatal or genetic factors might predispose some infants to perinatal brain injury, the data strongly suggest that events in the immediate perinatal period are most important in neonatal brain injury. These findings are important from management point of view as HBO therapy in the perinatal period may be of value in preventing the evolution of cerebral palsy.

Oxygen Therapy in the Neonatal Period

Following World War II, oxygen tents and incubators were introduced, and premature infants were given supplementary oxygen to improve their chances of survival, with levels up to 70% being given for extended periods. Epidemics of blindness due to retrolental fibroplasia followed in the 1950s, which led to a restriction of the level of supplemental oxygen to 40%. A reduction in the incidence of blindness followed, which appeared to confirm the involvement of oxygen in the development of the retinopathy. The link between the use of recurrent supplemental oxygen and the rise of retinopathy was rapidly accepted,

---

Table 22.1
Some Causes of Cerebral Palsy

Prenatal causes
Amniotic fluid embolus
Anoxia due to cord strangulation
Cerebrovascular accident in utero
Inadequate prenatal care
Maternal abdominal injury during pregnancy
Maternal cardiovascular disorders complicating pregnancy
Maternal drug or alcohol abuse or other toxicity (thalidomide, carbon monoxide)
Maternal infections, i.e., rubella, toxoplasmosis, herpes simplex, syphilis, cytomegalovirus
Maternal metabolic and endocrine disorders, i.e., diabetes, hyperthyroidism
Mitochondrial disruptions
Premature placental separation
Rh sensitization
Underdeveloped (low weight) fetus

Perinatal causes
Cerebrovascular accident at birth
Mechanical respiratory obstruction
Premature delivery, complications of delivery, low birth weight, respiratory distress
Trauma during labor/delivery, hemorrhage, use of forceps, breech delivery

Acquired cerebral palsy as a sequel of:
Anoxic ischemic encephalopathy resultant from near-drowning, near hanging, near-electrocution, cardiac arrest, etc.
Brain tumors
Infections of the nervous system: meningitis, encephalitis, brain abscess
Neurological complications of vaccination
Thrombosis or hemorrhage of the brain
Traumatic brain injury including shaken baby syndrome
Uncontrolled high fever

---

even though it was suggested that retrolental fibroplasia was produced by initially preconditioning a child to an enriched oxygen environment and then suddenly withdrawing the same: The disease occurred only after the child's removal from the high oxygen environment (Szewczyk 1951). It was also noted that retinopathy developed upon the withdrawal from the high level of oxygen, and that probably the best thing to do was to return the child to the oxygen environment (Forrester 1964). Under these circumstances, in many of the patients, the results were encouraging, and vision returned to normal. A slow reduction of oxygen and final return to the atmospheric concentration for several weeks was all that was needed to restore the vision. Thus, there is no rational basis for withholding oxygen therapy in the neonatal period. As mentioned in other chapters of this textbook, retrolental fibroplasia is not associated with HBO. Recent evidence in both animals and humans of HBO therapy in the neonatal period reinforces the concept that tonic exposure to elevated levels of oxygen with rapid withdrawal to more normal levels is responsible for retinopathy of prematurity, not the absolute level of oxygen exposure (see Chapter 32). Using both normal rats and a rat model of cerebral palsy, Calvert showed that doses of HBO as high as 3.0 ATA for 1 hour had no structural effect on the retina and showed no evidence of retinal neovascularization (Calvert et al 2004). In 60 neonates with hypoxic-ischemic encephalopathy a daily exposure to 1.4, 1.5, or 1.6 ATA HBO improved serum antioxidant levels, neurobehavioral scores, and decreased lipid peroxidation, while causing no retinal damage (Zhou et al 2008).

It is unfortunate that nearly all affected newborns today are deprived of appropriate oxygen therapy because of the fear that it will cause retrolental fibroplasia (see Chapter 32). Some observations indicate that since the practice of administration of high levels of oxygen has been abandoned, there is a rise in the incidence of cerebral palsy as compared to previous levels.

Treatment of Cerebral Palsy with HBO

The use of hyperbaric oxygenation in the pediatric patient was relatively common in Russia (see Chapter 29). HBO has been used in Russia for resuscitation in respiratory failure, for cranial birth injuries, and for hemolytic disease of the newborn. HBO was reported to reduce high serum bilirubin levels and prevent development of neurological disorders. In cases of respiratory distress, delayed use of HBO (12–48 h after birth) was considered useless. However, early use (1–3 h after birth) led to recovery in 75% of cases. The Italian physicians began treating the small fetus in utero in 1988 demonstrating a reduction of cerebral damage. Patients were hospitalized before the 35th week and hyperbaric treatments were given every 2 weeks for 40 min at 1.5. The fetal biophysical profile showed a remarkable improvement as soon as the second treatment.

Early use of HBO for neonatal resuscitation has been extensively used in China. A recent review of 20 randomized or quasirandomized controlled trials for HBO in HIE revealed a near uniformity of results. While the trials did not use rigorous methodology the reproducible findings were a reduction in mortality and improvement in neurological sequaelae, which are consistent with the results of animal studies (Liu et al 2006).

In the chronic phase, literature has been accumulating since 1989 for a beneficial effect of HBO in CP. At the conference "New Horizons for Hyperbaric Oxygenation" in Orlando, Florida, in 1989, results were presented of HBO therapy of 230 CP patients who had been treated in the early stages since 1985 in Sao Palo, Brazil (Machado 1989). Treatment consisted of 20 sessions of 1 h each at 1.5 ATA (100% oxygen), once or twice daily in a Vickers

monoplace chamber. A few of the children had exacerbation of seizures or developed seizures. The results showed significant reduction of spasticity: 50% reduction in spasticity was reported in 94.78% of the patients. Twelve patients (5.21%) remained unchanged. However, follow-up included only 82 patients, and 62 of these (75.6%) had lasting improvement in spasticity and improved motor control. The parents reported positive changes in balance and "intelligence with reduced frequency of seizure activity." Results of a continuation of this work in Brazil were presented by in 2001 at the 2nd International Symposium on Hyperbaric Oxygenation and the Brain Injured Child held in Boca Raton, Florida, to include 2,030 patients suffering from childhood chronic encephalopathy that had been treated since 1976, 232 of whom were evaluated with long-term follow-up; age ranged from 1 to 34 years. The improvements were noted as follows: 41.81% decreased spasticity, 18% noted global motor coordination improvement. Improvements were also noted in attention: 40.08%, memory, 10.77%, comprehension, 13.33%, reasoning, 5.60%, visual perception, 12.93%, sphincter control, 6.46%. It was concluded from this study that HBO therapy should be instituted as early as possible in such cases.

Another presentation at the 2nd International Symposium was a study by Chavdarov, Director of the Specialized Hospital for Residential Treatment for Rehabilitation of Children with Cerebral Palsy in Sofia, Bulgaria, where HBO had been considered an important part of the management of children with CP since 1997. This study included 50 children with distribution of various types as follows: spastic CP (n = 30), ataxic/hypotonic cerebral palsy (n = 8), and mixed cerebral palsy (n = 12). Measurements included motor ability, mental ability, functional development, and speech. Overall psycho-motor function (single or combined) improved in 86% of the patients following 20 HBO sessions at 1.5–1.7ATA lasting 40–50 min once daily.

The first North American case of CP treated with HBO was in 1992. The case was presented by Paul Harch at the Undersea and Hyperbaric Medical Society meeting in 1994 (Harch 1994). In 1995, Richard Neubauer began treating CP using HBO. Because of the growing worldwide anecdotal reports, a small pilot study of HBO therapy in cerebral palsy children was conducted in the UK in 1995, which showed similar improvements in a group of seriously brain-injured children and led to the foundation of the Hyperbaric Oxygen Trust, a charity to treat CP and the brain-injured children. The Trust, which has since changed its name to Advance, had treated over 350 patients, through 2003 though no scientific appraisals have been published. Positive anecdotal reports of its use in cerebral palsy started to accumulate. As more HBO treatment clinics for CP opened in the United States and Canada, further studies were conducted.

Published Clinical Trials

In 1999 the first pilot study in the use of HBO in CP was published (Montgomery *et al* 1999). This study involved 23 children (10 female, 15 male; age range 3.1 to 8.2 years) with spastic diplegia. Absence of previous surgical or medical therapy for spasticity was one of the prerequisites for inclusion as well as a 12-month clinical physiotherapy plateau. The study was performed at McGill University Hospital's Cleghorn Hyperbaric Laboratory in a monoplace chamber at 1.75 ATA (95% oxygen) for 60 min daily and at the Rimouski Regional Hospital in a multiplace chamber (60 min at 1.75 ATA twice daily) for 20 treatments in total. Assessments, pre- and post-treatment, included gross motor function measurement (GMFM), fine motor function assessment (Jebsen's Hand Test), spasticity assessment (Modified Ashworth Spasticity Scale) as well as parent questionnaire and video analysis. Results following treatment were an average of 5.3% improvement in GMFM and a notable absence of complications or clinical deterioration in any of the children. "Cognitive changes" were observed, but these were nonspecific. Video analysis was also positive. The obvious flaws of this study were the lack of placebo control and the application of two different HBO protocols. The assessment tools utilized also had inherent variations. Montgomery achieved improvement in CP children using 20 treatments at 1.66 ATA oxygen (1.75 ATA 95% O2)/60 min), but the children experienced rapid regression of neurological gains after cessation of treatment. The number of treatments was inadequate as the authors of this chapter had recommended 40 treatments at 1.5 ATA/60 min, because consolidation of the gains does not occur until 30 to 35 treatments. This first study, however, provided useful data regarding the potential efficacy of HBO therapy and provided the justification for a larger controlled, randomized study.

The results of just such a prospective, hyperbaric-air controlled, randomized multicenter study have been published "with intriguing results" (Collet *et al* 2001). This study included 111 CP children (ages 3–12 years) that were randomized into two groups: receiving either 1.75 ATA 100% oxygen or 1.3 ATA room air (the equivalent of 28% oxygen at 1 ATA) for 1 h for a total of 40 treatments. Gross and fine-motor function, memory, speech, language, and memory were assessed. Improvement in global motor function was 3% in the hyperbaric air group and 2.9% in the hyperbaric-oxygen-treated group. Although the results were statistically similar in both groups, the HBO-treated group had a more rapid response rate in the more severely disabled children. Cognitive testing was performed on a subset of the preceding study to investigate the effect of HBO on cognitive status of children with CP (Hardy *et al* 2002). Of the 111 children diagnosed with CP (aged 4 to 12 years), only 75 were suitable for neuropsychological testing, assessing attention, working memory, processing speed, and psychosocial functioning. The children received

40 sessions of HBO or sham treatment over a 2-month period. Children in the active-treatment group were exposed for 1 h to 100% oxygen at 1.75 atmospheres absolute (ATA), whereas the sham group received only air at 1.3 ATA. Children in both groups showed better self-control and significant improvements in auditory attention and visual working memory compared with the baseline. However, no statistical difference was found between the two treatments. Furthermore, the sham group improved significantly on eight dimensions of the Conners' Parent Rating Scale, whereas the active treatment group improved only on one dimension. Most of these positive changes persisted for 3 months. No improvements were observed in either group for verbal span, visual attention, or processing speed. Unfortunately, the Collet study increased the pressure to 1.75 ATA of 100% oxygen for 60 min (40 treatments) and to 1.3 ATA in the control group breathing air for 60 min, i.e., a 30% increase in oxygen for the controls. This dose of HBO had not been used previously in CP patients and was possibly an overdose (Harch 2001) and likely inhibited the HBO group's gains. Evidence for this was seen in the GMFM data where five of the six scores increased in the HBO group from immediate post HBO testing to the 3-month retest versus three of six scores in the controls. Some of the negative effects of 1.75 ATA likely had worn off by this time. Results of the Collet study showed significant improvements in both groups, but no difference between groups. The serendipitous flaw in the study was the 1.3 ATA air control group, which also improved significantly. This underscored the fact that the ideal dose of HBO is unknown in chronic pediatric brain injury, but it suggested that oxygen signaling may occur at very low pressures. Mild HBO therapy can be effective in improving SPECT as well as attention and reaction times (Heuser & Uszler 2001). Therefore, the beneficial effect in patients described by Collet and colleagues is probably related to the beneficial effects of slightly pressurized air rather than to the act of participating in the study. In addition a biphasic sham pressurization, which is highly recommended for a control group, was not used in this study. The duration of this study was only 2 months. Perhaps this length of time is not sufficient for evaluating neuropsychological effects of HBO in a chronic neurological condition.

The controversy regarding this study will undoubtedly take a long time to resolve, but it has already begun to raise some very important issues and some very important questions about the validity of "mild" HBO (1.3–1.35 ATA air or the same pressure supplemented with oxygen concentrator). The first issue is that 1.3 ATA ambient air was not an inert or true placebo, but had a real effect on the partial pressure of blood gases and perhaps other physiological effects as well. Compressed air at 1.3 ATA increases the plasma oxygen tension from 12.7 kPa (95 mmHg) to 19.7 kPa (148 mmHg), and the increase of a concentration of a reactive substrate by 50% is substantially notable. Rather than answer the question of effectiveness of HBO in CP the Collet study and its offspring Hardy (2002) substudy confused the scientific community not familiar with hyperbaric oxygen. The unequivocal finding of these studies is that both pressure protocols achieved statistically significant objective neurocognitive gains, a phenomenon that cannot be attributed to placebo. This reinforced the findings of the other noncontrolled studies in the chronic category above, and was strengthened by the studies using functional brain imaging as surrogate markers (Harch 1994a, Neubauer 2001, and Golden et al 2002).

The United States Army Study on Adjunctive HBO Treatment of Children with Cerebral Anoxic Injury

Shortly after the previous studies were begun, physicians at the US Army base in Fort Augusta, Georgia conducted a small study on functional outcomes in children with anoxic brain injury. Baseline and serial evaluations showed improvement in gross motor function and total time necessary for custodial care in nine children with CP. Eight volunteer (parental) subjects with varying degrees of CP and one near-drowning victim were included in this investigation. Of the CP cases studied, the mean age was 6.4 years (range 1.0–16.5 years), and the near drowning patient was 5.6 years of age seen 1 year post incident. Pretreatment evaluation included gross motor function (GMPM, lying, rolling, crawling and kneeling, sitting, standing and walking, running, and jumping), the Modified Ashworth Scale (MAS) for spasticity, rigidity, flexion/extension, the Functional Independence Measure for Children (WeeFIM) regarding self-care, sphincter control, transfers, locomotion, communication and social cognition, video, 24-h time measure, parental questionnaire, and single photon emission computerized tomography (SPECT) scanning. Testing was conducted every 20 treatments with the exception of SPECT and parental questionnaire which were completed at 40 and 80 sessions.

All subjects received 80 HBO treatments in a multiplace chamber (100% oxygen) at 1.70 ATA (60 min for each session) daily (Monday to Friday) for 4 months. Each patient served as his or her own control as compared to the baseline scores. Improvements in GMFM in the categories of lying and rolling, crawling and walking, sitting and walking, running and jumping were statistically significant (p < 0.05). The total time necessary for parental care also showed a statistically significant improvement (p < 0.03%) in reduction of custodial time required. In the parental questionnaire, overall improvement was indicated through the end of the study, including other assessments not included in the survey. Three children demonstrated improved swallowing function and were able to ingest a variety of liquids and foods; there was reduction in strabismus in two subjects, nystagmus was resolved in one participant, and one patient experienced complete resolution of a grade 3 vesi-

coureteral reflux, obviating the need for surgery. Unfortunately, the SPECT scan results were omitted due to multiple technical and procedural problems.

Overall improvement was 26.7% at 30 treatments, up to 58.1% at 80 treatments. Their conclusions were that HBO therapy seemed to effect overall improvement in CP (with little response in the near-drowning case), although the optimum number of treatments remained undetermined, since the improvements were noted at the end of the study. They advised further research and follow-up studies to determine the true potential of HBO for children with anoxic injury and CP.

The Indian Study of HBOT in CP

Based on multiple previous studies Drs. Sethi and Mukherjee in New Delhi conducted a randomized prospective trial of HBOT in CP (Sethi & Mukherjee 2003). Thirty subjects were randomly assigned to either standard occupational (OT) and physical therapy (PT) or HBO plus OT/PT. Children 2–5 years old with all types of CP were included and had a SPECT scan showing presence of recoverable penumbra. HBO patients received 40 HBO treatments at 1.75 ATA/60 minutes 6 days/week. Gross motor ability was measured using Norton's Basic Motor Evaluation Scale. While both groups improved significantly, the improvement in the HBO group was greater.

Unpublished Studies

The Cornell Study

Upon the urging of interested parents, Dr. Maureen Packard of Cornell University in New York City agreed to perform such a study. This study was randomized to immediate and delayed (6 months later) treatment with HBO (the delayed treatment group to serve as an untreated control group). Age range was 15 months to 5 years with moderate to severe CP and patients were given 40 1-h sessions at 1.5 ATA, once a day, 5 days a week for 4 weeks. The study population included 26 children with cerebral palsy secondary to prenatal insults, premature birth, birth asphyxia, and post-natal hemorrhage. The average age of enrollment was 30 months. Nine patients presented with cortical visual impairment. Assessment was neurodevelopmental, Bayley II (cognitive), Preschool Language Scale, Peabody Motor Scale, Pediatric Evaluation of Disabilities Inventory (PEDI), parental report of specific skills including mobility, self-care and social interaction. Final assessments were available on 20 subjects. The only side effects of the study were barotrauma in nine children requiring placement of a ventilation tube or myringotomy.

Assessments were performed at four time points: enrollment (T1), after the immediate group had received treatment (T2), prior to the delayed groups' HBO therapy 5 months after enrollment (T3), and after the delayed groups' treatment (T4). There was a significant difference (p < 0.05) in the improvement of scores on the mobility sub-domains for the time period T2 minus T1 in favor of the immediately treated group. For the period T4 minus T3 there was a trend favoring the recently treated delayed group and a trend in the social function subdomain in the more recent treated group. Parental diaries over the month of treatments demonstrated 83% marked improvement in mobility, 43% marked increase in attention, and 39% marked increase in language skills. Overall, there was some improvement in mobility in 91%, in attention in 78%, in language in 87%, and in play in 52%. One family saw no improvement and six families minimal improvement for a total of 30%. Five families (22%) reported major gains in skills, and 11 families reported modest gains (48%). Four of the nine children with cortical visual impairment had improvement in vision noted by families, vision therapists, and ophthalmologists. There was no statistical difference in Peabody or Bayley II scores on blinded assessment.

Their conclusions at 6-month post-interview were that although changes in spasticity may diminish over time, improvements in attention, language and play were sustained. "'This increase in attention is particularly important for children must be aware' in order to learn. This represents a direct impact on cognitive functioning. The main differences between HBO and traditional therapies are the rapid gains over time and the impact on cognitive skills, which, in general are not improved by physical, occupational and speech therapies." Results of this study have been published (Waalkes *et al* 2002).

Additional Studies

Studies of the use of mild HBO, hyperbaric air, supplemental oxygen, and higher pressures of HBO must be continued to eventually determine the ultimate benefits for cerebral palsy and to identify the subgroups of patients who may benefit from each. At the 2003 3rd International Symposium on Hyperbaric Oxygenation and the Brain Injured Child, a variety of these studies were presented from around the world. While the studies were of varied design rigor, the results were similar, showing benefit of HBOT in CP, regardless of the lower dose of HBOT employed. The most significant study to date, however, reviewed both published and unpublished studies of HBO in CP and compared published studies using the Gross Motor Functional Measures (GMFM) in HBO to traditional accepted therapies that used the GMFM (Senechal *et al* 2007). Compared to intensive physical therapy, dorsal rhizotomy, strength training, electrical stimulation, intrathecal baclofen, family-centered functional therapy, equine therapy, Bobath physical therapy, and other types of physical therapy HBO showed faster and more impressive improvements. Moreover, HBO was the only therapy to improve cognition and language. This study alone refutes the errant conclusion of the Collet study that the improvement in both groups of children was due to a parent-participation effect. The parent-participation effect as well as other "placebo"-type effects such as surgery, is clearly present in every one of the studies and therapies reviewed by Senechal. Such a dramatic effect with HBOT that simultaneously improved cognition and language is consistent only with a biological cause-effect relationship of HBO

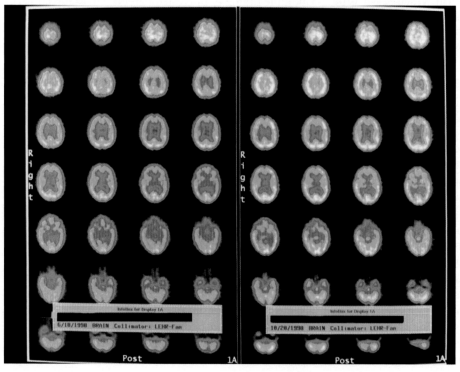

Figure 22.1
SPECT brain imaging transverse images of baseline pre-HBOT study on the left and after 80 HBO treatments on the right. Note the global increase in flow and change from heterogeneous to the more normal homogeneous pattern. Slices begin at the top of the head in the upper left corner and proceed to the base of the brain in the lower right corner of each study. Orientation is standard CT: the patient's left is on the viewer's right and vice versa with the patient's face at the top and the back of the head at the bottom of each image. Color scheme is white, yellow, orange, purple, blue, black from highest to lowest brain blood flow.

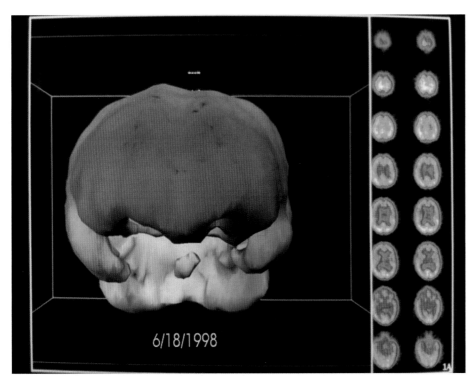

Figure 22.2
Three-dimensional reconstruction of baseline SPECT study in Figure 22.1 (study on left side). Note reduction in flow to both temporal lobes, inferior frontal lobes, and the brainstem (central round structure between the temporal lobes below the large colored area-frontal lobes).

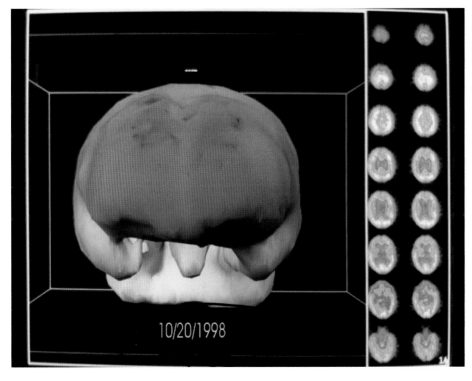

Figure 22.3
Three-dimensional reconstruction of SPECT after 80 HBO treatments (right hand study in Figure 22.1). Note the increased flow to the temporal lobes, inferior frontal lobes, and brainstem.

on CP and the entire brain, consistent with the total body immersion and effect of HBO in a chamber.

To date countless numbers of children with CP have been successfully treated with HBO worldwide. To the best of authors' knowledge no negative studies have been published. The medical and scientific community, however, continues to be misled by a misunderstanding of the science of HBO and its effects on chronic brain injury. In 2007, the scientific underpinning of HBO in chronic brain injury was partially elucidated in a study that represents the first ever improvement of chronic brain injury in animals (Harch *et al* 2007). This study demonstrated in a model of chronic traumatic brain injury that HBO could improve cognition and blood vessel density in a damaged hippocampus with a low pressure HBO protocol originally employed on chronic trauma, stroke, CP, and

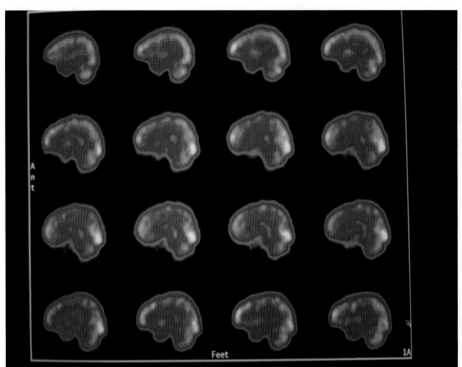

Figure 22.4
Sagittal slices of baseline SPECT brain imaging through the center of the brain. Note the heterogeneous pattern of blood flow. Slices proceed from the right side of the head in the upper left corner to the left side of the head in the lower right corner. The front of the brain (face) is on the left side and the back of the brain (back of the head) is on the right side of each slice.

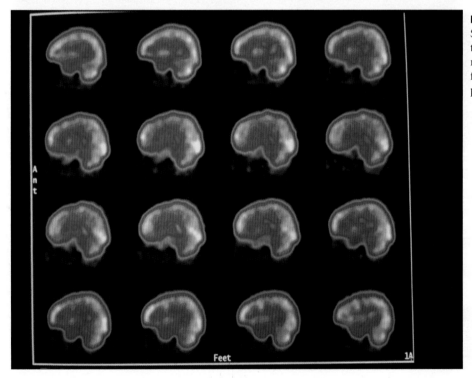

Figure 22.5
Sagittal slices of SPECT three hours after a single 1.5ATA/60 min HBO treatment. Note the generalized increase in flow and smoothing to a more normal pattern.

toxic brain injury patients in the early 1990s. The unusual nature of the study was its retrograde proofing of concept in animals after 18 years of clinical application of low-pressure HBO to chronic brain injury. Since HBO's effects on acute and chronic pathophysiology documented in this text and the scientific literature are generic effects that cross species boundaries, they can also be generalized to other types of chronic brain injury such as CP. Examples of the effect of HBO on brain blood flow and metabolism that is responsible for the observed clinical effects can be seen in the cases below from the Harch Hyperbaric Center in New Orleans.

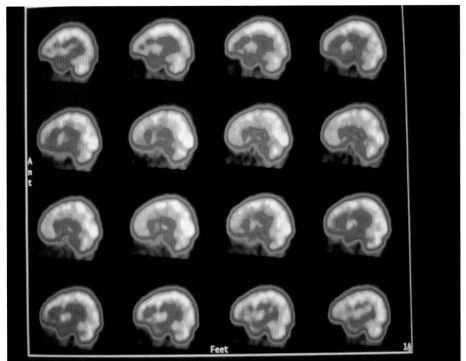

Figure 22.6
Sagittal slices of SPECT after 80 HBO treatments. Note the marked increase in flow and smoothing of the pattern compared to the baseline in Figure 22.4.

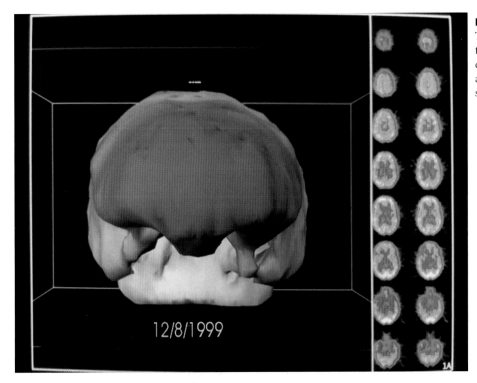

Figure 22.7
Three-dimensional surface reconstruction of SPECT in Figure 22.4. Note reduction in flow to the temporal lobes and coarse appearance of flow to the surface of the brain.

Case Reports

Patient 1: Cerebral Palsy

The patient is a 2-year-old boy whose twin died in utero at 14 weeks. He was delivered at term by vacuum extraction and developmental delay was detected at the age of 4–5 months. He was diagnosed as a case of cerebral palsy. At 2 years of age SPECT brain imaging was performed and showed a heterogeneous pattern of cerebral blood flow. The patient underwent a course of twice daily, 5 days/week HBO treatments in blocks of 50 and 30 treatments. At the conclusion of treatments he showed improvement in spasticity, speech, chewing/swallowing, cognition, and ability to sit in his car seat and stroller for prolonged periods. Repeat SPECT brain imaging showed a global improvement in

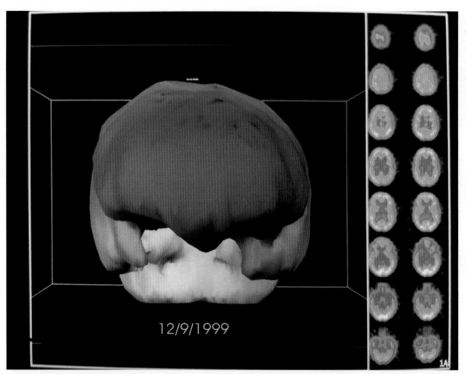

Figure 22.8
Three-dimensional surface reconstruction of SPECT in Figure 22.5. Note improvement in flow to the temporal lobes and slight smoothing of flow to the surface of the brain.

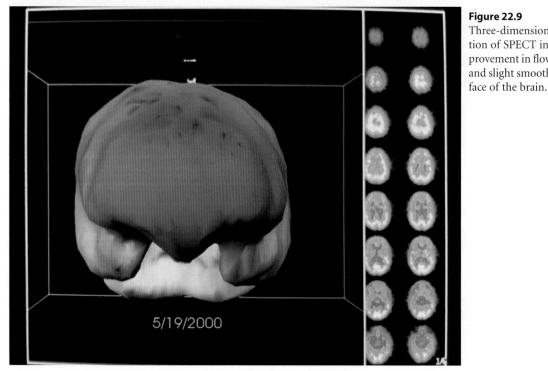

Figure 22.9
Three-dimensional surface reconstruction of SPECT in Figure 22.6. Note improvement in flow to the temporal lobes and slight smoothing of flow to the surface of the brain.

flow and smoothing to a more normal pattern consistent with the patient's overall clinical improvement. The two SPECT scans are shown side by side in Figure 22.1. Three-dimensional reconstructions of the two scans are shown in Figures 22.2 and 22.3.

Patient 2: Cerebral Palsy

The patient is an 8-year-old boy with a history of cerebral palsy. He had spastic diplegia secondary to premature birth from a mother with eclampsia. Patient was delivered by emergency Cesarean section at 27 weeks when his mother developed seizures. APGARS scores were 7 and 8. The patient spent 5 months in the hospital primarily because of feeding problems. The patient did not achieve normal milestones and developed infantile spasms at 2 years of age. Baseline SPECT brain imaging (Figure 22.4) showed a mildly/moderately heterogeneous pattern and reduction of blood flow. Three hours after a single HBO session at 1.5 ATA for 60 min, repeat SPECT showed global improvement and smoothing to a more normal pattern in Figure 22.5. The patient underwent a course of 80 HBO sessions (1.5 ATA/60 min) over the next 6 months in two blocks of treatment (twice daily, 5 days/week × 40, then once-daily 5 days/week × 40), and showed improvement in his impulsive inappropriate behavior, motor function, vision, and constipation. Repeat SPECT brain imaging reflected these neurological gains (Figure 22.6), showing generalized improvement in cerebral blood flow and pattern. Three-dimensional surface reconstruction of Figures 22.4, 22.5, and 22.6 are presented in Figures 22.7, 22.8, and 22.9, respectively. While there is a global increase in blood flow, the most significant relative increase in flow is to the temporal lobes as shown in the three-dimensional figures.

All SPECT brain imaging was performed on a Picker Prism 3000 at West Jefferson Medical Center. All scans were identically processed and three dimensional thresholds obtained by Phillip Tranchina. Pictures of the scans in the above figures were produced by 35 mm single frame photography under identical lighting and exposure conditions.

Conclusions

Cerebral palsy is the result of a large variety of causes, and it is difficult to design trials with subgroups of patients with similar pathomechanisms. The results of several studies have been presented including one controlled study that did not show improvement in neuropsychological status. A large number of patients have been treated, and some have been followed up for long periods to document improvement that can be correlated with imaging studies. Cognitive improvement is usually seen by the 40th treatment in patients with chronic neurological disorders such as CP (Golden *et al* 2002).

Controlled studies of HBO in CP should continue, but they may not resolve all the issues. The extensive experience of open clinical studies with some good results cannot be ignored. In a condition where there is nothing else to offer, HBO therapy is considered to be worth a trial. The concept of personalized medicine as described in Chapter 40 can be applied to HBO treatments in CP. One cannot recommend a standard protocol, but the ideal treatment schedule should be determined for each patient including the pressure, dose, and duration of treatment. It may be possible to identify responders early on in the treatment. Although molecular diagnostic procedures may be used in the investigation of patients with CP, genotyping and gene expression studies have not yet been done as a guide to treatment but this is a promising field for future investigation (Jain 2009).

23 HBO Therapy in Headache

C.E. Fife and J. Bookspan

Intractable headaches, particularly vascular headaches (including migraine), are a problem to manage. The role of hyperbaric oxygen in relieving headaches is discussed under the following headings:

Introduction

In the Stone Age, headaches were sometimes treated in South America by trephining holes in patient's skulls with flints "to let the demons out." Survivors with recurrent headaches underwent (even survived) repeat trephining, a practice that continued until the Middle Ages. In the ninth century British Isles, medicines against headache consisted of potions of "juice of elderseed, cow's brain, and goat's dung dissolved in vinegar."

Understandably, severe headache sufferers will do almost anything to relieve their terrible pain. Today more palatable and effective pharmaceutical treatments have been developed, although effectiveness may remain suboptimal for many, prompting investigations into other treatment modalities.

Vascular Headaches

Vascular headaches include migraine headaches with and without aura as well as cluster headaches. Migraine encompasses a group of severe, recurring headaches usually affecting one side of the head, accompanied by nausea, photophobia, sonophobia, and vomiting. In about 30–40% of migraineurs, there is an aura with transient neurological symptoms which precedes the attacks and last about 20 min. The aura of migraine is associated with focal reduction of cerebral blood flow which seem to be secondary to arteriolar vasoconstriction (Friberg et al 1994). The aura may include flashing or zigzag lights, lines, or dots, dimmed vision, tingling in the face or hands, weakness of an arm or leg, speech difficulties, and confusion. Migraine with aura used to be called "classic migraine." Migraine without aura used to be called "common migraine," as it is more common than migraine with aura. The name "migraine" derives from the Greek hemi-kranion, (contacted through usage to mikrania or megrem or migraine) meaning "half the head." Pain can be so severe that even the word meaning "depression or unhappiness" (megrems) comes from the Middle English variant of "migraine."

Cluster headaches occur mostly in men, presenting as a severely painful, unilateral and retroorbital characteristic pattern of pain, with lacrimation of one eye, lid drooping, papillary change and nasal stuffiness. Sufferers experience extreme bouts of pain on one side of the head for about an hour, one to three times per day. Often, the headaches occur at the same time each day, "clustered," hence the name, into periods of weeks or months, but may disappear for months to years, then recur. Sufferers may become irritable, pace, rock, and bang their heads against the wall during an attack. The pain can be so intense, that it has been called "suicide headache." Some cases become chronic and occur daily.

Epidemiology of Vascular Headache

Cluster headaches are rare, affecting less then 0.1% of the population and are more frequent in men. By comparison, about 10–20% of Americans experience migraine headaches, mostly in women with the young suffering more headaches than the elderly (Kaminski & Ruff 1991). Incidence of diagnosis of migraine has increased by nearly 60% in the last decade probably due to improved education about this disease. Headaches are painful and costly. Productivity lost through absenteeism and working at reduced levels of effectiveness ranges from an estimated $6.5 billion to $17.2 billion each year (Siegelman 1992).

Mechanisms of Vascular Headache

Ten to fifteen years ago, the prevailing theory was that migraine began with spasm of brain blood vessels. Today there is some evidence that migraine sufferers may have a lowered threshold to a "migraine generator" within the brain (Young 1997). One theory is that this generator is in the brainstem, involving serotonergic system of nerve cells. Another theory is that the aura, and aura-like phenomenon, begin in the cortex of the brain and start a cascade of events culminating in migraine pain, including inflammatory response of blood vessels surrounding the brain. The trigemino-vascular theory includes all these concepts (Moskowitz 1984).

Migraine pain was previously thought to result simply from vasodilation and pulsation of cerebral vessels. Ergotamine drugs and their derivatives, which were then the gold-standard of migraine pharmacologic agents, were thought to ease pain through vasoconstrictive properties. Current thinking is that migraine may involve, at least in part, an inherited abnormality of serotonin metabolism. Serotonin levels drop during a migraine attack. Anthony et al (1967) induced migraine using serotonin depleting drugs, and relieved the resulting migraine headache with intravenous serotonin. The migraine drug sumatriptan is now known to act, not only as a vasoconstrictive agent, but to stimulate subtypes of serotonin receptors responsible for controlling serotonin levels in the central synapses and vascular innervation. The drug DHE-45 (dihydroergotamine mesylate), another direct serotonin receptor agonist, also appears to act on a subtype of receptors that controls serotonin levels. DHE directly stimulates these serotonin receptors and turns the pain off (Starr 1992).

Other theories of etiology of classic migraine (migraine with aura) include the trigemino-vascular theory (Moskowitz 1984), spreading cortical depression hypothesis (Ferrari et al 1990), spreading depression as a characteristic of both classic and common migraine (Dalessio 1985), the combination of both spreading cortical depression (SCD) and potassium-induced vasoconstriction producing localized ischemia (Young & Van Vliet 1992), previous trauma (Borzyskowski 1989), and reduced ability to deaminate monoamines, particularly phenylethylamine, in susceptible individuals (McCulloch & Harper 1977). Olesen (1986) ruled out disturbances of adrenergic substances in blood as cause of migraine by intracarotid infusion of noradrenaline, adrenaline, and isoprenaline, with no headache-related effect. In contrast to this, Chang and Detar (1980) demonstrated enhanced vasoconstrictive response to catecholaminergic drugs. The increased sympathetic activity inherent in migraine with and without aura, affects the cerebral vasculature, neurons, and metabolism, increasing oxygen demand, which further worsens local hypoxia (Amery 1982). More recently, endothelin-1, a cerebral constrictor, has been implicated in SCD in animal models and appears to be associated with selective neuronal necrosis (Dreier *et al* 2007). It should be pointed out, however, that this process has not been substantiated in humans, although raised levels of endothelin-1 have been reported in the plasma of migraneurs compared to healthy controls in many studies.

Commonly Used Anti-Migraine Drugs

Abortive medications for migraine are shown in Table 22.1. These include sumatriptan (Imitrex), the newer synthesized "triptans," indomethacin, Cafergot, and corticosteroids. In cluster headache, subcutaneous sumatriptan is usually effective and well tolerated. Prophylactically, calcium channel blockers are effective. Intranasal capsaicin and leuprolide (a synthetic slow-release gonadotrophin-releasing hormone) may be useful. In chronic paroxysmal hemicrania, which clinically resembles cluster headache, indomethacin is effective for many (Stovner and Sjaastad 1995). Individual patients may respond to salicylates, naproxin, or prednisone (Brandt *et al* 1991).

Table 23.1
Commonly Used Anti-Migraine Drugs

Abortive agents for migraine
1. Nonsteroidal anti-inflammatory agents (NSAIDs) and acetaminophen
2. Ergot derivatives (ergotamine, dihydroergotamine, DHE-45 or dihydroergotamine mesylate, available in injectable form, and now as the nasal spray Migrainol)
3. Sumatriptan (Imitrex)
4. Isometheptene

Prophylactic agents
5. Beta-adrenergic blockers
6. Antidepressants
7. NSAIDs and acetaminophen
8. Divalproex sodium (Depakote)
9. Calcium channel blockers

Nonpharmacologic Approaches

Pharmacologic agents combating migraine and cluster headaches are generally effective with relatively few side effects, and are now usually self-administered, therefore, the need for treatment alternatives is relatively low. However, several factors illustrate the need for investigation and availability of other modalities.

Potential candidates for treatment with hyperbaric oxygen (HBO) therapy are those whose vascular headaches are unresponsive to oral or injected medications or accepted nutritional management involving avoidance of trigger foods. HBO can be considered for patients in whom have common pharmacologic agents are contraindicated, such as those with peripheral vascular disease, coronary artery disease or pregnancy or patients with substantial side effects to standard pharmacologic agents and in those with hypertension. Overuse of abortive agents, such as ergotamine, can lead to rebound effects, prompting the sufferer to take more medication, creating a vicious cycle of headaches and rebound headache that may continue for days or weeks or become chronic daily headaches. HBO might be useful for breaking such a cycle.

Rationale for Use of HBO in Migraine

The rationale for the use of HBO in migraine is based on two mechanisms of its action on the blood vessels: vasoconstriction and influence on other headache pathways.

Vasoconstriction

Exposure to HBO has been shown effective for both cluster and migraine headaches. One of the contributing mechanisms is assumed to be cerebral vasoconstriction in response to high oxygen tensions, invoked as a protective response against the effects of both hyperoxia and corresponding decreases in end-tidal carbon dioxide.

Hyperbaric oxygen provides much higher levels of blood oxygenation than normobaric oxygen, and presumably greater ability to constrict painfully dilated cerebral arteries. HBO has been used to combat cerebral edema, its effects decrease cerebral blood flow and increase cerebral oxygenation (Sukoff & Ragatz 1982).

Transcranial Doppler (TCD) is used in migraine research to determine blood flow velocity changes in cerebral arteries. Changes in vessel diameter are inferred from changes in velocity measurements. Using transcranial Doppler, Thomsen *et al* (1995) found decreased mean blood flow velocity, indicating an increase in middle cerebral artery cross-sectional area on the affected side during migraine without aura. Demarin *et al* (1994) found cerebral vasoreactivity to be within normal ranges in the majority of migraine patients, and that subjects experiencing migraine with aura were found to have a lower blood flow velocity (indicating vasodilation) compared to subjects without aura.

For evaluation of the effect of HBO, some modification of TCD technique was needed. Fife *et al* (1994, 1995) passed a Doppler probe through the HBO chamber's steel vessel hull via a custom fitted port. The Doppler image was projected into the chamber via a closed circuit camera and single lens projection television. Two examiners, one controlling the instrument panel outside the chamber and the other positioning the Doppler probe within the chamber, performed the study.

In studies sponsored by the National Headache Foundation, TCD examinations were carried out during hyperbaric exposures on 27 volunteers. Middle cerebral artery (MCA) signals were monitored in a series of separate exposures while subjects respired oxygen at sea level (1 ATA), 2 ATA and 3 ATA, after breathing the appropriate control gas (air, 10% oxygen/nitrogen, and 7% oxygen/nitrogen, respectively) via face mask. Mean flow velocity (MFV), pulsatility index (PI), blood pressure and pulse were recorded at 10 min intervals. As expected, there was no change in MCA MFV and PI between baseline (room air), 10% O_2 at 2ATA, or 7% oxygen at 3 ATA. This is consistent with the assumption that altering ambient pressure alone, without changing the inspired partial pressure of oxygen, has no measurable vascular effects. However, upon HBO exposure, all subjects demonstrated a statistically significant decrease in MCA MFV ($p = < 0.001$), and a significant increase in pulsatility. MCA MFV returned to baseline values almost immediately upon surfacing.

These findings are consistent with an increase in distal vascular tone caused by hyperoxic vasoconstriction. This decrease appeared greater at 3 ATA PO_2 than 2 ATA PO_2, suggesting that this vasoconstrictive effect may increase as PO_2 rises from 2 ATA to 3 ATA. However, a corresponding decrease in end-tidal CO_2 was noted during HBO exposure, a well described effect of oxygen breathing. A decrease in CO_2 is an even more potent vasoconstrictor than an increase in PO_2. When calculations were checked for this effect, nearly all of the changes in MCA velocity could have been accounted for on the basis of a decrease in CO_2. Thus, the mechanism of blood flow changes during HBO exposure may be related as much to carbon dioxide as to oxygen. However, it should be stressed that in migraneurs the proposed vasconstrictive response to the lowering of the pCO_2 may not be simple one. For example, a recent combined study of migraneurs and healthy controls utilizing TCD and NIRS (near-infrared spectroscopy) suggests that marked vasodilation as a functional response to an increase in pCO_2 during breath-holding protocols does not occur in migraneurs (Liboni *et al* 2007).

Effects of HBO on Other Headache Pathways

The effect of HBO is not limited to vasomotor change. Serotonergic pathways seem to be involved but the mechanisms has not been elucidated as yet.

Di Sabato *et al* (1997) assessed the therapeutic efficacy of HBO on serotonergic pathways in cluster headache patients. They studied serotonin binding to mononuclear cells before and after the treatment in study and control subgroups. Appearance of plateau in the binding curves in the HBO subgroup indicated that HBO could act as a serotonergic agonist.

Di Sabato *et al* (1996) assessed the effect of HBO exposure on substance P in the nasal mucosa of cluster headache patients. Substance P (for "pain") is a short-chain neuropeptide present in primary nociceptive neurons and serves to transmit pain impulses from peripheral nociceptive neurons to the central nervous system. Nasal mucosa samples were analyzed using blinded immunocytochemical methods. Compared to the placebo control group, the HBO group showed a significantly decreased immunoreactivity for substance P, indicating that "an influence on the content of peripheral neuropeptides could be involved in the mechanism of action of the beneficial effect of HBO on cluster headache." Busch (2003) investigated hyperbaric oxygen treatment for 120 patients who had migraine-only headache for at least two years before the study. Standardized migraine diary (intensity, duration, medication, vomiting) was documented for three months before treatment. Treatment was ten HBO sessions of 100% oxygen at 200 kPA max pressure for 40 min. At three months following treatment, the subgroup with migraine history of less than 10 years showed significantly reduced pain intensity, duration, headaches/per month, use of analgesics, and vomiting. Patients with a migraine history of 15 years or more showed no significant improvement. They hypothesize that HBO has long term influence on serotonin pathways. Their goal is therapeutic options for patients who cannot use tryptans or ergotamines.

Use of Oxygen in Migraine Treatment

The effect of inhalation of 100% normobaric oxygen on migraine is immediate and can be evaluated like that of any other headache medication (Jain 1989b). The varied nature and course of headache pain, the difficulty inherent in quantifying headache pain and outcomes, and the significant placebo effect in unblinded studies are some of the obstacles to performing well-designed, randomized, clinical trials, and interpreting headache treatment results.

Robbins (1996) reported oxygen inhalation to be "useful" in two of ten patients with menstrual migraine with features of cluster headache, although Evers and Husstedt

(1996) found no significant influence of oxygen inhalation on "chronic paroxysmal hemicrania." Shalkevich et al (1981) found hyperbaric oxygen relieved headache pain in patients with vertebral basilar headache. Isakov and Romasenko (1985) reported that HBO treatment relieved headaches in post-operative neurosurgical patients.

Myers and Myers (1995) compared efficacy of HBO to normobaric oxygen on "global headache severity" before and after exposure to oxygen treatment for a "typical" migraine attack. Twenty migraineurs were divided into a normobaric treatment subgroup of ten patients receiving 100% oxygen at 1 atmosphere of pressure, while the hyperbaric treatment subgroup of ten patients received 100% oxygen at 2 ATA. In the normobaric treatment subgroup, one of the 10 patients reported significant relief, while in the hyperbaric treatment subgroup, 9 of 10 found relief, a significant difference between groups. Normobaric subgroup patients who did not experience significant relief were administered HBO, with all nine experiencing significant relief.

In an unblinded study of 26 patients treated with HBO by Fife and Fife (1989), resolution of acute migraine pain was observed in 92% of patients. Pressure for HBO treatment ranged from 1.3 to 2.6 ATA. Twenty four patients obtained complete relief within 27 min. Both patients with facial hemiparesis had resolution of their neurological deficit during treatment. Average time to relief was 16 min. In a continuation of that unblinded study, Fife (unpublished data, 1993) treated 84 females and 16 males with acute migraine headache pain ($N = 100$) for a total of 211 HBO treatments at 1.6 ATA. Ninety-four patients reported relief of pain during treatment. Average duration to complete resolution was 35.33 min with a range of 8 to 74 min. In some instances subjects were relieved of pain before reaching 1.6 ATA. Additional compression to 2.3 ATA yielded no further improvement. Two patients could not tolerate pressure due to upper respiratory infections, one reported no relief, one felt worse and aborted treatment, and two patients discontinued the study due to time commitments. No subject obtained pain relief under hyperbaric air. It was observed that unless the pain was completely relieved, it would sometimes recur within a few hours. The mechanism of pain relief appears to be HBO-induced cerebral vasoconstriction, which counters the vasodilation causing the initial pain. These unblinded data suggest that while HBO does not cure migraine headache, it can break the cycle for a some patients. It was also noted that stress either slowed or prevented resolution of migraine headaches.

A subsequent double-blinded, randomized trial was sponsored by the National Headache Foundation and carried out at the University of Texas, Houston. Volunteers with a history of migraine, documented by neurological evaluation and in most cases xenon cerebral blood flow studies, were enrolled and oriented to the hyperbaric chamber prior to headache onset. Fourteen subjects, 6 males and 9 females, age 23 to 67 years, received either 100% oxygen at 2 ATA, or normoxic controlled gas, 10% oxygen/90% nitrogen (nitrox) at 2 ATA via a tight fitting, demand type face mask in a multi-place chamber. The subjects, the attendant and the physician were blinded as to the nature of the treatment gas. Subjects graded headache pain from 0–5 on a modified Blanchard pain inventory before and after a 45 min HBOT treatment. Treatment was initiated only for scores of 3 or more and in the absence of recent narcotic or other medication ingestion. Response was defined as a decrease of 2 or more grades. Of the 10 patients who received HBO initially, 7 (70%) obtained headache pain relief; 4 (29%) had no relief. None of 3 HBO failures responded to nitrox. Of the 4 receiving nitrox initially, 2 indicated that their headache had improved. One of 2 nitrox failures responded to HBO. The overall response to HBOT was 72%, and the overall response to nitrox was 29%. This study underscores the importance of controlled trials in headache research, where significant placebo effects can be observed.

In a blinded trial by Fife et al (1992), fourteen subjects with migraine documented by neurological evaluations and, in most cases by xenon cerebral blood flow studies as well, received either 100% oxygen at 2 ATA, or a normoxic controlled gas – 10% oxygen/90% nitrogen (nitrox) at 2 ATA. Subjects graded headache pain from 0–5 on a modified Blanchard pain inventory before and after a 45 min treatment. Treatment was initiated only for scores of 3 or more and in the absence of recent narcotic or other medication ingestion. Response was defined as a decrease of 2 or more grades. Ten patients received HBO initially, of which 7 (70%) obtained headache pain relief; 4 (29%) had no relief. Statistically significant results were not attained due to small sample size.

A recent double-blind, randomized controlled trial attempted to determine the prophylactic effect of HBO on number of hours per week that migraine patients recorded in a standardized diary (Eftedal et al 2004). The two treatments were three sessions of HBO (treatment group, 100% oxygen, 2 ATA, 30 minutes) or three sessions of hyperbaric air (control group, compressed air, 2 ATA, 30 minutes). Although there was a reduction in the number of headache hours reported by patients in the treatment group (n of 20) in comparison to the control group (n of 20), the difference was not significant, even though a weighting scheme was employed to test sensitivity of the results over the following 8 weeks. No differences in plasma endothelin-1 levels were observed between the groups. As the authors of this study indicate, although the relief obtained was not significant in the statistical sense, it is possible that, if the treatment plan had been optimized, the results might have been significant.

In one unreported case study by C. Fife, a migraneur with ptosis was able to open his eye after HBO treatment (Figure 23.1). The patient was a 52-year old white male with a history of basilar artery migraine attacks, thalamic infarctions and 3rd nerve palsy (Bickerstaff Syndrome). Infarctions were confirmed by MRI and the patient had com-

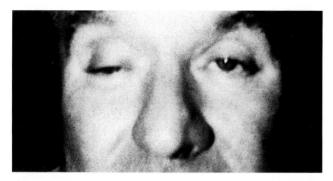

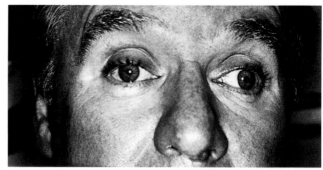

Figure 23.1
Patient with basilar artery migraine
Prior to HBO treatment. Note ptosis of the right eye due to partial III nerve palsy.

The same patient after treatment with HBO at 2 ATA for 2 h. Note that the patient is able to open his right eye (see text for comments)

plained of headaches intermittently for five days. He awoke pain free but with a partial third nerve palsy manifested as ptosis of the right eye, right medial rectus paresis, an ataxic gait and past pointing on finger-to-nose testing. Approximately 12 h after the onset of neurologic deficit, he underwent a HBO treatment at a pressure of 2ATA for 2 h. He was noted to have significant improvement but his ptosis did not resolve immediately following the treatment. He underwent two further treatments over a two day period, but noted no further improvement on subsequent exposures. HBO therapy was, therefore, discontinued. This case raises the question whether HBO may be useful for differentiation of transient ischemic attacks associated with migraine from fixed neurological deficits due to stroke. Use of HBO in stroke is the subject of considerable discussion currently and is dealt with in Chapter 18.

There are several unpublished anecdotal reports of decrease in frequency of migraine after undergoing HBO treatments but it would be difficult to demonstrate it conclusively in a condition as unpredictable in onset as migraine.

A very recent meta-analysis of 3 small clinical trials of HBO (Fife *et al* 1992; Hill 1992; Myers & Myers 1995) in the treatment of migraine headaches demonstrated unequivocal and good evidence for relief (mean RR: 5.97, 95% CI: 1.46–24.38) (Schnabel *et al* 2008). Although heterogeneity was not discussed, inspection of the Forrest plot suggests this is not likely to be a factor. The conclusion, therefore, would seem to be that HBO is efficacious in the treatment of migraine, and that previous trials that reported nonsignificant positive results were almost certainly limited by their relative small sample sizes.

Use of HBO for Treatment of Cluster Headache

Although normobaric oxygen treatment of cluster headaches can provide some relief, early results showed that the benefit is limited (Fogan 1985; Kudrow 1981). Di Sabato *et*

al (1993) compared HBO to placebo for the treatment of episodic cluster headaches. Six of seven patients in the HBO treatment subgroup experienced an improvement compared to none in the placebo treatment subgroup. Three of the six patients remained free from pain attacks for up to six days. The authors stated that their results indicate that HBO is effective in the case of a single attack of cluster headache, and might also be useful to prevent subsequent attacks. However, interpretation of the result of continued protection against repeat attacks must be weighed carefully, as a refractory period follows attacks, where further attacks cannot be induced (Krabbe 1986).

Pascual *et al* (1995) treated four cluster headache patients with "no clear response to pharmacological treatments using a 2-week HBO course." Two patients had reduced duration and frequency of cluster headache with benefits remaining for 2 and 31 days post treatment. Patient three had a reduced frequency of attacks only while patient four experienced no change.

Di Sabato *et al* (1997) compared the effect of HBO (n of 10) to that with environmental air (placebo control) treatments (n of 4) on patients with chronic cluster headache. The placebo control group experienced no change in number of attacks or analgesic consumption. The HBO group reported relief of symptoms.

Weiss *et al* (1989) reported a single case of a cluster headache treated with HBO in a patient with symptoms refractory to other treatments including normobaric oxygen inhalation. In both of two treatments pain was relieved at two atmospheres breathing 100% oxygen. Nilsson et al (2002) compared HBO to placebo in 16 patients, 12 with episodic and four with chronic cluster headache in a double-blind, placebo-controlled, cross-over study. Active treatment was conducted with 100% oxygen whereas placebo was 10% oxygen in nitrogen, corresponding to air at sea level. In both treatments gases were administered by mask in a multiplace hyperbaric chamber for 70 min at 250 kPa (2.5 ATA) in two sessions 24 h apart. Patients responded to both treatments and no difference between HBO and sham treatment was observed.

Predicting response to treatment in patients with cluster headaches is extremely difficult. For example, Schürks *et al* (2007a) investigated 246 patients using logistical regression models based upon personal, headache, and lifestyle characteristics, as well as outcome data (137 of 191 patients responded to triptans and 134 of 175 patients responded to oxygen) and found no significant factors. Investigators are hopeful that genetic studies might provide clues, but although the G1246A polymorphism in the hypocretin receptor 2 gene has been found significantly associated with cluster headaches, there appears to be no pharmacological relevance (Schürks *et al* 2007b).

Conclusions

Hyperbaric oxygen (HBO), for the treatment of vascular headaches, due to serotonergic or neurogenic mechanisms, seems to be effective and safe.

While the rationale for HBO treatment for vascular headache, particularly cluster headache, is sound and it is unlikely that patients would be harmed, the practical application is often limited. Hyperbaric (but probably not normobaric) oxygen may be useful in abortive management of migraine headache, however questions remain regarding optimal treatment pressure and duration of therapy, the cost/benefit ratio, lack of availability of hyperbaric centers for many patients, and the fact that some migraines run their course in a matter of hours. Also, little is known about optimum treatment pressure and potentially detrimental effects of oxygen that might develop at a particular pO_2. Treatment pressures which have been successful in unblinded trials of migraine headache have ranged from 1.6 to a maximum of 2.5 ATA. There is data to suggest that pressures greater than 1.5 ATA may increase cerebral lactate levels in the injured brain (Holbach *et al* 1977). However, there is no cerebral injury in migraine unless the complication of cerebrovascular ischemia occurs and pressures higher than 1.5 ATA may be well tolerated.

Many of the new migraine medications have 70% or better efficacy. Exceptions may lie in complicated migraine with neurologic deficits, and in those migraineurs refractive to established pharmacologic and nutritional interventions. The future for HBO may lie in treating migraine headaches that run for days with severe debility, for treating chronic daily headaches with migraine components, and for treatment and prevention of cluster headaches, which often take days or weeks to resolve, are extremely painful, and are less responsive to currently available medications.

Patients with chronic recurring vascular headache attacks benefit best from a continuous preventative treatment plans including medication; diet, exercise, and lifestyle changes, with exercise plus stress reduction techniques. This approach is better than relying on use of HBO (or other abortive interventions) treatment programs.

Editorial Comments

The authors have presented a straightforward review of their experience and review of the current literature indicting the usefulness of HBO in the management of migraine and cluster headaches. For clinical studies, the evaluation of relief of pain remains somewhat of a problem. This is the same situation as for the evaluation of various pharmaceuticals for migraine.

Wilson *et al* (1998) have used a visual analog pain scale, algometry, and manual palpation over tender areas to document relief of pain with HBO treatments. Resolution of tenderness and edema following both treatments was observable by manual palpation while algometry showed no differences between the two. Subjective pain was significantly decreased following HBO treatments but not following the control treatment (100% oxygen, no pressure). Results suggest that HBO treatment reduces migraine headache pain and that the patient's subjective assessment is the best indicator of relief.

Economic aspects of treatment of migraine with HBO need to be investigated. Reduction of medication use and their adverse effects would reduce the costs. Decreased frequency of attacks with less work missed would increase productivity. Finally, HBO may improve the quality of life of migraine sufferers.

24 HBO Therapy in Cardiovascular Diseases

K.K. Jain

HBO has been found to be useful in the management of myocardial ischemia, as an adjunct to cardiac surgery, and in improving the walking distance in ischemic limb pain. This chapter includes the following main sections:

Introduction

Normobaric oxygen therapy has been in use for many years in the management of ischemic heart disease (Jain 1989a). This chapter deals with the role of HBO in treating cardiovascular disorders. Some aspects of the pathogenesis of cardiovascular disease relevant to HBO will also be mentioned briefly.

It is well known that cardiovascular diseases are the leading cause of death in the Western countries, causing, for example, about 1 million deaths every year in the United States (half of the deaths due to all causes). About half of the deaths from cardiovascular diseases are due to coronary artery disease.

Pathophysiology

Risk Factors

The important risk factors for the cardiovascular diseases are arteriosclerosis, hypertension, hypercholesteremia, diabetes, and smoking.

Hypoxia, Hyperoxia, and Atherosclerosis

The major factor in coronary artery stenosis and occlusion is atherosclerosis. Hypoxia is a cause of atherosclerosis. Experimental studies have shown an enhancing effect of hypoxia (achieved by inhalation of low percentage oxygen) on the development of aortic atherosclerosis in cholesterol-fed rabbits, and reversal of this with the application of HBO. This occurs by direct action on the vessel wall and not by changes in the blood lipid concentration. Inhibition of diet-induced atherosclerosis in New Zealand White rabbits by HBO treatment is accompanied by a significant reduction of autoantibodies against oxidatively modified LDL-cholesterol and profound changes in the redox state of the liver and aortic tissues (Kudchodkar *et al* 2007). This antioxidant response may be the key to the antiatherogenic effect of HBO treatment.

Stillman (1983) carried out experiments on rabbits to assess the effects of changes in the inspired oxygen concentration on intimal healing. The aorta was stripped and the animals were kept in various normobaric oxygen concentrations (14%–40%) for up to 10 days. After 6 months nearly all the animals showed normal healing, but the progress of healing was different. Hypoxia appeared to cause more platelet adhesions, exaggerated media proliferation, and aberrant migration. This finding explains the unfavorable results of surgery if there is hypoxia. Formation of platelet mass on the surface of the intima of the traumatized vessel will cause local hypoxia that affects the cells

beneath the thrombus. Intimal hyperplasia at the site of vascular anastomosis is suppressed by steroids. HBO also has an immunosuppressive effect, and this may lead to a more orderly intimization.

There are two distinct oxygen-sensitive mechanisms in peripheral arteries, both of which regulate vascular tone. One mechanism is activated at high pO_2 values (10%–40%), and vasoconstriction induced by this mechanism is mediated by vascular prostaglandin synthesis. The other comes into effect at low pO_2 levels and is related to limitation of oxidative energy metabolism.

In addition to relieving the effects of tissue anoxia, attention has been directed to the pathogenesis and possible reversal of atherosclerotic lesions. Hypoxia induced by CO is an accepted risk factor in atherogenesis. It seemed likely that the reverse process, hyperoxia induced by HBO, may be of benefit in animals with induced atherosclerosis.

Alpha-tocopherol (vitamin E) decreases systemic oxidant stress. Concentration of free cholesterol in rabbits with experimentally induced hypercholesteremia has been shown to be reduced one and a half times by a combination of HBO and alpha-tocopherol effect.

Hyperbaric Oxygenation in Cardiology

Effect of Hypoxia, Hyperoxia, and Hyperbaric Environments on Cardiovascular Function

Feldberg and Zemfiresco (1969) investigated the effect of hypoxia and hyperoxia on the left chamber systole and contractility of the heart in 20 young healthy male volunteers. ECG, carotid sphygmogram, phonocardiogram, and acceleration ballistocardiogram techniques were used to record the changes. The authors concluded that acute hypoxia (8% oxygen) augments contractility, probably through an adrenergic mechanism. Under the influence of hyperoxygenation (100% oxygen) a vagotonic effect was observed. Both direct and indirect mechanisms are involved in these changes.

Hardenbergh *et al* (1973) studied cardiovascular changes in anesthetized dogs under hyperbaric conditions. Breathing air at 3 ATA had little effect on the physiological parameters, whereas breathing oxygen at 3 ATA depressed the heart rate and diminished the iliac blood flow as determined by the Doppler flowmeter. There was little effect on mean blood pressure. Breathing air at 5 ATA increased the blood pressure in all the animals and diminished the iliac artery flow as well as the heart rate. These observations are in agreement with other reports.

Murakhovsky and Lethova (1979) studied circulation parameters in ten subjects exposed to oxygen breathing at 20 mmHg. During the exposure there was a 27% decrease in cardiac output compared with controls. Those test subjects who were pretrained to the exposure showed the smallest reduction of cardiac output. The authors felt that this change is due not to any effect on the heart, but rather to peripheral vasoconstriction with increase of peripheral resistance and decrease of circulatory volume and venous return to the heart.

With exercise under hyperoxia, the peripheral vasoconstriction does not seem to play a role, as increased blood flow is required for the skeletal muscles. Fagraeus and Linnarson (1973) observed that exercise heart rate is markedly depressed in hyperbaric environments. This is due to the effect of raised oxygen partial pressure on the heart, both directly and also via parasympathetic stimulation of the heart. The cardiodepressive influences observed may be of importance in limiting the tolerance for heavy exercise in hyperbaric environments, particularly with normoxia. There was no mention of what the response may be with HBO.

Welch (1982) reviewed the literature on hyperoxia and human performance and concluded that there was no evidence of difference in cardiac output during heavy exercise under HBO, although there are reports of elevations of mean blood pressure (BP) and reduction of heart rate during exercise under hyperoxia.

Trefny and Svacinka (1969) studied the effect of hypoxia and hyperoxia on the quantitative ballistocardiogram in ten healthy male volunteers. They were exposed in a hypobaric chamber as well as in a hyperbaric chamber, where they breathed 100% oxygen at 1, 2, and 3 ATA. In hypoxia there was increase in minute cardiac force mainly due to increase of heart rate. There was a decrease of minute cardiac force under HBO due to decrease of heart rate and systolic force.

Kenmure et al (1972) studied the hemodynamic effects of oxygen at 2 ATA on healthy human subjects. Twenty healthy male volunteers breathed air at 1 ATA and oxygen at 2 ATA for 45 min successively at rest. Inhalation of oxygen at 2 ATA caused a 10% fall in cardiac index (mostly due to fall of heart rate). There was a 15% increase in systolic vascular resistance and an 8% decrease in left ventricular work. There was also a 3% rise in the mean arterial pressure.

Sventek and Zambranski (1985) tested the effect of 100% oxygen on the cardiovascular response to vasoactive compounds in the dog. The hyperoxic animals demonstrated a significant increase in the mean arterial pressure responsiveness to both angiotensin I and II (43%). The control dogs breathing ambient air showed no significant changes for any of the compounds tested. These data indicate that with 8 h of hyperoxia, the renin-angiotensin system's ability to influence cardiovascular function is augmented.

Metabolic Effects of HBO on the Heart

Mitochondrial respiratory rate is an essential component of myocardial function because it influences production of adenosine triphosphate during oxidative phosphorylation.

Mitochondrial phosphorylation depends upon oxygen tension. This is the key to understanding the pathophysiological processes that appear in the heart, such has hypoxia, ischemia, and the changes in the oxygen-carrying capacity. Gaudue et al (1982) studied the dependence of cardiac energy metabolism on the oxygen-carrying capacity of blood, using isolated perfused rat heart as a model. Oxygen supply became a limiting factor of mitochondrial respiratory rate in the absence of hemoglobin in the perfusate. Use of reconstituted blood permitted normal arterial oxygen pressure and enabled the maintenance of the physiological capacity of the cardiac energy metabolism.

Although not mentioned by Gaudue (1982) it may be possible to obtain the same effect using HBO instead of blood. Boerema et al (1959) have shown that with HBO (3 ATA), decreasing the hemoglobin concentration of pigs to less then 1.0% resulted in no ECG evidence of myocardial anoxia.

Miroshnichenko et al (1983) studied the effect of guanine nucleotides and HBO on cardiac adenine cyclase activity in rabbits with myocardial hypertrophy. They believe that this hypertrophy is the result of reduction of sensitivity of the adenylate cyclase system to hormonal action. This disturbance is normalized by HBO. Under HBO, guanine nucleotides participate in both the desensitization of adenosine cyclase to hormonal action and resensitization of this during HBO.

Bondarenko et al (1981) studied the influence of HBO on certain indices of tissue metabolism in patients with acute cardiac insufficiency. They found that the metabolic effects of HBO in patients with acute cardiac insufficiency are not secondary to changes of systemic circulation, but precede them due to direct action of hyperoxia on metabolic processes in the peripheral tissues. Moreover, improvement of regional blood flow and metabolism of peripheral tissues by HBO also exerts a beneficial effect on the systemic circulation thus breaking the vicious circle:

circulatory hypoxia → myocardial hypoxia → circulatory hypoxia

The above findings are confirmed by a decrease of both lactate level and metabolic acidosis, with an unchanged cardiac output. Further improvement in the hemodynamics of these patients is conditioned by a mechanism of compensation, including myocardial hypofunction, with removal of peripheral oxygen debt.

Role of HBO in Experimental Myocardial Infarction

Various studies of the effect of HBO on experimental myocardial infarction are shown in Table 24.1.

Vin et al (1986) studied the effect of HBO on experimental myocardial infarction in rabbits. ECG monitoring as

Table 24.1
Experimental Studies of the Effect of HBO in Myocardial Infarction

Authors and year	Experimental model	Results	Conclusions or comments
Smith and Lawson (1958)	Ligation of anterior descending coronary artery	Mortality in dogs breathing O_2 at 2ATA was 10% compared with 50%–60% mortality of dogs breathing air	HBO may reduce the mortality by protecting from ventricular fibrillation following myocardial infarction
Chardack et al (1964) Trapp and Creighton (1964)	Coronary artery ligation	Reduction of infarct size and reduction of ventricular fibrillation in HBO-treated animals	
Kline et al (1979)	Infarction	Excess lactate associated with ischemia disappeared with 100% oxygen at 3 ATA. Animals breathing room air continued to produce excess lactate.	Return to oxidative (aerobic) metabolism with HBO and reduction of myocardial ischemia
Kleep (1977)	Occlusion of the circumflex branch of the left coronary artery in sheep	Mortality of this procedure greatly reduced	
Demurov et al (1981)	Left coronary artery ligation in rabbits	HBO at 2 ATA for 1 H starting 30 min after occlusion	Partial restoration of myocardial contractility. Improvement of energy metabolism of the heart. Decrease of cAMP in ischemic areas. Increase of guanosine monophosphate in intact areas.
Efuni et al (1983)	Experimental myocardial infraction in rabbits. Combined use of HBO and antioxidants	Improvement of cardiac function	
Thomas et al (1990)	Dogs. Occlusion of left ant. descending coronary artery for 2 h. Myocardial injury was measured by histochemical staining.	4 groups: I. control, no treatment, II. HBO 2 ATA for 90 min, III. rt-PA only, IV. HBO + rt-PA simultaneously	Although HBO and recombinant tissue plasminogen activator (rt-PA) caused 35.9% 48.9% restoration of enzyme activity, maximal effect was obtained by combining both which reduces the extent of infarction.
Sterling et al (1993)	Open chest rabbit model of myocardial ischemia. A branch of left coronary artery was occluded for 30 min followed by 3 h of reperfusion. Infarction measured by tripheny tetrazolium staining.	Control group ventilated with 100% oxygen at 1 ATA. Treated animals with HBO at 2 ATA.	Animals exposed to HBO had smaller infarcts than controls. HBO given after 30 min of reperfusion had no protective effect.
Kim et al (2001)	Rats were intermittently exposed to 100% O_2 at 3 ATA for 1 h daily and then sacrificed after 24 h of recovery in room air. Isolated hearts were subjected to 40 min of ischemia and 90 min of reperfusion	HBO pretreatment enhanced enzymatic activity and gene expression of catalase, thereby significantly reducing infarct size after reperfusion.	HBO preconditioning may be developed as a new preventive measure for reperfusion injury in the heart
Spears et al (2002)	60-min balloon occlusion of the left anterior descending coronary artery in swine. Control groups consisted of autoreperfusion alone.	Intracoronary aqueous oxygen (AO) hyperoxemic perfusion for 90 min. Significant improvement in left ventricular ejection fraction at 105 min of reperfusion.	Intracoronary hyperbaric reperfusion with AO attenuates myocardial ischemia/reperfusion injury
Xuejun et al 2008	Rats with occlusion of the left anterior descending coronary artery. HBO pretreatment at 2.5 ATA for 60 min, twice daily for 2 days followed by 12 h of recovery in room air prior to the myocardial ischemic insult.	The infarct size of the HBO group was smaller than that of the control normoxic group. Capillary density, VEGF levels, and cell proliferation higher in HBO group.	HBO pretreatment accelerates angiogenesis and alleviates myocardial ischemia

well as postmortem examination of the heart was done after 3 weeks of HBO (2 ATA, 2 h daily). ECG changes cleared up in HBO-treated animals and postmortem examination showed only minimal histological changes. ECG changes (ST segment elevation) persisted in the untreated control animals and postmortem showed marked fatty degeneration of the myocardium.

Literature cited gives a somewhat favorable view concerning the role of HBO in myocardial infarction; other reports have been published that indicate no beneficial effect of HBO (Holloway *et al* 1965; Robertson 1966). Glauser and Glauser (1973) reviewed this conflict and tried to resolve it by analysis of the volume of tissue necrotized by vascular occlusion. This is considered in relation to the radius of the tissue supplied by the vessel before the occlusion. The volume of necrosis increases rapidly, as the cube of the original radius. The volume of tissue saved by breathing 100% oxygen at 3 ATA increases more slowly, as the square of the original radius. The percentage of the tissue thus saved varies according to the reciprocal of the original radius. Any phenomenon that produces multiple small infarcts will respond more favorably to HBO therapy than one large area of necrosis. This might possibly explain the variations in the results of different experiments where different sizes of infarcts were produced in different species of animals. In a clinical situation it can be predicted that HBO is more likely to be beneficial in a small vessel embolus, or in a thrombosis with multiple small infarcts, than in a single massive infarct.

An animal study was conducted by Thomas *et al* (1990) to test the hypothesis that combination of thrombolytic therapy and HBO would be more effective in reducing the size of myocardial infarction than either of these modalities alone. The study provided encouraging evidence for the validity of this hypothesis and both of these methods had a synergistic effect.

Clinical Applications of HBO in Cardiology

Acute Myocardial Infarction

Clinical features and principles of management. Myocardial infarction (MI) is one of the most common diagnoses in hospitalized patients in developed countries. Characteristic features are chest pain, ECG abnormalities and enzyme changes. Approximately 1.5 million myocardial infarctions occur each year in the United States. The mortality rate in acute infarction is about 30% with half of these occurring before the stricken individual can reach the hospital. Death usually occurs due to ventricular fibrillation. Silent myocardial infarctions may occur in 20–40% of cases who later develop clinically manifest MI. Diagnostic procedures are treadmill stress testing, thallium 201 scintigraphy, radionuclide angiography, two-dimensional echocardiography and ambulatory ECG monitoring (Holter).

Goal for the management of patients with suspected MI is rapid identification of patients who are candidates for reperfusion therapy. Current measures employed for reperfusion are intravenous thrombolytics, angioplasty (balloon or laser) and medications. Commonly used thrombolytic is tissue plasminogen activator (tPA). Other approved thrombolytics are streptokinase and anisoylated plasminogen streptokinase activator complex. The main goal is prompt restoration of patency of the occluded coronary artery to stop the life-threatening tachyarrythmias. Thrombolytic therapy can reduce the in-hospital death by 50% when administered within the first hour of onset of symptoms of MI. Primary percutaneous transluminal angioplasty (PTCA) is used in patients where prior angiography shows areas of narrowing or those with cardiogenic shock where immediate opening of the occluded artery is required. Pharmacologic measures are intravenous lidocaine for correction of ventricular tachyarrhythmia and potassium to correct auricular fibrillation. Other drugs used are aspirin, beta blocker and angiotensin converting enzyme inhibitors. There is evidence that theses agents reduce mortality. Calcium channel blockers are given to reduce the size of the infarct but results of clinical trials failed to establish this. Supplemental oxygen inhalation is given quite frequently to patients with MI.

The extent of the infarct size is the major determinant of prognosis in MI. A reduction of infarct size is the major therapeutic goal.

Normobaric oxygen in myocardial infarction. Arterial desaturation and hypoxemia following acute myocardial infarction has been documented for years and is worse in patients with heart failure. Traditionally inhalation of normobaric oxygen has been used. Koerner (1971) recommended oxygen concentrations below 50% for inhalation to counteract hypoxia. Kones (1974) recommended 100% oxygen inhalation. Decision to give oxygen can be made on the basis of pulse oximetry which measures oxygen saturation reliably (Wilson & Channer 1997). Here one is talking about correction of general hypoxia which affects other organs. The issue is focal hypoxia in the myocardium where systemic oxygen cannot diffuse easily because of vascular occlusion. It is unlikely that this method of oxygen administration can counteract myocardial hypoxia in face of vascular occlusion. Therefore, use of HBO in the management of patients with acute myocardial infarction has been investigated.

Role of HBO in myocardial infarction. Since there are localized areas of lack of oxygen in MI, there is a rationale for reperfusion of these areas with high concentrations of oxygen.

Cameron *et al* (1966) investigated the hemodynamic and metabolic effects of HBO in ten patients with acute myocardial infarction who breathed air, oxygen at atmospheric pressure, or oxygen at 2 ATA. Under HBO, systemic vascular resistance rose progressively, accompanied by some reduction in cardiac output and stroke volume, with little change in heart rate. In patients with raised lactic acid levels, there was a reduction of this parameter with HBO. The authors felt that HBO therapy may turn out to be of most value to patients with severe hypoxia, hypotension, and metabolic acidosis who have responded poorly to conventional therapy.

Thurston *et al* (1973) carried out the first randomized controlled investigation into the effects of HBO on mortality following recent myocardial infarction in 103 patients and in 105 controls treated by conventional methods in the same coronary care unit in London, England. Seventeen (16.5%) of the patients in the HBO group died, compared with 24 (22.9%) in the control group. Detailed analysis revealed that mortality in high-risk patients may be reduced by half by means of HBO. The only patients who survived cardiogenic shock were in the HBO group. The incidence of arrhythmias was lower in the HBO group and some of those were shown to disappear with HBO. The authors felt that the evidence in favor of HBO in the treatment of myocardial infarction was sufficiently strong to justify its use in selected patients where the facilities were available. This study was described again by Thurston (1977), and the comments appended to this publication, comprising a summary of the remarks of the discussants, are interesting and indicate the controversial nature of this topic.

Efuni *et al* (1984) used HBO in combined therapy of acute myocardial infarction in 30 patients. Pressure of 1.5–2 ATA was used for 60–90 min and the treatment course consisted of five to six sessions. All patients had acute myocardial infarction of the left ventricle with predominant damage of the anterior wall and duration of affliction ranging from 12 to 48 h. Patients with initial arterial hypoxemia ($n = 16$) showed a proven increase in arterial pO_2 from 64 ± 7 mmHg to 82 ± 5 mmHg following the first session and 86 ± 4 mmHg at the end of the course. Cardiac output and stroke volume tended to increase, the former mainly at the expense of the latter. Simultaneously there was a decrease in lactate:pyruvate ratio with fall of metabolic acidosis. The authors recommend HBO treatment in myocardial ischemia complicated by arterial hypoxemia.

Single photon emission computed tomography (SPECT) and thallium exercise scintigraphy have been used to document the improvement during the first week following myocardial infarction in 24 patients treated with HBO (Swift *et al* 1992).

Combination of HBO and thrombolysis. HBO in combination with thrombolysis has been demonstrated to salvage myocardium in acute myocardial infarction in the animal model. Therefore a randomized pilot trial was undertaken to assess the safety and feasibility of this treatment in hu-

man beings (Shandling *et al* 1997). Patients with an acute MI who received recombinant tissue plasminogen activator (rTPA) were randomized to treatment with HBO combined with rTPA or rTPA alone. Sixty-six patients were included for analysis. Forty-three patients had inferior acute MIs and the remainder had anterior acute MIs. The mean creatine phosphokinase level at 12 and 24 h was reduced in the patients given HBO by approximately 35% ($p = 0.03$). Time to pain relief and ST segment resolution was shorter in the group given HBO. There were two deaths in the control group and none in those treated with HBO. The ejection fraction on discharge was 52.4% in the group given HBO compared with 47.3% in the control group (difference not significant). The authors concluded that adjunctive treatment with HBO appears to be a feasible and safe treatment for acute MI and may result in an attenuated rise in creatine phosphokinase levels and more rapid resolution of pain and ST segment changes.

A randomized multicenter trial was conducted to further assess the safety and feasibility of this treatment in human subjects (Stravinsky *et al* 1998). Patients with acute MI treated with rTPA or streptokinase (STK), were randomized to treatment with HBO combined with either rTPA or STK, or rTPA or STK alone. Results indicate that treatment with HBO in combination with thrombolysis appears to be feasible and safe for patients with AMI and may result in an attenuated CPK rise, more rapid resolution of pain and improved ejection fractions. More studies are needed to assess the benefits of this treatment.

Chronic Ischemic Heart Disease (Angina Pectoris)

Ischemia here refers to lack of oxygen due to inadequate perfusion, which results from an imbalance between oxygen supply and demand. The most common cause of myocardial ischemia is atherosclerotic disease of the coronary arteries. Coronary artery disease is the most common, serious, chronic, life-threatening illness in the United States where there are about 11 million sufferers. Angina pectoris is due to transient myocardial ischemia. Management of ischemic heart disease starts with preventive measures such lowering of cholesterol and treatment of hypertension. Several vasodilators are used for the treatment of angina pectoris of which nitrates are the best known. Other agents are beta blockers and calcium channel blockers.

Smetnev *et al* (1979) treated 77 patients with chronic ischemic heart disease using HBO. Fifty-two of these had angina pectoris and 25 had multifocal postinfarction cardiosclerosis with insufficiency of systemic or pulmonary circulation. HBO in combination with drug therapy alleviated or arrested the symptoms of angina and corrected the central hemodynamics in the other patients.

Kuleshova and Flora (1981) discussed the rehabilitation phase of 233 patients with ischemic heart disease. All patients received physical therapy, autogenic training, massage, and therapeutic walking exercises. Group I ($n = 179$) received HBO while group II ($n = 54$) served as controls. HBO treatment was started on the 5th–10th day of admission with exposure to 1.5–2 ATA for 60 min daily. There was improvement of the general condition with relief of angina pectoris. Therefore, the rehabilitation measures in group I could be applied more intensively. There was clearance of arrhythmias in 72% of the patients in group I. Loading tests at the time of discharge from the hospital revealed that patients in group I adapted better to physical load. The range of activities in group II was limited. Therefore physical rehabilitation with HBO enhances the functional compensatory possibilities in cardiovascular disease.

Efuni et al (1984) conducted an isometric test prior to and after HBO sessions in 31 patients with chronic myocardial ischemia. It was shown that the isometric test could assess the HBO effect objectively in this situation. There was reduction in the severity of angina pectoris after HBO.

Goliakov et al (1986b) studied the effect of HBO on thromboelastogram, platelet aggregation, and prothrombin index in 40 patients with angina pectoris. There was a decrease of fibrinogen and fibrinogen degradation products, and adequate clinical effectiveness was seen in 84% of the patients. Eroshina et al (1986) showed that HBO improved myocardial contractility in patients with chronic ischemic heart disease.

The effect of HBO in reducing platelet aggregation and the serum fibrinogen content was shown to produce a favorable effect in 84% of the 40 patients with angina pectoris (Goliakov et al 1986a).

Cardiac Arrhythmias

Moderate sinus bradycardia is a common physiological response to HBO. This is due to marked increase in parasympathetic tone while breathing 100% oxygen at 2.5 ATA (Lund et al 2000). This level of HBO does not cause any cardiac arrhythmias. During the treatment of acute myocardial infarction with HBO various observers have noted an improvement of arrhythmias.

Allaria et al (1973) used HBO in a young patient with ECG abnormalities resulting from electrocution. The abnormalities cleared up. Zhivoderov et al (1980) noted disorders of rhythm and conductivity in 85% of 75 patients with myocardial infarction after the 15th day following the onset of the disease. HBO was used in 14 patients, and in 11 of these arrhythmias disappeared after 10–12 exposures. Isakov et al (1981b) used HBO in 31 patients with paroxysmal tachyarrhythmias in ischemic heart disease and concluded that the number and duration of paroxysms was reduced and that long-term remissions occurred. HBO also reduced the number of extrasystoles.

Zhivoderov et al (1982) applied HBO to 29 patients with ischemic heart disease (68.9%). In 17 patients there was disappearance of extrasystoles, which allowed the physical activity of the patients to be increased. There was no change in the acid-base balance resulting from the HBO treatment. Among another 28 patients where HBO was used along with antiarrhythmic drugs, improvement was seen in 21 cases (77.8%).

Goliakov et al (1986b) showed that there was improvement of ventricular extrasystoles in 67% of the coronary disease patients treated by HBO therapy. There was no change in 17% of the patients, and in 16% the arrhythmias increased.

Heart Failure

Acute myocardial infarction is a major contributing factor to heart failure, a chronic condition that is expected to increase in incidence along with increased life expectancy and an overall aging population. HBO has been shown to induce the production of heat shock proteins (HSPs) with a resultant protective effect. By augmenting the induction of endogenous HSPs, HBO may serve to repair and improve the function of failing hearts that have been damaged by myocardial infarction (Yogaratnam et al 2007).

Cardiac Resuscitation

Chen (1986) and Jiang (1986) studied the effect of HBO at 2 ATA on myocardial contractility during cardiac resuscitation applying external counter pulsation in dogs. Myocardial contractility was not affected, but cardiac output and carotid blood flow were increased significantly. There was a rise of arterial pAO_2 as well. Potentially HBO has applications during human cardiac resuscitation.

HBO as an Adjunct to Cardiac Surgery

Experimental Studies

Boerema (1961) was the first to report the use of a hyperbaric chamber in performing cardiac surgery. Meijne et al (1973) consider HBO to be indicated in palliative cardiac surgery for high-risk cases. They summarized the advantages as follows:

- Hypoxia or hypoxic bradycardia, which occur easily during compression of the lungs or impairment of the circulation, are much less severe.
- When flow is restored following inflow occlusion, optimal oxygenation is reached more rapidly because the low cardiac output phase is shorter.
- Cardiac resuscitation, when necessary during surgery, is markedly facilitated. Even when ventricular fibrillation occurs, defibrillation is very easy.

Bockeria and Zelenkini (1973) studied ECG changes in "dry" hearts of dogs under HBO and found that the best myocardial protection was achieved at 3.5 ATA for 60 min. Longer periods of HBO lead to oxygen intoxication. Preservation of the isolated heart for transplantation has been investigated by Todo *et al* (1974). Isolated canine hearts preserved by hypothermia and HBO at 3 ATA, as well as addition of magnesium as a metabolic inhibitor, showed no significant abnormality after 18–36 h.

Kawamura *et al* (1976) investigated the protective effect of HBO immediately after removal of an occluding ligation of a coronary artery in the dog. One group of dogs breathed room air and served as controls while the other group breathed 100% oxygen at 2 ATA before and after release of the coronary ligature. In the HBO group, the ischemic area was markedly reduced after reinstatement of the coronary blood flow. These dogs also had more stable hemodynamic conditions during operation, and ventricular fibrillation was suppressed. The authors considered HBO a useful aid in reconstruction of the acutely occluded coronary arteries. Richards *et al* (1963) investigated the role of HBO and hypothermia for suspended animation as an aid to open heart surgery. Anesthetized dogs were observed in a refrigerated hyperbaric chamber at 3 ATA. The authors concluded that the dogs could survive total circulatory arrest of up to 1 h with no gross evidence of central nervous system or myocardial damage. Accompanying acid-base disturbances were transient and reversible.

Ischemic reperfusion injury (IRI) occurs frequently in revascularization procedures such as coronary artery bypass graft (CABG). Conditioning of myocardial cells to an oxidative stress prior to IRI may limit the consequences of this injury. Preconditioning the myocardium with HBO before reperfusion has been shown to have a myocardial protective effect by limiting the infarct size post ischemia and reperfusion. Current evidence suggests that HBO preconditioning may partly attenuate IRI by stimulating the endogenous production of nitric oxide (NO), which has the ability to reduce neutrophil sequestration, adhesion, and associated injury, and to improve blood flow (Yogaratnam *et al* 2008). HBO preconditioning induced NO may play a role in providing myocardial protection during operations that involve an inevitable episode of IRI and protection of the myocardium from the effects of IRI during cardiac surgery.

Human Cardiac Surgery

Burakovsky and Bockeria (1977) reported on the resuscitative value of HBO in cardiac surgery. Deliveries have been conducted on women with cardiac disease in a hyperbaric chamber without any complications.

Bockeria *et al* (1977) described extracorporeal circulation under HBO. They performed 43 operations for conditions such as atrial and ventricular septal defects and Fallot's tetralogy. During perfusion, hemodynamic and biochemical indices were quite satisfactory. At 3 ATA,

performance of perfusions was possible without donor blood for the priming machine. The main danger of HBO was air emboli in the perfusate during decompression.

Bockeria *et al* (1978) analyzed changes in the total activity of lactic dehydrogenase (LDH), aspartic aminotransferase, and the isoenzyme spectrum of LDH in the plasma of patients with congenital heart defects. Some were operated on under HBO, others under normobaric conditions. The elevations of these enzymes as a result of trauma to the myocardium was less pronounced under HBO.

Gadzhiev (1979) investigated the dynamics of venous pressure in 80 patients during open heart surgery, where the heart was disconnected from the circulation (dry heart) using HBO. After occlusion of the vena cava, the blood was drained and subsequently autotransfused. HBO prevented disorders of the central nervous system in the intraoperative period. Burakovsky and Bockeria (1981) reported their experience of operations on the heart under conditions of HBO in 170 operations. HBO of 3–3.5 ATA allowed perfusion with hemodilution of 45%–55%. Induced diuresis rapidly restored the oxygen capacity of the blood and prevented hypoxic complications in the postoperative period.

Zelenkin and Gersimovskaya (1981) outlined the regimen of HBO for surgical treatment of patients with congenital cyanotic heart disease, based on their experiments on mongrel dogs. The appropriate value of HBO in every specific patient was calculated beforehand and controlled during the surgery. Pressure of 3.5 ATA was usually found to be optimal and the period of saturation was usually 30 min. Prolongation of this period was not accompanied by an increase of blood gas parameters. HBO was found to be a highly effective method of correction of gas metabolism problems in chronic arterial hypoxemia. Drawbacks of the method include the possibility of the development of acid-base equilibrium disturbances (hyperbaric acidosis) during long periods of saturation. Trizaminol was found to be the best drug for correction of this imbalance. Friehs *et al* (1978), of the University Clinic, Graz, Austria, reported that they performed 28 operations on congenital heart disease patients in a hyperbaric operating room and found this technique to be useful in:

- Heart operations like vascular ring, aortopulmonary shunt, and aortic isthmus stenosis with few collaterals
- High-risk operations on patients with coronary insufficiency
- Operations where blood transfusion is not permitted
- Operations with hypothermia and induced circulatory arrest: aortic or pulmonary valvotomy, and atrioseptectomy.

Li (1987b), from China, reported that his team carried out 48 open heart operations with extracorporeal circulation under HBO at 3 ATA with gratifying results. The operative procedures were similar to those outside the hyperbaric chamber. The advantage of HBO, according to the authors, is that the oxygen dissolved in the perfusing fluid is at a level 26.4 times the normal value, affording the myocardium additional protection against anoxia during the period of total occlusion of the ascending aorta. In ten cases, 800–1000 ml of blood was withdrawn from the inferior vena cava just before the institution of extracorporeal circulation. Hemoglobin was reduced to 3–4 g/100 ml and yet there was no sign of anoxia. Most of the hearts resumed beating spontaneously at the conclusion of the operation. This shows that blood can be highly diluted with no deleterious effect on the patient. Retransfusion of the withdrawn blood after surgery has the following advantages:

- Blood coagulation is hastened and postoperative oozing from the wound is reduced.
- Because of hemodilution, the internal organs are well perfused and microcirculation is improved.
- The perfusion rate can be reduced to 40–50 ml/kg/min. This reduces the damage to the blood cells during the period of extracorporeal circulation.

It may be pointed out that such a hemodilution can be performed safely only under HBO. The advantages of HBO as an adjunct to cardiac surgery can be summarized as follows:

- HBO increases the safe time of induced cardiac arrest under normothermia.
- HBO reduces the impact of hypoxic complications and metabolic disturbances associated with cardiac surgery.
- HBO enables surgery to be performed without blood transfusion in some cases.
- HBO is the treatment of choice for air embolism as a complication of cardiac surgery
- HBO has been found to be useful for the treatment of low-cardiac-output syndrome developing after cardiac surgery and associated with pulmonary hypertension.
- Pretreatment with HBO can reduce neuropsychometric dysfunction and also modulate the inflammatory response after cardiopulmonary bypass surgery (Alex *et al* 2005). However, further multicenter randomized trials are needed to clinically evaluate this form of therapy.

HBO in Preventive Cardiology

Prevention and Rehabilitation of Coronary Artery Disease

According to the animal research reports reviewed, atherosclerosis can be reversed with hyperoxia, but there are no clinical studies. It would be worthwhile to conduct a study on patients with angiographically proven coronary atherosclerosis, using HBO treatments on a long-term basis. This

could also be combined with a rehabilitation program using HBO for chronic myocardial ischemia.

Physical Training of Patients with Chronic Myocardial Insufficiency

These patients should ideally be trained in a hyperbaric chamber fitted with an ergometer. The hypothesis is that exercise leads to an increase in oxygen demand and lowers the threshold for angina. HBO increases this threshold and provides a longer duration of exercise. Exercise augments the cerebral blood flow and the interaction of improved mental function and improved physical health leads to a longer survival for these patients.

Conclusion and Comments

The role of hypoxia in the genesis of the consequences of coronary artery occlusion and myocardial infarction is well recognized. Oxygen therapy is generally accepted to be useful. The role of HBO in myocardial infarction is controversial: the bulk of animal experimental evidence favors the view that HBO has a beneficial effect in reducing the mortality and diminishing the size of the infarct. Among the clinical reports, that by Thurston *et al* (1973), which was a randomized double-blind study, remains the most important to date. According to this study, HBO is beneficial in acute myocardial infarction. The effect of HBO in reducing or reversing cardiac arrhythmias is not so important, as many useful drugs are available for this purpose.

The use of HBO as an adjunct to cardiac surgery remains confined to a few countries, notably Russia, where most of the papers reviewed have been published. Hyperbaric operating rooms have not become popular in the USA, where the operative mortality figures for cardiac surgery without HBO are lower than those reported with HBO in other countries.

HBO in Shock

Pathophysiology

The common denominator in shock, regardless of cause, is a failure of the circulatory system to deliver the chemical substances necessary for cell survival and to remove the waste products of cellular metabolism. This leads to cellular membrane dysfunction, abnormal cellular metabolism, and eventually cellular death. Some major causes of shock are:

- Decreased intravascular volume: acute hemorrhage, excessive fluid loss, and vasodilatation (relative hypovolemia)

- Cardiac conditions: acute myocardial infarction, myocarditis, acute valvular insufficiency, arrhythmias, and mechanical compression or obstruction
- Microvascular endothelial injury: burns, disseminated intravascular coagulation
- Cellular membrane injury: septic shock, anaphylaxis

Cardiac output is diminished in most states of shock; oxygen availability is reduced, and generally stagnant hypoxia ensues.

Oxygen Delivery by Blood

Hypoxia may reduce the rate of ATP synthesis, but it does not cause significant damage to mitochondrial membranes unless it is severe, sustained, and accompanied by ischemia, which also reduces the availability of other substrates. The mechanism by which ischemia and endotoxins have their adverse effect on mitochondrial function is not known.

There is little evidence that the shock state, except perhaps in its terminal stages, is associated with inability of the tissues to handle oxygen. Oxygen consumption of tissue cells falls in shock and the duration of anoxia is a measure of oxygen debt. There is a relationship between the duration of oxygen debt and survival.

Normobaric oxygen can correct arterial desaturation, but in some situations HBO is required to achieve normal oxygen saturation and even hyperoxia is necessary to reduce mortality (Ledingham 1969).

Traumatic and Hypovolemic Shock

Initial investigations of the effect of HBO in shock produced disappointing results. Subsequent experimental studies (Clark & Young 1965) showed that if HBO is administered during a period of hemorrhagic shock, the most striking observation is an elevation of arterial BP, which is due to a rise in peripheral arterial resistance rather than in cardiac output.

Ratlief et al (1976) have described myocardial zonal lesions that are pathognomonic of hypovolemic shock. This is a unique form of myocyte injury, which probably results from a combination of altered hemodynamics and inotropic stimulation accompanying hypovolemic shock. These lesions may have a role in the development of cardiac failure and loss of ventricular contractility. These lesions respond to HBO and are potentially reversible.

According to Kosonogov et al (1978) experimental and clinical investigations show a high degree of effectiveness of auxiliary perfusions in the treatment of traumatic shock. Use of HBO in the early postperfusion period increases the efficacy of resuscitative measures and stabilizes the good results achieved. Gross et al (1983a,b, 1984) produced hemorrhagic shock in animals and divided them into different

groups, which were treated under varying conditions of pressure. One group received 100% oxygen at 1 ATA, another group 100% oxygen at 2.8 ATA. The only common factor in the treatment was that each animal received lactated Ringer's solution in one series and a mixture of 10% dextrose and dextran-70 in another series. The authors found no significant differences in results with the addition of HBO in any of the groups.

Lischak et al (1987) demonstrated that HBO at 3 ATA improves the metabolic disturbances associated with experimental shock in guinea pigs induced by third degree burns. The use of HBO in conjunction with oxygen carrier blood substitutes is more promising in hemorrhagic shock and is discussed further in Chapter 24.

Cardiogenic Shock

Jacobson et al (1964) induced cardiogenic shock in dog experiments by microsphere embolization of the coronary vessels. In the control animals, mean central aortic pressure fell by 71%, cardiac output by 79%, and heart rate by 57%. With HBO at 3 ATA, mean central aortic pressure fell by only 28%, cardiac output by 43%, and heart rate by 10% following embolization. Survival was significantly greater in dogs exposed to HBO at 3 ATA; 65% of them were alive 24 h after myocardial infarction, compared with 23% of the control animals (breathing air at atmospheric pressure). Scheidt et al (1973) studied 73 patients with shock resulting from massive myocardial infarction, which they believed had evolved over a period of hours or sometimes even over a number of days. Based on the experimental evidence that infarcts can be prevented from extending by the use of various drugs and HBO, they recommended early intervention in patients with myocardial infarcts in order to prevent shock.

Kuhn (1974) described the clinical management of patients with cardiogenic shock. In those patients who have a low cardiac output and falling arterial pressure, circulatory support can be beneficial even though there is no shock. Various measures for this, such as left ventricle bypass via an interventricular drainage cannula, are carried out in conjunction with HBO to increase the oxygenation of the myocardium. Moderate hypothermia is added to reduce oxygen demand.

Barcal et al (1975) studied 18 patients to evaluate the effects of HBO therapy in cardiogenic shock complicated by the acute phase of myocardial infarction. This method achieved results equal to or better than those of the intra-aortic balloon counterpulsation technique or other methods. Success, according to these authors, depends upon early initiation of HBO therapy.

As far as cardiogenic shock is concerned, HBO appears to be a useful adjunct. There is, however, a paucity of well-documented clinical studies on this subject.

HBO in Peripheral Vascular Disease

Causes

The term peripheral vascular disease (PVD) usually refers to ischemic diseases of the extremities, mainly the legs. Various diseases that produce ischemia of the extremities are shown in Table 24.2.

Table 24.2
Diseases that Produce Ischemia in the Extremities

1. Arteriosclerosis obliterans
2. Thromboangiitis obliterans (Buerger's disease)
3. Sudden embolic or thrombotic occlusion of the artery to the limb
4. Traumatic arterial occlusion of an extremity
5. Miscellaneous arteriopathies
   – Vasculopathy resulting from drug abuse (intraarterial)
   – Granulomatous angitis
   – Allergic vasculitis
   – Collagen vascular disease

Arteriosclerosis obliterans denotes segmented arteriosclerotic narrowing or obstruction of the lumen in the arteries supplying the limbs. It is the commonest type of PVD and becomes manifest between the ages of 50 and 70 years. The lower limbs are involved more frequently than the upper limbs. Thromboangiitis obliterans is an obstructive arterial disease caused by segmental inflammatory and proliferative lesions of the medium and small vessels of the limbs. The etiology is unknown, but there is a strong association with cigarette smoking and autoimmune factors. There may be a genetic disposition to this disease; it is most prevalent between the ages of 20 and 40 years. Sudden occlusion of an artery to a limb may result from an embolus or thrombosis in situ. It occurs in 10% of cases of arteriosclerosis obliterans, but it is rare in thromboangiitis obliterans. The heart is the most frequent source of emboli in this syndrome; they may arise from a thrombus in the left ventricle.

Symptoms

Limb pain is the most frequent symptom of PVD. In the case of the legs, calf pain appears on walking a certain distance and disappears on rest. This is referred to as intermittent claudication. Pain at rest is a sign of severe PVD and occurs when there is a profound reduction in the resting blood flow to the limb. In sudden arterial occlusion, there may be numbness and weakness of the affected limb as well.

Signs

The arterial pulses distal to the site of obstruction are lost or reduced. The skin temperature is low and there may be pallor or reddish blue discoloration. There may be ulceration or gangrene of the affected extremity.

Pathophysiology of Limb Ischemia

Reduction of blood flow to a limb is due to stenosis of the arteries. Stenosis that decreases the cross-sectional area of an artery by less than 75% usually does not affect the resting blood flow to the limb; lesser degrees of stenosis may induce muscle ischemia during exercise. The presence or absence of ischemia in the presence of obstruction is also determined by the degree of collateral circulation. Some collateral vessels that are normally present do not open up until the obstruction occurs and may take several weeks or months to be fully developed. Vasodilatation in response to ischemia is the result of several mechanisms such as the release of vasodilating metabolites.

Biochemical Changes in Skeletal Muscle in Ischemia and Response to Exercise

A simple schematic overview of the energy metabolism of the skeletal muscles is shown in Figure 24.1. The fatty acids are introduced into the citric acid cycle and the mitochondrial respiratory chain by ß-oxidation. Decrease of glycogen content and succinic dehydrogenase activity has been observed in the muscles of the lower extremities in patients with circulatory disturbances.

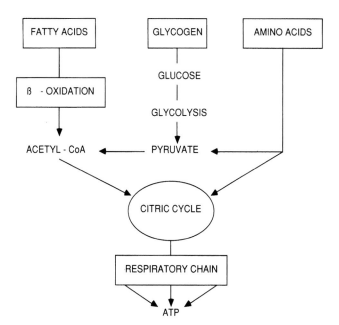

Figure 24.1
An overview of energy metabolism in skeletal muscles. The fatty acids are introduced into the citric cycle and the respiratory chain by ß-oxidation (From Reichman H *et al* 1988, reproduced by permission of the publisher: Georg Thieme Verlag, Stuttgart).

Henricksson *et al* (1980), after a study of enzyme activity, fiber types, and capillarity in the calf muscles of patients with intermittent claudication concluded that the low oxidation potential of the muscle was related to the low level of physical activity. Frequent episodes of ischemia were not considered to be stimuli for the glycolytic enzymes to adapt. A study by Bylund-Fellenius *et al* (1987) on leg muscle metabolism in patients with intermittent claudication led to somewhat different results. These authors found that patients with stable intermittent claudication had a spontaneous increase of inactivity of enzymes in the b-oxidation pathway for fatty acids, the citric acid cycle, and the respiratory chain in the gastrocnemius muscle tissue, as compared with matched controls.

During leg exercise, when the blood flow to the exercising muscles is limited and claudication develops, there was a more pronounced increase in the lactate content per unit of power in the patients compared with the controls. The fractional extraction of oxygen was higher in the patients, while the extraction of free fatty acids and glucose was similar to that in controls. A lower RQ during exercise in patients indicates that the endogenous fat was an important energy substrate. The results support the hypothesis that there is a beneficial effect of enzyme adaptation in maintaining an oxidative metabolism and that pain develops from hypoxia in certain fiber types.

Acute occlusion of a limb artery does not lead to complete ischemia due to collateral circulation. Sjöström *et al* (1982) studied human skeletal muscle metabolism and morphology after temporary incomplete ischemia resulting from aortic clamping during surgery for atherosclerotic occlusive disease of the aortic bifurcation. During the ischemic state, there were no significant changes in the muscle metabolism. After restoration of the blood flow, extensive morphological and metabolic changes were observed in the muscle biopsy tissue. The adenylate (ATP + ADP + AMP) and creatinine (Pcr + Cr) pools declined by 30%–40%, and the energy charge of the adenine nucleotides dropped significantly. The metabolic pool changes were closely related to the changes in lactate:pyruvate ratios. Signs of membrane disturbances such as fiber edema and swelling of mitochondria were seen in many muscle fibers. Type 2 fibers seemed to be selectively damaged.

An increased mitochondrial enzyme capacity in the skeletal muscle tissue is a well-documented adaptation to endurance training in humans, but the mechanism triggering this enzyme induction is not known. There is a parallel increase of key enzymes in the citric acid cycle and respiratory chain with physical training. The skeletal muscle of patients with peripheral vascular disease adapts in a similar way to endurance training by an increase in the activity of mitochondrial enzymes. Reduced blood supply to the muscle during exercise might generate the trigger for the induction of mitochondrial enzyme activity. Elander *et al* (1985) have demonstrated that, in a rat model, reduced blood flow induced by arterial ligation leads to an adaptive increase of citrate synthesis and cytochrome c oxidase, when intermittent muscle contractions were induced by electrical stimulation.

Lundgren *et al* (1988) have studied the exchange of amino acids in leg muscles during exercise in patients with arterial insufficiency. They demonstrated that a higher glutamine efflux and a correspondingly lower efflux of asparagine occurs in hypoxic leg muscles during exercise, compared with leg muscles during normal blood flow. This suggests an increase in the rate of amino acid oxidation in hypoxic muscles during exercise. Their results confirm that a normal resting balance of amino acids is restored within 10–20 min following interruption of exercise because of intermittent claudication. The membrane integrity, therefore, is not seriously affected by hypoxia due to arterial insufficiency.

Clinical and Laboratory Assessment of Patients with Peripheral Vascular Disease

During assessment of a PVD patient, it is important to rule out nonvascular causes of extremity pain such as intermittent claudication due to spinal cord stenosis. Clinical examination of the cardiovascular system with evaluation of the peripheral pulses and pressures in the distal arteries is an important part of clinical evaluation. Special laboratory diagnostic procedures are listed in Table 24.3.

Transcutaneous oxygen tension (tcpO$_2$) is a noninvasive method of measuring the tissue oxygen tension: the technique has been described in detail elsewhere (Jain 1989b). This test has been used to detect the presence or absence of peripheral arterial insufficiency. Bakay-Csorba *et al* (1987)

Table 24.3
Laboratory Procedures for the Evaluation of Peripheral Vascular Disease

1. Doppler flowmetry:detection of location of obstruction to blood flow
2. Venous occlusion plethysmography:measurement of rate of volume of arterial inflow into a limb after occlusion of the venous outflow
3. Transcutaneous oxygen tension (tcpO$_2$) measurement
4. Angiography:definite diagnosis and localization of pathology
5. Response to physical exercise; measurement of limits of performance

---

Table 24.4
Transcutaneous Oxygen Tension Measured with Changes in Arteriograms of Patients with Peripheral Vascular Disease

	Above knee	Below knee
Sensitivity	86%	91%
Specificity	20%	33%
Accuracy	69%	76%

compared the tcpO$_2$ measurements with changes in arteriograms of PVD patients. The results are shown in Table 24.4. These results show that ptcO$_2$ is more useful for the detection of femoral artery disease (below the knee) than iliac artery disease (above the knee).

Lusiani *et al* (1988) measured ptcO$_2$ on the dorsum of the foot in healthy subjects and found an average value of 71.2 ± 14.26 mmHg. In patients with PVD, these values were an average of 51.56 ± 26.38 mmHg; the deviations from the average were more marked than in normal subjects. Hence the accuracy of this test is limited: it can, however, be useful in assessing the response of a patient with PVD to exercise and HBO therapy. A more accurate method of measuring muscle tissue oxygen tension is a pO$_2$ histogram (Hauss & Spiegel 1987).

Table 24.5
Staging of Patients with Peripheral Vascular Disease
(after Fontaine)

Stage I:	Free from symptoms
Stage II:	Intermittent claudication
Stage IIa:	Walking distance over 200 m
Stage IIb:	Walking distance less than 200 m
Stage III:	Pain at rest
Stage IV:	Ulceration and gangrene

The staging system of Fontaine (Table 24.5) is usually followed to evaluate the progress and the results of treatment of PVD patients.

General Management of PVD Patients

The various methods that have been used for the management of PVD patients are listed in Table 24.6.

Table 24.6
Management of Patients with Peripheral Vascular Disease

1. **Medical management**
   Vasodilator drugs
   Platelet inhibitors: aspirin, dipyridamole, sulfapyrazine
   Drugs to improve hemorheology: pentoxyfylline
2. **Exercise therapy**
   Gradual intermittently increasing exercise
   Exercise with supplemental oxygen: normobaric or hyperbaric
3. **Surgery**
   Angioplasty; balloon catheter or laser
   Endarterectomy of the occluded vessel
   Vein bypass
   Teflon grafts
   Sympathectomy
4. **Prevention**
   Smoking cessation
   Control of risk factors for atherosclerosis

Drug Therapy

Most of the vasodilator drugs are no longer approved for use in PVD patients. The diseased vessels do not dilate; thus, these medications dilate the vessels in the healthy areas and cause a "steal" effect from the ischemic area.

The role of platelet-inhibiting drugs in PVD has not been defined. These drugs, of which aspirin is an example, remain the most widely used drugs in cardiovascular disorders.

Pentoxyfylline and cilostazol are the only two approved drug for ischemic pain due to PVD. The postulated mechanism of action is rheological. In a double-blinded, controlled study, Ehrly & Saeger-Lorenz (1988) showed that pentoxyfylline combined with exercise leads to an increase in pO$_2$ of the muscle as shown in a pO$_2$ histogram; there was no change in muscle pO$_2$ in the control subjects given normal saline and exercise.

Exercise Therapy

Exercise training appears to be an effective treatment for claudication, the primary symptom of peripheral arterial disease. Exercise-induced increases in functional capacity and lessening of claudication symptoms may be explained by several mechanisms, including measurable improvements in end thelial vasodilator function, skeletal muscle metabolism, blood viscosity, and inflammatory responses (Stewart *et al* 2002). This is currently the method of choice for managing patients with intermittent claudication who do not have surgically correctable lesions. Some patients, however, are not able to increase the walking distance by this approach alone and supplemental oxygen has been found to be helpful in these cases.

Surgery

A variety of surgical procedures is available. Endarterectomy, where the thrombus is removed, is usually done in acute occlusion. This procedure is less successful in small vessel occlusion. Where the stenotic lesion cannot be corrected, vein bypass or excision and replacement with a synthetic graft may be tried. Percutaneous balloon angioplasty is quite popular although the long-term results are controversial. Laser angioplasty and radiofrequency angioplasty are promising new techniques. Lumbar sympathectomy has been performed to release the alpha-adrenergic vasoconstriction. This procedure is performed rarely these days.

Role of HBO in the Management of Peripheral Vascular Disease

The various reasons given to explain the usefulness of HBO in PVD are summarized in Table 24.7. Tissue ischemia has

Table 24.7
Rationale for the Use of HBO in Peripheral Vascular Disease

1. **Relief of hypoxia**
   - HBO raises the low ptcO$_2$ in the marginally perfused ischemic/hypoxic tissues
   - HBO improves the cellular metabolism which has been impaired by hypoxia

2. **Relief of effects of ischemia: HBO is not a vasoconstrictor in ischemic tissues**
   - HBO reduces the incidence and extent of gangrene in the limbs
   - HBO helps in demarcating the line between viable and nonviable tissues as a guide to amputation where it is unavoidable
   - HBO promotes healing of ulcers due to vascular insufficiency
   - HBO helps the limb salvage in arterial trauma in patients who are (a) waiting for a surgical procedure, or those in whom (b) the surgical procedures have failed

3. **Relief of pain; the various mechanisms are**
   - Improved local circulation with decreased accumulation of algogenesic polypeptides
   - Secondary to relief of hypoxia
   - Secondary to antiedema effect of HBO
   - HBO increases the affinity of endorphins for receptor sites

4. **Increase of exercise capacity in combined HBO and exercise therapy**
   - HBO and exercise both improve hemorrheology and contribute to better perfusion of the ischemic limb
   - HBO improves the biochemical disturbances due to exercise and thus permits better physical performance
   - Exercise with resulting vasodilatation may prevent the vasoconstricting effect of HBO on arterioles in the nonaffected areas of the limbs

two primary effects – reduction of oxygen supply to the part, and retention of CO_2 and other products of tissue metabolism. It is difficult to modify the retention of toxic products, but the lack of oxygen can be compensated by HBO.

The most important of the beneficial effects of HBO in intermittent claudication treatment is the role in increasing walking capacity in patients who have reached a limit with simple gradually increasing exercise. This effect will be examined later in this chapter.

Experimental Studies

Bird and Telfer (1965) tested the effect of 100% oxygen on the blood flow to the arms of healthy young volunteers. At 1 ATA the reduction was 11.2%. At 2 ATA the reduction was 18.9%. After the HBO, the amount of available oxygen was increased even though the blood flow remained unchanged. The authors suggested that there was a homeostatic mechanism to keep the oxygen tensions constant.

This mechanism does not apply to the ischemic limb, where the oxygen tension is much below normal. The rate at which the oxygen diffuses from the blood through the capillary wall to the tissue fluids and the cells depends upon the gradient of the partial pressures between the plasma and the tissue cells.

Ackerman and Brindley (1966) showed that under HBO pO$_2$ tensions rise more than 5.6 times in the ischemic tissues compared with the normal tissues (Figure 24.2). Normobaric oxygen was shown to lead to a slight rise of pO$_2$ in the normal limb, but not in the ischemic limb. Stalker and Ledingham (1973) produced acute hind-limb ischemia in anesthetized dogs. Oxygen extraction and consumption rose initially, but then fell below the normal levels. HBO at 2 ATA did not influence the blood flow or the metabolic exchange. Kawamura et al (1978) conducted similar experiments to test the effects of HBO on hind-limb ischemia in dogs and concluded that oxygen does not act as a vasoconstrictor in hypoxic tissues until oxygen deficit is improved.

Schraibman and Ledingham. (1969) studied the effect of HBO and regional vasodilation in foot ischemia. They stated that the problem of the ischemia had not been solved by reconstructive surgery or sympathectomy, which benefits just over 50% of the patients. They measured foot blood flow in healthy volunteers and patients by means of strain gauge plethysmography. The resting blood flow was similar in normal subjects and patients with claudication, and showed a significant decrease with HBO. Resting blood flow was low in those with skin ischemia, but showed a significant increase with HBO when this was given in combination with an intravenous infusion of tolazoline hydrochloride (vasodilator). After sympathectomy neither HBO nor vasodilator produced any change in blood flow.

Kawamura et al (1978) investigated the effect of HBO on normal tissues and hypoxic tissues. Acute temporary ischemia was produced in the right hind limbs of dogs, while the left hind limbs served as a control. HBO at 2 ATA produced vasoconstriction in the normal limbs (control), whereas there was no vasoconstriction in the ischemic limbs until after the hypoxia had been corrected.

Following acute ischemia of a limb there are changes in microcirculation and interference with flow and transport. The integrity of membranes separating intravascular and extravascular spaces is impaired, and edema may result in ischemic muscle. Even when the circulation is restored, edema may persist or get worse. This can cause compression of capillaries and aggravation of ischemia, thus starting a vicious circle. Nylander et al (1985) produced edema in rats using a limb tourniquet to interrupt the circulation. HBO caused a significant reduction of postischemic edema, and this effect persisted 40 h after the last treatment. The authors considered HBO to be a useful adjunct to the treatment of acute ischemic condi-

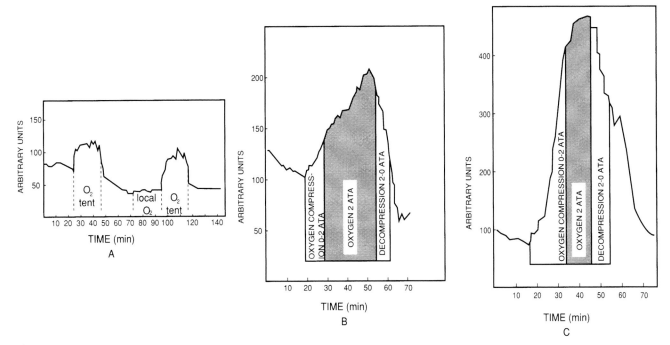

Figure 24.2
Oxygen tension in normal and ischemic tissues during hyperbaric therapy.*A*: Response of tissue pO_2 in normal limb to inhalation of oxygen at atmospheric pressure, and to a local oxygen-rich environment;*B*: Response of tissue pO_2 in normal limb to hyperbaric oxygen at 15 psig;*C*: Response of tissue pO_2 in ischemic limb to hyperbaric oxygen at 15 psig (Modified from Ackerman and Brinkley, 1966, by permission of the American Medical Association).

tions where surgical repair alone fails or is not adequate to reverse the condition.

Repeated HBO treatments in the postischemic phase have been shown to stimulate aerobic metabolism (Nylander *et al* 1987). Reduction of phosphorylase activity, which is a sensitive marker of muscle damage, is improved by HBO in the postischemic phase (Nylander *et al* 1988).

Review of Clinical Applications

Illingworth (1962) was the first to use HBO for peripheral vascular disease, and was able to salvage a few limbs after acute arterial injuries. He was the first to notice relief of pain in patients with thromboangiitis obliterans while undergoing HBO therapy. There was healing of skin ulcerations.

Stansell (1965) reported the effect of HBO in patients with atherosclerosis and incipient early gangrene of the lower extremities. It was noted that the gangrenous tissue was consistently rendered dry and the margins sharp and clearcut. The level of amputation required was usually lower than that necessary without the use of HBO.

Gorman *et al* (1965) described their experiences in the end stage of occlusive arterial disease in the lower extremities. In contrast to occlusion of proximal major vessels, these patients had involvement of small arteries and arterioles supplying the skin and subcutaneous tissues, where development of the collateral network is at a minimum.

Forty-eight such patients were treated with HBO at 3 ATA for 1 h daily. All of them had potential or incipient gangrene and all had undergone lumbar sympathectomy. The overall limb salvage and progression of ischemic process was not significantly altered by HBO in these cases. Microscopic examination of tissues at the margin of necrosis revealed less inflammatory reaction in HBO-treated patients than in controls, indicating an important relationship between hyperoxia and cellular response to injury.

Lukich *et al* (1976) studied the changes in tissue gas exchange and oxygen balance during HBO in patients with chronic thrombo-obliterating disease of the extremities. They reported that normalization of metabolic processes in ischemic tissues takes place, together with elimination of oxygen deficits and deviations in acid-base balance. Sakakibara *et al* (1985), from Japan, presented their experience with the use of HBO in 159 patients with chronic peripheral vascular disease seen over a period of 18 years. These included 109 cases of thromboangiitis obliterans, which has a high incidence in Japan. Of these cases, 69% had healing of their sores. Of the 43 patients with atherosclerotic occlusive disease, 70% had healing of their skin ulcers. The incidence of amputation required was decreased in all the patients.

Kostiunin *et al* (1985) analyzed the HBO treatment of 122 patients with advanced arterial occlusive disease of the lower extremities and showed that the effectiveness of HBO can be enhanced by combination with continuous intraar-

Table 24.8
HBO Treatment Results in Some Types of Vascular Pathologies

Type of pathology	Patients		Treatment results		
	(n)	Good		Satisfactory	No effect
Obliterative endarteritis	1684	1297		236	151
	100%	77%		14%	9%
Obliterative atherosclerosis	1537	1061		384	92
	100%	69%		25%	6%
Total	3221	2358		620	243
	100%	73.2%		19.3%	7.5%
Acute arterial insufficiency	18%	11		–	7
	100%	61%		39%	
Chronic venous insufficiency	163	72		48	43
	100%	44%		29.5%	26.5%
Trophic ulcers of vascular genesis	370	192		113	65
	100%	52%		30.5%	17.5%

terial infusions and lumbar sympathectomy. An important factor, according to them, is an increase of low cardiac output. Rosenthal *et al* (1985) presented three cases of infants with disseminated intravascular clotting involving peripheral arterial occlusions and gangrene of parts of the arms and legs. They were able, with HBO, to affect regression of the demarcation line of gangrene, and the amputations were minimized.

Baroni *et al* (1987) showed that HBO treatments reduced gangrene and the amputation rate in patients with diabetic gangrene. Fredenucci (1985) used HBO in treating arteriopathies of the limbs in 2021 patients treated between 1966 and 1983. Plethysmographic studies showed that blood flowed from the healthy areas (with vasoconstriction) to nonresponding hypoxic territories in 40% of the patients. The author felt that HBO is an important method of treatment of patients with asymptomatic arteriopathies.

Efuni *et al* (1985) believe that reduction of regional blood flow to 1.5 ml/min/100 g muscle tissue is the limit of HBO effectiveness. According to them, the primary reaction of ischemic tissues to HBO treatment is higher blood flow volume, which is due to opening of nonfunctioning capillaries, thus leading to a considerably larger oxygen diffusion area. HBO also improves the rheological properties of blood: fibrinogen concentration and plasma tolerance to heparin decrease, while fibrinolytic activity increases.

Efuni *et al* evaluated the degree of effectiveness of HBO treatment by polarography. In 70% of cases tissue pO_2 does not return to baseline for 1 h or more, as compared with a drop to normal values in the blood within 0.5 h. This "after effect" is due to reduction of tissue oxygen consumption after HBO treatment. There is some interrelationship between the duration of the after effect and the therapeutic effect of HBO, and this makes a fair prediction of the effects of HBO possible. The treatment is supplemented by vasodilators. The authors' 7-year expe-

rience with over 3,000 cases is summarized in Table 24.8. The best results were obtained in patients with chronic arterial insufficiency.

Visona *et al* (1989) treated patients in various stages of PVD and reported long-term improvement in more than 50% of the cases. Belov *et al* (1986) reported that HBO was 1.4 times more effective than conventional management in relieving symptoms of PVD.

Urayama *et al* (1992) studied the therapeutic effect of HBO in patients with chronic occlusive disease of the lower extremities in 50 patients. These patients had a variety of sequelae of limb ischemia: pain at rest, ulceration, etc. HBO was used at 2 ATA for 60 min and the number of sessions varied from 3–40. Five out of six patients with pain at rest were relieved. Necrosis or ulceration healed in 16 out of 30 patients. Transcutaneous oxygen tension was markedly increased during during HBO sessions and remained so for sometime afterwards. Lipid peroxide and SOD levels were not changed significantly by HBO treatments.

Kovacevic (1992) carried out a prospective placebo-controlled, double-blind study of the effect of HBO on atherosclerotic occlusive disease of the lower extremities in 65 patients. Treatment group (35 patients) was given HBO at 2.8 ATA, twice a day, for a total of 20 treatments during 2 weeks. The control group (30 patients) were given normoxic mixture (nitrox 7.5) to breathe in the hyperbaric chamber. Both groups maintained the conservative medical therapy and were advised to quit smoking. The treatment group showed improvement during the first three months as manifested by increase of pain free walking distance. The improvement persisted during the 6 month follow-up period.

HBO as an Adjunct to Exercise Therapy for Ischemic Leg Pain

Prior to 1989 there was no publication describing the use of ergometry under HBO for the rehabilitation of patients

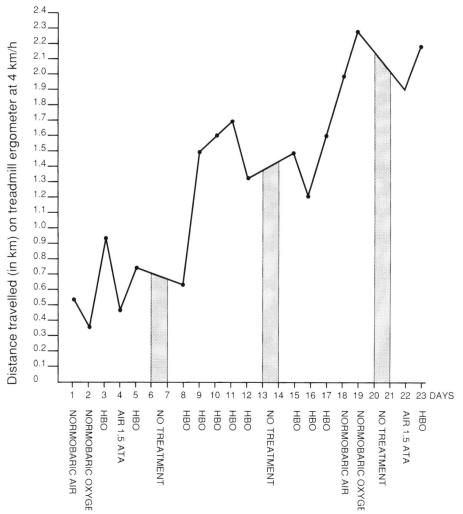

Figure 24.3
Treatment schedule of case no. 4 (Table 24.9). Pretreatment, days 1–4; posttreatment, days 18, 19, 22. 23: HBO, 100% hyperbaric oxygen, 1.5 ATA.

with ischemic leg pain. At first, normobaric oxygen supplementation was used (Jain 1989b). Those patients who could not make any further progress with bicycle ergometry breathing room air or 100% normobaric oxygen were selected for a pilot study using HBO at Fachklinik Klausenbach in Germany.

Four male patients, with varying degrees of limitation of walking due to ischemic leg pain, were treated with a combination of ergometry and HBO during the past 2 years. All of them had angiographic confirmation of arterial occlusion and of hemodynamic disturbance by plethysmography. All had been treated medically and all were in stable condition. None of them had had surgical treatment. Various medications including pentoxyfylline were maintained during our treatment.

All the patients underwent ergometric training on a treadmill installed in the hyperbaric chamber, with a computerized control outside. The speed, distance traveled, and time were recorded. The pressure used was 1.5 ATA for a 45-min session (10 min compression + 30 min of 100% oxygen at full pressure + 5 min decompression). The exercise was started at the completion of

the compression phase and stopped at the onset of leg pain, when the patient rested in the chamber until the session was completed. The control studies were ergometry in the chamber under normobaric air, hyperbaric air (1.5 ATA), and normobaric oxygen (100%). Laboratory studies included blood ammonia, lactate glucose, free fatty acids (FFA), and glycerin both before and after exertion during the first 4 days and last 4 days of the treatment (Figure 24.3). No treatments were done on weekends. No transcutaneous pO_2 measurements were taken, but arterial and venous pO_2 tensions were measured during the laboratory sessions.

The clinical results of training in the four patients are shown in Table 24.9.

One of the selection criteria of the patients was ability to do ergometry. This excluded the stroke patients with hemiplegia, who were treated in the chamber and showed improvement of the ischemic leg pain and improved capacity for walking. They performed leg exercises, but were not considered fit to proceed with the ergometry program.

All the treatments were given on an outpatient basis.

Table 24.9
Summary of the Results of Training in Four Patients with PVD Using Ergometry plus HBO

No.	Age stage	Diagnosis walking range	Before HBO treatment normobaric O$_2$	Maximum distance under HBO	Maximum distance sessions	No. of current condition	Remarks
1	70	Bilateral stenosis femorals, stage III; rest pains	150 m/3 min level 10 m at 25 W on 15° upgrade	Not done 400 m level	150 m with 15° upgrade	10	Relief of pain walks 3–4 km
2	51	Left femoral occlusion; stage IIa	605 m in 6 min	1074 m in 14 min	3166 m in 33 min	14	Ergometry in room air: 2285/24 min; 7 km mountain hike
3	66	Bilateral occlusive disease; stage IIa; myocardial and cerebrovascular insufficiency	529 m in 6 min	685 m in 9 min	1258 m in 20 min	10	Maintains improvement
4	49	Right femoral occlusion; stage IIa	526 m in 8 min	2358 m in 35 min	2250 m in 34 min	11	Maintains improvement (see Figure 24.3)

The first two patients were treated once a week and the last two on a daily basis except on weekends. This frequency was determined by the availability of the patients (retired or working) and the distance of their residence from the clinic. The protocol is still being modified. In patient no. 2, HBO sessions followed on the same days as sessions with room air. The protocol for patient no. 4 is shown in Figure 24.3. All four patients showed improvement of the distance they could walk on the treadmill ergometer. In spite of fluctuations in performance, there was overall improvement, as shown in Table 24.9. The laboratory results conformed to the pattern previously observed in healthy volunteers. Lactate and ammonia accumulation were less during exertion under HBO than under normobaric oxygen or in room air.

It is likely that HBO helped these patients to cross the "barrier" of limitation of walking, even though the vascular pathology was not reversed. The improvement in these patients was adequate to carry out the daily activities required for their jobs.

The number of HBO sessions (with exercise) should be guided by the "ceiling effect," i.e., when the performance under HBO is not significantly different from that while breathing normobaric oxygen or ambient air. At that point, HBO treatments serve no purpose and should be discontinued, and the patient should continue to exercise daily in room air.

Miscellaneous Arterial Conditions (Toxic and Allergic Arteriopathies)

Monies-Chass *et al* (1976) described the case of a child with allergic vasculitis due to penicillin affecting the limbs and abdominal wall. HBO was used successfully after failure of conventional treatment. The authors' explanation was that ischemia of the vessel wall leads to increased permeability with exudation of electrolytes, fluids, and proteins into the extracellular space, causing edema, which further aggravates ischemia. Fasciotomy does not help in this situation. HBO interrupted the circle of ischemia of vessel wall exudation compression of vessels aggravation of vessel wall ischemia.

De Myttenaere *et al* (1977) described a case of self-administration by injection of methylphenidate into the brachial artery by an addict. Intensive treatment started within 12 h and a combination of HBO, vasodilators, and stellate ganglion block saved the arm, with limited loss of the fingertips.

Ergotism can result from prolonged use of ergot-derived alkaloids in migraine. There is arterial constriction leading to peripheral ischemia and gangrene. Ergotamine may also cause toxic endothelial damage, either acute or chronic. Some cases recover after discontinuation of ergot and others improve with vasodilators. Merrick *et al* (1978) saw eight patients with ergotism after unsuccessful treatment using other methods. They were given HBO at 3 ATA for 1 h two to three times a day along with an epidural block for relief of pain due to ischemia of the limb. The treatment was successful in all cases.

HBO as an Adjunct to Peripheral Vascular Surgery

Eisterer and Staudacher (1971) found backflow during surgery on seven patients with severe vascular disease of the lower extremities. These patients were treated with multiple sessions of HBO after surgery, and the surgeons believed that this method saved the limbs in these patients. The authors pointed out that a single exposure to HBO without surgery is useless.

Monies-Chass *et al* (1976) presented a series of seven young men suffering from severe vascular trauma and acute ischemia of the limbs. Standard repair, though technically successful, failed to achieve satisfactory restoration of the circulation. HBO treatment of 2.8 ATA prevented the development of gangrene in all cases. The authors considered HBO a useful adjunct to reconstructive surgery in cases needing repair long after the injury.

The role of HBO in the treatment of ulcers caused by arterial insufficiency is reviewed in Chapter 15, and its use in limb edema in trauma and compartment syndrome is reviewed in Chapter 30.

Conclusions Regarding the Role of HBO in Peripheral Vascular Disease

Since the first observation by Illingworth (1962) on the effect of HBO in relieving pain due to limb ischemia, there has been no study to evaluate the effectiveness of HBO in patients where pain is the only symptom. Most of the reports in the literature deal with more serious cases, where there is gangrene or skin ulceration. HBO therapy is generally considered useful in the treatment of occlusive peripheral arterial disease and its role should be investigated further.

25 HBO Therapy in Hematology and Immunology

K.K. Jain

HBO has a useful role in certain hematological and immunological disorders. This chapter examines the following:

Introduction

This chapter will examine the important effects of hyperbaric oxygenation on the elements of the blood. The overall effect is improvement of hemorrheology, which is useful in many microcirculation disorders. The effect of HBO in lowering hematocrit and whole blood viscosity and increasing the RBC elasticity has been used in treating disorders of the inner ear. The effect of HBO on constituents of the blood and its applications in hematological disorders, which are rather limited, will be discussed in this chapter. Immunological effects of HBO are also considered as they involve the leukocytes.

Effect of HBO on Red Blood Cells

The major function of red blood cells is to transport hemoglobin, which in turn carries oxygen from the lungs to the tissues. They also contain carbonic anhydrase, which catalyzes the reaction between CO_2 and H_2O, and the product is transported in the form of bicarbonate ion (HCO_2) to the lungs.

Deformability

RBC are concave discs with a mean diameter of 8 μm and a maximum thickness of 2 μm at the periphery and 1 μm or less at the center. The average volume of the RBC is 83 μm³. As the RBC passes through the capillaries, it can be deformed into any shape. This deformability is an important determinant of whole blood viscosity, particularly in the microcirculation, where capillary diameter is smaller than the RBC diameter. This contributes to the inversion phenomenon – increased viscosity at the capillary level compared with larger vessels. The RBC can traverse a channel 14 μm long and 2.8 μm wide and can squeeze through a 0.5 μm opening between cells. The deformability of the RBC depends upon the normal hemoglobin structure, as well as adenosine triphosphate (ATP) stores. A normal RBC can undergo deformation without stretching the membrane or rupturing it. This ability of the RBC is an important factor in the microcirculation and tissue oxygen exchange.

Animals experimental studies of the effect of HBO on RBC deformability give conflicting results. Higher pressures usually transiently decrease the deformability. Pressures below 2 ATA usually increase the deformability. .Erythrocyte elasticity increases and hematocrit drops in healthy volunteers exercising under HBO at 1.5 ATA. This improves the ability of the RBC to navigate the capillaries and improve oxygenation of the tissues. The maximum ox-

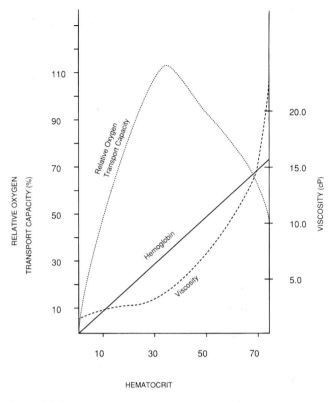

Figure 25.1

Relation of hematocrit, hemoglobin, and viscosity to relative oxygen transport capacity (From Hint H (1968) The pharmacology of dextran and the physiological background for the clinical use of Rheomacrodex and Macrodex. *Acta Anethesiol Belg* 19: 119–138).

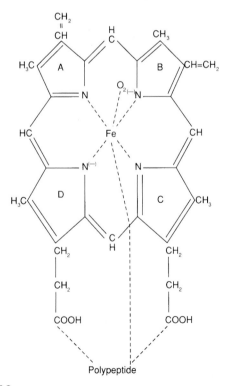

Figure 25.2

Basic structure of the hemoglobin molecule.

ygen delivery to the tissues is at a hematocrit level of 30%–33% (Figure 25.1), which is significantly lower than the normal hematocrit range of 36%–47% at sea level.

Oxygen Exchange

Oxygen transport requires diffusion of oxygen into the RBC and chemical combination with intracellular hemoglobin. Oxygen does not combine with the two positive valences of the ferrous iron in the hemoglobin molecule (Figure 25.2). Instead, it binds loosely with one of the six "coordination" valences of the iron atom. This is an extremely loose bond so that the combination is easily reversible. Furthermore, the oxygen does not become ionic oxygen, but is carried on to the tissues as molecular oxygen. There, because of the loose, readily reversible combination, it is released into the tissue fluids in the form of dissolved molecular oxygen rather than ionic oxygen.

Several factors, including RBC morphology and physiology, influence the rate of these processes. Cell size and shape define the surface area available for oxygen influx into the cytoplasm. Intracellular hemoglobin concentration determines the maximum amount of oxygen that can diffuse in and out of the cell, and changes in intracellular pH or organic phosphate concentration shift the rate of chemical reaction between oxygen and hemoglobin.

Studies of the kinetics of oxygen uptake of RBCs reveal that:

- The rate of oxygen uptake roughly depends on the second power of the surface area to volume ratio of the RBC, whereas the rate of release is much less dependent on these factors.
- The rate of RBC oxygenation is independent of the pH and internal 2,3-diphosphoglycerate (DPG) concentration, whereas the deoxygenation depends markedly on these conditions.

As pH is lowered or DPG concentration is raised, the overall oxygen affinity of the cell decreases sevenfold and oxygen release increased by the same extent. Under hyperoxic conditions, oxygen release reaches its maximum value at a partial pressure of 300 mmHg in resting cells, and 100–200 mmHg in flowing cells. The efficient release of oxygen from RBCs depends upon oxygen and oxyhemoglobin diffusion, as well as intracellular convection as a result of deformation of RBCs during flow.

The normal oxygen tension difference between RBCs and plasma is small, 6 mmHg or less. In anemia larger differences may exist between RBC pO_2 and plasma pO_2 because the diffusion of oxygen from the RBC lags behind tissue demand. Hemoglobin, which is outside the red cells (3%), enhances transfer and diminishes these differences.

Structure and Biochemistry

There are several changes in RBCs after exposure to HBO. Hemolysis and reduction of hematocrit may occur. Effects such as these may be related to alterations of membrane structures, which are largely composed of phospholipids and may undergo peroxidation. The levels of several phospholipids in plasma and RBCs is reduced following hyperoxygenation. Under hyperoxia there is a decrease in the RBC levels of ATP and DPG. This was accompanied by a decrease in the active RBC K^+ flux. It has already been mentioned (Chapter 5) that under hypoxic conditions the level of organic phosphates, particularly DPG, is increased. The decrease of ATP with hyperoxia may be due to inhibition of glycolytic enzymes. It may also be pointed out that it is the combined level of both DPG and ATP that are significant in determining the oxygen affinity of the hemoglobin.

Mengel *et al* (1965) reported a case of hemolytic anemia 2 days after exposure to HBO (2 ATA). They found that the patient's RBC resembled those of vitamin E deficient mice in terms of in vitro sensitivity to hydrogen peroxide. A mechanism of peroxide hemolysis and protection against it is shown in Figure 25.3.

The reduced glutathione (GSH) content of the intact erythrocytes is increased by 15% after HBO exposure, and remains so for 24 h after the cessation of therapy. The erythrocyte phospholipid fatty acid turnover is inhibited and this may be an early marker of oxygen toxicity. Meyerstein *et al* (1989) found that HBO at 3 ATA for 2 h does not affect the GSH content of the RBC.

In oxygen-induced seizures, morphological changes have been observed in RBC, which are likely the result of a decrease in the quantity of SOD. There are changes in the membrane that are likely due to free radical formation. These changes are not found in RBC's during epileptic seizures.

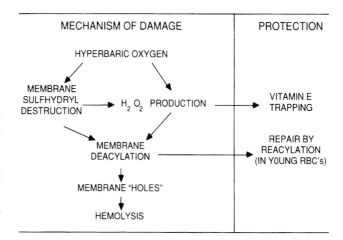

Figure 25.3
The mechanism of peroxide hemolysis and protection. Reacylation balances incorporation of plasma fatty acids in membrane phosphatidyl-ethanolamine (from Wirjosemito & Touhey 1988).

Landaw *et al* (1979) studied RBCs in rats continually exposed to 100% oxygen (pO_2 197–450 mmHg) for up to 105 days and noted no changes in RBC mass, plasma volume, or plasma iron turnover. Bairrington and Pryor (1969) stored hum an erythrocytes at 4°C for 22 days at a simulated depth of 2 ATA and found that they were more resistant to hemolysis caused by osmotic fragility than were erythrocytes stored at sea level for the same period. They proposed that the increased viability of the cellular membranes at depth was due to diminution of the metabolic rate and reduced binding of ATP and DPG to hemoglobin; the result was a conservation of energy metabolism with a more viable glucose transport and lipid synthesis mechanism.

Hemoglobin. Exposure to hyperoxia contributes significantly to reduced hemoglobin and increased ferritin concentrations. The changes may reflect a shift of iron from synthesis of hemoglobin in the bone marrow to storage in macrophages caused by a downregulation of hemoglobin synthesis, or an increased oxidative stress. The changes are too small to be of clinical significance with respect to HBO treatment (Thorsen *et al* 2001).

Erythropoiesis

The principal factor that stimulates RBC production is a circulating hormone called erythropoietin, most of which is formed in the kidneys. Tissue oxygen is the basic regulator of RBC production. Any condition that causes the quantity of oxygen transported to the tissues to decrease, increases the rate of RBC production. Increase of oxygen tension in the blood inhibits erythropoiesis and diminishes RBC production.

Voitkevich *et al* (1975) exposed rabbits to HBO at 2 ATA. The erythropoietic activity of the plasma was determined from the mitotic activity of a bone marrow culture in liquid medium containing colchicine. Erythropoietin disappeared from the plasma of the arterial and the venous blood, as well as from the kidneys. An erythropoiesis-inhibiting factor could be detected in blood outflow from the kidneys 24 h after exposure to HBO.

Voitkevich *et al* (1979) investigated the erythropoietin content of the plasma of the peripheral blood in volunteers exposed for the first time to the action of hyperbaric hyperoxia simulating diving. The pressure was 7 ATA and the breathing mixture was 25% O_2 + 15% He + 60% N_2, so that the pO_2 rose to 1400 mmHg. After 10 min the pressure was lowered to 2.5 ATA and decompression was continued so that the total procedure took 40 min. The concentration of erythropoietic factor in the plasma was markedly reduced 24 h after exposure, but no erythropoiesis-inhibiting factors were detected in the plasma.

Pierre (1964) showed suppression of erythropoiesis in mice exposed to HBO at 4 ATA for 24 h, but they could stimulate erythropoiesis by administration of exogenous erythropoietin. The fact that the RBC count does not increase in response to hypoxia or decrease in response to hyperoxia within 24 h, should be taken into consideration. These hyperbaric exposures should not result in a drop in the count of RBC unless the pressure is maintained for prolonged periods, which is not the case in clinical applications.

Effect of HBO on Leukocytes

Chen *et al* (1996) hypothesized that HBO caused a metabolic derangement in polymorphonuclear leukocytes that impaired the function of B_2-integrins. Isolated neutrophils from rats that had been exposed to 3 ATA oxygen for 45 min failed to exhibit B_2-integrin-dependent adherence to nylon columns or to fibrinogen-coated plates. Adherence was restored after cells were incubated with 8-bromo-cGMP, phorbol 12-myristate 13-acetate (PMA) or the reducing agent dithioerythritol. HBO was found to inhibit cGMP synthesis that normally occurred when cells were stimulated by passage through nylon columns, and exposure to PMA or dithioerythritol reestablished cGMP synthesis. Cells adherent to plastic plates synthesized cGMP when they were exposed to N-formyl-methionyl-leu-cine-phenylalanine (FMLP) or PMA. Neutrophils from rats exposed to HBO synthesized cGMP in response to PMA but failed to respond to FMLP, although hyperbaric oxygen did not alter the affinity of the FMLP receptor or its associated G protein. Dithioerythritol restored the cGMP synthetic ability of adherent neutrophils in response to FMLP. The authors concluded that hyperbaric oxygen inhibits B_2-integrin-dependent adherence because it impairs cGMP synthesis by activated neutrophils. In contrast to experimental data, repetitive exposure of human patients to hyperoxia does not influence human monocyte and lymphocyte functions (Jaeger *et al* 2002).

Effect of HBO on Platelets

A single exposure of isolated horse platelets to 100% oxygen at 2.2 ATA showed no detrimental effect on platelet biochemistry, and it does not cause overt oxidative stress *in vitro* (Shaw *et al* 2005). There are concerns about the cytotoxicity of oxygen to platelet function during prolonged HBO therapy. A study was conducted on patients scheduled for multiple HBO treatments in order to evaluate oxidative metabolism in platelets and platelet aggregation (Handy *et al* 2005). The capacity for oxidative metabolism (lactate ratio) in platelets was not affected by HBO, except in smokers, where it increased by the 20th HBO treatment.

There was also a 23% increase in platelet protein content and a 24% increase in arachidonic acid-dependent platelet activation. Collagen-dependent platelet aggregation was unaffected. Overall, there was no evidence that 20 HBO sessions caused adverse effects on platelet aggregation or oxidative metabolism in platelets or total antioxidant status of the plasma.

Effect of HBO on Stem Cells

Stem cells have two important characteristics that distinguish them from other types of cells. First, they are unspecialized cells that renew themselves for long periods through cell division. The second is that, under certain physiologic or experimental conditions, they can be induced to become cells with special functions such as myocytes (cells of the heart muscle) or the insulin-producing cells of the pancreas. In the embryo, these cells are the starting point for the development of the complete human being. In the adult body, stem cells are one of the mechanisms for the repair and renewal of some cells and tissues.

Embryonic stem cells (ESCs) are continuously growing stem cell lines of embryonic origin derived from the pluripotent cells of the inner cell mass or epiblast of the mammalian embryo. They may give rise to any cell type but not to an independent organism. Embryonic germ cell lines, established from primitive reproductive cells of the embryo, are functionally equivalent to embryonic stem cells. The distinguishing features of embryonic stem cells are their capacity to be maintained in an undifferentiated state indefinitely in culture and their potential to develop into every cell of the body. Their ability to develop into a wide range of cell types makes ESCs as a useful basic research tool and a novel source of cell populations for new therapies. Human embryonic stem cell (hESC) is a type of pluripotent stem cell derived from the inner cell mass of the preimplantation blastocyst produced by sperm-egg fertilization.

Further details of stem cells are described elsewhere (Jain 2009e). This chapter includes a brief description of role of stem cells in hematology and effect of HBO on stem cells. Autologous transplantation of hematopoietic stem cells (HSCs) from patients with genetic hematological disorders and immunodeficiencies could provide the same benefits as allogeneic HSC transplantation, without the attendant immunological complications. Autologous HSCs have been used as targets of gene transfer, with applications in inherited disorders, cell therapy, and acquired immunodeficiency. The types of cells include hematopoietic progenitor cells, lymphocytes, and mesenchymal stem cells (MSCs). Preclinical studies have been conducted in thalassemia, sickle cell anemia, Wiskott-Aldrich syndrome, and Fanconi anemia.

The bone marrow is home to MSCs that are able to differentiate into many different cell types. The effect of HBO on MSCs is poorly understood. Placental growth factor (PlGF) is an attractive therapeutic agent for stimulating revascularization of ischemic tissue. HBO has been shown to improve diabetic wound healing by increasing circulating stem cells. HBO mobilizes stem/progenitor cells by stimulating NO synthesis (Thom *et al* 2006). HBO induces PlGF expression in bone marrow-derived MSCs at least through the oxidative stress-related pathways, which may play an important role in HBO-induced vasculogenesis (Shyu *et al* 2008).

Effect of HBO Treatment on the Immune System

HBO has been reported to have both a stimulant as well as a depressant effect on the immune system, depending upon the pressure used and the experimental model.

De Graeve *et al* (1976) studied the effect of HBO (2 ATA, 5 h) on the thymus of adult rats. There was hyperplasia of the cortex after a transient depression. The newly formed thymic cells migrated and were stored in the red pulp of the spleen. The authors concluded that HBO has a stimulating effect on thymic cells and that this can be considered to belong to the general phenomenon of immune defence.

Lotovin *et al* (1981) reported a study of the problem of cellular and humoral activity under hyperoxia. They found that six sessions of HBO at 2.5 ATA resulted in an increase of T lymphocytes in guinea pigs. When pressure was raised to 5 ATA for 30 min, a form of oxygen toxicity occurred with depression of the functional activity of the T lymphocytes and a decrease in the cellular indices of immunity in the blood. The animals recovered from this 10 days after the exposure. In patients who were given 15 daily sessions of HBO at 2.5 ATA (60 min), the number of T lymphocytes increased 1.4-fold and that of B lymphocytes 2.8-fold. There was also an increase in all the immunoglobulins.

Feldmeier and Boswell (1987) analyzed a broad range of immune responses in nine healthy human volunteers exposed to 20 treatments of HBO at 2.4 ATA over 4 weeks. They found no effect on the immune system of these subjects.

Bitterman and Melamund (1993) studied the effect of a single exposure to HBO (2.8 ATA for 90 min) on blood mononuclear subset in healthy volunteers. Immediately after the exposure, a significant increase was observed in the percentage and absolute number of CD8 (suppressor/cytotoxic) T cells, with a concomitant decrease in the CD4 (helper/inducer) T cells as compared with controls. The result was a decreased CD4:CD8 ratio. A rise was also observed in the number of HLA-DR antigen-bearing cells with a transient increase in monocytes. These changes were only partially reversed 24 h following HBO exposure and suggest specific HBO-induced shifts and sequestration of T-cell subpopulations.

Biriukov *et al* (1988) observed that the number of lymphocytes is diminished after surgery and that HBO stimulates lymphocyte production and improves the patient's resistance against infections in the postoperative period.

Ulewicz and Zannini (1986) have reviewed the literature on the possible effect of HBO on pathological reactions of immunological hypersensitivity. Some of the evidence reviewed supports the beneficial effect of HBO on type I hypersensitivity reactions, i.e., anaphylactic reaction, by reducing the level of immunoglobulins IgE and IgG. This may also explain the beneficial effect of HBO observed in asthma. Reported increase of complement activity in the serum following HBO exposure may be of benefit in counteracting hypersensitivity reactions of types II and III. There is evidence also for the benefit of HBO on type IV hypersensitivity reactions.

HBO has been found to mitigate immune reactions, many of which are involved in rejection of allograft transplants, and thus offers a rationale for its possible use as an adjunct to help preserve and protect transplanted tissues (see Chapter 37). Rejection may involve both immunological reactions of the lymphoid system, or lymphoid-independent damage from trauma or other factors, including reperfusion injury. Lymphoid-induced damage involves cellular elements such as CD4 and macrophage cell types, as well as both proinflammatory and inhibitory cytokines. Cytokines such as TNFs and interleukins activate T-cells and macrophages, resulting in endothelial damage and its consequences. The immunosuppressive effects of HBO include suppression of autoimmune symptoms, decreased production of IL-1 and CD4 cells, and increased percentage and absolute number of CD8 cells (Al-Waili *et al* 2006). HBO normalizes cell-bound immunity and decreases the serum concentration of immune complexes. Studies have shown MHC class I expression to be altered when cultures were exposed to HBO, so as to become undetectable by monoclonal antibodies or cytotoxic T lymphocytes. In addition to its specific effects on the immune system, HBO improves tissue oxygenation, reduces free radical damage during reperfusion, maintains marginally ischemic tissue, and accelerates wound healing.

In conclusion, a great deal of work still needs to be done on the immunological aspects of HBO but it is important as it may explain the beneficial effect of HBO in infections, disorders of the immune system, and transplantation.

Effect of HBO Treatment on Plasma and Blood Volume

It has already been mentioned in Chapter 2 that enough oxygen (6 vol%) can be dissolved in plasma to support life.

The classical study on the subject of life without blood was made by Boerema *et al* (1959). The authors lowered the level of hemoglobin in young pigs to 0.4% by exchanging the blood for plasma by venesection. The animals breathing oxygen at a pressure of 3 ATA in the hyperbaric chamber lived for 45 min with a level of hemoglobin that would be incompatible with life at atmospheric pressure. These animals were kept alive virtually without any hemoglobin. ECG showed no changes, and the circulation and the blood pressure remained spontaneously normal. Recovery was uneventful after reinfusion of blood prior to decompression to the surface. Bokeria *et al* (1979) reported use of hemodilution up to 55%. HBO was able to provide adequate oxygenation during open heart surgery. Koziner *et al* (1981) replaced 94%–98% of the blood volume with dextran in cats and kept them alive for 8–9 h, breathing 100% oxygen.

The effect of hyperoxia on oxygen uptake (VO_2) during acute anemia is being re-examined experimentally. Chapler *et al* (1984) anesthetized dogs and ventilated them for 20-min periods with room air (normoxia), 100% oxygen (hyperoxia), and then normoxia again. Anemia was then induced by isovolemic dextran-for-blood exchange and the sequence of normoxia-hyperoxia-normoxia was repeated. Whole-body VO_2 and cardiac output rose following hypoxia during anemia. Both of these values fell following hyperoxia. The authors postulated that this could result from redistribution of the capillary blood flow away from exchange vessels in response to elevated pO_2. It was mentioned previously that hematocrit falls after exposure to HBO. Buxton *et al* (1964) reported that anesthetized dogs exposed to 3 ATA at 100% oxygen showed a marked elevation of hematocrit. This effect did not occur in controls kept at 1 ATA, splenectomized, or given buffering agents. The authors postulated that rise of hematocrit was due to splenic contracture. In evaluating this report, it must be borne in mind that dogs under pentobarbital anesthesia sequester up to 30% of blood volume in the spleen and release it into the circulation in response to catecholamines, which could result from the stress of HBO and/or anesthesia.

Use of HBO in Conjunction with Oxygen Carriers

In recently reported studies rats, subjected to loss of about half their blood volume causing respiratory arrest, were resuscitated by the intravenous infusion of 6% hetastarch in lactated electrolyte injection and HBO (Segal 2003). In the experiments, six of nine rats resuscitated with the plasma expander and treated with 100% oxygen at 2 ATA survived long term in comparison to survival of only one of the 11 rats given the same intravenous infusion but ventilated with 100% oxygen at atmospheric pressure. The results were statistically significant and confirmed previous experiments in which HBO had been shown to be advantageous in reviving rats following hemorrhagic shock causing a near-death condition. While hemorrhaging, and in the following period of respiratory arrest, all the animals' body temperatures declined. Restoring body temperature to normal by externally warming the animal was also an important feature of the resuscitation process.

Clinical Applications of HBO in Disorders of the Blood

Hypovolemia and Acute Anemia Due to Blood Loss

The average blood volume of a normal adult is approximately 5000 ml (3000 ml plasma + 2000 ml RBC). After an acute hemorrhage the body replaces plasma within 1–3 days, but a low concentration of RBCs persists. In chronic blood loss, a person cannot compensate and the hemoglobin can fall to dangerously low levels (severe anemia). The decrease in viscosity of the blood lowers the resistance to blood flow in the peripheral vessels. The peripheral vessels may dilate further due to the effect of hypoxia. The major impact is an increased workload on the heart and increased cardiac output. This may be able to sustain the individual at rest, but during exercise, which greatly increases the tissue demands on oxygen, it can lead to extreme tissue hypoxia with acute cardiac failure. The conventional treatment consists of whole blood or packed RBC transfusion and, if possible, correction of the cause.

There are problems with blood transfusion because of fear of contamination with HIV. There are difficulties in administering blood in some situations, particularly in patients who are Jehovah's Witnesses, since they do not accept any blood or blood component because of their religious beliefs. An alternative method for oxygenation of the blood is by oxygen carriers or blood substitutes.

HBO can temporarily meet the oxygen needs of the body in the absence of blood and has been termed "bloodless transfusion." Amonic et al (1969) reported the case of a Jehovah's Witness with gastric bleeding and a hemoglobin level of 2.2 g/100 ml who refused blood transfusion, but survived with HBO treatment.

Hart (1974) reported three patients who were dying of acute blood loss anemia and whom he treated successfully with HBO. All three had very low hemoglobin levels (2–3 g/100 ml), hematocrit of 10%–11.5%, and falling blood pressure, as well as a rising pulse rate. The treatment in all cases was limited to intravenous fluids, intramuscular iron-dextran, and HBO at 2 ATA for 60–90 min. HBO was repeated whenever the pulse rate rose above 120. All the patients improved dramatically, and in one case the hemo-

globin rose from 2 g to 8 g in 1 week of treatment. HBO can be used as an interim measure to save patients and improve their condition for more definite measures, such as surgical correction of the primary pathology or the cause of bleeding.

After this experience, Hart et al (1987) treated further 23 patients using HBO. Of the 26 patients, 6 patients who arrived in a decerebrate state with Hb of 3.8 g/dl and Hct of 10.5% died. The survivors had somewhat higher Hb (4.79 g/dl) and Hct (13.6%) on admission. Treatment was discontinued in the survivors when they no longer suffered from hypoxic sprue, postural hypotension, and when Hct was over 22% and Hb over 7 g/dl. The authors concluded that HBO may be useful in the treatment of acute blood loss anemia if applied early.

Treatment with HBO favorably affected recovery from moderate (30%) acute blood loss, in experimental animals resulting in lessened effects at 48 h and hastening recovery to baseline hemoglobin levels (Wright et al 2002). These results support the data gained from clinical experience treating extreme blood loss with HBO. It should be mentioned that the search for an ideal blood substitute or artificial blood continues. Under some circumstances, physically dissolved oxygen has advantages over chemically bound oxygen. Besides the necessary volume effects (iso-osmotic) and physiological bicarbonate concentration (prevention of dilutional acidosis), the solution should be shear-rate independent (having Newtonian behavior). Oxygen concentration at the given oxygen partial pressure should be at least 6 ml/dl. Such a blood substitute should be evaluated by means of the oxygen supply index:

$$\frac{(\text{oxygen concentration}) \times (\text{mean capillary oxygen pressure in mmHg})}{\text{viscosity}}$$

Hemolytic Anemia

Hemolysis of RBC may occur from a variety of causes, some of which are hereditary and others acquired. One example is sickle cell anemia. It is present in 0.3%–1.0% of West Africans and American blacks. RBC in this condition contain an abnormal hemoglobin called hemoglobin S. When this hemoglobin is exposed to a low concentration of oxygen, it is precipitated into long crystals inside the RBC. The crystals elongate the cell and give it the appearance of a sickle rather than a biconcave disc. The precipitated hemoglobin also damages the cell membrane so that the cells become highly fragile, leading to severe anemia. Such patients suffer a cycle called sickle cell disease crisis.

low oxygen tension in tissues → sickling → impairment of blood flow through the tissues → further decrease of oxygen tension

Once the process starts, it progresses rapidly, leading to a severe decrease of RBC mass and possible death. Oxygen has been used at the crisis stage to combat hypoxia, and the potential of HBO should be investigated. Patients with sickling hemoglobinopathies, including sickle cell trait, have an increased risk of permanent loss of vision following hyperemia caused by blunt trauma. RBC with hemoglobin S sickle more readily in the aqueous humor of the eye than in the venous blood, become trapped, and lead to secondary glaucoma. HBO at 2 ATA for 2 h was successful in reducing the number of sickle cells injected into the anterior chamber of the eyes in rabbits (Wallyn *et al* 1985).

HBO has also been used for hemolysis due to mismatched transfusion (Gonchar 1985).

Potential Benefits of HBO in Cerebrovascular Diseases Due to Blood Disorders

The relationship of the blood to the brain is quite apparent in cerebrovascular diseases. Primary RBC disorders cause cerebral ischemia by adversely affecting oxygen delivery or CBF. Hemoglobinopathies limit the binding and delivery of oxygen and cause altered erythrocyte shape and increased viscosity, as well as anemia. This moves oxygen delivery away from the apex of the parabolic curve (see Figure 25.1). Therapy of cerebral ischemia may be aimed at altering the viscosity or the properties of RBC in order to improve oxygen delivery. HBO, in addition to providing oxygenation, also improves blood rheology parameters such as Hct and RBC deformability. These may prove to be additional benefits to the useful role of HBO in combating cerebral ischemic and metabolic sequelae of stroke.

Li *et al* (1986) studied the hemorrheology of patients with cerebrovascular disease treated by HBO (2.5 ATA, 100% oxygen for 45 min, air break for 15 min, twice daily). They found that there was decrease of Hct and blood viscosity as well as of platelet aggregation. The oxygenation of the brain was improved in these cases without increasing the Hct.

Contraindication – Congenital Spherocytosis

In congenital spherocytosis the RBC are rigid and less deformable than normal. HBO is considered to be contraindicated because of the risk of increased hemolysis.

Wirjosemito and Touhey (1988) treated two patients with refractory leg ulcers (who also happened to suffer from congenital spherocytosis) by using HBO. No overt hemolytic complication occurred. The authors recommended the following precautions should patients with congenital spherocytosis need HBO treatment for another medical condition:

- Close monitoring of the hemogram, hemolysis parameters, and vitamin E levels
- Supplementary vitamin E
- Cessation of HBO therapy if there is any evidence of hemolysis

26 HBO Therapy in Gastroenterology

K.K. Jain

This chapter deals with a wide variety of HBO applications involving the gastrointestinal tract, including its use in dealing with:

Introduction

Hyperbaric oxygen (HBO) therapy has an important role in the management of gastrointestinal disorders. There are, however, few controlled studies. The rationale is the same as for the application of HBO in disorders of other systems: it counteracts ischemia and hypoxia, it promotes resistance to infections and healing of ulcers. An additional effect is the compression and reduction of volume of gases.

HBO in Peptic Ulceration

Pathophysiology and Rationale of HBO Therapy

A peptic ulcer is a mucosal lesion of the stomach or duodenum in which acid and pepsin play major pathogenic roles. The major forms of peptic ulceration are duodenal ulcer and gastric ulcer, both of which are chronic diseases caused by the bacterium *Heliobacter pylori*. In addition to the known causes, a few additional factors play a role in progression of ulceration. The gastric epithelium has mainly an aerobic metabolism and is dependent on a constant supply of oxygen for oxidative metabolism. Gastric mucosal ischemia is believed to be a factor in the pathogenesis of acute mucosal injury as occurs in patients with general medical or surgical illnesses (stress ulcers). It is not known whether reduction in blood flow contributes to the development of chronic gastric or duodenal ulcers. Most gastric ulcers occur on the lesser curvature, where there are fewer collateral vessels than on the greater curvature. Whether this anatomical difference leads to reduced blood flow at the lesser curvature has not been proven. Reduced blood flow, venous stasis or disturbances of microcirculation can lead to hypoxia. It has been shown experimentally that necrosis of the surface epithelium of the gastric mucosa starts at a pO_2 value of 9 mmHg in the dog (Efuni *et al* 1986). Studies on patients with gastric ulcers using endoscopic polarography show low pO_2 values near the ulcer margins. These values rise during the initial stage of healing or regeneration ("red scar" phase) and fall again later in the healing process ("white scar" phase).

Studies of Bowen and Fairchild (1984) point to perturbations in the subepithelial microcirculation concomitant with cellular hypoxia and inhibition of oxidative metabolism as common denominators of cellular injury. Due to functional arteriovenous shunting, there are focal areas of cellular hypoxia even when the total blood flow to the organ is normal or even increased. It is the more severely hypoxic areas in the fundus of the stomach that are susceptible to ulceration when exposed to gastric irritants such as acid and bile.

Efuni *et al* (1986) concluded that a hypoxic disorder with a fall of energy supply underlies ulcer formation and gave this as a rationale for the use of HBO therapy in patients with gastric ulcers. Earlier attempts to treat local hypoxia of the stomach ulcers by ingesting oxygen foams and oxygen cocktails given by gastric tube were not successful in raising the oxygen tension in the ulcerated areas.

HBO has an antibacterial effect (see Chapter 13). Part of the efficacy of HBO in peptic ulceration may be due to an antibacterial effect against *Heliobacter pylori*, although no studies have been done to demonstrate this. This is an area for further investigation. HBO promotes the healing of ulcers of skin and there is reason to believe that it will promote healing of mucosal ulcers as well. There is no evidence that HBO affects gastric acid secretion.

Experimental Studies in Animals

Koloskow and Dumurov (1986) induced gastric ulcers in rats using acetic acid (Okabe model). These lesions were morphologically similar to human gastric ulcers. After 10 days, HBO treatment was started at 2 ATA. One 45-min session was given daily for 10 days. In three of the 15 animals there was healing of the ulcer, and in the other 12 the appearance of the ulcer differed from that in controls. There was no necrotic material on the surface, but granular tissue appeared instead, and the ulcer margins showed signs of regeneration. In a second series HBO was given for 16 sessions. The ulcers healed, with formation of an overlying mucous membrane, in 60% of the animals in this group. The unhealed ulcers in the remaining animals were much smaller than those in the controls and were slit-like with no necrotic material at the base. Only 20% of the ulcers in the control animals healed spontaneously.

Clinical Assessment of HBO in Gastric and Duodenal Ulcer Patients

Perrins *et al* (1977) treated one gastric ulcer patient with ten daily 1-h sessions of HBO at 2 ATA. The ulcer healed completely. The case was never formally reported, and there are no clinical reports on this subject in the Western literature. All the studies quoted below are from Russia.

Lukich *et al* (1981) reported 92 patients with peptic ulcer in whom the lesions measured 0.2–2.0 cm in diameter. The progress was checked gastroscopically after 10–12 sessions of HBO treatment, and healing was complete in 65 patients with 10–12 treatments.

Komarov *et al* (1985) reported 132 patients. In 127 of these (94.9%), healing of the ulcer was confirmed by endoscopy. The average duration of the healing process was 21.7 ± 1.2 days in gastric ulcers and 20.2 ± 0.7 days in duodenal ulcers. Usually 10–15 treatments at 2 ATA sufficed, but in a few exceptional cases 30 treatments were required. The authors studied the gastrin content of the blood in 25 patients: it was 80.11 pg/ml before the treatment and 88.5 pg/ml afterward. Also, they observed increased mucous secretion and free hydrochloric acid secretion in the healing phase. This was interpreted as an increase in the basic function of the gastric mucous membrane. The ulcers healed in spite of this.

Efuni *et al* (1986) used HBO for treatment of peptic ulcer in 217 patients. The only drug therapy used as an adjunct was antacid, and this was stopped after the first week of daily HBO treatments. The number of HBO sessions ranged from nine to 17, each given at 2 ATA for 45 min. The healing time for the gastric ulcers was 19.7 ± 7 days and for the duodenal ulcers 19.3 ± 7 days. The healing was accompanied by improvement of symptoms such as pain. There was healing of 89.2% of the stomach ulcers and 95.8% of the duodenal ulcers.

The results were compared with those of a control group of 350 patients who had been treated with medications such as H2-receptor blockers. The HBO treatment shortened the healing of the ulcers by 7–28 days. Further HBO treatment helped the 39.2% of patients in the control group in whom ulcers persisted in spite of medical treatment. Efuni *et al* (1986) pointed out that one contraindication to HBO treatment is any suspicion of malignancy in the ulcer, as neoplasms may proliferate under HBO.

HBO in the Treatment of Intestinal Obstruction

Basic Considerations and Rationale of HBO Therapy

Intestinal obstruction can be divided into two categories:

- Paralytic ileus, where obstruction results from neural, humoral, or metabolic inhibition of bowel mobility. The most common causes are abdominal surgery, peritonitis, trauma, and intestinal ischemia.
- Mechanical ileus, where there is intestinal obstruction secondary to mechanical causes such as
  a) intrinsic, including tumors and inflammatory disease;
  b) extrinsic, including adhesions, tumors, and volvulus; and
  c) lumen obstruction, including foreign bodies and intussusception.

Obstruction may be partial or complete and the obstructed bowel may be viable or strangulated.

The composition of the gas in the nonobstructed human intestine is (Levitt 1971): 64% nitrogen, 0.69% oxygen 19% hydrogen, 8.8% methane, and 4% carbon dioxide.

After experimental intestinal obstruction, the factors that govern the diffusion rates of intestinal gases are (Cross & Wangensteen 1952):

1. The partial pressure gradient of the gases across the intestinal mucous membrane separating the bowel lumen and the blood.
2. The absorption coefficient of the gases in the blood.
3. The molecular weight (density) of the gases involved.
4. The area of surface contact between the gases and the permeable membrane.
5. The thickness of the membrane.
6. The diffusion velocity, which is inversely proportional to the square root of the molecular weight and directly proportional to its absorption coefficient in the medium in which it is diffusing.

The origin of intestinal gases in clinical and experimental bowel obstruction is shown in Figure 26.1.

Nitrogen leaves the bowel slowly because of its low diffusion velocity, based on its molecular weight and low absorption coefficient, and because blood and alveolar air are already saturated with nitrogen. Once nitrogen enters the bowel as swallowed air, it cannot be readily absorbed in significant amounts under the existing conditions. Since it is impossible to change the absorption coefficient of nitrogen, the only logical way to get rid of it is by changing its partial pressure gradient. This can be achieved by breathing 100% oxygen, or even more effectively by HBO.

The application of HBO therapy to bowel obstruction is based on the gas laws of Dalton and Boyle (see Chapter 2). It is the internal diameter of the distended bowel rather than the actual volume of the enclosed gas that determines the pathologic effects of overdistension, which lead to loss of contractility and jeopardizes viability by ischemia/hypoxia. There is a risk of peritonitis by transmural leakage or perforation. Boyle's law, as applied to bowel obstruction

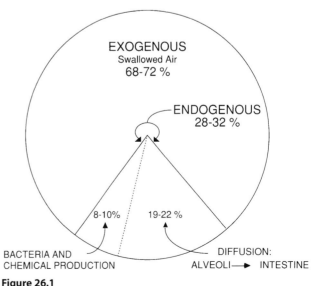

Figure 26.1
Intestinal gas origin in bowel obstruction.

or paralytic ileus, means that there will be a 50% reduction of the intestinal gas volume and the diameter of the intestinal lumen (a cylinder) will be decreased by 29% when the pressure is doubled from 1 to 2 ATA (Peloso 1982).

Experimental Studies in Animals

Cross described a series of experiments that demonstrated the efficacy of HBO therapy in dogs with mechanical closed loop obstruction (Cross 1954, 1965; Cross & Wangensteen 1952). In experiments involving the pressure/volume relationship, he studied the effects of increased atmospheric pressure on intestinal viability. In animals breathing air at ambient pressure, there was loss of viability in 70% of the obstructed loops, whereas, in animals breathing air at 2–4 ATA, only 10% of the obstructed loops lost their viability. This suggests that pressure, plus the 80% oxygen derived from the increased partial pressure, resulted in increased intestinal viability and survival in animals with closed loop obstructions. Although pressure alone reduced the volume of gas and luminal diameter within closed intestinal loops, addition of oxygen lead to the combined effect of diffusion and gas volume reduction.

Fritelli et al (1963) reproduced and substantiated Cross's results in similar animal models. Hopkinson and Schenk (1969) used HBO therapy at 2 ATA in long-term animal experiments and showed that it reduced mortality in animals with colon obstruction (17% vs 55% in controls).

Belokurov (1980) studied enzyme activities in the rat model of acute small bowel obstruction. The maximum fall of cytochrome oxidase and succinate dehydrogenase in the liver, kidney, and intestinal loops occurred after 72 h obstruction. Removal of obstruction alone failed to return the enzyme levels to normal. HBO therapy resulted in normal enzyme levels in all cases regardless of the time elapsed following obstruction. The author concluded that HBO plays a role in normalizing the enzyme activity, but the clinical implications of this observation are not as yet clear.

Secondary infection following intestinal obstruction increases morbidity. HBO has a beneficial effect as an antibacterial agent. In Wistar-albino rats HBO treatment at 2.5 ATA for 90 min daily for two days significantly reduced the endogenous bacterial overgrowth in the small intestine of rats following obstruction and prevented the bacterial translocation almost completely (Akin et al 2002).

HBO Therapy in Adynamic Ileus

Adynamic ileus is the most common cause of intestinal obstruction. It usually follows abdominal surgery but may occur after any peritoneal insult such as peritonitis and ret-roperitoneal hematoma. Other diseases such as pneumonia, myocardial infarction and electrolyte disturbances (potassium depletion) are associated with adynamic ileus. Intestinal ischemia, whether due to intestinal distension or as a result of vascular occlusion perpetuates this condition.

Stewart et al (1974) using the rationale based on the work of Cross, treated two critically ill patients with severe adynamic ileus with HBO at 2–2.5 ATA. Both improved but died later from their underlying illness. Watanuki et al (1970) reported excellent results after treating ten patients with postoperative paralytic ileus, using HBO for 60 min at 1–2 ATA. Ratner et al (1978) reported the results of HBO treatment of 216 patients with postoperative adynamic ileus. The duration of each treatment was 45–60 min at a pressure of 1.8–2.0 ATA and, this treatment was repeated 3–5 times. Sixty-four patients with adynamic ileus who were not treated with HBO served as controls and received only conventional therapy. There was a mortality of 30% in this group, compared with 16% mortality in the group treated by additional HBO therapy.

Grokhovsky et al (1978) treated 418 pediatric surgical patients with HBO. The pressures used were 1.8–2.2 ATA in younger children and 2.5–3 ATA in older children. Of these patients, 293 had peritonitis and the results were excellent in this group; postoperative morbidity was reduced from 50% to 10%, mortality from 14% to 7%, and the average hospital stay was reduced by 5 days. HBO was highly effective in 94% of the patients, less than optimal in 6%, and ineffective in 0.7%. For HBO therapy to be most effective, it should be instituted as soon as possible after surgery; it was ineffective if delayed by more than 5 days after surgery. This study failed to include controls, making an objective evaluation of the results difficult.

Loder (1977) treated 12 patients with adynamic ileus, ten of whom had this associated with infection. HBO was given from the 2nd to the 8th postoperative days at 2.5 ATA for 1 h twice daily. Eleven patients recovered after 4–10 h of compression. Loder recommended that if there is no improvement with nasogastric decompression and intravenous fluids, a course of HBO should be tried. Perrins et al (1977) reported similar results and attributed the improved circulation in the bowel wall and return of peristalsis to the rapid reduction in intestinal distension.

Belokurov and Medvedev (1976) investigated the effectiveness of HBO in 92 patients with diffuse peritonitis and adynamic ileus. They found that HBO promoted restoration of the motor emptying junction of the gastrointestinal tract and increased the peristalsis of the small intestine, as evidenced by electroenterographic data. Mamistov and Dildin (1976) treated 50 patients with peritonitis on the rationale that HBO controls intestinal paresis, metabolic disorders, and hypoxia. Recovery was achieved in 41 patients.

Saito et al (1977) used HBO (two to 12 2-h sessions at 2 ATA) in 24 patients with postoperative adynamic ileus, some of whom had lysis of adhesions of the intestines as a result of previous surgery. Twenty-four (75%) of these patients improved. The authors also investigated the effect of HBO on experimental paralytic ileus in dogs. They noted a reduction of the diameter of the distended intestine to half at 2 ATA. The pO_2 of the intestinal wall at 2 ATA rose to 13 times the preexposure value.

A retrospective review of postoperative paralytic ileus associated with abdominal surgery who underwent HBO therapy was undertaken to examine the efficacy of HBO therapy (Ambiru et al 2007). The overall resolution rates for patients receiving HBO was 92%. Among patients who were more than 75 years old, the therapies resolved 97% of cases of postoperative paralytic ileus. The mortality rate was 1.2% overall. Complications related to HBO therapy occurred in 3.8% of the admissions, and most of them were not serious. These results suggest that HBO therapy deserves further assessment for use in management of postoperative paralytic ileus.

HBO in Adhesive Intestinal Obstruction

Intestinal obstruction may occur because of adhesions formed as a result of abdominal surgery. Further surgery to relieve adhesions leads to the formation of further adhesions. A clinical trial was conducted to investigate the effects of HBO therapy on patients with adhesive intestinal obstruction who had failed to respond to more than 7 days of conservative treatment (Ambiru et al 2008). Patients were divided into groups according to the treatment and interval between the first day of the therapy and clinical symptoms of obstruction; tube decompression therapy within 7 days after appearance of clinical symptoms (Group I), clinical symptoms that have persisted for less than 7 days before the start of HBO therapy (Group II), and for more than 7 days (Group III). *Results:* The overall resolution and mortality rates in the cases of adhesive intestinal obstruction were 79.8% and 2.2% in Group I, 85.9% and 1.4% in Group II, and 81.7% and 1.6% in Group III, respectively. Group II had significantly better resolution rates than Group I. It is concluded that HBO therapy may be useful in management of adhesive intestinal obstruction associated with abdominal surgery, even in patients who fail to respond to other conservative treatments. HBO therapy may be a preferred option for treatment of patients for whom surgery should be avoided.

HBO in Chronic Idiopathic Intestinal Pseudo-Obstruction

Chronic idiopathic intestinal pseudo-obstruction is a syndrome in which symptoms of intestinal obstruction are present in the absence of mechanical obstruction. It is one of the disorders that is most refractory to medical and surgical treatment. Even when patients are given nutritional support, including total parenteral nutrition, obstructive symptoms seldom disappear. A case is reported of chronic idiopathic intestinal pseudo-obstruction, due to myopathy, in which hyperbaric oxygenation therapy was strikingly effective (Yokota et al 2000). HBO resulted not only in relief of the patient's obstructive symptoms but also in a rapid decrease of abnormally accumulated intestinal gas. This case suggests that HBO can be an effective therapy in the management of chronic idiopathic intestinal pseudo-obstruction.

HBO in Inflammations and Infections of the Gastrointestinal Tract

Inflammatory bowel disease is a general term for a group of inflammatory disorders of unknown cause involving the gastrointestinal tract. A typical example is ulcerative colitis and a variant of it called Crohn's disease. Various factors (genetic, immunologic and infectious) play a role in the pathogenesis even though the cause is unknown. Infectious diseases are also included in this section and the examples are pseudomembranous colitis and necrotizing enterocolitis.

Toxic Megacolon

Toxic megacolon is a rare but potentially lethal complication of idiopathic inflammatory bowel disease or infectious colitis, characterized by total or segmental nonobstructive colonic dilatation of at least 6 cm associated with toxicity. Initial treatment is medical with intravenous corticosteroids and surgery is done in emergency cases involving subtotal colectomy with end-ileostomy (Sheth & LaMont 1998). There is some rationale for trying HBO therapy in this condition as some of the antecedent conditions are amenable to HBO. HBO shows strong antiinflammatory effect in toxic colitis due to ulcerative colitis. It is considered to be the safest and most reliable nonsurgical method of treatment for patients with toxic colitis (Kuroki et al 1998).

Ulcerative Colitis

HBO was shown to be as effective as dexamethasone therapy as treatment for trinitrobenzenesulfonic acid-ethanol (TNBS-E)-induced distal colitis in rate (Atug et al 2008). HBO has been combined with conventional medical management in patients with chronic ulcerative colitis. HBO has also been used in the treatment of a patient with ulcerative colitis, refractory to conventional therapies (Buchman et al 2001). Therapy consisted of 30 courses of 100% oxygen at a pressure of 2ATA. Clinical remission was achieved and corticosteroids were successfully tapered off. Although favorable results were obtained, further study and research are required for this area of HBO application.

Pseudomembranous Colitis

Pseudomembranous colitis (induced by antimicrobial agents) is caused by a toxin-producing anaerobic organism, *Clostridium difficile*. The presence of the organisms and toxins upon assay is suggestive of the diagnosis that can be confirmed by proctoscopy and colonoscopy. Most of the cases of this disease are self-limiting. Vancomycin has produced symptomatic improvement in some cases. HBO therapy has been shown to be useful in the management of this disease, but further research is required.

Necrotizing Enterocolitis

"Necrotizing enterocolitis" is the English translation of the term "enterocolite nécrosante," from the French literature, which refers to necrosis of the intestine, usually following surgery. There are infective factors in the etiology, but mesenteric artery occlusion is excluded. In the English language literature, the term "necrotizing enteritis" refers to involvement of the bowel with gas gangrene.

Chevrel *et al* (1979) reported three cases of postoperative necrotizing enterocolitis; only one of these patients was treated by HBO and was the only survivor. Rathat (1979) reported this case in detail. The cause of this disease was considered to be prolonged distension of the intestine and anaerobic bacterial overgrowth resulting in mucosal ischemia. HBO not only reduced the volume of the distension but also improved the blood circulation of the intestine. The control of the anaerobic infection was also an important factor in the favorable outcome with HBO treatment.

Michaud *et al* (1989) used HBO in six cases of acute neonatal necrotizing enterocolitis. The rationale was to control the aerobic and anaerobic infection and to reduce the volume of intraperitoneal and intraluminal gases. HBO was administered via a helmet at 2 ATA for 1 h daily. Four of the six patients recovered in 6–9 days.

Radiation Enterocolitis

Delayed effects of radiation lead to ischemia and necrosis of the soft tissues due to obliterative endarteritis (see Chapter 16). In case of lesions of the mucous membranes, there is secondary infection as well. HBO has been shown to be beneficial in radiation-induced enteritis, colitis, and proctitis, and should be initiated in the ischemic, rather than the necrotic phase of the disease.

HBO in Pneumatosis Cystoides Intestinalis (PCI)

Pathophysiology

Pneumatosis cystoides intestinalis is a rare disease characterized by the presence of multiple intramural gas-filled cysts in the gastrointestinal tract. The cause is uncertain but the condition is most commonly diagnosed in patients who have chronic obstructive pulmonary disease, inflammatory bowel disease or collagen disease. The patients present with profound disturbances of bowel function. The choice of therapy depends upon the pathophysiology of the cyst.

The cysts vary in size from a few millimeters to 2 cm and may obliterate the bowel lumen. There are three theories of pathogenesis of this lesion. The mechanical theory states that the cyst is due to distortion of the intestinal mucosal barrier. Healing of the underlying disorder as well as the epithelial break could thus result in obliteration of the cyst. According to the bacterial theory, bacterial fermentation and hydrogen gas build-up lead to cyst formation. Antibiotics and/or HBO would be recommended here. Finally, the pulmonary hypothesis postulated that severe coughing produced alveolar rupture and pneumomediastinum with gas dissecting down to the retroperitoneal space and then along the perivascular spaces to the bowel wall.

Rationale for HBO therapy. The earlier treatment for this condition was normobaric oxygen therapy. There was some success and this led to the hypothesis that the cysts were created and maintained by anaerobic organisms which produce gas at a rate that exceeds the rate of absorption. The high tissue oxygen tension was supposed to kill the organisms. This theory has not been substantiated. Disadvantages of normobaric oxygen are that excessive amounts of 100% oxygen are required to be inhaled for prolonged periods and this may produce oxygen toxicity. In contrast to this HBO treatments are of shorter duration, are more effective, and lower the total pressure of gases in the surrounding tissues thus increasing the pressure gradient between the cysts and the tissues. The balance of pressure then favors diffusion and cysts will deflate.

Clinical experience. Mathus-Vliegen *et al* (1983) treated two patients with this condition by HBO, with rapid relief of symptoms and disappearance of the cysts. There were later recurrences. Masterson *et al* (1978) felt that HBO represented a significant advance in the treatment of pneumatosis cystoides intestinalis.

Iitsuka *et al* (1993) presented a case of PCI associated with nephrotic syndrome and long-term use of steroids. The patient improved with HBO treatment.

Grieve and Unsworth (1991) presented 8 patients with PCI who underwent 11 courses of HBO treatment. All patients responded with symptomatic relief. This was followed by 7 recurrences and 4 long-term cures. The authors concluded that HBO is effective for PCI provided it is continued provided it is continued till the cyst resolution and not just symptomatic relief.

Paw and Reed (1996) presented another case of PCI involving the small intestine which was diagnosed by barium meal and treated with HBO. The patient received HBO at 2ATA for 1 h/day/5 days a week for 2 weeks with improvement. The frequency of treatments was reduced to twice a week and then once a week. Relief was noted at the first treatment and the patient recovered completely with no recurrence. Repeat barium meal examination showed no evidence of recurrence of the lesions.

Several cases have been reported in the literature from Japan where HBO was used successfully for the treatment of PCI (Tomiyama *et al* 2003; Takada *et al* 2002; Shimada *et al* 2001; Iimura *et al* 2000; Togawa *et al* 2004). A case of systemic lupus erythematosus with enteritis and peritonitis who later developed pneumatosis cystoides intestinalis was treated successfully with a combination of intravenous cyclophosphamide, antibiotics, and HBO (Mizoguchi *et al* 2008).

HBO in Ischemic Disorders of the Intestine

Vascular accidents are rare in the intestine but when they occur they have serious consequences because of the toxic and infective nature of the bowel contents. Splanic ischemia can injure other organs such as the liver and pancreas. Restoration of the blood supply to the ischemic tissue leads to reperfusion injury mediated by free radical generation. Many of these patients are not candidates for surgical resection of the bowel and there is no satisfactory medical treatment. The mortality is high in these cases.

Experimental intestinal ischemia produced in dogs by vascular interruption (Van Zyl 1966) was treated by exposing animals to normobaric pressures (controls) and hyperbaric pressures (treated groups), breathing oxygen for periods up to 6 h. Gases were also administered by intestinal or respiratory routes. Bowel death occurred in all animals. All these modalities, including HBO, failed to preserve ischemic intestine without perfusion.

Takahashi *et al* (1987) presented the effect of HBO on experimental thrombosis of the mesenteric artery in dogs. HBO was given at 2 ATA for 75 min and repeated for 3 days

following the arterial ligation. Animals were sacrificed on the 3rd and the 7th postoperative days and changes in the infarcted intestine were observed. Hemorrhage, edema, and multiple ulcers were characteristic of the control animals but were less marked in the animals treated by HBO; as well, evidence of the repair process was seen in these animals. Microangiography revealed rich revascularization around the margins of infarction in HBO-treated animals. The authors concluded that HBO has the following benefits in mesenteric artery thrombosis:

- It minimizes the hemorrhagic and edematous changes of the infarcted intestine.
- It promotes revascularization and the repair process.

In experiments on rats with ischemic jejunal segments created by mesenteric vessel ligation, there was no significant difference in the rate of perforation of the intestine in HBO versus non-HBO groups (Dockendorf *et al* 1993). The authors concluded that HBO was only of limited value for the treatment of intestinal ischemia. In a rat model, HBO treatment reduces leukosequestration and neutrophil preactivation following intestinal ischemia-reperfusion (Tjarnstrom *et al* 1999).

There is no report of the use of HBO in human patients with acute occlusion of the superior mesenteric artery.

Use of Hyperbaric Therapy in Removal of Entrapped Intestinal Balloons

Intestinal tube balloons may get entrapped in the intestine and become markedly distended. The balloons can be punctured by passing needles percutaneously under radiographic control, but this technique is not always successful. Hyperbaric therapy facilitates removal of the balloons by decompressing them. Increasingly, the procedure of "gastric bubble" for obesity is being used. Some of these balloons may pass through the pylorus and become entrapped in the intestine.

Kulak *et al* (1978) reported four cases where a Kaslow gastrointestinal tube balloon was successfully removed with hyperbaric pressure to 4 ATA. Peloso (1982) reported the successful removal of a trapped Kaslow tube balloon that became distended and led to recurrence of intestinal obstruction. Following a single compression at 2.5 ATA for 60 min, the tube could be pulled out. Another successful removal of a gas distended tube balloon has been reported by Lautin and Scheinbaum (1987). D'Hemecourt and Stern (1987) reported the use of hyperbaric treatment (2 ATA, two sessions) to aid the successful passage through the intestine of a gastric bubble that had become entrapped in the proximal jejunum.

HBO in Acute Pancreatitis

Acute pancreatitis is thought to be due to autodigestion of the pancreas by activated enzymes. The commonest causes are chronic alcoholism and gallstones, and the most frequent symptom is abdominal pain. The main feature of this condition is pancreatic necrosis leading to sepsis, with both localized and systemic inflammatory response syndromes. Early pathophysiological changes of the pancreas include alterations in microcirculation, ischemia reperfusion injury, and leukocyte and cytokine activation. In about 50% of cases the attack is mild and the patients recover without any treatment, in 40% the attack is severe and they are quite ill, and 10% die. The use of HBO has been explored in severely ill patients.

Daily HBO therapy at 2.5 ATA in a rat model of acute pancreatitis, induced by pancreatic duct ligation, was effective in reducing the hemorrhage and acinar necrosis but was not sufficient to reduce edema and leukocyte infiltration (Festugato *et al* 2008).

Pallota *et al* (1980) treated nine patients with acute pancreatitis, four of whom had associated paralytic ileus. HBO resulted in improvement in all cases. Serum amylase fell on average from about 88 U/l initially to slightly less than half this level after the first treatment and was down to about 11 U/l in 72 h. A case of severe acute pancreatitis was treated by HBO therapy at a pressure of 2.5 ATA for 90 min given twice daily for a total of 5 days with improvement (Christophi *et al* 2007).

Pancreatic abscess is a late complication of severe acute pancreatitis and peripancreatic abscess may follow surgical exploration. Izawa *et al* (1993) treated five such patients with HBO which was effective in reducing fever, leukocytosis, serum amylase levels, and size of the abscess.

In a study from Russia, 25 patients with acute pancreatitis were examined to assess whether HBO was an efficient and safe adjunct to the standard treatment protocol (Anonymous 2008). The impact of HBO on oxygenation in the splanchnic area, homeostasis, oxidative stress, and intraabdominal hypertension was evaluated. A treatment group consisted of 11 patients treated twice a day for 3 days using a monoplace chamber under pressures of 1.7–1.9 ATA. Patients in the control group were managed in accordance with the standard treatment protocol. HBO improved oxygen delivery to the splanchnic area, positively affected homeostasis, and induced no significant complications. The outcome of patients treated with HBO was not described.

HBO in Diseases of the Liver

Effect of HBO on the Normal Liver

A number of investigators have studied the effect of HBO on the normal liver. Schaffner *et al* (1966) studied the effect of breathing pure oxygen at 1/3, 1, and 3 ATA for 1 week, 1 day, and 1 h respectively on the liver in experimental animals. Electron microscopy showed mitochondria crowding out the cytoplasmic reticulum and large pinocytic vacuoles near the sinusoidal surface. The authors felt that there was pulmonary toxicity in these animals and that it aggravated these changes by hypoxia.

Sutkovoi and Baraboi (1985) showed that lipoperoxidase, both in the blood and the liver of the rat, is activated by HBO at 1.8 ATA. Trytyshnikov (1986) noted that exposure of rats to HBO at 3 ATA for 60 min immediately after acute massive loss of blood prevented the depression of RNA and protein synthesis in the liver. Subsequent daily use of HBO at 0.5–3 ATA had a stimulating effect on the reparative plastic processes in the liver and increased survival. Mattle (1963) showed that exposure of rats to 3 ATA did not influence significantly the rate of ethanol elimination. Incubation of liver slices *in vitro* (under oxygen) showed a significant correlation between oxygen uptake and ethanol elimination.

Effect of HBO on Experimentally Induced Hepatic Disorders in Animals

Hogan and Ellisen (1966) found that HBO offers no protection against hepatic artery ligation in the dog. Mallet-Guy *et al* (1970) showed that arterioportal shunt causes lesions in the walls of the liver sinusoids in experimental animals. HBO led to slight improvement in the appearance of these lesions on electron microscopy.

Hill (1976) evaluated HBO in the treatment of abscesses produced by intraperitoneal injection of *Fusobacterium necrophorum* plus *F. nucleatum* or *Bacteroides fragilis* in mice. A group of animals were exposed to HBO at 2 ATA for 3 h daily. Autopsy revealed that the number of abscesses was significantly lower in the HBO-treated group than in the controls. This study has practical implications for the treatment of hepatic abscesses in patients.

Mininberg and Kvetnoy (1979) studied the effect of HBO on rats with hepatotoxicity induced by carbon tetrachloride. The liver tissue in treated animals showed a reparative process: necrosis was absent, and the activity of succinic dehydrogenase was increased, as was the quantity of glucagon. The functional activity of the liver chromaffin cells containing melantotin and serotonin was enhanced. Belokurov and Rybachov (1981) used HBO on 380 rats with mechanical jaundice. The basis for the favorable effect appeared to be elimination of oxygen insufficiency in the liver tissues with subsequent regeneration.

Korkhov *et al* (1981) noted that in animals with induced hepatic insufficiency, the morphological changes in the liver were characterized by mild dystrophy of the hepatocytes, insignificant accumulation of glycogen, and transient manifestations of fatty degeneration. Under the effect of HBO, oxygen tensions in the liver tissues were rapidly restored, with recovery from the changes.

In contrast to the beneficial effect of HBO in hepatic insufficiency, the regeneration of liver after hepatectomy is delayed at day 15 in rats exposed to oxygen at 2 ATA for 90 min daily (Di Giulio et al 1989).

Clinical Applications

Most of the clinical applications of HBO in liver disease are in the more severe forms, such as acute hepatic failure with encephalopathy. This condition usually results from viral hepatitis but may also follow exposure to hepatotoxic drugs.

Hepatic encephalopathy. Hepatic encephalopathy is a complex syndrome that occurs due to diverse liver disease and spontaneous or iatrogenic portosystemic venous shunting. Clinical manifestations range from subtle neuropsychiatric abnormalities to deep coma. The pathogenesis of hepatic encephalopathy remains unclear. It is partially attributable to toxic materials that are derived from the nitrogenous metabolism in the gut and bypass the liver through anatomic and function shunts. Ammonia, mercaptans, and aminobutyric acid (GABA) are some of the substances that are found in high concentration in the blood of patients with hepatic coma. Ammonia-induced changes in the nervous system include depletion of glutamic acid, aspartic acid, and adenosine triphosphate. While often present in increased amounts in the blood, the absolute concentrations of ammonia, ammonia metabolites, including glutamine, and mercaptans correlate only roughly with the presence or severity of encephalopathy.

Treatment is aimed at reduction of production or absorption of ammonia, increasing metabolism of ammonia in the tissues, reduction of false neurotransmitters (aromatic amino acids), inhibition of GABA-benzodiazepine receptors and correction of manganese deposits in basal ganglia (Riordan & Williams 1997). Orthotopic liver transplantation is increasingly used in treatment of patients with end-stage liver cirrhosis.

Reports of use of HBO in disorders of the liver are reviewed against this background. Aubert et al (1967) treated two patients in hepatic coma with HBO. The patients improved, but the author drew no conclusions and suggested further research in this area was necessary. Dordain et al (1968) found HBO to be successful in treating a case of hepatic coma due to viral hepatitis. Goulon et al (1971) found HBO useful in treating 16 patients with viral hepatitis associated with hepatic encephalopathy, and Tacquet et al (1970) found it useful in a case of acute hepatic failure with hepatic coma.

Blum et al (1972) treated four children in acute hepatic failure with exchange transfusion and in three of them also gave HBO. The neurological status and EEG improved with exchange transfusion, but HBO had no effect and produced some complications, including death of one of the patients. Laverdant et al (1971, 1973) treated patients with viral hepatitis by a variety of methods, including HBO, and concluded that no special treatment beyond basic resuscitation and correction of electrolyte and acid-base balance made any difference to the outcome of the disease.

Novikova and Klyavinsh (1981) considered improvement of oxygen delivery to the liver and the brain in viral hepatitis A and B to be of great importance. They used HBO at 1.8 ATA for 30 min, and the number of sessions required was three to 24. Fourteen patients with severe viral hepatitis, hyperbilirubinemia exceeding 10 mg%, and impairment of liver function were treated. Three of the patients were in hepatic coma. After three to four treatments hyperbilirubinemia was reduced, liver function tests improved, and the patients started to recover. In hepatic coma, the signs disappeared with five to seven treatments. Eventually all the patients recovered.

Orynbaev and Myrzaliev (1981) used HBO in the treatment of 96 children with viral hepatitis. A study of the long-term results showed residual symptoms of viral hepatitis in only 7% of the patients (a frequency four times lower than in the controls). Belokurov et al (1985) analyzed the causes of endogenous intoxication in 39 patients with acute hepatic insufficiency and identified 11 toxic compounds. They discussed the role of hemadsorption and HBO in eliminating the toxic products and found this approach to be useful.

Tsygankova et al (1986) treated 30 patients with acute hepatitis that developed with renal failure or after renal transplant. One-half of these patients were treated by conventional therapy and the other half by HBO. In the HBO group, 8–10 treatments at 1.5 ATA proved to be effective in reducing the pathological process as shown by immune homeostasis recovery.

Okihama et al (1987) used HBO in treating a patient with liver cirrhosis who developed hyperbilirubinemia after percutaneous transhepatic variceal obliteration and splenic artery embolization. HBO therapy was performed 33 times during 54 days, and the level of serum bilirubin was successfully reduced to 1.2 mg/dl, and other clinical findings also improved. This result suggests that HBO therapy may be worth trying in cirrhotic patients who have hyperbilirubinemia and liver failure.

HBO has been used in combination with plasma exchange and hemodialysis in a 3-year-old girl suffering from acute hepatic failure and coma (Ponikvar et al 1998). She received 9 HBO sessions each with 100% oxygen at 2.5 ATA for 90 min over a course of 1 month. Throughout the treatment, the patient was in good clinical, physical, and mental condition, but she was dependent on blood purification procedures. She was referred to a liver transplant center and successfully transplanted.

In conclusion, we may state that the reports of use of HBO in liver disease are all anecdotal and thus difficult to evaluate. There are several reports of the use of HBO in acute viral hepatitis, but practically no information on the effect of HBO on viruses. Most of the described effects of HBO are on the biochemical sequelae of liver disease. HBO has been found to be useful in hepatic encephalopathy. This may possibly be due to an ammonia lowering effect of HBO. There are no reports of the use of HBO in drug-induced hepatitis. It would be worthwhile to explore the use of HBO in this condition.

Conclusions Regarding the Use of HBO in Gastroenterology

The use of HBO in peptic ulcers appears to be a logical extension of its successful application in skin ulcers. Counteracting ischemia and hypoxia appears to be a reasonable rationale for using HBO to promote healing of peptic ulcers. A controlled study, however, is required. Antibacterial effect of HBO against *H. pylori* needs to examined in the laboratory. Although there are no double-blind random-ized studies, the sheer number of cases with peptic ulcer reported from Russia (over 500) with good clinical and laboratory documentation presents in favor of prescribing HBO for cases of refractory peptic ulcer.

The role of HBO in intestinal ischemia needs to be investigated further. HBO accelerates new vessel growth in ischemia by angiogenesis but the mechanism has not been defined. Role of HBO treatments done more frequent and for longer periods needs to be determined. Combination of HBO with free radical scavengers to avoid reperfusion injury also needs to be investigated. Observations may have to be made on human patients but controlled clinical trials are not practical for this condition.

Another area where the use of HBO is promising is intestinal obstruction. Although controlled studies of the treatment of patients with adynamic ileus are not well documented, clinical experience is extensive and is well documented. In patients who have adynamic ileus or bowel obstruction associated with adhesions, HBO may be considered appropriate as an adjunctive treatment along with nasogastric decompression and intravenous fluid therapy. If there is complete bowel obstruction with strangulation or impending perforation, surgery should not be delayed in order to use HBO therapy. Rather, such patients may be given supplemental HBO in the postoperative period. HBO be a useful adjunct to nonoperative therapy for intestinal obstruction when a patient's overall condition does not allow operative intervention.

27

HBO and Endocrinology

K.K. Jain

Reports on the use of HBO in the field of endocrinology are relatively few in number, and further studies appear to be warranted, especially in the areas of thyrotoxicosis and diabetes mellitus. The main sections here include:

Introduction

Changes in various endocrine organs have been reported under hyperbaric oxygenation (HBO). Edström and Röckert (1962) studied the effect of HBO on a number of endocrine organs and reported adrenal hypertrophy, decrease in the weight of the thymus, and increase in the weight of the thyroid. They concluded that the changes observed in the nervous and the endocrine systems represented nonspecific stress reactions. In a series of cases of vegetovascular dysfunction manifested by hypotension in adolescents and children with a history of perinatal disturbances of the central nervous system, functional activity of the pituitary-thyroid system normalized following HBNO treatment (Buriak 2001).

Thyroid Glands

Sjöstrand (1964) exposed rats to HBO at 6 ATA for 4–5 days and sacrificed them on the 6th day. In contrast to the results of previous investigators, the thyroid weight was found to be decreased but ^{131}I was increased. The author believed that this represented a specific effect of HBO on the thyroid.

Epinephrine/Norepinephrine

Hale *et al* (1973) studied the endocrinological and metabolic responses of healthy young men to a range of oxygen-rich and oxygen-poor gaseous environments (varying between 15% and 100% oxygen). The norepinephrine:epinephrine ratio (as index of catecholamine balance) varied directly with oxygen balance, ranging from 2:1 to 6:1. Norepinephrine and epinephrine act jointly in regulating regional blood flow – norepinephrine acting as a vasoconstrictor while epinephrine acts as a vasodilator in low concentrations and as a constrictor in high concentrations.

Nakada *et al* (1984) found increased adrenal epinephrine and norepinephrine in spontaneously hypertensive rats treated with HBO (2 ATA). Catecholamines have been described as facilitating oxygen toxicity and hence the rationale for experimental adrenalectomy for protection against oxygen toxicity in experimental animals (see Chapter 6).

Studies in divers have shown that HBO and hyperbaric air at 2.5 ATA do not induce a generalized hormonal stress reaction but induce an increase in endothelin-1 levels (Lund *et al* 1999).

Glucocorticoid Receptors

Golikov *et al* (1986a,b) studied the effect of a single exposure of HBO at 3 ATA for 5 h on glucocorticoid receptors in the lungs of rats. The level of these receptors was reduced to nearly half after the exposure. Twenty-four hours later the number of receptors in lungs had increased, while the blood cortisol level was reduced but was still a little higher than in the control animals.

Adrenocortical Function

Saito *et al* (1977a,b) showed that HBO (2 ATA, 35% oxygen, 90 min/day) increases adrenocortical function in rats. Casti *et al* (1993) studied the ACTH response in healthy adult male athletes after HBO exposure at 2.8 ATA for 1 h daily for 10 days. On day one (acute phase) ACTH level increased significantly whereas in the chronic phase (days 5–10), the values remained stable. No significant variations were found during hyperbarism with air. HBO, thus, has potential clinical application in the treatment of steroid dependency in patients with arthritis, possibly enabling withdrawal.

Prostaglandins

Walker *et al* (1980) studied the effect of hyperoxia on renal prostaglandin E_2 (PGE_2) excretion and diuresis in the dog. Hypoxia caused a 13% increase in renal blood flow, whereas hyperoxia caused a 5%–7% decline due to vasoconstriction. HBO at 1.8 ATA and 2.8 ATA caused a decrease in urinary flow of 61% and 70% respectively. The urinary PGE_2 declined by 61% at 2 ATA, 92% at 1.8 ATA, and 99% at 2.8 ATA. Plasma antidiuretic hormone (ADH) remained unchanged. The authors postulated that HBO antidiuresis may be a consequence of an increased medullary osmotic gradient secondary to reduced vasa recta blood flow, or may be due to a lowering of the normal functional antagonism between PGE_2 and ADH, so that influence of endogenous ADH is potentiated.

Mialon and Barthelemy (1993) studied the effect of HBO on prostaglandin synthesis in the cortex and striatum of the rat brain. Three groups were subjected to i) neurotoxic HBO at 6 ATA, ii) mild hyperoxia at 6 ATA room air, and iii) normoxia. Examination of brain samples after decapitation showed that release of 6-keto-PGF_{1a} was reduced significantly in the mild hyperoxia group.

Concentration of PGE values were restored to normal in gastric ulcer patients treated with HBO where previous treatment with H_2-blockers had reduced the PGE concentration (Serebrianskaia & Masenko 1993).

The contents of PGE_2 in alveolar bone and gingiva increases markedly in experimental peridontitis. The value of PGE_2 in alveolar bone and gingiva reduces markedly after HBO treatments at 2.5 ATA (Chen *et al* 2002).

Testosterone

Reduction of blood flow to the testes and a decrease in plasma testosterone have been observed in experimental animals under hyperbaric conditions. Röckert and Haglid (1983) reported that human divers also showed a decrease in plasma testosterone on exposure to 6 ATA. They also observed a reversible change in the rate of DNA synthesis in the testes of rats after exposure to hyperbaric air. Under conditions similar to clinical use of HBO (2–3 ATA daily, 90-min sessions), no changes were found in the testosterone concentration in serum or testes of rats after daily exposures to HBO for 58 days (Nakada *et al* 1986).

Clinical Applications

The only clinical applications of HBO in endocrinology are in disorders of the thyroid and in diabetes mellitus. All the clinical reports are from the USSR. None of the experimental evidence quoted above is relevant to the clinical applications.

Thyroid Disease

Shakarashvilli *et al* (1981) studied the effect of HBO on thyroid function in normal subjects and in patients with thyrotoxicosis. HBO (2 ATA, 60 min) was given daily for 10–12 days. The levels of thyrotropic hormone, triiodothyronine, and thyroxine were checked daily. They became normal after the HBO treatment regardless of whether the level before exposure had been normal, decreased, or increased. The therapeutic effect lasted an average of 1–1.5 months.

Droviannikova (1981) used HBO for preoperative preparation of patients with diffuse toxic goiter. The optimal course of treatment was found to be one 45- to 60-min session per day for 6–10 days. The pressure was selected by titration according to the pulse, blood pressure, and cardiac output of each patient, but did not exceed 2 ATA. As a result, tachycardia was eliminated. The circulating blood volume decreased by 10%–12% and the contractile action of the myocardium improved. There was no increase in the level of thyroid hormones in the blood. The authors concluded that HBO in combination with conventional drug therapy improved cardiovascular hemodynamics and reduced the period of preoperative preparation by 8–10 days.

Rakhmatullin and Hallev (1981) used HBO in the treatment of thyrotoxicosis crises in the postoperative period of patients with thyrotoxic goiter. The principal mechanism of postoperative complication was considered to be increased ejection of thyroid hormone into the circulation and emergence of hypoxia. HBO was used as preoperative preparation in 36 patients with toxic goiter. In eight of these patients HBO was required in the postoperative period for crises. In another series of cases from Russia, patients who underwent surgery for diffuse toxic goiter, recurrence of the disease was less in those who had undergone HBO therapy for preoperative preparation (Kariakin *et al* 1992).

Diabetes Mellitus

The effect of HBO has not been studied on experimentally induced diabetes in animals but there are reports of this application in human patients. Most of the human studies are in diabetic foot (see Chapter 15). The focus of this section is on the effect of HBO on systemic manifestations of diabetes mellitus.

Kakhnovski *et al* (1980a,b,c) noted improvement of cardiovascular complications in diabetic patients on using HBO therapy, and later (1981) reported HBO as an adjunct to diet and insulin in the treatment of moderately severe diabetes in 130 patients. The dosage of insulin was reduced by 4–38 units in 62.3% of the patients after treatment. The authors concluded that the hypoglycemic effect of HBO is due to inhibition of the effect of antiinsulin hormones (somatotropic hormone and glucagon) by HBO. There was also increased S-peptide secretion and tissue sensitivity to insulin due to correction of the acid-base balance.

Kakhnovskii *et al* (1982) also studied the indices of blood acid-base balance, glucose level, blood lactate and pyruvate concentration, and serum activity of malate dehydrogenase and lactate dehydrogenase, as well as of succinate dehydrogenase and glycerophosphate dehydrogenase in lymphocytic mitochondria. Diet and insulin therapy combined with HBO was accompanied by a rapid stabilization (within 12–18 days) of carbohydrate metabolism and good dynamics of all the tests. The results indicated a significant improvement in tissue metabolism – both glycolysis and the tricarboxylic cycle.

Ostashevskaia *et al* (1986) incorporated HBO in the treatment of juvenile diabetes and established high efficiency of the method for managing complications such as angiopathy, polyneuritis, and trophic changes in the tissues. Longoni *et al* (1987) treated 15 diabetic patients with HBO and found that insulin requirements were reduced in 11 of them. There was a concomitant improvement in the diabetic ulcers in these patients.

Epshtein *et al* (1988) treated 32 male patients with diabetes mellitus using HBO as a part of comprehensive management. They found that 10–14 sessions of HBO at 1.5–1.7 ATA for 40–50 min improved the carbohydrate metabolism, circulation in the lower extremities, and general condition of these patients. It was possible to reduce the dose of insulin and oral hypoglycemic agents in these patients. These authors recommended repetition of HBO courses every 6–8 months.

Transient hyperglycemia is common in patients with cerebrovascular accidents and is also a recognized risk factor for stroke. Hyperglycemia is more frequent in patients with an unfavorable outcome of stroke. This provides a rationale for the use of HBO in patients with stroke and high blood glucose levels

Apart from its effect on hyperglycemia, HBO has been used as an adjunct to pancreatic islet transplantation in diabetes mellitus. Peritransplant treatment of diabetic recipients by daily HBO sessions (2.4 ATA, 90 min) improves the outcome of the transplantation (Juang *et al* 2002).

Conclusions

In contrast to other areas of hyperbaric medicine, studies on the endocrinological aspect are scant. In view of the controversy regarding the effect of HBO on thyroid function, further experimental studies, as well as controlled trials on patients with thyrotoxicosis, should be carried out.

The idea of using HBO as an adjunct in the treatment of diabetes mellitus is a logical one. Fall in blood glucose has been observed in volunteers exposed to HBO. Controlled studies need to be done in diabetics to prove or disprove the beneficial effect of HBO. There is a lack of basic experimental studies assessing the effect of HBO in experimentally induced diabetes mellitus. HBO may also be a useful adjunct in reducing the transient hyperglycemia sometimes seen in cerebrovascular accidents. Diabetic patients who are given HBO for other indications should be carefully monitored for blood glucose, as the insulin requirements are usually reduced and the dosage needs to be readjusted. A calculation method devised by Dreval *et al* (1988) enables the effect of HBOin lowering the insulin requirement in diabetics to be assessed.

28 HBO and Pulmonary Disorders

K.K. Jain

This chapter reviews the modest number of applications in the area of pulmonary disorders, as well as important contraindications:

Introduction

Hyperbaric oxygen (HBO) therapy has a limited role in pulmonary disorders, which are usually treated by normobaric oxygen (Jain 1989b). Nonetheless, HBO has been used for a number of pulmonary conditions and these are reviewed in this chapter. Pulmonary oxygen toxicity and contraindications for the use of HBO will also be described.

Lung Mechanics and Pulmonary Gas Exchange

The physical and physiological aspects of gas exchange in the lungs under HBO have been discussed in Chapter 2.

Respiratory compliance is not changed when pressure is increased to 2 ATA on breathing air. Lung dynamics, however, fall by 15% in individuals breathing oxygen at a pressure of 2 ATA for 6–11 h. Hilpert *et al* (1973) studied the effect of on the lungs of six There are no significant changes in vital capacity, dynamic compliance, and maximum pulmonary pressure gradients of healthy subjects. breathing HBO at 2.8 ATA for 3 h

Gerbershagen *et al* (1977) performed pulmonary function studies on subjects breathing oxygen at 3 ATA for 90 min. They found a decrease of pulmonary compliance, which they attributed to absorption atelectasis, pulmonary vascular congestion, and edema. The oxygen diffusion capacity and diffusion pressure ratios were markedly reduced. The authors recommended a rest period of 36 h between exposures to allow recovery from these changes.

Adamiec *et al* (1975) investigated the respiratory effects of HBO at 2.4 ATA during treatment of patients with peripheral vascular disease. The HBO sessions were 90 min long and were repeated two to three times a week for 3 months. The authors found increased airway resistance, increased pulmonary elastance, decreased vital capacity and respiratory rate, and increased closing volume. These changes were completely reversible within 2 h of completion of the treatment.

To clarify the disparity in some of these findings among different investigators, it may be pointed out that there are individual variations in tolerance of HBO. Most HBO treatments are carried out at 1.5–2 ATA and the duration usually does not exceed 1 h. Within these limits no adverse effects have been observed on pulmonary function. If there are any adverse effects they certainly clear up within 24 h, which is the usual interval between treatments. According to some authors, the changes observed in the mechanics of respiration are early signs of oxygen toxicity.

Pulmonary Oxygen Toxicity

Pulmonary oxygen toxicity is more commonly seen with prolonged exposure to 100% normobaric oxygen (Jain 1989b). It is less of a problem during short exposures to HBO. Oxygen exposures at high pressures are limited by CNS rather than pulmonary intoxication because no pulmonary symptoms are reported by subjects who breathe oxygen at pressures ranging from 2.4–4 ATA until occurrence of neurological manifestations. Experimental observations regarding the toxicity of oxygen under normobaric and hyperbaric conditions are not comparable. Although the structural changes in the lungs produced by oxygen inhalation under normobaric and hyperbaric conditions are the same, and that the degree of change depends on the magnitude and duration of oxygenation.

Davis *et al* (1983) described the early reversible changes in the human alveolar structures induced by hyperoxia. Breathing 95% oxygen for 17 h caused a significant alveolar-capillary leak. These changes were reversible, but such alterations may induce processes that can result in fibrosis. One popular theory of the mechanism of lung toxicity suggests that high concentrations of oxygen are directly toxic to lung parenchyma, probably via toxic oxygen radicals.

Although the metabolism of lung connective tissue is unaffected by short-term exposure to HBO, the mechanism of toxicity is due, at least in part, to the effect of oxygen on surfactant synthesis. Oxygen inhibits enzymes involved in synthesis of surfactant and may also inhibit transport of surfactant to the alveoli.

Bergren and Beckman (1975) pointed out that an important causal mechanism involved in the development of lung injury is an initial increase in minimal surface tension due to increased intra-alveolar cholesterol. Ward and Roberts (1984) studied the effect of hyperoxia (breathing a concentration of oxygen higher than 95% for 48 h) on the newborn rabbit lung. Phosphatidylcholine synthesis, secretion, and uptake was impaired. This was consistent with the existence of multiple sites of action of hyperoxia on the pulmonary surfactant system in the newborn. This has serious implications for the premature infant with respiratory distress syndrome, for which oxygen may be administered. The pathological changes occurring in the lungs in response to hyperbaric oxygen are shown in Figure 28.1.

Eckenhoff *et al* (1986) showed that symptoms and pulmonary function changes consistent with early pulmonary oxygen toxicity (POT) occurred in 12 subjects exposed to 5 ATA air for 48 h, while none occurred in six subjects exposed to 5 ATA normoxic nitrogen-oxygen (6% O_2) for a similar period. All subjects eventually recovered completely.

Morphological changes in the lungs have been shown to depend on the degree and duration of oxygen pressure. Daily exposure to 2 ATA for 60 min for 2 weeks or 2.5 ATA

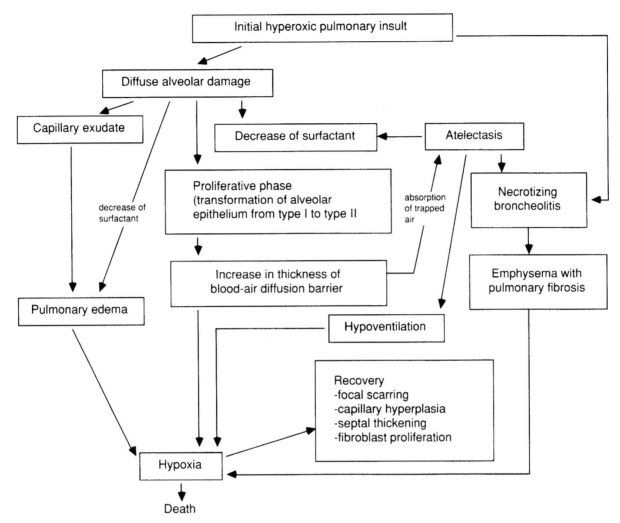

Figure 28.1
Sequence of events in pulmonary edema due to oxygen toxicity (Jain 1989).

for 1 week are considered to be the safe limits of HBO (Kharchenko *et al* 1986).

Alterations in pulmonary function that were observed in subjects breathing oxygen at 3.5 ATA for 3.5 h included small but significant decreases in several indices of both inspiratory and expiratory function (Clark *et al* 1991).

At higher inspired O_2 pressures, 2–3 ATA, pulmonary injury is greatly accelerated but less inflammatory in character, and events in the brain are a prelude to a distinct lung pathology. The CNS-mediated component of this lung injury can be attenuated by selective inhibition of neuronal nitric oxide synthase (nNOS) or by unilateral transection of the vagus nerve. Extrapulmonary, neurogenic events predominate in the pathogenesis of acute pulmonary oxygen toxicity in HBO, as nNOS activity drives lung injury by modulating the output of central autonomic pathways (Demchenko *et al* 2007).

Methods of prevention of oxygen toxicity have been discussed in Chapter 6. Lung toxicity can be prevented or minimized by alternation of HBO (2 ATA) and air-breathing.

Clinical Applications

Respiratory Insufficiency

Lukich *et al* (1978) treated by means of HBO at 1.3–1.5 ATA for 40–60 min. Sixteen patients with restrictive and obstructive disease of the lungs and respiratory insufficiency Arterial hypoxemia was eliminated, the acid-base balance became normal, and respiratory acidosis disappeared in all the patients.

The use of HBO in more severe forms of respiratory insufficiency has been investigated experimentally. Rogatsky *et al* (1988) showed that in Wistar rats with induced respiratory insufficiency HBO at 3 ATA for 2 h reduced the mortality and prevented the structural changes peculiar to the "wet lung" syndrome.

Jansen *et al* (1987) performed lung lavage under HBO conditions in two patients suffering from severe respiratory insufficiency in pulmonary alveolar proteinosis. Under these conditions, gas exchange was maintained and mixed venous partial pressure of oxygen and oxygen saturation showed increases to acceptable levels. This enabled the authors to limit the FiO$_2$ in order to extend the oxygen tolerance and to perform the lavage procedures more effectively. Both patients improved significantly and the authors concluded that the use of HBO in unilateral lung lavages is a useful procedure.

Most patients with chronic obstructive pulmonary disease (COPD) are treated with normobaric oxygen (Jain 1989b). Miller *et al* (1987) reassessed the role of hyperbaric air in the treatment of COPD. Patients with this condition were placed in a hyperbaric chamber of 1.25 ATA (air). Their arterial oxygen saturations were comparable to when they were breathing oxygen by nasal prongs at 2 l/min. The ability to exercise was improved under compressed air. The authors suggested hyperbaric air as an alternative to long-term O$_2$ therapy. No adverse effects were observed in their patients. It should be borne in mind that emphysema is a contraindication for HBO therapy. The pressure of 1.25 ATA may be safe for these patients, but those with emphysematous bullae should not go into a hyperbaric chamber.

Ivanova *et al* (1981) treated 89 bronchial asthma patients with HBO in addition to the conventional medical therapy. The treatment course consisted of 12 sessions. The effectiveness was evaluated by the decrease in dosage of the drugs used, frequency of asphyxial attacks, and indices of external respiratory function. Good results were obtained in 20 patients, and in a further 55 patients the results were considered satisfactory. No improvement was noted in the remaining patients.

Korotaev *et al* (1981) used HBO in 16 adult patients with bronchial asthma of infectious-allergic etiology. The medical management was supplemented by five to nine daily sessions of HBO at 1.5 ATA lasting 30–50 min each. Improvement was noted in half of the patients. The rest had been on steroids for long periods; attempts to wean them off steroid dependence by means of HBO treatment were not successful. The authors also treated four children with acute bronchospasm. Dyspnea was relieved during the HBO sessions.

Mikhailov (1982) stated that HBO was used in asthma in order to normalize various types of glucocorticoid metabolic disturbances associated both with the decreased synthesis of adrenocortical hormones and inactivation of glucocorticoids by blood transcortin and their reduced utilization. Normalization of glucocorticoid metabolism was maximal in patients with milder forms of asthma, and the best results were obtained in these cases.

Liu and Zhi (1986) treated 387 patients with bronchial asthma who were resistant to conventional treatment, using HBO at 2 ATA (80- to 90-min sessions with an air break of 10 min in the middle) for an average of 24 sessions. Good results (decrease in the frequency of asthma attacks and discontinuance of drug therapy) were obtained in 182 (47%) of the patients; satisfactory results (decrease in the dosage and frequency of use of medications) were observed in 163 patients (42%); and no effect was seen in 41 patients (11%).

Bronchitis

Efuni (1984) used HBO therapy in 92 patients with dust-induced bronchitis. There was improvement in 88.9% of the patients as determined by tolerance to physical exercise and blood gas measurements.

Inflammatory Processes of the Lungs

Ermakov and Barsky (1981) of the USSR investigated the effect of HBO on acute and chronic pneumonia. Three to five sessions at 1.5 ATA were used. The authors concluded that HBO had no adverse effects on the acute inflammatory processes and actually had some benefit in the chronic cases. They cautioned against the use of HBO in cases of hypercapnia. A pCO$_2$ value of 60 mmHg or above is considered to be a contraindication for the use of HBO unless the patient is on artificial ventilation.

A combination of HBO and antioxidants (unithiol and alpha-tocopherol) was used in a complex intensive therapy of 194 children, aged 3 days to 3 years, with severe pneumonias (Zhdanov *et al* 1991). HBO yielded excellent and good results in 75.8% of patients, was ineffective in 17% of cases, produced signs of oxygen toxicity in 7.2% of patients.

Pulmonary Embolism

Pulmonary air embolism occurs in inappropriate decompressions or clinical complications. Sudden lodging of air bubbles in the pulmonary circulation results in pulmonary hypertension, pulmonary edema, and deficiency in cardiopulmonary functions, which are often fatal without timely intervention. Burr and Trapp (1976) reported the case of a 20-year-old man who suffered a massive pulmonary embolism and underwent embolectomy with HBO support. The patient recovered and the authors felt that HBO had played an important role.

In venous air infusion induced acute lung injury in rats neither HBO therapy nor isoproterenol treatment was shown to effectively reverse the lung injury (Huang *et al* 2002). There is no report in the literature of HBO having been used on moderately severe cases of pulmonary embolism not requiring surgery.

Pulmonary Edema: Experimental Studies

Iazzetti and Maciel (1988) induced neurogenic pulmonary edema in rats by bilateral cervical vagotomy. The group of animals placed under HBO at 1.8 ATA for 325 min had less pulmonary edema than the controls breathing room air. Stewart *et al* (1988) induced smoke inhalation injury in rabbits and placed one group in a hyperbaric chamber breathing 100% oxygen at 2.5 ATA for 45 min. Pulmonary edema was less in the treated animals compared with controls breathing room air.

Although pulmonary edema is a feature of oxygen toxicity, it appears that some types, such as neurogenic and cardiogenic pulmonary edema, may be reduced by HBO therapy. Some smoke inhalation victims who are treated by HBO may experience relief through the beneficial effect on pulmonary edema. Administration of HBO (2.8 ATA for 45 min) inhibited adhesion of circulating neutrophils subsequent to smoke inhalation in rats (Thom et al 2001). HBO2 reduced pulmonary neutrophil accumulation whether used in a prophylactic manner, 24 h before smoke inhalation, or as treatment immediately after the smoke insult. The beneficial effect appears related to inhibition of neutrophil adhesion to the vasculature. Clinical studies are required to assess the effect of HBO in pulmonary edema in humans.

Contraindications

Nitrogen Dioxide Poisoning

Schechter et al (1975) produced nitrogen dioxide poisoning experimentally in dogs. Such poisoning carries high mortality due to lung edema and respiratory failure. The mortality and the pathological effects on the lungs were increased in animals treated with HBO compared with the controls. On this basis, the use of HBO in cases of human nitrogen dioxide poisoning is contraindicated.

Paraquat Poisoning

Rebello and Mason (1978) studied the lungs in 11 cases of death from paraquat poisoning and compared them to the lungs in cases of oxygen poisoning. They hypothesized that paraquat exerts its toxic action by sensitizing the lungs to oxygen at atmospheric pressure. HBO would thus be contraindicated in such a case. Locket (1973), however, indicated that HBO may be useful in cases of paraquat poisoning.

Emphysema

HBO has been suggested as a treatment adjunct in emphysema to lessen the trapped air, to oxygenate the blood without causing hypercapnia, and to alter the pulmonary perfusion. Chusid et al (1972) reviewed previous anecdotal reports of subjective improvement in such cases on the use of HBO and found that no objective data had ever been produced to support this claim. They treated five emphy-

sema patients with HBO and thoroughly investigated the pre- and post-HBO respiratory status by objective investigations. They found no improvement, and listed emphysema as a contraindication for HBO therapy.

Shock Lung

Although HBO is useful in the treatment of shock, it has been reported that serious respiratory distress, the so-called shock lung, can be aggravated by HBO. Ouda et al (1977) induced shock lung in rats by injection of endotoxins. They showed that the decrease of mucopolysaccharide of the alveolar epithelium and the decrease of phospholipid of the alveolar lining layer observed in endotoxic shock was prevented after 2 h of HBO at 3 ATA, but not after 4 h of HBO at the same pressure, which induces lung damage independent of endotoxin. They concluded that HBO treatment may be effective in endotoxin-induced damage if one observes the proper precautions. Ouda et al did not spell out the proper conditions for treatment of a human patient; we are not aware of any clinical reports of HBO use for shock lung, and it remains on the contraindication list.

Pneumothorax

Patients with pneumothorax will have problems during decompression and should not be placed in the hyperbaric chamber until a chest tube is placed, i.e., closed thoracotomy.

Conclusions

HBO therapy has no advantages over the normobaric oxygen therapy widely used in respiratory insufficiency. The main concern in the use of HBO for pulmonary disorders is the fear of aggravation of lung pathology by oxygen-induced pulmonary toxicity. Pulmonary toxicity is not a problem in patients with healthy lungs who receive HBO at up to 3 ATA for periods as long as 90 min once or twice daily.

There is no absolute or ideal indication for HBO in pulmonary disorders. Further research and controlled trials are required to assess the reported beneficial effect in asthma and bronchitis. It is worth noting that most of these treatments have been carried out at 1.5 ATA. Patients undergoing HBO treatment for other indications should be subjected to a thorough examination of the lungs supplemented by chest x-rays and pulmonary function studies. It must be remembered, of course, that pneumothorax and silent lung lesions are contraindications for HBO therapy.

29 HBO Therapy in Pediatric Surgery

S.A. Baydin

The chapter describes the experience in the use of HBO in a large pediatric surgical clinic in Russia.

Introduction

Experience with the successful use of HBO in treating different diseases in the adults formed the basis for the further investigation of its effectiveness in pediatrics.

Hutchison *et al* (1963) were the first to apply HBO in neonatology for the treatment of asphyxia of the newborn (see Chapter 33). Soon thereafter, techniques for the use of HBO in pediatric surgery and resuscitation were introduced (Bernhard *et al* 1964; Anokhin *et al* 1972). There are only few reports in the Western medical literature dealing with the treatment of diseases of children using HBO, even though its use in adult patients has expanded considerably. Vazquez and Spahr (1990) reported the use of HBO in four neonates with non-healing wounds. All wounds healed, and there were no complications of HBO therapy.

The first clinical experiments with HBO in pediatric practice began in our clinic in 1969, when a Moscow factory produced a monoplace chamber under the order of the Head of the Department of Pediatric Surgery and resuscitation of the 2nd Moscow Medical Institute, now called the Russian State Medical University. Since then we have performed about 30,000 HBO sessions on more than 4500 children (from newborn to 15 years old) having surgical pathology. About 5000 HBO sessions are carried out annually in our clinic.

As a result of clinical investigations, carried out both in our clinic and other clinics in Russia, indications for the use of HBO in pediatric surgery and intensive care have been defined and techniques for the of HBO use of HBO in children of different ages have been developed. We have evaluated the efficacy of HBO in comprehensive therapy for different surgical disorders of children. According to the presentations made at the Seventh International Congress of Hyperbaric Medicine at Moscow in 1981, HBO treatments have reduced the mortality from peritonitis and necrotizing enterocolitis (Baydin 1986). HBO has proven to be valuable as an adjunct in the management of crush injuries and scalping wounds, as well in as the postoperative management after plastic operations on the abdominal viscera in infants. Occasionally, HBO is a decisive factor in the outcome of resuscitation from cardiac and respiratory arrest.

Hyperbaric Chambers for Children

At present four types of monoplace chambers are used in Russia for children of different age-groups:

1. Chamber OKA-MT (Figure 29.1). This is a widely used bed type chamber for adults and grown children. Patients may be placed in different positions in this chamber, and the specific shape of the chamber enables a physician to get into it together with a patient and perform artificial ventilation with a breathing bag. This method is used because of the lack of special ventilators for children which can function under varying pressures. The control panel with desk is alongside the chamber. The chamber can be pressurized to 2 ATA. This chamber is comfortable and very reliable.

2. Chamber BLKS-301m (Figure 29.2). This chamber is designed for adults and grown-up children and can be

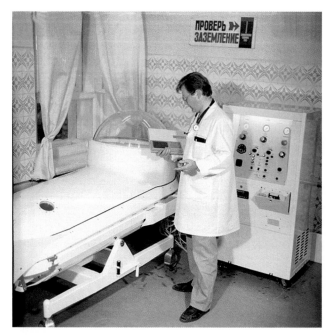

Figure 29.1
Monoplace chamber OKA-MT.

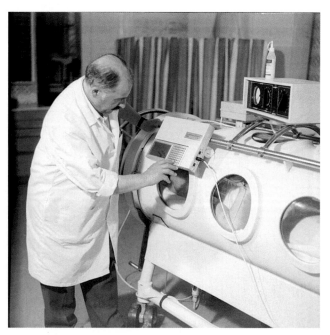

Figure 29.2
Monoplace chamber BLKS-301.

pressurized up to 4 ATA. The patient is placed on a sliding stretcher, which then is moved into a chamber. It is a reliable and durable chamber, and ventilators and respirators can be attached to it. A special system is provided to monitor the patient's condition during HBO sessions, which was designed by the Russian firm BION to enable selection of the proper regime of HBO treatment for a patient.

3. Chamber IRTISH-2MT. This is a new transportable chamber designed for use both in hospitals and under field conditions. This chamber can be pressurized to 3 ATA and has its own oxygen supply system, which suffices for 3 sessions without a refill. The chamber consists of two parts which telescope into each other, and it weighs only 90 kg and has special handles for carrying it. The IRTISH-2MT is comfortable enough for patients of different ages and is reliable and easy to operate. These features make it a suitable chamber for rendering urgent medical aid during catastrophes.

4. Chamber MANA-2 (Figure 29.3). This chamber is designed for newborns and children under the age of one year. It can be pressurized to 4 ATA and is very reliable. The patient's bed slides easily along special rails through which oxygen passes into the chamber. There is a special humidifier in this chamber for providing moisture, which prevents the toxic effect of oxygen on the respiratory tract of newborns.

All of these chambers are supplied with a special monitoring system B-OO1 M.

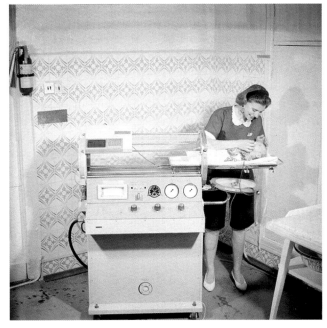

Figure 29.3
Monoplace chamber MANA-2.

Technique of Hyperbaric Oxygenation in Children

Preparation

This is important because of the anatomico-physiological and psychological aspects of children. Before they are placed into a chamber all children are examined by an otolaryngologist to detect otitis media or sinusitis, which are frequent intercurrent illnesses. There is less risk of barotrauma to the paranasal sinuses and middle ear in children than in adults. It is explained by the fact that in children the auditory tubes are relatively short and wide, so the process of pressure equalization in the middle ear cavity is easier than in adults. Paranasal sinuses as gas-containing cavities develop only by the fourth year of life. At that time nasal and auditory tube mucosa are liable to develop edema, which may cause barotrauma of the middle ear. To avoid possible otolaryngological complications patients are administered a 2% solution of ephedrine hydrochloride, 2 to 3 drops in each nostril. When carrying out HBO sessions in cases of rhinitis, sinusitis, and otitis it is advisable to clean the nasal meatus with a solution of epinephrine hydrochloride (1:1000). This procedure is effective and makes it possible to carry out HBO sessions in children with concomitant inflammatory diseases of the paranasal sinuses. Grown-up children should be taught to do self-inflation of the middle ear. Small children are given chewing gum or candy and babies are given a pacifier to suck on.

Thermoregulatory mechanisms are not well developed in infants and may lead to hyperthermia or hypothermia during the hyperbaric session; hyperthermia predisposes to oxygen toxicity. A physician should take into account the feeding schedule of the newborn while carrying on HBO sessions. It is not advisable to take an infant to a HBO session just after feeding, as regurgitating may interrupt the course of a session. It is better to begin HBO treatment, particularly in a monoplace chamber, 15 to 20 min after feeding.

Premedication

The main purpose of premedication should be to calm the child during HBO session, to reduce the risk of oxygen toxicity, and to optimize the effect of HBO. We administer an intramuscular injection of chlorpromazine hydrochloride (25%, 0.1 ml per year of age) to a child in satisfactory condition. The sedative effect of this drug suppresses the vomiting reflex and reduces the risk of oxygen toxicity.

Technique

The rate of compression in a HBO chamber should be $0.1 \, kg/cm^2$ per min using 100% oxygen. If children experience problems referable to the middle ear or the paranasal sinuses, it may be necessary to use compression with short stops at 1.25, 1.5, and 1.75 ATA or to decrease the rate of compression to $0.05 \, kg/cm^2$ per min. The process of compression must be accompanied by a careful monitoring of a patient's condition to detect any signs of hypersensitivity to HBO.

At present, different regimes of HBO pressures are used in pediatrics. There are some who use high-pressure HBO regimes, but many physicians consider 1.5 ATA to be adequate. Earlier on we used HBO at about 2.8 ATA for treatment of severe hypoxia and trauma of the central nervous system, but after reviewing our clinical experience and the results of functional investigations, we concluded that it is practically impossible to choose an optimal HBO regime for treatment of a certain disease because of the variations in the sensitivity of individual patients to HBO. We noted that use of pressures above 2 ATA often caused disturbance of cardiac rhythm (tachycardia, arrhythmia, and extrasystoles) while there was no increase of efficacy. The sensitivity of patients to oxygen may change during the procedure, and this may require adjustment of the HBO pressure.

On the basis of numerous investigations of the hemodynamic state under HBO, we have made some recommendations for choosing a proper HBO regime depending on the initial state of blood circulation, as shown in Table 29.1.

If the pressures presented in Table 29.1 are exceeded, there is a regression of the positive dynamics back to the initial state. This process is demonstrated most clearly by the dynamics of the reographic indices in patients with marked spasms of arterial vessels and hypocirculation, which are caused by infectious and/or inflammatory diseases and extensive injuries of the extremities. In these patients, during the compression phase of HBO, the hypertonicity of the arteries begins to disappear and blood perfusion of the limbs increases. At a pressure of 1.5 ATA, the index of vascular tone becomes nearly normal. Against this background there is statistically significant increase of blood perfusion by 24.4% as compared with the initial level. On increasing the pressure further, vascular tone does not change. However, the maximum tissue perfusion during the compression is reached at a pressure of 1.75 ATA, when it doubles. Further compression to 2 ATA causes a hypertonic reaction accompanied by the drop of the perfusion volume which requires the adjustment of HBO regime. Repeated application of pressure of 1.75 ATA results in the development of vascular dilation and an increase of blood perfusion. According to the available data, maximum balanced blood flow is achieved between 1.5 and 1.75 ATA. This is why we chose a regime with this range of pressures. During 40 min of application of this pressure, the rheo-

Table 29.1
Optimum HBO Regimes Based on Initial Hemodynamic State

Initial Hemodynamic State	Ideal HBO Pressure (ATA)
Disorders of Myocardial Contractility	
Energy-dynamic cardiac insufficiency:	
right heart ventricle	1.5–1.75
left heart ventricle	2.0
Hypodynamic myocardial reaction:	
right heart ventricle	1.75
left heart ventricle	2.0
Disturbances of Pulmonary Circulation	
Intrapulmonary hypocirculation	1.75–1.5
Hypertonicity of pulmonary vessels	1.5
Hypotonicity of pulmonary vessels	2.0
Circulatory Disturbances of Limbs	
Peripheral vasodilatation	2.0
Hypertonicity of arteries	1.75–1.5
Peripheral hypocirculation	1.75

Data were obtained with the polycardiographic method. Analysis of the phase structure of the systole of the right and the left ventricle was carried out separately. The state of the pulmonary circulation and that of the limbs was assessed by rheography before, during, and after HBO treatment.

gram indices do not change. On decompression the vascular tone increases but is less than it is initially. The state of circulation improves with successive sessions and as a rule normalizes by the eighth or ninth session. Based on these observations, we suggest the HBO regimes above for children with diseases caused mainly by hemodynamic disorders. However, it is not always possible to get a complete hemodynamic picture in urgent cases. Therefore, until these investigations can be completed, a pressure of 1.75 ATA should be used.

HBO treatment should be carefully prescribed for the patients with impaired adaptation. The pressure should be raised gradually, starting at 1.25 ATA, and increasing the pressure with successive sessions. Monitoring of the patient's condition during each session makes an individual approach possible. The simplest rule is not to use a pressure which may cause acceleration of the heart rate.

Duration of Exposure

As a rule, the maximum stay in the pressure chamber ranges from 40 to 60 min.

Decompression

The rate of planned decompression must not exceed $0.1 \, kg/cm^2$ per min. Grown children should be warned not to hold their breath during decompression to avoid the development of pulmonary barotrauma. Decompression is particularly difficult and dangerous for patients after plastic operations on the anterior abdominal wall. For these patients the rate of decompression should be reduced to 0.02 to 0.05 kg/cm^2 per min to avoid intestinal eventration caused by the expansion of the bowel gas during decompression. We have seen such complications after plastic operations for large ventral hernia. Increase of the routine duration of decompression by two to three times can prevent such complications.

Frequency of HBO Sessions

As a rule one session per day is adequate for the most patients. However, in cases of extensive wounds, severe circulatory disorders, and crush syndrome, the number of sessions per day should be increased to three during the first few days and then gradually reduced. A usual course of HBO treatment lasts 8 to 10 days, but this should be adjusted individually depending on the therapeutic effect and the patient's condition. Patients with a complete block of blood flow through the main arteries of extremities may require up to 56 HBO sessions, whereas two or three sessions are enough for patients with reflex spasms of arteries.

Monitoring

Bradycardia is one of the most important indices of HBO efficiency in children.

Slowing of the pulse rate is variable, but may be 30% of the initial rate. This simple sign helps to adjust the pressure and the duration of exposure to HBO. Tachycardia points to an inappropriate regime, and the pressure should either be reduced or the session discontinued.

We use the neonatal monitor M-512 (Corometriks, USA) and the Oxycardiorespirograph (Hellige, Germany). These monitors constantly record a cardiotachogram during the sessions at the rate of 1 cm per min, so that it is easy to follow the reaction of cardiac activity to the changing of HBO regime.

Recently, a special computerized monitoring system for HBO (SAM-3) has been introduced in Russia by BION. The analysis includes mathematical indices of cardiac rhythm adopted in Russia and enables the estimation of vegetative regulation of cardiac activity, as well as the reaction of the sympathetic and parasympathetic parts of the nervous system to HBO.

EEG is included in the monitoring system for patients with brain lesions.

Efficacy of HBO in Surgical Disorders of Children

The efficacy of HBO depends on many factors. The most important of these is the length of time that has elapsed from the onset of the disease to the start of HBO therapy. HBO is more effective at the initial stage of the disease, and delayed HBO therapy is less effective. The investigators of our Clinic of Pediatric Surgery and Intensive Care have studied the problem of estimation of the efficiency of HBO in different surgical diseases in children for more than twenty years. Besides the usual clinical investigations, we carried out studies of the blood circulation, respiration, bioelectric activity of brain, and myocytes of nonstriated muscles of the colon and small intestine. We have also investigated the dynamics of the acid-base state, blood gases, lactate and pyruvate, electrolyte balance, and dynamics of enzymes (succinate dehydrogenase, a-glycerophosphate-dehydrogenase of lymphocytes, alkaline phosphatase of neutrophils, superoxide dismutase, and catalase). The results were compared with those of a control group of patients.

We evaluated the effect of HBO in the following conditions seen in pediatric surgery:

1. Multiple trauma
2. Crush syndrome
3. Abdominal surgery in patients with purulent peritonitis
4. Post-operative paralytic ileus
5. Esophagoplasty using transposed intestine
6. Necrotizing enterocolitis
7. Megacolon

Multiple Trauma

About 30% of the patients undergoing HBO therapy were children with extensive multiple injuries who were in a serious condition with circulatory disturbances, hypoxia, and electrolyte disturbances. HBO therapy was given soon after primary surgical intervention. Blood circulation greatly improved in a damaged areas, cyanosis of skin grafts decreased or disappeared, and the skin regained the normal pink color. Rheography confirmed the increase of regional perfusion and normalization of vasotonicity. The amount of wound exudate decreased and there was return of sensation of pain in the injured extremity, indicating recovery of the sensory nerve endings. The efficiency of HBO in the comprehensive management of extensive wounds in children was investigated by us in 64 children who were divided into 2 groups: the main group (treated by HBO) and the control group (not treated by HBO), each consisting of 32 patients. We noted that as a result of HBO the period of wound clearance was reduced by 8 days and the period of wound epithelization by 6 days, which was statistically sig-

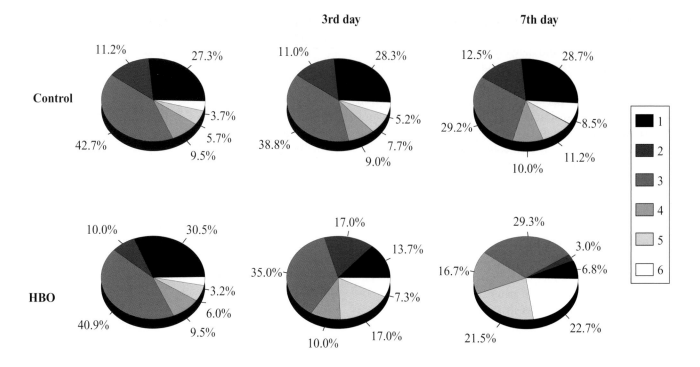

3rd day   **7th day**

1 – necrotic neutrophils, 2 – phagocytosed, 3 – other neutrophils,
4 – lymphocytes, 5 – macrophages, 6 – fibroblasts

Figure 29.4
Changes of cellular composition of wound exudate of patients having undergone HBO therapy.

nificant ($p < 0.05$). HBO produced a most pronounced effect on the patients' general condition, which improved considerably after three to five sessions. The hospital stay was reduced by 17 days in the HBO group. HBO treatment prevented the impairment of mitochondrial enzymes (succinate dehydrogenase and a-glycerophosphate dehydrogenase) during the treatment of extensive wounds. Against this background cells of wound exudate were functionally active and stable. The results of the investigation of wound imprints in the group are shown in Figure 29.4.

As shown in Figure 27.4, the wound imprints of the HBO group of patients on the third day of treatment (4–5 sessions) are characterized by statistically significant ($p < 0.02$) changes as compared with the initial values. There is reduction of the number of neutrophils by 19.4% and necrotic cells by 55.2% ($p < 0.05$). The number of phagocytosed cells increases by 1.5 times and that of macrophages by 2.8 times. Against this background the number of fibroblasts increases considerably. As a result of the HBO treatment, the period of wound clearance reduces and the wound process reaches the stage of proliferation quicker than in the control group.

After plastic operations on the skin in the main group, HBO reduced the necrotic areas of skin grafts two to three times as compared with the control group. In treatment of infected wounds, use of HBO reduced the period of prep-

aration of the patient for autodermoplasty by half compared with that required for the control group.

Crush Syndrome

Grave functional disorders of vital organs and reperfusion syndrome, often aggravated by HBO, make this group of patients the most difficult to treat. In spite of this, the role of HBO therapy in comprehensive intensive therapy is important in reducing the size of developing necrosis, and makes it possible to avoid amputation. Our method of use of HBO in this group, based on the experience of treating 18 patients after the earthquake in Armenia and 13 patients admitted to our clinic during the past years, has the following essential features:

1. HBO is included as early as possible in the comprehensive management of this condition. HBO sessions are carried out two to three times a day at a pressure of 1.7 ATA for 40 min. The treatment is continued till the clinical condition stabilizes.
2. Free radical scavengers including vitamin E are administered. Taking into account that HBO treatment is often accompanied by increasing endogenic intoxication, we carry out hemosorption and/or plasmopheres after HBO sessions.
3. Analgesics and sedatives are used as required.

Abdominal Surgery in Purulent Peritonitis

A study of the efficacy of HBO as a part of comprehensive management of purulent peritonitis was carried out in 127 children of various ages. The control group consisted of 118 patients whose comprehensive therapy did not include HBO. In the HBO group the number of postoperative complications was 2.8 times less and the period of postoperative wound healing 1.4 times shorter than in the control group. The duration of stay in intensive care and further hospitalization in the HBO group when compared with the control group were 1.6 and 1.2 times shorter respectively. In the HBO group the mortality was 4.6 times lower than in the control group.

Postoperative Paralytic Ileus

HBO eliminates postoperative intestinal paresis during the first few sessions. The efficiency of this method was assessed in 28 newborns with postoperative paralytic ileus of the first and second degrees who were operated on in our clinic for congenital intestinal obstruction. While studying the bioelectric activity of the intestine in these patients, we noted that the electrical activity of the bowel wall practically normalized after the third HBO session. In the control group the normalization of bioelectric activity of intestine took 2 days longer on an average. Use of three to four daily HBO sessions during the postoperative period shortened the time to appearance of defecation and the transfer of patients to an enteral diet by one day as compared with the control group. Improvement of the patient's general condition in the HBO group was noted 2.5 days earlier than in the control group. Mortality was 1.5 to 2 times lower in the HBO group than in the control group.

Esophagoplasty Using Transposed Intestine

HBO improved the viability of transposed parts of the intestine which were used for esophagoplasty. We noted that the first HBO session carried out just after the operation practically normalized the bioelectric activity of the transplanted intestine, indicating the normalization of oxygen balance in the smooth musculature of the intestinal wall.

Necrotizing Enterocolitis

We studied the results of the treatment of 75 newborns with necrotizing enterocolitis. In the group treated with HBO normalization of the principal clinical indices (defecation, intestinal peristalsis, patient's transfer to the enteral diet, acid-base balance, and blood gases) occurred,

on the average, 3 days earlier than in the control group. Mortality in the HBO group was 18.3% lower than that in the control group. In early stages of a disease, two to three HBO sessions were sufficient to restore passage of stools through intestine. In more advanced cases the number of HBO sessions required to obtain a beneficial effect was 10 or more. The number of HBO sessions required increased by 18.2% at the second stage and by 50% at the third stage of the disease. In the fourth stage, with intestinal perforative and peritonitis peritonitis, HBO was ineffective and bioelectric activity of intestine could not be restored.

Megacolon

We investigated 60 children with megacolon who needed surgery. In addition to disturbance of autonomic regulation of the viscera, these children showed a pronounced decrease of the activity of the main enzymes – superoxide dismutase (SOD) and catalase of peripheral blood – by $39 \pm 5\%$. These patients were at risk of developing postoperative complications. The patients were divided into two groups: the main group of patients, whose preoperative preparation included HBO therapy consisting of 8 to 10 sessions, and the control group of patients, who did not receive HBO. No HBO was used during the postoperative period in either of the groups. The results of our investigations showed that preventive HBO therapy increased SOD activity from $2.7 \pm 0.1\,\mu/mg$ Hb to $4.2 \pm 0.1\,\mu/mg$ Hb and catalase from 8.7 ± 0.1 catalase number to 12.7 ± 0.1 catalase number, which was considered to be statistically significant ($p < 0.05$). The enzyme activity of the group treated with HBO was considered to have normalized, whereas in the control group it remained reduced. According to endoscopic polarographic data an extreme disorder of the oxygen balance in the area of the operative intervention was not observed in the patients of the HBO group during the postoperative period. Clinical results of the preventive HBO course in patients with megacolon are presented in Table 29.2.

Table 29.2
Comparison of the HBO and the Control Groups of Children with Megacolon During the Postoperative Period

Factors Assessed	Control group	HBO group
Paralytic ileus	80%	10%
Number of days required for the restoration of passage through the intestine	4.2	2.5
Duration of stay in the intensive care unit	5.0	3.5
Presence of complications	35%	5%
Number of deaths	2	0

As shown in Table 29.2, HBO makes it possible to reduce statistically significantly ($p < 0.05$) the frequency of the appearance of different complications from 35% to 5% in postoperative period, to shorten the restoration period of the passage through intestine and the period of the patient's stay in the intensive care unit. In the control group there were two deaths, while in the group treated with HBO all of the patients recovered and were discharged from the hospital in satisfactory condition.

Conclusions

We have presented our experience in dealing with pediatric surgical problems by using adjuvant HBO therapy. There is evidence that HBO has contributed to a reduction of morbidity and mortality. We hope that it will encourage others to further investigate the potential uses of HBO in pediatric surgery.

30 Hyperbaric Oxygenation in Traumatology and Orthopedics

K.K. Jain

HBO has been shown to improve limb salvage in trauma, and facilitate the healing of fractures and reimplantation of body parts. Long-term HBO is an effective treatment of osteonecrosis. The key sections in this chapter are:

Introduction

Traumatology, by definition, has a multidisciplinary character and includes injuries of various systems of the body. In this chapter the focus is principally on musculoskeletal injuries and related orthopedic problems where hyperbaric oxygenation (HBO) has been used. Injuries to specific organs are discussed under the appropriate system, e.g., head injuries in Chapter 20 and traumatic shock in Chapter 23. Complications of trauma such as gas gangrene and osteomyelitis are described in Chapter 13.

The major role of HBO is considered to be in combating hypoxia – both local and general – that develops as a result of trauma. Therefore, HBO is an important auxiliary therapeutic measure in traumatology.

Crush Injuries

Crush injuries to the limbs present frequently in emergency departments. They may not be as apparent as open fracture dislocations or neurovascular injuries. If treatment of these lesions is delayed, irreversible changes may occur in the tissues.

The following criteria are used to define a crush injury:

- Two or more tissues (muscle, bone, other connective tissue, skin, nerve) must be involved.
- The injury must be severe enough to render the viability of the tissues questionable. If the tissues recover, functional deficits are likely.
- Severity of injury varies from minimal to irreversible with a partially viable gray zone between the two. Enhancing survival from injuries in the gray zone is the object of therapy.

Pathophysiology

The pathophysiology of crush injuries is illustrated in Figure 30.1. Trauma leads to death of tissue, which swells up (edema) and contributes to ischemia of the partially viable tissue. Ischemia is also a result of direct vascular injury. Ischemia and edema are parts of a vicious circle where hypoxia plays a central role. The partially viable tissue may recover if this circle is interrupted; otherwise, there is loss of function due to tissue damage. Edema of partially viable tissue may also affect the function of the adjacent normal tissue. Edema compounds the problem of ischemia, as it increases the diffusion distance from the capillary to the cell. With hypoxia, the tissues lose their ability to resist infection and repair themselves.

In a closed compartment, fluid pressure can rise higher than the capillary perfusion pressure, leading to ischemia of the tissues within the compartment. There is red cell clumping at the site of injury and this interferes with the microcirculation. Plasma may still go through the capillaries (no red cells), but normally it does not contain enough oxygen to sustain the tissues. Trauma may be direct or indirect. Direct trauma or crush injury may result from one of many causes. Indirect or closed trauma may occur from staying in one posture for a long time, such as in suicidal overdosage, or may be exercise-induced. Indirect trauma is also referred to as compartment syndrome.

Diagnosis

History and physical examination are important for making a diagnosis. During the examination five P's should be kept in mind: pain, paralysis, paresthesia, pallor, and pulselessness.

The most useful laboratory investigations are those measuring serum myoglobin, creatinine, potassium, and BUN. Urine may show myoglobinuria. Special investigations comprise the following:

- Measurement of compartment tissue fluid pressure.
- X-rays to detect fractures, cavitation, or air in soft tissues.
- Angiography, electromyography, and thermography for neurovascular assessment.

Treatment

Crush injury must be recognized immediately and treated aggressively. The basic therapy consists of management of the wound if present, treatment of any fracture, prophylactic antibiotics, and surgical debridement if required.

Role of HBO in Treatment

HBO is usually administered at 2–3 ATA and is an ideal adjuvant to the basic treatment for the following reasons:

- It counteracts the tissue hypoxia by elevating tissue pO_2.
- It reduces edema by vasoconstriction and reduction of blood flow. The latter is more than compensated by hyperoxia. By raising the oxygen dissolved in plasma tenfold, HBO creates a favorable diffusion gradient through the edema fluid and other barriers, such as blood, to the hypoxic cells. It breaks the vicious circle referred to in Figure 30.1 and allows the compromised tissues to survive in spite of deficient hemoglobin-oxygen delivery in low flow states.
- It promotes wound healing.
- It prevents infection.

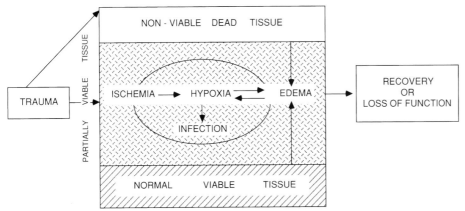

Figure 30.1
Pathophysiology of crush injury.

Most publications on this topic are uncontrolled studies and indicate that patients with crush injuries do better with HBO than they would have done without HBO under similar conditions. About 60% of the patients are reported to have a good response to HBO treatment. Controlled studies are difficult to perform under such condition.

Bouachour et al (1996) carried out a controlled study on 36 with crush injuries who were assigned in a blinded randomized fashion, within 24 h after surgery, to treatment with HBO (session of 100% O_2 at 2.5 ATA for 90 min, twice daily, over 6 days) or placebo (session of 21% O_2 at 1.1 ATA for 90 min, twice daily, over 6 days). All the patients received the same standard therapies (anticoagulant, antibiotics, wound dressings). Transcutaneous oxygen tension ($PtcO_2$) measurements were done before (patient breathing normal air) and during treatment (HBO or placebo) at the first, fourth, eighth, and twelfth sessions. The two groups (HBO group, $n = 18$; placebo group, $n = 18$) were similar in terms of age; risk factors; number, type or location of vascular injuries, neurologic injuries, or fractures; and type, location, or timing of surgical procedures. Complete healing was obtained for 17 patients in the HBO group vs. 10 patients in the placebo group ($p < 0.01$). New surgical procedures (such as skin flaps and grafts, vascular surgery, or even amputation) were performed on one patient in the HBO group vs. six patients in the placebo group ($p < 0.05$). Analysis of groups of patients matched for age and severity of injury showed that in the subgroup of patients older than 40 with grade III soft-tissue injury, wound healing was obtained for seven patients (87.5%) in the HBO group vs. three patients (30%) in the placebo group ($p < 0.05$). No significant differences were found in the length of hospital stay and number of wound dressings between groups. For the patients with complete healing, the $PtcO_2$ values of the traumatized limb, measured in normal air, rose significantly between the first and the twelfth sessions ($p < 0.001$). No significant change in $PtcO_2$ value was found for the patients in whom healing failed. The Bilateral Perfusion Index (BPI = $PtcO_2$ of the injured limb/$PtcO_2$ of the uninjured limb) at the first session increased significantly from 1ATA air to 2.5 ATA O2 ($p < 0.05$).

In patients with complete healing, the BPI was constantly greater than 0.9 to 2.5ATA O_2 during the following sessions, whereas the BPI in air progressively rose between the first and the twelfth sessions ($p < 0.05$), reaching normal values at the end of the treatment. The authors concluded that HBO was effective in improving wound healing, reducing repeat surgery and is a useful adjunct in the management of severe (grade III) crush injuries of the limbs in patients more than 40 years old.

In a systematic review of the literature, eight of nine studies showed a beneficial effect of HBO crush injury with only one major complication (Garcia-Covarrubias et al 2005). It was concluded that adjunctive HBO is not likely to be harmful and could be beneficial if administered early. Well-designed clinical studies are warranted.

Promptness in treatment is important in case of crush injury. If there is delay of more than 5–6 h and the extremity remains blue and swollen during this time, the prognosis for limb survival becomes poorer. Since oxygen tension remains elevated for only 1 h in the muscles and 3 h in the subcutaneous tissues following each HBO treatment, frequent treatments are necessary until the patient's condition is stabilized. The treatments can then be reduced in frequency, e.g., to once a week, until the patient is fully recovered.

Traumatic Ischemia

Various causes of acute peripheral vascular ischemia are listed in Table 30.1.

Vascular disease as a cause of limb ischemia is discussed in Chapter 24. The causes relevant to this chapter are direct compression, trauma, and compartment syndromes. Post-traumatic ischemic disturbances in the limbs are:

- Edema
- Disturbances of microcirculation
  - reduction of capillary perfusion
  - loss of endothelial integrity

Table 30.1
Causes of Acute Peripheral Vascular Ischemia

Cause	Comment and therapy suggestions
1. Allergic vasculitis	Adverse reaction to medicines. Discontinue offending agent.
2. Compartment syndrome	A vicious circle with acute muscle and nerve ischemia. HBO is beneficial.
3. Direct compression	Positional (secondary to overdose, stroke) fractures, tumors, or tourniquets. Removal of compression and treatment of the cause.
4. Direct traumas	Lacerations, vascular injury during surgery on limbs, gunshot wounds, and crush injuries. HBO is useful.
5. Ergot poisoning	Profound vasoconstriction, usually at the extremities.
6. Frostbite	Oxygenation of frostbitten tissues essential during rewarming process
7. Postvascular surgery	Usually flow problems or diffusion problems. HBO is useful.
8. Radiation vasculitis	Latent effect seen with radiation. HBO is useful.
9. Snakebite	Usually a chemical irritation rather than an ischemic problem
10. Thromboembolism	Arterial, immediate ischemia; venous congestion and delayed ischemia. HBO is useful.
11. Vascular diseases	Arteriosclerosis Buerger's disease Diabetes mellitus Precipitating causes Acute ischemias may be precipitated by injury, infection, or systemic problems.

- plugging of capillaries by leukocytes
- Reperfusion injury
  - formation of oxygen-derived free radicals
  - generation of leukotrienes
- Decreased level of adenosine triphosphate and creatine phosphate within muscle cells

Animals experimental studies have shown the beneficial effect of HBO on some of the disturbances listed above. Nylander *et al* (1985) used a tourniquet model of limb ischemia in the rat. In a group treated with HBO at 2.5 ATA for 45 min the edema was reduced significantly and this reduction persisted for 40 h after the treatment. The authors recommended the use of HBO as an adjuvant in treatment of acute ischemic conditions where surgical repair alone fails or is not sufficient to reverse the ischemic process. HBO treatments have been shown to enhance aerobic metabolism in the postischemic muscle. Reduction of phosphorylase activity, a sensitive marker for muscle cell damage, is prevented to a great extent by HBO treatment (Nylander *et al* 1988). HBO treatments have been shown to enhance the recovery of blood flow and functional capillary density in pressure-induced postischemic muscle tissue in the dorsal skinfold chamber in hamsters (Sirsjö *et al* 1993). Experiments in rats by Zamboni *et al* (1993) have shown that adherence of leucocytes in the ischemic venules following reperfusion is reduced by HBO at 2.5 ATA.

There is some concern that HBO may cause increase of free radical formation and aggravate reperfusion tissue injury. Nylander *et al* (1989) studied the effect of HBO on the formation of free radicals in the tourniquet model of ische-mia of the rat hind limb and used muscle biopsies with measurement of thiobarbituric acid reactive material which includes lipid peroxides and alkyds including malondialdehyde, a key intermediate in the formation of peroxides. Their results showed that HBO treatment at 2.5 ATA for 45 min had a favorable effect on the muscle tissue and did not cause increased lipid peroxidation in the skeletal muscle of rats.

Transcutaneous oxygen monitoring was shown to reflect tissue perfusion and advocated to predict the final outcome of major vascular trauma of the limb. Mathieu *et al* (1989) have shown that transcutaneous oxygen measurement at 2.5 ATA is a valuable, noninvasive adjunctive method for prediction of final outcome of major vascular trauma of the limbs.

Schramek and Hashmonai (1978) reported HBO treatment of seven soldiers with gunshot wounds of limb arteries in whom arterial repair did not reverse the ischemia. There was improvement in these patients and they were spared amputation. Shupak *et al* (1987) reported the use of HBO in 13 patients suffering from acute posttraumatic ischemia of the lower extremities. The average delay from the moment of injury to the institution of HBO therapy was 11 h and 53 min. Complete limb salvage was accomplished in eight cases (61.5%), and there was some improvement in four cases (30.7%). Only one case did not show any improvement.

Patients with pre-existing vascular disease are more susceptible to ischemia and more likely to suffer gangrene. Kuyama *et al* (1988) have treated such cases by a combination of repeated HBO treatments, sympathetic blocks, and anticoagulation in combination with reconstructive surgery. These authors found this combined approach to be quite effective in salvaging limbs.

Isakov *et al* (1979) explained the good results of HBO in severe trauma of the extremities on the basis of improved cardiac and respiratory functions, which further contribute to improved tissue oxygenation. This factor may be of importance in a victim of severe multiple injuries with cardiac and respiratory disturbances.

Compartment Syndromes

Compartment syndromes develop when pressures in the skeletal muscle compartments in the extremities are elevated enough to reduce capillary perfusion, resulting in ischemia, nonfunction, and necrosis of the tissues. Direct measurement of the compartment pressure enables quantitative assessment of the severity and outcome of this complication. A single pressure measurement, however, is not enough to indicate progression or resolution of the compartment syndrome. Fasciotomy is the accepted surgical treatment. The circulation is improved after fasciotomy, but the tissue damage is not always reversed. Controversy still exists regarding the pressure at which fasciotomy should be performed. HBO is expected to correct ischemia and edema which are important components of the pathophysiology of the compartment syndrome. HBO reduces the muscle damage significantly in experimentally produced compartment syndrome in dogs. HBO (three 1-h sessions at 3ATA) should be used in human compartment syndromes under the following conditions:

- If the patient has an elevated intracompartmental pressure in a range that borders on surgical decompression. Instead of just observing the patient for progression of symptoms, as is done conventionally, HBO may be used to prevent the progression. However HBO is not a substitute for decompression.
- As provisional treatment of compartment syndrome where surgery is indicated but there is delay in performing it. HBO may prevent further damage until surgery can be undertaken.
- In postoperative management of patients after surgical decompression if there is residual neurological deficit or muscle necrosis. HBO may improve the chances of recovery of marginally viable tissues.

Strauss *et al* (1986) reported that even if HBO therapy was delayed in the dog compartment syndrome models, there was significant reduction of edema and muscle necrosis in animals treated by HBO.

Skyhar *et al* (1986) have shown in experimental animal models that HBO reduces edema and necrosis of skeletal muscle associated with hemorrhagic hypotension.

Strauss *et al* (1987) reported a prospective study of 38 patients who were given HBO as an adjunct to the management of posttraumatic and iatrogenic skeletal muscle-compartment syndromes. In two-thirds of the patients, HBO was started after surgical decompression of the compartment because of threatened necrosis of the flaps and intracompartment tissues or the presence of a neuropathy. The results were resolution of the neuropathies, arrest of tissue necrosis, and absence of secondary infections. In the remaining one-third of patients HBO was started for symptoms and signs including elevated intracompartment pressure. No one in this group required surgical decompression and all recovered fully.

Fasciotomies performed for compartment syndrome and ischemic vascular disease often require closure in 2 to 4 weeks by skin graft. This leaves the patient with an unsightly scar and a limb with reduced strength. The use of vacuum-assisted closure (VAC) and HBO therapy quickly reduce the edema and permit earlier closure with adjacent skin. A study of three trauma patients with compartment syndrome, fasciotomies, and the use of the VAC and HBOT to close the fasciotomy wounds with adjacent skin reported closure of the fasciotomy wounds in 3 to 18 days (Weiland 2007). The simultaneous use of HBOT and VAC accelerates the reduction of edema in a synergistic fashion, permitting early closure of fasciotomy wounds.

High Pressure Water Gun Injection Injury

Accidental injection with a high pressure water gun in workers can cause extensive soft tissue injury with empyema. This is a painful condition and resolves slowly and sometimes with residual disability. Excellent results are described with use of HBO in such patients with immediate resolution of subcutaneous empyema, edema and pain. Two possible explanations have been offered for the effectiveness of this treatment:

1. Oxygen and carbon dioxide in the injected air are absorbed leaving nitrogen in the tissues which is similar to the situation in decompression sickness. HBO helps in the elimination of nitrogen.
2. HBO helps to alleviate ischemic limb pain.

Peripheral Nerve Injuries

Injuries of peripheral nerves are common. There are usually a part of traumatic injuries of extremities. Peripheral nerves may be crushed or severed. Injured nerves may have impairment of blood supply, oxygenation and edema which may set in a vicious cycle of further edema and hypoxia. Surgical techniques particularly with microsurgical

refinements have improved the rate of recovery in peripheral nerve injuries but some problems still remain. Nerve
regeneration is slow and sometimes erratic. Search continues for techniques to improve nerve regeneration and recovery after injury.

Rationale for the Use of HBO

In vitro fast axonal transport can be restored by administration of 95% normobaric oxygen to an anoxic nerve. It
has been speculated that HBO can provide optimal tissue
pO_2 tension for restore axonal transport and enable the
necessary delivery of materials to site of injury for regeneration to occur. Restoration of transportation would obviate the need for the natural compensatory response to
nerve injury by increased neurofilament concentration and
eventual formation of neuroma. HBO also reduced edema
in traumatized tissues and is expected to break the vicious
circle of edema leading to hypoxia and further aggravation
of edema with compression of the nerve fibers and ischemia. HBO counteracts tissue ischemia as well.

Experimental Studies

HBO has shown some promise to aid healing of mechanically damaged peripheral nerves where axonotmesis was
induced either by nerve transection or nerve crush. Nerve
regeneration has been documented by electrophysiological
studies. Bradshaw *et al* (1996) used oxygen environments
to study the regenerative effects of HBO on crushed sciatic
nerves in 30 adult male rabbits. Six different oxygen environments were used, and treatments were initiated 4 days
post injury. Transmission electron microscopy and light
microscopy were used to evaluate the regenerative morphology of crushed nerves. The morphology of crushed
nerves after 7 weeks of treatment with compressed oxygen
at 202, 242, and 303 kPa resembled normal uncrushed
nerves, with nerve fibers uniformly distributed throughout
the section. The treatment groups receiving 202 kPa compressed air, 100% normobaric oxygen, or ambient air did
not display morphologies similar to normal uncrushed
nerve. The nerves in these animals were edematous and
contained disarrayed nerve fibers. Myelination in the animals receiving 100% O_2 at high pressures resembled undamaged nerves. Collagen and blood vessels were more evident in the lower pressure/oxygen tension treatments than
in the animals receiving 100% O_2 at higher pressures. The
neurofilamentous material inside the crushed control axons was dense, whereas in the axons of animals treated with
compressed O_2 it was loosely packed. These differences in
morphology suggest that treatments consisting of 100% O_2
under pressure can accelerate a peripheral nerve's recovery
from a crush injury.

In contrast to the study of Bradshaw *et al* (1996), Santos
et al (1996) found no effect of HBO in accelerating regeneration of peripheral nerves. In their study, rat peroneal
nerves were transected and entubulated with a Silastic
channel. The experimental group was treated with HBO to
evaluate changes in acute edema, functional recovery, and
histology. HBO was administered with 100% O_2 at 2.5 ATA
for 90 min twice a day for 1 week and then four times a day
for 1 week. Acute edema changes based on nerve water
weight and transfascicular area measurements were greater
in injured than in uninjured nerves but demonstrated no
differences between HBO-treated and -untreated groups 2,
8 and 16 days after surgery. Functional evaluation with gait
analysis demonstrated significant changes between injured
and uninjured group 1, 3, 7, and 13 weeks after injury but
no differences between HBO-treated and -untreated
groups. Thirteen weeks after the initial injury, elicited muscle force measurements demonstrated no significant improvement from HBO treatment of injured nerves. Histologic evaluation of nerve area, myelinated axon number,
myelinated axon area, myelin thickness, and blood vessel
number and area revealed no significant differences between HBO-treated and -untreated groups. HBO was not
associated with improvement of nerve regeneration with
any of the outcome variables in this model. One explanation of this may be the technique of entubulation with
which might have prevented access of HBO to the site of
injury.

The effect of HBO treatment on regeneration of the rat
sciatic nerve was studied by Haapaniemi *et al* (1998). The
sciatic nerve was crushed with a pair of pliers and the animals were either left untreated or subjected to a series of
45-min exposures to 100% O_2 at 3.3ATA pressure at 0, 4,
and 8 h postoperatively and then every 8 h. Regeneration
was evaluated using the pinch-reflex test at 3, 4, or 5 days
following surgery and with neurofilament staining at 4
days. The regeneration distances at all time points were significantly longer in animals exposed to HBO treatment independent of the evaluation procedure. A short initial period of the same HBO treatment schedule, with no more
treatments after 25 h, appeared as effective as when treatments were maintained being given every 8 h until evaluation. The authors concluded that HBO treatment stimulates axonal outgrowth following a nerve crush lesion. A further study by the same authors, however, has shown that
HBO does not promote regeneration in traumatic peripheral nerve lesions. In a standardized models of nerve crush
injury as well as transection and repair, the animals were
treated postoperatively with 100% oxygen at 2.5 ATA pressure for 90 min and the treatment was employed twice daily
for 7 days (Haapaniemi *et al* 2002). The treatment was not
effective in the restoration of gait or the muscular strength
after 90 days. In another study using a similar model, exposure to 2.5 ATA HBO moderately enhanced early regeneration of the fastest sensory axons but it decreased the

number of regenerating axons in the injured nerves with compromised blood perfusion of the distal nerve stump (Bajrovic *et al* 2002).

Results of a study in rats suggest that functional recovery in transected peripheral nerves may be improved and accelerated by HBO following microsurgical repair (Eguiluz-Ordoñez *et al* 2006).

Clinical Applications

Use of HBO as an adjunct to peripheral nerve repair has also been explored clinically. Zhao (1991) obtained good results in 89.2% of the 54 patients with 65 nerve injuries repaired using HBO as a supplementary treatment. In 60 patients with similar injuries where HBO was not used good results were seen in only 73.2% ($p > 0.05$). In subgroups of patients with fresh injuries the results were not different in the two groups but HBO was significantly more beneficial in older cases.

Concluding Remarks

The most recent experimental studies do not support nerve crush injury or nerve transection and repair as indications for HBO treatment.

Fractures

Basic and Experimental Considerations

Most bone fractures heal spontaneously, but 3%–5% of them have delayed union or nonunion. This proportion may rise markedly in certain locations with compound comminuted fractures. The major cause of nonunion is interruption of blood supply at the ends of the fractures.

Lack of oxygen is considered to be a limiting factor in the healing of fractures. Multipotential precursors of fibroblastic origin form bone when exposed to increased oxygen tensions and compressive forces. If, instead, oxygen tensions are low, cartilage is formed. Cartilage is a relatively avascular tissue and its presence is noted at fracture sites in cases of nonunion. Low oxygen tensions are observed in healing fractures until the medullary canal is reformed. This is secondary to increased oxygen utilization associated with the fracture repair process.

Yablon and Cruess (1968) studied healing of fractured femurs in rats treated with 100% oxygen at 3 ATA for 1 h twice a day. By the 40th day the fractures treated with HBO had completely remodeled, while healing was just completed in the control animals. Microradiography showed abundant medullary canal and subperiosteal new bone in HBO-treated animals at a time when there was incomplete bony union in the control animals.

Coulson *et al* (1966) showed that rats treated at 3 ATA oxygen displayed a greater calcium ion uptake and lower fragility than air-breathing controls. Niinikoski *et al* (1970) demonstrated that 100% oxygen at 2.5 ATA for 2 h twice daily produced an increased callus formation in experimental fractures. There was increased accumulation of calcium, magnesium, phosphorus, sodium, potassium, and zinc, as well as accelerated collagen production compared with air-breathing controls.

Gray and Hamblin (1976) studied the effects of hyperoxia on bone in organ culture and noted that bone resorption was inhibited by exposure to 95% oxygen or HBO at 2 ATA. Hyperoxia also depressed new bone formation by osteoclasts. This finding contradicts the studies already quoted, and may stem from the absence of vital factors in the culture media.

Karapetian *et al* (1985) demonstrated that HBO at 2 ATA stimulates the repair of noninflamed mandibular fractures in rats, whereas HBO at 2.5 ATA hinders it. If, however, the bone wound is inflamed, HBO at 2.5 ATA is more effective for healing.

Tkachenko *et al* (1988) have shown that, in rabbits with experimental defects of the radius, HBO therapy results in the greatest activation of bone repair in the early period after trauma with the formation of osseus matrix. They recommended reduction of HBO exposure intensity at this stage.

Nilsson *et al* (1989) studied the effect of HBO on bone regeneration by inserting a bone harvest chamber in the rat tibia and rat mandible. Their results showed that HBO treatments caused a significant increase of bone mineralization in the implant, and that lamellar bone had invaded the implant as quantified by micro-radiography and microdensitometry.

Experimental studies in rats have shown once daily HBO treatments (2 ATA for 90 min) appeared to accelerate bone repair with vessel ingrowth whereas twice daily treatments retarded these processes (Barth *et al* 1990).

One serious obstacle to bone regeneration is migration of connective tissue from the surrounding soft tissues into the bony defect. Porous expanding membranes have been used to prevent the fibroblasts from entering the defect. Combination of this technique with HBO has been shown to produce better healing of mandibular defects in experimental animals as compared with HBO or membrane technique alone (Dahlin *et al* 1993).

Ueng *et al* (1998) investigated the effect of intermittent hyperbaric oxygen (HBO) therapy on the bone healing of tibial lengthening in rabbits. Twelve male rabbits were divided into two groups of six animals each. The first group went through 2.5 atmospheres absolute of HBO for 2 h daily, and the second group did not receive HBO. Each animal's right tibia was lengthened 5 mm using an uniplanar lengthening device. Bone mineral density (BMD) study was performed for all of the animals at 1 day before operation and at 3, 4, 5, and 6 weeks after operation. All of the animals were killed at 6 weeks postoperatively for biomechanical testing.

Using the preoperative BMD as an internal control, the authors found that the BMD of the HBO group was increased significantly compared with the non HBO group. The mean %BMD at 3, 4, 5, and 6 weeks were 69.5%, 80.1%, 87.8%, and 96.9%, respectively, in HBO group, whereas the mean %BMD were 51.6%, 67.7%, 70.5%, and 79.2%, respectively, in non-HBO group (two tailed t test, $p < 0.01$, $p < 0.01$, $p < 0.01$, and $p < 0.01$ at 3, 4, 5, and 6 weeks, respectively). Using the contralateral nonoperated tibia as an internal control, they found that torsional strength of lengthened tibia of the HBO group was increased significantly compared with the non-HBO group. The mean percent of maximal torque was 88.6% in HBO group at 6 weeks, whereas the mean percent of maximal torque was 76.0% in non-HBO group (two-tailed t test, $p < 0.01$). The results of this study suggest that the bone healing of tibial lengthening is enhanced by intermittent HBO therapy.

Clinical Experience

Strauss and Hart (1977) presented 20 patients with 24 long bone fractures treated by HBO. Primary healing occurred in 15 (75%) of the patients. The healing was 100% in cases where HBO was started within 10 days of the fracture. These are good results: the incidence of nonunion can be as high as 75% in displaced tibial fractures. The authors recommended the use of HBO when there is a significant risk of delayed union or nonunion.

Kolontai *et al* (1976) treated 295 patients with compound fractures of the long bones with a combination of local antibiotics, HBO (2–3 ATA), hypothermia, and surgery. They were able to reduce the complications, such as infections and nonunion, considerably.

Halva *et al* (1978) reported 142 cases of fracture dislocations in the region of the ankle where HBO was used as an adjunct to open or closed reduction and immobilization. Where treatment was started within 8 h of injury, good results were obtained in 90% of cases. This figure dropped to 60% when the treatment was started after a delay of between 8 h and 24 h. With a delay of more than 24 h the circulatory disturbances were not reversible.

Pseudoarthrosis is a pathological fracture with inadequate healing and false joint formation, which requires surgery such as bone grafting to correct it. Oriani *et al* (1982) used HBO as a useful adjunct to surgery both preoperatively and postoperatively in such cases, as well as in other nonhealing fractures.

HBO therapy in patients with defects of the long tubular bones contributes to shortening the period of rehabilitation. Based on the clinical evidence and cost analysis, medical institutions that treat open fracture and crush injuries are justified in incorporating HBO as a standard of care (Buettner & Wolkenhauer 2007).

Bone Fractures with Arterial Injuries

Blunt arterial injuries secondary to bone fractures are frequently associated with nerve, vein and soft tissue lesions. A delayed diagnosis or treatment is the main cause of high amputation rate. Porcellini *et al* (1997) described 34 patients who presented with acute arterial occlusion (15 cases), false aneurysms (13 cases) or arteriovenous fistulas (6 cases) of the extremity. Various procedures were performed to repair injured arteries, associated venous lesions were treated. External fixation of long bone fractures was made in 29 patients, before vascular reconstruction, to prevent further injury during orthopedic stabilization. Fasciotomies were made to treat compartmental where necessary. Hyperbaric oxygen therapy was applied in 7 patients to control bacterial contamination and improve wound healing. The authors emphasized that a multidisciplinary diagnostic and management strategy is required to improve limb and patient survival. HBO is an important component of such multidisciplinary strategies.

Traumatic Amputations and Reimplantations of Body Parts

After the establishment of blood circulation following reimplantation of a severed limb, the tissues of the implanted limb are apt to develop varying degrees of edema and degenerative changes due to anoxia. If these changes are not reversed, necrosis develops. The time limit of reimplantation at room temperature is 12 h and can be prolonged if the severed limb is preserved by hypothermia. HBO can help in reducing edema, improving microcirculation, reversing degenerative changes, and salvaging limbs reimplanted as long as 36 h after traumatic amputation.

Smith (1961) reported a case of near-avulsion of a foot treated by replacement and subsequent repeated exposures to HBO at 2 ATA. Although the foot had to be eventually amputated, a segment below the ankle survived. There are few reports in the literature about the use of HBO in reimplantation surgery.

Bao (1987) used HBO in reimplantation of severed limbs in 34 cases. The indications were:

- Prolonged anoxia or ischemia of the severed limb before reimplantation

- Failure of arterial anastomosis: vasospasm or thrombosis
- Microcirculatory disturbances with patent vessels.

Seventy percent of their reimplants survived with the use of intermittent hyperbaric therapy at 2.5 ATA. These are good results considering that many of their implants were severed as long as 36 h prior to implantation and kept at room temperature.

The most extensive experience in this area is that of Colignon (1987) who have used HBO in 371 cases with crush injuries and amputation of the limbs. Not only were the results of reimplantation by microsurgery good in terms of recovery of function, but the rate of complications such as infections and nonhealing was markedly reduced. Only one of their patients developed gas gangrene.

The results of reanastomosis of some severed body parts are usually poor. The reconstruction of a severed ear is a difficult procedure and the cosmetic results are poor. Neubauer *et al* (1988) have reported the use of HBO in successful reanastomosis of the severed ear in three cases. After the ear was sutured, HBO was used at 2.5 ATA for 90 min twice daily for 8-15 days.

HBO has even been used as an aid to penile reimplantation (McGough *et al* 1989).

Role of HBO in Battle Casualties

HBO therapy is a recognized form of treatment for certain emergencies in the United States Air Force (Cramer 1985). The use of HBO for decompression sickness was pioneered in the US Navy. The potential of HBO therapy for the injured soldier has been recognized (Workman & Calcote 1989) but hyperbaric chambers has not been used by US Armed Forces in the battlefield so far although these facilities were available on board US Navy ships during the Gulf wars (1991 and 2003). The Soviet Armed Forces used mobile field hyperbaric chambers for combat and chemical warfare casualties during the Afghanistan war (Gatagov 1982). A mobile multiplace chamber can be adapted for military use. Some injuries seen in the battlefield for which adjunctive HBO would be useful in an emergency are shown in Table 30.2.

During the war in Croatia (from May 1991 to December 1995), 67 patients with war injuries of the femoral vein and/or artery were treated at the Surgical Clinic of Split Clinical Hospital (Radonic *et al* 1997). Vascular repair was carried out of 70 arterial (28 isolated) and 49 venous injuries (six isolated). Intermittent HBO therapy was given to 18 of these patients with beneficial effect.

The injured soldier can be transported in a mobile hyperbaric chamber while receiving the emergency care. It

Table 30.2
Indications for the Emergency Use of HBO in the Battlefield

1. Crush injury
2. Air embolism
3. Decompression sickness – aviators and divers
4. Gunshot wounds of the vascular injuries with limb ischemia
5. Hemorrhagic shock and acute blood loss anemia
6. Thermal burns
7. Acute spinal cord injury
8. Acute head injury with cerebral edema (gunshot wounds)
9. Chemical weapon-induced injury
10. Cold injury: frostbite

is technically possible to install such a chamber in an airplane, helicopter or motor boat.

The use of HBO in treating the victims of nuclear fallout would be contraindicated as the effect of radiation would be enhanced (see Chapter 36) although HBO is useful in treating the late sequelae of radiation such as radionecrosis (see Chapter 16).

Effect of HBO on Osteogenesis

Various studies showing the effect of HBO in enhancing osteogenesis are quoted in the section of fractures. Makihara *et al* (1996) have shown a beneficial effect of intermittent HBO on osteogenesis in rachitic bone. The authors used 4-week old rats which were rendered rachitic by 1-hydroxyethylidene-1, 1-bisphosphonic acid disodium that exerts an inhibitory effect on deposition of calcium phosphate in bone. Radiologic and histologic findings indicated marked calcification in the center of the growth plate in rats treated with HBO.

HBO for Treatment of Osteonecrosis (Aseptic Necrosis)

Osteonecrosis is synonymous with aseptic or avascular necrosis of bone. These terms describe infarction of bone, presumably resulting from ischemia.

Several factors play a role in the pathogenesis of dysbaric osteonecrosis: intraosseous vessel obstruction by bubbles, platelet aggregation, fat embolism, and narrowing of the arterial lumen by bubble-induced myointimal thickening. The bone is vulnerable because of gas supersaturation of the fatty marrow and poor vascularization. Ischemia leads to hypoxia and impaired nutrition of bone, which leads to necrosis. The various causes of osteonecrosis are listed in Table 30.3.

Although osteonecrosis is an occupational hazard of commercial and navy divers, it is also a growing problem

Table 30.3
Causes of Osteonecrosis (Aseptic Avascular Necrosis)

1. Repeated exposure to compressed gases
2. Work at high altitudes
3. Medical conditions
   - Alcoholism
   - Arteriosclerosis
   - Alcaptonurea
   - Cirrhosis of the liver
   - Cushing's syndrome
   - Diabetes mellitus
   - Gaucher's disease
   - Gout
   - Hemoglobinopathies
   - Hepatitis
   - Rheumatic arthritis
   - Sickle cell disease
4. Prolonged steroid therapy
5. Trauma to hip; with or without fracture dislocation
6. Ionizing radiation injury
7. Idiopathic osteonecrosis

in recreational divers. It is found in individuals with no history of exposure to compressed gas environments. The bones usually involved are the humerus, femur, and tibia; the femoral head being the most common. The delay in onset of symptoms may be months to years following a decompression exposure. An idiopathic form of aseptic necrosis of the femoral head has also been described.

Lesions of the bone shaft are painless, but pain and disability are associated with juxta-articular lesions. Fracture and collapse of head of the femur may occur.

There is no satisfactory conservative treatment. The affected joints are immobilized. Surgical procedures consist of removal of necrotic tissue, replacement with bone graft, and immobilization. These measures have only a limited success. Therefore, HBO has been investigated as a treatment for this condition.

HBO therapy has been used in this condition with good results. The role of HBO in osteoradionecrosis is described in Chapter 16. Cases treated by HBO for osteonecrosis due to other causes are listed in Table 30.4.

The diagnosis and progress of this disease can be followed up with NMR (Figure 30.2). HBO therapy is usually given at 2.0 to 2.5 ATA and several treatment sessions may be required, even as many as 100. It is important that the treatment be adequate. Relief of symptoms alone is not a guide to cure. There must be radiological evidence of increase of bone density.

X-rays of the hip in another case of osteonecrosis of the hip are shown in Figure 30.3. There was reossification after HBO treatments.

Strauss and Winant (1998) have carried out a meta-analysis of survivorship in femoral head necrosis from previous studies and compared them with results from HBO treatment. Survivability of 8,567 hips was determined from meta-analysis of 86 studies. Treatment interventions that were analyzed were core decompression (CD), osteotomy, bone graft, HBO, HBO & CD, and no intervention. Survivability of hips with femoral head necrosis treated with HBO was as good as any other treatment intervention but combination therapies gave better results. The reported experience with HBO is limited. Prospective randomized studies and cost-benefit analyses are required for a more definite opinion regarding the suitability of HBO as a treatment for this condition.

Table 30.4
Reported Cases of Osteonecrosis Treated by Hyperbaric Oxygen Therapy (HBO)

Authors and year	Cases (n)	Diagnosis	HBO schedule	Results and comments
Baixe et al (1969)	41	Aseptic necrosis, various bones	2.8 ATA, (90 min)/day; average of 120 treatments	Improvement in all cases clinically as well as by X-rays
Sainty et al (1980)	9	Aseptic necrosis	2 ATA, 10–30 exposures	Pain relief in all cases but later recurrences; no X-ray improvement
Lepawsky et al (1983)	1	Aseptic necrosis, both femoral heads; wheelchair-bound	2.5 ATA; (90 min)/day; number of treatments?	Improvement both clinical and radiological; patient became ambulatory and remained so to follow-up 2 years later
Mao (1986)	44	Aseptic necrosis, various bones	2.8 ATA, (90 min); extended therapy?	Final results described as satisfactory
Neubauer et al (1989a)	1	Idiopathic aseptic necrosis, right femoral head	2–2.5 ATA, 90 min/day; total of 108 treatments	Full functional recovery with increase of bone density demonstrated on NMR (see Fig. 28.2); best documented case in literature
Scherer et al (2000)	12	Aseptic osteonecrosis following chemotherapy	HBO (2.4 ATA for 100 min, 38 sessions)	Retrospective study with evaluation by MRI. No beneficial effect in those treated by HBO.

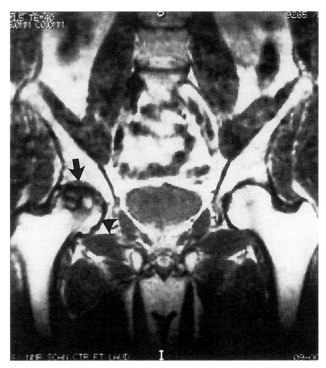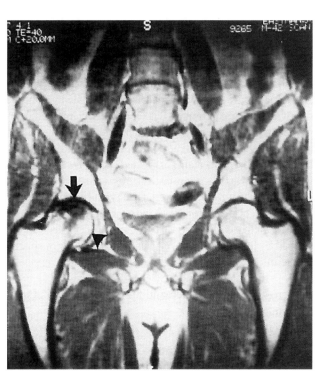

Figure 30.2

Left: Pre-HBO treatment NMR scan of right femur of a 41-year old male with diagnosis of aseptic necrosis. Intact hyaline articular cartilage (arrow) shows no evidence of femoral head collapse. Small medial area of high signal (arrowhead) shows normal fatty marrow. *Right:* Post-HBO treatment. Intact hyaline cartilage (arrow) overlies small ring-like zone of aseptic necrosis. Also, normal area of fatty marrow (arrowhead) is now larger (from Neubauer *et al* 1989a).

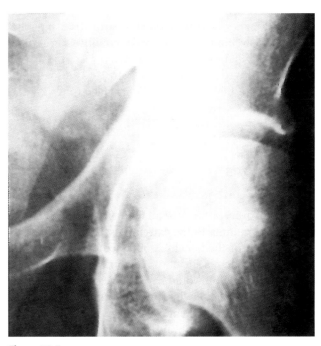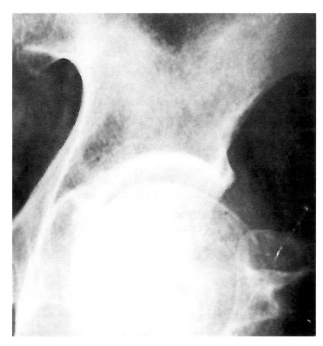

Figure 30.3

Left: Pretreatment x-ray of left femoral head showing aseptic osteonecrosis. *Right:* Post-HBO treatment (100 sessions) x-ray showing reossification (Photo courtesy of Dr. J H Baixe, Toulon, France).

Rheumatoid Arthritis

Basic Considerations

Rheumatoid arthritis is a systemic inflammatory disease of a chronic nature that is characterized primarily by a pattern of involvement of the synovial joints. The inflammatory process may involve soft tissues such as tendons, ligaments, and muscle, and may invade the bone. The etiology of the disease remains uncertain; suspected causes include immunological disturbances and infectious agents.

McCarty (1981) reviewed the available evidence in search of a rationale for HBO in the management of rheumatoid arthritis. Hypoxia of the arthritic patient is evidenced by low synovial pO_2 levels but these are not specific to rheumatoid arthritis. The causes of hypoxia are:

- Increased metabolic demand for oxygen by an inflamed joint.
- Decrease of blood flow to the joint by raised intraarticular pressure.

There is a fall in the synovial fluid of a rheumatoid knee joint after exercise. The hypoxic condition of many inflamed joints may be responsible for microinfarction of particulate collagens in joint fluid that are qualitatively and quantitatively identical to the collagens of synovial membrane.

HBO can suppress sterile inflammation due either to immunologic factors or microbial infection. Thus, arthritis induced in rats by injections of adjuvant is suppressed if HBO is started within 2 days after injection. Moreover, daily HBO therapy suppresses the inflammatory response even if given when the arthritis is fully developed (Warren et al 1979). Shakbazyan et al (1988) studied the effect of HBO (1.5 ATA and 3 ATA) on the development of clinical, immunological, and morphological manifestations of adjuvant arthritis in C57BL/6 mice. In comparison with the control group, HBO was found to inhibit the development of clinico-morphological manifestations of adjuvant arthritis and hindered the development of the process. The treatment was more effective in the early stages of the disease. Pressure of 3 ATA was more effective than 1.5 ATA, but toxic manifestations were seen with 3 ATA in the pulmonary vessels.

Clinical Applications

Kamada (1985) carried out laboratory examination of patients with rheumatoid arthritis undergoing HBO therapy.

Under HBO therapy, serum superoxide dismutase values increased and lipid peroxidase activity decreased. At the same time ESR and Lansbury's index showed a remarkable recovery. From these results, the authors suggested that HBO therapy may be an effective treatment for patients with rheumatoid arthritis.

Saikovsky et al (1986) have used HBO in treatment of 20 patients with rheumatoid arthritis and recommend it as an appropriate therapy when systemic symptoms such as ischemic neuropathy, arteritis, or Raynaud's phenomenon are present.

Davis et al (1988) conducted a pilot study in 10 patients with rheumatoid arthritis of which 8 received HBO treatments (100% oxygen at 2.5 ATA, ten 90-min sessions once a day on alternate days) and 2 sham treatments (breathing air at normal pressure). There was no remission of the disease during treatment period and authors concluded that further large scale double-blind trials to assess efficacy of HBO in rheumatoid arthritis were not worthwhile.

Lukich et al (1991) treated 35 patients with rheumatoid arthritis by HBO. Each patient received 21 sessions of HBO under 1.7 ATA for 40 min. Good clinical results, both immediate and late, were obtained. The effect of HBO on the immune system of the patients intensified the suppressive function of T-lymphocytes (especially in those with systemic manifestations of the disease), normalized cell-bound immunity and decreased the serum concentration in immune complexes.

Rui-Chang (1994) reported on the results of HBO treatment of 37 patients with rheumatoid arthritis using relief of pain and swelling with improved mobility as criteria of success. Nine patients (24.3%) recovered completely 19 (51.4%) improved markedly, and 6 (16.2%)showed slight improvement. Only 3 (8.1%) patients failed to respond.

Conclusions

HBO has proven to be a useful adjunct to surgery in the treatment of trauma to the extremities, particularly crush injuries. Most of the benefit is obtained by counteracting the effects of ischemia and anoxia commonly found in such injuries. Plainly HBO would have an even more important role to play in patients with multiple trauma. There is already evidence for the beneficial effects of HBO in head injuries (cerebral edema) and acute spinal cord injuries. Every large trauma center should have a hyperbaric facility, as it is vital to institute HBO therapy as soon as possible.

31 HBO Therapy in Otolaryngology

K.K. Jain

HBO is a valuable adjunctive treatment for sudden deafness and acute acoustic trauma. This chapter looks at:

Introduction

The role of hyperbaric oxygenation (HBO) therapy in oto-laryngology has mostly been investigational in the past, but its clinical applications in diseases of the inner ear are being increasingly recognized by physicians in the Federal Republic of Germany, Japan, and China. HBO has also proven to be useful in some diseases of the head and neck that partially overlap the domain of the otolaryngologist (Farri et al 2002). The application of HBO in the treatment of infections such as malignant otitis externa and osteomyelitis of the jaw is well recognized in the United States. Indications for the use of HBO are shown in Table 31.1.

Table 31.1
Indications for HBO Therapy in Ear, Nose and Throat Disorders as well as Relevant Areas of Head and Neck
(as practiced in Germany)

– Barotrauma
  Labyrinthine contusions
  Decompression sickness of inner ear
– Bone involvement in ENT area
  Osteomyelitis
  Osteonecrosis
– Hearing loss
  Acute acoustic trauma
  Drug-induced hearing loss
  Noise-induced hearing loss
  Postoperative hearing loss
  Retrocochlear hearing loss of unknown origin
  Sudden deafness
– Meniere's disease
– Otitis externa maligna
– Tinnitus
  Vertigo

Tinnitus

Tinnitus is the most common symptom associated with inner ear damage and it is estimated that more than 1% of the population of the Federal Republic of Germany (i.e., about 800,000 cases) suffers from disabling tinnitus and impairment of hearing. The yearly incidence of new cases is about 15,000.

Tinnitus may be acute or chronic. Chronic tinnitus is of more than a year's duration and is responsible for most of the cases. It is often part of a triad of hearing loss, vertigo and tinnitus because of the involvement of both cochlea and the vestibular apparatus in many of the disease processes. Various causes of tinnitus are shown in Table 31.2. Because of the subjective nature of the complaints, it is not possible to evaluate the symptom objectively but various scales are sued. In the visual analog scale, the patient patient depicts the loudness of the tinnitus.

Medical therapy of tinnitus is not satisfactory and HBO has been used. Using this method, Kau et al (1997) ob-

---

Table 31.2
Causes of Tinnitus

– Barotrauma
– Hypotension
– Ototoxic drugs
– Stress
– Vasculopathies of inner ear
– Vasomotor disorders
– Viral infections of the inner ear

---

served that in patients who had suffered from tinnitus for less than 3 months, excellent improvement was seen in 6.7% and noticeable improvement in 44.3% expressed by means of a visual analog scale. In 44.3% the tinnitus was described as unchanged. Patients who had had tinnitus for more than 3 months before HBO therapy showed a less favorable response to HBO. In none of the patients did the tinnitus disappear; 34.4% of the patients described a noticeable improvement in their complaints. A study from Germany has reported a improvement rate of 60–65% with HBO treatment in patients with tinnitus (Bohmer 1997). In another study from Germany, a total of 193 patients, having undergone primary intravenous hemorheologic therapy, were treated with HBO (Delb et al 1999). Tinnitus was evaluated before, after 10 sessions and after 15 sessions using a tinnitus questionnaire. Additionally, an audiometric examination was performed. Measurable improvements of the tinnitus occurred in 22% of the patients. The improvement rate decreased in those cases where the time from onset of tinnitus exceeded 40 days. It was concluded that hyperbaric oxygenation is a moderately effective additional treatment in the therapy of tinnitus after primary hemorheologic therapy, provided the time from onset of tinnitus is less than 1 month. In another study, HBO was prescribed to 20 patients who had had severe tinnitus for more than one year and who had already had other forms of tinnitus therapy with unsatisfactory results (Tan et al 1999). Four patients could not cope with hyperbaric pressure gradient. The effect of HBO was assessed using subjective evaluation and VAS scores before and after HBO. Follow-up continued until one year after treatment. Six patients had a reduction of tinnitus and accompanying symptoms, eight patients did not notice any change and two patients experienced an adverse effect. Any outcome persisted with minor changes until one year after treatment. The authors concluded that HBO may contribute to the treatment of severe tinnitus, but the negative effect on tinnitus should be weighed carefully.

Most of the studies which have shown the beneficial effect of HBO on tinnitus are uncontrolled. However, improvement of tinnitus has been documented in patients recovering from acute acoustic trauma following HBO treatment. A MEDLINE search from 1960–2007, yielding 22 studies of the effect of HBO on tinnitus, showed no significant effect in four prospective studies, but retrospective studies indicated greater improvement in tinnitus in acute cases compared with tinnitus episodes exceeding three months (Desloovere 2007). One study, however, showed significantly more improvement in patients with positive expectations before therapy (60.3%) compared with those with negative expectations (19%). Although there are indications of a better effect in acute cases, a major psychological component and a low risk of enhancement of the tinnitus should be considered. According to a systematic review of the literature, the significance of any improvement following HBO in a subjective rating of tinnitus could not be assessed because of poor reporting (Bebbett *et al* 2007). There were no significant improvements in hearing or tinnitus reported in the single study to examine chronic presentation (six months) of tinnitus. There was no evidence of a beneficial effect of HBO on chronic presentation of tinnitus, and the authors do not recommend routine use of HBO for this purpose.

Table 31.3
Causes of Sudden Deafness
1. Vascular
Thromboembolic disease
Labile hypertension or hypotension
Microcirculatory disturbances
2. Viral infections and postinfections
Autoimmunological disorders
3. Metabolic disorders
Hyperlipidemia
Diabetes
4. Toxic
Exposure to ototoxic drugs
Carbon monoxide poisoning
5. Diving injuries
Barotrauma
Decompression sickness of the inner ear
6. Miscellaneous
Rupture of the membrane of the round window
Intralabyrinthine membrane rupture
Stress

Sudden Deafness

Sudden hearing loss is a sensorineural hearing impairment, which develops over a period of few hours to a few days. The incidence of sudden sensorineural hearing loss has been reported to range from 5 to 20 per 100,000 persons per year. The most common forms of recent ear damage are sudden deafness and acute acoustic trauma. The conventional treatment of these conditions involves (a) infusions to improve microcirculation and (b) vasodilators. The effectiveness of these measures, however, remains unproven. Studies of Eibach and Börger (1980) indicate that these measures may be more harmful than beneficial. Experimental animal studies, for example, show that the cortilymph pO_2 decreases by 20% to 30% during exposure to infusions (Lamm & Klimpel 1989b). Some of the pioneering work referred in this chapter has been done by Pilgramm in Germany and described originally in his thesis (Pilgramm 1991).

The causes of sudden deafness are listed in Table 31.3. The pathogenesis of sudden deafness is not well understood: the oldest explanation of the disorder is that it is due to vascular insufficiency such as that resulting from occlusion of the labyrinthine artery; however, conclusive proof has never been provided. Animal experimental studies by Beck showed that the hair cells of the inner ear react in a uniform way to damage caused by such different agents as noise, viruses, ototoxic substances, and hypoxia. The hair cells first swell and lose their function. This effect is reversible in case of minor damage. In cases of severe damage or if the swelling persists for more than one year, the hair cells degenerate and are replaced by nonfunctioning endothelial cells.

The pathophysiology of ear damage in diving is described in Chapter 3. Clinically, one should differentiate between the hearing loss secondary to lesions such as an acoustic neuroma and those due to idiopathic disturbances of the inner ear.

Role of HBO in the Management of Sudden Deafness

Pioneer work on the role of HBO in disorders of the inner ear was done by Lamm in 1969 and Appaix *et al* (1970). Lamm and Klimpel (1971) reported 33 patients with diagnosis of hypoxia of the inner ear who improved after HBO therapy. Lamm and Gerstmann (1974) treated many inner ear disorders with HBO, but obtained the best results in 45 cases of sudden deafness. More than 90% of these patients showed an improvement of hearing, and in 40% of these a normal hearing was achieved. The therapeutic usefulness of HBO in sudden deafness was confirmed by other authors (Vincey 1978; Tarasiuk *et al* 1978; Ohresser *et al* 1980; Shu-Dong 1987). Most of the studies on this subject are uncontrolled. A summary of the controlled studies is shown in Table 31.4. From these studies it is concluded that HBO improves the results of the conventional treatment for sudden deafness, and best results are achieved if the treatment is started early after the onset of deafness. The spontaneous recovery rate, which is as high as 90%, makes the selection of patients for therapy and the evaluation of the results particularly difficult. This enthusiasm is not shared by the latest study from Japan (Nakashima *et al* 1998). If oxygen tension in the cochlea is reduced (as demonstrated by Fisch *et al* 1976), restoration of oxygen tension by HBO would be effective for the treatment of sudden deafness. HBO has been used successfully in the management of sudden deafness

Table 31.4
Controlled Studies of the Use of HBO in the Treatment of Sudden Deafness

Authors and year	Method	Patients (*n*)	Results
Goto *et al* (1979)	1. Standard treatment (vasodilators + steroids + vitamins) 2. Stellate ganglion block + HBO 3. Treatments 1 and 2 combined	22 49 20	Best results were obtained in group 3 where treatments were combined; those treated within 2 weeks showed an improvement of over 10 dB in hearing loss
Dauman *et al* (1985)	1. Steroids + vasodilators Total 2. HBO + hemodilution	43	First randomized controlled study; better results in the second group using HBO
Pilgramm *et al* (1985)	1. Hemodilution + vasodilators 2. Hemodilution + HBO	80	Statistically better results in group 2 in cases of acute sudden deafness
Takahashi *et al* (1989)	1. Standard, e.g., vasodilators 2. HBO (2 ATA, 1 h twice daily for 14–20 sessions added to the standard treatment)	316 ears 591 ears (900 cases)	No difference between the two groups in week of treatment, but improvement greater in the second group (with HBO) during the 2nd week
Nakashima *et al* (1998)*	1. Standard, e.g., vasodilators 2. HBO (2 ATA, 1 h twice daily for 14–20 sessions added to the standard treatment)	254 546	There were some cases where the hearing improved significantly after initiation of the HBO therapy. Because most of the patient in this series had poor outcome after basic treatment, the authors did not consider that it was worthwhile to compare the two groups.
Shiraishi *et al* (1998)	1. HBO 2. Stellate ganglion block 3. Oral vasodilator and vitamins	119	Therapeutic outcome in the HBO group was better than in the control group of 107 patients treated with various other therapies. Recovery rate of hearing in the HBO group was superior to that in the control group for those cases which had severe hearing loss at onset, had been seen more than 2 weeks after onset, and were resistant to other treatments.
Murakawa *et al* (2000)	1. HBO (2.5 ATA for 80 min daily) from 10 to 15 times. 2. Intravenous steroid, vitamin B12, prostaglandin E1, adenosine triphosphate, and low-molecular weight dextran.	522	Definite improvement in 34.9% (complete in 19.7%) and slight improvement in 58.1% of the patients. HBO given within 14 days from onset of SD was able to achieve hearing improvement in many cases unresponsive to the initial medical therapy even if given very early
Fattori *et al* (2001a)	1. Once-daily administration of HOB for 10 days in treatment group 2. Other group was treated for 10 days with an intravenous vasodilator	50	Within 48 h of the onset of SD, 30 patients were randomly assigned to HBO or intravenous vasodilator treatment. Patients in the HBO group experienced a significantly greater response to treatment than did those in the vasodilator group, regardless of age and sex variables.
Kestler *et al* (2001)	Primary HBO therapy compared to primary infusion therapy and no treatment in patients with SD of up to 3 weeks' duration	49	Neither the results of the infusion therapy nor those of the hyperbaric oxygenation surpass the rate of complete spontaneous remission.
Racic *et al* (2001)	100% oxygen at 2.8 ATA, for 60 min twice day, either until recovered or for a maximum of 30 sessions.	17	The average hearing level for all patients and for all five basic frequencies was 67.8 dB before therapy, in comparison with 21.6 dB after HBO therapy.
Aslan *et al* (2002)	1. Betahistine hydrochloride, prednisone, and daily stellate ganglion block. 2. HBO (4 ATA, 90 min) 4 treatments	25	Addition of HBO therapy to the conventional treatment significantly improved the outcome of SD compared to the control group of 25 patients who received the same basic treatment. HBO therapy is most useful in patients younger than 50 years, provides limited benefit in patients older than 50 years and no benefit in patients older than 60 years.
Inci *et al* (2002)	Patients unresponsive to medical treatment (steroids, vasodilators, Vit B) were given HBO (2.4 ATA), two sessions daily for the first three days, followed by a single daily session, to make 20 sessions of 90 min. Medications were continued during HBO treatment.	51	The mean hearing thresholds were 75.3 dB and 65.6 dB before and after treatment, respectively. Recovery was rated as complete in 3.9%, moderate 3.9%, mild in 37.25%, and as no recovery in 54.9%.
Muminov *et al* (2002)	1. Antioxidants 2. HBO (1.4 ATA for 40 min) 10 sessions	36 children	Improvement of sound perception at 5–25 dB in 72.2% patients. The highest effectiveness was seen in acute neurosensory hypoacusis.

Table 31.4 continued

Authors and year	Method	Patients (*n*)	Results
Narozny *et al* (2004)	Retrospective analysis of patients treated with HBO + corticosteroids, vasodilators, etc) *vs* those treated with drugs alone (81 subjects)	52	HBO at 2.5 ATA for 1 h daily for 5 d/wk. Improvement of hearing loss was statistically significantly better for HBO group.
Yan *et al* (2006)	Retrospective study of medical records of patients with sudden deafness treated by HBO vs non-HBO methods. Logistic regression was used in multivariate analysis.	236	Efficacy (hearing threshold elevated above 15 dB) ratio of HBO group comparing to the control group (non-HBO group), showed significant difference. It was concluded that HBO is effective for sudden deafness.
Dundar *et al* (2007)	Prospecti studymbined treatdical treatment alone in 25 subjects	52	In the HBO and medical treatment group, patients with tinnitus showed the highest hearing improvement but not in the medical treatment only group.

*Since this study is from Nagoya University, some of the patients in the study may be the same as in the previous report by Takahashi *et al* (1989).

based on the concept that pathogenesis may involve a reduction in cochlear blood flow and perilymph oxygenation (Domachevsky *et al* 2007). According to a systematic review of the literature, the use of HBO for early presentation of sudden sensorineural hearing loss (ISSHL) significantly improved hearing loss, but the clinical significance of the level of improvement is not clear (Bennett *et al* 2007). The routine application of HBO to these patients cannot be justified from this review. In view of the modest number of patients, methodological shortcomings, and poor reporting, this result should be interpreted cautiously, and an appropriately powered trial of high methodological rigor is justified to define those patients (if any) who can be expected to derive most benefit from HBO. There is no evidence of a beneficial effect of HBO on chronic presentation of ISSHL, and the authors do not recommend use of HBO for this purpose.

Rationale for HBO Therapy in Sudden Deafness

The rationale for this therapy is based on the following effects:

1. HBO increases the pO_2 in the inner ear. The experimental evidence for this has been provided by Lamm *et al* (1988). The insertion of oxygen-sensitive microelectrodes into the inner ears of guinea pigs led to a drop of pO_2 in the scala tympani. The animals were placed in the hyperbaric chamber and, after it was flooded with oxygen at normal pressure, pO_2 was noted to increase by 204%; when pressure was raised to 1.6 bar, pO_2 increased by 563% as compared with the original value. The increased oxygen supply corrects the hypoxia.
2. HBO improves hemorrheology and contributes to improved microcirculation. HBO not only lowers the hematocrit and whole blood viscosity, it also improves the erythrocyte elasticity.

Acute Acoustic Trauma

Acute acoustic trauma is defined as an acute impairment of hearing caused by sharp sounds like that of a gun going off near an unprotected ear. Sounds of moderate intensity as encountered in everyday life usually do not affect the oxygen tension within the cochlea, but high intensity sounds can reduce it. Important sequelae of acute acoustic trauma are.

- Failure of outside hair cells and then inside hair cells
- Rupture of cell membranes and decreased cochlear blood flow
- Decrease of hearing potentials corresponding to decrease of oxygen tension in the inner ear

Experimental Studies

Lamm *et al* (1977, 1982, 1987), in experimental studies in guinea pigs, investigated the effects of HBO on cochlear microphonics, action potentials of the auditory nerve, and brain-stem responses that had been damaged by short exposures to noise. The beneficial effect was variable and was seen in only 14 of 26 animals. Testing of postmortem cochlear microphonics after HBO treatment showed that oxygen can diffuse through the round window.

Pilgramm *et al* (1986) wrote that the impact of high levels of sound energy on an inadequately protected inner ear always results in the failure of the outside hair cells and the corresponding Deiters' supporting cells from the end of the first spiral to the middle of the second spiral. If the damage is pronounced, the inner hair cells will also fail. The damaged sensory cells will then be maintained in a transitional phase between regeneration and cell death. It is in this transitional phase that therapy has a chance. It was shown histologically that the alterations in the sensory cells, such as

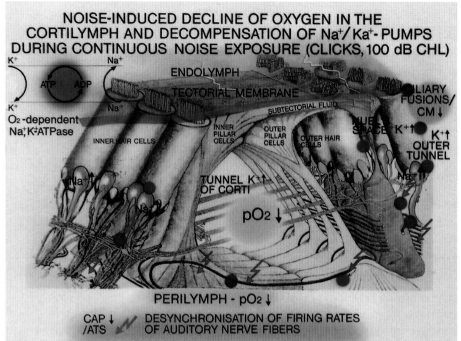

Figure 31.1

Noise-induced decline of pO2 in the fluid spaces of the inner ear, i.e., the perilymph and cortilymph.

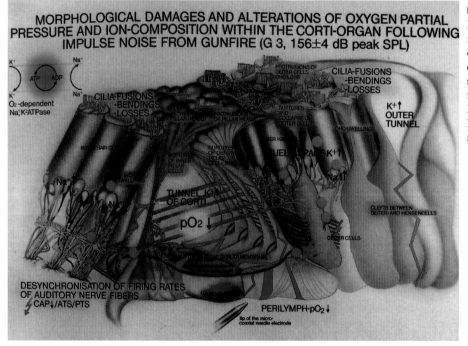

Figure 31.2

Morphological damage resulting from noise of gunfire, leading to intra- and extracellular ion imbalances, hearing damage, and decline of pO2 in the fluid spaces of the inner ear (Original photos from Bild-Atlas Innenohr, edition Duphar Pharma, retouched by Dr. K. Lamm, graphics by Atelier Gross, Hannover, reproduced by permission).

formation of cavernous nuclei, are the same as those resulting from anoxia. It was also shown in experimental animals that HBO has a beneficial effect in such a situation.

Lamm *et al* (1989a) exposed guinea pigs to a broad band of noise as well as impulse noise from gunfire. Some of the animals were treated with HBO at 1.5 ATA for 30 min after exposure to the noise.

Hearing potentials (cochlear microphonics or CM), and compound action potentials of the auditory nerve (CAP) were registered via the microaxial needle electrode for the polarographic measurements of pO2 directly in the inner ear (scale tympani). In all of the animals, pO2 decreased during the first 24 min of noise (broad band) exposure by more than one-third of the original values. Amplitudes of CM and CAP decreased by more than 20% to 25% of the original values. Treatment with HBO increased the pO2 in the inner ear by 70% of the original values and hearing potentials recovered during the therapy.

After exposure to the noise of the first 6–12 gunshots (G 3 of the German Army, 150–160 db), the pO2 in the inner ear initially increased slightly and then decreased by 20%–25% of the original values. The CM and CAP amplitudes were

Table 31.5
Clinical Studies of the Use of HBO in Acute Acoustic Trauma

Authors and year	Patients (n)	Cause	Results and comments
Lamm & Gerstmann (1974)	7	Noise damage	Only 4 obtained relief (2 complete and 2 partial); in 3 cases that did not improve treatment was started more than 8 weeks after onset
Demaertelaere & Van Opstal (1981)	50	Gunshot noise	HBO combined with vasodilators and explosion and antiflammatory drugs; better results with early treatment
Le Mouel et al (1981)	30	Diving accidents	Good results
Pilgramm & Schumann (1985)	22	Gunshot noise	Random allocation to 4 groups: therapy 1, 10% dextran-40 + 5% sorbitol; therapy 2, therapy 1 + 24 mg betahisine; therapy 3, therapy 1 + 10 HBO treatments; therapy 4, therapy 2 + 10 HBO treatments. Best results in groups 3 and 4. Patients with spontaneous recovery (48) excluded from the study. HBO shortens course of recovery and reduces relapse rate after improvement of hearing and tinnitus
Vavrina & Muller (1995)	78	Acute acoustic trauma from various causes	All subjects received saline or dextran (Rheomacodrex) infusions with Ginkgo biloba extracts and prednisone. Thirty-six patients underwent additional HBO 2 ATA for 60 min once daily. Both treatment groups were comparable as far as age, gender, initial hearing loss and prednisone dose are concerned. Treatment was started within 72 h in all cases. The average hearing gain in the group without HBO was 74.3 dB and in the group treated additionally with HBO 121.3 dB.
Ylikoski et al (2008)	60	acute acoustic trauma	HBO, given daily for 1–8 days, led to recovery of normal hearing at the end of the follow-up period in 42/60 compared with 24/60 in controls treated with normobaric oxygen

reduced by 40% and by a further 20% of the original values after six extra shots. HBO increased the pO_2 to 3.5-fold of the post-exposure values. Hearing also recovered.

Broad band noise increases the K^+ permeability in the transduction tissues of the inner ear, which have to be repolarized again by Na^+/K^+ pumps, which are dependent upon oxygen and energy. These pumps decompensate for lack of oxygen, which leads to an ion imbalance within the inner ear, which leads to structural changes reflected in decreased hearing potentials, as shown in Figure 31.1 (Lamm et al 1989b). In the case of impulse gunfire shots, these ion pumps decompensate for lack of oxygen while restoring the ion imbalance within the inner ear fluids, which had been disturbed by rupture of the cell membrane, as in Figure 31.2 (Lamm et al 1989a).

Cochlear blood flow, perilymphatic partial pressure of oxygen, cochlear microphonics, compound action potentials of the auditory nerve, and auditory brainstem responses were studied in noise-exposed guinea pigs during and after the several treatments (Lamm & Arnold 1999). A sustained therapeutic effect on noise-induced cochlear ischemia was achieved only by hydroxyethyl starch (HES), HBO + HES, and pentoxifylline. However, the best therapeutic effect on noise-induced hearing loss was achieved with a combination of HBO and prednisolone, followed by monotherapy with prednisolone or HES with the result that not only did the compound action potentials and auditory brainstem responses completely recover, the cochlear microphonics also showed significant improvement, although full recovery did not occur. All other therapies

were significantly less effective or did not improve noise-induced reduction of auditory evoked potentials.

In acute acoustic trauma, excessive noise exposure causes rupture of cell membranes and decreased cochlear blood flow. This leads to decreased oxygen tension in inner ear fluids and reduction of a variety of different oxygen-dependent cellular activities. HBO may help the cells suffering from hypoxia to survive. Kuokkanen et al (2000) exposed male Wistar rats to 60 impulses of 162-dB SPL from a 7.62-mm assault rifle equipped with a blank adaptor. After the exposure, 15 animals were given HBO treatment for 90 min daily for 10 consecutive days at 0.25 MPa. After a survival time of 4 weeks, auditory brainstem responses were measured and the left cochleae processed for light microscopy. The impulse noise caused permanent damage to the cochlea of all animals, with the most severe lesions in the lower middle coil, where a significantly smaller number of hair cells was missing in the HBO-treated group. The morphological damage was also reflected in function, as measured by auditory brainstem responses, which showed the greatest threshold shifts at 6.0, 8.0 and 10.0 kHz.

Clinical Studies

Lamm (1969) was the first to use HBO in vestibular disorders. Clinical studies of the use of HBO in acute acoustic trauma are summarized in Table 31.5. Most of the studies show that HBO therapy is useful in relieving tinnitus accompanying acute acoustic trauma, provided it is started within a few days following trauma. The only clinical study with negative effects is that of Kestler *et al* (2001) where the HBO was compared with infusion therapy but the two were not combined. Moreover the authors included patients with onset of sudden deafness up to 3 weeks prior to start of treatment. Perhaps the lesson from that study was to avoid the approaches followed by the authors. Many different pressures and durations of exposure are described in the literature. The following protocol is recommended:

- Institution of treatment within the first 3 days after the episode
- Ten exposures on 10 consecutive days at 2.5 ATA using 100% oxygen for 1 h.

Concluding Remarks About the Use of HBO in Hearing Loss

The published clinical data on this subject have been reviewed by Lamm *et al* (1998). Their conclusions are as follows:

- In case of patients with idiopathic sudden hearing loss, acoustic trauma or noise-induced hearing loss, 65% of those treated by multiple methods demonstrated a hearing improvement of 19 ± 4 dB. In 35% of the cases, no hearing improvement was detected independent of the drugs administered. This corresponds to the results obtained from placebo-treated patients who demonstrated a hearing improvement of 20 ± 2 dB in 61% of cases and no hearing gain in 39% of cases.
- A different set of results was obtained from patients with a hearing loss who were treated either with prednisolone or placebo. The percentage of patients who regained normal hearing in the placebo-treated group amounted to 31% and 38% and in the verum-treated group 50% and 78%. It may be concluded that a placebo therapy is equally effective to that of all nonsteroidal drugs. Problems arise when comparing non-treated patients since information on spontaneous remission rates differs greatly in the references, i.e., between 25–68% for spontaneous full remissions and 47–89% for spontaneous partial remissions. From a statistical point of view, 35% and 39% of patients experienced no success with non-steroidal drugs or placebo, respectively. These patients can still be helped with HBO therapy.
- In only 18 studies, the patients underwent primary HBO therapy. In all other 50 studies evaluated by the authors, with a total of 4, 109 patients suffering from idiopathic sudden hearing loss, acoustic trauma or noise-induced hearing loss and/or tinnitus, HBO therapy was administered as a secondary therapy, i.e., following unsuccess-

ful conventional therapy. If the onset of affliction was more than 2 weeks but no longer than 6 weeks, one half of the cases showed a marked hearing gain (in at least 3 frequencies of more than 20 dB), one-third showed a moderate improvement (10–20 dB) and 13% showed no hearing improvement at all. Four percent no longer experienced tinnitus, 81.3% observed an intensity decrease, 1.2% experienced an intensity increase of their tinnitus condition and 13.5% remained unchanged. If HBO therapy was administered at a later stage, but still within 3 months following onset of affliction, 13% showed a definite improvement in hearing, 25% a moderate improvement and 62% no improvement at all. 7% no longer suffered from tinnitus, 44% reported an intensity decrease, a similar percentage noticed no change and 5% a temporary deterioration of their tinnitus condition. If the onset of affliction was longer than 3 months up to several years, no hearing improvement can be expected in the majority of patients; however, one third of the cases reported an intensity decrease of tinnitus, 60–62% reported no change and 4–7% noticed a temporary intensity increase.

- In conclusion, HBO therapy is recommended and warranted in patients with idiopathic sudden deafness, acoustic trauma or noise-induced hearing loss within 3 months after onset of disorder.

Effect of HBO in Preventing Hearing Impairment from Chronic Noise Exposure

Hu *et al* (1991) carried out a series of experiments on guinea pigs to study the protective effect of HBO on hearing during chronic repeated noise exposure. A 1/3 octave band of noise centered at 1000 Hz was used for 1 h daily for 4 weeks. Groups of animals were exposed too to HBO at 2–3 ATA for 1 hr on alternate days. HBO was shown to markedly reduce the threshold shift and relieve cochlear damage. Further studies need to be done on this topic.

Miscellaneous Disturbances of the Inner Ear

Lamm *et al* (1977) studied the effect of HBO on CO-intoxicated guinea pigs. The microphonics recovered significantly faster from hypoxia than in animals treated by air alone (controls). When HBO was applied before CO exposure, the microphonics decreased less than under normal air breathing. Hyperoxia has also been shown to reduce the damage induced by combined carbon monoxide and noise exposure (Fechter *et al* 1988).

Lamm and Klimpel (1971) indicated that HBO should

be given within 8 weeks of the onset of inner ear ailments due to vascular causes. They believed that the mechanism of effectiveness was oxygenation of the cochlea through increased partial pressure of oxygen in the blood.

Rzayev (1981) tested the oxygenation of arterial blood in 100 caisson workers to ascertain the pathogenesis of work-related hearing disturbances. These workers were exposed to increased atmospheric pressures and vibration. There was decreased blood oxygenation and occult hypoxia, which could be correlated with the extent of hypoacusis. HBO produced more rapid normalization of hearing than did oxygen inhalation at normal pressure.

Patients with chronic (more than one year) impairment due to a variety of causes, such as ototoxicity of antibiotics, infections, and traumatic or occupational diseases, usually show poor results with HBO (Kozyro & Matskevich 1981; Lamm & Gerstmann 1974).

Neuro-otological Vascular Disturbances

Efuni *et al* (1980) used HBO in treating ten patients with cochleovestibular syndromes due to circulatory disturbances in the vertebrobasilar system. The results of treatment with HBO were compared with those of other methods and found to be superior. The effect of HBO was characterized by disappearance of vertigo and tinnitus. Eight of the patients showed improvement of hearing on audiograms.

Lyskin and Lebshova (1981) observed that disorders of the vertebrobasilar circulation give rise to diseases characterized by cochleovestibular syndromes due to impairment of the receptor inner ear. This may arise from impairment of the internal auditory artery or its branches, or as a "symptom at a distance" when vessels such as the anterior inferior cerebellar artery or the vertebral artery are occluded. Chronic or acute ischemia may give rise to impairment of the labyrinth, which responds to HBO. There was a considerable improvement of vertigo and hearing in 12 patients.

Kozyro and Matskevich (1981) obtained good results with HBO in 107 patients with transient ischemia of the vertebrobasilar territory and of the artery to the labyrinth. Their schedule was HBO at 1.5–2 ATA for 35–40 min with daily sessions for 8–10 days.

Guseinov *et al* (1989) treated 40 patients suffering from acute neurosensory hypoacusis of vascular etiology using combined HBO and drug therapy to improve microcirculation. One group was given HBO before drug therapy and the other group was given this treatment after drug therapy. Beneficial effects were more marked in the latter group and the explanation given was that drug therapy produced va-sodilatation, improved metabolism and counteracted the vasoconstricting effect of HBO

Menière's Disease

Menière's disease is recognized as a clinical entity. The classical triad of symptoms is roaring tinnitus, episodic vertigo, and fluctuating hearing loss.

A typical acute attack is followed by nausea, vomiting, and other vegetative symptoms. The classical triad is not always present. Characteristic histopathological lesion is endolymphatic hydrops. Disturbance of the quantitative relationship between the endo- and the perilymph is relevant to the pathogenesis. Further, a disturbance of the electrolyte composition of these two fluids leads to damage to the osmotic pressure regulation inside the membranous labyrinth. An endolymphatic hydrops results.

HBO reduces the hydrops both by increasing the hydrostatic pressure and by mechanically stimulating the flow of endolymph toward the duct and endolymphatic sac. In addition, an increase is seen in the amount of oxygen dissolved in the labyrinthine fluids and this contributes to recovering cell metabolism and restoring normal cochlear electrophysiological functions. Clinical studies of the use of HBO in Menière's syndrome and vertigo are summarized in Table 31.6. Although most of the authors have reported benefit from this therapy, the largest study failed to support this. One of the studies used controls but there has been no randomized study evaluating the use of HBO in Menière's disease.

Fattori *et al* (1996) investigated 45 patients suffering from Meniere's disease by submitted them to pressure chamber therapy: 20 with constant pressure (2.2 ATA, hyperbaric treatment) and 25 with continuous variations in pressure levels (from 1.7 to 2.2 ATA, alternobaric treat-

Table 31.6
Clinical Studies of Use of HBO in Menière's Disease

Authors and year	Patients (*n*)	Results and comments
Nair *et al* (1973)	7	Remission of nausea, dizziness, and inability to walk
Pavlik (1976)	42	Symptomatic relief with long-term use of HBO
Tjernström *et al* (1980)	46	Improvement of hearing in 21 patients
Kozyro & Matskevich (1981)	35	Good results
Qu Zhan-Kui (1986)	1000	No significant improvement
Fattori *et al* (1996)	45	More improvement in patients treated under varying conditions

ment). HBO therapy consisted of one session per day lasting 90 minutes for 15 days during the acute attacks followed by five consecutive sessions per month during a follow-up of two years. For a control group the authors treated 18 patients with 10% intravenous glycerol during the acute episode and 8 mg betahistine three times a day thereafter. They compared hearing loss, vertigo and tinnitus in the three groups 15 days after starting treatment and at the end of the follow-up, according to the criteria suggested by the 1995 Committee on Hearing and Equilibrium. They found no statistically significant differences in recovery from the cochlear-vestibular symptoms in the three groups at the end of the first 15 days of therapy, whereas hyperbaric and, in particular, alternobaric treatment permitted a significant control of the principal attacks of vertigo during the follow-up period. Hearing loss also showed a more significant and more persistent improvement in the patients treated with alternobaric oxygenation compared to the patients in the other two groups. At the end of a 4-year follow-up of these patients, hyperbaric treatment, and in particular alternobaric therapy, enabled a significant reduction in the episodes of dizziness as compared to the control group (Fattori et al 2001b).

Facial Palsy

Bell's palsy (idiopathic facial palsy) is unilateral facial paralysis of sudden onset. This term does not include lesions of the facial nerve caused by injury such as fractures of the base of the skull, infiltration by tumors, and as a complication of surgical procedures. The cause is not known, but there is disturbance of the facial nerve with swelling during its course in the facial canal leading to compression and ischemia of the nerve. It resolves spontaneously in 70 to 80% of cases, but the recovery may be prolonged and residual disability and disfigurement may persist. The outcome of the disease cannot be predicted during the first week and electrophysiological tests such as the nerve excitability test and electromyography show abnormalities only after this period. Various treatments used include corticosteroids and surgical decompression of the facial nerve. A less frequent cause of facial palsy is Ramsay-Hunt syndrome which is believed to be caused by reactivation of varicella zoster virus and the treatment for this condition has not explored as yet.

Treatment of Bell's palsy remains controversial. Surgical decompression has not produced any better outcome than spontaneous resolution of the palsy. Several prospective and retrospective studies suggest strongly that corticosteroids are beneficial but no definitive study has been done to prove the value of corticosteroids. Ramsy-hunt syndrome responds somewhat better to corticosteroids and also to acyclovir but the benefits have not been proven. The use of HBO has been explored in these conditions.

Litavrin et al (1985) reported on HBO as a part of multimodal therapy for Bell's palsy in 42 patients. A further 29 patients with a similar clinical picture were treated by conventional methods and served as controls. The authors concluded that the addition of HBO to other methods increases the efficacy of the treatment, and reduces the period needed for restoration of the function of the damaged nerve.

Nakata (1976) treated 66 patients with Bell's palsy using HBO. In 54 patients for whom the treatment was started within 2 weeks after onset, 45 (83%) recovered completely, 7 recovered partially, and 2 did not recover. All the patients whose EMG showed evidence of neuropraxia recovered completely. Those with incomplete denervation also recovered, but their recovery period was much longer. This pattern of recovery is better than could be predicted from the natural history of the disease, or as a result of other treatments such as steroids and surgical decompression.

Racic et al (1997) compared the therapeutic effects of HBO with those of prednisone treatment in 79 patients with Bell's palsy who were randomly assigned either to the HBO-treated group ($n = 42$) or to the prednisone-treated group ($n = 37$). The HBO group was exposed to 2.8 ATA of 100% oxygen for 60 min, twice a day, 5 days a week and was given a placebo orally. The prednisone group was exposed to 2.8 ATA of 7% O_2 (equivalent to 21% O_2 in air at normal pressure) following the same schedule as the HBO group; prednisone was given orally (total of 450 mg in 8 days). Subjects from both groups were treated in the hyperbaric chamber for up to 30 sessions or to complete recovery and were followed up for 9 months. At the end of the follow-up period, 95.2% of subjects treated with HBO, and 75.7% of subjects treated with prednisone recovered completely. The average time to complete the recovery in the HBO group was 22 days as compared to 34.4 days in the control group ($p < 0.001$). These results suggest that HBO is more effective than prednisone in treatment of Bell's palsy.

Makishima et al (1998) treated 12 patients with facial palsy and 11 patients with Ramsey-Hunt syndrome by a combination therapy consisting of HBO, stellate ganglion block as well as oral administration of a vasodilator (this combination therapy has also been used for sudden deafness). The period between the onset and start of treatment was longer than 3 days in most of the patients. Results were evaluated by a special grading system and showed satisfactory clinical results in 83.5% of Bell's palsy patients and 63.6% of Ramsay-Hunt patients. Total number of patients in this study is too small for statistical analysis and comparison with other studies. A definitive study on this topic remains to be done.

Otological Complications of HBO Therapy

These have been described in Chapter 8 but a brief mention will be made in this chapter of complications of HBO related to treatment for ENT indications. As in case of other indications, barotrauma, especially to the middle ear, remains the most common complication in this area with the reported rates varying between 5%–82%. Ueda et al (1998) have evaluated the incidence of complications in 898 patients who received HBO therapy at the University of Nagoya, Japan for various indications related to ENT. There was no evidence of barotrauma to the inner ear in any case. The overall incidence of barotrauma was 33.2% (577 of 1737 ears). Patients who developed barotrauma usually had poor Eustachian tube function. This observation can be used to predict barotrauma. The incidence of barotrauma was found to be unrelated to the extent of mastoid pneumatization.

Miscellaneous Conditions in Head and Neck Area

Malignant Otitis Externa

This syndrome was first described by Chandler (1968) and consists of an antibiotic resistant *Pseudomonas aeruginosa* infection of the external auditory meatus with osteomyelitis of the temporal bone. It usually affects patients with long-standing diabetes mellitus and a weakened immune system. Over 100 cases have been described in the literature. The overall mortality is 35%.

Lucente et al (1983) reviewed 16 patients and found that the spread of infection beyond the external auditory meatus can produce lethal invasive osteomyelitis. They recommend investigation of such patients by using radiological procedures such as tomography of the temporal bone and intensive management with antibiotics, surgery, and HBO. HBO has been recommended for this condition by other authors (Mader & Love 1982; Shupak et al 1989). In 1986, Pilgramm et al reviewed the literature on this subject and presented three cases with successful management using HBO. Davis et al (1992) treated 16 patients with malignant otitis externa with addition of a 30-day HBO course to antibiotic regimen. All of the patients recovered and remained free from infection and neurological sequelae during the follow-up from one to four years.

Advances in the diagnosis and treatment of malignant otitis externa during the past 20 years have improved substantially te prognosis of the disease. HBO potentiates the effect of antibiotic therapy. This condition should no longer malignant for the majority of the patients where the disease is diagnosed early and treated adequately (Hlozek et al 1989).

Bath et al (1998) reported a case of malignant otitis externa with optic neuritis that remained refractory to standard treatment but was cured by adjuvant HBO therapy. This is the only reported case that has survived this disease with optic neuritis.

Martel et al (2000) treated 22 patients over a period of four years; the causal organism was *Pseudomonas aeruginosa* in 87% of cases. The diagnostic work-up included a computed tomography scan and a technetium scintigraphy to confirm the diagnosis and assess extension of the disease. Medical treatment was used in most cases with parenteral antibiotic therapy with a third-generation cephalosporin (ceftazidime or ceftriaxone) and a fluoroquinolone (ciprofloxacin or ofloxacin) and, if there was no contraindication, HBO. A case has been reported of *Aspergillus flavus* malignant otitis externa, successfully treated with antifungal agents, surgical debridement, and HBO (Ling & Sader 2008). Adjunctive therapies, such as aggressive debridement and HBO, are reserved for extensive or unresponsive cases (Carfrae & Kesser 2008).

Aphonia Due to Chronic Laryngitis

James (1987) presented a case of aphonia due to chronic laryngitis, which resolved following a 4-day course of HBO at 2 ATA. The course of laryngeal edema was followed by laryngoscopy. The author pointed out that this case provided visual evidence that oxygen-induced vasoconstriction can be beneficial in long-standing edema by breaking the cycle of hypoxic edema and microcirculatory insufficiency.

Conclusions

The literature on the use of HBO in otorhinolaryngology is not very extensive. There is agreement that sudden deafness and acute acoustic trauma are good indications for HBO therapy, and that there is improvement of these conditions if the treatment is carried out soon after the onset of symptoms. HBO therapy does not displace but is adjunctive to conventional treatments. HBO has been used on a large scale for the treatment of tinnitus in Germany. It is effective in relieving tinnitus as a component of inner ear disorders, but whether this large scale use for tinnitus alone as a symptom is justified is questionable.

Most authors indicate lack of effectiveness of HBO in chronic anoxic conditions, and its use in Menière's syndrome is controversial. In symptoms secondary to ischemia, for example of the acoustic nerve, it is reasonable to suppose that HBO may be effective in the chronic stages, as the situation is comparable to that of ischemia in the brain.

Effectiveness in Bell's palsy has not been proven, although good results have been obtained in several series of patients. Malignant otitis externa is a good indication for the use of HBO as the effect of HBO in enhancing the effect of antibiotics is well documented. This therapy is well tolerated with minor complications and its use continues to be explored in several conditions of the head and neck.

32 HBO Therapy and Ophthalmology

Frank Butler, Jr, Heather Murphy-Lavoie, and K.K. Jain

There is significant evidence for the usefulness of HBO in the management of central retinal artery occlusion and some evidence of its usefulness for other ocular conditions.

Introduction

The eye and periocular tissues may benefit from hyperbaric oxygen therapy (HBOT) when affected with certain disorders. Several uses of HBOT in diseases of the eye have been reported over the years. Pertinent anatomy and physiology of the eye and the effects of hyperoxia on these will be reviewed. Following this will be a discussion of the ocular contraindications to HBOT and the reported clinical uses of HBO in ophthalmology.

Review of Pertinent Anatomy and Physiology of the Eye

In the process of producing the sensory experience that we perceive as vision, incident light passes through the cornea, the anterior chamber, the pupil, the posterior chamber, the crystalline lens, and the vitreous body before reaching the retina. The cornea provides approximately two-thirds of the refracting power required to focus light on the retina and the lens the other one-third. The anterior chamber, the posterior chamber, and the vitreous body are filled with noncompressible fluid, which means that the eye is not adversely affected by changes in pressure (barotrauma) unless a gas space exists adjacent to the eye (as with a facemask) or within the eye (as a result of surgical procedures or trauma).

The retina is comprised of nine distinct layers, with the photoreceptor cells as the outermost and the internal limiting membrane as the innermost layers (Regillo 2007). Light reaching the retina stimulates the photoreceptor cells, which results in stimulation of the ganglion cells. The confluence of the afferent portions of the ganglion cells (the nerve fiber layer) forms the optic disk. These cells then exit the eye as the optic nerve to carry visual stimuli back to the occipital cortex of the brain via the optic chiasm and the optic tract. At the middle and posterior aspects of the eye, the wall of the globe is composed of three main layers, the outermost fibrous sclera, the vascular uveal tract, and the innermost sensory retina. The uveal tract is further divided into the posterior choroid, the iris visible in the anterior portion of the eye, and the intermediate ciliary body.

Vision may be adversely affected by any factor that prevents light from reaching the retina or being sharply focused in the retinal plane. Vision may also be affected by injury to the retina, the occipital cortex, or the afferent neural tissues carrying visual stimuli between these two areas.

The arterial supply to the eye is provided by the ophthalmic artery, one of the branches of cavernous portion of the internal carotid artery. Some of the branches of the ophthalmic artery (lacrimal, supraorbital, ethmoidals, medial palpebral, frontal, dorsal nasal) supply orbital structures, while others (central artery of the retina, short and long posterior ciliaries, anterior ciliary arteries) supply the tissues of the globe (Cibis 2006). The central retinal artery enters the globe within the optic nerve and serves the inner layers of the retina through its branches. There are approximately twenty short posterior ciliary arteries and usually two long posterior ciliary arteries. The posterior ciliary vessels originate from the ophthalmic artery and supply the uvea, the cilioretinal arteries, the sclera, the margin of the cornea, and the adjacent conjunctiva. The long posterior ciliary arteries provide blood to the choroid and the outer layers of the retina. The short posterior ciliary arteries also supply the choroid. The anterior ciliary arteries also arise from the ophthalmic artery, supply the extraocular muscles, and anastamose with the posterior ciliary vessels to form the major arterial circle of the iris, which supplies the iris and ciliary body. The optic nerve receives its blood supply from various vessels as it progresses from the surface of the optic nerve head through the orbit, including branches of the central retinal artery, the posterior ciliary arteries, and branches of the ophthalmic artery. In approximately 15%–30% of individuals, a cilioretinal artery is present. This artery is part of the ciliary arterial supply but supplies the macular region of the retina, which subserves central vision.

The retina in the human eye has a dual blood supply, with the retinal circulation supplying the inner layers of the retina and the choroidal circulation supplying the outer layers under normoxic conditions. Normally, the choroidal circulation supplies the majority of the oxygen to the retina, with only the inner layers of the retina being oxygenated from the retinal circulation. Under normoxic conditions, approximately 60% of the retina's oxygen supply comes from the choroidal circulation. Animal models have shown that oxygen from the choroidal circulation diffuses in adequate quantity to the inner layers of the retina under hyperoxic conditions to maintain ganglion cell viability and retinal function even when retinal blood flow has been interrupted (Li 1996, Landers 1978, Patz 1955).

The cornea and lens are avascular structures. The cornea receives its oxygen supply both from the precorneal tear film and the anterior chamber of the eye, while the oxygen supply to the lens is provided by the aqueous and the vitreous (Cibis 2006).

If blood flow to the eye is unimpeded but oxygen delivery to the eye is impaired, such as is the case with hypobaric hypoxia, the retinal vessels respond by dilating and ocular blood flow is markedly increased (Butler 1992). The retinal vessels respond in a similar manner with the hypoxia of CO poisoning (Resch 2005).

Many vision-threatening eye diseases are accompanied by elevated levels of vascular endothelial growth factor (VEGF). VEGF is a homodimeric soluble glycoprotein growth factor specific for endothelial cells. This substance is produced normally and is essential for normal embryonic angiogenesis. Chronic retinal hypoxia, however, results in elevated levels of VEGF that triggers neovascularization in the retina, optic disk, and iris. Elevated levels of VEGF also cause increased vascular permeability that may produce loss of vision through macular edema. VEGF isoform 164 has been found to be an important isoform in the pathogenesis of early diabetic retinopathy (Ishida 2003). A number of agents have been developed to block the effect of VEGF and are now being used to combat a variety of ocular conditions (Butler 2008).

Ocular Oxygen Tension

Most of the information on oxygen tension in the normal eye is based on animal experiments. Oxygen tension in the vitreous humor (80–90 mmHg) is higher than in the anterior chamber (50 mmHg). The cornea, the lens, and the vitreous humor are mostly avascular. The basic facts include the following:

1. The corneal epithelium utilizes atmospheric oxygen.
2. Oxygen can diffuse across the cornea, and, interestingly, the rate is equal both inward and outward.
3. The lens consumes 0.2–0.5 ml oxygen/min.
4. The retina carries out its oxygen exchange exclusively through the retinal and the choroidal vessels.
5. The ratio of tissue pO_2 when breathing 100% oxygen to tissue pO_2 when breathing air is 2.6:3.4 for both the vitreous and the aqueous humors. This is much higher than the similar ratio for other tissues (2.1:2.3), and accounts for the increased susceptibility of the eye to the effects of hyperoxia.

Physiology of the Eye in Hyperoxic Conditions

Because the retina has a dual blood supply as described above, hyperoxygenation may enable the choroidal blood supply to supply the oxygen needs of the entire retina. Since central retinal artery obstructions are often transient, this phenomenon may enable the retina to survive the period of occluded blood flow. The studies published by Landers demonstrate that this is possible in cat and rhesus monkey models. When the authors of that study occluded the retinal artery and ventilated the animals with 100% oxygen at one ATA, a normal or increased oxygen tension was produced in the inner layers of the retina. They noted that at an arterial oxygen tension of 375 to 475 mmHg provided a normal or increased inner retinal oxygen tension, even with the central retinal artery occluded (Landers 1978). Breathing 100% oxygen at one atmosphere has been shown to restore the visual evoked response (VER) to normal despite an occluded retinal arterial circulation. A normal VER requires that all layers of the retina are functioning normally

and indicates the inner retinal layers were adequately oxygenated in this model (Landers 1978).

Hyperbaric oxygen is well known to cause vasoconstriction of the retinal vessels (Yu 2005, Vucetic 2004, Polkinghorne 1989, Nichols 1969 NEJM, Frayser 1967, Anderson 1965a, Saltzman 1965, Haddad 1965, Jacobson 1963). As the partial pressure of oxygen is increased to 2.36 and 3.70 ATA, the retinal vessels become progressively smaller (Frayser 1967). Both retinal arterioles and venules are affected (Saltzman 1965). At 30 pounds per square inch gauge pressure (PSIG) partial pressure of oxygen, which produces an arterial oxygen tension of approximately 1,950 mmHg, the retinal arterioles have been reported to decrease 19% in diameter (Anderson 1965a). Vucetic noted a retinal arteriole constriction of 9.6% and a retinal venule constriction of 20.6% after 90 minutes of 2.5 ATA partial pressure of oxygen. Ten minutes after the hyperoxic exposure, the vessels had returned to 94.5% and 89.0% of their primary size, respectively (Vucetic 2004).

Hyperoxic retinal vasoconstriction has led some authors to theorize that there is a decrease in retinal oxygenation in hyperoxic conditions (Herbstein 1984). This is not the case. Retinal venous hemoglobin oxygen saturation was found to increase from 58% breathing room air to 94% at 2.36 ATA, indicating that the hyperoxygenated choriocapillaris is supplying enough oxygen to more than offset any decrease in oxygen supply caused by retinal vasoconstriction at elevated partial pressures of oxygen (James 1985, Frayser 1967). Jampol demonstrated that hyperbaric oxygen at 2 ATA in a primate model markedly increased the preretinal oxygen tension, indicating higher inner retinal oxygen levels under hyperoxic conditions (Jampol 1987). Dollery has also confirmed that a hyperoxygenated choroid can supply the oxygen requirements of the whole retina (Dollery 1969). Saltzman noted that while retinal vasoconstriction occurs under hyperoxic conditions, the appearance of bright red blood in the retinal veins indicates that the increase in oxygen transport during hyperoxia more than compensates for any reduction in retinal blood flow resulting from vasoconstriction (Saltzman 1965).

Pressure with the fingertip applied on the lateral aspect of the eye through the lid raises intraocular pressure and typically causes a dimming of vision in less than 5 seconds. This phenomenon is believed to be due to retinal ischemia induced by the elevated intraocular pressure. Hyperbaric oxygen administered at 4 ATA extends the interval from pressure application to dimming of vision to 50 seconds or more. (Note that this partial pressure of oxygen will rapidly produce toxic effects on the central nervous system and is not used in standard clinical practice) (Carlisle 1964).

Jampol also found that normobaric oxygen delivered to the corneal surface of rabbits increased the pO_2 in the anterior chamber from 63.5 to 139.5 mmHg. Hyperbaric oxygen at 2 ATA presented to the corneal surface of air breathing rabbits further raised the anterior chamber pO_2 to 295.2 mmHg (Jampol 1988, Jampol 1987).

Hyperoxia (air at 3 ATA) has been reported to cause a decrease in intraocular pressure from 15.3 mmHg to 12.3 mmHg in 14 volunteers over a mean time of 38 minutes. 100% oxygen administered at one atmosphere also produced a significant decrease in intraocular pressure from 14.8 to 12.7 mmHg. The exact mechanism of the decrease in pressure was not clear (Gallin-Cohen 1980). Hyperoxic vasoconstriction is one potential mechanism for the observed decrease. Note that intraocular pressure measurements in hyperbaric environments typically describe the difference between the intraocular tissues and the external environment, not the absolute pressure which increases with the ambient environment (Butler 2008).

Retinal Circulation Under Normoxia, Hypoxia, and Hyperoxia

The central artery of the retina supplies oxygen to the inner layers of the retina. Oxygen to the outer layers of the retina is supplied by the choroidal circulation. It has no capillaries, but it is extremely vascular tissue with a blood flow of 1200 ml/100 g tissue/min, in contrast to the retinal blood flow of 166 ml/100 g/min. There is an overlap between the retinal and the choroidal circulations. Under conditions of air breathing the choroid supplies oxygen to 60% of the retina, but with retinal artery occlusion it has the remarkable potential to oxygenate the whole thickness of retina (Dollery et al 1969).

The response of the retinal circulation to hyperoxia is similar to that of the cerebral circulation, but the retinal blood flow in response to 100% oxygen results in a diminution several times that of the cerebral blood flow.

Saltzman et al (1965) photographed the optic fundus in eight volunteers breathing air or oxygen at 1–3.72 ATA during quiet respiration and hyperventilation. HBO resulted in marked attenuation of both arterioles and venules, and the smallest retinal vessels disappeared completely. The normal color difference between the arteries and the veins was lost. These changes occurred during the first 5 min exposure and were reversed by 1 min of breathing air. Hyperventilation with accompanying hypercapnia was not associated with significant decreases in vessel caliber. These studies indicated a major vasoconstricting action of oxygen on the retinal circulation. The arterial color of the vein suggested that there was a significant increase in retinal tissue oxygen content during HBO.

Dollery et al (1965) measured the caliber of retinal arterioles and veins from color photographs of the ocular fundus in normal males breathing gas mixtures with oxygen pressures varying from 160 to 1520 mmHg. The mean percentage change in diameter varied approximately linearly with the log

of the inspired pO_2. The smallest measurable arterioles decreased by 30.2% when inspired pO_2 was 760 mmHg, and by 40.3% when it was raised to 1520 mmHg. Breathing 7% CO_2 completely inhibited the vasoconstriction brought about by inspired pO_2 of 710 mmHg.

Fallon et al (1985) used the blue field entropic technique to measure macular blood flow in healthy volunteers breathing room air under conditions of hypoxia or hyperoxia. They also measured retinal artery and vein diameter in a computerized digital system. Under isocapnic hypoxia there was an average 38% increase of blood flow, and an increase in diameter of 8.2% and 7.4% in retinal arteries and veins respectively. In hyperoxia the blood flow fell by an average of 35% and retinal artery and vein diameter decreased by 5.6% and 10% respectively. This technique has potential value in determining blood flow changes in pathologic states thought to cause hypoxia, such as diabetes mellitus and sickle cell disease. Vasoconstriction of both arterioles and venules during prolonged hyperoxia has been recorded by Hague et al (1988).

Riva et al (1986) studied the regulation of local oxygen tension and blood flow in the inner retina during hyperoxia in miniature pigs. They established an association between changes in local periarteriolar pO_2 and retinal blood flow in response to breathing 100% oxygen. Oxygen is an important factor in the regulation of retinal blood flow, and its effects on the vessel wall, whether direct or indirect, appeared to be aimed at maintaining a constant inner retinal pO_2.

Adverse Effects of Hyperoxia

Retinal Oxygen Toxicity

Oxygen can be directly toxic to the tissues of the eye (Clark 2003). Oxygen at 1 ATA has not been shown to produce adverse ocular effects in adult humans. Oxygen at this partial pressure typically results in pulmonary toxicity before the eye is affected (Kinney 1985). As early as 1935, Behnke reported a reversible decrease in peripheral vision after oxygen breathing at 3.0 ATA (Behnke 1935). Lambertsen and Clark and their colleagues also observed a progressive decrease in peripheral vision associated with hyperoxic exposures (Lambertsen 1987, Nichols 1969). A decrease in peripheral vision was noted after approximately 2.5 hours of oxygen breathing at 3.0 ATA in a dry chamber. This decrease was progressive until oxygen breathing was discontinued. The average decrement in visual field was 50%. Recovery was complete in all subjects after 45 minutes of air breathing (Lambertsen 1987). A decrease in ERG amplitude was noted as well, but did not correlate directly with the size of the visual field defect and returned to normal more slowly after the termination of the hyperoxic exposure (Lambertsen 1987). Visual acuity and visual cortical evoked responses remained normal in all subjects. A 4-hour exposure to 1 ATA of oxygen, in contrast, produced no change in visual acuity or visual fields (Miller 1958). The changes in visual field noted above probably represent a form of retinal oxygen toxicity rather than CNS oxygen toxicity in that they are predictable, evolve slowly, and resolve slowly after the discontinuation of the hyperoxic exposure. Retinal oxygen toxicity is not commonly reported as a complication of HBOT, but the incidence may be underreported since visual fields are not typically performed during the course of HBOT and any defects present would be expected to resolve shortly after a return to normoxia. Moreover, repetitive HBOT is almost always administered at 2.0 to 2.5 ATA and for shorter exposure times than those that have been documented to cause retinal oxygen toxicity.

Retinal oxygen toxicity has been further explored in animal models. Hyperbaric oxygen administered in severe enough exposures results in photoreceptor cell death preceded by attenuation of the electroretinogram (Bridges 1966, Noell 1962). Beehler exposed dogs to hyperoxia (680 to 760 mmHg of oxygen) continuously for 72 hours. All animals were either dead at the end of the exposure or died shortly thereafter due to pulmonary complications. 50% of the animals were found to have ocular lesions as a result of this exposure. The observed findings included bilateral retinal detachments, corneal haze, chemosis, and hyphema (Beehler 1963). Four-hour exposures of rabbits to 3 ATA of oxygen or 40–48 hours of exposure to 1 ATA of oxygen resulted in destruction of the retinal photoreceptor cells (Nichols 1969b, Noell 1962). Sodium-potassium ATPase has been shown to be inhibited by hyperbaric oxygen and may be a factor in retinal oxygen toxicity (Ubels 1981).

Hyperoxia is especially toxic to the immature retina, causing vasoconstriction and subsequent failure of normal vascularization in the retinas of infants given high doses of supplemental oxygen (Patz 1965). Retrolental fibroplasia was first described in 1942 (Terry 1942). It became the leading cause of blindness in preschool children in the 1950s (Beehler 1966). Following the determination that hyperoxia was the major causative factor in this disorder, the incidence of retrolental fibroplasia was greatly reduced (Butler 2008).

Lenticular Oxygen Toxicity

Hyperoxic Myopia

Progressive myopic changes are a known complication of repetitive HBOT treatments (Fledelius 2002, Thom 1997, Ross 1996, Clark 1993, Anderson 1987, Palmquist 1984, Anderson 1978, Lyne 1978). The rate of myopic change has been reported to be approximately 0.25 diopters per week, and this change was progressive throughout the course of

HBOT (Anderson 1978). Hyperoxic myopia is generally attributed to oxidative changes causing an increase in the refractive power of the lens, since studies have shown that axial length and keratometry readings did not reveal a corneal curvature or axial length basis for the myopic shift (Fledelius 2002, Anderson 1987, Anderson 1978, Lyne 1978). Reversal of the myopic shift after discontinuation of HBOT usually occurs within 3–6 weeks, but may take as long as 6–12 months (Thom 1997). In his series of 26 patients exposed daily to 2.5 ATA oxygen for 60 minutes with an additional 30 minutes each of oxygen during compression and decompression, Lyne noted that the rate of myopic change was about 0.5 diopters a month, with the change being progressive throughout therapy and slowly reversible after HBOT was completed. Two patients were observed to have a myopic shift of 5.5 diopters (Lyne 1978).

The partial pressure of oxygen in HBOT typically varies from 2.0–3.0 ATA depending on the treatment protocol used, but hyperoxic myopia has also been reported in a closed-circuit mixed-gas scuba diver at a PPO2 of 1.3 ATA, a lower partial pressure of oxygen than those typically used in HBOT (Butler 1999). The myopic shift noted above resolved over a one-month period after finishing the series of hyperoxic SCUBA dives (Butler 2008).

Hypermetropic changes after HBOT exposures have also been reported (Evanger 2006, Fledelius 2004).

Fledelius *et al* (2002) recorded changes in refraction and refractive parameters associated with a standard HBO treatment protocol consisting of a 95 min session at > 95% oxygen at 2.5 ATA given daily up to a total of 30 sessions. Refraction was determined subjectively assessed by keratometry and by A-scan axial ultrasound measurement. The refractive changes associated with HBO were found to be smaller than reported previously in the literature. No significant change in axial eye length measurements was found, and keratometry readings reflected only minimal change, although this was statistically significant. Therefore it is most likely that lens changes, whether in internal refractive indices or curvatures, accounted for the transitory shift toward more myopic/less hyperopic values.

Cataract

Cataract formation has been reported by Palmquist and his co-authors in patients undergoing a prolonged (150 or more exposures) course of daily HBOT therapy at 2.0–2.5 ATA (Palmquist 1984, Palmquist 1986). Seven of fifteen patients with clear lenses at the start of therapy developed cataracts during their course of treatment. Fourteen of these fifteen patients received a total hyperbaric oxygen treatment time of between 300 and 850 hours. All of the patients developed myopia during treatment. Seven of the 15 patients with clear lenses before the treatment developed cataracts and reduced visual activity during the treatment. The authors considered myopic change to be an early sign of increasing nuclear cataract. The lens opacities noted were not completely reversible after HBOT was discontinued. Gesell and Trott reported *de novo* cataract formation in a 49-year-old woman who underwent 48 HBOT treatments for chronic refractory osteomyelitis of the sacrum and recurrent failure of a sacral flap (Gesell 2007).

Hyperoxic myopia and subsequent cataract formation may be considered to represent two points on the continuum of severity of lenticular oxygen toxicity. The high success rate of modern cataract surgery makes cataract formation an easily manageable complication of HBOT, and this side effect is not necessarily an indication to discontinue therapy if the patient's clinical indication for continuation of HBOT is strong enough (Butler 2008).

Retrolental Fibroplasia

Retrolental fibroplasia is a retinopathy of prematurity and was considered to be a toxic effect of oxygen on the retina of the immature infant leading to blindness. This condition still occurs, although rarely, even though oxygen is not routinely administered for long periods in high concentrations in the neonatal period. Its use is guided by transcutaneous oxygen tension ($tcpO_2$) determinations. One of the explanations given for the pathogenesis of this condition was that hyperoxygenation leads to constriction of the growing vessels and degeneration of endothelium and neovascularization around ischemic areas. Vitamin E has been shown to have some protective effect against this complication in the premature infant. Retrolental fibroplasia has not been reported as a complication of HBO in adult humans. It is now believed that variations of $tcpO_2$ in the first two weeks of life is a significant predictor of retinopathy of prematurity (Cunningham *et al* 1995).

Ricci *et al* (1989) exposed newborn Wistar rats to normobaric oxygen (80%) for 5 days after birth. They developed retinopathy with marked peripheral retinal neovascularization. Similar animals given HBO (1.8 ATA) did not develop any peripheral retinopathy. The authors concluded that, in the newborn rat, hyperbarisms provides a protective action against the toxic effects of oxygen supplementation on immature retinal vessels (Ricci, 1995).

Ocular Contraindications to Hyperbaric Oxygen Therapy

While the presence of impaired vision itself may be a contraindication to commercial or recreational diving, it is not a contraindication to receive HBOT. The prescribed convalescent period prior to resumption of diving activity after ocular surgery should typically not be relevant to HBOT (except as noted below), since the potential for facemask barotrauma and water intrusion into an ocular operative site will not be present in a hyperbaric chamber. Glaucoma is also not a contraindication to HBOT, despite the presence of elevated ambient (and intraocular) pressures (Butler 1995). Oxygen has actually been shown to reduce intraocular pressures slightly (Gallin-Cohen 1980).

The following ocular conditions remain contraindications to HBOT:

1. Presence of a hollow orbital prosthesis. Individuals who have had an eye removed typically have a prosthesis placed in the orbit. There are reports of pressure-induced collapses of hollow silicone orbital implants at depths as shallow as 10 feet (Isenberg 1985). Most ocular implants used presently, however, are not hollow and should not be considered a contraindication to diving or HBOT. A hollow orbital prosthesis is a relative contraindication and should not prevent HBOT required to preserve life, neurological function, or vision in the fellow eye (Butler 2008).

2. Presence of an intraocular gas bubble. Intraocular gas is used in selected cases by vitreoretinal surgeons as a means to maintain juxtaposition of the retina to the retinal pigment epithelium and by anterior segment surgeons to maintain juxtaposition of Descemet's membrane to the posterior corneal stroma. Gas in the eye may result in intraocular barotrauma during compression or a CRAO during decompression and is a contraindication to exposure to changes in ambient pressure (Butler 2007). Intraocular gas bubbles expand even with the relatively small decreases in ambient pressure entailed in commercial air travel (Kokame 1994, Mills 2001). This expansion causes an increase in intraocular pressure (Kokame 1994, Lincoff 1989) and may cause sudden blindness at altitude due to a pressure-induced closure of the central retinal artery (Kokame 1994, Polk 2002). Jackman has shown that intraocular bubbles in a rabbit model result in a dramatic decrease in intraocular pressure during compression followed by a marked increase in intraocular pressure upon return to one atmosphere as the bubble expands (Jackman 1995).

One important exception to the rule of intraocular gas bubbles contraindicating HBOT is gas bubbles in the eye that may occur as a manifestation of decompression sickness. Recompression and HBOT should be undertaken in this instance with the expectation that the normal volume of the anterior chamber, posterior chamber, and vitreous prior to the formation of the gas bubble due to inert gas supersaturation will prevent compression barotrauma. Resolution of the intraocular bubbles and inert gas supersaturation during HBOT would be expected to prevent an expanding gas phase on decompression and a secondary rise in intraocular pressure.

Intraocular gas bubbles may also be present with intraocular gas gangrene. HBOT is recommended for this disorder as well, although the bubble dynamics during HBOT might be different in this instance from those seen with inert gas supersaturation (Butler 2008).

Pre-HBOT Ocular Examination

If HBOT is indicated on an emergent basis for an ocular indication for HBOT, such as central retinal artery occlusion (CRAO), DCS, or arterial gas embolism (AGE), delays for ophthalmic consultation and detailed eye examination may result in worsening of the patient's clinical condition and are not indicated. Visual function should be quantified in an expedited manner while awaiting recompression using rapidly performed measures such as emergency department visual acuity charts, color vision plates, Amsler grids, near-vision cards, ability to read printed material, and confrontation visual fields. Some of these methods may also be used to follow visual function inside the chamber during HBOT should it be a multiplace facility. Some may be useful even through the window of a monoplace chamber as well.

If ocular signs or symptoms were part of the indication for HBOT, an eye examination by an ophthalmologist as outlined above should be conducted as soon as feasible after recompression (Butler 2008).

HBO in the Treatment of Diseases of the Eye

The authors can recommend without reservation that HBOT be used for the indications listed in the primary indications section of Table 32.1. The evidence is less strong yet promising for the indications listed under secondary indications. The indications listed in the last section may have a theoretical basis for efficacy of HBOT but have the weakest level of evidence to support their use.

Recommended Indications

Discussions of decompression sickness with ocular signs and symptoms, arterial gas embolism with ocular signs and symptoms, ocular gas gangrene, necrotizing soft tissue and fungal infections involving the orbit/periorbital tissues, carbon monoxide poisoning with visual sequelae, radiation optic neuropathy, and compromised periorbital skin grafts and flaps will be covered in those individual chapters.

Central Retinal Artery Occlusion

The visual outcome of arterial occlusive diseases of the retina depends on the vessel occluded as well as the degree and

---

Table 32.1
Conditions in Ophthalmology

Recommended indications
- Decompression sickness with ocular signs and symptoms
- Arterial gas embolism with ocular signs and symptoms
- Central retinal artery occlusion
- Ocular Gas Gangrene
- Necrotizing soft tissue and fungal infections involving the orbit/periorbital tissues
- Carbon monoxide poisoning with visual sequelae
- Radiation optic neuropathy
- Compromised periorbital skin grafts and flaps
- Scleral ischemia or necrosis

Potential indications
- Anterior segment ischemia (especially post-operative)
- Ischemic optic neuropathy
- Ischemic Central Retinal Vein Occlusion
- Branch Retinal Artery Occlusion (esp with central visual loss)
- Cystoid Macular Edema with Central Retinal Vein Occlusion
- Cystoid Macular Edema with Post-surgical Inflammation
- Cystoid Macular Edema with intrinsic inflammatory Disorders
- Refractory Pseudomonas keratitis
- Pyoderma gangrenosum of the orbit

Other reported uses
- Toxic Amylopia (eg. Quinine toxicity)
- Retinitis Pigmentosa
- Macular Hole Surgery
- Diabetic retinopathy
- Uveitis
- Keratoendotheliosis
- Sickle cell hyphema
- Retinal detachment (includ. associated sickle cell disease)
- Glaucoma

---

location of the occlusion. The type of occlusion (thrombosis, embolus, arteritis, or vasospasm) may also affect the outcome (Hayreh 2005, Stone 1977). The classic presentation of CRAO is sudden painless loss of vision in the range of light perception to counting fingers. Vision at the "no light perception" level usually indicates an occlusion at the level of the ophthalmic artery with a resulting absence of blood flow to either the retinal or the choroidal circulation (Regillo 2007). On dilated fundoscopic exam, patients with CRAO will display a whitish appearance of the macula due to the opaque and edematous nerve fiber and ganglion cell layers. A cherry red spot is often present in the fovea, but this finding may be absent, especially when there is an occlusion of the ophthalmic artery. Cilioretinal arteries are part of the ciliary (not retinal) arterial supply and supply the area of the retina around the macula (central vision area.) If a cilioretinal artery is present, central vision may be preserved in the presence of a CRAO, but the peripheral visual fields are typically severely decreased (Butler 2008).

In the largest published series of CRAO patients, Hayreh describes the outcome of this condition without HBOT. He found that patients with cilioretinal arteries had much better visual outcomes than those who did not. In those patients without cilioretinal arteries, 80% had a final visual outcome of count fingers or less and only 1.5% of individuals obtained a final vision of 20/40 or better (Hayreh 2005).

Natural spontaneous recanalization eventually takes place after CRAO (Duker 1988, David 1967). In relatively few cases, however, does this reperfusion lead to an improvement of vision, presumably because the retinal tissue has been irreversibly damaged during the ischemic period (Duker 1988). The retina has the highest rate of oxygen consumption of any organ in the body at 13 ml/100 g/min and is therefore very sensitive to ischemia (Hertzog 1992).

As with oxygen administration at one ATA, HBOT must be started within the time interval that retinal tissue can still recover. There is a point beyond which ischemic tissue can no longer recover even if reperfusion occurs (Li 1996). Hayreh et al occluded the ophthalmic artery of rhesus monkeys for varying periods of time. Retinas that went more than 105 minutes without blood flow showed permanent damage. If the duration of occlusion was less than 97 minutes, the retinas recovered their normal function (Hayreh 1980). Treatment of CRAO should be aimed at promptly supplying oxygen to the ischemic retina at a partial pressure sufficient to maintain inner retinal viability until restoration of central retinal artery blood flow occurs.

Traditional treatment regimens for CRAO have been aimed at promoting downstream movement of the embolus by lowering intraocular pressure and producing vasodilatation. These measures include ocular massage, anterior chamber paracentesis, intraocular pressure-lowering medications, carbogen, and aspirin (Regillo 2007, Hertzog 1992, Duker 1988, Stone 1977). These treatment modalities have been largely unsuccessful (Neubauer 2000, Duker 1988, Stone 1977). The American Academy of Ophthalmology Basic and Clinical Science Course states that "the efficacy of treatment is questionable" (Regillo 2007). More recently studied treatment modalities include thrombolytic agents (Petterson 2005, Weber 1998) and surgical removal or the embolus or thrombus (Garcia-Arumi 2006, Tang 2000). Hayreh stated recently that no currently used therapy is efficacious for CRAO (Hayreh 2005). Acute obstruction of the central retinal artery without HBOT typically results in severe, permanent visual loss (Hayreh 2005, Duker 1988).

Supplemental normobaric oxygen therapy may be successful in reversing retinal ischemia in CRAO. In order to be effective, the administration of supplemental oxygen must be continued until retinal arterial blood flow has resumed to a level sufficient to maintain inner retinal function under normoxic conditions. If ischemia and cellular hypoxia have resulted in cell death of the inner layers of the retina, vision will not return when blood flow is re-established (Mangat 1995).

Butler reported a patient who suffered acute loss of vision in his only seeing eye and presented approximately one hour after vision loss. His vision was 20/400 and he had fundus findings of a CRAO. He was treated with oxygen administered by reservoir mask at one atmosphere in the emergency department and his vision quickly improved to 20/25. After approximately 5 minutes, the supplemental oxygen was discontinued, whereupon vision equally quickly returned to 20/400. This process was repeated several times to confirm the beneficial effect of the supplemental oxygen with the same results. The patient was then hospitalized, anticoagulated, and maintained on supplemental oxygen for approximately 18 hours, after which time his central retinal artery presumably recanalized, because at this point removal of the supplemental oxygen no longer caused a decrease in vision. He was discharged with a visual acuity of 20/25 in his only seeing eye (Butler 2007). In similar cases, Patz reported improvement in two CRAO patients given oxygen at 1 ATA. One patient received oxygen after a four-hour delay to therapy and improvement from 4/200 to 20/70 was maintained after supplemental oxygen therapy was discontinued 4 hours later. The second patient improved from no light perception to 20/200 after a delay to treatment of 90 minutes and maintained this improvement when oxygen was discontinued 3 hours later. In both patients, early discontinuation of oxygen was followed by deterioration of vision within minutes. Improved vision was restored when oxygen breathing was resumed shortly thereafter. This phenomenon was observed several times in both patients (Patz 1955).

The study published by Augsberger and Magargal in 1980 emphasized the importance of prompt oxygen treatment to successful outcome. They used paracentesis, ocular massage, carbogen (95% oxygen and 5% CO_2), acetazolamide, and aspirin to treat 34 consecutive cases of CRAO. Twelve of the 34 patients were successfully treated, with 7 of the 12 having been treated within 24 hours of onset of symptoms. The longest delay to treatment after which treatment was considered successful was 72 hours. The average delay to therapy in the patients with successful outcomes was 21.1 hours, compared to 58.6 hours in those who did not improve. Carbogen inhalation was conducted for 10 minutes every hour during waking hours and 10 minutes every 4 hours at night and continued for 48-72 hours (Augsberger 1980).

Stone et al reported two patients with CRAO of greater than 6 hours duration treated with intermittent carbogen at one ATA, retrobulbar anesthesia, and anterior chamber paracentesis. The first patient had vision loss of 6 hours duration. His vision improved from hand motion to 20/20 on the above therapy, with carbogen being administered for 10 minutes every hour. The second patient presented 8 hours after onset of visual loss and had improvement from finger counting to 20/25. Carbogen was administered 10 minutes every hour for 48 hours (Stone 1977).

Carbon dioxide is added to the oxygen in carbogen for its vasodilatory effect in an effort to counter hyperoxic vasoconstriction. If the mechanism of improved oxygenation to the retina is diffusion from the choroidal circulation; however, then the addition of carbon dioxide should not be required to improve oxygenation. Unlike retinal blood flow, choroidal blood flow is not significantly affected by changes in oxygen tension (Yu 2005, Li 1996).

Another case report described a patient with angiographically documented obstruction of both the central retinal artery and his temporal posterior ciliary artery (Duker 1988). He presented after 5 hours of visual loss with minimal light perception vision. In addition to ocular massage, anterior chamber paracentesis, timolol, and acetazolamide, he was given carbogen for 10 minutes every hour around the clock. His vision did not improve significantly during his three days of hospitalization, but improved spontaneously approximately 96 hours after onset of vision loss. Vision in the affected eye was documented to be 20/30 one week after discharge. Although the authors of this case report do not necessarily ascribe his recovery to any one of treatments used, the role of supplemental oxygen in maintaining retinal viability until spontaneous recanalization occurred must be considered, since only rarely do patients with CRAO have a spontaneous improvement in vision (Duker 1988).

Supplemental oxygen at one atmosphere may not successfully preserve retinal function in CRAO. This intervention did not reliably prevent inner retinal hypoxia in a rat model when the retinal circulation was occluded by laser photocoagulation (Yu 2007). If normobaric supplemental oxygen is not successful in restoring vision in a CRAO patient, emergent HBOT should be considered.

HBOT has been successful when normobaric hyperoxia has failed to restore vision in CRAO. Phillips reported a 71-year-old white female patient with CRAO in whom surface oxygen was ineffective in reversing "total vision loss" of approximately 2 hours duration (Phillips 1999). The patient was then compressed to 2.8 ATA breathing 100% oxygen on a U.S. Navy Treatment Table 6. As she passed 15 feet during her descent, light perception was restored and at the end of her first air break at 2.8 ATA, she reported full return of vision. She was discharged with a visual acuity of 20/30 in her only seeing eye. A 2+ afferent papillary defect noted prior to treatment had resolved after treatment (Phillips 1999).

Treatment of CRAO should be aimed at promptly supplying oxygen to the ischemic retina at a partial pressure sufficient to maintain inner retinal viability until restoration of central retinal artery blood flow occurs. The ophthalmology literature includes cases in which patients with CRAO have regained significant vision even when treatment was delayed for periods of up to two weeks (Matsuo 2001) with the strongest evidence for symptomatic improvement in cases with less than 12 hours of delay (Wein-

berger 2003, Li 1996, Yotsukura 1993, Beiran 1993, Hertzog 1992). In the clinical setting of CRAO, residual retinal arterial blood flow may be detected by fluorescein angiogram (Augsberger 1980, David 1967). This may help to explain the great variability in visual outcome observed with different time delays until treatment. The studies by Hayreh quoted above that noted irreversible retinal damage after 105 minutes entailed complete occlusion of the ophthalmic artery, the most severe model of ocular vascular occlusion and one that may not be frequently encountered in the clinical setting.

Papers that discuss treatment options for CRAO patients with duration of symptoms of several weeks or longer would be expected to have a minimal chance of improvement, yet there are some patients who are reported to improve even after this prolonged time interval, although details of the level of improvement were limited in this study (Hirayama 1990).

Murphy-Lavoie et al. (2004) reviewed the records of 16 patients treated with HBOT for CRAO (2.0 ATA of oxygen 90 minutes twice daily for 2–3 days, then once daily until reaching clinical plateau. Eleven of the 16 showed improvement with HBOT. Four of the five patients who showed no improvement had a delay to presentation of more than 24 hours (Murphy-Lavoie, 2004).

Hertzog reported a series of 17 patients with CRAO treated with HBOT. They retrospectively divided patients into four treatment groups based on the time from symptom onset to HBOT and noted that HBOT seemed useful in preserving visual function when applied within 8 hours from the onset of visual impairment. The patients in this study were treated with 105 minutes of oxygen at 2.0 ATA three times a day until they ceased to show improvement in visual acuity, or for 3–4 days if no improvement occurred, receiving a mean of 29.3 hours of HBOT early in the study and 34.6 hours later in the study. The authors point out that the phrase "time is muscle" used in management of myocardial infarctions can be changed to "time is vision" in CRAO (Hertzog 1992). Takeuchi reported a patient with central retinal artery occlusion occurring after a long surgical procedure to fuse the lumbar spine. Immediate treatment with urokinase, PGE1, stellate ganglion block, and HBOT resulted in improvement of the affected eye (Takeuchi 2001).

In 2001, Beiran published a retrospective study of 35 patients treated with HBOT compared to 37 matched controls from another facility where hyperbaric oxygen was not available (Beiran 2001). All patients were treated within 8 hours of symptom onset and none of the patients included in the trial had a cilioretinal artery. The patients in the hyperbaric group received oxygen at 2.8 ATA for 90 minutes twice a day for the first three days and then once daily until no further improvement was seen for 3 consecutive days. In the hyperbaric group, 82% of the patients improved compared to only 29.7% of patients in the control group. Improvement was

Table 32.2
Treatment of Retinal Artery Occlusions: Literature Summary

Authors and year	CRAO/BRAO	Therapy	Delay to Tx	Initial VA	Final VA	Total Patients (n)	Cases Improved (n)
Gool & Jong 1965 (36)	BRAO CRAO CRAO BRAO	HBOT: 3 ATA, anticoagulants, Complamin	5 days 2 days Unknown (< 24 h) 10 days	1.5% nil 125% 1.6%	100% nil 125% imp VF 1.6%	4	2
Haddad & Leopold 1965 (28)	CRAO	HBOT	Unknown	NLP CF	NLP CF	2	0
Anderson et al 1965 (13)	BRAO CRAO BRAO	HBOT, Retrobulbar lidocaine, ocular massage, nicotinic acid	"several hours" 40+ h 6+ days	CF 2–3 ft 20/25 20/200	20/20 20/25 imp VF Unknown	3	2
Takahashi et al 1977 (37)		HBOT: 2.5 ATA Ocular Massage Paracentesis Vasodilator	1–6 days	Graph	Graph	9	9
Pallota et al 1978 (38)	CRAO	HBOT: 2.8 ATA		NLP	10/10	1	1
Sasaki et al 1978 (39)	CRAO	HBOT, Stellate ganglion block				10	7
Szuki et al 1980 (40)	CRAO	HBOT				6	6
Krasnov et al 1981 (41)	CRAO	HBOT				39	22
Zhang & Cao 1986 (42)	CRAO	HBOT				80	49
Desola 1987 (43)	CRAO	HBOT				20	11
Miyake et al 1987 (15)	CRAO (53) BRAO (19)	HBOT @ 2ATA or 3ATA, varied vasodilators, stellate ganglion block, 2% carbocaine	18 h to 15 days, all but 3 within 12 days	Graph	Graph	72	32
Kindwall & Goldmann 1988 (44)	CRAO	HBOT				14	7
Hirayama et al 1990 (48)	CRAO	HBOT; mixtures of urokinase, steroid, bifemelane HCL	< 1 month	Graph	Graph	11	15
Hertzog et al 1992 (8)	CRAO	HBOT: 1.5–2.0 ATA; mixtures of Timolol maleate 0.5%, acetazolamide, paracentesis, carbogen, vasodilator, steroids, ocular massage, retrobulbar anesthesia	< 8 h > 8, ≥ 24 h > 24 h All patients	Graph	Graph	19	14
Beiran et al 1993 (32)	CRAO	HBOT: 2.5 ATA, ocular massage, SL nifedipine, oral glycerol	2: < 100 min 1: occluding 1: 6 h	LP HM CF 2 m HM	6/20 6/6 6/9 CF 60 cm	4	4
Yotsukura et al 1993 (16)	CRAO	HBOT, ocular massage, IV urokinase, & 2/15 with IV prostaglandin	3 h to 6 days	Graph	Graph	15	8
Li et al 1996 (3)	BRAO OS BRAO OD (15 months later)	HBOT: 2.32 ATA HBOT: 2.82 ATA	< 24 h < 24 h	20/200 CF 2ft	20/25 20/25	2	2
Phillips et al 1999 (30)	CRAO	100% surface O2 HBOT: 2.4 ATA	< 2 h	NLP	20/30	1	1
Aisenbrey et al 2000 (45)	CRAO (8) BRAO (10)	HBOT: 240kPa, ocular massage, paracentesis, IV acetazolamide		Graph	Graph	18	12

Authors and year	CRAO/BRAO	Therapy	Delay to Tx	Initial VA	Final VA	Total Patients (n)	Cases Improved (n)
Matsuo 2001 (34)	BRAO (OU)	HBOT, IV prostaglandin, urokinase	4 days	20/30 20/600	20/15 20/400	2	2
Beiran et al 2001 (33)	CRAO (29) BRAO (6)	HBOT: 2.8 ATA; mixtures of ocular massage, retrobulbar block, timolol, acetazolamide, paracentesis	< 8 h	Graph	Graph	35	29
Weinberger et al 2002 (46)	CRAO	HBOT, ocular massage, antiglaucoma eyedrops	4–12 h	Graph	Graph	21	13
Murphy-Lavoie et al 2004 (12)	CRAO BRAO	HBOT: 2.0 ATA	6 h–4 days	Graph	Graph	16	12
Imai et al 2004 (47)	BRAO	HBOT, stellate ganglion block	2 days	CF	0.08	1	1
TOTAL						405	261
% IMPROVED							65%

Note: see full graphs of patient results in original papers.

defined as reading at least three lines better on Snellen chart compared to admission. The mean visual acuity for the hyperbaric group at discharge was 20/70 (Beiran 2001).

Reports that describe failure of HBOT in CRAO sometimes fail to even note the elapsed time from symptom onset to HBOT (Haddad 1965) and HBOT in these cases may have been started well after the time window for successful treatment had passed. Miyake reported on 53 cases of CRAO and 19 branch retinal artery occlusions treated with HBOT over a 13-year period. He found no significant difference between time to treatment and response to HBOT; however, only 3 of these patients received HBOT within 24 hours of symptom onset, which places most of his patients outside the time window in which improvement from HBOT is most likely to occur. Overall 44% of his patients showed improvement of at least two levels on the visual acuity scale after treatment with HBOT despite this delay to treatment. Unfortunately, no distinction was made between patients with cilioretinal arteries and those without (Miyake 1987).

Failure of HBOT has been reported in one case of CRAO in which there was angiographic documentation of a complete obstruction of the involved ophthalmic artery. There must be an intact choroidal circulation for HBOT to reverse the vision loss in CRAO (Mori 2007).

The case series and case reports noted above document that some patients with CRAO can be treated successfully with hyperoxia, either at 1 ATA or with HBOT. HBOT is a low-risk therapeutic option with demonstrated good results in treating CRAO if treatment is begun prior to the retina suffering irreversible ischemic damage and there is an intact choroidal circulation. There are no alternative therapies with similarly favorable outcomes (Hayreh 2005, Neubauer 2000, Hayreh 1982).

The devastating vision loss that CRAO entails when left untreated calls for an aggressive approach to employing HBOT for this disorder. Triage nurses should be aware that sudden painless loss of vision of less than 24 hours duration is an emergency that requires immediate attention. Patients with documented or suspected CRAO of less than 24 hours duration should receive supplemental oxygen at the highest fraction attainable immediately (Murphy-Lavoie in press, Butler 2007, Duker 1988, Perkins 1987, Augsberger 1980, Stone 1977, Patz 1955). Emergency HBOT should be undertaken if this intervention is not rapidly effective in improving vision. The patient should be maintained on supplemental oxygen at the highest possible FIO2 until HBOT is begun, and then treated with the step-wise protocol outlined in "emergency HBOT for acute vision loss" (Table 32.3). Ocular massage and topical ocular hypotensive agents may also be employed as adjuncts. While there are some case reports of patients presenting after 24 hours from onset of vision loss obtaining benefit from HBOT, the majority of cases do not respond when treated beyond this point (Butler 2008, Murphy-Lavoie 2004, Yotsukura 1993, Hertzog 1992, Miyake 1987, Augsberger 1980, Anderson 1965b).

Reports of treatment of CRAO by HBO are summarized in Table 32.2.

Potential Indications

Scleral Necrosis

Pterygium is an actinic condition in which an area of fibrotic tissue extends from the conjunctiva onto the cornea. The disorder is often progressive and may cause ocular discomfort, cosmetic issues, and interference with vision if it is allowed to extend into the visual axis. Pterygium surgery has a recurrence rate as high as 46% unless preventive measures are incorporated into the surgical excision (Sebban 1990). Preventive measures include beta irradiation, cauterization, topical steroids, thiotepa, mitomycin-C, and conjunctival autograft (Bayer 2002). Irradiation may result in a small-vessel obliterative endarteritis followed by tissue ischemia and fibrosis. Scleral necrosis is a potentially blinding complication of both beta irradiation and mitomycin-C therapy, since the necrosis may lead to perforation of the globe and endophthalmitis with devastating visual consequences (Butler 2008).

Adjunctive HBOT has been shown to reverse this process. One paper reported a patient who developed severe scleral necrosis following pterygium surgery and beta radiation and who was not responding to conventional therapy that included topical antibiotics, topical steroids, lubricants, and patching. HBOT (2 ATA for 90 minutes daily × 14 days) was employed and resulted in marked improvement, first noted after four treatments. The patient went on to make a complete recovery (Green 1995). Mitomycin-C may also induce a similar condition and another case report noted that a patient who developed scleral necrosis after mitomycin-C and had likewise deteriorated on conventional therapy was given HBOT (2.5 ATA for 90 minutes daily × 24 days) made a remarkable recovery with improvement noted after day 5 (Bayer 2002).

This section reviews ocular indications for HBOT for which a strong physiological basis for the usefulness of HBOT exists and/or for which case reports have been published documenting success with HBOT in managing these disorders. As noted previously, although rapid return of vision is a valuable indicator of efficacy when treating ocular disorders with HBOT, the failure of vision to normalize rapidly does not necessarily indicate a lack of success, especially in disorders such as central retinal vein occlusion and branch retinal vein occlusion, where macular hemorrhage may prevent immediate return of vision.

Postoperative Anterior Segment Ischemia

Strabismus surgery entails detaching selected extraocular muscles from the globe and re-attaching them in a slightly different location to improve the alignment of the eyes. Anterior segment ischemia (ASI) is an uncommon but potentially serious complication of this surgery. It is seen in approximately 1 out of every 13,000 strabismus operations (de Smet 1987). Blood supply to the anterior segment of the eye is provided by the long posterior ciliary arteries (approximately 30%) and the anterior ciliary arteries which travel anteriorly in the rectus muscles (approximately 70%) (Saunders 1994). ASI results from the anterior ciliary vessels being disrupted as the extraocular muscles are surgically detached and repositioned. The first pathological specimen diagnosed with ASI was obtained in 1954 from a 76-year-old

male who developed a blind, painful eye after retinal detachment surgery in which the lateral rectus muscle was disinserted. The changes seen on histology were consistent with ischemic damage (Saunders 1994). ASI is typically seen when three or more extraocular muscles are operated on in the same procedure, but may occur with two-muscle surgery (Murdock 2001). Children have virtually no risk of developing this complication, while adults with cardiovascular disease are at higher risk (Saunders 1994).

Patients with ASI present with pain and decreased vision several days after their surgery. Eye examination may reveal striate keratopathy, iris atrophy, immobile pupil, posterior synechiae, cataract, and anterior uveitis with cells and flare in the anterior chamber (Saunders 1994, Pfister 1991).

Systemic and topical steroids are used to treat ASI. Most patients have good recovery of visual acuity with steroid therapy. Cycloplegics are often used to decrease the pain of ciliary spasm that may accompany ASI (Murdock 2001, Saunders 1994). Performing strabismus surgery in stages, so that collateral circulation has a chance to develop between surgeries, may help to prevent ASI; using botulinum toxin as an alternative or adjunct to rectus muscle surgery for strabismus is also an effective preventive measure (Saunders 1994).

HBOT has been shown to increase the oxygen tension in the anterior chamber (Jampol 1987) and therefore has promise as a way to treat anterior segment ischemia. In a 1987 paper, believed by the authors to be the first report of the use of HBOT to treat anterior segment ischemia, de Smet and his colleagues noted that HBOT (2.5 ATA O_2 for 90 minutes a day, delivered with 5-minute air breaks after each 30 minutes, for 7 days) was successful in treating a patient who presented with anterior segment ischemia. Systemic steroids were withheld from this individual because of a history of tuberculosis (de Smet 1987). HBOT may be a good option for individuals with severe ASI that does not respond to steroids or for individuals in whom steroids are contraindicated (Butler 2008).

Ischemic Optic Neuropathy

Nonarteritic ischemic optic neuropathy (NAION) is one of the most widespread visually disabling diseases in the middle-aged and elderly population (Hayreh 2008, Matthews 2005, Olver 1990). It typically presents as acute unilateral vision loss affecting patients over 50 years of age. It is characterized by optic disk edema, disk margin hemorrhages, and altitudinal visual field loss in which the inferior field is preferentially affected. This pattern of injury is related to the blood supply to the laminar and retrolaminar optic nerve, which is derived from the short posterior ciliary arteries via the circle of Haller and Zinn, which also has contributions from the choroidal vessels (Olver 1990). Most of the blood supply for the prelaminar region of the optic nerve head comes from the short posterior ciliary arteries rather than the peripapillary choroid (Olver 1990) NAION typically results from perfusion insufficiency in the short posterior ciliary arteries leading to infarction of the retro-laminar portion of the optic nerve.

Risk factors for NAION include hypertension, diabetes, nocturnal hypotension, and a small-cup-to-disc ratio (Desai 2005). It has also been associated with the use of erectile dysfunction medications (Hayreh 2007). The fellow eye of NAION patients is often sequentially affected. Involvement of the second eye occurs within 3 years in approximately 43% of NAION patients.

Treatments employed in the past for NAION have included optic nerve sheath decompression, high-dose steroids, levodopa, carbidopa, and neuroprotective agents, without any of these modalities being reliably effective to date (Matthews 2005, Desai 2005, Arnold 1996).

The potential for oxygenation of the optic nerve from choroidal branches of the Circle of Haller and Zinn offers a theoretical basis for the efficacy of HBOT in NAION. Reducing intra-axonal optic nerve ischemia and its resultant edema may also interrupt the cycle of microvascular compromise that is thought to occur within the structurally crowded optic disks of patients with NAION (Arnold 1996).

One study reported two NAION patients treated with HBOT (2 ATA for 90 minutes once a day for 18 sessions) and noted improvement in both vision and visual field (Bojic 2002). HBOT was undertaken 3–5 months after the onset of symptoms. The same author had previously published a case series that documented the results of HBOT (2.8 ATA oxygen for 60 minutes twice a day for the first three patients, then 2.0 ATA oxygen for 90 minutes daily for the remaining patients for a total of 14–30 sessions) in nine patients with NAION who had previously been unsuccessfully treated with steroids. He noted that four patients with optic disc atrophy (a sign of long-standing disease) had no improvement with HBOT while 5 other patients without optic atrophy had marked improvement in visual acuity and/or visual field at 6-month follow-up. The time between the onset of symptoms and the initial HBOT session ranged from 21 to 84 days (Bojic 1994). A third study from the same first author documented a series of 21 patients (with some overlap from the previous papers) in which 11 control patients were treated with corticosteroids, while the study group received steroids but also got HBOT (2.8 ATA O_2 for 60 minutes twice a day for the first three patients, then 2.0 ATA O_2 for 90 minutes daily for the remaining patients for a total of 14–30 sessions). The time between the onset of symptoms and the initial HBOT session ranged from 7 to 84 days. Six of the ten HBOT patients experienced a marked improvement in visual function, and all of these patients save one had continuation of this benefit at 6-month follow-up. The authors note that spontaneous improvement in NAION is unusual. Patients with optic atrophy obtained no benefit from HBOT, while those in whom optic atrophy was not evident did display improvement (Bojic 1995).

HBOT was used in a 66-year-old woman who presented with a 4-day loss of vision OD. Presenting vision was finger-counting in that eye. She had lost vision in her left eye 3 months previously from an episode of NAION. Fundus examination showed the disk edema and disk margin hemorrhages of NAION. She was treated with HBOT (2.5 ATA oxygen for 90 minutes × 5 sessions). Vision improved from finger counting to 6/24 after the second session. No further improvement in vision was observed in the 3 subsequent HBOT sessions, but this improvement remained stable over one year of follow-up. The authors note that (1) visual acuity OD before treatment was declining and that this decline stopped and vision began to improve immediately after starting HBOT; (2) final vision was definitely better in the treated eye that in the untreated fellow eye; and (3) the patient was legally blind when she entered the chamber, but was not when she left (Beiran 1995).

Arnold reported that 22 eyes of 20 patients with NAION treated with hyperbaric oxygen (2.0 ATA for 90 minutes twice a day for 10 days) had no beneficial effect compared to 27 untreated controls. Patients were included in this study if they presented within 21 days after their onset of visual loss. The authors' earliest treatment break-out group in these studies was 9 days or less from onset of symptoms and they noted that treatment initiated within 72 hours might have been more effective (Arnold 2002, Arnold 1996).

Arterial hypotension associated with blood loss during surgery and hemodialysis may also cause ischemic optic neuropathy. Hemodialysis is occasionally associated with dramatic unilateral or bilateral visual loss (Keynan 2006, Wells 2004). The etiology of the visual loss in hemodialysis is believed to be hypotension-induced NAION (Cuxart 2005, Wells 2004, Buono 2003), but other reported etiologies for visual loss in this setting include cerebral infarction (Wells 2004), a Purtscher's type retinopathy (Arora 1991), and posterior ischemic optic neuropathy (Buono 2003). HBOT has been associated with immediate and dramatic return of vision to baseline in a patient who suffered bilateral blindness during hemodialysis. The authors emphasize that early HBOT should be considered for acute visual loss during or immediately after hemodialysis (Keynan 2006).

Some 15% of individuals with NAION have been reported to suffer an attack on NAION in their fellow eye during 5-year follow-up (Newman 2002). Because of the significant potential for NAION to occur in the second eyes of individuals who have already lost vision in the first eye due to this disorder, these patients should be warned to be alert for any decrease in vision in the second eye so that they can seek medical attention promptly and HBOT can be employed in an effort to prevent permanent vision loss.

Arteritic ischemic optic neuropathy (AION) is a related disorder characterized by ischemic damage to the optic nerve associated with giant cell arteritis. The visual loss in this disorder is typically more severe and immediate treatment with high-dose systemic steroids is required to prevent a high percentage of vision loss from occurring in the fellow eye shortly after the index eye (Hayreh 2003b, Hayreh 1998). Long-term tapering and maintenance steroid administration is required to prevent recurrence (Hayreh 2003b). No reports were found of HBOT being employed in AION, but there is a theoretical basis for efficacy in this type of ischemic optic neuropathy as well (Butler 2008).

Ischemic Central Retinal Vein Occlusion

Central retinal vein occlusion (CRVO) is a relatively common cause of visual loss. Ischemic CRVO with neovascular glaucoma is the single most common cause of surgical removal of the eye in North America (Boyd 2002). Risk factors for this disorder include glaucoma, older age, male gender, systemic vascular disorders, and hyperviscosity syndromes such as multiple myeloma (Glacet-Bernard 1996). CRVO may also be seen, however, in young adults with no known systemic disease or ocular problems (Fong 1993). The hallmarks of CRVO are four-quadrant retinal hemorrhage and distended retinal veins. An afferent pupillary defect and severe vision loss are typical of the ischemic variety of CRVO.

Vision loss in CRVO may result from macular ischemia, the development of persistent macular edema, and neovascular glaucoma (Mohamed 2007). A complicating factor in discussing treatment for CRVO is the need to determine whether one is dealing with ischemic or nonischemic CRVO. Making this determination may be a clinical challenge, but is crucial because the two entities have significantly different natural histories and outcomes. Nonischemic CRVO does not cause neovascularization and typically has a more benign course, with final visual acuity dependent primarily on the presence and degree of macular edema. Two-thirds of patients with nonischemic CRVO have final visual acuities of 20/40 or better with no treatment. Some eyes with nonischemic CRVO, however, may progress to ischemic CRVO (Hayreh 2003a, Glacet-Bernard 1996). 54% of initially nonischemic CRVO eyes were reported in one paper to subsequently develop retinal ischemia (Glacet-Bernard 1996). With ischemic CRVO, there is permanent ischemic damage to the macular ganglion cells, so there is little chance of improvement in visual acuity (Hayreh 2003a). There is also a significant risk of anterior segment neovascularization, with neovascular glaucoma resulting in 40–50% of cases (Hayreh 2003a). Differentiation between ischemic and nonischemic CRVO may be more difficult than the application of the commonly used criteria of 10 disk diameters of retinal nonperfusion on IVFA (Hayreh 2003a). The degree of macular ischemia has been found to be a more significant factor affecting the outcome of retinal venous occlusion than macular edema (Miyamoto 1995). It is important to differentiate ischemic from nonischemic CRVO when considering invasive therapies such as radial optic neurotomy (Bhatt 2004).

The pathophysiology of CRVO is different in several important respects from CRAO. First, the obstruction of the CRV is chronic and is not characterized by the relatively early recanalization and restoration of blood flow seen in CRAO. Hayreh notes: "In both types of CRVO, the retinopathy spontaneously resolves after a variable period. There is marked inter-individual variation in the time that it takes to resolve; it is usually faster in younger than older people" (Hayreh 2003a). Secondly, the tissue hypoxia produced by CRVO often does not lead to rapid retinal cell death, as CRAO does. This allows the ischemic retinal cells to produce the vascular endothelial growth factors responsible for the neovascularization that is a feature of CRVO, but not typically CRAO. Third, the nonischemic version of CRVO does not produce macular ganglion cell death, but causes visual loss through macular edema.

The natural history of CRVO has been described by the CRVO Study Group. Visual acuity outcome was found to be largely dependent on visual acuity at presentation, with 65% of individuals presenting with VA 20/40 or better maintaining that level of acuity for the 3-year follow-up period. Individuals with vision 20/200 or less had an 80% chance of having vision at that level or worse at the end of the study. Patients with intermediate levels of visual acuity on presentation had a more variable outcome (CRVO Study Group 1997). This paper also noted that one-third of the eyes that were initially nonischemic CRVOs converted to ischemia in the course of the study.

Multiple interventions have been proposed for CRVO. Therapy is often aimed at preventing or reversing the neovascularization that can result in glaucoma, chronic eye pain, and loss of the eye (CRVO Study Group 1997). One study postulated that CRVO constitutes a neurovascular compartment syndrome at the site of the lamina cribosa and proposed relieving this pressure by performing a radial incision at the nasal part of the optic nerve head. The authors subsequently did 107 radial optic neurotomies and found that the majority of patients showed rapid normalization of the morphologic fundus findings, with an improvement in VA. The authors noted that surgery performed more than 90 days after the occlusion produced little improvement (Hasselbach 2007). Another paper studying this technique in 5 patients produced less successful results (Weizer 2003).

Other reports on the therapeutic options for CRVO have been less encouraging, especially with regard to reversing vision loss. Treatments employed in the management of CRVO have included anticoagulants, fibrinolytics, intravitreal corticosteroids, acetazolamide, isovolemic hemodilution, antivascular endothelial growth and angiostatic agents, panretinal photocoagulation (PRP), grid pattern photocoagulation, laser-induced chorioretinal anastamosis, and endovascular thrombolysis (Madhusudhana 2007, Mohamed 2007, Feltgen 2007, Shahid 2006, CRVO Study Group 1995). There have been several reports of success in treating CRVO with low-molecular weight heparin (Lee 2006) and the anti-VEGF agent bevacizumab (Spandau 2006, Boyd 2002).

None of the interventions described above will be useful in restoring vision if the retinal cells have already been irreversibly damaged by hypoxia prior to therapeutic intervention. The primary benefit of HBOT in ischemic CRVO, then, would be to maintain retinal viability while interventions to return normal retinal venous outflow are accomplished or spontaneous resumption of flow occurs, although the longer period required for spontaneous resumption of venous flow makes waiting for spontaneous resolution of the impaired retinal blood flow a more problematic choice than in CRAO.

Can HBOT reverse the acute retinal ischemia seen in ischemic CRVO? A recent case report in UHM described a 43-year-old male with CRVO. Onset of symptoms was two days before presentation. The authors describe the case as an ischemic CRVO with macular edema and retinal hemorrhages, although visual fields were reported to be normal. He was treated with HBOT at 2.4 ATA for 90 minutes on the day of presentation. Vision improved in the affected eye from 20/200 to 20/30 after the first two HBOT treatments. Vision was reported to gradually deteriorate in the time period after HBOT and then to improve again with the next treatment. This observation is an important one because it suggests that the acute administration of HBOT can reverse the retinal cell hypoxia caused by the venous infarct of CRVO, presumably because of the ability of oxygen to diffuse from the anatomically distinct choroidal circulation that is not affected by the retinal venous occlusion. Daily HBOT treatment was continued for 30 treatments, then treatment was decreased to 2–3 treatments per week for a total of 60 treatments. Final visual acuity was 20/20 in the affected eye, a remarkable outcome for ischemic CRVO (Wright 2007). Another report was of a USAF aircraft navigator who presented with a nonischemic CRVO that progressed to an ischemic CRVO. He was treated with HBOT early in the course of his disease with return of vision to normal. His vision was reported as being 20/17 two years later (Johnson 1990). Less favorable results using HBOT to treat CRVO were reported by Miyamoto, but there was no information available about the time interval after onset of the CRVO before HBOT was undertaken in these two studies (Miyamoto 1995, Miyamoto 1993). Gismondi and colleagues reported the use of HBOT to manage CRVO in 3 patients and concluded that it was a useful treatment modality for this disorder (Gismondi 1981). HBOT has been mentioned as one of the major therapeutic options in managing CRVO (Greiner 1999). Kiryu and Ogura (1996) reported 12 patients with macular edema in retinal vein occlusion who received HBO treatment. Median visual acuity improved from 20/100 to 20/25 ($p = 0.002$). Clinically significant improvement (2 lines or more) was achieved in 10 cases (83%). Evaluation of the inward permeability coefficient of the blood-retinal barrier using vitreous fluorophotometry showed no significant alteration in the permeability.

In summary, there is a strong theoretical basis for HBOT to be useful in managing ischemic CRVO and there are case reports documenting success with this treatment modality. As with CRAO, there is likely a time window beyond which HBOT is less effective, but this time window is not well-defined. HBOT may be most effective when used with other measures designed to expedite the restoration of venous outflow. The optimum HBOT treatment regimen for CRVO is not well defined, but both reversal of acute macular ischemia and prevention of neovascular complications from chronic retinal hypoxia should be considered, as should the possible beneficial effects of HBOT on eventual outcome even if visual acuity is not improving acutely because of macular hemorrhage. Outcome measures that should be considered in HBOT for ischemic CRVO should include as a minimum visual acuity, visual fields, and the impact of HBOT on the development of neovascularization and neovascular glaucoma. Although rapid return of vision is a valuable indicator of efficacy when treating ocular disorders with HBOT, the failure of vision to normalize rapidly does not necessarily indicate a lack of success. This is especially true in disorders such as CRVO, where macular hemorrhage may prevent immediate return of vision. If HBOT is effective in prevent hypoxic cell death, vision may improve when the hemorrhage resolves, as has been reported in the hypoxic vasculopathy of high-altitude retinal hemorrhages (Lang 1997).

The role of HBOT in nonischemic CRVO is less clear, considering the more favorable visual prospects in this entity even when untreated (Butler 2008).

Branch Retinal Artery Occlusion with Central Vision Loss

The presentation of branch retinal artery occlusion (BRAO) is more variable than that of CRAO. If the occluded artery does not supply the central or paracentral visual areas, the occlusion may be clinically silent. 24 of 30 patients with BRAO reported in one paper had visual acuities of 20/40 or better (Yuzurihara 2004). Another study noted that almost 90% of 201 patients with BRAO had visual acuities of 20/40 or better (Ros 1989). Even when visual acuity is not affected, however, there is typically a permanent visual field defect in the area served by the infarcted retina (Regillo 2007). Neovascular complications of BRAO are unusual but do occur (Yamamoto 2005).

BRAO is seen on ophthalmoscopy as a localized area of whitish opacified retina, although this may develop over the course of hours to days (Regillo 2007). The embolus causing the BRAO may be visible on examination.

Vision loss in BRAO may occasionally be severe. Mason reported a series of 5 patients with BRAO and severe loss of central vision. He used transluminal neodymium:YAG embolysis to disrupt the embolus and restore flow. All 5 patients had visual acuities ranging from 20/25 to 20/40 the first day after the procedure (Mason 2007).

If vision loss is severe, HBOT may also have a role in the management of this disorder, with many of the same considerations that applied to CRAO. HBOT must be applied before the affected retina has been irreversibly damaged to have any beneficial effect. A 67-year-old woman with rheumatoid arthritis presented with decreased vision in both eyes for 4 days. Visual acuity in the right eye was 20/30 and 20/600 in left. She was found to have an occlusion of the superotemporal branch of the retinal artery in both eyes. She was also noted to have arterial sheathing and large cotton-wool patches around both optic discs. IVFA findings were delayed filling of the superotemporal retinal artery in the right eye, no filling in the superotemporal artery in the left eye, and segmental absence of filling in peripheral branches of other major retinal arteries in both eyes. She was treated with HBOT, prostaglandin E1, and urokinase for 2 weeks and had improvement of her vision to the 20/15 level in the right eye and 20/300 in the left (Matsuo 2001).

Another case series reported 10 patients with BRAO who were treated with HBOT (30 minutes at 2.4 ATA for three sessions on the first day, twice a day on the second and third day, and once daily for at least another 4 days) in addition to ocular massage, paracentesis, and IV acetazolamide. The authors noted that HBOT seems to be beneficial for visual acuity in eyes with BRAO (Aisenbrey 2000).

In another report, a 32-year-old man with a rectal carcinoid and iron-deficiency anemia presented two days after the onset of vision loss. He was found to have a visual acuity of count-fingers in his left eye and fundus findings consistent with BRAO to include milky-white edema in the posterior pole except for the upper temporal area and a cherry-red spot at the fovea. He was treated with stellate ganglion block, HBOT, and ferrous sulfate, but vision improved only minimally (Imai 2004).

Cystoid Macular Edema (CME) Associated with Retinal Vein Occlusion

Cystoid macular edema (CME) is the cystic accumulation of fluid in the macula. Gass originally described CME as the leakage of fluid from perifoveal capillaries that was low in lipid and protein (Gass 1966) with secondary polycystic expansion of the extracellular spaces (Gass 1985). CME frequently complicates occlusion of a central or branch retinal vein. If the edema is severe or chronic, it may cause permanent visual loss and retinal damage (Coscas 1984). CME rates after retinal vein occlusions (RVO) of between 30 and 60% have been reported (Quinlan 1990, Gutman 1984, Coscas 1984, Hayreh 1983, Greer 1980). CME may result from retinal capillary engorgement in RVO with the increase in hydrostatic pressure driving fluid out of the retinal capillaries (Dick 2001) or from increased capillary permeability (Vinores 1997) or a combination of these two mechanisms.

CME patients typically present with decreased vision, metamorphosia (image distortion) or scotoma. Slit-lamp exam findings include loss of the foveal depression, retinal thickening and/or multiple cystoid spaces. Fluorescein angiographic examination in CME shows early foveal leakage with expansion and coalescence over time. In later phases, a "flower-petal" pattern of hyperfluorescence is seen as a result of the accumulation of dye within the cystoid spaces.

Multiple interventions have been attempted for the treatment of RVO-associated macular edema. Medical treatments have included the use of carbonic anhydrase inhibitors (CAI), anti-VEGF agents and topical or intravitreal steroids (Schaal 2007, Rabena 2007, Iturralde 2006, Tamura 2005, Rosenfeld 2005, Antonetti 2000, Gardner 1999, Nauck 1998a, Nauck 1998b, Cox 1988, Marmor 1982).

Intravitreal triamcinolone has been shown to improve vision in CME from BRVO and nonischemic CRVO (Park 2005, Jonas 2005, Ozkiris 2005, Avitabile 2005, Williamson 2005, Chen 2004, Bashshur 2004, Ip 2004, Greenberg 2002, Jonas 2002). However, in most cases the effect was not sustained and required repeat injections for recurrent edema. Potential complications of intravitreal steroid injections include an increase in intraocular pressure, cataract formation, endophthalmitis, injection-related vitreous hemorrhage and retinal detachment.

A surgical option for BRVO is pars plana vitrectomy (PPV) with lysis of the common adventitial sheath at the site of the affected crossing vessels, thereby relieving the venous compression and potentially reducing hydrostatic pressure and CME (Osterloh 1988). The ability of PPV with sheathotomy to improve visual acuity and CME after BRVO has been supported by other reports (Kumagai 2007, Mason 2004, Mester 2002, Shah 2000, Shah & Sharma 2000, Opremack 1999). There are also studies that question its efficacy (Cahill 2003, Le Rouic 2001). Yamamoto *et al* reported that both PPV and PPV with sheathotomy reduce CME and improve visual acuity but showed no statistical difference between the two forms of treatment (Yamamoto 1997).

Grid argon laser photocoagulation for CME after RVO is different from previously described PRP in that the laser spots are smaller and delivered with a lighter intensity only within the affected region. This therapy is thought to work by improving RPE barrier function (CRVO Study Group 1994) or reducing retinal ischemia (Molnar 1985). Significant side effects of grid laser treatment include paracentral scotoma and inadvertent treatment of the fovea with central vision loss.

The Central Retinal Vein Occlusion Study Group evaluated the effect of grid laser photocoagulation on visual acuity for patients with CME associated with ischemic or nonischemic CRVO. They reported angiographic reduction of the CME, but no improvement of visual acuity and therefore did not recommend grid laser treatment for CRVO patients (CRVO Study Group 1994).

The Branch Retinal Vein Occlusion Study Group found a benefit from grid laser photocoagulation in patients with BRVO of more than 3 months duration, macular edema and visual acuity of < 20/40 (BRVO Study Group 1984). Some additional reports have supported the efficacy of grid laser treatment for BRVO-associated macular edema (Blankenship 1973, Campbell 1973, Krill 1971), while others did not (Shilling 1984, Wetzig 1979). Grid laser photocoagulation is currently the only intervention for BRVO-associated macular edema that is supported by Level I evidence. Grid laser photocoagulation is not indicated for predominantly ischemic maculopathy after RVO (Tranos 2004, CRVO Study Group 1994). Miyamoto noted that the severity of macular ischemia better determines visual prognosis after HBOT than the degree of macular edema (Miyamoto 1995).

A number of reports have shown HBOT to be of benefit in RVO-associated CME (Jansen 2004, Krott 2000, Kiryu 1996, Miyamoto 1995, Miyake 1993, Miyamoto 1993, Mandai 1990, Ogura 1987). HBOT for BRVO-associated CME has been noted to have a more favorable outcome than for CRVO (Miyamoto 1995, Miyamoto 1993). In many reports, visual acuity has been noted to improve rapidly upon the initiation of HBOT, even when other treatment modalities were previously attempted (Jansen 2004, Krott 2000, Kiryu 1996, Miamoto 1995, Miamoto 1993, Miyake 1993, Ogura 1987). Some of these studies reported an improvement of foveal leakage on fluorescein angiogram that correlates to the visual improvement (Miamoto 1995, Miamoto 1993, Roy 1989, Ogura 1987), whereas others show improved visual acuity despite continued macular edema by IVFA testing (Miyake 1993, Xu 1991). Hyperoxic vasoconstriction may produce a decrease in RVO-associated CME through reduction of retinal blood flow and decreased retinal venous pressure. HBOT may also reduce the production of VEGF and thereby decrease retinal vascular permeability. Xu and Huang (1991) carried out a prospective study of the effect of HBO on 14 eyes with cystoid macular edema secondary to retinal vein occlusion. Visual acuity improved 2 to 6 lines (average 3.6) after HBO treatment while there was no improvement in the control group. There was no reduction of leakage from perifoveal capillaries or enhancement of vision prior to improvement of the fundus.

There are potential benefits of HBOT over grid laser photocoagulation. Laser treatment may cause a permanent scotomas and this therapy is not undertaken for 3 months after the RVO to avoid its potential complications in those patients who might spontaneously resolve. HBOT offers a relatively safe treatment option for the 3-month timeframe after disease onset and may be repeated if necessary without any permanent visual consequences. If no improvement has been noted with HBOT, grid laser could be added as an adjunct after three months has elapsed.

As with intravitreal injections of steroids and anti-VEGF agents, there are reports of CME recurrence after HBOT (Miyake 1993, Ishida 1989, Roy 1989), sometimes with vision regressing back to pre-treatment levels and at other times with only slight regression from the improved vision obtained after HBOT (Butler 2008).

Cystoid Macular Edema Associated with Postsurgical Inflammation

CME may complicate surgical procedures such as cataract extraction, Nd: YAG capsulotomy, and panretinal photocoagulation. CME occurs in approximately 1% of cataract extraction patients, but the incidence may be as high as 20% if the surgery is complication by posterior capsule rupture and vitreous loss (Tranos 2004).

Available therapy for postsurgical CME includes nonsteroidal anti-inflammatory agents (NSAIDs), carbonic anhydrase inhibitors, steroids (topical, intravitreal, and periocular), and immunomodulators (Tranos 2004).

HBOT may be a valuable adjunct to the management of patients whose CME does not respond to the above measures or in whom side effects have required discontinuation of therapy. Pfoff and Thom reported on five patients with chronic CME documented by decreased visual acuity to the 20/40 level or worse and findings consistent with CME on IVFA. All patients had undergone cataract extraction/IOL implantation 7–11 months prior to HBOT (2.2 ATA oxygen for 1.5 hours twice a day for 7 days, then 2 hours once a day for the next 14 days). All 5 patients showed significant improvement in visual acuity with only mild regression upon follow-up, whereas three control patients treated with prednisolone acetate and indomethacin drops did not improve over a 3-month treatment period (Pfoff 1987). The authors proposed that vasoconstriction of the perifoveal capillaries serves to bring the damaged endothelial junctional complexes closer together, allowing them to repair themselves and thereby prevent further leakage (Pfoff & Thom 1987).

Ishida et al reported 12 eyes of CME treated with HBOT (2 ATA O_2 for 60 minutes daily for 2–4 weeks). Eight of the cases resulted from BRVO and four from cataract surgery. Seven of the eyes had an improvement in vision as a result of the HBOT (Ishida 1989).

Cystoid Macular Edema Associated with Intrinsic Inflammatory Disorders

Intraocular inflammation may result from localized ocular disorders as well as in association with systemic inflammatory disorders (HLA-B27-associated inflammation, sarcoid, tuberculosis, Lyme disease). Chronic CME is the most common cause of significant visual loss in patients with intraocular inflammation. The pathogenesis of CME in uveitis is not completely understood, but may result from dysfunction of either the inner or the outer blood-eye barrier. Untreated uveitic CME tends to cause progressive injury to the macula (Coma 2007).

Treatment options for CME associated with intrinsic inflammatory disorders include the agents noted above for post-surgical CME (Coma 2007, Tranos 2004). Anti-VEGF agents have been used with success in this disorder. Five of 13 patients with uveitic CME refractory to other treatments treated with intravitreal bevacizumab had an improvement of vision of 2 or more lines (Coma 2007).

HBOT may be useful in this disorder as well. Miyake treated two patients with poor vision from CME; one was from a CRVO and the other from sarcoid uveitis. HBOT was administered at 2 ATA O_2 for 60 minutes and then 3 ATA for 60 minutes twice a day for 25 days. The author noted that (1) both patients improved markedly with HBOT; (2) both patients had recurrence of CME when HBOT was discontinued; (3) both patients also improved on acetazolamide therapy; and (4) the pattern of macular hyperfluorescence improved with acetazolamide, but not with HBOT, leading him to suggest that the two therapies had different mechanisms of action (Miyake 1993).

HBOT (2 ATA O_2 for 60 minutes daily × 14 to 17 days) was found to provide little lasting benefit in 11 eyes with CME secondary to uveitis, but it was noted that one individual with uveitis of recent onset obtained a sustained visual improvement from the HBOT (Okinami 1992).

HBOT (3 ATA oxygen for 75 minutes five times a week for 5 weeks) was used to treat a 46-year-old woman with bilateral posterior uveitis and vitritis. She had previously been treated with high-dose steroids, acetazolamide, cyclosporine, and grid laser therapy without success. Her vision prior to HBOT was 20/200 OD and 20/80 OS. HBOT resulted in visual improvement to 20/100 OD and 20/40 OS (Suttorp-Schulten 1997). Although the HBOT had to be repeated to provide continued benefit in this patient, when one eye is legally blind and the other has impaired vision, repeated HBOT may be a very useful therapeutic option when other treatment modalities have been unsuccessful (Butler 2008).

Refractory Pseudomonas Keratitis

Chong described a 30-year-old white female with culture-proven soft contact lens-associated *Pseudomonas keratitis* who was getting progressively worse despite topical, oral, and intravenous antibiotics. On her third day after admission, she was begun on a course of HBOT (2.0 ATA for 90 minutes daily). She began to improve after the addition of HBOT to her treatment regimen and 24 hours after her first HBOT treatment, her vision had improved from count fingers to 6/24. The HBOT was continued for 2 more days with progressive improvement and the patient was discharged after 6 days with a visual acuity of 6/9. Her vision subsequently improved to 6/6 (Chong 2007).

Pyoderma Gangrenosum of the Orbit

Pyoderma gangrenosum is an uncommon inflammatory skin disorder associated with inflammatory bowel disease and arthritis. It is characterized by its bluish color, exquisite painfulness, and potential to cause extensive tissue necrosis. It is uncommon in the periocular region, but Newman reported a case in which the lower lid lesion became extremely painful and relentlessly progressive, destroying orbital tissue, perforating the cornea, and eventually requiring evisceration of the eye. Oral and intralesional steroids, improved control of underlying diabetes, and oral clofazimime all failed to produce clinical improvement. The author used four HBOT sessions before her evisceration (2 ATA oxygen for 3 × 30-minute oxygen breathing periods separated by two 10-minute air breaks) and followed with 10 sessions of HBOT after the surgery. The patient recovered after the surgery and HBOT sessions and the author considered HBOT a valuable adjunct in the management of this challenging patient (Newman 1993).

Other Reported Uses

This section contains a number of ocular indications for HBOT for which a theoretical basis for the usefulness of HBOT exists and/or case reports have been published documenting the use of HBOT in managing these disorders. The evidence for these indications was considered to be less strong than that for the disorders listed in the previous two sections.

Toxic Amblyopia

Toxic amblyopia is a reduction in visual acuity secondary to a toxic reaction in the optic nerve. It can be caused by many toxins including lead, methanol, chloramphenicol, digoxin, ethambutol, and quinine. In severe cases it can lead to blindness. Bilateral amaurosis (loss of vision) is a common finding in quinine toxicity, typically occurring when serum levels are over 10mg/liter (Boland 1985, Dyson 1985). Visual loss usually occurs within 24 hours of ingestion of a toxic dose. Tissue hypoxia is thought to be a factor in this disorder, but direct retinal toxicity may be causative as well. Although the natural course is usually return of vision, permanent visual loss may occur (Wolff 1997, Bacon 1988).

Kern *et al* (1986) treated four patients with toxic amblyopia using HBO at 2 ATA. Improvement in vision was obtained in three of the four patients. Ocular quinine toxicity typically involves a partial or total and often permanent loss of vision. Apart from gastric lavage and oral administration of activated charcoal, current treatment modalities are of doubtful efficacy. Two patients with quinine amaurosis were treated with hyperbaric oxygen (HBO) in an effort to increase oxygen delivery to the retina (Wolff *et al* 1997). Visual outcomes in these patients were evaluated. Two patients had bilateral no light perception vision and dilated, nonreactive pupils within hours of ingesting 13–15 g of quinine in addition to other drugs. Following initial oral charcoal administration, HBO therapy was used. Within 17 h after quinine ingestion, both patients underwent HBO therapy at 2.4 ATA with 100% O_2 for 90 min. Both patients had return of visual acuity to 20/20 in both eyes less than 24 h after treatment. Follow-up visual fields revealed constriction and paracentral scotomas bilaterally. HBO may represent an additional or alternative, and perhaps safer, method of treatment for toxic amblyopia (Butler 2008).

Retinitis Pigmentosa

Retinitis pigmentosa (RP) is a heterogeneous group of retinal disorders characterized by slowly progressive degeneration of the photoreceptor cells (the rods and cones). Although the majority of RP cases are inherited as X-linked or dominant, approximately 40% of cases are isolated, with no other family members affected. Metabolic factors within the retina may also contribute to the progression of cell death (Yu 2005). The early stage of RP is often detectable only by the presence of an abnormal electroretinogram. (ERG) Loss of visual field occurs later, with the peripheral field being affected first. Affected individuals lose visual field at rates of 4 to 18% per year (Baumgartner 2000). Symptoms progress from light/dark adaptation difficulties to progressive loss of peripheral vision until only a central tunnel of vision remains.

It has been suggested that HBOT may be useful in slowing the progress of RP. Algan *et al* (1973) advocated the use of HBO for retinitis pigmentosa and macular degeneration. Bojic *et al* (1988) treated four patients with HBO at 2 ATA (90-min sessions daily). Visual acuity improved significantly in three of the four patients after 30 sessions of HBO. Chacia *et al* (1987) reported improvement of visual acuity in a patient with retinitis pigmentosa and macular edema. Another study showed a statistically significant improvement or stability in ERG in 24 patients who received HBOT (2.2 ATA for 90 minutes on a tapering regimen from five times a week for one month to one week a month for 11 months to one week every 3 months for the balance of 2 years) compared to controls (Vingolo 1999). This improvement in retinal ERG did not correlate with an improvement in visual acuity, but this would not be expected when HBOT is performed before the disease has reached end-stage, since the loss of vision moves from peripheral to central with the central island typically being the last sector of the visual field extinguished.

Skogstad reported a 26-year-old man with RP treated with HBOT (2.4 ATA of oxygen for 97 minutes five days a week × 4 weeks) and noted that he had improvement of his lateral vision at the conclusion of therapy (Skogstad 1994).

Oxidative stress, however, has been implicated as potentially contributing to the degenerative process and antioxidant supplements proposed as one possible therapeutic approach to RP. Baumgartner believes that HBOT is likely to be associated with considerable risk of increased oxidative damage to the retina in RP patients. Additionally, HBOT given acutely is unlikely to arrest the process of a disease that is chronic and progressive (Baumgartner 2000).

Visual Field Defects Following Macular Hole Surgery

Macular holes are caused by traction on the retina produced by fibrous attachments to a detaching vitreous body. Vitreoretinal surgery is indicated in some cases to close these holes. One of the complications of this surgery is temporal visual field defects (TVFD). A study reported that 7 patients with TVFD following macular hole surgery were treated with HBOT while a control group of 5 patients were not. The preoperative VF determined by kinetic perimetry was considered to be 100%, and the VF following HBO therapy was compared with that standard. In all five patients who had no HBO therapy, VF defects were unchanged, while the VF recovered remarkably in all patients treated with HBO therapy. The VF recovered to 81.7 ± 16.7% of the preoperative VF after 3 days of HBO, and to 91.6 ± 15.8% months after HBO therapy. Since the cause of VF defect is likely to be chorioretinal circulation disturbance during surgery, HBO improves VF by activating the retinal cells. The authors conclude that HBO is useful in the treatment of VF defect after macular hole surgery. Unfortunately, visual acuity itself was unchanged despite HBOT (Kuroki 2002).

Diabetic Retinopathy

Diabetic retinopathy (DR) is the leading cause of blindness for Americans in the 20–64-year-old age group. The underlying pathophysiology is believed to be an endothelial vasculopathy characterized by loss of pericytes and basement membrane thickening caused by sustained exposure to hyperglycemia (Butler 2008). Vision loss in diabetic retinopathy can be caused by retinal edema, retinal or optic nerve neovascularization, and/or ischemic macular changes. Elevated levels of vascular endothelial growth factor (VEGF) have been found in both the proliferative and nonproliferative types of diabetic retinopathy (Ishida 2003).

Treatment options for DR and diabetic macular edema (DME) include blood sugar control, laser PRP, grid laser therapy, intravitreal triamcinolone, and intravitreal anti-VEGF agents. Hyperbaric oxygen therapy is most likely to be of benefit early in the disease as a method of reducing edema and reversing ischemia.

Improvement of a patient with DME from 20/125 in the right eye and 20/320 in the left to 20/63 and 20/160 respectively was noted after HBOT. A decrease in foveal thickness from 620u/580u to 233u/305u accompanied the improvement in vision. The HBOT was administered in 14 sessions over 1 month. (The pressure and times of the HBOT were not mentioned in the article.) DME recurred several times in the succeeding months, but each time improved after repeat HBOT. The authors attributed the success of HBOT in this patient to either the hyperoxygenation of the macular tissue or constriction of the retinal vessels (Averous 2006).

A total of 22 eyes of 11 patients with DME were treated with 2 ATA of oxygen for one hour twice a day for two weeks and then once a day for the third week. Visual acuity improved by two lines or more in 15 eyes (68%) after HBOT. The improvement in vision diminished over time but at the end of follow-up was still better than pre-treatment. Static visual perimetry was also noted to improve in 76% of eyes (Ogura 1988).

Krott reported a series of 5 patients (seven eyes) with macular edema (3 diabetics, 1 with CRVO, and 1 with BRVO) treated with HBOT (2.4 ATA oxygen for 30 minutes per day × 10–30 treatments). At 15-month follow-up, the mean increase in visual acuity was 3.5 lines after HBOT. Other treatments for macular edema were employed as well (laser, acetazolamide, hemodilution), but HBOT was used after most other approaches had failed (Krott 2000).

Haddad reported no improvement in three patients with "advanced diabetic retinopathy" treated with HBOT (between 2 and 3 ATA for periods of 1 hour each) and noted that none of these three patients demonstrated any appreciable change in visual acuity, retinal pathology, or visual fields (Haddad 1965). Winstanley (1963) tried 100% oxygen at 1–3 ATA on three patients with diabetic retinopathy, but observed no changes on fundoscopy.

Dudnikov *et al* (1981) noted that hypoxia of the eye tissues is a characteristic of diabetic retinopathy. They used HBO therapy on 35 patients with diabetic retinopathy. Posttreatment angiography showed reduction of venous congestion and improvement of hemodynamics. In some patients the authors noted ischemic edema zones in areas of neovascularization. They drew no conclusions but continue with further investigations.

A major issue in treating this very common disorder with HBOT is its chronicity. HBOT would likely have to be undertaken on a long-term basis to provide a sustained benefit.

HBOT likely aids in acute episodes of edema but cannot reverse the more chronic permanent changes of necrosis nor can it prevent edema from recurring once HBOT is stopped (Butler 2008).

Uveitis

One report of a rabbit model of uveitis noted that hyperbaric oxygen was as effective as topical steroids used alone in treating this disorder and enhanced the efficacy of topical steroids when the two modalities were used together (Ersanli 2005).

Secondary Keratoendotheliosis

Corneal endothelial dysfunction ranging from mild postoperative corneal edema to bullous keratopathy and opacification of the cornea (secondary keratoendotheliosis) may occasionally complicate cataract removal surgery, although this complication has been reduced by currently used phacoemulsification techniques and the routine use of viscoelastics during cataract surgery. Recupero reported that hyperbaric oxygen therapy produced improved visual acuity in all 12 of the study patients compared to improvement in only 33% in the 21 control patients (Recupero 1992).

Vitullo *et al* (1987) have reported on the treatment of 32 patients with corneal disorders using HBO at 2.8 ATA. The various corneal diseases included were keratitis, keratoconus, traumatic injuries, and ulcerations. HBO was found to be beneficial in most of these cases.

As a rationale for the use of HBO, these authors have stated that tissue edema, hypoxia, and ischemia in these conditions are improved by hyperoxygenation.

The presence of a soft lens on the anterior surface of the cornea for prolonged periods interferes with the oxygenation of the cornea, and leads to anoxia and edema predisposing to the formation of corneal ulcers. Polse and Mandell (1976) produced striae on the posterior surface of the cornea in volunteers; the striae were then reversed by the use of HBO.

Complications of Sickle Cell Disease

Patients with sickle cell disease experience obliteration of retinal arterioles and venules and develop areas of retinal avascularity. This may result in proliferative vitreoretinopathy, which in many cases progresses to retinal hole formation and retinal detachment. These patients do very poorly with standard scleral buckling procedures to repair their detachments, with anterior segment ischemia nullifying what would otherwise be successful surgery (Freilich 1973, Freilich 1972). In experimental retinal detachment, retinal hypoxia caused by the separation of the retina from its normal source of nutrients is a factor in inducing the death of photoreceptor cells. Supplemental normobaric oxygen at 70% was found to reduce cell death in a cat model of retinal detachment (Mervin 1999). Oxygen in this model was also found to limit the proliferation and hypertrophy of Muller cells that is responsible for the proliferative vitreoretinopathy that may complicate retinal detachment surgery (Lewis 1999).

Freilich and his colleagues performed three scleral buckling procedures in a hyperbaric chamber with the patient breathing 100% oxygen at 2 ATA. The percentage of sickled red blood cells in one patient decreased from 10% at the start of the procedure to 3.5% at the end of 2 hours of hyperoxia. All patients treated using this unique surgical approach had anatomical success (no recurrence of

Table 32.3
Emergency HBO in Patients with Acute Vision Loss: Selection Criteria

HBOT is indicated as an emergency measure in patients who present with acute vision loss and meet the following criteria:

- Presentation within 24 hours of vision loss
- Corrected visual acuity 20/200 or worse
- Visual acuity still 20/200 or worse with pinhole testing
- Age > 40
- No pain associated with the vision loss
- No history of acute onset of flashes or floaters prior to vision loss
- No history of recent eye surgery or eye trauma

Notes: 1. HBOT should be administered in all cases if the loss of vision was associated a recent exposure to a hyperbaric environment or unpressurized high-altitude conditions. 2. HBOT should be administered in all cases if the history is suggestive of radiation optic neuropathy or for vision loss that occurs during or immediately after hemodialysis. 3. Consultation with an ophthalmologist is desirable if it can be obtained without delaying HBOT. 4. Acute, painless, severe vision loss should be referred as an emergency to an ophthalmologist in all cases so that additional patients may be identified for whom HBOT might be beneficial (Butler 2008).

the detachment) and improvement in their vision 6 to 12 months after their surgery (Freilich 1973, Freilich 1972). Five additional patients reported by the same author using hyperoxic conditions for surgery likewise produced good results (Freilich 1975). The author subsequently provided 2-year follow-up on these 8 patients and reported that their retinas had all remained completely attached and that no new retinal tears had developed. Visual acuity improved in all 6 of the patients who had had a decrease preoperatively (Freilich 1977). The author concludes that this remarkable success in these difficult surgical cases "merits the continued use of this technique in these difficult cases of detachment of the retina" (Freilich 1977).

Hyphema is another complication of sickle cell disease, and HBO has been advocated as a treatment for this condition on the basis of experimental evidence (Wallyn *et al* 1985).

Glaucoma

Glaucoma is a chronic and progressive disorder characterized by elevated intraocular pressure, damaged optic nerve heads, and lesions in the visual fields. Elevated intraocular pressure is only one of the symptoms of this disease, and although it can be lowered by medications, visual field deficits may persist. There are several theories of the etiology of glaucoma; one is that ischemia, resulting from insufficient vascularization of the pericapillary choroid and of the optic nerve head, is one of the primary causes of glaucoma lesions. Bohne *et al* (1987) recorded

retinal potentials to pattern-reversal stimuli while intraocular pressure was artificially elevated. In glaucoma patients the amplitude of potentials decreased at higher perfusion pressures than in healthy subjects. These data indicate that the dysfunction of ganglion cells is likely caused by a diminished retinal perfusion and therefore a reduced oxygen supply of the inner retinal layer. Hyperbaric oxygen therapy does not significantly lower intraocular pressures (Gallin-Cohen 1980); however, it may be theoretically useful in decreasing edema and ischemia.

Bojic *et al* (1993) conducted a double-blind, placebo-controlled study on 111 subjects to test the effect of HBO on visual fields and intraocular pressure in patients with open angle glaucoma. Two groups were formed at random: an experimental group of 91 and a control group of 20 patients. The experimental group was divided into 4 subgroups according to the number of HBO sessions at 2 ATA for a duration of 90 min: 30 sessions (31 patients), 20 sessions (20 patients), 15 sessions (20 patients) and 10 sessions (20 patients). There was improvement in visual fields in all treatment groups, except the 10 treatment group, whereas, there was none in the control group. There was no change in intraocular pressure in any of the patients. The authors recommend that a 20-session treatment should be given initially and if the visual fields improvement value reaches 50%, HBO treatments should be repeated. Popova and Kuz'minov (1996) treated 35 patients (64 eyes) with primary open-angle glaucoma by HBO combined with antioxidants. Repeated courses were administered during 5 years. Stabilization of the visual function was attained in 80% patients. Follow-up of controls (34 patients – 66 eyes) showed stabilization of the visual function in only 35% cases.

Emergency HBO in Patients with Acute Vision Loss

Patients who present with acute painless loss of vision have a differential diagnosis that includes CRAO, retinal detachment, CRVO, BRVO, BRAO, choroidal neovascularization with subretinal hemorrhage, vitreous hemorrhage, and ischemic optic neuropathy. It may take several hours to several days and an ophthalmology consult to establish a definitive diagnosis for the vision loss. In the interim, whatever potential that may exist to restore vision with HBOT might be lost.

Considering that at least five of the relatively common ocular disorders producing acute, painless loss of vision have the potential to benefit from HBOT, the authors propose the following approach to managing patients with acute loss of vision:

1) Patients who present with acute painless loss of vision of recent onset should be triaged as *"emergency."*

2) Visual acuity should be checked immediately. If vision with the patient's current glasses or contact lenses is 20/200 or worse, cannot be improved significantly with pinhole, and the patient meets the other selection criteria listed in Table 32.3, then he or she should be considered for emergency HBOT.

3) The patient should then be started immediately on supplemental oxygen at one atmosphere at the highest possible inspired fraction of oxygen.

4) If vision is restored by oxygen at 1 ATA and HBOT is not necessary, maintain on oxygen at an inspired fraction sufficient to maintain the improvement in vision until ophthalmologic consultation can be obtained. Titrate continued supplemental oxygen as clinically appropriate thereafter.

5) If visual acuity does not improve to near baseline within five minutes after starting supplemental oxygen and there are no contraindications to HBOT, refer for emergency HBOT. Maintain supplemental oxygen until HBOT is initiated. Even though vision has not responded to the normobaric oxygen, the increased oxygenation produced by this intervention may be helpful in maintaining retinal viability until HBOT is initiated.

6) Compress to 45 FSW on 100% oxygen.

7) If no response within 5 minutes, compress to 60 fsw and perform a USN Treatment Table 6. (Note: If DCS or AGE is diagnosed, follow the USN dive manual treatment protocols.)

8) Upon surfacing from the HBOT, the patient should be referred to an ophthalmologist as an emergency.

9) The decision regarding further management should be made by the ophthalmologist and a hyperbaric consultant working in concert.

10) In general, if vision improves with HBOT, the treating physicians should titrate HBOT to effect using the guidelines noted in the sections above as general guides. Note that several consecutive days of Treatment Table 6's are sufficient to result in a significant incidence of pulmonary oxygen toxicity. Twice daily treatment with intervening supplemental oxygen may be required acutely (Butler 2008).

Conclusions

HBOT has not traditionally been used widely as a treatment modality in the management of ocular disorders. There are a number of ocular indications, however, in which HBOT may reverse profound vision loss. The authors recommend prompt aggressive HBOT for the indications listed when vision loss is severe and the patient presents within the appropriate time frame. Further studies will help to define which ocular disorders are best treated with HBOT, the critical time window for each, and the optimal treatment dosing (Butler 2008).

33 Hyperbaric Oxygenation in Obstetrics and Neonatology

K.K. Jain

HBO has been applied safely during pregnancy. It has a role in the management of neonatal hypoxis. The major sections of this chapter include:

Introduction

Careful consideration must be given to use of hyperbaric oxygenation (HBO) during pregnancy. Pregnant women can benefit from HBO treatment of obstetrical disorders and associated medical conditions. There is no evidence that pregnancy is a contraindication for HBO treatment of the mother but some concern has been expressed about effects on the fetus and possible congenital malformations.

HBO and Risk of Congenital Malformations

Grote and Wanger (1973) exposed pregnant rabbits on the 9th day of gestation to oxygen pressures of 1.5 or 2 ATA for 5 h. The mother rabbits were sacrificed on the 29th day. Fetuses were removed and uteri studied for resorption, and the evidence showed increases in the resorption rate and number of congenital malformations.

Bimes et al (1973) exposed pregnant rabbits daily to HBO (2 ATA) for periods of 1–2 h. On the 27th day or the 30th day of pregnancy cesarean sections were performed. The weight of all fetuses was found to be about half normal. The brain was the only organ not affected consistently. The dimensions of the long bones were reduced, particularly at the diaphysis. Glycogenic and lipid overload and delay of endochondral ossification of long bones were observed.

Yusa (1981) studied the effect of oxygen on chromosomes in bone marrow. No aberration was noted in chromosomes as a result of exposure to normobaric oxygen, but significant abnormalities (breakage and gap) were noted in mice exposed to HBO at 3–4 ATA. Malformations (umbilical hernia and abnormalities of the coccyx) were noted in some newborns when the mother was exposed to HBO at 2.5 ATA for 2 h on the 5th and 8th days of gestation, and in all the newborns of animals exposed to HBO daily.

In a controlled experimental study, pregnant Fischer rats were exposed to HBO at 3.2 and 4.2 ATA (90 min daily) for 5 days (Sapunar et al 1993). The embryos in the HBO group did not show any congenital malformations but showed reduced weight as compared with sham-treated control animals.

There are no studies describing the extrapolation of these studies to humans, but it is presumed that exposure to HBO in the earlier months of human pregnancy carries the risk of abortion and congenital malformation. The immature cells of the nervous system would be expected to be more susceptible to the toxic effects of oxygen, but malformations of the nervous system have not been described. More experimental studies on this subject are required.

Role of HBO in Obstetrics

Experimental Studies

Maillot et al (1979) tested HBO therapy in a placental insufficiency model in the rat. HBO was used at 2.5 ATA for 2 h and resulted in definite improvement.

Chaika et al (1981) studied the effect of HBO on the functional state of the hypothalamo-hypophysio-adrenal system (HHAS) in pregnant rats and their fetuses under conditions of experimentally induced chronic hypoxia. The HHAS was found to react actively to pregnancy, to hypoxia of the mother as well as of the fetus, and to HBO action. Hypoxia in the pregnant led to deficiency of corticosteroids, which caused intense discharge of hypothalamic corticotropin and subsequent activation of the adreno-hypophysial adrenocorticotropic hormone according to the feedback principle. The functional state of the HHAS varied in pregnant rats with experimental myocardial dystrophy treated by means of HBO at pressures of 3, 2, and 1 ATA.

Morin et al (1988) exposed pregnant ewes to 100% oxygen at 3 ATA for 20 min. This exposure increased the pulmonary oxygen tension in the fetuses from 20 ± 1 to 54 ± 9 mmHg. It increased pulmonary blood flow from the fetal to the newborn values from 31 ± 3 to 295 ± 20 ml/kg/min. Pulmonary arterial pressure did not change during hyperoxygenation.

Clinical Applications

Various conditions in which HBO has been used in pregnant women are listed in Table 33.1. Part of this list is based on practice in Russia as there is very limited use of HBO in obstetrical disorders in the Western countries.

Table 33.1
Conditions in Which HBO Has Been Used During Pregnancy

Obstetric disorders
Threatened abortion
Fetal hypoxia
Toxemias of pregnancy
Late gestation

Medical disorders complicating pregnancy
Diabetes
Heart disease
Carbon monoxide poisoning
Air embolism
Status epilepticus

Threatened Abortion

HBO was employed alone and in combination with drugs acting on the hypothalamo-hypophysio-ovarian system by Pobedinsky *et al* (1981) in 158 women with threatened abortion and fetoplacental insufficiency. They were able to prolong the pregnancy.

Electrophoretic properties of syntrophoblast proteins are distinctly altered under conditions of fetoplacental insufficiency of endocrine origin. HBO treatments have been shown to prevent the impairment of the membrane protein composition (Pogorelova *et al* 1983).

Fetal Hypoxia

A cesarian section has been performed in a hyperbaric chamber (2 ATA) on a comatose female who developed generalized convulsions; death was thought to be imminent (Ledingham *et al* 1968). Fetal distress was rapidly relieved at 2 ATA with the mother breathing 100% oxygen via endotrachial tube. Despite inspired oxygen concentration of 1500 mm Hg, the arterial oxygen tension was only 430 mm Hg and the uterus remained cyanosed. However, a healthy female infant with an Apgar score of 9 was delivered. Aksenova *et al* (1981) used HBO for prevention of fetal hypoxia and hypotrophy in 230 pregnant women (70 with heart disease, 70 with nephropathy, 70 with fetoplacental insufficiency, 10 with anemia, and 10 with hypertension). HBO was used at 1.5–1.8 ATA for 40–50 min per session, and 10–12 sessions were given in the second and third trimesters of pregnancy; 120 women with similar pathology were managed without HBO and served as controls. Signs of hypoxia and hypotrophy abated or disappeared, and the condition of newborn children in the experimental group was much better than that of those in the control group.

Toxemias of Pregnancy

Drel *et al* (1981) used HBO to treat 92 pregnant women suffering from nephropathy of stages I–III. The nephropathy improved along with improvement of catecholamine metabolism.

Late Gestation

Tereshin and Charushnikova (1985) noted that the serum levels of di- and triglycerides which declined in late gestation returned to normal under HBO therapy.

Diabetes

Zhdanov *et al* (1981) treated pregnant women with diabetes by means of HBO at 1.4–1.8 ATA. Three to four courses, each consisting of six to ten sessions of 45–60 min, were given during the pregnancy. There was a general improvement of the condition with normalization of blood glucose and a decrease in the levels of xanthine and guanine-the rise of the latter was a characteristic of hypoxia. Control of diabetes was achieved in 92% of cases, and all the patients progressed to full-term pregnancies and gave birth at 37–38 weeks of gestation.

Korobova *et al* (1981) pointed out that a high content of histamine in the blood of pregnant diabetic women may play an important role in the pathogenesis of circulatory hypoxia jeopardizing the fetal life due to hypoxia. They gave HBO at 1.2–1.6 ATA for 45 min. After an initial rise, the histamine value dropped to 37% of the original level after the seventh HBO session. This fall coincided with a considerable improvement in the patient's condition.

Management of Pregnancy and Delivery in Women with Heart Disease

HBO has been used extensively in Russia for the management of pregnant women with congenital as well as acquired heart disease.

Molzhaninov *et al* (1981) used HBO in the management of 170 pregnant women with heart disease, and labor was conducted under HBO (1.5–2 ATA). The hypoxic condition of the mother as well as the fetus was counteracted in each case, and no complications were reported.

Vanina *et al* (1981) used HBO during labor in 54 patients with cardiopulmonary pathology. In 28 women the delivery was vaginal, and in 26 cases cesarean section was performed. The indication for HBO was arterial hypoxia, that is, pO_2 below 70 mmHg. Pressure of 2 ATA was used. Two women died as a result of complications of cardiac disease. Three infants died, one as a result of multiple congenital anomalies and two due to prematurity. The rest were discharged home in good condition.

Vanina *et al* (1977) observed labor in a patient with acute myocardial infarction in the 32nd week of pregnancy. Successful delivery by cesarean section under 3 ATA of HBO was performed at the 36th–37th week of pregnancy.

Use of HBO for Medical Conditions in Pregnancy

Roman *et al* (2002) reported the first case of a pregnant woman presenting with a paradoxical air embolism due to accidental removal of a central venous catheter. Secondary right hemiplegia associated with a confused state justified emergency HBO therapy, which was followed by complete neurological recovery. The authors assess risk situations of gas embolism during pregnancy and puerperium, as well as indications and fetal effects of hyperbaric oxygen therapy.

Acute Carbon Monoxide Poisoning During Pregnancy

If indicated, HBO can be used for the treatment of a pregnant mother (see Chapter 12). Abboud *et al* (2001) reported two cases of moderate maternal poisoning during the third trimester of pregnancy. They underwent HBO therapy at 2.5 ATA for 90 min and were delivered at term. In one case the newborn presented an antenatal ischemic cerebral lesion probably due to carbon monoxide poisoning.

Applications of HBO in Neonatology

Various techniques of oxygen administration to infants have been described by Jain (1989b). Cartlidge and Rutter (1988) have shown that raising the ambient oxygen concentration can raise the paO$_2$ of premature infants by 8.9 mmHg (mean figure). Transdermal oxygen can supplement oxygen delivery to premature infants with poor pulmonary gas exchange, but the absorption is not adequate in full-term infants.

The first report in the English language literature on the use of HBO in neonates was published in the *Lancet* in 1963 by Hutchinson *et al* These authors resuscitated apneic newborns by means of HBO (1–3 ATA) at 2–38 min after birth. The effects were described as dramatic, with improvement of skin color and of cardiovascular as well as respiratory function. Thirty-five of the 65 neonates so treated survived. Barrie (1963) criticized Hutchinson *et al* in the same issue of the *Lancet*, stating that the mortality of 46% was too high. The problem of neonatal asphyxia is different from that of respiratory arrest in an adult. In the neonate the lung alveoli are not fully open and oxygen would not diffuse through the lungs. The possibility of absorption of oxygen through the skin and the mucous membranes of the respiratory tract was considered, but such absorption cannot be adequate. This subject was discussed by Hertel (1964), who advised against the use of HBO in such situations unless the improvement in oxygenation of these infants could be verified by blood gas analysis. Placing an

infant in the hyperbaric chamber restricts the other methods of resuscitation. This method has not gained popularity. A number of papers, all by Russian authors, were presented on this topic at the Seventh International Congress of Hyperbaric Medicine in Moscow in 1981. The consensus at that congress was that inclusion of HBO in intensive care of asphyxic infants reduces the post-hypoxic sequelae. HBO was used for resuscitation in respiratory failure, for cranial birth injuries and for hemolytic disease of the newborn. HBO was reported to reduce high serum bilirubin levels and prevent development of neurological disorders. In cases of respiratory distress, delayed use of HBO (12–48 h after birth) was useless. Early use (1–3 h after birth) led to recovery in 75% of cases.

Cartlidge and Rutter (1988) expressed their concern that use of a hyperbaric chamber would make direct access to an infant impossible. This objection has been answered by James (1986), who points out that the infants should be treated in a multiplace chamber with all the facilities of modern pediatric intensive care, including intubation and controlled ventilation. Intubation and ventilation with pulsed high dose oxygen, to rapidly establish normal tissue oxygen values in the brain and cause vasoconstriction, may well prove to be the key factor in the control of periventricular hemorrhage in neonates, where the high water content inevitably poses a barrier to oxygen diffusion.

Rosasco *et al* (1972) improvised a Chamberland autoclave as a hyperbaric chamber for infants and used it to treat very sick postoperative pediatric surgical patients. The pressure used was 1.5 ATA and oxygen flow of 7 l/min was maintained to reduce the CO$_2$ concentration in the chamber. Thirteen infants varying in age from 1 day to 11 months were treated by HBO, following operations for conditions such as intestinal perforation (with peritonitis) and hypertrophic pyloric stenosis. Twelve of these patients survived; the only death was an infant with mesenteric artery thrombosis.

The use of HBO in pediatric surgery is discussed in Chapter 29.

Conclusions

The potential of HBO in obstetrics is exciting. The results of the large number of deliveries conducted in the hyperbaric chamber in Russia indicate the safety of this technique. Caution should be exercised in the introduction of HBO in resuscitation of newborn infants. The role of HBO in disorders of pregnancy needs to be verified thoroughly by controlled studies.

34 Hyperbaric Oxygenation in Geriatrics

K.K. Jain

HBO has been found to be useful in a number of disorders common in elderly patients, but it of course cannot reverse the aging process. The main topics of this chapter are:

Introduction

Geriatrics has now become a recognized medical specialty as the number of elderly in Western societies has grown and the life span has continued to increase. It is expected that by the year 2000, one in seven residents of the USA will be over the age of 65. Aging is not a disease but certain diseases are associated with aging. Hyperbaric oxygenation (HBO) has an important role to play in the practice of geriatric medicine, as many of the indications for the use of this therapy that have already been discussed are more common in the elderly.

Physiology of Aging

Theories of Aging

Multiple factors, including the inborn aging process, genetic defects and environmental agents, participate in the aging process and sequence of changes with aging is shown in Figure 34.1. There are more than 300 theories to explain the aging phenomenon (Jain 2001). The most well-known of these states that aging may be due to deleterious, irreversible changes produced by free radical reactions. This theory will be described here.

Free Radicals and Aging

The free radical theory of aging, postulated first by Harman in 1954, remains the most popular and widely tested theory of aging. It is based on the chemical nature and ubiquitous presence of free radicals. Despite the actions of antioxidant nutrients, some oxidative damage will occur, and accumulation of this damage throughout life is believed to be a major contributing factor to aging and disease. Oxidative stress and production of free radicals tends to increase with aging whereas the body's natural antioxidant defenses decline.

The free radical theory of aging postulates that a single common process, modified by genetic and environmental factors, is responsible for the aging and death of all living cells. The theory was extended in 1972 with the suggestion that life span was largely determined by the rate of free radical damage to the mitochondria (Harman 1999). This theory suggests the possibility that measures to decrease the rate of initiation or the chain length of free radicals, may decrease the aging changes. Supporting evidence for the free radical theory of aging is as follows:

1. Studies on the origin of life and evolution indicate that free radical reactions were involved in these processes.
2. Studies of the effect of ionizing radiation on living things where the damage occurs through generation of free radicals.
3. Life span experiments in which endogenous free radical reactions were counteracted by dietary manipulations.
4. Studies on several organisms as diverse as yeast, the roundworm *Caenorhabditis elegans* and the fly *Drosoph-*

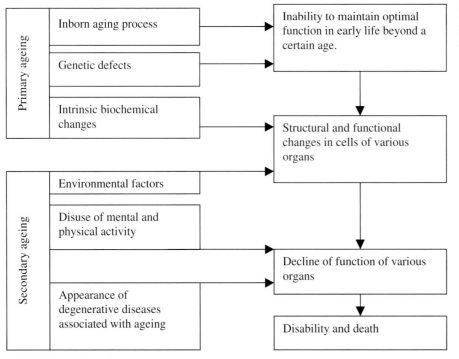

Figure 34.1
Sequence of changes with aging. Reproduced by permission.

ila melanogaster show a strong link between genetic defects in the body's oxidative-stress-response mechanisms, and dramatic lifespan extensions.

5. Mammalian species with a higher rate of formation of mitochondrial superoxide radical have a shorter life span than species with a lower rate of formation of these radicals.

6. Studies that implicate free radical reactions in the pathogenesis of diseases such as atherosclerosis, Alzheimer's disease and cancer which are more common in the elderly.

However, it is not known why free-radical damage does not adversely affect certain cells such as gonadal germ cells. Although its appeal derives from a long-standing body of supporting correlative data, the free radical theory was more rigorously tested only recently. Ongoing researches in the study of free radical biochemistry and the genetics of aging have been at the forefront of this work. Transgenic approaches in invertebrate models with candidate genes such as superoxide dismutase (SOD) involved in the detoxification of reactive oxygen species (ROS) have shown that the endogenous production of ROS due to normal physiologic processes is a major limiting factor for life span. Genes involved in ROS detoxification are highly conserved among eukaryotes; hence, the physiologic processes that limit life span in invertebrates are likely to be similar in higher eukaryotes.

The increased life span caused by certain mutations in the nematode *C. elegans* has been interpreted in terms of two metabolic theories of aging: the oxidative damage theory and the rate of living theory. New findings support the former, but not the latter interpretation.

Hypoxia and Aging

Aging is also viewed as a manifestation of hypoxia. The acquisition and use of oxygen involves a series of steps, each subject to change with aging, as shown in Table 34.1.

The subject of hypoxia and aging has been discussed in detail by Jain (1989b). Most studies of blood gas determinations have shown a linear regression of arterial pO_2 with aging. Blom *et al* (1988) found that mean paO_2 was 95 mmHg (12.67 kPa) in those between the ages of 30 and 50. It dropped during successive decades until it was 77 mmHg (10.20 kPa) in those over the age of 70. The oxygen saturation, however, did not differ significantly in various age groups.

Table 34.1
The Oxygen Conductance System (from Kenny RA, 1985, Physiology of Aging. Clin Geriat Med 1:37–59)

Process	Factors involved
Ventilation: ability to maintain a supply of air to the alveoli	*Thoracic compliance *Lung compliance *Airway resistance *Vital capacity *Timed ventilatory function, e.g., maximum voluntary ventilation *Closing volume *Chemoreceptor drive to ventilation
Diffusion: movement of gas from the terminal bronchioles bulk flow creases into the alveolar sacs; movement of gases across the alveolar membrane	*Length of terminal airways *Size of the alveolar sac *Area of the alveolar membrane Thickness of the membrane Alveolar pO_2
Uptake: uptake of the available oxygen by blood flowing in the pulmonary capillaries	*Pulmonary perfusion rate *Shunting of blood *Ventilation/perfusion ratio Hemoglobin concentration Association characteristics of hemoglobin
Delivery: distribution of the available oxygen to the tissues	*Tissue perfusion rate *Dissociation characteristics of hemoglobin *Tissue pO_2
Diffusion: movement of the oxygen from the tissue capillary to the active cell	*Capillary density, i.e., proximity to cell *Nature of the interstice Pressure gradient for oxygen Myoglobin concentration
Utilization: metabolism of oxygen in the cell	*Intracellular enzyme systems *Intracellular enzyme systems
*Changed by aging	

Changes in the Brain with Aging

Morphological Changes

The most striking change in the brain with age is a loss of volume and weight. Most of the tissue loss takes place over the cerebral cortex, with more taking place over the frontal lobes and less over the parietal and temporal lobes and basal ganglia. With modern anatomical techniques, it is possible to determine the relative volume of gray and white matter of the brain. Atrophy involves mostly the gray matter, both cortical and subcortical. Cortical atrophy, as well as ventricular enlargement indicating a loss of cerebral substance with advancing age, have been shown on CT studies. The loss of neurons has been estimated to be about 50,000 per day past the age of 20 years (Jain 2003g). When it does occur, age-related neuronal loss has no satisfactory explanation. Cell integrity is maintained by the exchange of neurotropic hormones or growth factors as well as by the functional activity. Trophic factors within the brain maintain the integrity of various neuronal populations and an age-related loss of specific trophic factors may contribute to the selected dropout of individual neuronal elements in large neural networks. Compensation of this neuronal loss may occur by synaptic growth (reactive synaptogenesis). Old nerve cells seem to retain the ability to modify their synaptic endings and partially compensate for reduced surface density of contact zones by expanding the size of the surviving junctions. Precise morphometric studies show that the total number of neurons in the human brain does not change with aging if pathological processes are excluded (Haug 1985). The decrease in brain size is counterbalanced by an increase in neuron density. The number of synaptic contacts usually varies with the number of dendritic spines.

Cerebral Blood Flow and Metabolism in Aging

Using a Xenon-133 technique, several investigators have reported a decrease in the mean gray matter cerebral blood flow with aging, whereas the white matter cerebral blood flow remains stable with advancing age. Cerebral metabolism is not disturbed significantly with aging as far as glucose and oxygen utilization are concerned but it is not possible to exclude occult disorders of the brain in the elderly. Changes in cerebral metabolic rate for glucose are more clear-cut in dementias. The aging brain is more susceptible to metabolic insults. One study suggests that the structural and functional changes that occur in vessels in the aging brain impair the ability of cerebral microcirculation to optimally deliver nutrients and oxygen to the brain, affecting the mitochondrial ability to respond to anoxia (Zarchin *et al* 2002).Role of Hypoxia in the Decline of Mental Function with Aging

McFarland (1963) theorized that the aging process involves a diminished capacity of the central nervous system to use oxygen. He compared the decline of mental function resulting from aging with that resulting from hypoxia.

Schulze and Jänicke (1986) studied the effect of aging on the ability to adapt to normobaric hypoxia (10%) in the rat. There was a decline in behavior regarding food and fluid intake and spontaneous activity, but physiological parameters of the blood (blood gases and hematocrit) did not change. The authors concluded that although there is impairment of functional activity with hypoxia in aging, the metabolic capacity is not totally exhausted.

Applications of HBO in Geriatrics

Rationale

Although hypoxia accompanies the aging process and HBO can counteract hypoxia, there is no evidence that HBO can halt or reverse the aging process. If one accepts the free radical theory of aging and also the free radical theory of the mechanism of oxygen toxicity, then HBO would be contraindicated, as it would aggravate the tissue damage by oxygen free radicals. There is no clinical or experimental evidence that this is so. In the first place, HBO is not used

for the treatment of aging as such, and second, the pressures usually used (1.5–2 ATA) do not produce oxygen toxicity. Some degree of protection is afforded by the administration of antioxidants, such as vitamin E, to patients receiving HBO therapy.

The main object of HBO is to counteract tissue hypoxia and improve the metabolism. Both of these are important in disturbances of the brain, which constitute a major portion of the problems in geriatric patients treated by HBO.

Indications

Elderly patients may suffer from any of the conditions discussed in previous chapters where HBO has been found to be useful (with some obvious exceptions such as obstetrics and decompression sickness). The major indications are shown in Table 34.2. It should be noted that ischemia is a common factor in all the indications listed in this table. Changes in mental function occur frequently in patients with cardiovascular disease over the age of 60. Decline of mental activity is also common in hospitalized patients.

Table 34.2
Major Indications for HBO Therapy in Geriatric Patients

1. Cerebrovascular insufficiency with neurological deficits such as hemiplegia
   As an aid to physical therapy and rehabilitation
   As prophylaxis against recurrence of acute episodes of stroke
2. Disorders of cognition, such as mild to major dementia secondary to vascular insufficiency
3. Peripheral vascular disease
4. Chronic myocardial ischemic disease

Role of HBO in Rehabilitation of Elderly Patients

The role of HBO in rehabilitation is described in Chapter 35. Rehabilitation of elderly patients, particularly those with neurological disabilities, is a challenge. The capacity for physical exercise is reduced in these patients. HBO may not increase the physical performance in healthy adults, but it improves the physical performance capacity in those limited by pain and paralysis or spasticity. Physical therapy in such patients can be carried out in a hyperbaric chamber (see rehabilitation of stroke patients, Chapter 18).

HBO in the Management of Decline of Mental Function with Aging

HBO does not increase the mental performance in otherwise healthy and active elderly persons. Studies of Talton *et al* (1970) showed that focused attention, alertness, motor coordination, and the facility to deal rapidly with symbolic material do not improve in the "normal" healthy elderly

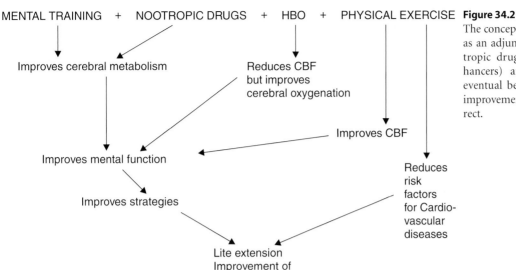

Figure 34.2

The concept of hyperbaric oxygenation as an adjunct to mental training, nootropic drugs (cerebral metabolic enhancers) and physical exercise. The eventual benefit of life extension and improvement of quality of life is indirect.

during HBO exposure at 2.8 ATA. HBO does not have any effect in primary degenerative dementias, but it improves mental function in patients with cerebrovascular insufficiency. HBO is part of a multidisciplinary approach to the patient with decline of mental function with aging. It is combined with brain jogging (mental exercises), physical exercise, and nootropic medications (to improve cerebral metabolism).

One technique of mental exercise (Jain *et al* 1988) was found very useful to counteract mental decline with aging. Physical exercise has been known to reduce the age-related decline in aerobic capacity and increase the life expectancy. It should also be stressed that physical exercise has an important role in improving cerebral circulation and function. Exercising skeletal muscles has been shown to release ATP in quantities sufficient to alter cerebral blood flow (CBF) and increase cerebral metabolism during exercise. It has been shown using the ^{131}Xe method that exercise increases regional CBF in areas of the brain as specific as the prefrontal, somatosensory, and primary areas of the motor cortex. Hollmann found that exercise at 25 watts and 100 watts increases CBF by 15% and 25% respectively (Hollmann 1987).

Thus exercise may prevent or postpone a commonly existing cycle: disuse decreases metabolic demands in the motor and somatosensory brain tissue, which decreases the need for circulatory flow, which in turn may result in neuronal dysfunction, leading to disuse of brain tissue, and so on. The concept of mutually interacting beneficial effects of brain jogging, physical exercise, and nootropic drugs (cerebral metabolic enhancers) as adjuncts to HBO therapy in the elderly is shown in Figure 34.2. Physical exercise improves mental function, increased mental activity improves physical performance, and both together increase the life span. There is evidence that persons who are mentally active live longer. Mentally active persons develop better strategies for survival after myocardial infarction.

Whether the decline in the oxidative capacity of the human brain with aging can be postponed by chronic physical exercise is not established, but theoretical evidence indicates that it is possible. HBO improves the metabolic disturbances associated with hypoxia.

Safety of HBO Treatments in the Elderly

HBO is generally considered to be safe in the aged persons unless they have a medical contraindication. Some conditions such as cataracts occur more frequently in the elderly. Oxidation could account for the lipid compositional changes with loss of transparency that are observed to occur in the lens with age and cataract. Animal experimental evidence indicates that increased lipid oxidation and hydrocarbon chain disorder correlate with increased lens nuclear opacity in the in vivo HBO model (Borchman *et al* 2000).

Conclusions

HBO has proven to be helpful in geriatrics, and its most useful role is in vascular insufficiency syndromes. Since elderly inactive patients also suffer from mental decline in the absence of organic disease of the brain, a combination of HBO, nootropic drugs, brain jogging (mental exercises), and physical therapy is maximally effective for geriatric patients. If the genetic programming theory of aging is true, one cannot extend the life span, but one can help the patient achieve the maximal age determined for him or her at an optimal level of mental and physical functioning.

There is no evidence that oxygen, whether normobaric or hyperbaric, given alone by any technique, can "rejuvenate" elderly people.

35 HBO as an Adjuvant in Rehabilitation and Sports Medicine

K.K. Jain

HBO is a valuable adjunct in the rehabilitation of chronic diseases and treatment of sports injuries. The chapter discusses:

Introduction

Physical therapy is an essential part of rehabilitation in many chronic diseases and in dealing with the sequelae of cerebrovascular insufficiency and myocardial ischemia, as well as in many neurological disabilities. Physical exercise in various forms is an important component of physical therapy and preventive medicine programs. Hyperbaric oxygenation (HBO) has also proven useful in many medical problems, such as infections and gangrene. There has been very little work on the combination of HBO and physical exercise.

Exercise physiology – under normoxia, hypoxia, and hyperoxia – has been discussed in Chapter 4, which should be read in conjunction with this chapter. The role of HBO in the treatment of various disorders has been considered in the appropriate chapters. Important points that are relevant to rehabilitation are repeated here.

Rehabilitation is a multidisciplinary undertaking to aid the functional recovery of patients and their integration into society. It has an important role to play in all branches of medicine, and particularly so in neurological disorders; rehabilitation is not only physical but psychological as well.

Rehabilitation uses the techniques of physical medicine, and currently these include ultraviolet light, electrotherapy, and ultrasound. HBO can be added to these. Traditionally, rehabilitation therapy has followed recovery from an acute illness. In some cases rehabilitation measures should already start during the acute phase of an illness and should also aim at preventing further recurrences of the disease process.

Role of HBO in Rehabilitation

Indications

The conditions in which HBO has been found to be a useful adjunct to rehabilitation are shown in Table 35.1.

Advantages

The combination of HBO (1.5 ATA) with physical therapy has the following advantages.

Biochemical improvement. Excess concentrations of lactate, pyruvate, and ammonia, particularly in older people, are detrimental to fitness and contribute to fatigue, and there is significant increase of these substances during exercise. HBO reduces this.

Increase of capacity for strenuous exercise. HBO allows more strenuous and prolonged exercise than is possible un-

der normobaric conditions. This is of particular advantage in the rehabilitation of chronic ischemic heart disease patients, for treatment of mild hypertension, and for lowering blood lipids.

Neurological disorders. The role of HBO in the rehabilitation of stroke patients is described in Chapter 18. The rationale for HBO in stroke rehabilitation is summarized in Table 35.2. HBO is beneficial in the acute stages of head injury with cerebral edema, and the evidence for HBO therapy in the rehabilitation of the head-injured patient is summarized in Table 35.3. Rehabilitation starts when the patient has regained consciousness and can be moved. The usefulness of HBO in the management of spinal cord injury is described in Chapter 20, and its role in intensive rehabilitation is summarized in Table 35.4.

HBO has been found useful in the rehabilitation of patients with postoperative neurological deficits. In many neurological conditions, where the effect of HBO on the course of the disease remains uncertain, rehabilitation is greatly facilitated by conducting physical therapy during an HBO session, for example, in cases of multiple sclerosis and muscular dystrophy. The physical performance capacity of neurologically disabled patients is thus improved.

Table 35.1
Conditions in Which HBO is a Useful Adjunct to Rehabilitation

- Stroke
- Peripheral vascular disease
- Head injury
- Toxic encephalopathy, e.g., CO poisoning
- Multiple sclerosis
- Paraplegia
- Sports injuries
- Coronary heart disease

Table 35.2
Rationale of Use of HBO in Stroke Rehabilitation

- Activates dormant neurons in the penumbra zone
- Relieves spasticity
- Facilitates movements
- Improves motor power
- Reduces stroke recurrences
- Increases physical and mental exercise capacity

Table 35.3
Role of HBO in the Rehabilitation of Head Injury

- Decreases cerebral edema in acute stage
- Decreases spasticity
- Accelerates recovery
- Improves cognitive function recovery in combination with brain jogging
- Relieves post-traumatic headaches

Table 35.4
HBO in Rehabilitation of Paraplegia

- Relieves spasticity
- Improves vital capacity
- Increases exercise capacity
- Decreases hyperammonemia resulting from exhaustive exercise

---

Table 35.5
HBO in Rehabilitation of Myocardial Ischemia

- Improves exercise capacity
- Prevents recurrence of ischemic episodes
- Decreases BP in hypertensives
- Long-term use reverses atherosclerosis

Table 35.6
Benefits of Exercise Under HBO in Patients with Ischemic Leg Pain

- Increases painless exercise capacity
- Relieves pain both at rest and on activity
- Reduces biochemical disturbances resulting from exercise of ischemic muscles
- Counteracts the vasoconstricting effect of HBO
- Improvement is maintained after cessation of HBO when the ceiling effect is reached

---

Table 35.7
Benefits of HBO in Sports Injuries

- Reduces swelling and pain in acute stage
- Speeds up recovery and return to active training
- Improves fracture healing
- Aids recovery from exhaustion and collapse

Myocardial infarction. There is some controversy regarding the usefulness of HBO in acute myocardial infarction. Exercise therapy is popular for the rehabilitation of patients who have recovered from acute episodes. Most of the beneficial effects of HBO in cardiovascular disease are associated with increased capacity for physical exercise. This is particularly true in cases with hypertension, where exercise therapy has been shown to reduce blood pressure. The role of HBO in the rehabilitation of myocardial ischemia is shown in Table 35.5.

Peripheral vascular disease. The role of HBO in the management of peripheral vascular disease has been described in Chapter 23. Exercise therapy for patients with ischemic leg pain is facilitated by the use of HBO in situations where it is possible to extend the limit of performance by the use of normobaric oxygen. A treadmill controlled by the patient can be installed in a hyperbaric chamber for training therapy for those suffering ischemic leg pain. The benefits of exercise under HBO conditions are summarized in Table 35.6.

HBO for Treatment of Sports Injuries

HBO has an important role in the acute management of trauma (see Chapter 30). The rehabilitation of an injured athlete should start right after the injury. The benefits of HBO in the rehabilitation of sports injuries are summarized in Table 35.7. Since the use of HBO was recommended in the Handbook of Hyperbaric Oxygen Therapy (precursor of this textbook) 20 years ago, HBO has been applied widely in the treatment of sports injuries. Some of the experiences have been reported in scientific journals and some studies have been carried out to evaluate the beneficial effect.

The potential benefits of HBO for sports injuries appear to be a blunting of initial injury, possibly by controlling the neutrophil adhesion and release of oxygen free radicals as well as an enhancement of healing processes requiring oxygen-like collagen formation and phagocytosis (Staples & Clement 1996).

Borromeo et al (1997) conducted a randomized double-blind study of 32 subject with acute ankle sprains to compare treatment with HBO at 2 ATA ($N = 16$) (treatment group) with treatment using air at 1.1 ATA ($N = 16$) (control group) in a hyperbaric chamber. Each group received three treatments at their respective pressures: one for 90 min and two for 60 min each. Mean age, severity grade, and time to treatment were similar in both groups. The change from initial to final evaluation was significantly greater in the treatment group. Subjective pain index fell significantly with HBO as compared to the fall with air treatment. No differences were noted in passive or active range of motion when comparing HBO treatment with air treatment. Time to recovery was the same in both groups. Regression analysis to determine the influence of time to treatment, initial severity of injury, HBO, and age showed no effect of HBO treatment on time to recovery. Although this study did not show any lessening of the time of recovery, there was a reduction of the pain index.

HBO treatment has been reported to reduce post-injury swelling in animals, and in humans. Positive results have also been reported regarding tissue remodeling after injuries involving bones, muscles and ligaments with improved recovery.

HBO as an Adjunct to Sports Training

The effect of HBO on physical performance has been discussed in Chapter 4. There is no evidence that HBO can extend the limits of physical performance in normal healthy adults. Recovery from exhausting physical exercise is, however, hastened in line with the faster recovery from biochemical disturbances.

The role of oxygen inhalation in physical exercise was examined by Jain (1989b). There is no conclusive proof that oxygen inhalation can extend human physical performance. As well, oxygen is a drug and its use may not be permitted by some sports organizations, particularly the International Olympic Committee. Exercise under HBO conditions may have its limits, as strenuous exercise with rise of body temperature may predispose to oxygen toxicity. We have used HBO to aid exercise in neurologically disabled patients without any complications although their exercise capacity is somewhat limited. In normal healthy volunteers, no problems have been seen in carrying out nonexhaustive physical exercise. Further investigations are needed to determine the effects of exhaustive exercise under HBO conditions by trained athletes.

HBO is not a panacea for all pains and aches associated with sports. Delayed onset of muscle soreness after intensive training is one of the commonest complaints, particularly among those not conditioned to heavy exercise. This can occur in the absence of any direct trauma or injury to bones and ligaments. Byrnes et al (1998) tested 21 college students without a history of recent weight training who followed a strenuous program of eccentric weight lifting to establish muscle soreness on the dominant arm that was allowed to recover for 14 days. Subjects were then randomized to 3 groups:

1. Control ($n = 8$)
2. Preventive treatment with one session of HBO at 2.4 ATA for 120 min administered within 2 h of the injury and followed by four subsequent sessions ($n = 6$).
3. Regenerative treatment by 4 HBO treatments beginning 24 h after injury ($n = 7$).

All subjects were tested for creatine phosphate kinase as a marker of muscle injury and MRI for muscle imaging, before the exercise and at intervals throughout the study period. There were no significant differences between the three groups. The authors concluded that HBO started immediately post-exercise or applied 24 h later did not significantly alter the course of delayed onset of muscle soreness.

Future Prospects

Several professional athletic teams, in the fields of hockey, football, basketball, and soccer, utilize and rely on HBO as an adjuvant therapy for numerous sports-related injuries acquired from playing competitive sports (Babul & Rhodes 2000; Dolezal 2002). HBO treatment has effectively increased recovery from fatigue. This was clearly seen at the Nagano Winter Olympics, where sports players experiencing fatigue were successfully treated, enabling the players to continue performing in the games (Ishii et al 2005). However, there is still a paucity of publications on the value of HBO for sports injuries. With the expansion of the use of HBO in rehabilitation, the construction of special rehabilitation facilities with HBO capabilities is foreseen. The most convenient method would be to have the whole physical therapy room pressurized and 100% oxygen administered during the exercises. Such a construction is technically possible and economically feasible.

The role of HBO in sports medicine should be investigated further. At present, HBO is a useful aid in the rehabilitation of sports injuries. Whether it can improve the training and performance of athletes remains to be proven.

36 The Role of HBO in Enhancing Cancer Radiosensitivity

K.K. Jain

Hypoxia generally makes curing some tumors more difficult, and HBO appears to be the best complement to help radiotherapy be more effective. This discussion here is organized around the following points:

Introduction

Studies concerned with the relationship between oxygen tension and the effect of radiation in humans can be traced back to 1910 (Dische 1983). It has long been recognized that hypoxia influences the response of cells and tissues to radiation. Biological evidence for this was gathered in the 1950s, and HBO was introduced into radiotherapy by Churchill-Davidson et al (1955). The technique developed by this team required a special radiotherapy unit and general anesthesia. Reducing the pressure from 4 ATA to 3 ATA, and the avoidance of general anesthesia, have made the technique simpler.

Hypoxia has been noted in malignant tumors (Gray et al 1953). Anemia is common in the cancer population and is suspected to contribute to intratumoral hypoxia. Thomlinson and Gray (1955) showed that the corded structure of some tumors could be explained in terms of diffusion gradients of oxygen. At a specific distance from individual blood vessels the tumor cells die, leaving cords or cuffs of viable cells around the blood vessel, enclosed in pockets of tumor cells. The recently dead cells are adjacent to the outer edge of the viable cord, and the long-dead cells at greater distances. The radius of the cord, as measured in histological sections, was shown to be similar to the calculated diffusion distance for oxygen. It was postulated that one or two cell layers adjacent to necrosis would contain hypoxic but viable cells and hence be radioresistant.

The oxygen tension inside the tumor has been reported to be as low as 8 mmHg. It drops to even lower figures as the tumor enlarges and may drop to zero in the necrotic center of the tumor. Hypoxia increases the resistance of cancer to radiotherapy. With oxygen tension at zero, the amount of radiation required to be effective is three times that required with normal oxygen tension. Various approaches to coping with hypoxia in cancer include:

- Fractionation of total radiation dose to shrink the tumor and to allow tumor cells to reoxygenate in the intervals between sessions of radiotherapy.
- Oxygenation. This is usually achieved by HBO at 2–3 ATA. It is questionable if breathing 100% oxygen at normobaric pressure can be effective. Oxygen carrying solutions have also been used to improve oxygenation of the tumors.
- Modification of oxygen unloading capacity of the hemoglobin
- Hypoxic cell sensitizers: metronidazole and misonidazole. These substances substitute for oxygen and act similarly to oxygen to "fix" the radicals. They kill the hypoxic cells that survive irradiation.
- Correction of anemia may be a worthwhile strategy for radiation oncologists to improve tumor hypoxia and im-

prove response to radiotherapy as well as survival (Harrison et al 2002).

The theoretical basis for the use of HBO as an adjunct to radiotherapy is as follows:

- A number of proliferating cells in many tumors are under severely hypoxic or anoxic conditions.
- The reproductive integrity of such cells is substantially more resistant to damage by radiation than that of cells oxygenated to normal physiological levels.
- The larger the number of cells that lose their reproductive capability, the greater the chance of cure or palliation.

More than a quarter of century ago, opinions on this topic were as follows. Glassburn et al (1977) stated: "It has not been demonstrated unequivocally that radiation under hyperbaric oxygen is superior to well fractioned, well conceived conventional radio-therapy . . . well controlled studies especially in early stage disease are still necessary. It would be worthwhile to undertake such trials especially with tumors of the head and the neck which constitute the most promising site of tumor for study. As others have noted, even 5–10% improvement in survival would mean many lives saved." Russian investigators were more enthusiastic about the role of HBO in radiotherapy. Sergeev et al (1977) concluded: "Hyperbaric oxygen employed in radiotherapy increases the rate of neoplasm damage and reduces the rate of recurrences . . . No rise in percentage of distant metastases was noted in cases irradiated under hyperbaric oxygenation."

To demonstrate the effectiveness of HBO in increasing the radiosensitivity of tumors, one must show that it improves either the therapeutic ratio or the therapeutic efficiency. The radiation therapeutic ratio is the relation between the damage caused in the tumor and the damage caused to normal tissues exposed to the same dose of radiation under the same physiological conditions. The therapeutic ratio for a specified dose of radiation will be increased by HBO if the oxygen enhancement ratio (OER) for the tumor exceeds that of the normal tissues. This is easy to achieve in small tumors but is difficult in large tumors because of the vasoconstriction produced by HBO. The term "radiation therapeutic ratio" should be used in reporting data on treatment with HBO, systemic radiation sensitizers, and whole body hyperthermia. The term "radiation efficiency" should be used if local hyperthermia is applied to the tumor to increase the local effectiveness of treatment with HBO.

Another factor to be considered is the increase in tissue perfusion following radiation. Radiation biologists and oncologists have disputed the importance of hypoxic cells in clinical radiotherapy. Hypoxic tumor cells in animals do impair the radiation response of animal tumors, but it is questionable whether hypoxic cells persist following reoxy-

Table 36.1
Experimental Studies of the Effect of HBO on Tumor Radiosensitivity

Authors and year	Experimental design	Results
Fujimura (1974)	Rabbits with implanted VX2 maxillary carcinoma. Two groups: – Experimental. Radiotherapy under HBO – Control. Radiotherapy without HBO	1. Tumor disappeared in 53% of the experimental group as compared to 13% in control group. 2. DNA synthesis inhibited more markedly in the experimental than in the control group.
Ihde *et al* (1975)	Study of effects of various durations of exposure to air and HBO on incorporation of tritiated thymidine into DNA of B 16 melanoma in mice.	Depression of incorporation of thymidine into DNA under HBO indicating reduction of tumor growth.
Wiernick and Perrins (1975)	Study of rectal biopsies of patients with rectal carcinoma undergoing radiotherapy under HBO.	A more extensive depression of pericryptal fibroblasts under HBO with radiation than under air. No difference after recovery.
Milas *et al* (1985)	Study of sensitivity of 4-day, induced pulmonary micrometastases of murine fibrosarcoma to ionizing	Radiation sensitivity increased 1.13 times under HBO. radiation. radiation under HBO.
McDonald et al (1996)	Twenty Golden Syrian hamster cheek-pouch carcinomas were induced with an established chemical carcinogen. Half of these underwent 30 HBO sessions (2.81 ATA/1 h) while the other half served as controls.	At necropsy, animals receiving HBO therapy had significantly smaller tumors and fewer metastases.
Kalns *et al* (1998)	Carcinoma prostate cell monolayers grown under normoxic conditions were exposed to cisplatin, taxol or doxorubicin for 90 minutes under HBO (3 ATA 100% oxygen) or normal pressure air.	HBO decreased the rate of growth, and increased sensitivity to anticancer agents but the effects were cell line dependent

genation that occurs with increased perfusion following each radiation fraction. The use of bioreducible markers to positively label zones of viable hypoxic cells within solid tumors and to predict for tumor radioresistance is now possible. Several hypoxic markers have been identified and their selective binding within tumors has been measured by both invasive and non-invasive assays (Chapman *et al* 1998).

The focus of this chapter is on the role of HBO in tumor hypoxia and radiation therapy. As an alternative to radiation, antiangiogenic approaches are being developed to target tumor vasculature to prevent tumor growth. Hypoxia-mediated gene therapy is another approach. Modified quinone-based bioreductive drugs retain their potent cytotoxic effects under hypoxic conditions and can be delivered, selectively, to hypoxic tumors (McNally *et al* 2002). Although antiangiogenic therapy alone can suppress the growth of established tumors, it can also potentiate the effects of radiation and chemotherapy. Because the latter treatments depend on adequate blood flow to the tumor to deliver oxygen and drugs, respectively, antiangiogenic therapy to reduce the tumor blood supply would interfere with this delivery. It is recommended that the antiangiogenic treatment should follow rather than precede a combination of radiation or chemotherapy with HBO (Jain 2004). There is no evidence that HBO stimulates tumor angiogenesis.

Experimental Studies of the Radiosensitizing Effect of HBO

The radiosensitizing ability of 100% normobaric oxygen has been investigated in mouse mammary carcinoma using a variety of fractionated regimens and indicate that oxygen can play an important role in the management of cancers where hypoxia may limit the effect of radiotherapy (Rojas *et al* 1990). Some experimental studies of the effects of HBO on radiosensitivity of cancer are listed in Table 36.1.

Brizel *et al* (1997) have assessed tumor growth after exposure to radiation plus either HBO, carbogen or carbogen/nicotinamide and the relationship between pretreatment tumor oxygenation and growth time. R3230Ac carcinomas were grown in the flanks of F344 rats. Animals were randomized to one of seven radiation treatment groups: sham irradiation or irradiation plus room air, HBO (100% O_2/3 ATA), nicotinamide, carbogen, carbogen/nicotinamide or HBO/nicotinamide. Tumors received 20 Gy in a single dose. Irradiation with HBO, HBO/nicotinamide and carbogen/nicotinamide increased growth time relative to room air. HBO was significantly more effective than carbogen/nicotinamide. Growth times for all tumors exposed to HBO were longer than those of the most fully oxygenated tumors (no baseline pO_2 values < 10 mmHg) not exposed to HBO. These results suggest that HBO may improve radiation response by additional mechanisms separate from overcoming the oxygen effect.

Clinical Studies of HBO as Radiation Sensitizer

Carcinoma of the Cervix

The first pilot study involving the use of HBO as an adjunct to the radiotherapy of carcinoma of the cervix (stages III and IV) was published by Johnson in 1965. The author suggested that HBO might improve the survival of patients treated without intracavitary radiation and that any difference might be small if intracavitary radiation were added to HBO.

Watson *et al* (1978) reported the results of the British Medical Research Council (MRC) randomized clinical trial of HBO in the radiotherapy of advanced cancer of the cervix. A total of 320 cases were contributed by four radiotherapy centers in the United Kingdom. The use of HBO re-

sulted in improved local control of the tumor and extended survival. The benefit was greatest in patients under the age of 55 with stage II disease. There was a slight increase in radiation morbidity, but it seemed that the benefit of HBO outweighed this factor and that there was genuine improvement of the therapeutic ratio. A randomized controlled trial of HBO in the radiotherapy of Stage IIb and III carcinoma of cervix was performed between 1971 and 1980 (Dische *et al* 1999). HBO gave no benefit in the treatment of patients with stage IIb and III carcinoma of the cervix treated with radiotherapy using two fractionation regimes. There was evidence for an increase in late radiation morbidity when treatment was given in hyperbaric oxygen rather than in air and when, using 10 fractions, a total dose of 45 rather than 40 Gy was achieved. The issue remains controversial – randomized trials have not settled it. Currently though, the interest in HBO as an adjunct to radio-

Table 36.2
Clinical Studies of HBO as an Adjunct to the Radiotherapy of Head and Neck Cancer

Authors and year	Diagnosis and type of study	Results
Glanzmann *et al* (1974)	Malignant tumors of oropharynx and laryngopharyn. Combined radiation and HBO. Results compared with literature reports of treatment by radiation alone.	Improvement observed in the healing quotient in advanced tumors particularly those of the oropharynx.
Sealy *et al* (1977)	Head and neck cancer. Random allocation to treatment by radiotherapy alone or combined with HBO.	Higher death rate in HBO group but less local recurrences and longer life span.
Nelson and Holt (1978)	Advanced head and neck cancer. Three groups; 1. Cobalt radiotherapy 2. Cobalt radiotherapy plus HBO 3. Radiotherapy + HBO + microwave hyperthermia	Group　Resolution rate　3-year survival 1　36.5%　19% 2　62.5%　29% 3　94.0%　54%
Sause *et al* (1979)	Squamous cell carcinoma of head and neck. Randomized. 1. Treated in air. 250 rads, 4 times/2. Total 6250 rads. 2. Treated under HBO. 480 rads × 13 sessions = 6250 rads	Better tolerance of radiotherapy in immediate results were not different.
Churchill-Davison *et al* (1973)	Squamous cell carcinoma of head and neck with metastases in cervical lymph nodes. Treated by HBO and radiotherapy and compared with patients treated previously by conventional surgery and radiation.	No improvement in survival rate
Darialova *et al* (1985)	Laryngeal cancer. Randomized. Method of mean fractionation to overcome tumor hypoxia and to raise selective radiosensitivity.	In the group with HBO plus radiation: 1. Less frequent radiation reactions 2. Less metastases
Henk (1986)	Head and neck cancer. Prospective controlled trial to compare effects of 10 fractions of radiotherapy under HBO versus 30 fractions under air.	No difference in tissue effects between the 2 groups but survival rate was higher and recurrences less in HBO group.
Denham *et al* (1987)	Squamous cell carcinoma arising from: anterior two-thirds of the tongue, oropharynx, hypopharynx, supraglottic larynx. Radiotherapy under HBO versus air.	5-year survival was higher in the HBO group than in the group treated in air but the difference was not significant.
Whittle *et al* (1990)	Glottic cancer. Retrospective analysis of 397 patients. 240 treated in air and 157 under HBO.	Local tumor control rate showed significant improvement in favor of HBO: Stage 1, 10%; Stage II, 37%; Stage III, 73%
Haffty *et al* (1999)	Randomized trial on 48 patients evaluating HBO at 4 ATA in combination with hypofractionated radiation therapy in patients with locally advanced squamous cell carcinoma of the head and neck (SCCHN).	Long-term outcome from this study demonstrates substantial improvements in response rate with the use of HBO.

therapy of carcinoma of the cervix has declined. In a retrospective analysis of patients in MRC trials, anemic patients (hemoglobin less than 10 g%) treated with blood transfusion and HBO had a better local tumor control than those treated in air (Dische *et al* 1983).

Head and Neck Cancer

Lee *et al* (1996) have reviewed the rationale and results of clinical trials that utilize hypoxic sensitizers or cytotoxins in the treatment of head and neck carcinoma. Since the mid-1970s, clinical research in overcoming tumor hypoxia was mainly centered on the use of nitro-imidazoles as hypoxic cell sensitizers. However, the results from several major clinical trials remain inconclusive. Hypoxic cytotoxins, such as tirapazamine, represent a novel approach in overcoming radioresistant hypoxic cells. Tirapazamine is a bioreductive agent which, by undergoing one electron reduction in hypoxic conditions, forms cytotoxic free radicals that produce DNA strand breaks causing cell death. *In vitro* and *in vivo* laboratory studies demonstrate that tirapazamine is 40 to 150 times more toxic to cells under hypoxic conditions as compared to oxygenated conditions. However, HBO trials for head and neck cancer, conducted since 1970s, have demonstrated that HBO improved local control and survival rates in patients with head and neck cancer receiving radiotherapy. Combination of HBO with radiotherapy is considered to be useful for the following reasons:

- It allows a more uniform kill by improving the oxygenation, and therefore the radiosensitivity, at the cellular level.
- It is useful as an adjunct to surgical repair after radiation.

Other studies to evaluate HBO as an adjunct to radiotherapy are listed in Table 36.2. The number of patients in these studies varied from 50 to 120.

It has been shown that HBO enables the reduction of preoperative radiation. This makes no difference in the immediate postoperative results but has the following advantages:

- Reduction of period of preoperative radiation and the interval between its discontinuance and the operation.
- Increase in the rate of primary wound healing because of fewer radiation effects on the skin and the soft tissues.
- Less impairment of the lymphocyte function.

In conclusion it may be stated that most of the studies show some advantage of using radiotherapy in combination with HBO.

Carcinoma of the Lung

Cade and McEwen (1978) concluded from the results of a controlled trial on the effect of HBO plus radiotherapy in 281 patients that in cases of squamous cell tumors treated by large fractions of radiotherapy (3600 rads in six fractions), the survival rate was 24.6% in the HBO group compared with 12.4% in the air group.

Carcinoma of the Bladder

Kirk *et al* (1976) treated 27 patients suffering from carcinoma of the bladder with radiotherapy (4 MeV linear accelerator) and HBO (3 ATA). There was a high incidence of rapid onset of high dose effects. The authors felt that to achieve maximal effect the maximum value of the cumulative radiation effect was required. It appears that this is difficult to achieve in such cases. Cade *et al* (1978) carried out a randomized clinical trial sponsored by MRC (Medical Research Council, UK) of HBO in carcinoma of the bladder in 241 patients. No benefit from the use of HBO was seen, and this study was abandoned. In a more recent study, 61 patients with locally advanced bladder carcinoma were treated using a Phase II trial delivering radiotherapy to the bladder with inhalation of carbogen alone in 30 patients and the addition of oral nicotinamide prior to radiotherapy with carbogen (normobaric 95% oxygen, 5% carbon dioxide) in 31 patients (Hoskin *et al* 1999). The results from these 61 patients were compared with those from two earlier attempts at hypoxic sensitization: the second MRC HBO trial in patients with bladder carcinoma and a Phase III trial of misonidazole with radiotherapy in patients with bladder carcinoma. Although there was no difference between the HBO and misonidazole trials, when compared with the two earlier series there was a large, statistically significant difference in favor of those patients receiving carbogen with or without nicotinamide for local control, progression free survival, and overall survival. Although the advantage for the carbogen group may be explained in part by changes in radiotherapy practice over the period of the three studies the improvement in local control is sufficiently great to support the hypothesis that hypoxia is important in modifying the control of bladder carcinoma using radiation therapy. Further evaluation of accelerated radiotherapy, carbogen, and nicotinamide in patients with bladder carcinoma is needed in a Phase III trial.

Malignant Melanoma

Sealy *et al* (1974) treated 22 malignant melanoma patients with large fractions of cobalt and HBO. Half of the lesions responded favorably to the treatment, including metastases. The authors concluded that radiotherapy, probably in combination with HBO, should receive more consideration in the treatment of malignant melanoma.

Malignant Glioma

The results of radiotherapy combined with HBO in 9 patients with malignant glioma were compared with those of radiotherapy without HBO in 12 patients (Kohshi *et al* 1996). This is the first report of a pilot study of irradiation immediately after exposure to HBO in humans. All patients receiving this treatment showed more than 50% regression of the tumor, and in 4 of them, the tumors disappeared completely. Only 4 out of 12 patients without HBO showed decreases in tumor size, and all 12 patients died within 36 months. So far, this new regimen seems to be a useful form of radiotherapy for malignant gliomas. Beppu *et al* (2003) added HBO to IAR therapy (Interferon-beta, ACNU as nimustine hydrochloride and radiotherapy), which is a common therapy for malignant glioma in Japan. Although there was a good initial response in patients with residual tumors. The addition of HBO did not increase the survival time but this is a problem specific to malignant glioma. Because HBO/IAR therapy could be applied to patients with poor prognostic factors, short treatment period, and acceptable toxicity, the authors recommend a prospective randomized trial to assess the benefit of this therapy.

Advantages of HBO as an Adjunct to Radiotherapy

HBO is considered to be the most effective method for counteracting tumor hypoxia for enhancing the effect of radiotherapy on cancer). This approach has been shown to be effective in only some types of cancer. Concern has been expressed about the danger to the normal tissues of the body from the excessive free radical generation with HBO. In fact, the damage to the normal tissues is reduced by oxidation of cofactors in the peroxidation process. The advantages of HBO combined with radiotherapy are:

- HBO is also a useful therapy for radiation-induced necrosis of normal tissues.
- In a controlled study of patients with head and neck cancer treated by radiation with or without HBO, the survival was shown to be higher in the HBO group. The greatest advantage was seen in the less advanced tumors).
- In experimental bladder tumor, tissue oxygen tension has been shown to be higher in the bladder trigone region (Nakada 1988). HBO was shown to enhance the effect of combined chemotherapy and radiotherapy in this model (Akiya *et al* 1988).

Drawbacks of HBO as Adjunct to Radiotherapy of Cancer

1. HBO is effective only if hypoxia is present.
2. HBO is not effective in the presence of metastases. It is certain that small metastatic lesions are hypoxic. Concern has been expressed that HBO may enhance the growth of metastases.
3. If tumor vessels are occluded either spontaneously or therapeutically in an attempt to necrose the tumor, oxygen cannot penetrate the surviving hypoxic cells.
4. In the case of some tumors where the intercapillary distance is 125 μm, about 20% of the tumor cells are hypoxic (Vaupel *et al* 1988). Even if 1% if these survive the treatment, the tumor would grow back again. To eradicate the tumor completely would require further therapy beyond the tolerance limits of the body.
5. Oxygen toxicity. Protective agents such as vitamin E and magnesium can reduce it.
6. HBO is contraindicated in patients with acute radiation sickness as it may aggravate the symptoms.

Combination of Other Methods with HBO and Irradiation For Cancer

Hyperthermia

Tumors can be destroyed by raising the core temperature to 42°–43°C by various devices. The mechanism of this treatment is based on the fact that cancer cells are heated preferentially by heat application due to lower vascularity in the tumor compared with the surrounding normal tissue. When this method is used in conjunction with radiation therapy or chemotherapy, higher partial pressures of oxygen in the tumor result in increase in tumor cell damage. Maguire *et al* (1988) have studied the oxygen profile of a tumor spheroid model and stated that the more broadly based the thermal radiation, the greater is the tendency to a rise of oxygen tension in the tumor.

General warming of the body, which is sometimes referred to as hyperthermia, involves temperatures of only 38.5°C. This causes vasodilatation and increases oxygen uptake in the body. Hyperthermia has been used either before or after HBO sessions. Thermal enhancement has been shown to be greater by hyperthermia given before irradiation compared with the reverse sequence (Urano *et al* 1988).

Hypothermia

Lowering of body temperature is associated with reduced metabolism of the tissues and reduced oxygen consumption by the tumors. If the blood supply to a hypothermic tumor can be maintained, then the hypoxic fraction of the cells should be reduced and the radiation response increased. This hypothesis has been tested with radiation under HBO and increased tumor response has been demonstrated (Nias *et al* 1988).

Sealy *et al* (1986) have suggested a combined approach for radiosensitization using hypothermia and HBO. Hypothermia causes reduction of oxygen utilization and hence a better redistribution of oxygen. The authors treated 31 patients in whom radiosensitivity was achieved by the use of hypothermia and HBO (3 ATA). Of the 29 patients in whom the treatment was completed, 27 had full regression of the tumors. The major problems of this technique are the logistics of combining the three modalities and the complications of hypothermia.

Vasodilators

Vasodilators increase the blood flow to the tumor but may cause a steal phenomenon. The use of vasodilators to counteract the vasoconstricting effect of HBO has been suggested by Sealy *et al* (1986), but has not been tried experimentally or clinically.

Induced Anemia and Red Cell Infusion

This procedure has been shown to increase the effectiveness of radiation therapy under HBO (Rojas *et al* 1987). Sealy *et al* (1989) showed improved 21-month survival of patients with cervical cancer undergoing radiation therapy when anemia was induced by venesection. Mice with transplanted tumors and anemia induced by iron-deficient diet showed decreased radiosensitivity when treatment was given in air whereas HBO was successful in overcoming increased resistance to radiation (McCormack *et al* 1990).

Radiation Sensitizing Agents

Combination with nitroimidazoles improves the efficacy of radiation therapy and its effectiveness may be enhanced further by combining with treatment of induced anemia (Sealy 1991).

Use of Perfluorochemicals as Oxygen Carriers

These are highly fluorinated organic compounds which can dissolve large volumes of oxygen and this property can be enhanced under hyperbaric conditions. Fluosol-DA and HBO (3 ATA) combination has been shown to increase the radiation response of malignant cells in rat rhabdomyosarcoma. The proportion of the severely hypoxic cells in the tumor is reduced to less than 1.5% of the original number (Martin *et al* 1987). Treatment with Fluosol-DA combined with breathing 100% oxygen has been shown to be an effective adjuvant to radiation therapy and chemotherapy in several animal tumor systems (Teicher *et al* 1988).

Dowling *et al* (1992) demonstrated the safety of combined use of Fluosol with HBO (3 ATA) in a pilot study on patients with malignant glioma of the brain. Adverse reactions have been reported, and the safety of currently available preparations of perfluorochemicals should be viewed with caution (Lowe 1987).

Perfluorooctylbromide (Oxydent) has been shown to increase radiosensitivity of experimentally induced sarcoma of mice and warrants further study as an adjunct to cancer chemotherapy (Rockwell *et al* 1992).

Antineoplastic Agents

Combination of antineoplastic agents and HBO induces dual injury to the mitochondrial respiration and cell membranes. HBO can be added to regimes combining radiotherapy with chemotherapy. Concomitant HBO enhances the effects of 5-fluorouracil on malignant tumors (Takiguchi *et al* 2001). However, no clinical trials have been done to evaluate this combination.

Photodynamic Therapy

Use of HBO in photodynamic therapy of tumors has been suggested by Jirsa (1990). Combination of hematoporphyrin derivatives and laser radiation has been used for treatment of cancer. Addition of HBO to this regimen speeds up the photodynamic reaction processes by raising the transmission efficiency of light energy, increasing the quantum amount of oxygen, and extending the effective distance radius of oxygen (Dong *et al* 1986).

Conclusions

Machin *et al* (1997) have reviewed the survival outcome from the randomized Phase III trials in solid tumors published on behalf of, or in collaboration with, the Cancer Therapy Committee (CTC) of the British Medical Research Council over a 30-year period to 31 December 1995. In all, 32 trials, involving over 5000 deaths in more than 8000 patients, have been published. Tumor types have included bladder, bone, brain, cervix, colon and rectum, head and neck, kidney, lung, ovary, prostate and skin. The MRC trials have made an impact on both clinical practice and research activities. Trials of HBO have defined the biological activity of this approach, and the appropriate dose of radiotherapy in patients with brain tumors has been found.

There is considerable evidence for the presence of hypoxia in human tumors. Vascular insufficiency has been demonstrated on histopathology of the tumors, direct oxygen measurements, and mapping of hypoxic areas by imaging techniques. It appears that hypoxia is probably responsible for failure to cure some tumors such as squamous cell carcinoma but, even within tumors of the same type and stage, hypoxia does not occur to the same extent. Response to modifying agents also depends upon whether hypoxia is acute or chronic. New methods to detect hypoxic tumor cells (hypoxic cell stains) are being developed. The future prospects for the control of those tumors where hypoxia is a problem appear to be good.

A systematic search of the literature was conducted for randomized controlled trials of HBO for radiosensitization incacer, and pooled analyses were made of predetermined clinical outcomes (Bennett *et al* 2008). Nineteen trials involving 2286 patients contributed to this review. There is some evidence that HBO improves local tumour control and mortality for cancers of the head and neck, and local tumour recurrence in cancers of the uterine cervix. These benefits may only occur with unusual fractionation schemes. There were methodological and reporting inadequacies of the studies included in this review and more research is needed.

Of the various adjuvants to radiotherapy, HBO appears to be the best. It can be combined with other radiation enhancers. The effect of HBO in enhancing radiosensitivity is most pronounced in head and neck tumors. The objectives of future research projects to assess the role of HBO in cancer radiotherapy should be:

- To determine the effect of increasing oxygen tension on the radiosensitivity of a tumor model in animal experiments, where variable factors such as tumor pathology, size, location, etc. are eliminated.
- To identify the mechanism of radiosensitivity-enhancing action of oxygen. The current hypothesis is that "HBO, by increasing oxygen tension in the hypoxic tumor, increases its susceptibility to free radicals, which are generated in excess by the combined HBO and radiation." To prove this would require monitoring of oxygen tension in the tumor as well as measurement of free radicals in the tissues.
- To determine the most effective and safest measures that combine HBO and radiotherapy.
- Comparison of HBO with carbogen (95% oxygen + 5% carbon dioxide) as an adjunct to radiation therapy.

37 HBO Therapy and Organ Transplants

H.A. Wyatt

HBO has been used for preservation of organs prior to transplant. It has a beneficial effect on ischemia-reperfusion injury, which is a significant problem in organ transplant. Use of HBO is recommended in patients prior to transplant procedures.

Introduction

There are several good reasons to believe that HBO may play a role in transplant medicine as it has often been used successfully as an adjunct in treating wound infections in heart and lung transplants, and several studies have explored the use of HBO to increase the length of time that harvested organs may be stored prior to transplantation (Guimaraes *et al* 2005). However, the most important reason to think that HBO may play a beneficial role in organ transplantation is that significant ischemia-reperfusion injury (IR) occurs in all deceased donor organ transplants – as well as in some of those from live donors. In fact, in renal transplants, IR is the leading contributor to the development of delayed graft function (Gandolfo & Rabb 2008). In pancreas transplants, graft pancreatitis is one of the main complications. Free-radicals generated by IR are predominantly responsible for the development of the pancreatitis (Albendea *et al* 2007). In liver transplant, reactive oxygen species are a major cause of hepatocellular injury during transplantation (Zwacka *et al* 1998). In lung transplantation, IR is a major source of early mortality (de Perrot *et al* 2003).

The usefulness of HBO in ameliorating IR is well documented. This attenuation of IR injury underlies many of the approved and off-label treatment indications of HBO. By blocking the CD11/18 (beta-2 intergrin)-mediated neutrophil adhesion in the post-capillary venules, HBO also blocks the formation of oxygen free radicals, inflammatory cytokines, and interleukins, which in turn protects the vascular endothelium, prevents the disruption of the endothelial basement membrane, and protects against microcirculatory failure.

As with some other recent HBO applications, the idea of using HBO in organ transplants is not a new one. Several studies to investigate potential roles for HBO in transplant medicine were conducted in the early 1970s. However, despite promising results, these were not translated from the laboratory to the clinic. Recently, however, there has been a resurgence in interest in the use of HBO. There are also several patents on file for hyperbaric chambers designed to reduce reperfusion injury for organ preservation.

The significance of IR injury in various organ transplants led to a great deal of research into possible methods to ameliorate the problem. Several studies involving various organ transplant models examined the effect of inhaled carbon monoxide in reducing chemokine activation from IR (Kaizu *et al* 2007, Kohmoto *et al* 2006, Neto *et al* 2004). The use of a known toxin to prevent injury – when a safe and convenient alternative with documented effectiveness exists – makes little clinical sense.

While IR injury plays a major role in acute transplant problems, rejection issues arise from lymphoid tissue activation as well. The importance of immunosuppression in transplant recipients is well known. There are a number of different immune mechanisms involved in transplant rejection. These can include CD4, macrophage, and MHC-1 expression. MHC-1-related chain A antibodies seem to be associated with an increased frequency of acute rejection and decreased donor graft survival (Morales-Buenrostro & Alberu, 2008). HBO is known to decrease the number of CD4 cells, inhibit expression of MHC-1, and inhibit cytokine production that would otherwise lead to an increase in macrophage activation (Al-Waili *et al* 2006).

Lung Transplants

Ischemia-reperfusion injury to the lung following transplant is a well-known complication (de Perrot *et al* 2003). It has been demonstrated that the ischemia-reperfusion injury in lung transplantation is the result of a biphasic process involving the leukocytes from both the donor and the recipient (Fiser *et al* 2001). Currently, one method of decreasing IR injury is to use a heart-lung bypass machine with a leukocyte depleting filter to remove leukocytes from the recipient's blood prior to reperfusion (Kurusz *et al* 2002). One HBO treatment effectively inhibits leukocyte adhesion for at least 24 hours. It would therefore be possible to treat the donor, once the decision to harvest the organ has been made and a recipient identified, prior to harvesting the organ. Given the short treatment time, the recipient could receive an HBO treatment pre-op, while the donor lungs are being evaluated. This would have the effect of suppressing both donor and recipient leukocyte adhesion.

HBO has been used to treat other complications arising from lung transplant as well. These include sternal osteomyelitis (Mills & Bryson 2006), respiratory infection, acute peripheral embolism, and arterial gas embolism (Higuchi *et al* 2006). In all cases, HBO was shown to be a safe and effective therapy for these complications.

A small pilot study examining the effects of HBO on pulmonary function in patients suffering from chronic transplant rejection was initiated in New Orleans in 2005, but was disrupted by a natural disaster. However, some of the initial findings in the small group of end-stage patients were promising. For this study, four patients in the terminal stages of chronic lung transplant were enrolled to receive daily HBO. All patients had regular follow-up by a lung transplant team at a local teaching hospital. Although the study was disrupted by Hurricane Katrina in 2005, three of the four patients reported subjective improvements in their pulmonary function, and in two patients improvement of their pulmonary function tests were also documented. Of the four, only one had received the full study course of 40 HBO treatments. The other two had received 10 and 12 treatments, respectively. The single patient to complete the initial phase of the trial had achieved a 10% increase in

FVC, despite having had a continuous decline in lung function over the previous year, and he also experienced a near doubling of his exercise tolerance. It is worth noting that all of the patients in this study were in the end-stages of chronic rejection with very poor prognoses.

The relative ease with which HBO therapy can be delivered, even to a patient on mechanical ventilation, the short treatment duration, and the duration of the treatment effect seem to indicate that this treatment could be easily integrated into the transplant surgery protocol. The relatively low potential for harm to the recipient from HBO further increases the attractiveness of this therapy.

Pancreas Transplants

Graft pancreatitis is one of the main post-operative complications of pancreas transplantation. Studies using a porcine model have demonstrated the role of lipid peroxidation, which occurs after graft reperfusion, in the development of pancreatitis (Albendea et al 2007).

While there are no current studies evaluating the degree of donor vs. host leukocyte contribution to pancreatic injury, it is not unreasonable to assume that both immune systems play a role as they do in the lung model.

Animal studies of islet cell transplantation have demonstrated a beneficial effect of peritransplant HBO on the survival and function of the transplanted islet cells (Juang et al 2002). This study also examined the effect of HBO treatment regimen on the functional outcome of the transplant. It was found that in all cases HBO improved functional measures. However, those rats that received twice daily treatment beginning 14 days prior to transplant and continued through post-operative day 28 showed not only improved function, but also a greater beta-cell mass than any of the other regimens including once daily treatment.

Renal Transplants

The role of IR in renal injury during transplantation is well documented and is the main cause of intrinsic acute renal failure as well as a major cause of early renal dysfunction in cadaveric transplants (Gandolfo & Rabb 2008). A number of methods have been tried to decrease the amount of IR injury sustained by the kidneys. Machine perfusion has been used with some reduction in delayed graft function, although no difference in graft survival was found 1 year following transplant (Wight et al 2003). HBO has been tested in conjunction with various perfusates in transportable chambers to increase the preservation time and decrease IR injury (Inuzuka et al 2007, Rubbini et al 2007). The results

have been promising, with organs demonstrating significant preservation of function for up to 48 hours.

Liver Transplants

IR injury also plays a major role in acute hepatic damage following transplant. It has been shown that this damage is the result of neutrophils (Ramaiah & Jaeschke 2007), oxygen free-radicals (Muralidharan & Christophi 2007), and cytokines (Colletti et al 1996, Zwacka et al 1998). Unlike some of the other organs discussed, the use of HBO in liver transplant has been more extensively researched. In addition to the suppressive effects that HBO has on the IR injury, it has also been considered as a possible adjunct treatment in post-transplant hepatic artery thrombosis and primary graft dysfunction (Castro e Silva et al 2006). In this case report, two patients were treated with HBO, one having developed hepatic artery thrombosis and the other a primary graft dysfunction. In both cases, the patients' liver function studies began to normalize soon after HBO was initiated.

Another aspect of liver transplant is the development of IR injury to the lung after liver transplant. Chemokines released secondary to hepatic IR injury are reported to be responsible for the development of IR injury in the lung of liver transplant recipients (Colletti et al 1995). The use of HBO on the donor and recipient to ameliorate the development of IR in the transplanted liver would disrupt this pathway, potentially protecting not only the transplanted liver, but also the recipient's lung.

Another area in which HBO has been evaluated is in the case of small-for-size liver grafts. Because of the perennial shortage of organs, techniques that allow the donation of a portion of the organ from a living donor have been developed. Initially, this involved donation of the smaller, left-lobe of the liver into the recipient. However, the left lobe is often significantly smaller than the right and had been found to be insufficient to meet the metabolic demands of some of the recipients. As a result, some teams began using the larger right lobe. This technique, however, imposes more surgical stress on the donor and cannot be used if the remaining left lobe amounts to less than 30% of the donor's total liver volume. Several groups have examined the effect of HBO on the regeneration and function of liver grafts. One group examined the use of HBO pretreatment on rats, which then underwent either a 70% or 90% hepatectomy (Nori et al 2007). The rats pretreated with HBO had more graft growth and better graft function than controls. Similar results have been reported previously on liver regeneration in rats after undergoing 15% hepatectomy (Kurir et al 2004). Additionally, Kurir's group found that the liver lobules in the HBO treated rats were more histologically normal by light microscopy than those of controls. These findings suggest that the use of HBO may improve recipient outcome and decrease the risk to donors in living donor liver transplant.

Miscellaneous Transplants

In addition to the organ systems discussed above, many animal studies have been performed to valuate the effect of HBO on transplantation of organs such as thyroid (Talmage & Dart 1978), small bowel (Inuzuka *et al* 2007, Sasaki & Joh 2007, Guimaraes *et al* 2005), and skin (Jacobs *et al* 1979). In all cases, investigators found a beneficial effect of the use of HBO with respect to graft survival and function. In these cases, the improved outcomes appear to be related to the inhibition of chemokine formation as the result of attenuation of the IR injury present in the non-HBO transplant groups.

Clinical Application

HBO can be used at three distinct points in the transplant process: in the treatment of the donor in the case of living or heart-beating but brain-dead donors, in the organ storage process, and in the treatment of the recipient prior to, and possibly after, surgery. The treatment of the donor should inactivate the donor white cell component, whereas the treatment of the recipient attenuates the recipient response during the reperfusion phase. The use of HBO during cold-storage, especially in conjunction with organ perfusion may help ameliorate any donor component in cadaveric transplants as well as increase tissue viability in cases where prolonged storage is anticipated.

The optimal treatment protocol would need to be determined clinically; however, our understanding of the mechanisms by which HBO blocks IR injury in its current applications would suggest that even a single treatment of both donor and recipient within 24 hours of surgery may offer significant protection. Further post-op treatments of the recipient may offer additional benefit.

Conclusions

In view of the results obtained in the many animal studies, and the well understood pathways by which IR induces injury and the mechanisms by which HBO is known to block this injury, it seems reasonable to conclude that HBO may be an effective adjunct to the transplant process. Given the chronic organ shortage and the deleterious effects of IR on acute and chronic graft function, the addition of HBO to several steps in the transplant process has the potential to significantly improve the success of organ transplant without significant risk to the recipient or undue stress on the donor. This is true whether the donor is brain-dead or living. In the case of cadaveric transplant, the use of HBO during storage coupled with HBO treatment of the recipient should also prove beneficial.

The low complication rate and favorable side-effect profile of HBO render it a safe adjunct, while the ease with which treatment can be delivered and the short time required to deliver it should make it relatively easy to integrate into the transplant protocol. It is anticipated that this will be a fertile area for future clinical research.

38 Anesthesia in the Hyperbaric Environment

E.M. Camporesi

F = Although the use of anesthesia in the HBO environment is unusual, several clinical indications do exist, though especially diligent attention to technique is required. The key topics in this chapter are:

Historical Perspective

The administration of general anesthesia in the hyperbaric environment was first described by Paul Bert in 1878. His aim was to use nitrous oxide in anesthetic doses and to be able to provide adequate oxygenation. Through the use of elevated pressure he reported this successful endeavor, his results were confirmed by Tindal in 1941, and were reconfirmed by Smith *et al* (1974).

In the 1940s and 1950s cardiac surgical techniques clearly outgrew life support technology. Interest in the surgical treatment of congenital heart malformations grew rapidly after Blalock performed the first successful procedure for tetralogy of Fallot in 1944. When surgical correction of the septal and valvular abnormalities was attempted, the intracardiac portions of the procedures had to be done under hypothermia and cardiopulmonary arrest, as this provided a motionless heart. Limitations to this technique were primarily the short times of total circulatory arrest (less than 10 min) without significant ischemic CNS sequelae. General anesthesia under hyperbaric oxygenation (HBO) provided an added degree of protection and increased the safe cardiac arrest time up to 30 min. Several groups have reported their experiences with anesthesia under hyperbaric conditions, including Smith (1965) at Massachusetts General Hospital, Boerema (1961) in Holland, and McDowell (1966) at the Royal Infirmary in Glasgow. Anesthesia was usually achieved and maintained through the use of nitrous oxide, halothane, or methoxyflurane.

In the mid 1960s a practical cardiopulmonary bypass machine was perfected for wider use. With the introduction of safe cardiopulmonary bypass pumps, cardiac surgery no longer needed to be performed in the hyperbaric chamber. Carotid endarterectomy had also been performed under hyperbaric conditions but this practice fell into disfavor, as it was never firmly demonstrated to be beneficial.

A landmark report from a committee headed by Severinghaus (1965) reviewed the practice of anesthesia under hyperbaric conditions. No recommendations on choice of anesthetic were made in this report; rather, the advantages and disadvantages of commonly used techniques were presented. However, it was stated that intravenous techniques could prove especially useful in the hyperbaric setting.

Present Indications

Nowadays, anesthetic care may be required at increased pressure for the following indications:

- Anesthesia delivered for the treatment of various conditions that produce transient hypoxemia, such as whole lung lavage (usually performed at 2–4 ATA).

- Delivery of anesthesia as a result of emergency surgical procedures required on a patient involved in a diving accident, which might occur while at pressures of up to 35 ATA (depth of saturation in deepest commercial diving).

Winter *et al* (1976) described the phenomenon of pressure reversal of barbiturate anesthesia in mammals. They observed the reversal of barbiturate anesthesia in rats at pressures of 103 ATA. However, the clinical relevance of these findings proved of limited value, since therapeutic pressures of HBO do not exceed 6 ATA. A comprehensive review of this argument appeared later (Kendig & Cohen 1977). Continuing studies, however, in the areas of high pressure physiology have extended the range of pressures tolerated by humans. The deepest exposure recorded for a human is at 69 ATA, and was achieved during a study of physiological responses to exercise (Salzano *et al* 1984) at Duke University Hyperbaric Center.

Physical Considerations Concerning Anesthetic Gases Under Pressure

Modern vaporizers work by forcing a gas, usually oxygen, at a known flow rate through a sintered bronze disk at the bottom of a pool of liquid anesthetic. The amount of anesthetic agent delivered to the patient depends on four factors:

- The particular vapor pressure of the agent (a function of the polarity of the agent, i.e., Van der Waals forces)
- The temperature of the liquid
- The flow of gas through the liquid, and
- The dilution of the anesthetic vapor with by-pass oxygen flow to constitute the desired concentration for delivery.

The key point in calculating the required flows at various ambient pressures is that the vapor pressure of a liquid remains constant with variations in ambient pressure (Morris 1952). For example, the vapor pressure of halothane at 20°C is 243 mmHg. According to Dalton's law of partial pressures, saturated halothane vapor at 1 ATA (760 mmHg) will contain 32% halothane (243/760), while at 4 ATA (3040 mmHg) the same halothane partial pressure will produce a concentration of 8% (243/3040). The amount of carrier gas required to dilute the saturated vapor to the desired inspired concentration (0.5% to 1%, at the clinically useful doses) remains constant with changing ambient pressure. If the desired inspired partial pressure is 7.6 mmHg (1% halothane at 1 ATA), then each volume of saturated vapor must be diluted with 32 volumes of carrier gas at 1 ATA, or with 8 volumes at 4 ATA (which represents the same number of molecules).

Few empirical observations in this area used the Fluotec vaporizer at pressure and measured actual concentrations of gas delivered at different dial settings (McDowell 1987). The Fluotec vaporizer works by directing a stream of gas over a surface of liquid anesthetic and diluting the total gas output. McDowall found that the particular vaporizer tested would deviate at low settings (0.5% to 1%), by delivering nearly twice the anesthetic gas concentration while at two atmospheres. Gas concentrations did not vary significantly from 1 ATA at higher settings (from 2% to 4%).

Flowmeters/rotameters are also affected by pressure, as they measure the flow of a gas on the principle that flow past a resistance is proportional to the pressure gradient. Density is the key variable, especially at high flow rates. Viscosity is a more significant variable at low rates, when the shape of the resistance is tubular. At increased ambient pressure the approximate correction factor is:

$$F_1 = F_0 \times \sqrt{d_0/d_1}$$

where F_1 represents the flow at ambient pressure, F_0 the indicated flow, d_0 the density at 1 ATA, and d_1 the density at present ATA.

For example, at 4 ATA:

$$F_1 = F_0 \times 1/4$$

Therefore,

$$F_1 = 0.5\, F_0$$

This calculation is a good correction estimate if one assumes that the supply line pressure gradient between the chamber and the outside is kept constant.

Physiological Considerations

The major alterations of increased barotrauma pressures are reflected in the respiratory, the cardiac, and the central nervous systems.

Exposure for 24 h to high levels of oxygen (90% to 100%) at 1 to 2 ATA can result in rapid damage to the mucosa of the tracheobronchial tree, manifested by hyperemic mucosa, increased secretions, and atelectasis. This might be of special importance in the patient with reactive airway disease or chronic obstructive pulmonary disease. Airway irritation could complicate endotracheal intubations, because of increased tendency to laryngospasm.

In chronic obstructive pulmonary disease, and any other pulmonary process that narrows the caliber of the airways, increased secretions and increased work of breathing at increased ambient pressure may lead to severe ventilatory difficulties. In addition, pulmonary bullae and other slow exchange zones, as well as mucus plugging, may cause a disastrous problem during decompression as they can lead to parenchymal rupture, pneumothorax, or air embolism secondary to barotrauma.

A reduction in vital capacity has been measured as an index of atelectasis, which correlates with the length and pressure of oxygen exposure and is predicted by empirical units, i.e., units of pulmonary toxicity dose (UPTD) (Clark & Lambertsen 1971). Reductions of vital capacity reverse within hours after termination of oxygen exposure (Don et al 1970; Hickey et al 1973).

Loss of pulmonary surfactant has been described after exposure to HBO. It is not clear whether peroxidation of surfactant plays a significant role in its destruction, but it is clearly demonstrated that surfactant production is inhibited. There is evidence, especially in practice, that adequate humidification of inspired gases protects against some of these pulmonary problems, especially airway irritation (Miller et al 1987). The work of breathing is increased at increased ambient pressures. This is a result of increased turbulent flow due to high gas density. These pressure-induced changes can be minimized by using the largest possible endotracheal tubes.

Cardiovascular Effects

It has been demonstrated that significant peripheral vasoconstriction occurs with the exposure to high blood oxygen tensions. Barratt-Boyes and Wood (1958) showed in humans that while the peripheral vasoconstriction does occur, the pulmonary vascular resistance was decreased. Because of the peripheral vasoconstriction one should avoid giving medications through intramuscular or subcutaneous routes.

Vasoconstriction can also occur in coronary vessels. A number of studies have demonstrated that coronary blood flow is significantly decreased during exposure to HBO. Krishnamurti et al (1971) reported two patients who suffered myocardial infarction while being treated with HBO (one of them died). Patients with significant obstructive coronary disease should be approached cautiously, especially in the delivery of a general anesthetic under HBO.

Some studies have demonstrated that cardiac output can be reduced by as much as 12% during hyperbaric hyperoxia. Probably as a result of increased afterload, no significant changes in contractility have been demonstrated, in a sophisticated dog model exposed to 3 ATA O_2 (Savitt et al 1994).

Central Nervous System

Oxygen is also a potent cerebral vasoconstrictor that affects pial as well as cerebral arterioles. This principle becomes important when treating patients with closed head injuries, as one would expect a protective effect of oxygen on neural

Table 38.1
Pharmacokinetic Parameters for Meperidine (M) and Pentobarbital (P) under Normal and Hyperbaric Conditions (Mean ± SD)
(from Kramer *et al* 1983a,b)

Parameter/Drug	1 ATA	2.8 ATA	6 ATA
$t_{1/2}$ (min)/M	60.40 ± 43.6	44.90 ± 22.7	55.70 ± 17.5
$t_{1/2}$ (h)/P	4.49 ± 1.11	4.88 ± 1.89	6.08 ± 2.29
CLT (ml/(min/kg))/M	75.20 ± 49.8	84.40 ± 37.4	75.40 ± 40.0
CLT (ml/(min/kg))/P	2.82 ± 0.32	3.69 ± 1.23	2.67 ± 0.85
V (l/kg)/M	4.56 ± 2.06	5.18 ± 2.77	5.54 ± 1.63
V (l/kg)/P	1.11 ± 0.37	1.44 ± 0.42	1.29 ± 0.24

No statistically significant differences between different pressures were noted.

structures in patients with closed head injuries or intracranial masses. Although few data on this subject are available, it is possible that seizure threshold may be reduced during general anesthesia in patients who are already at higher risk for seizures. Such patients should have prophylactic anticonvulsant medications before exposures to HBO at high pressures (3 ATA or above) under anesthesia.

The ability of the attending personnel in the chamber to make sound clinical decisions may be impaired while exposed to breathing air at high pressure. Inert gas narcosis is a well described phenomenon in humans breathing air at increased atmospheric pressure. Although not always a significant problem, inert gas narcosis can be observed at pressures of 2 ATA and greater. Nitrogen narcosis is not unpleasant and it has been compared to alcohol intoxication. The affected individual may also experience drowsiness and euphoria and judgment can be impaired. The severity of nitrogen narcosis is directly proportional to the pressure to which a patient is exposed. Patients are usually not at risk since they are breathing high oxygen levels.

Pharmacokinetics in the Hyperbaric Environment

There is only a small volume of data concerning the pharmacokinetics of i.v., anesthetics in the literature. A few studies have been performed with specific agents using animal models. Drugs studied include meperidine and pentobarbital. No significant differences were observed in the half-life, volume of distribution, or plasma clearance of the drugs when pentobarbital and meperidine were measured at 2.8 or 6 ATA. Despite the fact that absolute pharmacokinetic values for the dog differ considerably from those of humans, these observations support the concept that intravenous anesthetic agents commonly used at 1 ATA can be judiciously administered at pressures of 2 to 6 ATA (Table 38.1).

Pressure reversal was addressed by Kramer *et al* (1983a, b) who showed no significant differences in the pharmacokinetics of pentobarbital when given at 1, 2.8, or 6 ATA. In

addition, one does not observe this phenomenon in practice, especially at 2.8 ATA. Pressure reversal could play a role if anesthesia is being delivered at much greater depths (e.g., > 50 ATA).

Intravenous Anesthesia

Ross *et al* (1977) were one of the first groups to advocate intravenous anesthesia for use in the hyperbaric chamber. This was a result of considering the problem of anesthetic gas pollution while delivering gaseous anesthetics at pressures of up to 35 ATA. Li *et al* (1987b) reported the successful use of ketamine anesthesia in 48 patients undergoing open heart surgery while having oxygen administered at 3 ATA. Camporesi and Moon (1987b) reported on the use of ketamine and benzodiazepines along with muscle relaxants in the delivery of anesthesia to patients undergoing therapeutic lung lavages. Approximately 20 patients have been treated with this anesthetic regimen without complications.

Practical Aspects of Anesthesia in the Pressure Chamber

Noise

During decompression and compression, the air entering or escaping the chamber generates a significant level of noise, which can interfere with auscultation or the ability to hear equipment alarms. These traveling times are precisely when the anesthetist must be especially alert of the condition of the patient. Most complications in anesthetic management occur during these chamber pressure changes.

Airway Equipment

Laryngoscopes are not greatly affected by pressure as long as the battery handle is vented and can exchange gas at pressure. Sealed batteries have been shown to function adequately up to 35 ATA. Endotracheal tubes should be of the largest size appropriate for the patient, as when pressure rises, turbulent flow increases and will cause an increase in airway resistance and increasing ventilatory work. Tracheal tube cuffs should be filled with saline rather than air, since water is incompressible and the danger of volume variations in the cuff with changing ambient pressure is avoided.

Ventilators

It is imperative to minimize the amount of electrical equipment in the hyperbaric chamber where oxygen partial pressures are high and the danger of fire and explosion are very real.

Ventilators driven by compressed air are desirable. One must keep in mind that these ventilators function through a pressure differential of about 50 psi. Therefore, as long as the supply line is adjusted to maintain this differential gradient above ambient pressure, the ventilators should work well at pressure, although they will exhibit somewhat lower peak flow rates.

Another consideration is the rate of oxygen leakage from the ventilator. This must be kept to a minimum, as standard operating procedure for multiplace hyperbaric units dictates that the ambient concentration of oxygen should not exceed 23%. This can be achieved by choosing a ventilator with an inherently low oxygen leak and by scavenging and venting outside the chamber. Oil lubrication presents a high risk of fire. Lubrication used for the ventilator should be compatible with high oxygen tensions (e.g., tetrafluoroethylene polymer based lubricants).

Moon *et al* (1986) reported the use of the Monaghan 225 ventilator under hyperbaric conditions. He found that this ventilator, after minor modifications, provided adequate ventilatory support at pressures of up to 6 ATA.

Monitoring

Because anesthesia is not commonly practiced under hyperbaric conditions, it is not administered according to set rules or special dosage tables that correct for pressure. Rather, the anesthesiologist must titrate the agents used to effect. This makes the importance of good monitoring paramount. Monitoring should include the usual monitors for vital signs. The need for accurate blood pressure readings and access for arterial blood sampling would suggest that an arterial line should be in place prior to any procedure that will require prolonged anesthesia under hyperbaric conditions.

Arterial oxygen measurements present a problem in the chamber. When a sample is drawn and passed through a lock to the surface, gas bubbling may occur during decompression, and the time that the sample remains in transit is also critical. Most blood gas analyzers used in clinical practice are not calibrated to measure oxygen tensions as high as those observed during hyperbaric therapy, therefore oxygen content is only an approximation when it is measured outside the chamber. A direct solution to the problem is to maintain blood gas measuring equipment in the chamber or in a lock pressurized to the same pressure as the therapeutic chamber. The disadvantage of this approach is that although accurate blood gas measurements can be performed at pressure, trained personnel must remain available in the chamber to carry out the measurements. Pulse oxymetry can also be monitored by splicing cables through chamber walls. Its use has been of value when treating patients with high pulmonary shunts, in order to increase ambient partial pressure of O_2 until there is restoration of high SO_2 levels. A respiratory mass spectrometer can be set up outside the chamber with a sampling line traversing the wall of the chamber in order to monitor the actual concentrations of O_2, CO_2, N_2, or N_2O inhalation agent continuously.

At usual therapeutic pressures (2.8 ATA) CNS oxygen toxicity is rarely a problem. If prolonged exposure to high oxygen tension or unusual depths are to be used EEG should be monitored, especially when muscle paralysis impedes the visual recognition of seizures. Since convulsions are often the first signs of CNS toxicity, the EEG would be the only way to detect a seizure in an adequately paralyzed patient. Electrical activity from the ECG must be monitored as usual, but the monitor itself will usually remain outside the chamber, since it most often uses a CRT based display. The monitor must remain visible to the attendants inside the chamber through a porthole window. The leads are passed through a pressure tight access to the outside of the chamber. Recently, a variety of flat-screen display monitors have been used to record digital and analog signals during the pressure phase.

Defibrillation is possible during the phase of pressure in the hyperbaric chamber. Martindale *et al* (1987) reported the use of an R2 defibrillator adaptor on a Life Pak 6S unit. Self adhering pads were used in order to reduce the danger of fire caused by sparking between defibrillator paddles. As with ECG monitors, the defibrillator unit must be kept outside the chamber and wires passed through the chamber wall and attached to the patient. Standard defibrillator paddles can be used if care is taken to make good paddle-skin contact through the use of a low resistance gel, and the paddles are positioned far enough from each other to prevent arcing across the paddles.

A neuromuscular transmission monitor can be used in the chamber without fear of fire or explosion as the amperage delivered is quite low. Any electrical equipment to be used inside the hyperbaric chamber must be flushed with nitrogen (N_2) in order to provide an inert gas atmosphere in case of spark generation.

Conclusions

Anesthesia is not usually performed in the hyperbaric chamber but there are a few indications for its use in life-saving hyperbaric therapy. Attention to detail is paramount while delivering anesthesia under hyperbaric conditions. I recommend that, where possible, i. v., anesthesia should be used. Ketamine and benzodiazepine, along with a muscle relaxant, have been proven to be very useful for induction and maintenance of anesthesia under hyperbaric conditions. Inhalation agents almost always leak into the operating environment and are avoided because of their possible effects on the operating team. An anesthetics should be delivered to be effective at pressure and not with any preconceived formulations. At pressures up to 6 ATA, pressure reversal of anesthesia should induce only minor changes from surface treatment.

It is best to induce anesthesia while the patient is at 1 ATA and, after adequate anesthesia is obtained, perform bilateral myringotomies to avoid middle ear equilibration problems. This has been proven to be better than induction of anesthesia at depth, because the patient is more comfortable if the compression phase is avoided.

A nasogastric tube should be used in every instance in order to drain expanding gastrointestinal air which is introduced by masking at depth. It will expand to several times the original volume and cause a number of mechanical problems, including ventilatory difficulty and desaturation. If a gas is used, a volatile agent would be preferable to nitrous oxide, especially for prolonged anesthesia, as there is risk of the development of decompression sickness.

An anesthetist may be involved in the transfer of patients requiring HBO treatment. The problems of low-altitude helicopter transfer or transport to a hyperbaric facility of patients with decompression sickness via fixed wing in a pressurized aircraft cabin, risk of dehydration and the use of sedation are reviewed in a book chapter (Bratteboe & Camporesi 2001).

Finally, the anesthetist is an important member of the interdisciplinary team for acute hyperbaric oxygen therapy in a medical center where the other members are emergency room physicians and surgeons and where intensive care therapy is required. Some of the hyperbaric emergencies such as air embolism may arise during surgical procedures and require monitoring by the anesthetist and well participation in the treatment if such an event should occur.

39 HBO in Emergency Medicine

K. Van Meter and P.G. Harch

Hypoxemia and ischemia are the underlying pathologies in many of the conditions seen in an emergency department. In addition to resuscitation and other emergency treatments, hyperbaric oxygen increasingly plays a vital role in the management of these patients. This topic is discussed under the following headings:

Introduction

Timely resuscitation by augmentation of oxygen delivery to tissue damaged by ischemia is key to many emergency medicine interventions in sickness and injury . Further, the prompt attempt to lessen reperfusion injury and necrosis after initial resuscitative clinical success should not be forgotten. Finally, the patient, once past the initial resuscitative effort, followed by restorative oxygenation, should receive maintenance oxygenation as needed to optimize the chance of continued recovery. In other words, one of the major purposes of an emergency department is to first assure proper oxygen delivery to many of its sick and injured. The oxygen delivery must be adjusted to maximize therapeutic effect in the emergency medicine interventional phases of resuscitation and restoration, and the maintenance phase of patient management.

Oxygen delivery to tissue has been described in Chapter 2. Oxygen delivery is dependent on cardiac output. Oxygen delivery to tissue is given by the following formula:

$$\text{Oxygen delivery} = \text{cardiac output} \times \text{arterial oxygen content}$$
(Shannon & Celli 1991)

Table 39.1 shows data on a hypothetical adult possessing a hemoglobin level of 15 grams per decaliter. The assumption is made that the patient would have been placed by whole body exposure to differing barometric pressures with varying surface equivalent fraction of inspired oxygen (SEFIO$_2$). The potential oxygen delivery values assuming a cardiac output of 5 liters/min and an oxygen saturation of hemoglobin of 100% are calculated (Table 39.1). Note that the arterial oxygen content achieved by systemic HBO inhalation is in the range of that provided by fluorocarbons (Table 39.2).

It is not a certain that oxygen delivery to ischemic tissue always has the full benefit of 1.34 ml oxygen carriage per gram of hemoglobin. Hemoglobin's release of oxygen to peripheral ischemic tissue is relative to plasma tempera-ture, CO_2 content, hydrogen ion concentration and di-phosphoglycerate levels (Table 39.3). The dissolved oxygen in the plasma fraction is more independent of the above tabulated variables and more dependent upon ambient pressure.

Oxygen, if successfully delivered to mitochondria, becomes a powerful electron acceptor as it attaches to the end of the cytochrome chain. Essentially, electrons, as they are stripped off the atoms in the chemical structures of the nutrient source of fats, carbohydrates and protein, plummet down an elegant cytochrome chain within mitochondria to a receptive oxygen diatomic molecule (O_2 liganded to cytochrome aa$_3$) as shown in Figure 39.1. As the electrons

---

Table 39.2
Comparison of Arterial Oxygen Content Achieved by Systemic HBO Inhalation and that Provided by Fluorocarbons

Oxygen content of the arterial blood (15 g/dl Hb)	
SEFIO$_2$ 300% (3 ATA)	26.8 vol%
SEFIO$_2$ 400% (4 ATA)	29.0 vol%
SEFIO$_2$ 600% (6 ATA)	33.5 vol%
90% wt/vol Perflubron (4 ml/kg or fluorocrit 3.8%) SEFIO$_2$ 100% (1 ATA)	22.6 vol% (Rockwell 1991) (Wahr 1996)
20% wt/vol Fluosol DA (15 ml/kg or fluorocrit 4%) with SEFIO$_2$ 100% (1 ATA)	24.1 vol% (Fischer 1986)

Table 39.3
Characteristics of the Oxyhemoglobin Dissociation Curve (Sigmoidal Curve with the Ordinate Representing mmHg pO2 and the Abscissa Representing Percentage Saturation of Hemoglobin)

Shifts curve to left	DPG↓ · CO$_2$↓ · Δ↓ · H$^+$ conc.↓
Shifts curve to right	DPG↑ · CO$_2$↑ · Δ↑ · H$^+$ conc.↑

Δ = temperature, DPG = diphosphoglycerate

Table 39.1
Oxygen Delivery Based on Ambient Pressure and Inhaled Oxygen Fraction of the Breathing Mix

Breathing mix	Atmosphere	fsw	SEFIO$_2$ Exposure	PaO$_2$	Dissolved Plasma Vol% O$_2$	CaO$_2$	Oxygen Delivery (ml/min)
air	1.0 ATA/Abs	0	21%	150 mmHg	0.3 vol%	20.4 vol%	57.12 ml/min
100% O$_2$	1.0 ATA/Abs	0	100%	673 mmHg	2.0 vol%	22.1 vol%	1105 ml/min
100% O$_2$	1.5 ATA/Abs	16.5	150%	1053 mmHg	3.2 vol%	23.3 vol%	1165 ml/min
100% O$_2$	2.0 ATA/Abs	33	200%	1433 mmHg	4.3 vol%	24.4 vol%	1220 ml/min
100% O$_2$	2.4 ATA/Abs	45	240%	1737 mmHg	5.2 vol%	25.3 vol%	1265 ml/min
100% O$_2$	2.8 ATA/Abs	60	280%	2041 mmHg	6.1 vol%	26.2 vol%	1310 ml/min
100% O$_2$	3.0 ATA/Abs	66	300%	2193 mmHg	6.6 vol%	26.8 vol%	1334 ml/min
100% O$_2$	4.0 ATA/Abs	99	400%	2955 mmHg	8.9 vol%	29.0 vol%	1447 ml/min
100% O$_2$	5.0 ATA/Abs	132	500%	3713 mmHg	11.1 vol%	31.2 vol%	1562 ml/min
air	6.0 ATA/Abs	165	126%	958 mmHg	2.9 vol%	23.0 vol%	1149 ml/min
100% O$_2$	6.0 ATA/Abs	165	600%	4473 mmHg	13.4 vol%	33.5 vol%	1676 ml/min

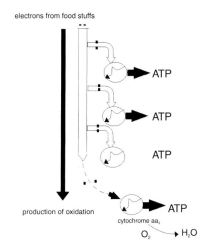

Cytochrome aa₃ liganded
Oxygen as the ultimate electron sink

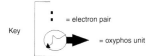

Figure 39.1
Cytochrome aa₃ liganded oxygen as the ultimate electron sink.

fall in energy level as they traverse down the cytochrome chain, energy is tapped to empower "Oxphos" units to make ATP. The ATP, among many things, runs membrane ion pumps (ionophores) to maintain acid base and electrolyte balance (deDuve 1984).

Non-delivery of oxygen wrecks the human machine

functionally, then structurally, as evidenced by the almost instant loss of consciousness and neurologic damage which occurs by asphyxiating inhalation of 100% N_2 or by inhalation of high levels of H_2S, HCN or CO which bind to cytochrome aa₃ stopping short the oxidative flow of electrons.

Indications for Emergency Use of HBO

Approved indications for HBO which are considered to be an emergency are shown in Table 39.4.

Often the patient's entry into the medical system for these conditions does not follow regular hours. As a result, these patients enter the system through the emergency department. Emergency medicine, especially in the United States, is a specialty brought into existence by public demand rather than preexistence of a discrete specialty of skills or knowledge. In fact specialists are, more often than not, equally (if not more) skilled in the management of medical emergencies in their respective specialties. The number of emergency department visits has rather steadily increased in the United States despite the United States Federal Government's effort to increase the number of primary care clinician by favorable reimbursement. The American public has voted in legislation giving the patient the right to determine a medical emergency (Prudent Lay Person Laws). The United States Federal Government has produced strong regulations (EMTALA = Emergency Medical

Table 39.4
The 1996 Approved Indication List for Hyperbaric Oxygen Therapy for the American College of Hyperbaric Medicine (ACHM)/Undersea and Hyperbaric Medical Society (UHMS) and the European College of Hyperbaric Medicine (ECHM) (Camporesi 1997)

ACHM/UHMS	ECHM
1. *Arterial Gas Embolism (see Chapter 11)	1. *Arterial Gas Embolism (see Chapter 11)
2. *Acute Decompression Illness (see Chapter 10)	2. *Acute Decompression Illness (see Chapter 10)
3. *Acute Carbon Monoxide Poisoning (see Chapter 12)	3. *Carbon Monoxide Poisoning (see Chapter 12)
4. *Acute Necrotizing Infection(See Chapter 13)	4. *Soft Tissue Necrotizing Infection (see Chapter 13)
5. *Acute Thermal Burns (see Chapter 15)	5. *Thermal Burns (see Chapter 15)
6. *Acute Crush Injury, Compartment Syndrome, Other Traumatic Ischemias (see Chapter 30)	6. *Post Anoxic Encephalopathy (see Chapter 19)
7. *Gas Gangrene (clostridial myonecrosis) (see Chapter 13)	7. *Acute Ischemia (Traumatic or Vascular) (see Chapter 23)
8. *Compromised Graft or Flap Preservation (see Chapter 15)	8. **Ischemic Lesions in Diabetes (see Chapter 15)
9. *Intracranial abscesses (see Chapter 20)	9. **Ischemic Atherosclerotic Lesion (see Chapter 15)
10. **Enhancement of Selected Problem Wounds (see Chapter 15)	10. *Ocular Ischemia (see Chapter 32)
11. Chronic Refractory Osteomyelitis (see Chapter 15)	11. Chronic Osteomyelitis (see Chapter 13)
12. Osteoradionecrosis, Soft Tissue Radiation Necrosis (see Chapter 16)	12. Radionecrosis (see Chapter 16)
	13. *Acute Hearing Loss (see Chapter 31)

*Emergency condition. **Treatment of these wounds may be considered to be an emergency when exacerbations threatening loss of limb exist.

Treatment and Active Labor Act) to direct hospitals and physicians to not shirk their duty of medical evaluation of all patients regardless of their ability to pay and regardless of the initial trivialness of a complaint when the patients present to an emergency department. To date, this remains an unfunded mandate. Collectable reimbursement for emergency medical services, accordingly, range from 15 to 45% of charges, whereas other specialties in the U. S. often enjoy reimbursement of 45% to 90%. The reimbursement constraints and legal directives to see and treat all comers properly and effectively has placed rather amazing evolutionary operational stresses on emergency departments. Fast Tracks have been developed to move less complicated and less severe cases more quickly. Managed care, while initially accusing emergency medicine of being cost-ineffective, has embraced it with increasing enthusiasm, because the advantage of low marginal cost of seeing extra patients on a timely basis can be passed on to managed care. Managed care's reaction to emergency medicine might reflect some interesting features that are inherent to emergency medical services. Hospitals have slowly come to realize that emergency departments are in fact a front porch to the public. Many progressive hospitals have architecturally expanded and embellished their emergency departments. Many hospitals have enclosed or internalized these "front porches" to make the emergency department patient waiting room the de facto hospital lobby.

The marginal cost of seeing one more emergency patient in a day is extremely low. The emergency department is a technological work bench with a full range of equipment not available in a private office or clinic. Emergency departments have sophisticated risk management and quality management institutionally in place. The spectrum of clinical intervention ranges from the application of the Ottowa Rules (Stiell 1994) for economic fast evaluation of ankle sprains, all the way to the use HBO in resuscitation of a CO-intoxicated patient on ventilator because of cardiopulmonary arrest. Procedural skills and equipment needed for resuscitators, once available only in non-emergency department areas of the hospital, have tended to become especially available in the emergency department. An example is the procedural skill of rapid sequence intubation (RSI) to protect a patient's airway. This skill has moved from the exclusivity of the Anaesthesia Department to being a routinely performed skill by emergency physicians in the emergency department. The same trend is just starting to merge for focus-limited diagnostic ultrasonography and HBO therapy. Increasingly, emergency departments are being staffed by board-certified, residency-trained emergency physicians. Increasingly, emergency medicine residency programs are adopting residency training rotations in focus-limited ultrasonography and fellowships in hyperbaric medicine.

The emergency department is open 24 h a day and is legislated by popular demand to be egalitarian in kindness,

skill and attention given to all patients at its door. Health care providers in the emergency department are increasingly in-serviced to be "Disneyesque" in demeanor by being a "health care cast," offering respectful attentions to all patients. The recent development of two specialty units within the emergency department in the U. S. has added a curious dimension to emergency medical services. One of these – observation units – run by emergency departments have allowed serious or unclear patient cases to be managed aggressively with fast-moving diagnostics and interventions, within the first 24 h of presentation to the hospital health care team. Again, managed care has picked up on the cost saving potential of this approach. The other – Hyperbaric Units – contained within emergency departments take advantage of the economy of having a doctor automatically present. The U. S. Center for Medicaid and Medicare Services (CMS) requires a physician to be physically present on site during a hyperbaric treatment to enable reimbursement for both Part B (physician services) and Part A (equipment, disposable medical supplies, technician, nursing service, and houseplant use). Recently CMS has allowed reimbursement for the emergency physician to multitask for physician coverage of hyperbaric patient treatments for chambers in the emergency department. This is most fitting, for across its broad spectra of care, emergency medicine is in fact operationally a multitasking specialty in every respect.

The emergency use of HBO often requires multiple treatments, both scheduled and unscheduled, as needed over 24 h. The patient condition can be clinically static, e.g., the management of a diabetic foot wound. At other times treatments can be dynamically complicated, e.g., the critical care of a ventilator-supported patient with Fournier's gangrene who is being staged for serial debridement operations. Again, traditionally, the emergency physician is at comfort with treating stable, non-urgent patients alongside severely unstable and complicated cases.

Finally, issues of continuity of care are rapidly improving in emergency medicine. With electronically recorded medical information, emergency medicine is moving from episodic, disconnected care to medical intervention, informationally connected to both past and future primary and specialty medical care on any one patient. In fact, emergency medicine is fast becoming a vital link in American primary medical care. In the same way, emergency department based hyperbaric medicine units have utilized electronic patient records to include electronically recorded wound pictures and treatment plans to maintain consistency in hyperbaric patient care from shift to shift.

In the United States, the prehospital emergency medical base station medical control is well worked out using the "911" entry into the hyperbaric medical system of the country by calling the DAN (Divers Alert Network) hot line. It is intended that HBO be used in planned, controlled, and prospective human trials in stroke intervention in the

United States. These stroke trials will utilize a similar "call 911 stroke" emergency medical service (EMS) telephone number. EMS HBO therapy will be discussed further in the section on emergency medicine management of decompression illness and arterial gas embolism.

Promising yet investigational medical conditions which show improvement with the emergency use of hyperbaric oxygen are:

a) thrombolysis in acute myocardial infarct (see Chapter 24; Shandling 1997)
b) acute stroke (see Chapter 18)
c) acute head injury (see Chapter 20)
d) cardiopulmonary arrest
e) hanging (See Chapter 19)
f) near drowning (See Chapter19)
g) vascular headaches (see Chapter 23)

Tissue Ischemia as Common Factor For Emergency Medical Indications

One possible common factor for many of the emergency medical indications is acute or recurrent tissue ischemia, the resuscitation of which initiates reperfusion injury in an anatomic construct of tissue injury zones. The anatomic construct of injury involves a zone of necrosis surrounded by a penumbral zone of injured but viable tissue surrounded by a zone of reactive hyperemia. Some of the past attempts to clarify injury pattern along these lines are shown in Table 39.5.

In summary, oxygen has a dose dependent effect in reduction of ischemic inflammation immediately in the post-injury period. Improving oxygen delivery to the zone of stasis (penumbra) supports or boosts viability of ischemic and dysfunctional but viable cells. Possibly, improved oxygen delivery to the zone of hyperemia (luxury perfusion) may suppress some of the inflammation in this zone of reaction to injury.

In convalescence, during recovery from injury, improved oxygen delivery aids in the resorption of the zone of coagulation (umbra) (see Figure 39.3, entry 3). Periodic pulsed administration of improved oxygen delivery induces wound contraction and soft tissue substitution into resorbing necrotic portions of ischemic wounds (a wound healing process termed "creeping") (Van Meter 1997). This underlies the rationale for "tailing" hyperbaric treatments after initial resuscitative HBO therapy in acute ischemic tissue injury.

During convalescence, "tailing" hyperbaric treatments may induce continuing recovery in the acute penumbra as it converts to the "ex-penumbra." Already, pulsed, improved oxygen delivery afforded by HBO "tailing" treatments has been demonstrated to up-regulate m-RNA directed induction of platelet derived wound healing factor

Table 39.5

Historical Attempts in Literature to Characterize Acute or Recurrent Ischemic Injury by Anatomic Zones of Injury to Include Equivalents of: Zone of Necrosis (Umbra) Surrounded by Zone of Injured but Viable Tissue Cells (Penumbra) Surrounded by Reactive or Hyperemic Tissue

Acute burns:	(Zone of Coagulation/Zone of Stasis/Zone of Hyperemia)
	Jackson D. Br J Surg 1952;40:588–596.
Acute crush injury:	(Zone of Necrotic Devitalized Tissue/"Gray Zone" of Viable but Failing Tissue/Zone of Hyperemia)
	Strauss M. Topics in Emergency Medicine 1984;6(1):9–23.
Acute stroke:	(Infarction/Ischemic Penumbra/Luxury Perfusion)
	Astrup J. Stroke 1981;12:723–725.
Acute myocardial infarct:	(Zone of Necrosis/Ischemic Boundary Zone/Hyperemic Margin)
	Cox JL. Am Heart J 1968;76(5):650–659.
Acute exacerbated chronic nonhealing Diabetic foot wound:	(Necrotic Dead Space/Non Physiologic O_2 Gradient/Cellulitic Hyperemic Wound Margin)
	Van Meter K. Chronic Wound Care in Krasner D and Kane D (Eds.) Health Management Publications, Inc., PA, 1997:260–275.
Focal CNS decompression illness or arterial gas embolism:	(Necrotic Central (Umbra), Idling neurons (Penumbra), Hyperemic Border) Van Meter K. Treatment of Decompression Illness, 45th UHMS Workshop, Moon R and Sheffield PJ (Eds.) Kensington, MD; 1996 203–243.

receptor sites in recovering ischemic tissue – the wound penumbra (Yu *et al* 1996; Zhao *et al* 1994). By pulsing wound penumbra with improved oxygen delivery, apoptosis may be limited by alteration of the redox potential of cytochrome C leached out of mitochondria into the cytosol. Oxidized cytochrome C may prevent the induction of the CASPASE injury cascade or arrest its progression whereas reduced cytochrome C may enhance or initiate it as shown in Figure 39.2 (Li 1997).

The effect of improved oxygen delivery in the resuscitation, restoration and maintenance of tissue damaged by ischemia is schematically represented in Figure 39.3.

In the past, the emergency medical use of HBO has been described to effectively take advantage of Bigelowian flow of plasma through injured microvasculature stricken by endothelial derangement and occluded by formed blood element debris (Bigelow 1964). In a HBO-treated patient, the plasma stream provides for adequate oxygen delivery to satisfy tissue oxygen demand (Boerema *et al* 1960).

Various mechanisms of oxygen-dependent wound repair mechanisms that are facilitated by HBO and described prior to 1985 are shown in Table 39.6. Effects of HBO on

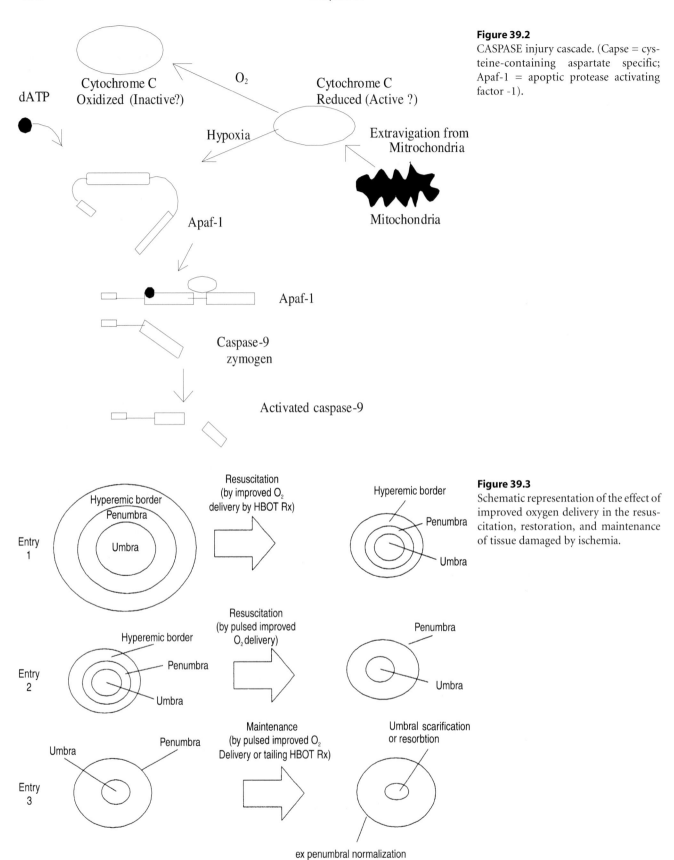

Figure 39.2
CASPASE injury cascade. (Capse = cysteine-containing aspartate specific; Apaf-1 = apoptic protease activating factor -1).

Figure 39.3
Schematic representation of the effect of improved oxygen delivery in the resuscitation, restoration, and maintenance of tissue damaged by ischemia.

Key: HBOT Rx = hyperbaric oxygen therapy

Table 39.6

Mechanisms of Oxygen-Dependent Wound Repair that are Facilitated by Hyperbaric Oxygen Therapy (Described Prior to 1985)

1. Enhancement of fibroblast replication, migration and collagen elaboration (Silver 1973).
2. Enhancement of endothelial replication and migration over unepithelialized wound surface (Perrin 1967).
3. Enhancement of osteoblastic and osteoclastic bone reparation (Strauss 1987).
4. Assistance of migration of macrophages into the zone of injury by steepening the oxygen concentration gradient between the wound penumbra to wound umbra. (Marx 1988).
5. Enhancement of angiogenesis of microvasculature in ischemic wounds (Knighton 1981).
6. Enhancement of nonspecific but effective bacterial killing by polymorpho-nucleocytes and macrophages by oxygen dependent production of hypo-chlorous acid (Klebanoff 1980; Batoir 1984; Weiss 1989).
7. Medical decompression of compartment syndrome by induction of arterial vasoconstriction in a compartment to provide more room for plasma flow. This arterial vasoconstriction has been verified not to compromise tissue oxygenation in musculoskeletal compartments (Byrd 1965; Strauss et al 1987) and in closed head injury (Sukoff et al 1967).

Table 39.7

Rationale of HBO Therapy in Conditions with Ischemic Tissue Injury (Publications Since 1985)

1. Truncation of lipid peroxidation after reperfusion of ischemic tissue by altering free radical formation which favors hydroperoxide radical formation which act as quenching radical to react with lipid radicals to form non radical products (Thom & Elbuken 1991).
2. Reduction of leukocyte adhesiveness to endothelial surface in reperfused microvasculature of ischemic tissue by stopping production of b_2 integrins on the surface of the leukocyte for approximately 8 h (Zamboni 1996; Thom 1993b).
3. Potential for enhancement of endogenous thrombolysis of thrombosed microvasculature of ischemic microcirculation by provision of oxygen to marginated leukocytes to enable them to produce hypochlorous acid, which reacts with plasma tissue plasminogen activator inhibitor shield to lessen inactivation of endogenous leukocyte plasminogen activator in micro milieu surrounding endothelial adherent leukocytes (Weiss 1989; Lawrence & Luskutoff 1986).
4. Up regulation of m-RNA specific for elaboration of platelet derived wound factor receptor sites in wounds for platelet derived growth factor (Yu et al 1996).
5. Enhancement of vasodilation in arterioles (within at least a 15 micron distance of post capillary venules encumbered by endothelial adherent leukocytes on reperfusion after prolonged venule occlusion) by reversal of otherwise persisting vasoconstriction at least in muscle (Zamboni 1993).

the injured tissues of a patient are: (1) improves oxygen dependent tissue repair and (2) "medical decompression" of compartment syndromes. Since 1985, delivery of HBO to patients with ischemic injured tissue has been based on the rationale shown in Table 39.7.

Table 39.8

Classification of Therapeutic Interventions in CPR and ECC3 (from Standards for Cardiopulmonary Resuscitation (CPR) and Emergency Cardiac Care (ECC). *JAMA* 1992; 268:2199–2241).

1.	Class I	A therapeutic option that is usually indicated, always acceptable, and considered useful and effective.
2.	Class II	A therapeutic option that is acceptable, is of uncertain efficacy, and may be controversial.
	Class IIa	A therapeutic option for which the weight of evidence is in favor of its usefulness an efficacy.
	Class IIb	A therapeutic option that is not well established by evidence but may be helpful and probably is not harmful.
3.	Class III	A therapeutic option that is inappropriate, is without scientific supporting data, and may be harmful.

Use of HBO in Cardiopulmonary Resuscitation (CPR)

Oxygen is the primary drug in modern resuscitation of cardiopulmonary arrest patients. Supplemental oxygen should be used during cardiopulmonary emergencies as soon as it is available and in the highest possible concentration. The use of supplemental oxygen in resuscitation fits into a system of classifying recommendations in interventional resuscitation pharmacology proposed by the American Heart Association (Table 39.8).

Supplemental O_2 in resuscitation is a Class I agent (a therapeutic option that is indicated, always acceptable, and is considered useful and effective). Classically, cardiopulmonary resuscitation of patients is done under normobaric conditions, allowing only a maximum of 100% oxygen to be administered. For humans, dose response curves for use of 100% oxygen at increased atmospheric pressure by hyperbaric exposure have not as yet been developed.

Currently, hyperbaric oxygen administered to a patient in cardiopulmonary arrest may be considered as a Class II(b) agent (a therapeutic option that is not well established by evidence, but may be helpful and probably is not harmful).

Interestingly, one might wonder if a fraction of inspired oxygen at 100% (F_{IO2} 100%) in normobaric conditions is a Class I agent, just how far along the way from a Class I agent on the way to a Class IIb agent is a surface equivalent of inspired oxygen (in a hyperbaric environment) of 105% (SEF_{IO2} 105%).

Standard External Versus Open Chest CPR

In the latter part of the 1950s modern standard external cardiopulmonary resuscitation (SE-CPR) and advanced cardiac life support (ACLS) emerged as a way to deliver oxygen to the mitochondria of a victim of cardiopulmonary arrest. Specifically, external defibrillation for ventricular fibrillation, mouth-to-mouth ventilation, and closed chest cardiac massage (or SE-CPR) merged into CPR/ACLS. Ironically, SE-CPR/ACLS replaced open chest cardiac massage CPR(OC-CPR), which up until that point had provided the cardiopulmonary arrest patients a better outcome. Unfortunately, the combined SE-CPR/ACLS approach to resuscitation has demonstrated no improvement in patient outcome over that achieved when it was first introduced nearly fifty years ago. Resuscitation using SE-CPR is not as effective as that achieved with OC-CPR (Heller 1990) and resuscitation rates can be as low as 0 to 5% (see Table 39.9).

Table 39.9
Survival (%) Related to Response Times for SE CPR/ACLS

Time to SE CPR (min)	Time to ACLS (min)		
	< 8	8–16	> 16
0– 4	43%	19%	10%
4– 8	26%	19%	5%
8–12	–	6%	0%

Abbreviations: SE = standard external, CPR = cardiopulmonary resuscitation, ACLS = advanced cardiac life support system

---

Role of HBO in CPR

Enhancement of patient oxygen delivery by hyperbaric oxygenation (HBO) may be a productive way to implement better patient outcome as SE-CPR/ACLS is applied to cardiopulmonary arrest patients.

In CPR/ACLS, central venous oxygen content as measured indirectly by central venous O_2 saturation, is receiving increased attention as a indicator of patient outcome (Snyder *et al* 1991). Cardiopulmonary arrest patients with persistent central venous O_2 saturations of less than 30% have no chance of recovery of spontaneous circulation and survival. All of cardiopulmonary arrest patients with a central venous oxygen saturation of greater than 72% recovered spontaneous circulation (Rivers *et al* 1992).

Tissue oxygenation is sensitive to changes in both convective and diffusive oxygen transport, which is not apparent under normal circumstances because oxygen is not present in excess (Douglas 1994). Cardiopulmonary arrest leads to hypoxia, which can be corrected by HBO. Hyperbaric oxygen can produce central venous oxygen saturations of 100%, even in shock, and is capable of increasing both convective oxygen transport and diffusive oxygen transport.

Animal Experimental Studies

The role of HBO in resuscitation was investigated in guinea pigs (Van Meter *et al* 1988). Cardiac arrest was induced with intravenous injection of 2 cm^3 of iced 1% KCl followed by 2 cm^3 of iced normal saline concurrently with cross clamping tracheostomy tubes for 15 min. By continuous EKG monitoring, all animals were found to be asystolic or in fine ventricular fibrillation at 15 min. Cardiac arrest was induced in a hyperbaric chamber and resuscitation was done in the same chamber, whether it was pressurized or not. All animals had abdominal compression-chest compression CPR/ACLS after 15 min of cardiopulmonary arrest . The animals were maintained at 34°C (± 1.5°C) by a heating pad servo-linked to a rectal temperature probe. Initially, during CPR/ACLS, all animals received 0.5 cm^3 of 1/10,000 epinephrine intravenously administered by an internal jugular line and, thereafter, 0.25 cm^3 of 1/10,000 epinephrine intravenously every 10 min.

Forty-two animals were divided into six groups for purposes of post-arrest resuscitation: three groups were ventilated during resuscitation with air at 1, 2.8, and 6 ATA, and three groups were ventilated with 100% oxygen at 1, 2.8, and 6 ATA. The animals were graded by success at initial post-resuscitation survival and mean post-resuscitation survival time. Results are shown in Table 39.10.

In all of the animals in the 6 ATA oxygen group and six of seven of the animals in the 6 ATA air group, asystole or fine ventricular fibrillation reverted to normal sinus

---

Table 39.10
Hyperbaric Oxygen as an Adjunct in Advanced Cardiac Life Support System-Study in Guinea Pigs After 15 Minutes of Cardiopulmonary Arrest (from Van Meter *et al* 1988)

Initial Post-Resuscitation Survival			Mean Post-Resuscitation Survival Time		
Pressure ATA	Air	O_2	Pressure ATA	Air	O_2
1	1/7	3/7	1	0.2 h	7.2 h
2.8	2/7	6/7	2.8	0.5 h	10.3 h
6	5/7	5/7	6	4.9 h	13.4 h

1/7 means that one animal out of seven survived.

rhythm rapidly on their way to compression. In all groups, whether compressed or non-compressed, the animals responded better to oxygen than to air at each respective pressure. Inhalation of pure oxygen itself is considered to be anti-arrhythmic. This work was next conducted in an open chest swine model in a controlled, randomized, prospective trial at the Baromedical Research Institute (BRI) in New Orleans, and similar results were achieved (Van Meter *et al* 2008) The animals were defibrillated by a human resuscitator at 1, 2, and 4 ATA while the animal was placed on oxygen. Perhaps, in the instance of the animals exposed to 4 ATA, oxygen diffuses through endocardial cardiac chamber surface into the ischemic cardiac conducting system during cardiopulmonary arrest. In this open chest swine model, return of spontaneous circulation is achievable after 25 min normothermic, non-intervened upon cardiopulmonary arrest. Cardiac compressions, fixed low dose intravenous epinephrine and ventilation with SEF_{IO2} 400% produced encouraging results in this randomized, controlled animal trial (Figure 39.11).

In this study, initial success was defined as return of spontaneous circulation (ROS) with production of a mean arterial pressure (MAP) greater than 75 mmHg and sustained ROS at a MAP greater than 50 mmHg at 2 h post resuscitation. Clearly resuscitation rates were better in the animals resuscitated at 4 ATA on oxygen than those resuscitated at either 1 or 2 ATA on oxygen. Brain lipid peroxidative change was likewise more ameliorated in the 4 ATA group (Van Meter 1999, 2001a).

Cardiopulmonary arrest upon resuscitation with return of spontaneous circulation imposes a global reperfusion injury upon a patient. HBO therapy may immediately provide enough oxygen delivery to the cerebral and systemic circulation to attenuate biochemical injury cascades. There is theoretical concern that HBO may aggravate the free radical mechanisms implicated in reperfusion injury, but this has not been substantiated. On reperfusion of ischemic tissue, hyperbaric oxygen has been demonstrated to lessen leukocyte endothelial adherence in microvasculature by modifying B_2 integrins (Thom 1993b). Likewise, on reperfusion of ischemic tissue, HBO, which is more effective than normobaric oxygen, promotes the conversion of xanthine oxidase to dehydrogenase (Thom 1990). Oxygen provided to thrombosed microvasculature promotes endogenous thrombolysis by preventing the inactivation of leukocyte plasminogen activator by the plasma anti-plasminogen activator shield. Ample provision of oxygen to thrombosed microvasculature allows polymorphonuclear leukocytes to elaborate hypochlorous acid, which reacts with the methionine-rich plasma anti-tPA shield protein. Leukocyte tPA, which is sparse in methionine, is spared (Weiss 1989). In simple terms, well-oxygenated thrombosed microvasculature undergoes endogenous thrombolysis more readily if the partially thrombosed microvasculature has an ample oxygen supply.

In animal experimental studies, HBO has been demonstrated to accelerate neurologic recovery after cerebral ischemia (see Chapter 18). Likewise, hyperbaric oxygen alone and hyperbaric oxygen with tPA have been demonstrated to accelerate myocardial recovery in animal myocardial infarct models (see Chapter 24). Hyperbaric oxygen has been applied clinically in serial daily fashion to ameliorate central nervous system injury from ischemic insult as a post-injury "tailing" of treatments. Serial low-dose hyperbaric oxygen has been demonstrated to immunomodulate lymphocytes (see Chapter 25). Perhaps this use of hyperbaric oxygen will be applied to lessen the neurologic injury and improve the quality of life after successful resuscitation of patients suffering cardiopulmonary arrest in the future. Saving life is not the only goal of medicine; rather it is saving a life to be lived as a person (Miller 1993). Case 5 in the following section illustrates the use of HBO as an adjunct to CPR in preventing neurological injury.

Further experimental work in animals is needed, followed by controlled, randomized, prospective human trials. Institutional Review Board (IRB) approved consent for treatment in clinical resuscitation trials must respect the autonomy of the unresponsive patient. IRB-approved, presumed consent may be used provided that the previously FDA approved drug be used in a dose response trial. In the instance of oxygen in ACLS use, one solution would be to draw the choices together – for resuscitation oxygen breathing mix to be considered a Class IIb agent closely approximating a Class I agent. For oxygen, this could be accomplished initially with a SEF_{IO2} of 110% by means of hyperbaric oxygen, compared with a F_{IO2} of 100% in normobaria, with presumed consent. If 110% SEF_{IO2} were found to improve patient outcome over and above F_{IO2} of 100%, then the patient dose response with presumed consent could be advanced to explore the advantage of a SEF_{IO2} of 120% compared with a SEF_{IO2} of 110%. Accordingly, a dose response curve for use of hyperbaric oxygen in SE-CPR/ACLS could be obtained, all with presumed consent. Animal experimental work substantiated preliminarily in acute focal ischemia of the CNS after stroke as well as in global ischemic insult of the CNS after cardiopulmonary resuscitation (Rosenthal *et al* 2003) that oxygen concentration is less injurious in the sequence arranged in order of least (1st) to most (3rd) reperfusion injury.

1st (3 ATA O_2) $SEFIO_2$ 300%
2nd (1 ATA air) $SEFIO_2$ 21%
3rd (1 ATA O_2) $SEFIO_2$ 100%

For evaluation and management of CPR/ACLS in the future it will be important to perform real-time monitoring of oxygen tissue delivery to obtain information for the servo-control F_{IO2} administered during resuscitation of a victim of cardiopulmonary arrest. Clinically, transcutaneous pO_2 electrodes and intravenous fiber-optically connected optodes for oximetry have been used to evaluate human

Table 39.11
Interventions and Monitoring Possible "at depth" with a Critical Care Patient in Hyperbaric Chamber

Monoplace Hyperbaric Chamber	Multiplace Hyperbaric Chamber
1. Ongoing intravenous access for infusion of fluid and drugs and for blood sampling with or without infusion pumps*	1. Ongoing intravenous access for infusion of fluid and drugs and for blood sampling with infusion pumps**
2. Functioning indwelling arterial and central venous lines for manometry (to include Swan-Ganz wedge pressures and cardiac pacing catheters)*	2. Functioning indwelling arterial and central venous lines for manometry (to include Swan-Ganz wedge pressures and cardiac pacing catheters)**
3. Serial mechanized sphygmomanometry monitoring* (Meyer *et al* 1990)	3. Serial mechanized sphygmomanometry monitoring
4. Subarachnoid manometry*	4. Subarachnoid manometry**
5. ABG retrieval (Dooley *et al* 1990)	5. ABG retrieval**
6. Electrocardiographic electroencephalographic and other neuroelectrophysiologic manometry*	6. Electrocardiographic, electroencephalographic and other neuro electrophysiologic monitoring
7. Intravascular oximetry and digit pulse oximetry*	7. Intravascular oximetry and digit pulse oximetry**
8. Mechanical ventilation with PEEP*	8. Mechanical ventilation with PEEP**
9. CPAP*	9. CPAP**
10. Rectal or intravascular thermistry*	10. Rectal or intravascular thermistry**
11. Capnometry*	11. Capnometry**
12. NG tube and foley catheter for U/O*	12. NG tube and foley catheter for U/O**
13. At depth transcutaneous PO_2 monitoring*	13. At depth transcutaneous PO_2 monitoring**
14. At depth x-rays (Dauphinee 1985)	
15. At depth cardioversion or defibrillator (see this chapter, HBOT ATLS Section)	
16. Emergency myringotomy on descent (see this chapter, H_2S poisoning case report)	
17. At depth chest tube insertion (Van Meter 1991)	
18. At depth endotracheal intubation (Van Meter 1991)	
19. Anstadt ventricular assist device/open chest thoracotomy (see HBOT/ACLS section of this chapter)	
20. External cardiac compressions manually or mechanically (see HBOT/ACLS case report, this chapter)	

*Sheffield & Piwinski 1983; *Weaver 1991

response to resuscitation of cardiopulmonary arrest. Optical spectroscopy also may play a role in non-invasively monitoring brain tissue oxygen delivery in CPR/ACLS, in an effort to develop more effective treatment of cardiopulmonary arrest.

The hyperbaric chamber has been modified to allow conventional resuscitation of critically injured patients. Table 39.11 shows monitoring devices and interventions currently used routinely in both monoplace and multiplace chambers (Weaver 1991; Moon & Camporesi 1991). It is now possible to reproduce in multiplace or monoplace chambers all medical care and attentions necessary for critically ill or injured patients in a well-equipped emergency department.

Because all of the approved medical indications for both ACHM/UHMS listed previously in this chapter (see Table 39.4) have been thoroughly covered elsewhere in this textbook, details on the pathophysiology that makes them amenable to hyperbaric oxygen treatment will not be discussed in this chapter. Rather, seven cases will be presented to demonstrate the interaction of the emergency department with the prehospital EMS and the medical care: a diver affected with dysbarism, one case of severe CO intoxica-

tion, two chemists with severe H_2S poisoning, one diver with acute blood loss from exsanguination from a duodenal ulcer arterial bleed, and one diver with severe arm crush injury and missed decompression,. An additional case of hyperbaric management of barotrauma and cardiopulmonary arrest will also be presented.

Case Studies of Medical Emergencies Treated with HBO

Case 1: Prehospital EMS and Emergency Department Management of Decompression Illness/Arterial Gas Embolism (DCI/AGE)

On 16 June 1996, a 60-year-old woman performed a single 60 feet sport SCUBA dive for 54 min off the west coast of Florida. She made an in-water stop of 15 feet for 4 min. She was a choreographer and dance team instructor and had maintained an excellent physical condition by jogging every day. She neither drank, smoked, or used recreational drugs. Shortly after surfacing, she experienced bilateral arm pain and hypesthesia caudally from the axillary level down. She had scapular pain and clonic jerks of her lower extremities which were easily elicitable. She was unable to stand due to weakness and instability. The boat from which she was diving had no available oxygen and her transport to land took 2 h. Upon reaching land, while awaiting helicopter transport, paramedics placed her on oxygen by non-rebreathing mask with reservoir (O_2 with NRM with R). She was transported for approximately 15 min at under 500 feet altitude to a hospital-based emergency department with a multiplace hyperbaric unit. Approximately 3 h after surfacing, she was begun on a USN TT6 with O_2 extensions. She had some improvement of scapular pain but no signif-

icant change in her condition. Approximately 24 h later she was begun on a USN TT6A with O_2 extensions with little improvement. Approximately 21 h later she was begun on a US N TT6 with extensions, again with little improvement. The decision was made to transport her to a hospital based emergency department experienced with saturation hyperbaric oxygen treatment for refractory cases of DCI/AGE. She was transported by a Lear jet while on O_2 with NRM with R by one atmosphere. At the new facility, the patient began a RN TT71 treatment table with nitrox 60/40 (nitrogen 60%/oxygen 40%) breathing mix at 165 fsw at an approximate 52 h after surfacing from her injurious dive. The chamber was injected with nitrogen to bring environmental O_2 to a SEFIO$_2$ of 35%. At 165 fsw after several nitrox

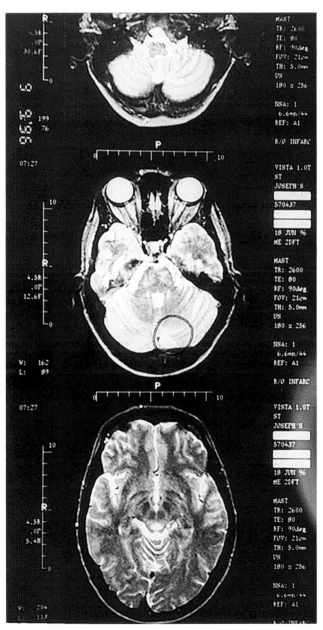

Figure 39.4
Cerebellar infarct by MRI.

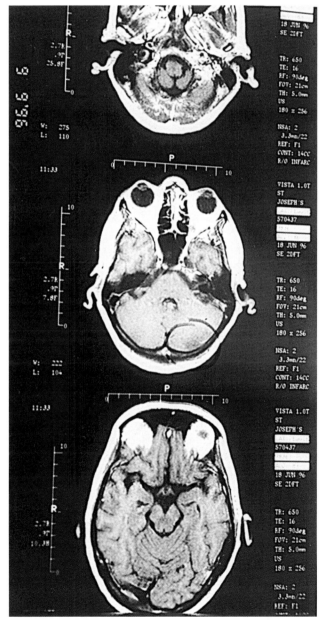

Figure 39.5.
Occipital lobe infarct by MRI.

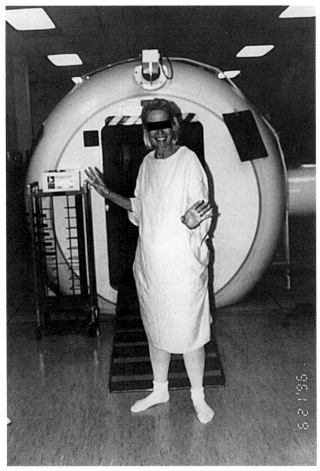

Figure 39.6
The patient exiting chamber from 165 fsw "quasi saturation" treatment table in ambulatory state at the JESMC Emergency Department Chamber in New Orleans, LA.

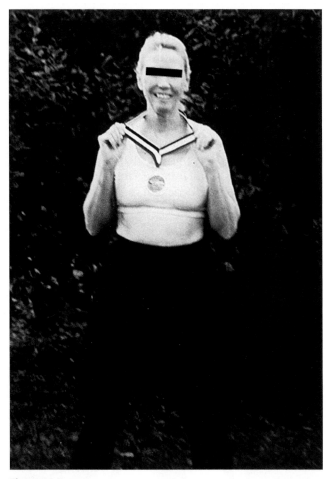

Figure 39.7
The patient after recovery and returning to pre-injury activity, 8 months post-injury.

60/40 30 min breathing periods, her symptoms began to improve.

The patient continued to improve and over the next 72 h gradually came to surface on a RN 71 profile (the patient's ascent was held at a stop each day between 1600 and 1800 and between 0000 and 0600) with intermittent nitrox 60/40 breathing periods deeper than 60 fsw and with 100% O_2 breathing periods from 60 fsw to surface. She surfaced in an ambulatory and completely alert state. She was discovered by MRI to have an ischemic region in her cerebellum (Figure 39.4) and cortical occipital lobes (Figure 39.5). She

> **Table 39.12**
> **Post-diving Accident, Prehospital Information Should Include Patient's Age, Depth, Time and Profile of Injurious Dive; Reporting of the Case Should Include the Items Listed**
>
> - Evolution
> - Manifestation
> - Time of onset
> - Gas burden
> - Evidence of barotrauma

was given six 33/90 tailing hyperbaric oxygen treatments and her unstable gait improved. Now, two years after this event, she runs and dances and has productively re-entered her choreographic career. She has no residual injury (Figures 39.6 and 39.7).

Discussion

The patient exemplifies that all is not known that could be known about treatment of decompression illness and arterial gas embolism. Immediate post injury one atmosphere high concentration reoxygenation is advocated. The Divers Alert Network (DAN) in the United States urges the availability of high pressure oxygen flasks with oxygen administration equipment on all diving operations. It is not unusual to see even quite severe symptoms of DCI/AGE ameliorate favorably with this early treatment approach. Cautious but complete hydration should be carried out orally if the patient is tolerant, but parenterally if the patient is not. The Divers Alert Network should be called (+1 919–685–8111) for needed advice in the United States (or its equivalent in other countries). The patient should

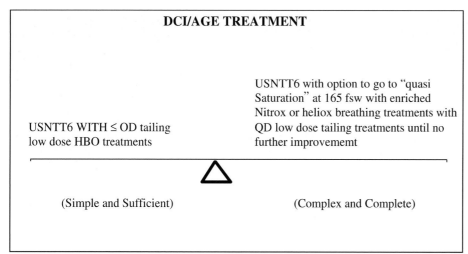

Figure 39.8
Balancing the uncertainty in treatment of decompression illness.

be transported to hyperbaric chamber for recompression and hyperbaric oxygenation. The prehospital essential emergency data set (EEDS) which should be conveyed to DAN and to the receiving emergency department should be along the lines shown in Table 39.12 and as advocated by Gorman (1990).

The ideal treatment table for human decompression illness and arterial gas embolism is not known. In fact, no human controlled, prospective, randomized trial exists to prove if the outcome of DCI or AGE patients is better if treated with or without HBO, let alone with different hyperbaric treatment regimens (Flynn 1991). Further, no controlled, prospective, randomized trial exists to prove if DCI or AGE patients have a better outcome if treated with just a few (<5) or many (>5) low dose tailing HBO treatments after an initial definitive deeper HBO treatment (Flynn, 1991). The uncertainty is summarized in Figure 39.8.

Several hyperbaric clinicians have reported cases where USN TT6's did not resolve DCI/AGE injury, to be followed with resolution or improvement with a 165 fsw treatment table delayed as long as 72 h after the "failed" USN TT6's (Kol et al 1993a; Lee et al 1991: Van Meter 1996). The 165 fsw tables incorporate enriched nitrox or heliox breathing periods at 165 fsw with stays often at 165 fsw of longer than 30 min with conservative decompression thereafter to surface. In our experience in New Orleans, the USN TT6A during decompression can itself cause DCI in the non-injured tender or recurrence of symptoms of DCI in the injured diver.

In fact, there is no firmly established time period beyond which hyperbaric treatment of residual injury from DCI/AGE has definitely been found to be effective. It is not unusual to observe untreated symptoms present up to a week resolve by an initial recompression (Kizer 1982; Myers 1985). For all cases with residual neurologic injury after an initial recompression treatment for DCI/AGE, the JESMC Department of Emergency Medicine and Hyperbaric Unit in New Orleans, Louisiana, has averaged 17 "tail-

ing" hyperbaric oxygen treatments (Van Meter 1996) and the Duke University, F.G. Hall Laboratory's Clinical Hyperbaric Unit in Durham, North Carolina, has averaged 13.7 "tailing" hyperbaric oxygen for similar cases (Davis et al 1994).

One thing is certain, no favorable O_2 source should be bypassed in the push to have the patient recompressed. This includes surface O_2 inhalation and monoplace chamber oxygen administration if multiplace chambers are distant and transport to them would delay treatment.

Case 2: Severe Carbon Monoxide Intoxication and Hyperthermia

On 6 April 1997, a 22-year-old woman was found unconscious in a closed garage where the temperature was 130°F because of a housed running car. She was intubated by paramedics and brought unconscious and hypotensive to the East Ascension Hospital Emergency Department in Gonzalez, Louisiana, and was parenterally hydrated, cooled and given a HBO treatment (modified monoplace USN TT6) while on ventilator. She then had a CT scan of the brain and was found to have ischemic change in the basal ganglia bilaterally. She was transferred in unresponsive coma to the Emergency Department at Charity Hospital (MCLNO) in New Orleans from where she was transferred across town to the Emergency Department at JESMC. There, she was treated while still on ventilator with a USN TT 6. She became more responsive at a depth at 60 fsw in the multiplace chamber at the JESMC ED but relapsed to coma at surface. She was weaned from the ventilator after 2 weeks. She was given a tailing series of 33/90 HBO treatments daily for a total of 110 at no charge in a fully consented entry (her parents consented for her) in an IRB approved longitudinal case series for investigational use of HBO therapy in severe brain injury. She was awake enough at depth on the 49th tailing hyperbaric

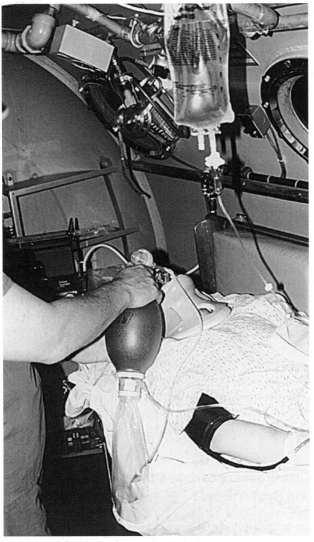

Figure 39.9A
Patient on ventilator in multiplace chamber at JESM Dept. of EM, New Orleans, LA.

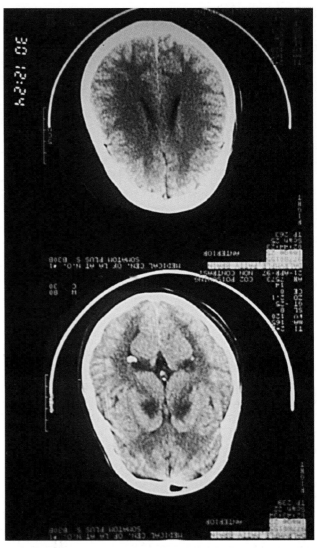

Figure 39.9B
Initial brain CT scan at HBO unit after initial treatment in the ED HBO unit at EAPH Gonzalez, LA, exhibiting basal ganglia ischemia.

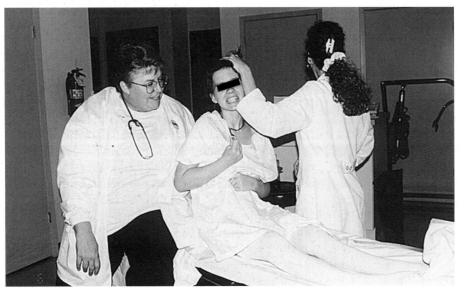

Figure 39.9C
Patient receiving HBO tailing treatments at EPC in monoplace chamber in New Orleans, LA.

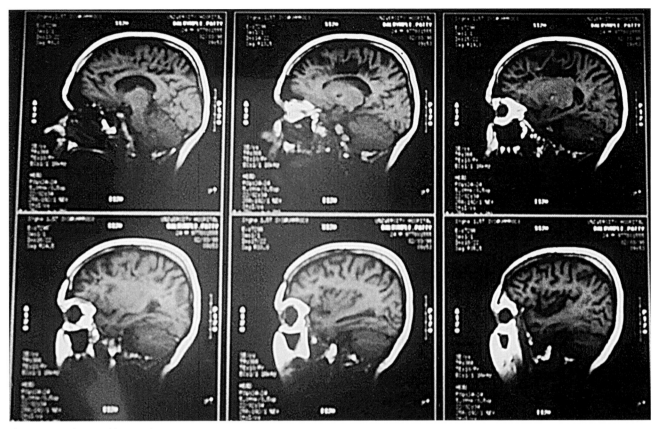

Figure 39.9D (top and bottom)
Follow-up MRI of patient at one year revealing subcortical white matter cystic degeneration and periventricular leukoencephalopathic change.

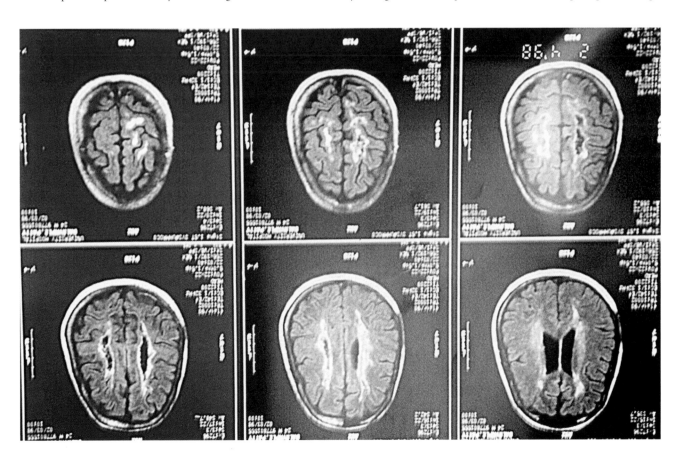

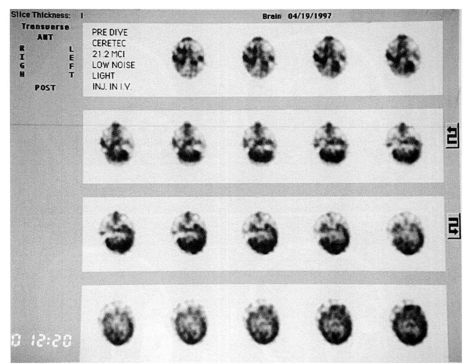

Figure 39.9E
Initial ECD SPECT brain scan (transverse section) with marked perfusion/perfusion/metabolic defects.

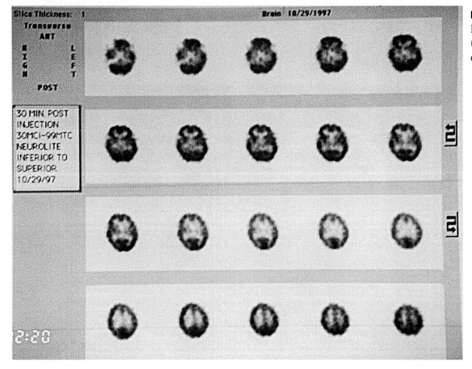

Figure 39.9F
Follow-up ECD SPECT brain scan (transverse section) with amelioration of metabolic defects.

treatment to say "stop!" out loud. She relapsed on surface but within a week was conversant with monosyllabic words and responses persisting at surface. She was quadriplegic (paresis of upper extremities and paraplegia of lower extremities) with contractures of the extremities. Over the next 61 treatments, she gradually began to move her limbs with return of strength as well as coordination and dissipation of contractures. She became conversant and recovered short-term memory. At the time of last examination she laughed and talked lucidly. She was able to feed and clothe herself and enjoys her two children. She took her first steps with the aid of a foot drop splint for her left lower extremity at exactly one year post-injury. This case is illustrated in Figure 39.9.

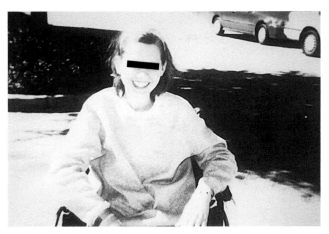

Figure 39.9G
Improvement post HBO treatment series at total of 110 treatments.

Discussion

Clinically, the optimal dose and duration of HBO therapy after CO intoxication is not known. Anywhere from 8 to 20% of patients with severe CO intoxication develop neurologic sequelae (Grinker 1926). The expeditious use of HBO therapy seems to limit the development of neurologic residual injury in some reported human trials. Goldfrank's *Textbook of Toxicologic Emergencies,* the Bible in toxicology for most emergency physicians, currently states that, "although HBO therapy cannot be recommended in every victim of carbon monoxide poisoning, it is a relatively safe treatment that should be considered in all serious exposures" (Tomaszewski 2002, Weaver *et al* 2002).

This patient's tailing HBO treatments stopped when her progress plateaued. Perhaps the patient's penumbra areas of CNS injury were improved by the neurotrophic effect (or a signaling effect) of pulsed increased O_2 delivery to her central nervous system afforded by HBO therapy. In animal models subjected to both CO and hypotensive insult, HBO has been demonstrated to truncate lipid peroxidation (Thom & Elbuken 1991) and to prevent leukocyte adhesion in the CNS microvasculature (Thom 1993b).

The period after the CO intoxication during which the residual injury remains receptive to amelioration by tailing HBO therapy is not known. Reports in the literature indicate that the residual injury from CO intoxication improves with tailing low dose HBO therapy begun even up to a year post-exposure in some cases (Van Meter *et al* 1994; Dean *et al* 1993; Neubauer 1979).

Cases 3 and 4: Severe H₂S poisoning

On 29 April 1998, a 29-year-old male chemical plant worker (BB) was adding pentasulfide pellets to alcohol in a "closed" batching vat into which CO_2 was being added to keep the exothermic reaction under control. A rotten egg odor was emitted and he ran from the vat, collapsing while running to land face first on a steel deck. He was apneic and unresponsive. A 32 year male co-worker (TS) came to his side to assist BB but collapsed on top of him. While the pressurized CO_2 was cut off to the batching vat, a third worker with self-contained breathing apparatus attempted mouth-to-mouth ventilation on BB after both BB and TS were pulled to safety. Paramedics placed the now breathing but comatose patients on O_2 with NRM with R and transported the patients to the nearest hospital emergency department. TS began to have seizures shortly before arriving in the ED and BB began to have seizures shortly after arriving in the ED. Both were intubated by RSI and placed on mechanical ventilation with continuance of paralysis by pancuronium . The patients were given 300 mg of sodium nitrite (10 ml of 3% N_2NO_2 solution) to produce methemoglobinemia and were transported to the JESMC HBO₂ Emergency Department, New Orleans, where they were treated on a USN TT 6. Emergencies myringotomies were performed on both patients in the chamber on descent. During the second O_2 period (still on ventilator) both patients woke up. The time from poisoning to the treatment time with the USN TT 6 was 5.6 h. In the chamber, TS became more lucid, was cooperative and could be taken off ventilator, extubated, and put on a Duke hood. BB became combative and was re-sedated and re-paralyzed with pavulon and kept on ventilator. Four hours after the USN TT6, BB woke up in the ICU and was extubated. Both were treated on low doses (33/90 HBO) treatments twice daily for following two days. BB was later diagnosed to have a perilymphatic fistula and had prophylactic pressure equalization tubes placed to allow further HBO treatment. These low dose treatments were reduced to 45/60 BID but the patients reported feeling worse so the treatments were reduced to 33/90 four times daily where both of the patients reported improvement.

Post injury symptomatology included headaches, incoordination of gait and trouble concentrating. TS had clonus on ankle jerk on the left which disappeared by two weeks. While TS's symptoms dissipated with time, BB's symptoms persisted and BB was returned to a four times daily course of 0.15 mPa/60 min HBO treatments tapered to once a day treatments. At this schedule gradual improvement was noticeable to the patient, his wife and the treating physicians. Cases 3 and 4 are illustrated in Figure 39.10.

Initially both patient's C-spine x-rays and urine toxicologies were negative. (TS's CT of the brain without contrast was negative and BB's CT scan of the brain without contrast evidenced diffuse cerebral edema.) At the time of this writing, both patients have recovered completely.

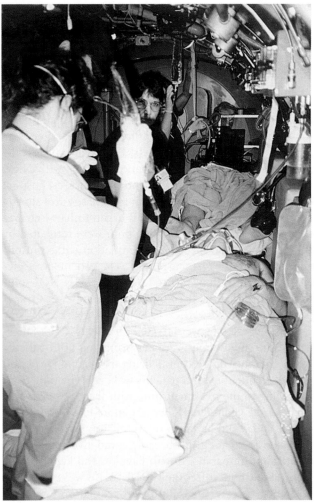

Figure 39.10A
6.5 hours after H₂S intoxication and still comatose and unresponsive, patients BB and TS after being intubated and being placed on ventilators in the multiplace HBO chamber at JESMC Department of Emergency and Hyperbaric Medicine, New Orleans, LA.

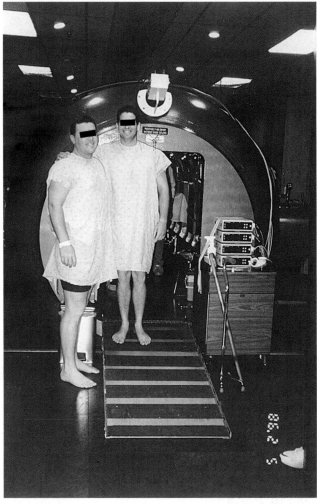

Figure 39.10B
Both patients on the following day after completing a low dose tailing HBO treatment at JESMC Department of Emergency and Hyperbaric Medicine, New Orleans, LA.

Discussion

Goldfrank's *Textbook of Toxicologic Emergencies* states: "The potential benefits of nitrite therapy and HBO therapy should be considered for seriously ill patients exposed to hydrogen sulfide" (Kerns 2002). It is ironic that the standard therapy of production methemoglobinemia by administration of sodium nitrite (to produce a sulf-methemoglobin to pull H₂S into inaccessibility from tissue mitochondria cytochrome liganding) in itself reduces hemoglobin's ability to carry O₂. In H₂S poisoning, HBO therapy may in part treat the decrement in O₂ carriage caused by iatrogenic creation of methemoglobinemia.

While HBO therapy has been used to effectively treat H₂S poisoning experimentally in animals and incidentally in humans (case reports), the optimal dose or duration of HBO therapy in H₂S poisoning is not known (Whitecraft 1985; Smilkstein *et al* 1985; Bitterman *et al* 1986). As with CO poisoning, HBO therapy even when delayed, has been reported to lessen persisting neurologic symptoms by tailing of HBO treatments (Pontani *et al* 1998).

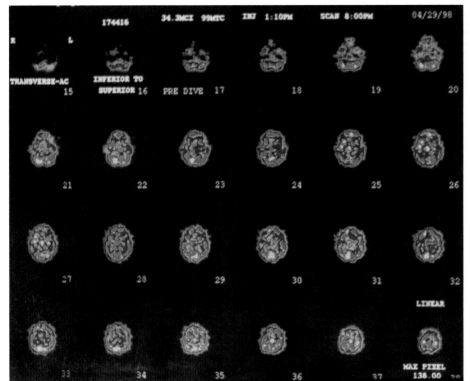

Figure 39.10C
Patient BB. SPECT scan transverse sections pre initial HBO treatment and immediately after and in convalescence.

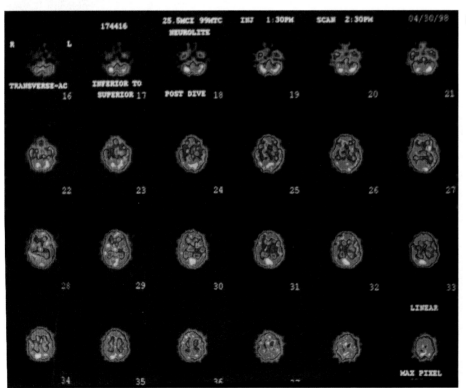

Figure 39.10C (continued)

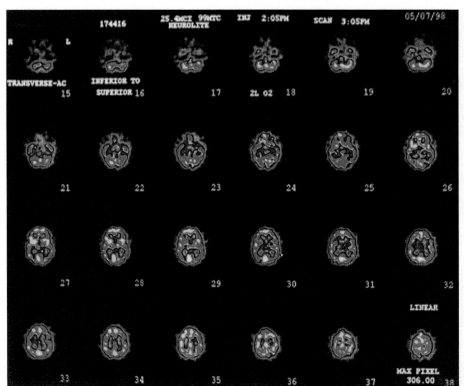

Figure 39.10C (continued)

Figure 39.10C (continued)

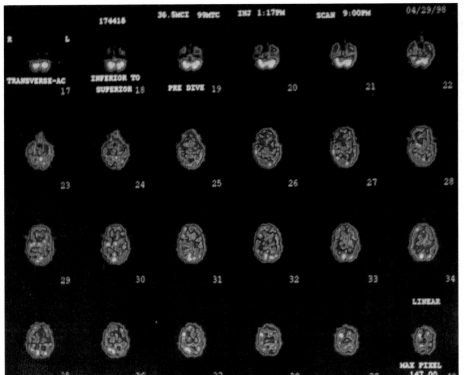

Figure 39.10D
Patient TS. SPECT scan of transverse sections pre initial HBOT and immediately after and in convalescence.

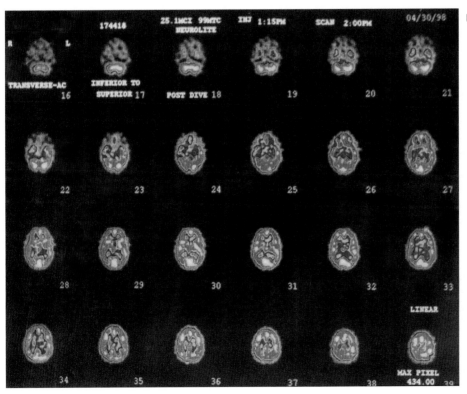

Figure 39.10D (continued)

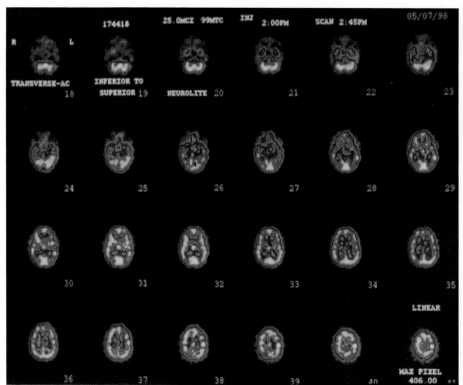

Figure 39.10D (continued)

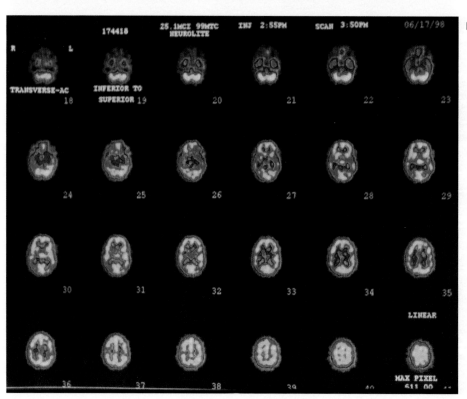

Figure 39.10D (continued)

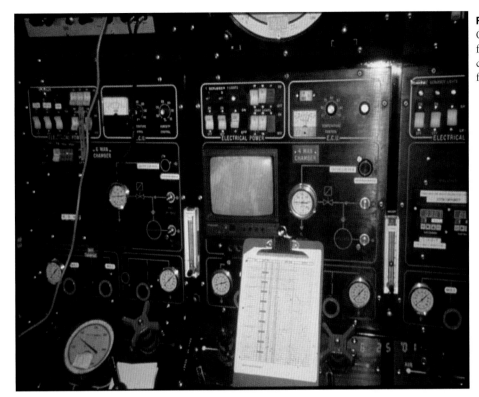

Figure 39.11
Control console shack on diving ship for saturation hyperbaric dormatory chamber depicting diver patient at 660 fsw storage on central television screen.

Case 5: Use of HBO in Resuscitation of Acute Blood Loss Anemia

On 12 May 2001, a 42-year-old commercial diver engaged in a saturation dive with storage at 660 foot sea water with working excursions to 750 feet sea water (Figure 39.11 and Figure 39.12). His recent routine medical diving clearance hemoglobin was 47 g/dL. Previously healthy, the diver was surprised to find himself especially fatigued on this operation. He was curiously short of breath without provocation. On more than one occasion, near syncopal episodes punctuated his work. In his storage dormitory chamber, on 22 May 2001, he diaphoresed, copiously stooled melena and syncoped. He was confused upon regaining consciousness. On 23 May 2001, in an increasingly confused and obtunded state, he again profusely diaphoresed and had massive hematemesis. A diver medical technician (DMT) locked down to the 660 fsw chamber depth to attempt intravenous access. The patient was placed on continuous 0.24 mPa O_2 by mask (built-in breathing system [BIBS], which constituted a securely fitting oral-nasal mask with breathing gas scavaging system). The marked intravascular contraction in the patient disallowed successful intravenous access after an approximate 30 attempts by the DMT. The DMT could not obtain a blood pressure on the patient, but he could feel a feeble carotid rapid pulse. The bidirectional motility of the patient's gastrointestinal tract precluded effective oral hydration. The DMT was instructed to implement extremity hypodermocleisis with normal saline at multiple

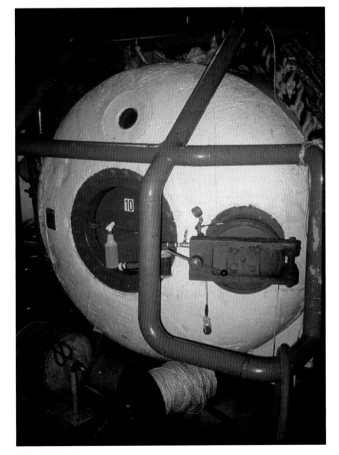

Figure 39.12
Saturation dormatory hyperbaric system containing the duodenal ulcer blood patient aboard commercial diving ship.

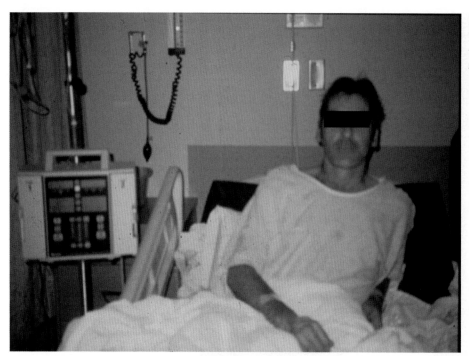

Figure 39.13
Recovered patient in land-based hospital after decompression from heliox saturation.

extremity sites. This parenteral fluid loading method effectively returned the patient to a normotensive state with mild tachycardia. The normal saline was continued by hypodermocleisis short of producing clinically taught extremity compartment syndromes. The 0.24 mPa O_2 breathing periods were administered by BIBS mask for periods of 20 min spaced by normoxic chamber atmosphere breathing periods (heliox with < 0.23 MB O_2). These O_2 breathing periods with normoxic breathing breaks were given in rounds of four titrated to relief of patient confusion or hypotension.

The patient began taking oral fluids with tolerance and retention. Next, oral hematenics (iron and B-complex vitamins), bouillon broth, and glucose supplement clear fluids were tolerated and retained. Routine decompression from storage depth to surface commenced as supplemented by the close interval cyclic 0.24 mPa O_2 breathing periods before described. The diving support vessel made landfall. The patient walked out of the chamber upon surfacing, and land-based paramedics placed intravenous lines and placed him on precautionary supplemental oxygen for transport to an emergency department. There the patient had a hemoglobin of 4.7 g/dL and was transfused 6½ matched units of packed red blood cells over time. The patient had diagnostic endoscopy to reveal a 3 mm duodenal ulcer which had eroded a small vessel which was now hemostatic. Helicobacter pylori sampling was positive. With oral antibiotic regime, the patient went on to completely resolve the duodenal ulcer as confirmed by endoscopic examination. The recovered patient is shown in Figure 39.13.

Discussion

In acute blood loss anemia, oxygen debt can be calculated by estimating a patient's expected oxygen consumption minus calculated oxygen delivery over time.

1. Oxygen Content of Arterial Blood (CaO_2):
   CaO_2 = (grams Hg/dL × 1.34 ml × 0% O_2 Hgb) + (0.003 × mm pO_2) (Van Slyke & Neill 1924)
2. Oxygen Delivery (DO_2):
   a. Cardiac Index (CI) = Cardiac Output (CO) ÷ Body Surface Area (BSA)
   b. BSA = Square root of the quantity: height in inches × weight in pounds ÷ 3131
   c. DO_2 = CI × CaO_2 (Chance & Chance 1988)
3. Oxygen Consumption (VO_2):
   VO_2 = CO (CaO_2 – CvO_2) × time (Fick 1870)
4. Oxygen Debt = expected oxygen consumption over time or for a 2.8 m^2 surface (56/h) – oxygen delivery over time (or DO_2)

Critical care specialists have established estimated predictors of clinical outcome in seriously injured or ill patients by calculation of patient oxygen debts in one atmospheric patient care settings. Patients may amass acutely reversible oxygen debt of 9 L/m^2 without sustaining residual organ injury. If a patient's oxygen debt exceeds 22 L/m^2, then multiorgan failure (MOF) is likely. If an oxygen debt of 33 L/m^2 occurs, then death is likely (Shoemaker *et al* 1988).

Using the formulas above, the patient would have assuredly accumulated an oxygen debt in excess of 22 L/m^2 (and perhaps even have exceeded 33 L/m^2). The patient in fact recovered completely without any detectable CNS, myocardial, hepatic, intestinal, or renal residual injury. The patient went on to be a successful land-based housing renovation contractor.

More and more, hyperbaric oxygen therapy is being considered as an effective treatment modality to reduce oxygen deficit in acute illness or injury (Van Meter 2003). Preliminary pilot work was conducted at the Baromedical Research Institute in New Orleans utilizing a swine model to examine the difference between resuscitating an exsanguinated animal (40% blood loss over 15 minutes) with a $SEFIO_2$ of 100% (normobaric oxygen) versus $SEFIO_2$ 400% (hyperbaric oxygen). The animals were monitored for continuous mean arterial pressure (MAP) by indwelling arterial catheter, and for brain tissue oxygen by a poloragraphic oxygen tissue tension catheter passed through a cranial burr hole. The MAP in the animals fell to zero, and the brian oxygen tension level fell to 10 mmHg from a pre-experimental oxygen tension of 30 mmHg. The animals then received an IV bolus of D5 Ringers solution of 3 cc per cc of shed blood while inhaling 100% oxygen at one atmosphere. The animals regained a suboptimal MAP while remaining diaphoretic and tachycardic. Brain pO_2 then dropped to 10 mmHg to 0 mmHg. The animals thus treated uniformly died in short order. Animals with this treatment that were then promptly taken to 60 fsw of pressurization in a hyperbaric chamber regained normal MAP, ceased diaphoresis, and normalized heart and breathing rates when ventilated with 100% oxygen. Even though the animals were acutely and profoundly anemic, their brain pO_2 rose to 30 mmHg. After 50 minutes at 60 fsw the animals were retransusfed their anticoagulated, shed blood. The animals were then brought to surface to survive indefinitely without discernable impairment. A controlled randomized prospective trial is now in progress to expand on the initial findings of this pilot study.

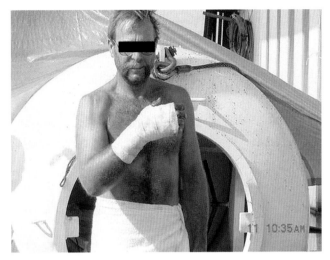

Figure 39.14
Patient exiting the deck decompression chamber after completion of a USN TT 7.

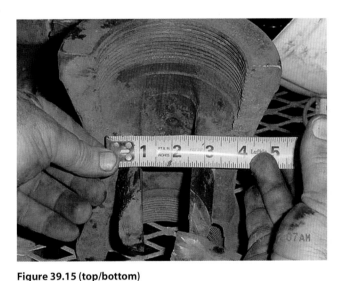

Figure 39.15 (top/bottom)
"Bivalved" valve casing after it was removed from patient's forearm. Note that orifice is 1½ inches wide.

Case 6: Use of HBO in Severe Extremity Crush Injury

On 9 October 2002, a 32-year-old commercial diver began a dive to 189 fsw with intended surface oxygen decompression to incorporate a deck decompression chamber. When the diver reached the Gulf bottom, he held on to the casing of a valve attached to the end of a long run of an underwater hydrocarbon pipeline. He opened the quarter turn ball valve in the valve casing and his right hand forcibly drew into the pipeline to his mid-forearm. The channel in the ball of the valve was 1½ inches wide. In retrospect the pressurized hydrocarbon pipeline was at a lesser pressure than that of the 189 fsw pressure of the natural Gulf bottom. The relative vacuum in effect morphed the diver's hand much like soft plastic stock pulled into a vacuum mold. His

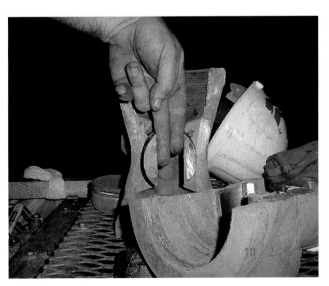

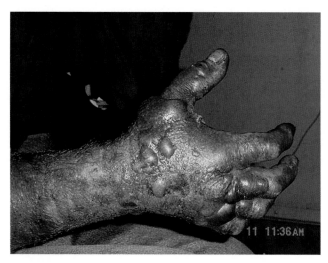

Figure 39.16
The blistered hand and forearm of patient is shown after removal of the valve. The tight tourniquet time was twelve hours.

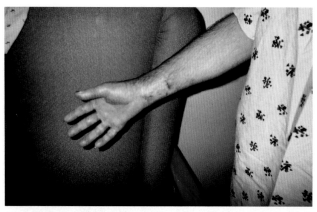

Figure 39.17
Patient two months after accident with nearly full functional recovery of forearm and hand.

extremity was not degloved. Rather the skin envelope was disrupted only partly at the base of his thumb. His radius and ulna had a cross-section greater than that of the channel in the ball of the valve through which his hand and forearm were drawn. He aerobically exercised at great length and time to pull his arm out to free his left arm and to mitigate intense pain. A stand-by diver came down to assist him. A carborundom hydrolic rotary cutter could not be used to cut the pipe for concern of exploding the hydrocarbon content of the line. The stand-by diver used a hand hacksaw to arduously begin a cut through the thick schedule steel pipeline.

The base station diver medical service physician was advised of the problem when the injured diver had an approximate 75-min bottom time at 189 fsw. The choice to cut the diver's arm or cut the pipe to free the diver to forestall the accumulation of disabling bottom time became an additional pressure for consideration in medical direction. No published U. S. Naval surface oxygen decompression air ta-

ble existed for the diver's depth or time at this point in the accident. Before the pipe was cut and the diver could be freed, 120 min of bottom time accumulated for the stand-by diver and 310 min of bottom time occurred for the injured diver. The water temperature was 40°F. The divers had unheated wet suits. Published U. S. Navy exceptional air exposure tables would have required 11 h of in-water decompression for the stand-by diver and 15 h of in-water decompression for the injured diver.

The New Orleans Way Out Emergency Decompression Rule (NO Way Out Decompression Rule) used often in the past for complicated decompression for cardiopulmonary resuscitation research dives and emergency treatment of seriously injured divers was utilized. The rule is explained in the discussion section of this case report. A fresh stand-by diver was sent down to assist the diver and free up the first stand-by diver. By use of the NO Way Out Decompression Rule, the first stand-by diver was first brought to surface as the "test case" to then finish necessary surface oxygen decompression with a USN Table 6 without problem. Next the freed up injured diver, still with cut off pipe and valve attached to his arm, was brought to surface utilizing the NO Way Out Decompression Rule for decompression profile. For life salvage, the patient needed surface oxygen decompression additionally. For limb salvage, the diver needed the valve casing cut off his hand and forearm. To accommodate this, the patient was put on a U. S. Navy Treatment Table 7 (USN TT 7) for required surface oxygen decompression and "tailing" HBO treatment thereafter for the extremity crush injury (Figure 39.14). The USN TT 7 allowed ample air saturation soaking time to use mechanical cutters at depth in the chamber to arduously cut the valve casing off the diver's arm (by "bivalving" the valve) in a compressed air environment rather than the nearly continuous oxygen breathing environment required by a USN TT 6 (Figure 39.15). The diver had distal extremity pulses intact after removal of the valve but had blisters (see Figure 39.16). The diver was up to date with tetanus toxoid immunization. Once in the deck decompression chamber, he was given a shot of ceftriaxone and oral doxycycline and oral levofloxacin. His blistered arm and forearm (reperfusion injury) was copiously buttered with mupirocin ointment and dressed with cotton gauze strip dressing.

The diver came to surface and had serial low-dose (0.24 mPa/90 min) BID tailing HBO treatments at a multiplace hyperbaric medicine unit. At two months post-accident, the diver had regained an approximate 80% mechanical function of his right extremity; at four months he was nearly completely recovered (Figure 39.17).

Discussion

At 189 fsw for a very prolonged bottom time, the uninjured stand-by diver and the injured diver faced life-threatening emergency decompression. No published surface supplied

Table 39.13
Stand-by Diver (189 fws/120 min): Heliox Surface O₂ Decompression Tables Modified by "2 + 2 and/or O₂" NO ED Rule [210 fsw/120 min Longest Allowed Published Bottom Time]

- In-water Nitrox (60/40) breathing mix
  100/7
  90/8
  80/18
  70/23
  60/23
- In-water O₂ breathing
  50/16
  40/99
- 3-min surface interval
  → USN TT6

Table 39.14
Injured Diver (189 fws/190 min): Heliox Surface O₂ Decompression Tables Modified by "2 + 2 and/or O₂" NO ED Rule [240 fsw/120 min Longest Allowed Published Bottom Time]

- In-water Nitrox (60/40) breathing mix
  120/7
  110/3
  100/12
  90/17
  80/19
  70/23
  60/23
- In-water O₂ breathing
  50/16
  40/99
- 3-min surface interval
  → USN TT7

air surface oxygen decompression tables existed at the time of this accident. The 40°F water temperature and injury level for the patient made the U. S. Navy exceptional air exposure decompression tables very dangerous.

The NO Way Out Decompression Rule mentioned earlier allowed the use of published U. S. Navy heliox surface oxygen decompression tables. These tables were supplemented by padded decompression to address the extreme cold exposure with marked physical exhaustion present. The NO Way Out Decompression Rule also addresses the inapplicability of applying heliox decompression to an air dive.

Specifically, the NO Way Out Decompression Rule allows padding of published tables by adding on to the table to be used 2 [units of 10 fsw to depth] plus 2 [2 of 10-min units of bottom time] and/or supplemental in-water oxygen decompression further supplemented by a USN TT 6 for surface oxygen decompression. Specifically each 10-min time or 10-foot depth overrun can be substituted by nitrox 60/40 breath on water stops by adding on one deeper water stop supplemental nitrox breathing before the 50 fsw in-water oxygen breathing water stop.

The USN heliox table applied to both the stand-by diver and the injured diver as modified by the NO Way Out Decompression Rule is given in Tables 39.13 and 39.14, respectively.

The rule allows for substituted decompression elements to be added if published tables do not extend to required depths of all bottom times. For the stand-by diver, in lieu of having published table times that went beyond 120 min, a 140 min bottom time would be achieved by adding 60/40 nitrox breathing at two in-water decompression stops deeper then 50 fsw. In the instance of the injured diver, the

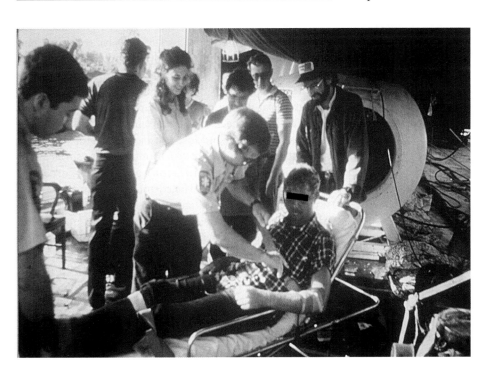

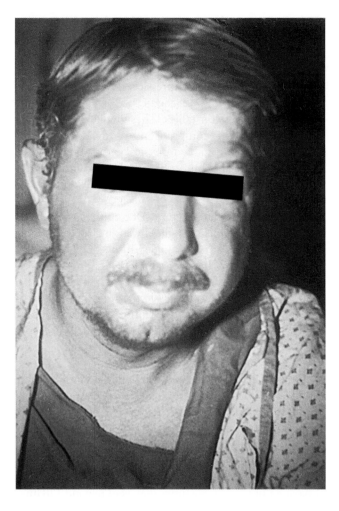

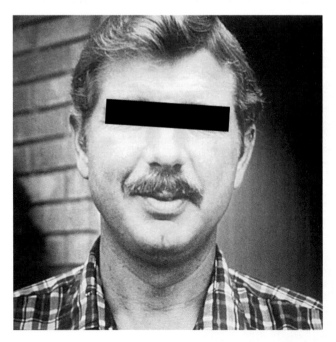

bottom time exceeded the maximum allowable published bottom time of 120 min (the 120 min published fell short of the actual bottom time of 310 min by 70 min). 20 min thereof were converted to 20 feet in theoretically added padded depth and 50 min were padded by nitrox 60/40 breathing on at least 5 in-water stops deeper than 60 fsw.

It is noted that the USN heliox surface oxygen decompression tables incorporate oxygen breathing on in-water stops at 50 and 40 fsw remained unchanged.

The rule has been checked by one of the acknowledged contributors (Vasquez 2003) by the use of the NOBEN-DEM (US Naval Diving Manual Volume 2 and 3, revision 4, March 2001) computer program and Zwart's Advanced Decompression Tables (*http://scuba-doc.com/NOBEN-DEM.pdf*). This approach has been established to provide safe, sufficient, and not excessive decompression in emergency decompression for unanticipated prolonged bottom times on air dives.

Case 7: Use of HBO as an Adjunct to CPR Following Barotrauma

RP, a 35-year-old commercial male diver, dove on surface supplied air to 83 fsw for 25 min in the Mississippi River in approximate 29°C. His task was to airlift sand off a sunken river tugboat. His work was brought abruptly to a halt when his helmet was accidentally sucked into the intake of the airlift. His DESCO® hard helmet became caught on a compressed air injector elbow joint inside the intake orifice of the airlift, preventing him from being sucked in entirely up the airlift conduit. The airlift applied a forceful differential suction to the helmet neck dam of his "diving dress," and severely barotraumatized his head and neck. He opened fully the free-flow air supply valve to his helmet. The oronasal mask within his helmet rippled "in the wind" of the high velocity air supply that air compressors topside were forcing down his umbilical air supply line to keep up with the relative vacuum that was produced by disruption of the seal of his neck dam by the airlift. In the rarified air, he became hypoxic and lost consciousness. Topside crews shut off the airlift and he was brought to the surface by a stand-by diver. On the surface, on a working support barge, his helmet was removed. His edematous, ecchymotic head was barotraumatized sufficiently to hide the location of his mouth. The patient was not breathing and a pulse could not be obtained as he was placed supine in upright position on the inner circumference of a small deck decompression chamber. Chest compressions without mouth-to-mouth ventilation were begun and he slowly descended to 165 fsw on oxygen supplied by a oxygen mask (built-in breathing system mask without overboard dump) strapped to his face over what was assumed to be his mouth. Chest compressions without ventilation were continued. He received a surface equivalent fraction of inhaled oxygen (SEFIO$_2$) of 600% for 10 min before he woke up to pull off the oxygen mask himself. Some 22 min elapsed from the time he was sucked into the airlift until the time he had CPR with O$_2$ administration. The injured diver was ascended with periodic HBO breathing periods of SEFIO$_2$ of 300% on a treatment table which would resemble the USN TT 8 developed years later. It was noted that the diver's swollen, ecchymotic head and neck appeared purple/black during air breaks but during hyperbaric oxygen breathing periods with SEFIO$_2$ of 300% his skin would turn tomato red as the extravasated dermal extravascular hemoglobin would become saturated with oxygen.

The diver made an uneventful recovery after therapeutic air saturation decompression supplemented by enriched nitrox breathing periods. Neurologic examination, as well as psychometric and neuroelectrophysiologic testing upon exiting the chamber, did not reveal any abnormalities. The case is illustrated in Figure 39.18. At the time of this publication, some twenty-five years later, he is fully intact without impairment and is self-employed as a fine furniture and cabinet-maker.

Potential Future Uses of HBO Therapy in Emergency Medicine

As mentioned earlier in this chapter, HBO therapy has had both promising animal and human controlled randomized trials reported in the literature which indicate improvement with thrombolysis and HBO therapy in acute myocardial infarct (Thomas *et al* 1990; Shandling *et al* 1997). Likewise, hangings (Mathieu *et al* 1987) and near drownings (Shn-Rong 1995) have had encouraging responses to HBOT, as shown in published human case reports.

Multicenter controlled prospective randomized trials of HBO therapy in hyperacute stroke are planned (see Chapter 18). A future arm of the trial may even have paramedics enroll patients at the site of their ictus in the community by response with a hyperbaric chamber aboard an ambulance. The concept of having immediate HBO in the prehospital phase using van or ambulance transportable hyperbaric chamber is not so new. The French proposed the same in the late 1800s in Paris to address an epidemic of CO poisonings (Bert 1878) and the British in the 1960s used a Vickers monoplace chamber aboard an ambulance to resuscitate acute myocardial infarct patients in transport to the hospital (Smith 1962; Moon *et al* 1964). The Paracel transport chamber, the Drager transportable treatment chamber, and, more recently, the inflatable transport chamber have become shelf items that could be transported by land or air ambulances for the EMS (Van Meter *et al* 1992; Van Meter *et al* 1999).

The Academic Emergency Medicine Committee Task Force on prehospital management of stroke has recently published a recommendation that patients be given "low flow" oxygen in the field instead of higher concentrations of FIO$_2$ of 100% achievable by high flow mask administration (Pepe *et al* 1998). This reflects the clinical intrigue we face as we progress to the next century to unravel the oxygen dosing paradoxes in emergency medicine in an attempt to improve our patients' outcome in illness and injury.

Acknowledgments

We would like to acknowledge the Baromedical Research Institute in New Orleans, LA and our colleagues Diana Barratt, MD, James Moises, M.D., Paul Staab, M.D., Heather Murphy-Lavoie, MD, and Fred Kriedt, Ph.D. We also wish to acknowledge Johnny Vazquez, M.D. and Julie Anderson, M.D. for their evaluation and assistance in the write-up of the crush injury and acute blood loss case reports. We also wish to express our appreciation to Stephanie Dudenhefer and Sylvia Cusimano for their assistance in preparation of this manuscript.

40 Hyperbaric Medicine as a Specialty: Training, Practice, and Research

K.K. Jain

HBO therapy will likely become more widely used in the future. This chapter discusses a number of the specific developments which can be expected in this regard. The key sections are:

Introduction

Hyperbaric medicine is not universally recognized as a full specialty, although the American Board of Hyperbaric Medicine has started to award certification. Most of the contemporary experts in hyperbaric medicine have another primary medical specialty. Only a small number of physicians devote their full time to hyperbaric medicine, and there are only a handful of professors of hyperbaric medicine.

The time has now come for hyperbaric medicine to be recognized as a full medical specialty. Further development and research can best be carried out by dedicated, full-time physicians. Chairs should be established for hyperbaric medicine at the university level.

Because new techniques in medicine come in and go out of fashion with the passage of time, medical specialties should not be created on the basis of techniques. Hyperbaric medicine is more than a technique for administering oxygen under pressure. It is total care of the patient with emphasis on the pathology that can be corrected by hyperbaric oxygenation (HBO). Normobaric oxygen therapy can be prescribed by any physician, anywhere, and sometimes by nonphysicians as well, but HBO is restricted to use by those who have special training and experience with this method of treatment. This therapy can only be carried out in a hyperbaric chamber.

Relation of Hyperbaric Medicine to Other Medical Specialties

Historically, hyperbaric medicine is an offshoot of diving medicine, which itself is not recognized as a full medical specialty. Diving medicine has assumed importance due to the large navies, increasing recreational diving and offshore oil drilling. Some of the physicians involved in diving medicine have background training in environmental and occupational medicine, but they have developed an interest in hyperbaric medicine because the treatment of decompression sickness involves use of HBO.

The primary specialties of physicians who are currently active in hyperbaric medicine vary greatly and do not necessarily correlate with their clinical interests within hyperbaric medicine. The primary specialties of these physicians are internal medicine (with its subspecialties), general surgery (with subspecialties such as orthopedics, neurosurgery, plastic surgery, and chest surgery), anesthesia, and emergency medicine.

Locating the hyperbaric facility within some other restricted specialty in a general hospital has some disadvantages such as the following:

- There may not be enough work load within the specialty to keep the hyperbaric facility in full use.
- Some departments may be reluctant to send their patients to another department.

Ideally the hyperbaric medicine service should be an independent department available for service to patients and their physicians from other departments in the hospital.

Training in Hyperbaric Medicine

Most of the present generation of hyperbaric physicians are self-taught or have some training by preceptorship. There are no residency training programs in hyperbaric medicine as such, but there are 4-year programs in diving medicine in Europe that include training in hyperbaric medicine. One year fellowships in hyperbaric medicine have been available in some hyperbaric centers in the USA.

If hyperbaric medicine is recognized as a specialty, the following should be the requirements of a training program in the discipline.

Admission Requirements

Graduation in medicine followed by 2 years of graduate training in medicine or surgery. Special cases would be those with training in a specialty or those who have been in general medical practice for some years.

Training Program: 3 Years

First Year: Basic Subjects of Research

The following should be used as a guideline for making up the training schedule for this year:

- A research project involving HBO; animal experiments or clinical investigation.
- Instruction in physiology relevant to hyperbaric medicine.
- Hyperbaric technology; study of function of various chambers and ancillary equipment.

Those with previous research experience in hyperbaric medicine can be exempted from this year and receive their basic instruction during the next year of clinical work.

Clinical Experience

Two years of residency in a recognized hyperbaric center. The training may be divided between two training centers affiliated with a training program. Private practice clinics may be used to supplement university hospital based training. Balanced exposure to acute as well as chronic conditions with a good mix of clinical material.

Optional Extra Training

Extra training or fellowship for one year should be used for advanced training in a special area such as neurological rehabilitation, treatment of burns, or management of decompression sickness, in an institution that specializes in such activities. An advanced research project may be carried out during this year. This fellowship would be suitable for those planning academic careers in hyperbaric medicine.

Examinations

These should be conducted by specialty boards in hyperbaric medicine at the end of the training period. The examination should have written, and additional oral or practical parts. The written examination should be designed to test the knowledge of basic subjects relevant to hyperbaric medicine as well as of the theory of hyperbaric medicine. An oral examination would be the most important factor in deciding on certification of the candidate.

For those who are certified in internal medicine or general surgery, the training program should be reduced to two years – one year of basic studies and one year of clinical training. Those with some experience in hyperbaric medicine may be allowed to take their examinations after one year of fellowship.

The training should be conducted in approved centers and the number of trainees should be limited. The aim should be to produce specialists of a high caliber who will advance hyperbaric medicine.

Practice of Hyperbaric Medicine

This should be hospital-based or at least affiliated with a hospital. Several methods of developing a hyperbaric medical service have been described (Persels 1987, Kindwall 1992). A sample development plan for a hyperbaric medical program is shown in Table 40.1.

Key referral specialties for the hyperbaric program include orthopedic surgery, oral and maxillofacial surgery, radiation oncology, plastic surgery, infectious diseases, and emergency medicine. The pattern of practice in each country is guided by local socioeconomic factors. The indications for HBO vary in each country (see Chapters 8 and 38). The most stringent list of indications is that of the Undersea and Hyperbaric Medical Society (1986) in the USA.

Table 40.1

Sample Development Plan Outline for a Hyperbaric Medicine Program (Persel 1989)

1. Develop an in-house hyperbaric medicine program steering committee (to consist primarily of members of key referring specialties)
2. Program kick-off
   Hyperbaric expert to speak to medical staff 30 to 60 days before accepting patients
3. Opening coverage
   Open house for administrative and medical staff of host institution
   Media announcements
   Review for technical detail
   Stress referral nature of program
4. Orientation programs
   In-house
   Community
   Insurance carriers
5. On-going exposure
   Tours of facility
   Human interest stories
   Individual and small group presentations by physician(s)
6. Hyperbaric medicine training courses
   Develop nursing and technical personnel pool
   Spread knowledge of hyperbaric medicine in the community
7. Brochures and mailing pieces
   Patient brochure
   Physician's and surgeon's guides
   Mail to key physician specialties every 6 months
   Update wound photography every year

Economic Aspects

Economic aspects of the practice of medicine are important in some countries. The cost-effectiveness of HBO for a disease has become a criterion for approval of this treatment in the USA. Many of the clinical studies using HBO deal with this aspect and HBO has been shown to be a cost-effective treatment for the following conditions:

- Non-healing wounds
- Chronic osteomyelitis
- Osteoradionecrosis
- Burns
- Gas gangrene
- Diabetic foot

Some of the reasons for this cost-effectiveness are:

- HBO reduces the length of hospitalization
- HBO obviates the need for surgical procedures in many cases.

Although the initial cost of equipment for hyperbaric medicine is high, the operational costs can be kept low in a mul-

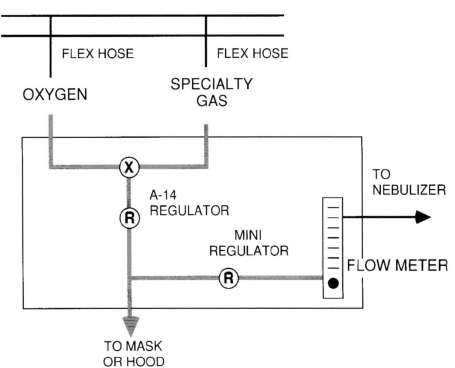

Figure 40.1
Protocol respirator unit for double-blind studies. (From Workman and Cramer 1987).

tiplace chamber that is run to full capacity with nonacute cases.

Most of the medical care in the USA is provided by physicians in private practice, and the insurance companies may refuse payment for methods of treatment that are not yet recognized in conventional medicine, or where the cost is much higher than any benefit obtained.

Research in Hyperbaric Medicine

Most of the current indications for HBO are based on evidence obtained from uncontrolled clinical trials. There are few of the randomized, double-blind, and controlled studies that are emphasized these days before recognition of any new therapeutic method or for reevaluation of older well-established methods.

Limiting factors for research in hyperbaric medicine are as follows:

1. Basic pathophysiology of several disorders treated with HBO is not well understood.
2. Animal models of some diseases do not adequately represent human illnesses. There are species differences in response to HBO so that the animal results cannot always be extrapolated to humans.
3. Blinding is difficult in controlled trials with HBO.
4. In life-threatening illnesses such as air embolism and decompression sickness, it would be unethical to deny a patient HBO treatment in a controlled trial. Clinical trials would essentially be limited to conditions which are

not a threat to the patient's life or those where HBO is an adjuvant treatment.

5. Financial support for clinical trials in hyperbaric medicine is very slim. Although HBO is a drug, it does not have a commercial sponsor. For new pharmaceuticals, the manufacturers support the high cost of clinical trials which are necessary to get the drugs approved for general use.
6. Shortage of patients for trials in any individual medical center. This limitation can be overcome by multicenter studies but it is more difficult to implement a uniform HBO protocol than it is in case of pharmaceuticals.

Clinical Trials. The general methods of conducting controlled studies are well known to medical clinical investigators. There are basically three types of clinical trials with HBO:

1. Patients receive HBO as a primary treatment and controls do not receive HBO.
2. HBO is an add-on therapy to conventional medical treatment and controls receive no HBO.
3. HBO treatment is compared with sham treatment in a hyperbaric chamber.

All three methods may be combined in a trial which has several groups.

One of the problems in carrying out these studies is that in the usual setting of a hyperbaric chamber, the control patient and the investigator would not be blind to the nature of the experiment. To overcome this difficulty, Workman and Cramer (1987) described a technique for randomized controlled studies. The protocol respirator unit used for these studies is shown in Figure 40.1. This allows the patient to breathe a specific mixture of gases known only to an umpire, but not known to the patient or the investigator. All the control patients breathe a mixture of 8.9% oxygen and 91.1% nitrogen on the assumption that at a pressure of 2.4 ATA, it is equivalent to breathing air. Those in the experimental group breathe 100% oxygen at the same pressure. The drawbacks of this method are:

- Possible undesirable side effects of nitrogen under pressure (Thomas *et al* 1976)
- Possible decompression sickness in the control group
- Errors in gas mixture; if 100% nitrogen is breathed, the consequences can be disastrous

Equipment for double-blind studies is commercially available (Dräger AG, Lübbock, FRG).

There are some situations in which controlled studies on a large number of patients cannot be done. Even when such studies are done they do not necessarily resolve the issues. Careful documentation in a small patient population with longitudinal studies may prove more useful.

Ethical Aspects of Clinical Trials with HBO. It would be unethical to deprive a patient of HBO in a life-threatening situation where HBO has shown to be effective in uncontrolled studies. There are ethical objections to double-blind studies in the case of patients for whom HBO therapy has been shown to be nearly 100% effective in well-conducted uncontrolled clinical trials. An example of this is the physical therapy for chronic post-stroke patients under simultaneous HBO. The difference between the patients treated with HBO and those treated outside is so great that any controlled study on these patients may have to be called off. The response to HBO in these patients is reproducible on multiple applications and the benefit persists with prolonged therapy. Another situation where a controlled study would be unethical is in life-threatening situations such as CO poisoning and gas gangrene. Extensive clinical trials in several countries over the past several years have established the superiority of results in these illnesses when HBO is added to the conventional therapy. Apart from the decreased mortality, there is improvement of quality of life in patients treated with HBO. If controls were to be deprived of this, they cannot be compensated for it by crossing over at a subsequent date to the HBO group, for then it may be too late.

Ideally, clinical trials should be based on solid basic experimental research in animals. In conditions where there is no suitable animal model, it may be ethical to conduct controlled clinical trials without previous animal data.

Clinical trials should be designed with professional statistical input and the results whether positive or negative should be considered valuable information. To ignore these principles would be considered unethical.

Basic Research in HBO. A panel of HBO experts (Gail 1991) have identified the need for research in the following areas:

1. Study of basic molecular and chemical biology of oxygen and understanding the physiology of oxygen transport.
2. More precise tools for measuring detailed organ function and cellular pO_2 in particular.
3. Understanding cellular responses and cell-cell interactions in both hypoxia and hyperoxia, especially in the injured state.
4. Need for controlled clinical research based on basic research.

Perhaps there should be a study of the variable response of different species to HBO, which could then serve as a guide to researchers as well as to readers who want to compare the result of different studies. Important areas where research is required are identified in various chapters of this book. Some important topics are listed in Table 40.2.

Table 40.2
Important Areas for Research in Hyperbaric Medicine

Basic Research
- Monitoring of the level of free radicals in normal as well as hypoxic conditions and determining the effect of HBO on both
- Determination of mitochondrial oxygen tension and the effect of HBO on it

Animal Experiments
- Toxic encephalopathies

Studies on Human Volunteers
- Effect of physical exercise under HBO
- Pharmacokinetics of commonly used drugs under hyperbaric conditions

Studies on Human Patients
- Patients with AIDS encephalopathy
- Superior mesenteric artery thrombosis
- Treatment of adverse effects of drugs
  - Hepatotoxicity
  - Toxic epidermal necrolysis
- Treatment of acute mountain sickness

Longitudinal Studies (long-term follow-up)
- Rehabilitation of patients in chronic post-stroke stage as an adjunct to physical therapy
- Multiple sclerosis
- Cerebral palsy
- Anoxic encephalopathies
- Ischemic leg pain as an adjunct to exercise

Controlled Clinical Trials
- Acute stroke
- Migraine
- Acute spinal cord injury
- Acute severe head injury
- Diabetes mellitus

Conclusions

Hyperbaric oxygenation has become a recognized treatment for a number of disorders, although its role in many other conditions remains experimental, controversial, or simply unknown to the medical profession at large. The main indications for HBO as the primary therapy are decompression sickness, air embolism, and CO poisoning. In all other disorders where it has been used it remains an adjunctive therapy. There is a rational basis for HBO therapy in disorders, where hypoxia plays an important role in the pathophysiology. Clinical results in many of these indications have been excellent although controlled studies are lacking.

As a drug, hyperbaric oxygen has a specific effect on the structure and the function of the human body both in health and disease. It has a defined range of effectiveness that varies according to the disorder under treatment. It is the drug with the longest list of indications, but it is not a panacea. Like other drugs, it has certain contraindications, as well as toxic and overdose effects.

In contrast to the restricted list of indications recommended by the Undersea and Hyperbaric Medical Society, application of HBO in various disorders that span most systems of the body have been described in this book. Less than half of these indications are recognized – the others are experimental or speculative. Evidence has been provided from the literature with brief comments at the end of each chapter. The central nervous system disorders and their rehabilitation constitute the most important indications and therefore proportionately more space has been allocated to these problems.

The Future

HBO will play a greater part in the practice of medicine in the future. Availability of hyperbaric chambers in every major medical facility in the developed countries is foreseen by the end of the first decade of 21st century. Already, there is greater awareness of this form of therapy among physicians and patients. A considerable amount of research work still needs to be done to place hyperbaric medicine on a sound scientific basis.

Role of Hyperbaric Oxygen in the Multidisciplinary Healthcare Systems of the Future

Modern medicine is increasing in complexity. The pathophysiology of most of the diseases is not fully understood. Several established treatments are empirical. Increasing activity in molecular biological approach to diseases is indicating that only a minority of the disease genes discovered fit in with the concept of one gene the one disease phenom-

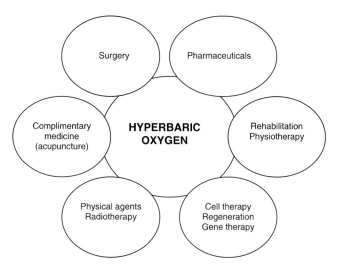

Figure 40.2
Important components of the multidisciplinary approach to disease management and relation to hyperbaric oxygen.

enon. Several of the common diseases are polygenic and multifactorial in origin. Increasing numbers of risk factors are being identified.

This has implications for treatment. Even if a single cause of the disease is identified (e.g., mutation in a gene), correction of this defect, even if possible, is usually not enough. The patient may need to control risk factors and therapies to give relief and aid recovery from the damage done by the disease process. As more methods of treatment become available, medicine is assuming a multidisciplinary form. It is a rare patient who receives only one medicine. The increasing number of options require a discussion of the choice of treatments and integration of treatments in the best interests of the patients. A simplified concept of the relationship of some forms of treatment to HBO is shown in Figure 40.2. Mainstream medicine and those who practice it have contact with practitioners of other forms of therapy. Complementary medicine is gaining increasing popularity. Acupuncture has been combined with HBO. Most physicians have no objection to their patients receiving this form for minor self-limiting diseases or for those where no treatment is available. Cell therapy, particularly involving the use of stem cells, can be combined with HBO. New technologies to facilitate regeneration can be combined with HBO for repair of fractures and wound healing. Gene therapy, on the other hand, is being developed for some serious and previously incurable diseases. The role of physical therapy and rehabilitation in patient care is increasingly recognized.

The role of HBO in a multidisciplinary approach is shown in Figure 40.3. The level of importance for HBO depends upon the level of evidence available. Only examples are given, with no effort to compile an exhaustive list of diseases for which HBO has a rational basis. Simply because no other treatment is available for a condition is no argument for giving priority to HBO for a condition.

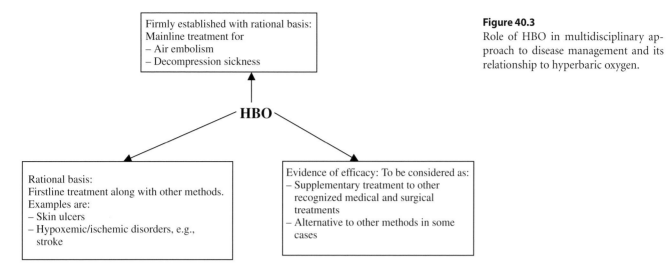

Figure 40.3
Role of HBO in multidisciplinary approach to disease management and its relationship to hyperbaric oxygen.

However, HBO may be tried on an individual case by case basis.

Hyperbaric Oxygen and Personalized Medicine

There are individual variations in therapeutic response to HBO therapy as well as development of adverse effects. Pressure and duration of treatment need to be tailored to individuals. This approach is in line with the current thinking about personalized medicine, which aims to tailor or individualize the treatment for each patient depending on various variables, the most important of which is the genotype (Jain 2002). It is conceivable that the individual sensitivity of a patient to hyperbaric oxygen can be predicted by genotyping (Jain 2009i).

41 Hyperbaric Medicine in the United States

Thomas M. Bozzuto

Hyperbaric medicine is practiced throughout the world, but the indications vary. HBO developments in the United States are described.

Introduction

The early history of hyperbaric medicine in the United States has been partially covered in Chapter 1. The first organization formed to encompass this specialty was the Undersea Medical Society (UMS), which was primarily devoted to diving medicine, as the original name indicated prior to addition of the word hyperbaric. Later, in order to include the practice of clinical hyperbaric medicine, the name of the society was changed to Undersea and Hyperbaric Medical Society (UHMS). As of 2008, there are seven chapters of the parent organization including one in Latin America and one in Brazil. There are 1,853 UHMS members as of 2008, and approximately 20% of its membership is international. In 1992, the first board certification examination in the subspecialty of Undersea Medicine was offered by the American Board of Preventive Medicine. Ten physicians took the examination. It then went dormant until 1998. The name of the examination was then changed to Undersea and Hyperbaric Medicine to reflect the increase in clinical hyperbaric medicine practice, and in 2000, the American Board of Emergency Medicine began offering the same subspecialty board certification. Currently, subspecialty certification is available through both Specialty Boards.

The first organization of physicians devoted to hyperbaric medicine was the American College of Hyperbaric Medicine (ACHM) which was founded in 1983 by Drs. Richard Neubauer, Charles Shilling, William Maxfield and J.R. Maxfield. The current president of the College is Dr. Jeffrey A. Niezgoda. A key figure in the development of hyperbaric medicine in the United States was Dr. Edger End. He carried out the earlier trials of HBO in CO poisoning. He is also the inventor of SCUBA gear and the use of liquids as an oxygen substitute for respiration while diving, among numerous other innovations. He was a visionary who predicted that the use of HBO would extend beyond treatment of wounds into other clinical applications, particularly in diseases of the nervous system. Drs. End and Neubauer published a paper on the use of HBO in stroke in 1980. Dr. Neubauer applied and investigated the use of HBO in neurological disorders such as stroke, multiple sclerosis and hypoxic encephalopathies. He also pioneered the use of SPECT scan in evaluating the effect of HBO in stroke. Other applications of SPECT are in reassessing the late effects of decompression sickness on the brain.

As of the last edition of this book, there were approximately 350 hyperbaric centers operating in the United States, 90% of which are hospital-based with more than one hyperbaric chamber. Most of the hyperbaric chambers in the United States were monoplace chambers. In the year 2008, the number of hyperbaric facilities has increased to 800–900, with approximately 50–70 multiplace chambers and roughly 2300–2400 monoplace chambers (assuming an average of three monoplace chambers per facility), but the figures for the breakdown into various categories are not available.

In an effort to raise the quality of care provided to the hyperbaric patient, the Undersea and Hyperbaric Medical Society (UHMS) established a clinical hyperbaric facility accreditation program in 2001. The objectives of the program is to ensure that clinical hyperbaric facilities:

- Are staffed with the proper specialists who are well-trained,
- Use quality equipment that has been properly installed and maintained, and being operated with the highest level of safety possible,
- Provide high quality of patient care,
- Maintain the appropriate documentation of informed consent, patient treatment procedures, physician involvement, etc.

Since the first survey in September 2002, the UHMS has surveyed 90 programs across the country, and 82 have maintained their initial accreditation. The UHMS plans to seek recognition from the Joint Commission as a complementary accrediting body once 100 programs are actively accredited. At the present time, accreditation is voluntary in all states except for Utah. The Utah Medicaid Program Office requires UHMS specific accreditation to be reimbursed for hyperbaric oxygen therapy by that program.

There is a growing international interest in hyperbaric facility accreditation. The UHMS is working with representatives from Brazil, Mexico, Australia, New Zealand, Singapore, Sweden, and others to establish accreditation programs in these respective countries. The first international facility accreditation was awarded recently to Dr. Roberto Bammann and the staff of the Medicina Hiperbarica Zona Sul, Hospital Nossa Senhora de Lourdes, Sao Paulo, Brazil.

American College for Hyperbaric Medicine

The American College of Hyperbaric Medicine (ACHM) continues to serve as a medical specialty society for physicians practicing hyperbaric medicine. There are about 800–900 hyperbaric facilities in the US. In the US, ACHM works to deliver support and services to nearly 200 physicians in 40 states, many of whom practice clinical hyperbaric medicine. A small number of physicians from outside the United States also belong to the organization. One of the most important roles of the College involves responding to events impacting the field. Advocacy efforts help create a cohesive group of clinical hyperbaric physicians. Functions and goals of the ACHM are:

- **Development of Hyperbaric Medicine as a Specialty.** A goal of the College is to develop an image of hyperbaric medicine as a distinct medical specialty. In support of that goal, it represents hyperbaric physicians before organized medicine bodies, supports certification of experienced hyperbaric physicians, sponsors special events for hyperbaric fellows, and maintains an active publications program. Among other things, the College publishes hyperbaric protocols and a directory of clinical hyperbaric physicians. There is also an examination process to certify specialists in hyperbaric Medicine in the United States and in other countries. There is also Fellowship recognition for certified hyperbaric physicians who are members of the College and have made significant contributions to the field.

- **Representing Hyperbaric Medicine Specialists.** For over eight years, ACHM Executive Committee members have represented hyperbaric physicians before the Specialty and Service Society (SSS) of the American Medical Association. The SSS represents the interests of a broad spectrum of medical specialties before the policy-making body of the AMA, which is known as the House of Delegates. The ACHM also maintains liaison with the American Hospital Association.

- **Specialist Certification.** A certification program, which includes an examination, helps to create an identifiable group of expert hyperbaric physicians. Most of the nearly 80 hyperbaric physicians who earned certification are now required to be recertified every 10 years. Recertification includes successfully sitting for a certification examination, as well as completing 100 hours of continuing medical education credits every decade.

- **A New Examination.** The American Professional Wound Care Association (APWCA) was contacted about 2 years ago by members of the American College of Hyperbaric Medicine (ACHM), who expressed their opinion that there was a need for a certification process in wound care available to their members that was physician oriented. After reviewing options, they concluded that the APWCA was the most appropriate organization for them to work with. An adhoc committee was established with key members of both organizations to investigate the concept further. It found that there is a growing need for some formal process to distinguish those who are skilled in the art and science of wound care. An examination construction committee was established with members from the two professional societies. This gave a tremendous jump start to the creation of a physician certifying exam. While the APWCA has supported this initiative at many levels and will continue to endorse the examination, a separate testing organization will administer the certification process. The exam was first to be offered on Friday, June 6, during the 2008 Congress of the World Union of Wound Healing Societies (June 4–8, in Toronto Canada). The development of this physician exam is a first step toward the long-term goal of achieving specialty recognition of wound care by the American Board of

Medical Specialties, the American Osteopathic Association, and the Council of Podiatric Medical Education.

- **Reimbursement for Hyperbaric Treatments.** In recent years, the ACHM successfully worked together with a consortium of hyperbaric groups (International Hyperbaric Medical Association, Undersea Hyperbaric Medical Society, Hyperbaric Oxygen Therapy Association) to resolve a serious funding crisis that threatened to close as many as 80 percent of the hyperbaric chambers in the US. In the end, hospital-based facilities received increased Medicare fees for their services. College officers often work to assure adequate reimbursement for hyperbaric treatments and represent hyperbaric physicians before bodies that determine reimbursement policies for hyperbaric medicine. They provide information at the request of such bodies. College officials are now working to increase Medicare payment rates to hyperbaric physicians.

In early 2003, ACHM was pressing the Centers for Medicare and Medicaid Services (CMS) to "appropriately adjust the overhead expensive RVU (relative value unit) of the CPT Code 99183 (physician attendance and supervision of hyperbaric oxygen therapy) to accurately reflect the high overhead of 24 h availability of hyperbaric medical services and high physician costs of providing this service, and to appropriately adjust the total RVU of CPT 99183 to accurately reflect the requirement for constant attendance and supervision during the hyperbaric oxygen therapy session as mandated by Medicare guidelines."

The ACHM asked CMS to increase reimbursement rates to physicians because of the significant overhead involved in on call duties, treating indigent patients and emergency treatments.

After a reimbursement battle lasting more than four years, CMS recently increased payments for "facilities" fees to hospitals with hyperbaric centers. Hopefully the move will stop closures of US hyperbaric centers. Over a dozen ceased operations while the new policy was being developed.

The crisis arose over the proposal by CMS predecessor, the Health Care Financing Administration (HCFA) to stop paying for an important hyperbaric indication. Effective the spring of 2000, HCFA had announced plans to end payments for using hyperbaric oxygen therapies to prepare compromised wound beds for skin grafts. To resolve the crisis, a delay was requested, and another hyperbaric organization, the Undersea and Hyperbaric Medical Association (UHMS) proposed that HCFA create a new indication, ischemic wound. ACHM supported this proposal.

While CMS refused to create an indication for "ischemic wound," officials said they would reconsider this policy if more evidence were presented. A final Medicare policy on payments for diabetic wounds of the lower extremities (DWLE) was published in December 2002 and took effect

April 1, 2003. The preparation of scientific data by hyperbaric physicians and submission to CMS helped produce the favorable final DWLE policy.

Medicare officials agreed to pay for treatment of DWLE for patients at hospital facilities who meet strict guidelines. Criteria include (1) patients who have Type I or Type II diabetes and have a lower extremity wound due to diabetes, (2) patients who have a wound classified as a Wagner Grade II or higher, and (3) patients who have failed an adequate course of standard wound therapy. It will not pay for treating DWLE with hyperbaric oxygen as an initial treatment. The benefit category for HBO therapy (DWLE) was hospital outpatient services, physician services, or incident to physician services. In practice this means freestanding centers are paid no technical fees for DWLE or other CMS approved indications. Freestanding centers only receive physician fees for services provided, although freestanding centers' physician fees are slightly higher to compensate for the loss of technical fees.

Another crisis arose this past year when Blue Cross/ Blue Shield circulated an (internal) assessment of hyperbaric treatments, leading to some historically well-documented treatments being labeled as investigational and therefore not reimbursable. One of the most significant of these is radiation injury, which accounts for approximately 40%–60% of all hyperbaric treatments rendered in the United States. For most hyperbaric programs, loss of the revenue generated from this therapy would lead to program closure, as they would no longer be self-supporting. The ACHM is already seeing a "chilling" effect as hospitals are postponing entry into the field of hyperbaric medicine until the full impact of the BCBS decision is assessed. In the meantime, chamber sales and program startups are decreasing steadily. The College initiated a Radionecrosis Registry, whereby facilities could enroll and electronically submit their data, which will be collected, deidentified, and submitted to third-party payors. This radionecrosis registry will serve as the basis for reporting outcomes, success rates, and cost savings when compared with historical controls and the natural course of the disease in patients without hyperbaric therapy. At the present time, three states (Idaho, Pennsylvania, and Hawaii) are affected by the BCBS central office recommendation for nonpayment of these services. Over the next 12 months, the remaining 47 states will make their own determinations. So far, the registry as reached over 1000 cases making it the largest study ever conducted in hyperbaric medicine. As this book goes to print, we were notified that Blue Cross and Blue Shield have reversed their non-payment decision for radiation injuries (soft tissue radionecrosis and osteoradionecrosis).

Indications for Use of Hyperbaric Oxygen. Hyperbaric medicine represents an emerging medical specialty whose scientific basis, while supported by over 6,000 studies, continues to be explored. The College supports use of hyperbaric therapy for the 14 indications approved by Medicare and those published in the Undersea and Hyperbaric Medical Society's Hyperbaric Oxygen Committee Report. It also supports research into investigational uses of hyperbaric oxygen therapy.

Out of the list of UHMS approved indications referenced in Table 8.1, Medicare (and most other insurance companies) in the United States does not reimburse for Exceptional Blood Loss Anemia, Intracranial Abscess, or Thermal Burns. For problem wounds, they will only reimburse for Diabetic Wounds of the Lower Extremity which have failed a course of conventional therapy of at least 30 days as referenced in the Medicare guidelines CIM 35-10.

42 Hyperbaric Medicine in Japan

H. Takahashi and H. Yagi

The development of hyperbaric medicine in Japan had a rather late start compared to Europe and USA but a faster rate of development. The status of hyperbaric medicine in Japan is discussed under the following headings:

History of Hyperbaric Medicine in Japan

Before World War I, research on hyperbaric medicine in Japan was focused mainly on the environmental physiology of Ama diving or the industrial hygiene of caisson workers. In 1958, Saitoh in Chiba reported favorable results of hyperbaric air therapy for stroke and attributed the effect to increased oxygen content in the blood. This may be considered the dawn of hyperbaric medicine in Japan (Sakakibara 1986). Clinical work in hyperbaric medicine started in 1963 when Furuta of Tokyo University presented a paper at a thoracic surgical meeting in Japan on his experience of designing a hyperbaric surgical theater and a hyperbaric recovery room.

In 1965, a group of thoracic surgeons at Sopporo Medical University presented a paper titled "A study on hyperbaric oxygen therapy." These two groups in Tokyo and Sapporo may be called the founders of hyperbaric medicine in Japan. Parallel to this in 1963, Sakakibara at Nagoya University initiated a series of clinical investigations of hyperbaric oxygen therapy which led to the installation of the world's largest hyperbaric chamber at Nagoya University (see Chapter 7). Many new indications for HBO were developed there. This was followed by installation of multiplace chambers at Osaka and Kyoto Universities. The first workshop on hyperbaric medicine was held in Tokyo in 1966 and was followed by formation of the Japanese Society for Hyperbaric Medicine (JSHM) in 1969.

During the long history of hyperbaric medicine in Japan, five fatal chamber fires have taken place to-date (Table 42.1). In 1969, JSHM Safety Committee published the first edition of Safety Guidelines for HBO. The aim was to prevent chamber fires through carelessness and this document has been updated many times to keep up with the changing social customs (Japanese Society for Hyperbaric Medicine 1995).

In 1982, JSHM launched the Educational Course in Hyperbaric Medicine for hyperbaric nurses and engineers. In 1981, the *Japanese Journal of Hyperbaric Medicine*, the official journal of JSHM started to publish quarterly.

Table 42.1
Chamber Fires in Japan

Year	Chamber type	No. victims	Cause of fire
1967	Monoplace	1	Metal pocket warmer
1969	Multiplace	4	Uncertain (electrical?)
1989	Monoplace	1	Metal pocket warmer
1993	Monoplace	1	Metal pocket warmer
1996	Monoplace	2	Chemical pocket warmer

Indications for HBO Approved by the JSHM

Currently 20 disorders are accepted as indications for HBO therapy according to the guidelines of JSHM (Table 42.2). They are divided into two groups: emergency and nonemergency indications. Emergency means acute and serious hypoxic disorders and are absolute indications for HBO. Nonemergency implies chronic disorders in which HBO is recommended as an adjunct to other established effective treatments. This group also includes some investigative indications.

Table 42.2
Currently Accepted Indications for Hyperbaric Oxygen Therapy as Recommended by the JSHM

Emergency (acute) indications:
1. Acute carbon monoxide and other gas-induced intoxications, including delayed intoxications
2. Gas gangrene
3. Air embolism and decompression sickness
4. Acute peripheral vascular disorders:
   a) Severe burn injury and frostbite
   b) Combined with large crush injury or massive vascular damage
5. Shock
6. Myocardial infarction and other coronary insufficiencies
7. Consciousness disorders and brain edema after brain embolism or severe cranial injury
8. Acute and severe hypoxic disorder of brain
9. Paralytic ileus
10. Acute obstructive disorders of the retinal artery
11. Sudden deafness
12. Severe spinal cord disorders

Non-emergency (chronic) indications:
1. Malignant neoplasms, combined with radiation or chemotherapy
2. Peripheral circulatory disorders with refractory ulcers
3. Skin grafts
4. SMON (Subacute myelo-opticoneuropathy)
5. Motor paresis, as the later sequelae of cerebrovascular attack, severe cranial injury or craniotomy
6. Delayed syndromes in carbon monoxide intoxication
7. Spinal cord neuropathy
8. Osteomyelitis and radiation necrosis

Distribution and Number of Hyperbaric Chambers in Japan

At the end of fiscal year 1997 (March 31st), the total number of hyperbaric chambers in Japan was 815, of which 758 were monoplace (93%) and 57 multiplace (7%). These chambers are located at 617 medical facilities. The distribution of these chambers is shown in Table 42.3.

Table 42.3
Distribution of Hyperbaric Chambers in Japan

Area of Japan	Hospitals	Monoplace	Multiplace	Subtotal
Hokkaido	91	147	2	149
Toh-hoku (North Japan)	42	47	4	51
Kantoh (Tokyo Metropolitan)	187	233	18	251
Chubu (Central Japan)	85	104	7	111
Kansai (Osaka, Kyoto, Kobe)	36	36	6	42
Chugoku	31	32	4	36
Shikoku	13	13	1	14
Kyushu, Okinawa	132	146	15	161
Total	617	758	57	815

Chambers are distributed uniformly all over Japan. However, multiplace chambers are located rather densely especially around Tokyo and Kyushu areas. Within Tokyo metropolitan area, Chiba and Kanagawa prefectures are included. In Chiba there are seven, and in Kanagawa four multiplace chambers are in use. Also, in the Fukuoka prefecture in the Kyushu area there are four active multiplace chambers; they belong to a national university hospital, a private medical college, an emergency medical center and a key local community hospital. The total number of clinical chambers is still increasing and one of the remarkable tendencies is that, every year, at least one university hospital introduces a new multiplace chamber.

Current Status of Research and Academic HBO Centers in Japan

In the early 1970s, two important new indications for HBO therapy were developed and established in Japan. These involve sensory organ disorders, sudden deafness and retinal artery embolism, and are accepted widely now. We have improved our knowledge of clinical types of these conditions that are suitable for HBO therapy and the timing of treatment for optimal results (Miyake *et al* 1972). Further clinical investigations in ophthalmology have opened another new indication – cystoid macular edema (CME) – which is often associated with diabetes, uveitis, and retinal venous embolism. Ophthalmologists at the University of Nagoya have shown that combined use of HBO land diuretics can improve disturbed visual acuity in most of the cases (Miyake *et al* 1993).

In oral and maxillofacial region, a new trial is in progress, mainly at the Universality of Nagoya. Although clinical experience is still limited, administration of HBO before and after the implant surgery has facilitated the integration of the implanted fixture. This application of HBO

has improved the management of irradiated or grafted tissue (Ueda *et al* 1993).

A group of urologists at the University of Nagoya is trying to administer HBO routinely for patients undergoing urological plastic surgery. HBO is considered to enhance the wound healing in these cases and also suppresses bacterial infections which often result in fistula formation as post-surgical complication (Tsuji 1992).

Orthopedic surgeons are now conducting fundamental research to establish the basic background for HBO in their specialty. They are attempting to clarify the effect of HBO on bone metabolism. One of important key issues is whether HBO can improve senile degenerative changes in bone tissue (Iwase *et al* 1996).

Neurosurgeons at the University of Occupational and Environmental Health in Kitakyushu and Kagoshima University are conducting elaborate research to demonstrate the combined effect of HBO, chemotherapy and radiation on malignant gliomas of the brain. Among the HBO indications list of JSHM, cancer therapy has been considered as investigative but this method is being applied with encouraging results (Kohshi *et al* 1996; Hirakawa 1996).

Cost-Benefit Issues of HBO Therapy in Japan

Health insurance is compulsory in Japan and almost all medical costs relevant to HBO are covered by health insurance carriers, the Japanese government, local government and non-government health insurance carriers operated by non-profit organizations. All the medical costs in Japan are determined by Japanese Government, Ministry of Health and Welfare, and are revised usually every two years. According to the recent version of medical costs guidelines, HBO costs are as follows:

1. Emergency indications only up to 7 days after onset
   i) 5,000 points (1 point = 10 Yen) per day for monoplace chamber
   ii) 6,000 points per day for multiplace chamber
2. Non-emergency indications (seven days after onset)
   200 points per day for both mono- and multi-place chambers.

Many people urge that the big gap between emergency and non-emergency indications is an issue that should be looked into in the near future and proper adjustments should be made. Another problem is serious decompression sickness which requires a special recompression table and hyperbaric personnel are forced to work long hours outside the routine program.

Future Prospects

Historically, Japanese hyperbaric medicine has emphasized clinical applications, and fundamental research to provide a scientific background for clinical indications has tended to be delayed. By conducting more basic investigations, many new indications will be established in the future. One of the most important goals of HBO therapy is to participate in cancer therapy; the combination of hyperbaric medicine and oncology is an attractive new horizon.

An important issue to be clarified is the biological safety of the hyperbaric oxygenated environment for the human beings. There are numerous scientific papers that have described the effect of HBO on microorganisms at tissue and cell level, but few have dealt with the effects of HBO on human patients. As HBO is a method of treatment for patients on a daily basis in a high pressure oxygenated environment, it is important to prove that it is a safe therapeutic maneuver. Finally, the combination of hypo- and hyperbaric medicine seems to be opening new gateways for many incurable diseases.

43 Hyperbaric Medicine in the Rest of the World

K. K. Jain

Hyperbaric medicine is practiced throughout the world, but the indications vary. As examples, HBO developments in various countries are described here as well as the world distributors of hyperbaric facilities.

Introduction

The practice of medicine varies around the world and so does hyperbaric medicine. It was considered appropriate to include a brief description of trends in the practice of hyperbaric medicine around the world. It was not possible to include all the countries. Only those countries outside of the United States where hyperbaric medicine is practiced on a significant scale are included. A brief description of hyperbaric medicine in United States was given in Chapter 41. This chapter will briefly describe the current state of hyperbaric medicine in Germany, Russia and China. HBO in Japan is described in detail in Chapter 42.

Hyperbaric Medicine in Germany

Germany has played an important part in the development of modern hyperbaric medicine, particularly in the applications for neurological disorders. Important work in this area was done in the late 1960s and early 1970s at the University Neurosurgical Clinic, Bonn, by Professor K.H. Holbach and colleagues, of whom Prof. Wassmann continued this work. The author (KKJ) had an opportunity to work with this team. HBO was applied to patients with head injuries and stroke and the important contribution was the response to HBO for selecting patients for extra-intracranial bypass operation. This application of HBO did not spread in clinical practice for the next decade when the group in Bonn moved to other centers and followed other interests in neurosurgery. In 1980s research was done into the applications of HBO for inner ear disorders, particularly sudden deafness. In 1986, the author returned to Germany and during the following three years had a chance to work on the clinical applications of HBO in a rehabilitation clinic. This is where the work on treatment of chronic stroke patients was carried out. In 1989, there were only four active hyperbaric chambers for clinical HBO therapy in Germany.

In recent years there has been a rapid expansion of hyperbaric facilities in Germany and in 2008 there are approximately. These are all multiplace chambers (monoplace chambers are not approved in Germany currently) and over 50,000 patients were treated in the year 2007. Most of these patients (about 85%) are treated on an ambulatory basis for indications related to the inner ear (tinnitus and hearing loss). Most of these chambers are outside of university centers and are mostly business enterprises with little research activity. Efforts are being made to expand the indications to other areas and some of these chambers may be used for the treatment of patients in acute stroke trials that are planned in conjunction with US centers.

Hyperbaric Medicine in China

The first Chinese hyperbaric chamber was built in 1964 by Dr. Wen-ren Li, Hyperbaric medicine has developed rapidly in China during the past decade and there are now over 18000 hyperbaric chambers in the country. The total staff including physicians, nurses, technicians and research scientists is over 35,000. The number of patients treated yearly with HBO exceeds 2.5 million. Apart from the routine practice, research is being carried out on the mechanisms of action of HBO and its role in the management of the following conditions:

- Stroke
- Persistent vegetative state
- Autoimmune diseases
- Cancer
- Rejection in transplants

Indications and contraindications for hyperbaric oxygen in China are shown in Table 43.1.

Table 43.1
Indications for HBO in China, Chinese Society of Hyperbaric Oxygen Medicine

Emergency indications, first line
1. Acute CO poisoning and its delayed neurological sequelae
2. Acute decompression sickness
3. Acute air embolism
4. Acute cerebral dysfunction after cardiopulmonary resuscitation (electric injury, drowning, hanging)
5. Anaerobic infections (Gas gangrene, tetanus, etc)
6. Shock
7. Chemical and gas poisoning (hydrogen sulfide, petroleum gas etc)
8. Acute retinal artery occlusion
9. Acute cerebral edema and pulmonary edema
10. Crush injury and its syndrome
11. Acute peripheral circulatory failure
12. Severe spinal cord injury.

Second line indications, adjunctive
1. Coronary heart disease
2. Myocardial infarction
3. Myocarditis
4. Bronchial asthma and asthmatic bronchitis
5. Ischemic cerebrovascular disease
6. Migraine
7. Bell's palsy
8. Peripheral nerve injuries and neuropathies
9. Mountain sickness
10. Brain trauma
11. Brain tumor, post-operative
12. Cerebrovascular disease, post-operative
13. Multiple sclerosis
14. Epilepsy
15. Reimplantation of severed limb, post-operative

16. Myelitis
17. Bone fractures and non-union of fracture
18. Aseptic osteonecrosis
19. Chronic skin ulcer
20. Congenital heart disease surgery
21. Coronary artery bypass operation
22. Paralytic ileus
23. Peripheral vascular disease
24. Chilblain
25. Burns
26. Cosmetic surgery, post-operative
27. Post skin grafting
28. Sudden deafness
29. Acoustic deafness
30. Vertigo
31. Retinal venous thrombosis
32. Central serous retinopathy
33. Retinal concussion
34. Optic atrophy
35. Diabetic retinopathy
36. Viral encephalitis
37. Infectious hepatitis
38. Chronic hepatic insufficiency
39. Peptic ulcer
40. Ulcerative colitis
41. Sports injuries
42. Radiation injury
43. Pharmaceutical and chemical intoxications
44. Pityriasis rosea
45. Shingles
46. Erythema nodosum
47. Periodontal disease
48. Recurrent aphthous ulcer
49. Cancer (combined with radiotherapy and chemotherapy)
50. Pneumonia in children
51. Neonatal asphyxia
52. Fetal distress
53. Cerebral palsy in children

Investigative indications
1. Meningitis
2. Arrhythmia
3. Chronic heart failure
4. Glaucoma
5. Manganese poisoning
6. Autoimmune diseases
7. Diabetes mellitus
8. Radiation-induced vasculitis
9. Cervical spondylopathy
10. Mycosis
11. Parkinson's disease
12. Senile dementia
13. Pyocephalus
14. Progressive myodystrophy
15. Rheumatoid arthritis
16. Adult respiratory distress syndrome
17. Childbirth in women with heart disease
18. Habitual abortion

Absolute contraindications
1. Untreated pneumothorax and mediastinal emphysema

2. Active bleeding and hemorrhagic disease
3. Positive reaction to oxygen tolerance test
4. Tuberculous cavitation in lungs and hemoptysis
5. Second degree heart block

Relative contraindications
1. Severe upper respiratory tract infection
2. Severe pulmonary emphysema and bullae of lungs
3. Severe sinusitis
4. Untreated malignant tumor
5. Detachment of retina
6. Sick sinus syndrome
7. Bradycardia
8. Otitis media suppurativa
9. Eustachian tube occlusion
10. Hypertension

Hyperbaric Medicine in Russia

Russia has extensive hyperbaric facilities. There are over 60 centers with hyperbaric facilities and approximately 1300 hyperbaric chambers are currently in use. Russia had one of the longest lists of indications for hyperbaric oxygen therapy. These indications are shown in Table 43.2.

Table 43.2
Hyperbaric Oxygen Indications in Russia

Vascular diseases
    Arterial obstructions in the limbs before and after surgery (embolism, traumas, thrombosis)
    Arteriosclerosis
Gas embolism in the blood vessels
Ulcers caused by defective blood circulation
Cardiac disorders
    Heart strain
    Heart rhythm disturbances
    Irregular heartbeat
    Paroxysmal extrasystole
    Cardiac insufficiency
    Cardiosclerosis decompensation
    Cardiac insufficiency after heart surgery
    Heart contraction disturbances
    Cardio-pulmonary insufficiency
Pulmonary disorders
    Lung abscess before and after surgery
    Nonspecific chronic lung affections with cardiopulmonary insufficiency signs
Gastrointestinal disorders
    Stomach and duodenal ulcers
    Intestinal obstruction
Liver diseases
    Acute viral hepatitis
    Hepatic encephalitis
    Liver cirrhosis
    Obstructive jaundice
    Hepatic insufficiency after resuscitation
    Toxic hepatitis

Table 43.2 (continued)

Central nervous system diseases
    Cerebral gas embolism
    Brain ischemia
    Cranial traumas
    Posthypoxic encephalopathy
    Botulism
    Cervical spinal cord trauma
Eye disorders
    Acute retinal ischemia
    Retinal dystrophy
    Diabetic retinopathy
    Optic neuritis by methanol intoxication
Endocrine disorders
    Diabetic arteriopathy
    Diabetic ulcers and polyneuritis
    Toxic goitre
Facial and maxillary pathology
    Paradontosis
    Facial phlegm
    Maxillary osteomyelitis
    Necrotic gingivitis and stomatitis
    Facial actinomycosis
Orthopedics
    Fractured limbs with blood circulation disturbances
    Fractures in an arteriopathic or diabetic patient
    Delayed fracture union
    Osteomyelitis
Obstetrics
    Abortion by placental ischemia
    Threatened abortion due to endocrine disorders
    Placental hypoxia
    Fetal hypoxia
    Pregnancy neuropathy (stage 1, 2)
    Pregnancy with immunological disorders
    Pregnancy complications by extragenital pathology
    Cardiac malformation: acquired or congenital
    Diabetes
    Pregnant or delivered mothers in critical state
    Coma after eclampsia
Diseases of newly born
    Asphyxia during delivery
    Cerebrovascular disturbance
    Hemolysis
General surgery infections
    General septic abscess unresolved in spite of incision
    Infectious peritonitis with surgical removal of initial lesion
Wound pathology
    Clostridial infection
    Wound abscess in spite of drainage
    Prophylactic treatment of wound infected after open trauma
    Granular wound
    Wound with superficial burn
    Postsurgery wound
Exogenous poisoning
    Carbon monoxide poisoning
    Cyanide poisoning
    Chloroxide poisoning
    Organic phosphate poisoning

World Distribution of Hyperbaric Facilities

Some idea of the quantity of hyperbaric medical facilities in the world can be obtained by a review of the statistics regarding the distribution of hyperbaric chambers in various countries. Accurate information on this subject is difficult to obtain, but the available figures are shown in Figure 43.1. The largest number of chambers are located in China (about 1800) and Russia with 1300 chambers is next. Europe has about 475 hyperbaric chambers, and the distribution of these is shown in Figure 43.2. The number of chambers does not necessarily correlate with the number of patients or the number of treatments given. There is no separation of multiplace and monoplace chambers in the statistics.

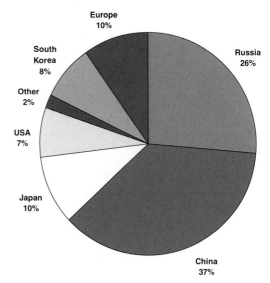

Figure 43.1
World distribution of hyperbaric chambers.

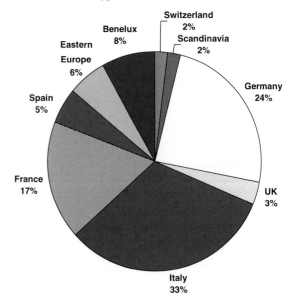

Figure 43.2
Distribution of hyperbaric chambers in Europe.

PART III:
APPENDIX,
BIBLIOGRAPHY,
INDEX

44 Appendix: Diagnostic Imaging and HBO Therapy

P.G. Harch, R.A. Neubauer[†], J.M. Uszler, and P.B. James

Diagnostic imaging plays an important role in diagnosis of diseases of the CNS. It is even more important in assessing the effects of HBO on hypoxic/ischemic lesions of the brain. Various techniques that are relevant to HBO include single photon emission computerized tomography (SPECT), positron emission tomography (PET), functional magnetic resonance imaging (MRI), and MR spectroscopy. For practical purposes, SPECT using hexamethylpropyleneamine (HMPAO) or ethyl cysteinate dimer (ECD) is the most practical and widely used diagnostic procedure in combination with HBO therapy. This technique is illustrated in this appendix.

In the past 20 years single photon emission computerized tomography (SPECT) has matured with the development of hexamethylpropyleneamine oxime (HMPAO), ethyl cysteinate dimer (ECD), and receptor specific agents (Maziere 1993). The resolution on triple-head SPECT systems is now 6–9 mm (Holman & Devous 1992) and counting statistics are excellent, but semiquantitative, i.e., HMPAO and ECD underestimate high flow (Heiss 1990 and Ishizu 1996, respectively) and HMPAO overestimates low flow (Heiss 1990) compared to PET.

Ready availability, expanding applications, long shelf-life of the agents, computer-assisted evaluation methods, and the known coupling of brain blood flow and metabolism in chronic brain injury (Meyer *et al* 1968, Kuhl *et al* 1980, Obrist *et al* 1984) have popularized SPECT in recent years, but its unique advantage resides in its ability to image the uncooperative patient, e.g., pediatric, combative, or demented patients. Since the radiopharmaceuticals are fixed in brain on first pass and are independent of subsequent brain activity, thus giving a freeze-frame snapshot of brain blood flow at the time of injection that can be imaged later, an uncooperative patient can be sedated after tracer injection and not alter the picture of brain blood flow acquired later.

Positron emission tomography (PET) is the current gold standard for measurement of cerebral blood flow, metabolism, and receptor activity. PET exploits the annihilation geometry of positrons that results in the emission of two high energy gamma rays at 180 degree angles (Gilman 1998). PET is technically much more demanding than SPECT and because of high costs, limited availability, and the requirement of a nearby or on-site cyclotron to produce ultra-short half-life radiopharmaceuticals it remains a research and clinical tool at university centers.

The number of additional functional imaging modalities has steadily increased in the past 10 years. The armamentarium now includes functional magnetic resonance imaging (fMRI) and MR spectroscopy (MRS) – (Potchen 1991), diffusion weighted MRI (DWI) with or without perfusion MRI, Xenon enhanced CT, and CT perfusion. For an excellent review of these in stroke please see (Latchaw *et al* 2003). To our knowledge most have not been employed in sequence with one or more HBO treatments.

The most important application of functional imaging to hyperbaric oxygen (HBO) therapy has been the attempt to capture the effect of a single or multiple hyperbaric treatments on brain blood flow, metabolism, or function. The first attempt employed EEG (Holbach 1977f) while all subsequent investigations have used SPECT in an effort to visualize idling neurons (Neubauer 1990) or recoverable brain tissue in a functional ischemic penumbra (Neubauer *et al* 1989b, 1992c, 1995a, 1998, 2001, Harch 1992, 1994b, 1996, Golden *et al* 2002, Miura *et al* 2002).

The basic technique involves SPECT imaging with Iodo-amphetamine (IMP), HMPAO, or ECD before and after

HBO treatment in full or split-dose fashion. The full dose technique is a two day procedure with baseline SPECT imaging the first day, a single HBO treatment later that day or the following day, and repeat SPECT imaging at least 24 h (four half-lives of technetium, the SPECT tracer) after the first SPECT, and ideally 2 or more hours after HBO treatment. The split-dose technique is a one day procedure that uses a single full SPECT dose of radiotracer divided in weighted or equal parts with imaging before and shortly after a single HBO treatment. Because of the requirement for special subtraction software (Hashikawa 1994) to eliminate the confounding visual effects of the two superimposed split doses the split-dose method has been infrequently used in the clinical setting.

Regardless of full or split-dose, the generally observed response has been a global increase in flow and a redistribution of flow from higher to lower flow areas to give a visual appearance of smoothing or homogeneity (see cases 1–4 in Chapter 19). The effect appears to be non-specific since it has been documented in a variety of neuropathologies (vide supra), but may be dependent on timing of the SPECT injection after the HBO exposure.

In the first years of investigation of this technique a few select patients were injected with SPECT tracer within a few minutes of exit from 1.5 ATA hyperbaric treatments while on room air (Figure 44.1B) or supplemental high flow oxygen (Figures 44.2C & 40.2D) to see if the effect first described by Neubauer *et al* (1990) was a direct or indirect effect of oxygen.

It appeared from these and a multitude of other cases that the effect was an indirect action of HBO treatment and that if patients were injected too soon after chamber exit (Figure 44.1B) or while on supplemental oxygen (Figures 43.2C and 44.2D) after chamber exit hyperoxic vasoconstriction was disproportionately recorded; this hyperoxic vasoconstrictive effect on normal brain is even more pronounced in normal individuals (Figures 44.3C and 44.3D). The exact explanation of the delayed improved brain blood flow to ischemic regions following a 1.5 ATA HBO treatment is unclear, but acutely may be due to reverse steal from higher flow more normal vascular beds to ischemic beds as the higher flow beds vasoconstrict in response to hyperoxia (Figures 44.2C & 44.2D), increased perfusion to passive damaged cerebral vascular beds as a result of increased peripheral vascular resistance and widened pulse pressure (Chapter 2), increased flow demanded by HBO-stimulated increased metabolism in the ischemic territory, or some other explanation. However, as the time period after HBO treatment lengthens and hyperoxic vasoconstriction wanes the Neubauer Effect is best explained by the latter mechanism (Figures 44.4A and 44.4B).

This phenomenon was recently (delete this word) rigorously evaluated in patients with chronic brain contusions and normal subjects by one of the authors (PGH) and colleagues with statistical parametric mapping analysis of

SPECT (Barrett *et al* 1998). Improvement in SPECT was shown in patients with brain contusions but not the normal subjects.

This SPECT technique to visualize the ischemic penumbra and the capacity of injured brain to respond to repetitive HBO treatment is still in its infancy. Specifically, the sensitivity and specificity, exact timing of SPECT post-HBO treatment, the question of timing in different neuropathologies, whether the degree of improvement in brain blood flow post-HBO treatment is predictive of the magnitude of subsequent functional outcome, and the degree of transience/permanence to the effect of a single or multiple HBO's are all unknown. Since the publication of the third edition of this text the final question has been partially addressed. The animal studies (Harch *et al* 1996) both demonstrated persistence of cerebrovascular changes in chronic injured rat brains three to six weeks after the 80th HBO. Vascularity was decreased in normal brain and increased in damaged brain. The degree of transience and permanence to these changes have been observed in a number of patients treated with HBO by author PGH over the past years. An example is shown in Patient 1, Figures 44.5 A-1. The series of scans shows an improvement in brain blood flow and pattern to a more normal pattern with each course of HBO and a partial regression after completion of the second course of HBO. Concomitantly, the patient improved symptomatically, on physical exam, and after the third course of HBO, on psychometric testing.

Author PGH has noted this pattern of partial regression post HBO treatment and improvement after reintroduction of HBO in a variety of other patients he has followed over the years, particularly those with toxic brain injury. SPECT has recorded changes in blood flow consistent with the patients' clinical conditions. It appears that blood flow is redirected to damaged areas or metabolism/flow are increased transiently to these areas, consistent with the finding in the animal model (Harch *et al* 1996) where brain vascularity was decreased in normal brain and increased in damaged brain. This phenomenon implies a manipulation of brain blood flow and metabolism that requires some schedule of ongoing HBO to maintain the effect. In other words, low-pressure HBO appears to behave like a simple drug for part of its non-trophic effect consistent with the definition of HBO given in the introduction to Chapter 19. Mechanistic answers as well as answers to the other questions posed above will require further research, clinical experience, and application of functional imaging to HBO.

Acknowledgment

All images in Figures 44.2–44.4 were obtained on a Picker Prism 3000 Triple-head Nuclear Scanner by technologist Phil Tranchina, West Jefferson Medical Center, Marrero, Louisiana. Pictures were taken by author, PGH, with a 35 mm camera on tripod. Images in Figures 44.5 A-J orig-inated from an ADAC dual-head camera and were photos of color laser prints taken by a 5.2 megapixel digital camera on a tripod. Since the transverse images on laser print were not available for all of the scans the sagittal orientation was chosen for most of these figures. The photos were then adjusted to reduce glare. As a result, some of the scans appear brighter than others with a slightly different background. The color scale for blood flow was not altered, however, and remains the same throughout the sequence of scans.

Patient 1: The patient is a 29-year-old white male who experienced carbon monoxide poisoning from a propane-powered forklift operating in a 40 × 50 ft. room for 4 h. The patient complained of a moderate headache and mild nausea. He was taken to a nearby emergency room and given surface oxygen for approximately 6 h and was then transferred to a hyperbaric unit where he underwent a single 3.0 ATA multiplace CO table 9 h after extrication. CO level drawn 3 h after extrication while on oxygen was 24.1%. Past medical and social history are significant for one pack/day smoking and significant polypharmacy drug abuse habits; the drug use ended 2 months before the CO exposure. Over the ensuing 3 days the patient developed delayed neuropsychiatric syndrome (DNS) of carbon monoxide poisoning with headaches and a variety of cognitive symptoms. Physical exam revealed mild balance abnormalities and a Folstein Mini-Mental Status score of 26; score was 30 after his first HBO three days earlier. The patient was imaged with SPECT in Figure 44.5A and underwent a course of HBO at 1.5 ATA/60 daily twice a day for 40 treatments with steady clinical improvement. Three hours after the second HBO treatment and 17 h after injection of the first SPECT in Figure 44.5A, SPECT was repeated in Figure 44.5B, showing a more normal pattern of flow, consistent with partial amelioration of his symptoms. Seven days after the conclusion of HBO SPECT was obtained in Figure 44.5C, demonstrating an improvement in flow and pattern of flow, again consistent with clinical improvement. To highlight the change from baseline the scan in Figure 44.5C is registered on the pixel scale for the scan in Figure 44.5A and presented in Figure 44.5D. The doses of radiopharmaceutical (HMPAO), conditions of injection, time from injection to scanning, and processing are identical for every scan in this case presentation.

In the subsequent weeks the patient experienced a recurrence of symptoms. Because of complications in obtaining further HBO the patient was treated pharmacologically with minimal effect on his condition. At the request of the patient and others injured in the mass exposure (23 persons) the author (PGH) began a third course of HBO at 1.5 ATA/90 daily, beginning 4 months after the final HBO and SPECT from the second course of treatment. SPECT was repeated in Figure 44.5E before this third course of HBO and demonstrated a florid deterioration in amount (note maximum pixel count) and pattern of blood flow compared to the last scan after HBOT in Figure 44.5C, but an improvement in pattern compared to the patient's first scan seen in Figure 44.5A. This scan was consistent with the clinical condition in that the patient was better now than before the second course of HBO when he was experiencing DNS – but worse than after his peak clinical experience from the second course of HBO. For easier comparison the scan in Figure 44.5E is registered on the pixel scale of the scan in Figure 44.5A and presented in Figure 44.5F. The patient underwent a single HBO at 1.5 ATA/90 and SPECT repeated in Figure 44.5G. Note the improvement in pattern with minimal increase in flow (maximum pixel count increased from 230 to 239). The patient proceeded through 34 additional HBO treatments. At the conclusion of this third round of HBO he was clinically better and showed an improvement in neuropsychological testing compared to the identical testing 4 months earlier at the initiation of HBO.

A Repeat SPECT 2 days after the 35th HBO treatment is featured in Figure 44.5G and again tracks the patient's clinical condition. SPECT of Figure 44.5G is placed on the same pixel scale as the baseline scan in Figure 44.5A (before the second round of HBO) and Figure 44.5E (before the third course of HBO) and presented in Figures 44.5H and 44.5I, respectively. Throughout this patient's clinical course the SPECT tracked the clinical condition.

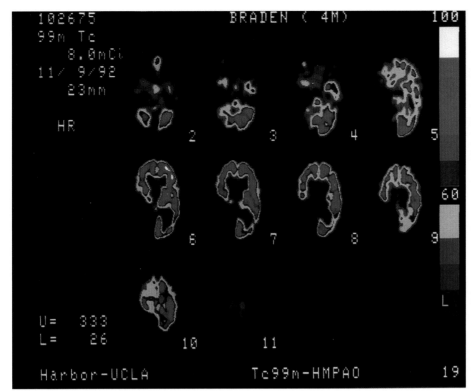

Figure 44.1A
Transverse HMPAO SPECT brain images of 4-year-old boy, 2 years after severe traumatic brain injury baseline study. Color code bar is on the right with highest brain blood flow white and lowest blue. Orientation is base of brain in left upper corner to vertex in second image of third row.

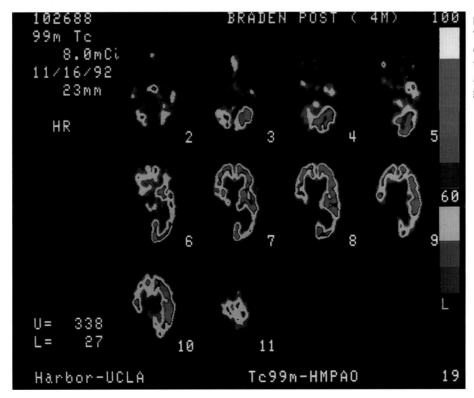

Figure 44.1B
Transverse HMPAO SPECT brain images of patient in Figure 44.1A, injected with tracer 5 min after exit from first 1.5 ATA/90 min HBO treatment. Note global decrease in brain blood flow.

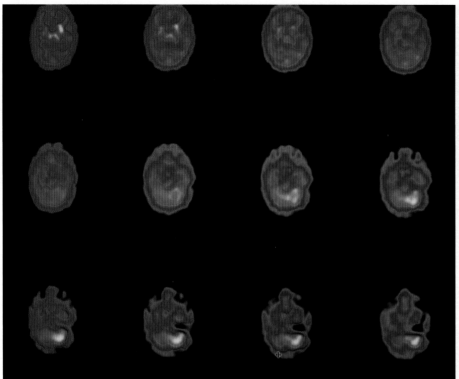

Figure 44.2A
Selected transverse HMPAO SPECT brain images of 49-year-old male, one month after brain decompression sickness and 1 day after second HBO treatment. Note multiple defects, especially the right cerebellum. Orientation is from cephalad in left upper corner to base of brain in right lower corner. Patient's right is on reader's left, identical to CT convention. Color code is bright white yellow, highest flow, to blue/black, lowest flow.

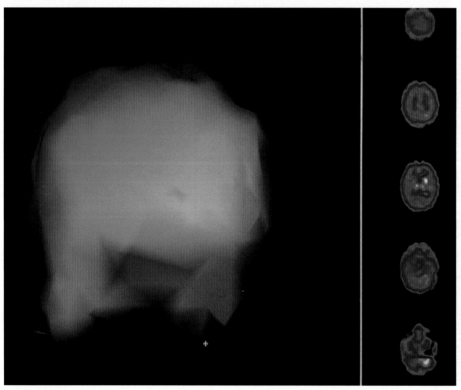

Figure 44.2B
Three dimensional surface reconstruction, posterior view, of scan in Figure 44.2A. Note decrease in right cerebellum.

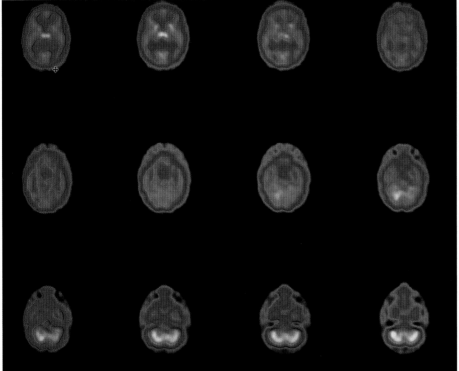

Figure 44.2C
Selected transverse HMPAO SPECT brain images of patient in Figure 2A injected with tracer 30 min after 1.5ATA/90 min HBO treatment while on high flow oxygen by non-rebreathing mask. Note improvement in right cerebellum while flow is decreased in left occiput, a reverse steal phenomenon.

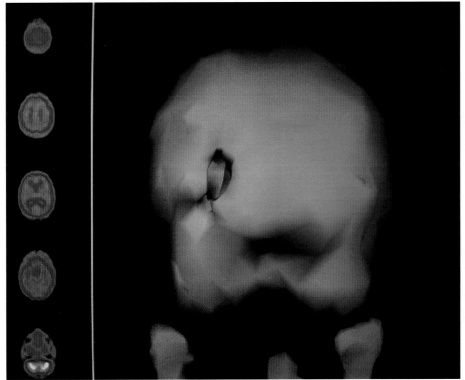

Figure 44.2D
Three dimensional surface reconstruction of scan in Figure 44.2C. Note normalization of flow to right cerebellum and decrease in left occiput.

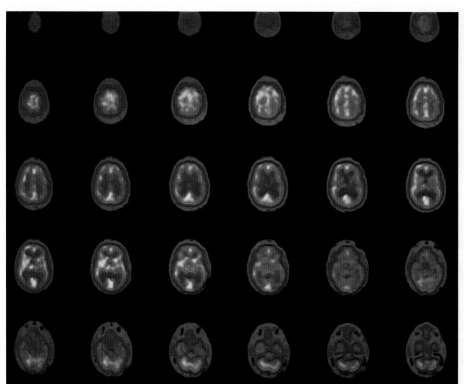

Figure 44.3A
Transverse HMPAO SPECT brain images of 47 year old normal male ex-smoker with no history of brain injury.

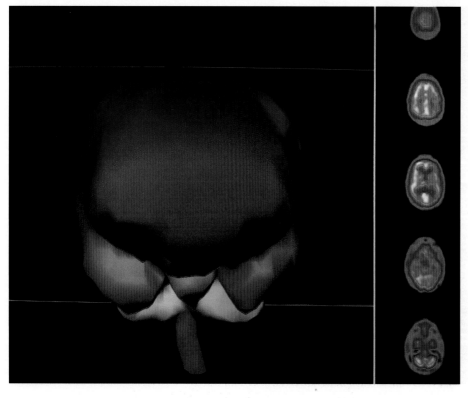

Figure 44.3B
Three dimensional surface reconstruction of scan of Figure 44.3A, frontal facial view.

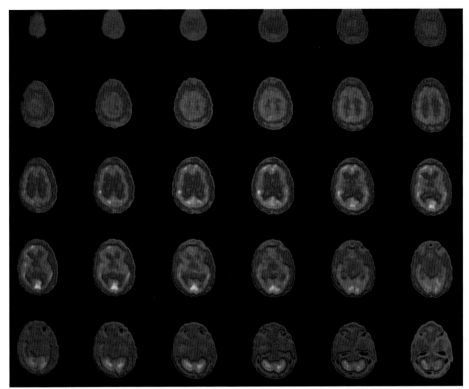

Figure 44.3C
Transverse HMPAO SPECT brain images of patient in Figure 44.3A injected with tracer 30 min after a 1.5 ATA/90-min HBO treatment while on high flow oxygen by non-rebreathing mask. Note global decrease in brain blood flow.

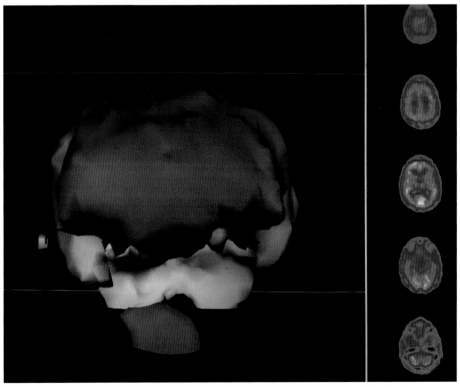

Figure 44.3D
Three dimensional surface reconstruction of scan in Figure 44.3C, frontal facial view. Note global decrease in brain blood flow with appearance of focal defects and coarseness of the cortical surface.

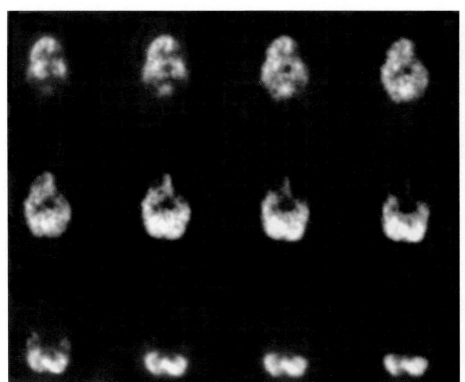

Figure 44.4A
Selected transverse ECD SPECT brain images of 3-year old cerebral palsy boy, baseline study.

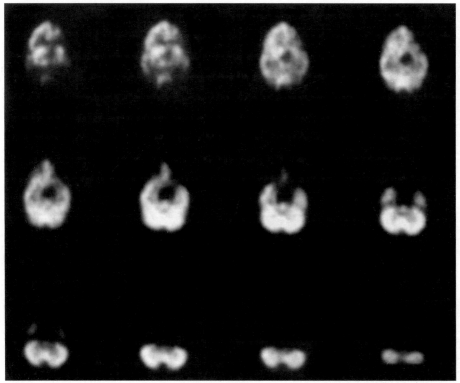

Figure 44.4B
Selected transverse ECD SPECT brain images of patient in Figure 44.4A injected 22 h after 1.5 ATA/60-min HBO treatment. Note global improvement and smoothing of brain blood flow.

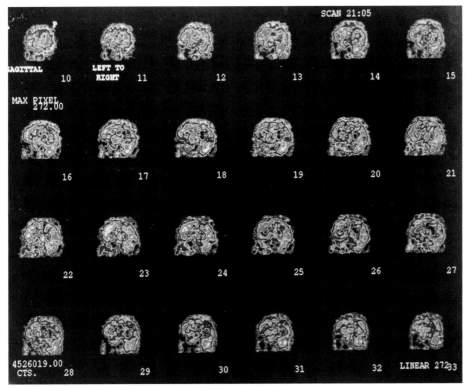

Figure 44.5A
HMPAO SPECT brain imaging, sagittal slices, on 4/28/1994, 3 days after single HBO for acute CO poisoning. Slices proceed from the left side of the brain in the upper left corner to the right side in the lower right corner. Color scale is yellow, red, green, deep blue, purple, black from highest to lowest flow. Maximum pixel count to which the scan is scaled is recorded in the figure. Note the diffusely heterogeneous flow to the cortex in both hemispheres.

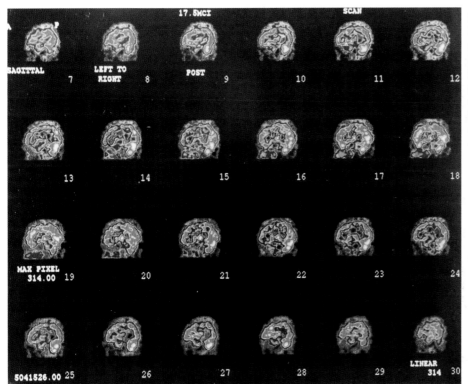

Figure 44.5B
HMPAO SPECT brain imaging, sagittal slices, on 4/29/1994, 3h after second HBO in the previous 24 h and 17 h after injection for previous SPECT scan. Note generalized smoothing of blood flow towards a more normal pattern with filling in of some of the abnormally reduced areas of the cortex in Figure 44.5A, especially on rows 1 and 4.

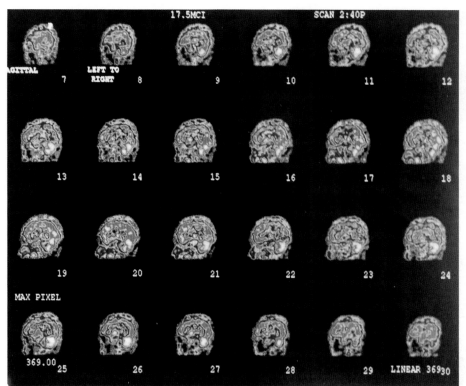

Figure 44.5C
HMPAO SPECT brain imaging, sagittal slices, on 15 June 1994, 7 days after the 40th HBO treatment. Note the generalized smoothing as well as improvement in overall level of flow (max pixel 369 vs. 272 in Figure 44.5A).

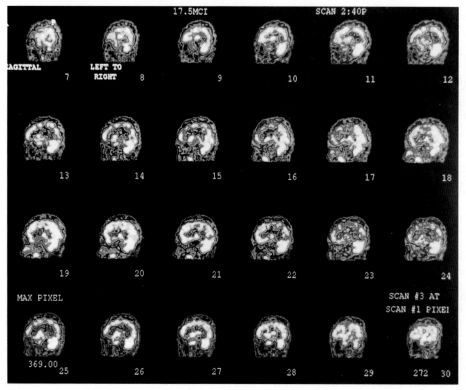

Figure 44.5D
HMPAO SPECT brain imaging, sagittal slices, of scan in Figure 44.5C registered on the pixel scale of scan in Figure 44.5A. Note the generalized increase in flow.

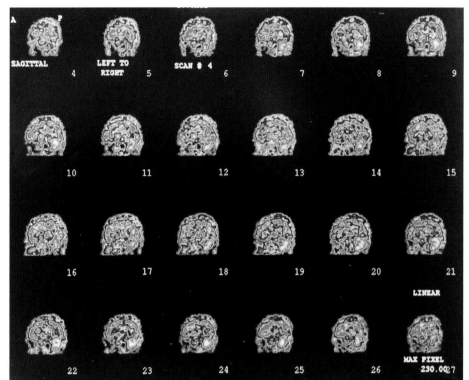

Figure 44.5E

HMPAO SPECT brain imaging, sagittal slices, on 10/19/1994, nearly 4½ months after previous HBOT and SPECT brain scan in Figures 44.5C and D. Note the deterioration in overall flow (max pixel 230) and pattern (heterogeneity on all rows). Patient now on flexeril, ativan, mepergan forte, paxil, atenolol, mellaril, and clonidine

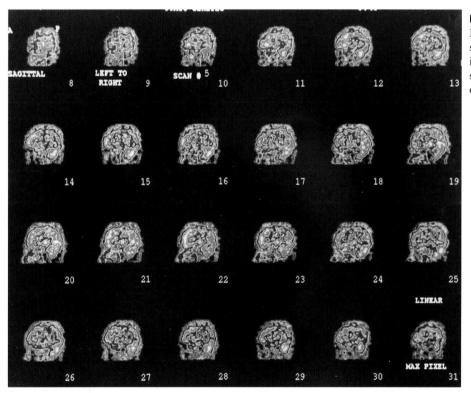

Figure 44.5F

HMPAO SPECT brain imaging, sagittal slices, on 10/21/1994, after first HBOT in third course of HBOT. Note slight smoothing of pattern, but no change in overall flow.

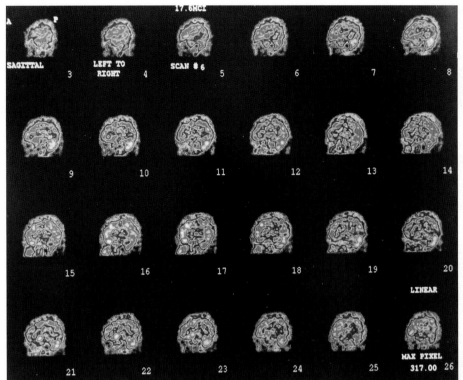

Figure 44.5G
HMPAO SPECT brain imaging, sagittal slices, on 15 December 1994, 2 days after 35th HBOT in third course of HBOT. Note generalized smoothing and overall increase in brain blood flow.

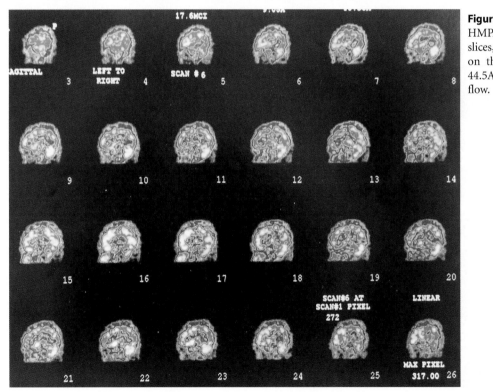

Figure 44.5H
HMPAO SPECT brain imaging, sagittal slices, of scan in Figure 44.5G registered on the pixel scale of scan in Figure 44.5A. Note the generalized increase in flow.

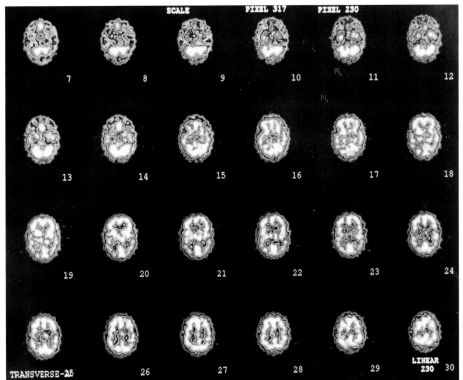

Figure 44.5I
HMPAO SPECT brain imaging, transverse slices, of scan in Figure 44.5G registered on the pixel scale of scan in Figure 44.5E. Note massive increase in flow.

45

Bibliography

A

Abbot NC, Beck JS, Carnochan FMT *et al* (1994) Effect of hyperoxia at 1 and 2 ATA on hypoxia and hypercapnia in human skin during experimental inflammation. *J Appl Physiol* 77: 767–773.

Abboud P, Mansour G, Lebrun JM *et al* (2001) Acute carbon monoxide poisoning during pregnancy: 2 cases with different neonatal outcome. *J Gynecol Obstet Biol Reprod (Paris)* 30: 708–711.

Abelsohn A, Sanborn MD, Jessiman BJ, Weir E (2002) Identifying and managing adverse environmental health effects: 6. Carbon monoxide poisoning. *CMAJ* 166: 1685–1690.

Abramovich A, Shupak A, Ramon Y *et al* (1997) Hyperbaric oxygen for carbon monoxide poisoning. *Harefuah* 132: 21–24, 71.

Ackerman NB, Brinkley FB (1966) Oxygen tensions in normal and ischemic tissues during hyperbaric therapy. *JAMA* 198: 142–145.

Adamiec L, Kaminski B, Kwiatkowski H *et al* (1975) Hyperbaric oxygen in treatment of acute carbon monoxide poisoning. *Anaesth Resusc Intensive Ther* 3: 305–313.

Adamic R (1975) Das Verhalten der arteriellen Blutgase. *Med Welt* 26: 142–148.

Agir H, Mersa B, Aktas S, Olgac V (2003) Histologic effects of hyperbaric oxygen therapy administered immediately after or two hours after ischemia-reperfusion injury: a rat abdominal skin flap model. *Kulak Burun Bogaz Ihtis Derg* 10: 18–124.

Aharon-Peretz JS, Adir Y, Gordon CR *et al* (1993) Spinal cord decompression sickness in sport diving. *Arch Neurol* 50: 753–756.

Ahlbom HE (1941) Results of radiotherapy of hypopharyngeal cancer at Radium-hemmet, Stockholm. *Acta Radiol* 22: 155–171.

Aisenbrey S, Krott R, Heller R *et al* (2000) Hyperbaric oxygen therapy in retinal artery occlusion. *Ophthalmologe* 97: 461–467

Akgül EO, Cakir E, Ozcan O *et al* (2007) Pressure-related increase of asymmetric dimethylarginine caused by hyperbaric oxygen in the rat brain: a possible neuroprotective mechanism. *Neurochem Res* 32: 1586–1591.

Akimov GA, Lobzin VS, Sapov IA *et al* (1985) Assessment of the efficiency of hyperbaric oxygen therapy in early forms of cerebrovascular disorders. *Neurosc Behav Physiol* 15: 13.

Akin ML, Uluutku H, Erenoglu C *et al* (2002) Hyperbaric oxygen ameliorates bacterial translocation in rats with mechanical intestinal obstruction. *Dis Colon Rectum* 45: 967–972.

Akiya T, Nakada T, Katayama T *et al* (1988) Hyperbaric oxygenation for experimental bladder tumor. *Eur Urol* 14: 150–155.

Akman MN, Loubser PG, Fife CE *et al* (1994) Hyperbaric oxygen therapy: implications for spinal cord injury patients with baclofen infusion pumps. Case report. *Paraplegia* 32: 281–284.

Aksenova TA, Ezbov LS, Titchenko LI *et al* (1981) Hyperbaric oxygen in prevention and treatment of fetal hypoxia and hypotrophy. In Yefuny SN (Ed.) *Proceedings of the 7th international congress on Hyperbaric medicine.* USSR Academy of Sciences, Moscow, pp 361.

Aksoy FG (2003) MR imaging of subclinical cerebral decompression sickness (2003) *Acta Radiol* 44: 108–110.

Albendea CD, Miana-Mena FJ, Garcia-Gil A, Fuentes-Broto L, Martinez-Ballarin E, Berzosa C, Gonzalvo E, Garcia JJ (2007) Ischemia-reperfusion induces lipid peroxidation in the transplant of the pancreas in pigs. *XXXIV Congress of the Spanish Society for Physiological Sciences* Vol 190, Supplement 655: P113.

Alex J, Laden G, Cale AR *et al* (2005) Pretreatment with hyperbaric oxygen and its effect on neuropsychometric dysfunction and systemic inflammatory response after cardiopulmonary bypass: a prospective randomized double-blind trial. *J Thorac Cardiovasc Surg* 130: 1623–1630.

Algan B, Benichoux R, Marchal H (1973) First personal results of the application of hyperbaric oxygen in eye diseases. *Bull Soc Belge Ophthalmol* 163: 183–194.

Allaria B, Decio B, Libutti M (1973) Electrocution and hyperbaric oxygen therapy: a case with electrocardiographic changes from electrocution cured by hyperbaric oxygen therapy. *Anesteziol Reanimatol* 14: 167–172.

Allen DB, Maguire JJ, Mahdavian M *et al* (1997) Wound hypoxia and acidosis limit neutrophil bacterial killing mechanisms. *Arch Surg* 132: 991–996.

Alleva R, Tomasetti M, Sartini D *et al* (2008) alpha-Lipoic acid modulates extracellular matrix and angiogenesis gene expression in non-healing wounds treated with hyperbaric oxygen therapy. *Mol Med* 14: 175–183.

Alves OL, Daugherty WP, Rios M (2004) Arterial hyperoxia in severe head injury: a useful or harmful option? *Curr Pharm Des* 10: 2163–2176.

Al-Waili NS, Butler GJ, Beale J *et al* (2005) Hyperbaric oxygen in the treatment of patients with cerebral stroke, brain trauma, and neurologic disease. *Adv Ther* 22: 659–678.

Al-Waili NS, Butler GJ, Petrillo RL, Carrey Z, Hamilton RW (2006) Hyperbaric oxygen and lymphoid system function: A review supporting possible intervention in tissue transplantation. *Technol. Health Care* 14(6): 489–498.

Ambiru S, Furuyama N, Aono M *et al* (2007) Hyperbaric oxygen therapy for the treatment of postoperative paralytic ileus and adhesive intestinal obstruction associated with abdominal surgery: experience with 626 patients. *Hepatogastroenterology* 54: 1925–1929.

Ambiru S, Furuyama N, Kimura F *et al* (2008) Effect of hyperbaric oxygen therapy on patients with adhesive intestinal obstruction associated with abdominal surgery who have failed to respond to more than 7 days of conservative treatment. *Hepatogastroenterology* 55: 491–495.

Amery, WK (1982) Brain hypoxia: the turning-point in the genesis of the migraine attack? *Cephalalgia* 2: 83–109.

Amonic RS, Cockett AT, Lorhan PH, Thompson JC (1969) Hyperbaric oxygen therapy in chronic hemorrhagic shock. *JAMA* 208: 2051–2054.

Anderson B, (1978) Hyperoxic myopia. *Trans Am Ophthalmol Soc* 7: 116–124.

Anderson B, Heyman A, Wahlen RE (1965) Migraine like phenomenon after decompression from hyperbaric environments. *Neurology* 15: 1025–1040.

Anderson B, Shelton DL (1987) Axial length in hyperoxic myopia. In Bove AA, Bachrach AJ, Greenbaum LJ (Eds.) *Ninth International Symposium on Underwater and Hyperbaric Physiology*. Bethesda, MD: Undersea and Hyperbaric Medical Society, pp 607–611.

Anderson DC, Bottini AG, Jagiella WM *et al* (1991) A pilot study of hyperbaric oxygen in the treatment of human stroke. *Stroke* 22: 1137–1142.

Andrews BT, Weinstein PR (1990) Protection from cerebral ischemia by hyperoxygenation. In Weinstein PR, Faden AI (Eds.) *Protection of the Brain from Ischemia*. Williams and Wilkins, Baltimore, pp 207–212.

Angibaud G, Ducasse JL, Baille G, Clanet M (1995) Potential value of hyperbaric oxygenation in the treatment of post-radiation myelopathies. *Rev Neurol (Paris)* 151(11): 661–6.

Anokhin MI, Ostreikov IF, Kazansky DD, Baydin SA (1972) HBO experience in postoperative period in children. *Bull USSR Acad Med Sci*, 7: 17–21.

Anonymous (2008) Use of hyperbaric oxygenation as a component of intensive care in acute pancreatitis and its impact on homeostasis and intensity of oxidative stress. *Anesteziol Reanimatol* 3: 49–53.

Anthony M, Hinterberger H, Lance JW (1967) Plasma serotonin in migraine and stress. *Arch Neurol* 16: 544–552.

Antonetti DA, Wolpert EB, DeMaio L, Harhaj NS, Scaduto RC (2000) Hydrocortisone decreases retinal endothelial cell water and solute flux coincident with increased content and decreased phosphorylation of occluding. *J Neurochem* 80: 667–677.

Arieli R, Gutterman A (1997) Recovery time constant in central nervous system O2 toxicity in the rat. *Eur J Appl Physiol* 75: 182–187.

Arieli R, Yalov A, Goldenshluger A (2002) Modeling pulmonary and CNS O(2) toxicity and estimation of parameters for humans. *J Appl Physiol* 92: 248–256.

Armon C, Deschamps C, Adkinson C *et al* (1991) Hyperbaric treatment of cerebral air embolism sustained during an open-heart surgical procedure. *Mayo Clin Proc* 66: 565–571.

Arndt S, Aschendorff A, Echternach M, Daemmrich TD, Maier W (2008, May 10) Rhino-orbital-cerebral mucormycosis and aspergillosis: differential diagnosis and treatment. *Eur Arch Otorhinolaryngol* doi:10.1007/s00405-008-0692-y.

Arnold AC, Hepler RS, Lieber M *et al* (1996) Hyperbaric oxygen therapy for nonarteritic anterior ischemic optic neuropathy. *Am J Ophthalmol* 122: 535–541.

Arnold AC, Levin LA (2002) Treatment of ischemic optic neuropathy. *Seminars in Ophthalmology* 17: 39–46.

Arntzenius AKW (1887) *De pneumatische Therapie*. Scheltema and Holkema, Amsterdam.

Artru F, Chacornac R, Deleuze R (1976a) Hyperbaric oxygenation for severe head injuries. *Eur Neurol* 14: 310.

Artru F, Philippon B, Gauf, Berger M, Deleuze R (1976b) Cerebral blood flow, cerebral metabolism and cerebrospinal fluid biochemistry in brain-injured patients after exposure to hyperbaric oxygen. *Eur Neurol* 14: 351–364.

Ashamalla HL, Thom SR, Goldwein JW (1996) Hyperbaric oxygen therapy for the treatment of radiation-induced sequelae in children. The University of Pennsylvania experience. *Cancer* 77: 2407–2412.

Aslan I, Oysu C, Veyseller B, Baserer N (2002) Does the addition of hyperbaric oxygen therapy to the conventional treatment modalities influence the outcome of sudden deafness? *Otolaryngol Head Neck Surg* 126: 121–6.

Associated Pres (2008) Doctors to reassess guidelines on "chronic Lyme" disease cure. Available at: http://ap.google.com/article/ALeqM5hokteRVeiNb790jgYZB9xIeY45ewD90DPT7G0. Accessed May 27, 2008.

Astrup J, Siesjö BK, Symon L (1981) Thresholds in cerebral ischemia; the ischemic penumbra. *Stroke* 12: 723–725.

Atochin DN, Fisher D, Demchenko IT, Thom SR (2000) Neutrophil sequestration and the effect of hyperbaric oxygen in a rat model of temporary middle cerebral artery occlusion. *Undersea Hyperbaric Med* 27: 185–190.

Atug O, Hamzaoglu H, Tahan V *et al* (2008) Hyperbaric oxygen therapy is as effective as dexamethasone in the treatment of TNBS-E-induced experimental colitis. *Dig Dis Sci* 53(2): 481–485.

Aubert L, Arroyo H, Malavaud A (1967) Note sur le traitement du coma hépatique par l'hyperoxie hyperbarique. *Marseille Med* 104: 357–362.

Augsburger JJ, Magargal LE (1980) Visual prognosis following treatment of acute central retinal artery obstruction. *Br J Ophthalmol* 64: 913–917.

Austin F (1993) Maintenance of infective *Borrelia burgdorferi* Sh-2–82 in 4% oxygen – 5% carbon dioxide in vitro. *Canadian J Microbiol* 39: 1103–1110.

Averous K, Erginay A, Timsit J *et al* (2006) Resolution of diabetic macular edema following high altitude exercise. *Acta Scandinavia Ophthalmologica* 84: 830–831. (letter)

Avitabile T, Longo A, Reibaldi A (2005) Intravitreal triamcinolone compared with macular laser grid photocoagulation for the treatment of cystoids macular edema. *Am J Ophthalmol* 140: 695–702.

Ayan F, Sunamak O, Paksoy SM *et al* (2005) Fournier's gangrene: a retrospective clinical study on forty-one patients. *ANZ J Surg* 75: 1055–1058.

B

Babul S, Rhodes EC (2000) The role of hyperbaric oxygen therapy in sports medicine. *Sports Med* 30: 395–403.

Bacon P, Spalton DJ, Smith SE (1988) Blindness from quinine toxicity. *Br J Ophthalmol* 72: 219–224.

Bacha S, Annane D, Gajdos P (1996) Iatrogenic air embolism. *Presse Med* 25: 1466–1472.

Badalian LO, Dunaevskaya GN, Sitnikov VF (1975) The treatment of patients with progressive dystrophy. *Zh Nevropatol Psikhiatr* 75: 1317–1323.

Badr AE, Yin W, Mychaskiw G, Zhang JH (2001a) Effect of hyperbaric oxygen on striatal metabolites: a microdialysis study in awake freely moving rats after MCA occlusion. *Brain Res* 916: 85–90.

Badr AE, Yin W, Mychaskiw G, Zhang JH (2001b) Dual effect of HBO on cerebral infarction in MCAO rats. *Am J Physiol Regul Integr Comp Physiol* 280: R766–770.

Baiborodov BD (1981) Some peculiarities in application of hyperbaric oxygenation during the treatment of acute respiratory insufficiency in newborn infants. In Abstracts VII Int Cong HBO Medicine, Moscow September 2–6, p 368.

Bairrington JD, Pryor WH (1969) Increased storage life of whole blood under increased barometric pressure: a feasibility study. *Am J Med Technol* 35: 337–344.

Baixe JH (1978) Bilan de onze annees d'activite en medicine hyperbare. *Med Aer Spatiale Med Subaquatique Hyperbare* 17: 90–2.

Baixe JH, Bidart J, Nicolini JC (1969) Treatment of osteonecrosis of the femoral head by hyperbaric oxygen. *Bull Med Subhyp* 1: 2.

Bajrovic FF, Sketelj J, Jug M *et al* (2002) The effect of hyperbaric oxygen treatment on early regeneration of sensory axons after nerve crush in the rat. *J Peripher Nerv Syst* 7: 141–148.

Bakay-Csorba PA, Provan JL, Ameli FM (1987) Transcutaneous oxygen tension measurements in the detection of iliac and femoral arterial disease. *Surg Gynecol Obstet* 164: 102–104.

Baker B (1992) Use of an implantable infusion pump in the multiplace hyperbaric chamber. *Undersea Biomed Res* 19: 63.

Bakker DJ (1988) Clostridial myonecrosis. In Davis JC, Hunt TK (Eds.) *Problem wounds – role of oxygen.* Elsevier, New York, pp 153–172.

Bakker DJ (2000) Hyperbaric oxygen therapy and the diabetic foot. *Diabetes Metab Res Rev* 16 (Suppl 1): S55–8.

Balentine JD (1982) *Pathology oxygen toxicity.* Academic, New York.

Ball R (1993) Effect of severity, time to recompression with oxygen, and retreatment on outcome in forty-nine cases of spinal cord decompression sickness. *Undersea Hyperbaric Med* 20: 133–145.

Balzan M, Cacciottolo JM, Casha A (1993) Intestinal infarction following carbon monoxide poisoning. *Postgrad Med J* 69: 302–303.

Bao JYS (1987) Hyperbaric oxygen therapy in re-implantation of several limbs. In Kindwall EP (Ed.) *Proceedings of the 8th international congress on hyperbaric medicine.* Best, San Pedro, pp 182–186.

Barcal R, Emmerova M, Sova J *et al* (1975) Hyperbaric oxygen therapy of cardiogenic shock in the acute stage of myocardial infarction. *Cas Lek Cesk* 114: 259–262.

Barcroft J (1920) Anoxemia. *Lancet* 11: 485.

Bardin H, Lambertsen CJ (1970) A quantitative method for calculating pulmonary toxicity. Use of "unit pulmonary toxicity dose" (UPTD). Institute for Environmental Medicine Report. University of Pennsylvania, Philadelphia.

Barnes MP, Bates D, Cartlidge NEF *et al* (1985) Hyperbaric oxygen and multiple sclerosis: short term results of a placebo-controlled, double-blind trial. *Lancet* ii: 297–300.

Barnes MP, Bates D, Cartlidge NEF *et al* (1987) Hyperbaric oxygen and multiple sclerosis: final results of a placebo-controlled, double-blind study. *J Neurol Neurosurg Psychiatry* 50: 1402–1406.

Baroni G, Porro T, Faglia E *et al* (1987) Hyperbaric oxygen in diabetic gangrene treatment. *Diabetes Care* 10: 81–86.

Barratt-Boyes BG, Wood EH (1958) Cardiac output and related measurements and pressure values in the right heart and associated vessels, together with the analysis of the hemodynamic responses to inhalation of high oxygen mixtures in healthy subjects. *J Lab Clin Med* 51: 72–90.

Barrett K, Harch P, Masel B *et al* (1998) Cognitive and cerebral blood flow improvements in chronic stable traumatic brain injury induced by 1.5 ATA hyperbaric oxygen. *Undersea Hyperbaric Med* 25: 9 (abstract).

Barrie H (1963) Hyperbaric oxygen in the resuscitation of neonates. *Lancet* ii: 1223.

Barth E, Sullivan T, Berg E (1990) Animal model for evaluating one repair with and without adjunctive hyperbaric oxygen therapy: comparing dose schedules. *J Invest Surg* 3: 387–392.

Bashshur ZF, Ma'luf RN, Allam S, Jurdi FA, Haddad RS, Noureddin BN (2004) Intravitreal triamcinolone for the management of macular edema due to nonischemic central retinal vein occlusion. *Arch Ophthalmol* 122: 1137–1140.

Bass BH (1970) The treatment of varicose leg ulcers by hyperbaric oxygen. *Postgrad Med J* 46: 407.

Bast-Pettersen R (1999) Long-term neuropsychological effects in non-saturation construction divers. *Aviat Space Environ Med* 70: 51–57.

Bath AP, Rowe, JR, Innes AJ (1998) Malignant otitis externa with optic neuritis. *J Laryngol Otol* 112: 274–277.

Batoir BM (1984) Oxidants from Phagocytes: agents of defense and destruction. *Blood* 64(5): 959–966.

Baugh M (2000) HIV: reactive oxygen species, enveloped viruses and hyperbaric oxygen. *Medical Hypotheses* 55: 232–238.

Baumgartner WA (2000) Etiology, pathogenesis, and experimental treatment of retinitis pigmentosa. *Med Hypotheses* 54: 814–824.

Baydin SA (1986) Pediatrics. In Efuni SN (Ed.) *Hyperbaric oxygenation: A Manual.* Meditsina, Moscow, pp 325–341.

Bayer A, Mutlu FM, Sobaci G (2002) Hyperbaric Oxygen Therapy for Mitomycin C-Induced Scleral Necrosis. *Ophthalmic Surg Lasers* 33: 58–61.

Bayne C (1978) Acute decompression sickness: 50 cases. *J Am Coll Emerg Physicians* 7: 351–354.

Bean JE, Lingnell J, Coulson J (1945) Effects of oxygen at increased pressure. *Physiol Rev* 25: 1.

Bean JE, Lingnell J, Coulson J (1971) Regional cerebral blood flow oxygen tension and EEG in exposure to oxygen at high pressure. *J Appl Physiol* 31: 235.

Beard RR, Wertheim GA (1967) Behavioral impairment associated with small doses of carbon monoxide. *Am J Public Health* 57: 2012–2022.

Beehler CC (1964) Oxygen and the eye. *Aeromed Rev* 3: 1–21.

Beehler CC, Newton NL, Culver JF, Tredici T (1963) Ocular hyperoxia. *Aerospace Med* 34: 1017–1020.

Behara AK, Hildebrand E, Szafranski J *et al* (2006) Role of aggrecanase 1 in Lyme arthritis. *Arthritis Rheum* 54: 3319–3329.

Behnke AR, Forbes HS, Motley EP (1936) Circulatory and visual effects of oxygen at 3 atmospheres pressure. *Am J Physiol* 114: 436–442.

Beiran I, Goldenberg I, Adir Y, Tamir A, Shupak A, Miller B (2001) Early hyperbaric oxygen therapy for retinal artery occlusion. *Eur J Ophthalmol* 11: 345–350.

Beiran I, Reissman P, Scharf J, Nahum Z *et al* (1993) Hyperbaric oxygenation combined with nifedipine treatment for recent onset retinal artery occlusion. *Eur J Ophthalmol* 3: 89–94.

Beiran I, Rimon I, Weiss G, Pikkel J, Miller B (1995) Hyperbaric oxygenation therapy for ischemic optic neuropathy. *Eur J Ophthalmol* 5: 285–286.

Belley R, Bernard N, Côté M, Paquet F, Poitras J (2005) Hyperbaric oxygen therapy in the management of two cases of hydrogen sulfide toxicity from liquid manure. *CJEM* 7: 257–261.

Belokurov MI, Stepankov AA, Kirsanov BI (1988) Hyperbaric oxygenation in the combined therapy of comatose states in children. *Pediatriia* (2): 84–87.

Belokurov, YN (1980). The influence of hyperbaric oxygenation on the activity of succinated hydrogenase and cytochrome oxidase of visceral organs in intestinal obstruction. *Anesteziol Reanimatol*, 5, 44–46.

Belokurov YN, Medvedev VF (1976) Restoration of gastro-intestinal motility in patients with diffuse peritonitis in conditions of hyperbaric oxygenation. *Klin Khir* 5: 22–25.

Belokurov YN, Rybachkov VV (1981) Possibilities of hyperbaric oxygen treatment under conditions of hepatic insufficiency. In *Proceedings of the 7th international congress on hyperbaric medicine, Moscow,* Sept 2–6.

Belokurov YN, Rybachkov VV, Pankov AG (1985) Endogenous toxicity on acute hepatic failure and ways of eliminating it. *Vestn Khir* 134: 60–64.

Belov KV, Isakov YV, Alyabaiev VS (1986) Efficacy of hyperbaric oxygenation in ischemia of the lower extremities. *Khirugiia* (Mosk) 12: 69–72.

Bennett M, Heard R (2001) Treatment of multiple sclerosis with hyperbaric oxygen therapy. *Undersea Hyperb Med* 28: 117–122.

Bennett M, Heard R (2004) Hyperbaric oxygen therapy for multiple sclerosis. *Cochrane Database Syst Rev* 1: CD003057.

Bennett MH, Kertesz T, Yeung P (2007) Hyperbaric oxygen for idiopathic sudden sensorineural hearing loss and tinnitus. *Cochrane Database Syst Rev* 1: CD004739.

Bennett PB, Elliot DH (Eds.) (2003) *The Physiology of Diving Medicine, 5th ed.* WB Saunders, London.

Bennett M, Feldmeier J, Smee R, Milross C (2008, Jul 18) Hyperbaric oxygenation for tumour sensitisation to radiotherapy: A systematic review of randomised controlled trials. *Cancer Treat Rev* doi:10.1016/j.ctrv.2008.01.001.

Ben-Yishai Y, Diller L (1973) Changing of atmospheric environment to improve mental and behavioral function. *NY State J Med* 73: 2877–2880.

Ben-Yishai Y, Diller L, Reich T *et al* (1978) Can oxygen reverse symptoms of senility? *NY State J Med* 78: 914–919.

Beppu T, Kamada K, Nakamura R *et al* (2003) A phase II study of radiotherapy after hyperbaric oxygenation combined with interferon-beta and nimustine hydrochloride to treat supratentorial malignant gliomas. *J Neurooncol.* 61: 161–170.

Bergö GW, Engelsen B, Tyssebotn I (1993) Unilateral frontal decortication changes in cerebral blood ldistribution during hyperbaric oxygen exposure in rats. *Aviat Space Environ Med* 64: 1023–1031.

Bergö GW, Tyssebotn I (1999) Cardiovascular effects of hyperbaric oxygen with and without addition of carbon dioxide. *Eur J Appl Physiol Occup Physiol* 80: 264–75.

Bergren DR, Beckman DL (1975) Hyperbaric oxygen and pulmonary surface tension. *Aviat Space Environ Med* 46: 994–995.

Bernachhi A, Myers R, Trump BF *et al* (1984) Protection of hepatocytes with hyperoxia against carbon tetrachloride-induced injury. *Toxicol Pathol* 12: 315–323.

Bernard C (1857) *Lecons sur les effets des substances toxiques et medicamenteuses.* Paris: Bailliere.

Bernhard WF, Frittele G, Jane ES *et al* (1964) Surgery under hyperbaric oxygenation in infants with congenital heart disease. *Circulation* 29: 91.

Bernhardt TL, Goldman RW, Thombs PA, Kindwall EP (1988) Hyperbaric oxygen treatment of cerebral air embolism from orogenital sex during pregnancy. *Crit Care Med* 16: 729–730.

Bert P (1878) *La pression barométrique. Recherches de physiologie expérimentelle.* English version Barometric pressure republished by the Undersea Medical Society, Bethesda, (1978).

Bertin E (1855) *Etude clinique de l'emploi et des effets du bain d'air comprimé dans le traitement de diverses maladies.* Baillière, Paris.

Bhatt UK (2004) Radial optic neurotomy in retinal vein occlusion. *Am J Ophthalmol* 137: 970–971.

Biersner RJ, Hall DA, Linaweaver PG (1976) Associations between psychological factors and pulmonary toxicity during intermittent oxygen breathing at 2 ATA. *Aviat Space Environ Med* 47: 173–176.

Bigelow WG (1964) The microcirculation. *Can J Surg* 7: 237–249.

Bimes C, Guilhem A, Mansat A *et al* (1973) Modifications staturales et pondérales des foetus nés de lapines soumises à l'oxygène hyperbare durant la gestation. *Bull Assoc Anat* 57: 443–456.

Bird AD, Telfer ABM (1965) Effect of hyperbaric oxygen on limb circulation. *Lancet* 13: 355–356.

Biriukov IB, Tsygankova ST, Bronskaia LK, Namazbekov BK, Akimova NI (1988) Immunological indicators as the criteria of prognosis and treatment of nonspecific diseases of the lungs and pleura. *Vestn Khir* 140: 10–13.

Bitterman H, Melamud Y (1993) Delayed hyperbaric treatment of cerebral air embolism. *Israel J Med Sci* 29: 22–26.

Bitterman N, Eilander E, Melamed Y (1991) Hyperbaric oxygen and scopolamine. *Undersea Biomed Res* 18: 167–174.

Bitterman N, Talmi Y, Lerman A *et al* (1986) The effect of hyperbaric oxygen on acute experimental sulfide poisoning in the rat. *Toxicol Appl Pharmacol* 84: 325–328.

Blanco YC, Farias AS, Goelnitz U *et al* (2008) Hyperbaric oxygen prevents early death caused by experimental cerebral malaria. *PLoS ONE* 3: e3126.

Blankenship GW, Okun E (1973) Retinal tributary vein occlusion. History and management by photocoagulation. *Arch Ophthalmol* 89: 363–368.

Bleiberg B, Kerem D (1988) Central nervous system oxygen toxicity in the resting rat: Postpponement by intermittent oxygen exposure. *Undersea Biomed Res* 15: 337–352.

Blogg SL, Loveman GA, Seddon FM *et al* (2004) Magnetic Resonance Imaging and Neuropathology Findings in the Goat Nervous System following Hyperbaric Exposures. *Eur Neurol* 52: 18–28.

Blom H, Mulder M, Verweij W (1988) Arterial oxygen tension and saturation in hospital patients: effect of age and activity. *Br Med J* 297: 720.

Blum D, Viart P, Szliwowski HB, Thys JP *et al* (1972) Exchange transfusion and hyperbaric oxygen in the treatment of children with acute hepatic failure. *Helv Paediatr Acta* 27: 425–436.

Boadi WY, Thaire L, Kerem D *et al* (1991) Effects of dietary supplementation with vitamin E, riboflavin and selenium on central nervous system oxygen toxicity. *Pharmcol Toxicol* 68: 77–82.

Bockeria LA, Khapy KH, Gazhiev AA *et al* (1977) Extracorporeal circulation under hyperbaric oxygenation. In Smith G (Ed.) *5th international congress on hyperbaric medicine.* University of Aberdeen Press, Aberdeen, pp 189–197.

Bockeria LA, Sokolova NA, Ladynima EA, Gadzhiev AA (1978) Enzyme determinants as a check on adequacy of body defences during heart operations under hyperbaric oxygenation. *Anesteziol Reanimatol* 3: 45–49.

Bockeria LA, Zelenkini MA (1973) Electrocardiographic changes during exclusion of the heart from the circulation under hyperbaric oxygenation and hypothermia (in Russian). *Eksp Khir Anestesiol* 18: 80–84.

Boerema I (1961) An operating room for high oxygen pressure. *Surgery* 47: 291–298.

Boerema I, Meyne NG, Brummelkamp WH *et al* (1959) Life without blood. *Arch Chir Neer* 11: 70–83.

Boerema I, Meyne NG, Brummelkamp WK *et al* (1960) Life without blood: a study of the influence of high atmospheric pressure and hypothermia on dilution of blood. *J Cardiovasc Surg* 1; 133–146.

Bohlega S, McLean DR (1997) Hemiplegia caused by inadvertent intra-carotid infusion of total parenteral nutrition. *Clinical Neurology and Neurosurgery* 99: 217–219.

Bohmer D (1997) Treating tinnitus with hyperbaric oxygenation. *Int Tinnitus J* 3: 137–140.

Bohne BD, Klatt A, Reimann J, Kästner R (1987) Die Sauerstoffversorgung des vorderen Sehnervenbereiches bei künstlicher Augeninnendruckerhöhung. *Z Klin Med* 42: 1795–1797.

Bojiæ L, Cerovski B, Buæan K, Zuljan I, Kuzmaniæ B, Kovaceviæ H. Andric D (1995) Hyperbaric oxygen for the treatment of nonarteritic anterior ischemic optic neuropathy. *Arch Med Croatica* 49: 133–136.

Bojiæ L. Kovaceviæ H, Andriæ D, Karaman-Kraljeviæ K, Cagalj S (1994) The effects of hyperbaric oxygen on visual functions in ischemic optic neuropathy. *Arh Hig Rada Toksikol* 45: 19–24.

Bojic L, Ivanisevic M, Gosovic G (2002) Hyperbaric oxygen therapy in two patients with non-arteritic anterior optic neuropathy who did not respond to prednisone. *Undersea Hyperbaric Med* 29: 6–92.

Bojic L, Kovacevic H, Andric D *et al* (1993) Hyperbaric oxygen dose of choice in the treatment of glaucoma. *Arh Hig Rada Toksikol* 44: 239–247.

Bokeria LA, Krutik IG, Khapyi KK *et al* (1979) The characteristics of EEG, ECG and hemodynamics in artificial circulation with hemodilution under hyperbaric oxygenation. *Anesteziol Reanimatol* 4: 23–28.

Boland ME, Roper SMB, Henry JA (1985) Complications of quinine poisoning. *Lancet* 1(8425): 384–385.

Bondarenko AV, Rodionov VV, Moscolova LA (1981) Influence of hyperbaric oxygenation on certain indices of tissue metabolism in patients with acute cardiac insufficiency. *Anesteziol Reanimatol* 6: 30–34.

Borchman D, Giblin FJ, Leverenz VR *et al* (2000) Impact of aging and hyperbaric oxygen in vivo on guinea pig lens lipids and nuclear light scatter. *Invest Ophthalmol Vis Sci* 41: 3061–73.

Borromeo CN, Ryan JL, Marchetto PA *et al* (1997) Hyperbaric oxygen therapy for acute ankle sprains. *Am J Sports Med* 25: 619–625.

Borruat FX, Schatz NJ, Glass JS *et al* (1993) Visual recovery from radiation-induced optic neuropathy: role of hyperbaric oxygenation. *J Clin Neuroophthalmology* 13: 98–101.

Borzyskowski M (1989) Migraine, epilepsy, post-traumatic syndromes, and spreading depression. *Developmental Medicine & Child Neurology* 31: 682–689.

Boschetti M, De Lucchi M, Giusti M *et al* (2006) Partial visual recovery from radiation-induced optic neuropathy after hyperbaric oxygen therapy in a patient with Cushing disease. *Eur J Endocrinol* 154: 813–818.

Boschetty V, Cernoch J (1970) Aplikace Kysliku za pretlaku u nekterych neurlogickych onemocneni. *Bratisl Lek Listy* 53: 298–302.

Bouachour G, Cronier P, Gouello JP *et al* (1996) Hyperbaric oxygen therapy in the management of crush injuries: A randomized double-blind placebo-controlled clinical trial. *J Trauma* 4: 333–339.

Bouhanick B, Verret JL, Gouello JP *et al* (1998) Necrobiosis lipoidica: treatment by hyperbaric oxygen and local corticosteroids. *Diabetes Metab* 24: 156–159.

Boveris A, Chance B (1978) The mitochondrial generation of hydrogen peroxide. *Biochem J* 134: 707–716.

Bowen JC, Fairchild RB (1984) Oxygen in gastric mucosal protection. In Allen A *et al* (Eds.) *Mechanisms of mucosal protection in the upper gastrointestinal tract.* Raven, New York, pp 259–266.

Boyd SR, Zachary I, Chakravarthy U *et al* (2002) Correlation of increased vascular endothelial growth factor with neovascularization and permeability in ischemic central vein occlusion. *Arch Ophthalmol* 120: 1644–1650.

Bradshaw PO, Nelson AG, Fanton JW (1996) Effect of hyperbaric oxygenation on peripheral nerve regeneration in adult male rabbits. *Undersea Hyperbaric Med* 23: 107–113.

Brady CE, Cooley BJ, Davis JC (1989) Healing of severe perineal and cutaneous Crohn's disease with hyperbaric oxygen. *Gastroenterology* 97: 756–760.

Brandt T, Paulus W, Pollmann W (1991) Cluster headache and chronic paroxysmal hemicrania: current therapy. *Nervenarzt* 62: 329–39.

Bratteboe G, Camporesi EM (2001) Diving injuries and hyperbaric medicine. In Søreide E, Grande CM (Eds.) *Prehospital Trauma Care,* Marcel Dekker Inc, New York, pp 639–656.

Bray P, Myers RAM, Cowley RA (1983) Orogenital sex as a cause of non-fatal air embolism in pregnancy. *Obstet Gynecol* 61: 653.

Bridges WZ (1966) Electroretinographic manifestations of hyperbaric oxygen. *Arch Ophthalmol* 75: 812–817.

Brizel DM, Hage WD, Dodge RK *et al* (1997) Hyperbaric oxygen improves tumour radiation response significantly more than carbogen/nicotinamide. *Radiat Res* 147: 715–720.

Broderick J, Brott T, Kothari R *et al* (1998) The greater Cincinnati/Northern Kentucky stroke study. *Stroke* 29: 415–421.

Broome JR, Smith DJ (1992) Pneumothorax as a complication of recompression therapy for cerebral arterial gas embolism. *Undersea Biomed Res* 19: 447–455.

Brott T, Adams HP, Olinger CP (1989) Measurement of acute cerebral infarction: a clinical examination scale. *Stroke* 20: 864–870.

Broughton G (1997) Management of brown recluse spider bite to the glans penis. *Military Medicine* 161: 627–629.

Brown SD, Piantadosi C A (1990) In vivo binding of carbon monoxide to cytochrome c oxidase in rat brain. *J Appl Physiol* 68: 604–610.

Brummelkamp WD, Hogendijk J, Boerema I (1961) Treatment of anaerobic infections (clostridial myositis) by drenching the tissues with oxygen under high pressure. *Surgery* 49: 299.

Brvar M, Mozina H, Osredkar J *et al* (2003) The potential value of the protein S-100B level as a criterion for hyperbaric oxygen treatment and prognostic marker in carbon monoxide poisoned patients. *Resuscitation* 56: 105–9.

Buchman AL, Fife C, Torres C, Smith L, Aristizibal J (2001) Hyperbaric oxygen therapy for severe ulcerative colitis. *J Clin Gastroenterol* 33: 337–9.

Buettner MF, Wolkenhauer D (2007) Hyperbaric oxygen therapy in the treatment of open fractures and crush injuries. *Emerg Med Clin North Am* 25: 177–188.

Bulkley BH, Hutchins GM (1977) Myocardial consequences of coronary artery bypass graft surgery: The paradox of necrosis in areas of revascularization. *Circulation* 56(6): 906–913.

Buono LM, Foroozan R, Savino PJ, Danesh-Meyer HV, Stanescu D (2003) Posterior ischemic optic neuropathy after hemodialysis. *Ophthalmology* 110: 1216–1218.

Burakovsky VI, Bockeria LA (1977) The resuscitative value of HBO in cardiac surgery and cardiology. In Smith G (Ed.) *6th international congress on hyperbaric medicine*. University of Aberdeen Press, Aberdeen, pp 184–188.

Burakovsky VI, Bockeria LA (1981) Experience of operating on the heart under conditions of hyperbaric oxygen. In *Proceedings of the 7th international congress on hyperbaric medicine*, Moscow, Sept. 2–6.

Buras JA, Stahl GL, Svoboda KK (2000) Hyperbaric oxygen downregulates ICAM-1 expression induced by hypoxia and hypoglycemia: the role of NOS. *Am J Physiol Cell Physiol* 278: C292–302.

Buriak VN (2001) Effects of hyperbaric oxygenation on the dynamics of clinical manifestations and deviations in the functional state of the pituitary-thyroid system in hypotensive type vegetovascular dysfunction in adolescents who had perinatal effects on the central nervous system. *Lik Sprava* 2: 46–9.

Burk RF, Reiter R, Lane JM (1986) Hyperbaric oxygen protection against carbon tetrachloride hepatotoxicity in the rat. *Gastroenterology* 90: 812–818.

Burkhardt KK, Hall AH, Gerace R (1991) Hyperbaric oxygen treatment for carbon tetrachloride poisoning. *Drug Safety* 6: 332–338.

Burr LH, Trapp WG (1976) Pulmonary embolism: surgery in a hyperbaric chamber. *J Thorac Cardiovasc Surg* 72: 306–308.

Burt JT, Kapp JP, Smith RR (1987) Hyperbaric oxygen and cerebral infarction in the gerbil. *Surg Neurol* 28: 265.

Butler FK (1991) Decompression sickness presenting as optic neuropathy. *Aviat Space Environ Med* 62: 346–350.

Butler FK (1995) Diving and Hyperbaric Ophthalmology. *Survey of Ophthalmology* 39: 347–366.

Butler FK (2007) The Eye in the Wilderness. In Auerbach PS (Ed.) *Wilderness Medicine*. St Louis, Mosby; Fifth Edition.

Butler FK, Hagan C (2008) Ocular complications of hyperbaric oxygen therapy. In Neuman and Thom (Eds.) *Hyperbaric Oxygen Therapy* (in press).

Butler FK, Hagan C, Murphy-Lavoie H (2008) Hyperbaric oxygen therapy and the Eye. *Undersea Hyper Med* (in press).

Butler FK, Harris DJ, Reynolds RA (1992) Altitude Retinopathy on Mount Everest 1989. *Ophthalomology* 99: 739–746.

Butler FK, White E, Twa M (1999) Hyperoxic Myopia in a Closed-Circuit Mixed-Gas SCUBA Diver. *Undersea Hyperb Med* 26: 41–45.

Butler WP, Topper SM, Dart TS (2002) USAF treatment table 8: treatment for altitude decompression sickness. *Aviat Space Environ Med* 73: 46–9.

Buxton JT, Stallworth JM, Bradham GB (1964) Hematocrit changes under hyperbaric oxygen. *Am Surg* 30: 18–22.

Bylund-Fellenius AC, Elander A, Lundgren F (1987) Effects of reduced blood flow on human muscle metabolism. In Okyayuz-Baklonti I, Hudlicka O (Eds.) *Muscle ischemia – functional and metabolic aspects*. Wolff, Munich, pp 75–88.

Byrnes W, Robinson D, Stevens B *et al* (1998) The effect of hyperbaric oxygen on the delayed onset of muscle soreness as quantified by magnetic resonance imaging. *Undersea Hyperbaric Med* 25: p 10 (abstract).

C

Cade IS, McEwen JB (1978) Clinical trials of radiotherapy in hyperbaric oxygen at Portsmouth, 1964–76. *Clin Radiol* 29: 333–338.

Cade IS, McEwen JB, Dische S *et al* (1978) Hyperbaric oxygen and radiotherapy: a Medical Research Council trial in carcinoma of the bladder. *Br J Radiol* 51: 876–878.

Cahill MT, Kaiser PK, Sears JE, Fekrat S (2003) The effect of arteriovenous sheathotomy on cystoid macular edema secondary to branch retinal vein occlusion. *Br J Ophthalmol* 87: 1329–1332.

Cakovska A, Nejedla P, Holikova A, Dendis M (2002) Positive findings of *Borrelia burgdorferi* in *Culex (Culex) pipiens pipiens* larvae in the surrounding of Brno city determined by the PCR method. *Ann Agric Environ Med* 9: 257–259.

Calabro F, Jinkins JR (2000) MRI of radiation myelitis: a report of a case treated with hyperbaric oxygen. *Eur Radiol* 10: 1079–84.

Calhoun KH, Shapiro RD, Stiernberg CM *et al* (1988) Osteomyelitis of the mandible. *Arch Otolalyngol Head Neck Surg* 114: 1157–1162.

Calverley RK, Dodds WA, Trapp WG *et al* (1971) Hyperbaric treatment of cerebral air embolism: a report of a case following cardiac catheterization. *Canad Anaesth Soc J* 18: 665–674.

Calvert JW, Cahill J, Yamaguchi-Okada M, Zhang JH (2006) Oxygen treatment after experimental hypoxia-ischemia in neonatal rats alters the expression of HIF-1alpha and its downstream target genes. *J Appl Physiol* 101(3): 853–865.

Calvert JW, Cahill J, Zhang JH (2007) Hyperbaric oxygen and cerebral physiology. *Neurol Res* 29: 132–141.

Calvert JW, Yin W, Patel M, Bader A, Mychaskiw G, Parent AD, Zhang JH (2002) Hyperbaric oxygenation prevented brain injury induced by hypoxia-ischemia in a neonatal rat model. *Brain Research*: 951(1): 1–8.

Calvert JW, Zhang JH (2005) Hyperbaric oxygenation restores energy status following hypoxia-ischemia in a neonatal rat model. *FASEB Journal* 19(4,S–1): A481.

Calvert JW, Zhou C, Zhang JH (2004) Transient exposure of rat pups to hyperoxia at normobaric and hyperbaric pressures does not cause retinopathy of prematurity. *Exp Neurol* 189: 150–161.

Cameron AJV, Hutton I, Kenmure ACF. Murdoch WR (1966) Haemodynamic and metabolic effects of hyperbaric oxygen in myocardial infarction. *Lancet* I: 833–837.

Campbell CJ, Wise GN (1973) Photocoagulation therapy of branch vein obstructions. *Am J Ophthalmol* 75: 28–31.

Capes JP, Tomaszewski C (1996) Phrophylaxis against middle ear barotraumas in US hyperbaric oxygen therapy centers. *AM J Emerg Med* 14: 645–648.

Carfrae MJ, Kesser BW (2008) Alignant otitis externa. *Otolaryngol Clin North Am* 41: 537–549.

Carlisle R, Lanphier EH, Rahn H (1964) Hyperbaric oxygen and persistence of vision in retinal ischemia. *J App Physiol* 19: 914–918.

Carlson S, Jones J, Brown M *et al* (1992) Prevention of hyperbaric-associated ear barotrauma. *Ann Emerg Med* 21: 1468–1471.

Cartlidge PH, Rutter N (1988) Percutaneous oxygen delivery to the premature infant. *Lancet* 1: 315.

Caruso VG, Winkelman PE, Correia MJ *et al* (1977) Otologic injuries in divers: clinical studies on nine commercial and two sports divers. *Laryngoscope* 77: 508.

Casti A, Orlandini G, Vescovi P (1993) Acute and chronic hyperbaric oxygen exposure in humans: effects on blood polyamines, adrenocorticotropin and beta-endorphin. *Acta Endocrinol Copenh* 129: 436–441.

Castro e Silva O, Sankarankutty AK, Martinelli AL, Souza FF, Teixeira AC, Feres O, Mente ED, Olivers GR, Akita R, Muglia V, Elias J Jr, Ramalho LN, Zucoloto S (2006) Therapeutic effect of hyperbaric oxygen in hepatic artery thrombosis and functional cholestasis after orthotopic liver transplantation. *Transplant Proc* 38(6): 1913–1917.

Catron PW, Dutka AJ, Biondi DM *et al* (1991) Cerebral air embolism treated by pressure and hyperbaric oxygen. *Neurology* 41: 314–315.

Centers for Disease Control and Prevention (2007) Lyme disease – United States, 2003–2005. *Morb. Mortal Wkly Rep* 56: 573–576.

Central Retinal Vein Occlusion Study Group (1994) Evaluation of grid pattern photocoagulation for macular edema in central vein occlusiton. *Ophthalmology* 102: 1425–1433.

Central Retinal Vein Occlusion Study Group (1997) Natural History and clinical management of central vein occlusion. *Arch Opthalmol* 115: 486–491.

Chacia N, Combes AM, Romdane K, Bec P (1987) Maculopathy in typical retinitis pigmentosa a propos of 33 cases. *J Fr Ophthalmol* 10: 381–386.

Chaika VA, Elsky VN, Borodin AD (1981) The effect of hyperbaric oxygen on the functional state of HHAS in pregnant rats and their fetuses. In Yefuny SN (Ed.) *Proceedings of the 7th international congress on hyperbaric medicine.* USSR Academy of Sciences, Moscow, p 369.

Champion WM, McSherry CK, Goulion D (1967) Effect of hyperbaric oxygen on the survival of pedicled skin flaps. *J Surg Res* 7: 583.

Chan EC, Brody B (2001) Ethical dilemmas in hyperbaric medicine. *Undersea Hyperb Med* 28: 123–130.

Chan J, Flynn J (2004) The immunological aspects of latency in tuberculosis. *Clin Immunol* 100: 2–12.

Chance B, Erecinska M, Wagner M (1970) Mitochondrial responses to carbon monoxide toxicity. *Ann NY Acad Sci* 174: 193–204.

Chance EM, Chance B (1988) Oxygen delivery to tissue: calculation of oxygen gradient in the cardiac cell. *Adv Exp Med Biol* 222: 69–75.

Chandler JR (1968) Malignant external otitis. *Laryngoscope* 78: 1257.

Chang CF, Niu KC, Hoffer BJ *et al* (2000) Hyperbaric oxygen therapy for treatment of postischemic stroke in adult rats. *Exp Neurol* 166: 298–306.

Chang CH (1977) Hyperbaric oxygen and radiation therapy in the management of glioblastoma. *NCI Monogr* 47: 163–169.

Chang EA, Detar R (1980) Oxygen and smooth muscle contraction revisited. *American Journal of Physiology* 238: H716–H728.

Chapler CK, Cain SM, Stainsby WN (1984) The effects of hyperoxia on oxygen uptake during acute anemia. *Can J Physiol Pharmacol* 62: 809–8124.

Chapman JD, Engelhardt EL, Stobbe CC *et al* (1998) Measuring hypoxia and predicting tumor radioresistance with nuclear medicine assays. *Radiother Oncol* 46: 229–37.

Chardack WM, Gage AA, Frederico AJ *et al* (1964) Reduction by hyperbaric oxygenation of the mortality from ventricular fibrillation following coronary artery ligation. *Circ Res* 15: 497–502.

Charneau J, Bouachour G, Person B *et al* (1991) Severe hemorrhagic radiation proctitis advancing to gradual cessation with hyperbaric oxygen. *Dig Dis Sci* 36: 373–375.

Chen Q, Banick PD, Thom SR (1996) Functional inhibition of rat polymorphonuclear leukocyte B2 integrins by hyperbaric oxygen is associated with impaired cGMP synthesis. *J Pharmacol Exp Ther* 276: 929–933.

Chen SD, Lochhead J, Patel CK, Frith P (2004) Intravitreal triamcinolone acetonide for ischemic macular edema caused by branch retinal vein occlustion. *Br J Ophthalmol* 88: 154–155.

Chen T, Lin S, Liu J *et al* (2002) Effects and mechanism of hyperbaric oxygen on prostaglandins in alveolar bone and gingival of experimental periodontitis in animal. *Zhonghua Kou Qiang Yi Xue Za Zhi* 37: 228–230.

Chen WT (1986) *Studies of myocardial contractility and hemodynamic changes under 2 ATA combining with external counterpulsation.* Presented at the 5th Chinese congress on hyperbaric medicine, Fuzhow, China, Sept. 26–29.

Cheshire WP Jr, Ott MC (2001) Headache in divers. *Headache.* 41: 235–247.

Chevrel JP, Guterman R, Rathat C *et al* (1979) Entérocolites aigues nécrosantes: à propos de trois observations. *Sem Hop* 55: 897–904.

Cho S-H, Lee DH, Yeun DR (1986) Incidence of carbon monoxide intoxication. *J Korean Med Assoc* 29: 1233–1240.

Choi IS (1983) Delayed neurologic sequelae in carbon monoxide intoxication. *Arch Neurol* 40: 433–435.

Choi IS, Lee MS (1993) Early hypoperfusion of technetium-99 m hexamethylprophylene amine oxime brain single photon emission computed tomography in a patient with carbon monoxide poisoning. *Eur Neurol* 33: 461–464.

Chong R, Ayer CJ, Francis IC, Coroneo MT, Wolfers DL (2007) Adjunctive hyperbaric oxygen in pseudomonas keratitis. *Br J Ophthalmol* 91: 560–561.

Christophi C, Millar I, Nikfarjam M *et al* (2007) Hyperbaric oxygen therapy for severe acute pancreatitis. *J Gastroenterol Hepatol* 22: 2042–1046.

Chuba PJ, Aronin P, Bhambhani K *et al* (1997) Hyperbaric oxygen therapy for radiation-induced brain injury in children. *Cancer* 80: 2005–2012.

Churchill-Davidson I, Metters JS, Foster CA, Bates TD (1973) The management of cervical lymph node metastases by hyperbaric oxygen and radiotherapy. *Clin Radiol* 24: 498–501.

Churchill-Davidson I, Sanger C, Thomlinson RH (1955) High pressure oxygenation and radiotherapy. *Lancet* I: 1091.

Chusid EL, Maher GG, Nicogossian A *et al* (1972) The effect of a pressurized environment (hyperbaric chamber) on pulmonary emphysema. *Am J Med* 53: 743–747.

Cianci P, Lueders H, Lee K *et al* (1989) Current status of adjunctive hyperbaric oxygen in the treatment of thermal burns. In Schmutz J, Bakker D (Eds.) *Proceedings of the 2nd Swiss symposium on hyperbaric medicine.* Foundation for Hyperbaric Medicine, Basel.

Cianci P, Williams C, Lueders H *et al* (1989) Adjunctive hyperbaric oxygen therapy reduces length of hospitalization in thermal burns. *J Burn Care Rehabil* 10: 432–435.

Cianci P, Williams C, Lueders H *et al* (1990) Adjunctive hyperbaric oxygen in the treatment of thermal burns: an economic analysis. *J Burn Care Rehabil* 11: 140–143.

Ciaravino ME, Friedell ML, Kammerlocher TC (1996) Is hyperbaric oxygen a useful adjunct in the management of problem lower extremity wounds? *Ann Vasc Surg* 10: 558–562.

Cibis, GW, Beaver HA, Johns K *et al* (2006) Basic and Clinical Science Course: Fundamentals and Principles of Ophthalmology. *American Academy of Ophthalmology, San Francisco*: 38–40.

Cimsit M, Ilgezdi S, Cimsit C, Uzun G (2007) Dysbaric osteonecrosis in experienced dive masters and instructors. *Aviat Space Environ Med* 78: 1150–1154.

Clark JM (1974) The toxicity of oxygen. *Am Rev Respir Dis {Suppl}* 10: 40–50.

Clark JM, Jackson RM, Lambertson CJ *et al* (1991) Pulmonary function in men after oxygen breathing at 3.0 ATA for 3.5 h. *J Appl Physiol* 71: 8788–885.

Clark JM, Lambertsen CJ (1971) Pulmonary oxygen toxicity: a review. *Pharmacol Rev* 23: 37–133.

Clark JM, Thom S (2003) Oxygen under pressure. In Brubakk AO, Neuman TS (Eds.) *Bennett and Eliott's Physiology and Medicine of Diving*. London: WB Saunders, pp 358–418.

Clark RG, Young DG (1965) Effects of hyperoxygenation and sodium bicarbonate in hemorrhagic hypotension. *Br J Surg* 52: 704.

Clarke D, Gerard W, Norris T (2002) Pulmonary barotrauma-induced cerebral arterial gas embolism with spontaneous recovery: commentary on the rationale for therapeutic compression. *Aviat Space Environ Med* 73: 139–46.

Clements KS, Vrabec, Mader JT (1998) Complications of tympanostomy tubes inserted for facilitation of hyperbaric oxygen therapy. *Arch Otolaryngol Head Neck Surg* 124: 278–280.

Coe JE, Hayes TM (1966) Treatment of experimental brain injury by hyperbaric oxygenation. A preliminary report. *Am Surg* 32: 493–495.

Colignon M, Carlier A, Khuc T *et al* (1987) Hyperbaric oxygen therapy in acute ischemia and crush injuries. In Marroni A, Oriani G (Eds.) *Proceedings of the 13th annual meeting of the European Undersea Biomedical Society*, Palermo, Italy, Sept 9–12.

Colignon M, Lamy M (1986) Carbon monoxide poisoning and hyperbaric oxygen therapy. In Schmutz J (Ed.) *Proceedings of the 1st Swiss symposium on hyperbaric medicine*. Foundation for Hyperbaric Medicine, Basel, pp 51–68.

Collet JP, Vanasse M, Marois P *et al* (2001) Hyperbaric oxygen for children with cerebral palsy: a randomised multicentre trial. HBO-CP Research Group. *Lancet* 357: 582–586.

Colletti LM, Kunkel SL, Walz A, Burdick MD, Kunkel RG, Wilke CA, Strieter RM (1995) Chemokine expression during hepatic ischemia/reperfusion induced lung injury in the rat. *J Clin Invest* 95: 134–141.

Colletti LM, Kunkel SL, Walz A, Burdick MD, Kunkel RG, Wilke CA, Strieter RM (1996) The role of cytokine networks in the local liver injury following hepatic ischemia/reperfusion in the rat. *Hepatology* 23(3): 506–514.

Coma MC, Sobrin L, Onal S, Christen W, Foster CS (2007) Intravitreal bevacizumab for treatment of uveitic macular edema. *Ophthalmology* 114: 1574–1579.

Contreras FL, Kadekaro M, Eisenberg HM (1988) The effect of hyperbaric oxygen on glucose utilization in a freeze-traumatized rat brain. *J Neurosurg* 68: 137.

Cope C (1961) The importance of oxygen in the treatment of cyanide poisoning. *JAMA* 175: 1061–1064.

Corkill G, Van Housen K, Hein L, Reitan J (1985) Videodensimetric estimation of the protective effect of hyperbaric oxygen in the ischemic gerbil brain. *Surg Neurol* 24: 406.

Cormio M, Robertson CS, Narayan RK (1997) Secondary insults to the injured brain. *J Clin Neurosci* 4(2): 132–148.

Corning JL (1891) The use of compressed air in conjunction with medical solutions in treatment of nervous and mental affections. *Medical Records*, 40: 225.

Coscas G, Gaudric A (1984) Natural course of nonaphakic cystoid macular edema. *Surv Ophthalmol* 28(Suppl): 471–484.

Coulson DB, Ferguson AB, Diehl RC (1966) Effect of hyperbaric oxygen on healing femur of the rat. *Surg Forum* 17: 449.

Courtiere A, Reybaud J, Camilla C *et al* (1991) Oxygen-induced modifications of benzodiazepine receptors and D$_2$ dopamine receptors in the rat under hyperoxia. *Free Rad Res Comm* 15: 29–34.

Courville CB (1959) Multiple sclerosis as an incidental complication of a disorder of lipid metabolism: close resemblance of the lesions resulting from fat embolism to the plaques of multiple sclerosis. *Bull Neurol Soc* 24: 60–75.

Cowan F, Rutherford M, Groenendaal F *et al* (2003) Origin and timing of brain lesions in term infants with neonatal encephalopathy. *Lancet* 361: 736–742.

Cox SN, Hay E, Bird AC (1988) Treatment of chronic macular edema with acetazolamide. *Arch Ophthalmol* 106: 1190–1195.

Cramer FS (1985) Care of the injured soldier: a medical readiness role for clinical hyperbaric oxygen therapy. *Milit Med* 150: 372–375.

Crisomoto E, Duncan PE, Propst M *et al* (1987) Evidence that amphetamine with physical therapy promotes recovery of motor function in stroke patients. *Ann Neurol* 23: 94.

Cross FS (1954) Effect of increased atmospheric pressures and the inhalation of 95% oxygen and helium oxygen mixtures on the viability of the bowel wall and the absorption of gas in closed loop obstructions. *Surgery* 36: 1001–1026.

Cross FS (1965) Hyperoxic treatment of experimental intestinal obstruction. *Dis Chest* 47: 374–381.

Cross FS, Wangensteen OH (1952) Effect of increased atmospheric pressures on the viability of the bowel wall and the absorption of gas in closed loop obstructions. *Surg Forum* 3: 111–116.

Cunningham S, Fleck BW, Elton RA *et al* (1995) Transcutaneous oxygen levels in retinopathy of prematurity. *Lancet* 346: 1464–1465.

Cuxart M, Matas M, Picazo M *et al* (2005) Acute bilateral visual loss in a hemodialysed patient. *Nefrologia* 25: 703–705. (Spanish)

D

D'Hemecourt PA, Stem W (1987) Dislodged gastric bubble. *J Hyperbaric Med* 2: 233–234.

D'Olhaberriague L, Litvan I, Mitsias P *et al* (1996) A reappraisal of reliability and validity studies in stroke. *Stroke* 27: 2331–2336.

Dahlin C, Linde A, Röckert H (1993) Stimulation of early bone formation by the combination of osteoporotive membrane technique and hyperbaric oxygern. *Scand J Plastic Reconstruct Surg* 27: 103–108.

Dalessio DJ (1985) Is there a difference between classic and common migraine? What is migraine, after all? *Archives of Neurology* 42: 275–276.

Dauman R, Cros AM, Poisot D *et al* (1985) Treatment of sudden deafness: first results of a comparative study. *J Otolaryngol* 14: 49–56.

David HN, Balon N, Rostain JC, Abraini JH (2001) Nitrogen at raised pressure interacts with the GABA(A) receptor to produce its narcotic pharmacological effect in the rat. *Anesthesiology* 95: 921–7.

David NJ, Norton EWD, Gass JD, Beauchamp J (1967) Fluorescein angiography in central retinal artery occlusion. *Arch Ophthalmol* 77: 619–629.

Davis FM, Glover PW, Maycock E (1990) Hyperbaric oxygen for cerebral air embolism occurring during cesarian section. *Anesth Intensive Care* 18: 403–405.

Davis JC (1977) Refractory osteomyelitis of the extremities and the axial skeleton. In Davis JC, Hunt TK (Eds.) *Hyperbaric oxygen therapy*. Undersea Medical Society, Bethesda, pp 217–277.

Davis JC (1981) Soft tissue radiation necrosis: the role of hyperbaric oxygen. *HBO Rev* 2: 153–170.

Davis JC (1987) The use of adjuvant hyperbaric oxygen in treatment of the diabetic foot. *Clin Podiatr Med Surg* 4: 429–437.

Davis JC (1989) Hyperbaric oxygen therapy. *J Intensive Care Med* 4: 55–57.

Davis JC, Dunn JM, Heimbach RD (1988) Hyperbaric medicine; patient selection, treatment procedures and side effects. In Davis JC, Hunt TK (Eds.) *Problem wounds: the role of oxygen*. Elsevier, New York pp 225–235.

Davis JC, Gates GA, Lerner C *et al* (1992) Adjuvant hyperbaric oxygen in malignant external otitis. *Arch Otolaryngol Head Neck Surg* 118: 89–93.

Davis JC, Heckman JD, DeLee JC *et al* (1986) Chronic nonhematogenous osteomyelitis treated with adjuvant hyperbaric oxygen. *J Bone Joint Surg* 68A: 1210–1217.

Davis JC, Landeen JM, Levine RA (1987a) Pyoderma gangrenosum: skin grafting after preparation with hyperbaric oxygen. *Plast Reconstr Surg* 79: 200–207.

Davis JC, Sheffield PJ, Schuknecht L *et al* (1977) Altitude decompression sickness: hyperbaric therapy results in 145 cases. *Aviat Space Environ Med* 48: 722–730.

Davis TRC, Griffiths ID, Stevens J (1988) Hyperbaric oxygen treatment for rheumatoid arthritis: failure to show worthwhile benefit. *Brit J Rheumatology* 27: 72 (letter).

Davis TRC, Holloway IT, Pooley J (1990) Effect of exposure to compressed air and elevated oxygen levels on bone blood flow in the rabbit. *Undersea Biomed Res* 17: 201–211.

Davis WB, Rennard SI, Bitterman PB *et al* (1983) Pulmonary oxygen toxicity: early reversible changes in human alveolar structures induced by hyperoxia. *N Engl J Med* 209: 878–883.

de Duve C (1984) *A guided tour of the living cell*. Scientific American Library, New York, pp 102–118.

De Graeve PH, Bimes C, Barthelemy R *et al* (1976) Histological modifications of the guinea pig thymus subjected to hyperbaric oxygen. *Bull Assoc Anat* (Nancy) 60: 663–667.

De Haan R, Horn J, Limburg M *et al* (1993) A comparison of five stroke scales with measures of disability, handicap and quality of life. *Stroke* 24: 1178–1181.

De Myttenaere S, Heifetz M, Shilansky H *et al* (1977) Different treatments used in a case of gangrene due to accidental intraarterial injection of methylphenidate (Ritalin). *Anesth Analg* 34: 405–410.

dePerrot M, Liu M, Waddell TK, Keshavjee S (2003) Ischemia-reperfusion-induced lung injury. *Am J Respir Crit Care Med* 167(4): 490–511.

De Smet MD, Carruthers J, Lepawsky M (1987) Anterior segment ischemia treated with hyperbaric oxygen. *Can J Ophthalmol* 22: 381–383.

Dean BS, Verdile VP, Krenzeloc EP (1993) Coma reversal with cerebral dysfunction recovery after repetitive hyperbaric oxygen therapy for severe carbon monoxide poisoning. *Am J Emerg Med* 11: 616–618.

Delb W, Muth CM, Hoppe U, Iro H (1999) Outcome of hyperbaric oxygen therapy in therapy refractory tinnitus. *HNO* 47: 1038–45.

Delektorsky VV, Antonyev AA, Nomoeva TN (1987) Ultrastructural changes in the mitochondria in scleroderma patients in the course of hyperbaric oxygenation. *Vestn Dermatol Venerol* 11: 20–27.

Demaertelaere L, Van Opstal M (1981) Treatment of acoustic trauma with hyperbaric oxygen. *Acta Oto Rhino Laryngol Belg* 25: 303–314.

Demarin V, Rundek T, Podobnik-Sarkanji S *et al* (1994) A correlation of 5-hydroxytriptamine and cerebral vasoreactivity in patients with migraine. *Functional Neurology* 9: 235–245.

Demchenko IT, Boso AE, Natoli MJ *et al* (1998) Measurement of cerebral blood flow in rats and mice by hydrogen clearance during hyperbaric oxygen exposure. *Undersea Hyperbaric Med* 25: 147–152.

Demchenko IT, Boso AE, Whorton AR, Piantadosi CA (2001) Nitric oxide production is enhanced in rat brain before oxygen-induced convulsions *Brain Res* 917: 253–61.

Demchenko IT, Luchakov YI, Moskvin AN *et al* (2005) Cerebral blood flow and brain oxygenation in rats breathing oxygen under pressure. *J Cereb Blood Flow Metab* 25: 1288–1300.

Demchenko IT, Oury TD, Crapo JD, Piantadosi CA (2002) Regulation of the brain's vascular responses to oxygen. *Circ Res* 91: 1031–1037.

Demchenko IT, Welty-Wolf KE, Allen BW, Piantadosi CA (2007) Similar but not the same: normobaric and hyperbaric pulmonary oxygen toxicity, the role of nitric oxide. *Am J Physiol Lung Cell Mol Physiol* 293: L229–L238.

Demchenko IT, Welty-Wolf KE, Allen BW, Piantadosi CA (2007) Similar but not the same: normobaric and hyperbaric pulmonary oxygen toxicity, the role of nitric oxide. *Am J Physiol Lung Cell Mol Physiol* 293: L229–L238.

Demurov EA, Vesilieva NN, Kakhnovskaya VB *et al* (1981) The effect of hyperbaric oxygenation on some indices of neurohormonal regulation, metabolic and heart contractile function under conditions of acute occlusion of the coronary artery. In Yefuny SN (Ed.) *Proceedings of the 7th international congress on hyperbaric medicine*. USSR Academy of Sciences, Moscow, p 273.

Denham JW, Yeoh EK, Wittwer G *et al* (1987) Radiation therapy in hyperbaric oxygen for head and neck cancer at Royal Adelaide Hospital – 1964 to 1980. *Int J Radiat Oncol Biol Phys* 13: 201–208.

Dennog C, Hartmann A, Frey G *et al* (1996) Detection of DNA damage after hyperbaric oxygen (HBO) therapy. *Mutagenesis* 11: 605–609.

Desai N, Patel MR, Prisant LM, Thomas DA (2005) Nonarteritic anterior ischemic optic neuropathy. *J Clin Hypertens* 7: 130–133.

Desloovere C (2007) Hyperbaric oxygen therapy for tinnitus. *B-ENT* 3(Suppl 7): 71–74.

Desola J (1987) Hyperbaric oxygen therapy in acute occlusive retinopathies. In Schmutz J (Ed.) *Proceedings of the Ist Swiss symposium on hyperbaric medicine*. Foundation for Hyperbaric Medicine, Basel, pp 333.

Desola J, Escola E, Moreno E *et al* (1990) Combined treatment of gas gangrene with hyperbaric oxygen, surgery and antibiotics. National multicenter collaborative study. *Med Clin (Barcelona)* 94: 641–650.

Dexter F, Hindman BJ (1997) Recommendations for hyperbaric oxygen therapy of cerebral air embolism based on a mathematical model of bubble absorption. *Anesth Analg* 84: 1203–1207.

Di Guilio C, Innocenti P, Loffredo B et al (1989) Hyperbaric hyperoxia and rat's hepatic regeneration. *J Hyperbaric Med* 4: 27–31.

Di Piero V, Cappagli M, Pastena L et al (2002) Cerebral effects of hyperbaric oxygen breathing: a CBF SPECT study on professional divers. *Eur J Neurol* 9: 419–21.

Di Piero V, Lenzi G, Collice M et al (1987) Long term non-invasive single photon emission computed tomography monitoring of perfusional changes after EC/IC bypass surgery. *J Neurol Neurosurg Psychiat* 50: 988–996.

Di Pretoro L, Forti G, Adami V (1968) Effet dell'iperbarismo e dell'ossigeazione iperbarica sul circolo cerebrale. *Acta Anaesthesiol (Padova)* 19 (Suppl 9): 73–84.

Di Sabato F, Fusco BM, Pelaia P et al (1993) Hyperbaric oxygen therapy in cluster headache. *Pain* 52: 243–245.

Di Sabato F, Giacovazzo M, Cristalli G et al (1996) Effect of hyperbaric oxygen on the immunoreactivity to substance P in the nasal mucosa of cluster headache patients. *Headache* 36: 221–223.

Di Sabato F, Rocco M, Martelletti P et al (1997) Hyperbaric oxygen in chronic cluster headaches: influence on serotonergic pathways. *Undersea Hyperbaric Medicine* 24: 117–122.

Dick JSB, Jampol LM, Haller JA (2001) Macular edema. In Ryan SJ, (Ed.) *Retina.* St. Louis: Mosby, pp 973–985.

Dietrich WD (1990) Influence of amphetamine treatment on somatosensory function of the normal and infarcted brain. *Stroke* 21(suppl III): III-147-III-150).

Dinser R, Jendro MC, Schnarr S, Zeidler H (2005) In vitro susceptibility testing of Borrelia burgdorferi sensu lato isolates cultured from patients with erythema migrans before and after antimicrobial chemotherapy. *Antimicrob Agents Chemother* 49: 1294–301.

Dirnagl U (1993) Cerebral ischemia: the microcirculation as trigger and target. In Kogure K, Hossmann KA, Siesjö (Eds.) *Progress in brain research V. 96 Neurobiology of ischemic brain damage.* Elsevier, Amsterdam, pp 49–65.

Dische ST (1983) The clinical use of hyperbaric oxygen and chemical hypoxic cell sensitizers. In Steel GG, Adams GE, Peckham M (Eds.) *The biological basis of radiotherapy.* Elsevier Scientific, Amsterdam, pp 225–237.

Dische S, Saunders MI, Sealy R et al (1999) Carcinoma of the cervix and the use of hyperbaric oxygen with radiotherapy: a report of a randomised controlled trial. *Radiother Oncol* 53: 93–8.

Dockendorf BL, Frazee RC, Peterson WG et al (1993) Treatment of acute intestinal ischemia with hyperbaric oxygen. *South J Med* 86: 518–520.

Doctor N, Pandya S, Supe A (1992) Hyperbaric oxygen therapy in diabetic foot. *J Postgrad Med* 38: 112–114.

Dolezal V (2002) Hyperbaric oxygen therapy in athletic injuries. *Cas Lek Cesk* 141: 304–306.

Dollery CT, Bulpitt CJ, Kohner EM (1969) Oxygen supply to the retina from the retinal and choroidal circulations at normal and increased arterial oxygen tensions. *Invest Ophthalmol Vis Sci* 8: 588–594.

Dollery CT, Hill DW, Mailer CM et al (1965) Response of retinal blood vessels to changes in respiratory gas pressures. *J Physiol* (Lond) 177: 70.

Dolmierski R, Maslowski J, Matousek M et al (1988) EEG changes under hyperbaric conditions: spectral analysis during simulated diving. *Acta Neurol Scand* 77: 437–439.

Domachevsky L, Keynan Y, Shupak A, Adir Y (2007) Hyperbaric oxygen in the treatment of sudden deafness. *Eur Arch Otorhinolaryngol* 264: 951–953.

Don HF, Wahba M, Cuadrado L et al (1970) The effect of anesthesia and 100% oxygen on the functional residual capacity of lungs. *Anesthesiology* 32: 521–529.

Donaghy MP, Yasargil MG (1967) *Microvascular surgery,* Thieme, Stuttgart.

Dong GC, Gao SZ, Zha GY et al (1986) *Experimental study of effect of HBO-laser-HpD on animal-transplanted tumor.* Presented at the 5th Chinese conference on hyperbaric medicine, Fuzhow, China Sept 26–29.

Dooley J, Schirmer J, Slade B et al (1996) Use of transcutaneous pressure of oxygen in the evaluation of edematous wounds. *Undersea Hyperbaric Med* 23: 167–174.

Dooley JLW, Mehm WJ, Jennings CA et al (1990) Modification of an automated vascular diagnostic system for hyperbaric use. *Undersea Biomed Res* 17: 247–251.

Dordain M, Humbert G, Robert M, Leroy J et al (1968) Coma hépatique par hépatite virale avec succès par l'oxygène hyperbare. *Sem Hop* 44: 1617–2622.

Douglas M (1994) Tissue oxygen transport: lessons from muscle and brain. *Sem Hematol* 31: 102–111.

Dowling S, Fischer JJ, Rockwell S (1992) Fluosol and hyperbaric oxygen as an adjunct to radiation therapy in the treatment of malignant gliomas: a pilot study. *Biomater Artif Cells Immobilization Biotechnol* 20: 903–905.

Dreier JP, Kleeberg J, Alam M, Major S, Kohl-Bareis M, Petzold GC, Victorov I, Dirnagl U, Obrenovitch TP, Priller J (2007) Endothelin-1-induced spreading depression in rats is associated with a microarea of selective neuronal necrosis. *Exp Biol Med (Maywood)* 232: 204–213.

Drel IK, Molzhaninov Ev. Samsonenko RA (1981) Effect of hyperbaric oxygenation on catecholamine metabolism in the placenta in late toxemia of pregnancy. *Akush Ginekol (Mosk)* 16–29.

Dreval AV, Dreval TP, Lukicheva TI (1988) Two-dimensional parameter of the kinetics of glucose in the assessment of the efficacy and prognosis of therapy of diabetes mellitus. *Ter Arkh* 60: 20–24.

Droghetti L, Giganti M, Memmo A, Zatelli R (2002) Air embolism: diagnosis with single-photon emission tomography and successful hyperbaric oxygen therapy. *Br J Anaesth* 89: 775–778.

Droviannikova IP (1981) Hyperbaric oxygen in the complex treatment of patients with diffuse toxic goiter. In Yefuny SN (Ed.) *Proceedings of the 7th international congress on hyperbaric medicine.* USSR Academy of Sciences, Moscow, p 372.

Ducassé JL, Celsis P, Marc-Vergnes JP (1995) Non-comatose patients with acute carbon monoxide poisoning: hyperbaric or normobaric oxygenation? *Undersea Hyperbaric Med* 22: 9–15.

Dudgeon DL, Kellogg Dr, Gilchrist GS et al (1971) Purpura fulminans. *Arch Surg* 103: 351–358.

Dudnikov LK, Kakhovsky IM, Molokanova SP (1981) Hyperbaric oxygenation in complex treatment of diabetic retinopathy. In Yefuny SN (Ed.) *Proceedings of the 7th international congress on hyperbaric medicine.* USSR Academy of Sciences, Moscow, pp 305–306.

Duker JS, Brown GC (1988) Recovery following acute obstruction of the retinal and choroidal circulations. *Retina* 8: 257–260.

Dunbar EM, Fox R, Watson B et al (1990) Successful treatment of venous air embolism with hyperbaric oxygen. *Postgrad Med J* 66: 469–470.

Dundar K, Gumus T, Ay H et al (2007) Effectiveness of hyperbaric oxygen on sudden sensorineural hearing loss: prospective clinical research. *J Otolaryngol* 36: 32–37.

Dunn JE (1974) *An evaluation of HBO, hypocapnic hyperventilation and methyl prednisolone therapy in cold induced cerebral swelling.* Paper presented at the 5th international congress on hyperbaric medicine, Simon Fraser University, Burnaby, Canada.

Dunn JE, Connolly JM (1966) Effects of hypobaric and hyperbaric oxygen on experimental brain injury. In Brown IW, Cox BG (Eds.) *Hyperbaric medicine.* National Research Council, Washington, pp 447–454.

Duplessis CA, Fothergill D (2008) Investigating the potential of statin medications as a nitric oxide (NO) release agent to decrease decompression sickness: a review article. *Med Hypotheses* 70: 560–566.

Dutka AJ, Kochanek PM, Hallenbeck JM (1989) Influence of granulocytopenia on canine cerebral ischemia induced by air embolism. *Stroke* 20: 390–395.

Duydu Y, Üstündag A, Aydin A *et al* (2006) Increased sensitivity to mitomycin C-induced sister chromatid exchange in lymphocytes from patients undergoing hyperbaric oxygen therapy. *Environ Mol Mutagen* 47: 185–191.

Dyer J, Millac P (1996) Late deterioration after decompression illness affecting the spinal cord. *Br J Sports Med* 30: 362–363.

Dyson EH, Proudfoot AT, Prescott LF, Heyworth R (1985) Death and blindness due to overdose of quinine. *Br Med J* 291: 31–33.

E

EC/IC Bypass Study Group (1985) Failure of extracranial-intracranial arterial bypass to reduce the risk of ischemic stroke: results of an international, randomized trial. *N Engl J Med* 313: 1190–1200.

Eckenhoff RG, Osborne SF, Parker JW, Bondi KR (1986) Direct ascent from shallow air saturation exposures. *Undersea Biomed Res* 13: 305–316.

Edlow JA (2002) Erythema migrans. *Med Clin North Am* 86: 239–260.

Edmonds C (1985) Hearing loss with frequent diving (deaf divers). *Undersea Biomed Res* 12: 315–320.

Edmonds C (1985) *Diving and subaquatic medicine.* Butterworth Heinemann, London, pp 392–400.

Edsberg LE, Brogan MS, Jaynes CD, Fries K (2002) Topical hyperbaric oxygen and electrical stimulation: exploring potential synergy. *Ostomy Wound Manage* 48: 42–50.

Edström JE, Röckert H (1962) The effect of oxygen at high pressure on the histology of the central nervous system and the sympathetic nervous system. *Acta Physiol Scand* 55: 255–263.

Edwards AE, Hart GM (1974) Hyperbaric oxygenation and the cognitive functioning of the aged. *J Am Geriatr Soc* 22: 376–379.

Edwards DF, Chen Y-U, Diringer MN (1995) Unified Neurological Stroke Scale is valid in ischemic and hemorrhagic stroke. *Stroke* 26: 1852–1858.

Eftedal OS, Lydersen S, Helde G, White L, Brubakk AO, Stovner LJ (2004) A randomized, double blind study of the prophylactic effect of hyperbaric oxygen therapy on migraine. *Cephalagia* 24: 639–644.

Efuni SM (1984) Effect of combined treatment including hyperbaric oxygenation on bronchitis. *Sov Med* 9: 8–12.

Efuni SN, Kudryashev Ve, Rodionov VV, Belefsky YV *et al* (1984) Significance of the isometric test in the objective assessment of the efficacy of hyperbaric oxygenation in coronary heart disease. *Kardiologiia* 24: 77–80.

Efuni SN, Levashova AS, Lyskin GI (1980) Hyperbaric oxygenation in the treatment of the cochleovestibular system. *Sov Med* 5: 45–49.

Efuni SN, Pogromov AP, Jegorov AP (1986) The use of hyperbaric oxygen in the treatment of gastric and duodenal ulcers. In Schmutz J (Ed.) *Proceedings of the 1st Swiss symposium on hyperbaric medicine.* Foundation for Hyperbaric Medicine, Basel pp 212–221.

Eguiluz-Ordoñez R, Sánchez CE, Venegas A *et al* (2006) Effects of hyperbaric oxygen on peripheral nerves. *Plast Reconstr Surg* 118: 350–357.

Ehler WJ, Bonney CH, Lam KW, Cissik JH (1987) Hyperbaric induction of ocular hyperuricosis. *J Hyperbaric Med* 2: 89–73.

Ehler WJ, Marx RE, Kiel J *et al* (1991) Induced regression of oral carcinoma by oxygen radical generating systems. *J Hyperbaric Med* 6: 111–118.

Ehrly AM, Saeger-Lorenz K (1988) Einfluss von Pentoxifyllin auf den Muskelgewebesauerstoffdruck von Patienten mit Claudicatio intermittens vor und nach fussergometrischer Belastung. *Med Welt* 39: 739–744.

Eibach H, Börger U (1980) Therapeutische Ergebnisse in der Behandlung des akuten akustischen Traumas. *Arch Otorhinolaryngol* 226: 177–186.

Eisterer H, Staudacher M (1971) Die Anwendung der hyperbaren Sauerstoffkammer in Verbindung mit gefässrekonstruktiven Massnahmen. *Chirurg* 42: 187–190.

Elander A, Idström JP, Schersten T *et al* (1985) Metabolic adaptation to reduced muscle blood flow. I. Enzyme and metabolite alterations. *Am J Physiol* 249: E63–E69.

Elkharrat D, Raphael JC, Korach JM *et al* (1991) Acute carbon monoxide intoxication and hyperbaric oxygen in pregnancy. *Inten Care Med* 17: 289–292.

Eltorai I, Montroy R (1991) Hyperbaric oxygen therapy leading to recovery of of a 6-week comatose patient afflicted by anoxic encephalopathy and posttraumatic edema. *J Hyperbaric Med* 6: 189–198.

Eltorai IM, Hart GB, Strauss MB (1984) Osteomyelitis in the spinal cord injured: a review and a preliminary report on the use of hyperbaric oxygen. *Paraplegia* 22: 17–24.

Eltorai IM, Hart GB, Strauss MB *et al* (1987) Does hyperbaric oxygen provoke occult carcinoma in man? In Kindwall EP (Ed.) *Proceedings of the 8th international congress on hyperbaric medicine.* Best, San Pedro, pp 18–29.

Emerson TS, Keiler J (1998) Pattern shift visual evoked potential screening for HBO2 in mild-to-moderate carbon monoxide poisoning. *Undersea Hyperbaric Med* 25: 27–32.

Emhoff TA, Myers RA (1987) Transcutaneous oxygen measurements and wound healing in diabetic patients. In Kindwall EP (Ed.) *Proceedings of the 8th international congress on hyperbaric medicine.* Best, San Pedro, pp 309–313.

End E, Long CW (1942) HBO in carbon monoxide poisoning. I. Effect on dogs and guinea pigs. *J Ind Hyg Toxicol* 24: 302–306.

Engler RL, Dahlgren MD, Peterson A *et al* (1986) Accumulation of polymorphonuclear leukocytes during 3-h experimental myocardial ischemia. *Heart Circ Physiol* 20: H93–H100.

Epshtein BV, Nishchenko VF, Timchenko PM (1988) Hyperbaric oxygenation in the comprehensive treatment of patients with diabetes mellitus. *Vrachebnoe Delo* 1: 65–66.

Epstein J, van der Meij E, McKenzie M *et al* (1997) Postradiation osteonecrosis of the mandible: A long-term follow-up study. *Oral Surg Oral Med Oral Pathol Oral Radiol Endod* 83: 657–662.

Ermakov EV, Barksy RL (1981) Hyperbaric oxygen in cases of inflammatory diseases of the lungs. In Yefuny SN (Ed.) *Proceedings of the*

7th international congress on hyperbaric medicine. USSR Academy of Sciences, Moscow, p 290.

Ersanli D, Karadayi K, Toyran S *et al* (2005) The efficacy of hyperbaric oxygen for the treatment of experimental uveitis induced in rabbits. *Ocul Immunol Inflamm* 13: 383–388.

Ersohina VA, Gasilin VS, Goliakov VN *et al* (1986) The effect of hyperbaric oxygenation on the indicators of the functional status of the myocardium in patients with ischemic heart disease. *Kardiologii* 26: 61–65.

Eschenfelder CC, Krug R, Yusofi AF *et al* (2008) Neuroprotection by oxygen in acute transient focal cerebral ischemia is dose dependent and shows superiority of hyperbaric oxygenation. *Cerebrovasc Dis* 25: 193–201.

Esclamado RM, Larrabee WF, Zel GE (1990) Efficacy of steroids and hyperbaric oxygen on the survival of dorsal skin flaps in rats. *Otolaryngol Head Neck Surg* 102: 41–44.

Esterhai, JL, Jr, Clark JM, Morton HE *et al* (1986) Effect of hyperbaric oxygen exposure on oxygen tension within the medullary canal in the rabbit tibial osteomyelitis model. *J Orthop res* 4: 330–336.

Esterhai, JL, Jr, Pisarello J, Brighton, CT *et al* (1987) Adjunctive hyperbaric oxygen therapy in the treatment of chronic refractory osteomyelitis. *J Trauma* 27: 763–768.

Esterhai, JL, Jr, Pisarello J, Brighton, CT *et al* (1988) Treatment of chronic refractory osteomyelitis with adjunctive hyperbaric oxygen therapy. *Orthop Rev* 17: 809–815.

Evers S, Husstedt IW (1996) Alternatives in drug treatment of chronic paroxysmal hemicrania. *Headache* 36: 429–432.

F

Faglia E, Favales F, Aldeghi A *et al* (1996) Adjunctive systemic hyperbaric oxygen in treatment of severe prevalently ischemic diabetic foot ulcer – A radomized study. *Diabetes Care* 19: 1338–1343.

Fallon BA, Keilp JG, Corbera KM *et al* (2008) A randomized, placebo-controlled trial of repeated IV antibiotic therapy for Lyme encephalopathy. *Neurology* 70: 992–1003.

Fallon TJ, Maxwell D, Kohner EM (1985) Retinal vascular autoregulation in conditions of hyperoxia and hypoxia using the blue field entoptic phenomenon. *Ophthalmology* 92: 701–705.

Fang GC, Xu GH, Wang FM (1986) Clinical significance of monitoring blood carboxyhemoglobin. *J Hyperbaric Med* 1: 233–238.

Farmer JC, Thomas WG, Preslar M (1971) Human auditory responses during hyperbaric helium-oxygen exposures. *Surg Forum* 22: 456–458.

Farri A, Pecorari GC, Enrico A, Sartoris A (2002) Hyperbaric oxygen therapy application in otorhinolaryngology and head and neck surgery: state of the art and review of literature. *Acta Otorhinolaryngol Ital* 22: 227–34.

Fasano VA, Nunno T, Urciuoli R *et al* (1964) First observations on the use of oxygen under high atmospheric pressure for treatment of traumatic coma. In Boerema I, Brummelkamp WH, Meijne NG (Eds.) *Clinical applications of hyperharic oxygen. Proceedings of the 1st international congress on hyperbaric medicine.* Elsevier, Amsterdam, pp 168–173.

Fattore L, Strauss RA (1987) Hyperbaric oxygen in the treatment of osteoradionecrosis: A review of its use and efficacy. *Oral Surg Oral Med Oral Pathol* 63: 280–286.

Fattori B, Berrettini S, Casani A *et al* (2001a) Sudden hypoacusis treated with hyperbaric oxygen therapy: a controlled study. *Ear Nose Throat J* 80: 655–660.

Fattori B, De-Iaco G, Vannucci G *et al* (1996) Alternobaric and hyperbaric oxygen therapy in the immediate and long-term treatment of Meniere's disease. *Audiology* 35: 322–334.

Fattori B, Nacci A, Casani A *et al* (2001b) Oxygen therapy in the long term treatment of Meniere's disease. *Acta Otorhinolaryngol Ital* 21: 1–9.

Fechter LD, Young JS, Carlisle L (1988) Potentiation of noise induced threshold shifts and hair cell loss by carbon monoxide. *Hear Res* 34: 39–48.

Feldberg B, Zamfiresco NR (1969) Changes of heart dynamics in hypoxia and hyperoxia. *Pflugers Arch* 312: R21.

Feldmeier JJ, Boswell RN (1987) The effect of hyperbaric oxygen on the immunologic status of healthy human subjects. In Kindwall EP (Ed.) *Proceedings of the 8th international congress on hyperharic medicine.* Best, San Pedro, pp 41–46.

Feldmeier JJ, Hampson NB (2002). A systematic review of the literature reporting the application of hyperbaric oxygen prevention and treatment of delayed radiation injuries: an evidence based approach. *Undersea Hyperb Med* 29: 4–30.

Feldmeier JJ, Heimbach RD, Davolt DA *et al* (1993a) Hyperbaric oxygen as an adjunctive treatment for severe laryngeal necrosis: a report of nine consecutive cases. *Undersea Hyperbaric Med* 20: 329–335.

Feldmeier JJ, Heimbach RD, Davolt DA *et al* (1993b) Hyperbaric oxygen aand the cancer patient: aa survey of practice patterns. *Undersea Hyperbaric Med* 20: 337–345.

Feldmeier JJ, Heimbach RD, Davolt DA *et al* (1994) Does hyperbaric oxygen have a cancer-causing or -promoting effect? A review of the pertinent literature. *Undersea Hyperbaric Med* 21: 467–475.

Feldmeier JJ, Heimbach RD, Davolt DA *et al* (1996) Hyperbaric oxygen as an adjunctive treatment for delayed radiation injuries of the abdomen and pelvis. *Undersea Hyperbaric Med* 23: 205–213.

Feldmeier JJ, Lange JD, Cox SD *et al* (1993c) Hyperbaric oxygen as a prophylactic or treatment for radiation myelitis. *Undersea Hyperbaric Med* 20: 249–255.

Feldmeier JJ, Heimbach RD, Davolt DA *et al* (1998) Hyperbaric oxygen as an adjunct in the treatment of delayed radiation injuries of the extremities. *Undersea Hyperbaric Med* 25: 9 (abstract).

Feltgen N, Junker B, Agostini H, Hansen LL (2007) Retinal endovascular lysis in ischemic central retinal vein occlusion. *Ophthalmology* 114: 716–723.

Ferguson BJ, Hudson Wr, Farmer JC (1987) Hyperbaric oxygen therapy for laryngeal radionecrosis. *Ann Otol Rhinol Larngol* 96: 1–6.

Fernau JL, Hirsch BE, Derkay C *et al* (1992) Hyperbaric oxygen therapy: effect on middle ear and eustachian tube function. *Laryngoscope* 102: 48–52.

Ferrari, MD, Odink J, Bos KD *et al* (1990) Neuroexcitatory plasma amino acids are elevated in migraine. *Neurology* 40: 1582–1586.

Ferrari MD, Saxena PRS (1993) On serotonin and migraine: a clinical and pharmacological review. *Cephalalgia* 13: 151–165.

Festugato M, Coelho CP, Fiedler G *et al* (2008) Hyperbaric oxygen therapy effects on tissue lesions in acute pancreatitis. Experimental study in rats. *JOP* 9: 275–282.

Fick A (1870) über die Messung des Blutquantums in den Herzventrikeln. *S.B. Phys-Med Ges, Würzburg,* v. 16.

Fife C, Powell M, Sutton T *et al* (1995) Transcranial doppler evaluation of the middle cerebral artery during hyperbaric hyperoxia. *Symposium on Cerebral Hemodynamics,* The Institute of Applied Physiology & Medicine, February.

Fife CE, Buyukcakir C, Otto GH *et al* (2002) The predictive value of transcutaneous oxygen tension measurement in diabetic lower extremity ulcers treated with hyperbaric oxygen therapy: a retrospective analysis of 1,144 patients. *Wound Repair Regen* 10: 198–207.

Fife CE, Meyer JS, Berry JM *et al* (1992) Hyperbaric oxygen and acute migraine pain: Preliminary results of a randomized, blinded trial. *Undersea and Hyperbaric Med* 19(S): 106–107.

Fife CE, Powell MG, Sutton TE *et al* (1994) Transcranial doppler evaluation of the middle cerebral artery from 1 ATA to 3 ATA PO2. *Undersea and Hyperbaric Med* 21(S): 77 (abstract).

Fife CE, Sallee DS, Gray L *et al* (1989) Prognostic value of brain CT after HBO in severe CO poisoning. *Undersea Biomed Res* 16: 19.

Fife WP, Fife CE (1989) Treatment of migraine with hyperbaric oxygen. *Journal of hyperbaric Medicine* 4: 7–15.

Finderle Z, Cankar K (2002) Delayed treatment of frostbite injury with hyperbaric oxygen therapy: a case report. *Aviat Space Environ Med* 73: 392–394.

Firlik AD, Kaufmannm Wechsler LR (1997) Quantitative cerebral blood flow determinations in acute ischemic stroke. Relationship to computed tomography and angiography. *Stroke* 73: 2208–2213.

Fisch U, Murata K, Hossli G (1976) Measurement of oxygen tension in human perilymph. *Acta Otolaryngol* (Stockholm) 81: 278–282.

Fischer BH (1969) Topical hyperbaric oxygen treatment of pressure sore and skin ulcers. *Lancet* I: 405–409.

Fischer BH (1975) Treatment of ulcers on the legs with hyperbaric oxygen. *J Dermatol Surg* 1: 55–58.

Fischer BH, Marks M, Reich T (1983) Hyperbaric oxygen treatment of multiple sclerosis. A randomised placebo-controlled double-blind study. *N England J Med* 308: 181–186.

Fiser SM, Tribble CG, Long SM, Kaza AK, Cope JT, Laubach VE, Kern JA, Kron IL (2001) Lung transplant reperfusion injury involves pulmonary macrophages and circulating leukocytes in a biphasic response. *J Thorac Cardiovasc Surg* 121: 1069–1075.

Fitch W (1976) Anesthesia for carotid artery surgery. *Br J Anaesth* 48: 791–796.

Flam F, Boijsen M, Lind F (2008 May 29) Necrotizing fasciitis following transobturator tape treated by extensive surgery and hyperbaric oxygen. *Int Urogynecol J Pelvic Floor Dysfunct* doi:10.1007/s00192-008-0653-4.

Fledelius HC, Jansen EC, Thorn J (2002) Refractive change during hyperbaric oxygen therapy. A clinical trial including ultrasound oculometry. *Acta Ophthalmol Scand* 80: 188–90.

Flynn ET (1991) *Hyperbaric oxygen therapy, a critical review*, UHMS, Bethesda, MD, Camporesi EM, Barker A, (Eds.), pp 55–74.

Fogan L (1985) Treatment of cluster headache. A double-blind comparison of oxygen v air inhalation. *Arch Neurol* 42: 362–363.

Folio LR, Arkin K, Butler WP (2007) Frostbite in a mountain climber treated with hyperbaric oxygen: case report. *Mil Med* 172: 560–563.

Fong AC, Schatz H (1993) Central retinal vein occlusion in young adults. *Surv Ophthalmol* 37: 393–417.

Fontaine JA (1877) Effets physiologiques et applications thérapeutiques de l'air comprimé Germer-Baillière, Paris.

Formai C, Sereni G, Zannini D (1980) *L'ossigenterapia iperbarica nel trattamento della sclerosi multipla*. Presented at the 4th Congresso Nazionale di medicina subacqua ed iperbarica. Naples, Italy, Oct 24–26.

Forrester RM (1964) Oxygen, cerebral palsy and retrolental fibroplasias. *Dev Med Child Neurol* 186: 648–650.

Frayser R, Saltzman HA, Anderson B, Hickam JB, Sieker (1967) The effect of hyperbaric oxygenation on retinal circulation. *Arch Ophthalmol* 77: 265–269.

Fredenucci P (1985) Oxygénothérapie hyperbare et artériopathies. *J Mal Vasc* 10 {Suppl A}: 166–172.

Freilich D, Seelenfreund MH (1973) Hyperbaric oxygen, retinal detachment, and sickle cell anemia. *Arch Ophthalmol* 90 (2): 90–93.

Freilich DB, Seelenfreund MH (1972) The use of hyperbaric oxygen in the treatment of retinal detachment in patients with sickle cell disease. *Isr J Med Sci* 8: 1458–1461.

Freilich DB, Seelenfreund MH (1975) Further studies in the use of hyperbaric oxygen in retinal detachment with sickle cell anemia. *Mod Probl Ophthalmol* 15: 313–317.

Freilich DB, Seelenfreund MH (1977) Long-term follow-up of scleral buckling procedures with sickle cell disease and retinal detachment treated with the use of hyperbaric oxygen. *Mod Probl Ophthalmol* 18: 368–372.

Friberg L, Olesen J, Lassen NA *et al* (1994) Cerebral oxygen extraction, oxygen consumption, and regional cerebral blood flow during the aura phase of migraine. *Stroke* 25: 974–979.

Fritelli G, Bernhard WF, Tank ES, Gross RE (1963) A study of ileus underhyperbaric conditions. *Surg Forum* 14: 376–377.

Fujimura E (1974) Experimental studies on radiation effects under high oxygen pressure. *J Osaka Dent Univ* 19: 100–108.

Fukaya E, Hopf HW (2007) HBO and gas embolism. *Neurol Res* 29: 142–145.

G

Gadzhiev AA (1979) Prevention of venous hypertension on the dry heart under hyperbaric oxygenation. *Grudn Khir* 5: 7–10.

Gail DB (1991) Hyperbaric Oxygen Therapy: NHLB Workshop Summary. *Am Rev Resp Dis* 144: 1414–1421.

Gajendrareddy PK, Sen CK, Horan MP, Marucha PT (2005) Hyperbaric oxygen therapy ameliorates stress-impaired dermal wound healing. *Brain Behav Immun* 19: 217–222.

Gallin-Cohen PF, Podos SM, Yabionski ME (1980) Oxygen lowers intraocular pressure. *Invest Ophthalmol Vis Sci* 19: 43–48.

Gamache FW, Myers RAM, Ducker TB, Cowley RA (1981) The clinical application of hyperbaric oxygen therapy in spinal cord injury: a preliminary report. *Surg Neurol* 15: 85–87.

Gandolfo MT, Rabb H (2008) Ischemia-reperfusion injury: Pathophysiology and clinical approach. In Ashan N (Ed.) *Chronic Allograft Failure: Natural History, Pathogenesis, Diagnosis and Management*. Landes Bioscience, pp39–47.

Garcia-Arumi J, Martinez-Castillo V, Boixadera A, Fonollosa A, Corcostgui B (2006) Surgical embolus removal in retinal artery occlusion. *Br J Ophthalmol* 90: 1252–1255.

Garcia-Covarrubias L, McSwain NE Jr, Van Meter K, Bell RM (2005) Adjuvant hyperbaric oxygen therapy in the management of crush injury and traumatic ischemia: an evidence-based approach. *Am Surg* 71: 144–151.

Gardner TW, Antonetti DA, Barber AJ, Leith E, Tarbell JA (1999) The molecular structure and function of the inner blood-retinal barrier. Pennsylvania State Retina Research Group. *Doc Ophthalmol* 97: 229–237.

Gass JD, Anderson Dr, Davis EB (1985) A clinical, fluorescein angiographic, and electron microscopic correlation of cystoid macular edema. *Am J Ophthalmol* 100: 82–86.

Gass JDM, Norton EDW (1966) Cystoid macular edema and papilledema following cataract exgtraction: a fluorescein fundoscopic and angiographic study. *Arch Ophthalmol* 76: 221–224.

Gatagov B (1982) Possibility of hyperbaric oxygen at medical evacuation. *Slages Mosk Vogenno-Med Zh* 5: 16–19.

Gaudue Y, Martin JL, Teisseire B, Duruble M, Duvelleroy MA (1982) The dependence of cardiac energy metabolism on oxygen carrying capacity. *Biochem Med* 28: 324–339.

Gaziev D, Baronciani D, Galimberti M *et al* (1996) Mucormycosis after bone marrow transplantation: report of four cases in thalassemia and review of the literature. *Bone Marrow Transplant* 17: 409–414.

Gelderd JB, Fife WP, Bowers DE, Deschner SH, Welch DW (1983) Spinal cord transection in rats: the therapeutic effects of dimethyl sulfoxide and hyperbaric oxygen. *Ann NY Acad Sci* 911: 218–233.

Gerbershagen HU, Kuffner H, Rocker H (1977) Lungenmechanik und pulmonaler Gasaustausch nach hyperbarer Oxygenierung. *Anaesthesist* 26: 433–452.

Gesell LB, Trott A (2007) De novo cataract development following a standard course of hyperbaric oxygen therapy. *Undersea Hyperb Med* 34: 389–392.

Giblin FJ, Schrimscher L, Chakrapani B, Reddy VN (1988) Exposure of rabbit lens to hyperbaric oxygen in vitro: regional effects of GSH level. *Invest Ophthalmol Vis Sci* 29: 1312–1319.

Gibson AJ, Davis FM, Ewer T (1991) Delayed hyperbaric ooxygen therapy for carbon monoxide intoxication-two case reports. *NZ Med J* 104: 64–65.

Gillis MF, Peterson PL, Karagianes MT (1968) In vivo detection of circulating gas emboli associated with decompression sickness using the Doppler blood flow detector. *Nature* 217: 965–967.

Gilman S (1998) Imaging the brain. First of two parts. *N Engl J Med* 338: 812–820.

Gilman SC, Colton JS, Dutka AJ (1988a) Release of dopamine from striatal synaptosomes: high pressure effects. *Undersea Biomed Res* 15: 13–18.

Gilman SC, Colton JS, Hsu SC *et al* (1988b) Pressure suppresses serotonin release by guineapig striatal synaptosomes. *Undersea Biomed Res* 15: 69–77.

Gismondi A, Micalella F, Metrangolo C *et al* (1981) Treatment of cerebral ischemia with hyperbaric oxygen therapy. *Minerva Med* 72: 1417.

Glacet-Bernard A, Coscas G, Chabanel A *et al* (1996) Prognostic factors for retinal vein occlusion. *Ophthalmology* 103: 551–560.

Glantz SA (1992) Experiments when each subject receives more than one treatment. In *Primer of bio-statistics* McGraw-Hill, New York, pp 278–319.

Glanzmann C, Magdeburg W, Bash H *et al* (1974) The results of radiotherapy of malignant tumours in the oropharynx and hypopharynx under hyperbaric oxygenation. *Strahlentherapie* 148: 16–23.

Glassburn JR, Brady LW, Plenk HP (1977) Hyperbaric oxygen in radiation therapy. *Ann Cancer* 39: 751–765.

Glauser SC, Glauser EM (1973) Hyperbaric oxygen therapy: size of infarct determines therapeutic efficacy. *Ann Intern Med* 78: 7–80.

Gleissner MW, Spantzel T, Bucker-Nott HJ, Jorch G (2003) Risk factors of retinopathy of prematurity in infants 32 to 36 weeks gestational age. *Z Geburtshilfe Neonatol* 207: 24–8.

Gliner JA, Horvath SM, Mihevic PM (1983) Carbon monoxide and human performance in a single and dual task methodology. *Aviat Space Environ Med* 54: 714–717.

Golden Z, Golden CJ, Neubauer RA (2006) Improving neuropsychological function after chronic brain injury with hyperbaric oxygen. *Disabil Rehabil* 28(22): 1379–1386.

Golden ZL, Neubauer R, Golden CJ *et al* (2002) Improvement in cerebral metabolism in chronic brain injury after hyperbaric oxygen therapy. *Int J Neurosci* 112: 119–31.

Goldstein LB (1998) Potential effects of common drugs on stroke recovery. *Arch Neurol* 55: 454–456.

Goliakov VN, Eroshina VA, Zimin YV, Semiletova VI (1986a) Hemostasis in patients with ischemic heart disease during hyperbaric oxygenation. *Klin Med (Mosk)* 64: 92–95.

Goliakov VN, Zimin IV, Eroshina VA, Gasilin VS, Efuni SN (1986b) Effect of hyperbaric oxygenation on extrasystole in ischemic heart disease patients. *Kardiologiia* 26: 45–49.

Golikov PP, Rogatsky GG, Nikolaeva NY (1986b) Glucocorticoid receptors in the lungs in hyperbaric oxygenation. *Patol Fiziol Eks Ter* 2: 32.

Golikov VN, Eroshina VA, Zimin IV (1986a) Hemostasis in ischemic heart disease patients undergoing hyperbaric oxygenation. *Klin Med* 64: 92–95.

Gonchar DI (1985) Hyperbaric oxygenation and hemoperfusion in intensive therapy of posttransfusion blood hemolysis. *Anesteziol Reanimatol* 4: 32–34.

Goodhart GL (1994) Patient treated with antidote kit and hyperbaric oxygen survives cyanide poisoning. *South Med J* 87: 814–6.

Gool J, Jong H (1964) Hyperbaric oxygen treatment in vascular insufficiency of the retina and optic nerve. In Ledingham IM (Ed.) *Proceedings of the 2nd international congress on clinical and applied hyperbaric medicine.* Livingstone, Edinburgh, pp 447–460.

Goplen FK, Grønning M, Irgens A *et al* (2007) Vestibular symptoms and otoneurological findings in retired offshore divers. *Aviat Space Environ Med* 78: 414–419.

Gordillo GM, Roy S, Khanna S *et al* (2008) Topical oxygen therapy induces vascular endothelial growth factor expression and improves closure of clinically presented chronic wounds. *Clin Exp Pharmacol Physiol* 35: 957–964.

Gordman DF, Browning DM (1986) Cerebral vasoreactivity and arterial gas embolism. *Undersea Biomed Res* 13: 317–355.

Gorman DF (1990) A proposed classification of the decompression illness. In Francis TJP, Smith DJ (Eds.) *Describing Decompression Illness.* UHMS Workshop, Alverstoke, UK, UHMS, Bethesda MD, pp 6–9.

Gorman DF, Clayton D, Gilligan JE *et al* (1992) A longitudinal study of 100 cases consecutive admissions for carbon monoxide poisoning to the Royal Adelaide Hospital. *Anesth Intens Care* 20: 311–316.

Gorman JF, Stansell GB, Douglas F (1965) Limitations of hyperbaric oxygenation in occlusive arterial disease. *Circulation* 32: 936–939.

Goto F, Fujita T, Kitani Y *et al* (1979) Hyperbaric oxygen and stellate ganglion blocks for idiopathic sudden hearing loss. *Acta Otolaryngol* 88: 335–342.

Gottlieb SF (1963) The possible role of hyperbaric oxygen in the treatment of leprosy and tuberculosis. *Dis Chest* 44: 215–217.

Gottlieb SH, Neubauer RA (1988) Multiple sclerosis: its etiology, pathogenesis and therapeutics. *J Hyperbaric Med* 3: 143–164.

Goulon M, Barois A, Bapin M *et al* (1969) Intoxication oxycarbonée et anoxie aigue par inhalation de gaz de charbon et d'thydrocarbures. *Ann Méd Interne (Paris)* 120: 335–349.

Goulon M, Rapin M, Barois A (1971) Trial treatment of severe viral hepatitis with hyperbaric oxygenation (apropos of 16 cases). *Ann Med Interne (Paris)* 122: 93–98.

Gray DH, Hamblin DL (1976) The effects of hyperoxia upon bone organ culture. *Clin Orthop Relat Res* 119: 225–230.

Gray LH, Conger AO, Ebert M *et al* (1953) The concentration of oxygen dissolved in tissues at the time of irradiation as a factor in radiotherapy. *Br J Radiol* 26: 638–648.

Green MO, Brannen AL (1995) Hyperbaric oxygen therapy for beta-radiation-induced scleral necrosis. *Ophthalmology* 102: 1038–1041.

Greenberg PB, Martidis A, Rogers AH, Duker JS, Reichel E (2002) Intravitreal triamcinolone acetonide for macular edema due to central retinal vein occlusion. *Br J Ophthalmol* 86: 247–248.

Greenwood TW, Gilchrist AG (1973) Hyperbaric oxygen and wound healing in postirradiation head and neck surgery. *Br J Surg* 50: 394.

Greer DV, Constable IJ, Cooper RL (1980) Macular edema and retinal branch vein occlustion. *Aust J Ophthalmol* 8: 207–209.

Gregorevic P, Lynch GS, Williams DA (2001) Hyperbaric oxygen modulates antioxidant enzyme activity in rat skeletal muscles. *Eur J Appl Physiol* 86: 24–7.

Greiner KH, Lang GE (1999) Risk-adapted management of central vein occlusions. *Ophthalmologe* 96: 736–740. (German)

Grieve DA, Unsworth IP (1991) Pneumatosis cystoides intestinalis: an experience with hyperbaric oxygenation. *Aust NZ J Surg* 61: 423–426.

Grigoryeva AV, Kasantzeva MV *et al* (1992) Effect of different doses of hyperbaric oxygenation on cortical neurons of rats with experimental brain ischemia. *Biulleten Eksperimentalnoi Biologii I Meditsiny* 113(4): 419–421.

Grinker RR (1926) Parkinsonism following carbon monoxide poisoning. *J Neuro Ment Dis* 6d: 18–28.

Grokhovsky VI, Mogiliak OL, Bonovik PI (1978) Five-year experience using hyperbaric oxygenation in pediatric surgery. *Klin Khir* 6: 66–70.

Gross DR, Dodd KT, Welch DW *et al* (1984) Hemodynamic effects of 10% dextrose and of dextran 70 on hemorrhagic shock during exposure to hyperbaric air and hyperbaric hyperoxia. *Aviat Space Environ Med* 55: 1118–1128.

Gross DR, Moreau RM, Chaikin BN *et al* (1983b). Hemodynamic effects of lactated Ringer's solution on hemorrhagic shock during exposure to hyperbaric air and hyperbaric hyperoxia. *Aviat Space Environ Med* 54: 701–708.

Gross DR, Moreau RM, Jabor M *et al* (1983a) Hemodynamic effects of dextran 40 on hemorrhagic shock during hyperbaria and hyperbaric hyperoxia. *Aviat Space Environ Med* 54: 413–419.

Grossman AR (1978) Hyperbaric oxygen in the treatment of burns. *Ann Plast Surg* 1(2): 163–171.

Grossman AR, Grossman AJ (1982) Update on hyperbaric oxygen and treatment of burns. *Hyperbaric Oxygen Rev* 3: 51–59.

Grote W, Wanger WD (1973) Malformations in rabbit embryos after hyperbaric oxygenation. *Klin Wochenschr* 51(5): 248–2250.

Gruber RP, Brinkley FB, Amato JJ *et al* (1970a) Hyperbaric oxygen and pedicle flaps, skin grafts and burns. *Plast Reconstr Surg* 45: 24–30.

Gruber RP, Heitkamp DH, Lawrence JB etal. (1970b) Skin permeability to oxygen and hyperbaricoxygen. *Arch Surg* 101: 60–70.

Gu ZZ (1985) Effect of oxygen at various pressures on intracranial pressure. *Chung Hua Shen Ching Ching Shen Ko Tsa Chih* 18: 17–20.

Guang-bo X, Bing-xue Y, Xiao-zhong W *et al* (1991) Stroke in urban and rural areas of China. *Chinese Medical Journal* 104: 697–704.

Gudewicz TM, Mader JT, Davis CP (1987) Combined effects of hyperbaric oxygen and antifungal agents on the growth of Candida albicans. *Aviat Space Environ Med* 58: 673–678.

Guernsey LM, Clark JM (1981) Hyperbaric oxygen therapy with subtotal extirpation surgery in the management of radionecrosis of the mandible. *Int J Oral Surg* 10(suppl 1): 168–177.

Guimaraes FAG, Taha MO, Simoes MJ, Moino CAA, Santos IV, Amador JC, Santos RA, Queiroz RB, Amaro RR, Jesus MAS, Caricati-Neto A (2005) Use of hyperbaric oxygenation in small bowel preservation for transplant. *Transplant Proc* 38(6): 1796–1799.

Gunther A, Manaenko A, Franke H *et al* (2004) Hyperbaric and normobaric reoxygenation of hypoxic rat brain slices-impact on purine nucleotides and cell viability. *Neurochem Int* 45(8): 1125–1132.

Gupta R, Vora N, Thomas A *et al* (2007) Symptomatic cerebral air embolism during neuro-angiographic procedures: incidence and problem avoidance. *Neurocrit Care* 7: 241–246.

Guseinov NM, Konstantinova NP, Lukich VL *et al* (1989) Our experience in the hyperbaric oxygenation treatment of patients with acute sensorineural hearing disorders of vascular etiology. *Vestnik Otorinolaryngologii* 4: 76–79.

Gusev EI, Kazantseva NV, Nifontova LA *et al* (1990) Mechanisms of the therapeutic effects of hyperbaric oxygenation in minor differential pressures in stroke. *Zh Nevropatol Psikhiatr* 90: 34–40.

Guskov EP, Shkurat TP, Shimanskaja EI *et al* (1990) Genetic effects of hyperbaric oxygen therapy. *Mutation Research* 241: 341–347.

Gutman FA, Zegarra H (1984) Macular edema secondary to occlusion of retinal veins. *Surv Ophthalmol* 26: 462–470.

Guy J, Schatz NJ (1986) Hyperbaric oxygen in the treatment of radiation-induced optic neuropathy. *Ophthalmology* 93: 1083–1088.

Guyton AC (1986) *Textbook of physiology*. Saunders, Philadelphia.

H

Haapaniemi T, Nylander G, Kanje M (1998) Hyperbaric oxygen treatment enhances regeneration of the rat sciatic nerve. *Exp Neurol* 149: 433–438.

Haapaniemi T, Nishiura Y, Dahlin LB (2002) Functional evaluation after rat sciatic nerve injury followed by hyperbaric oxygen treatment. *J Peripher Nerv Syst* 7: 149–54.

Haddad HM, Leopold IH (1965) Effect of hyperbaric oxygenation on microcirculation: use in therapy of retinal vascular disorders. *Invest Ophthalmol* 4: 1141–1151.

Haffty BG, Hurley R, Peters LJ (1999) Radiation therapy with hyperbaric oxygen at 4 atmospheres pressure in the management of squamous cell carcinoma of the head and neck: results of a randomized clinical trial. *Cancer J Sci Am* 5: 341–347.

Hague S, Hill DW, Crabtree A (1988) The calibre changes of retinal vessels subject to prolonged hyperoxia. *Exp Eye Res* 47: 87–96.

Hai YU, Tian RL, Pan XW, Luan Z, Song LW (2002) Effects of hyperbaric oxygen on brain bFGF and bFGF mRNA expression of neonatal grafts after hypoxia/ischemia injury. In James T. Joiner (Ed.) *Proceedings of the 2nd International Symposium on Hyperbaric Oxygenation for Cerebral Palsy and the Brain Injured Child* Best, San Pedro, pp 57–65.

Haldane JS (1907) *Admiralty report on deep water diving.* London HMSO CN 1549.

Hale HB, Williams EW, Ellis JP (1973) Human endocrine-metabolic responses to graded oxygen pressures. *Aerospace Med* 44: 33–36.

Halouzka J, Wilske B, Stunzner D, Sanogo YO, Hubalek Z (1999) Isolation of *Borrelia afzelii* from overwintering *Culex pipiens* biotype molestus mosquitoes. *Infection* 27: 275–277.

Halva ZD, Koziel M, Zoch V (1978) Die Anwendung der Hyperbaroxie bei Sprunggelenksverletzungen. Application of hyperbaric oxygen in ankle joint injuries (English abstracts). *Beitr Orthop Traumatol* 25: 324–327.

Hamblin DL (1968) Hyperbaric oxygen: its effect on experimental staphylococcal osteomyelitis in rats. *J Bone Joint Surg (Am)* 50: 1129–1141.

Hamilton RW, Sheffield PJ (1977) Hyperbaric chamber safety. In Davis JC, Hunt TR (Eds.) *Hyperbaric oxygen therapy*, Undersea and Hyperbaric Medical Society, Bethesda, pp 47–60.

Hammarlund C, Svedman C, Svedman P (1991) Hyperbaric oxygen treatment of healthy volunteers with u.v.-irradiated blister wounds. *Burns* 17: 296–301.

Hamour A, Denning DW (1996) Hyperbaric oxygen therapy in a women who declined colostomy. *Lancet* 348: 197.

Hampson NB *et al* (1994) Central nervous system oxygen toxicity during hyperbaric treatment of acute CO poisoning: comparison of treatment pressures. *Undersea Hyperbaric Med* 21(Suppl): #1.

Hampson NB (1998) Treatment of mechanically ventilated patients poisoned with carbon monoxide: Is "hyperbaric oxygenation" achieved. *Undersea Hyperbaric Med* 25: 17 (abstract).

Hampson NB, Dunford RG, Kramer CC *et al* (1995) Selection criteria utilized for hyperbaric oxygen treatment of carbon monoxide poisoning. *J Emerg Med* 13: 227–31.

Hampson NB, Simonson SG, Kramer CC *et al* (1996) Central nervous system oxygen toxicity during hyperbaric treatment of patients with carbon monoxide poisoning. *Undersea Hyperbaric Med* 23: 215–219.

Handschel J, Brüssermann S, Depprich R *et al* (2007) Evaluation of hyperbaric oxygen therapy in treatment of patients with osteomyelitis of the mandible. *Mund Kiefer Gesichtschir* 11: 285–290.

Handy RD, Bryson P, Moody AJ *et al* (2005) Oxidative metabolism in platelets, platelet aggregation, and hematology in patients undergoing multiple hyperbaric oxygen exposures. *Undersea Hyperb Med* 32: 327–340.

Hansbrough JF, Piacentine JG, Eiseman B (1980) Immunosuppression by hyperbaric oxygenation. *Surgery* 87: 662–667.

Hao M, Yu CK (1987) An outline of hyperbaric oxygen therapy in treatment of ischemic cerebrovascular disease in China. *J Chin Med Univ* 16: 56–58.

Harch PG (1996) Late treatment of decompression illness and use of SPECT brain imaging. In Moon RE, Sheffield PJ (Eds) *Treatment of Decompression Illness, 45th Workshop of the Undersea and Hyperbaric Medical Society.* UHMS, Kensington, pp 203–242.

Harch PG (2000) Generic inhibitory drug effect of hyperbaric oxygen therapy (HBOT) on reperfusion injury (RI). *Euro J Neurology* 7(Suppl 3): 150.

Harch PG (2001) The dosage of hyperbarcic oxygen in chronic brain injury. In Joiner JT (Ed.), *The proceedings if the 2nd International Symposium on Hyperbaric Oxygenation for Cerebral Palsy and the Brain-Injured Child.* Best Flagstaff, AZ, pp 31–56.

Harch PG, Gottlieb SF, Van Meter K *et al* (1994) HMPAO SPECT brain imaging and low pressure HBOT in the diagnosis and treatment of chronic traumatic, ischemic, hypoxic and anoxic encephalopathies. *Undersea Hyperbaric Med* 21 (suppl) (abstract).

Harch PG, Kriedt C, Van Meter KW, Sutherland RJ (2007) Hyperbaric oxygen therapy improves spatial learning and memory in a rat model of chronic traumatic brain injury. *Brain Research* 1174: 120–129.

Harch PG *et al* (1996) Use of HMPAO SPECT for assessment of response to HBO in ischemic/hypoxic encephalopathies. In Jain KK *Textbook of hyperbaric medicine* (2nd ed). Hogrefe & Huber: Seattle, pp 480–491.

Harch PG, Kriedt CL, Weisend MP, Van Meter KW, Sutherland RJ (2001) Low pressure hyperbaric oxygen therapy induces cerebrovascular changes and improves complex learning/memory in a rat open head bonk chronic brain contusion model. *Undersea Hyperbaric Med* 28(Suppl): 28–29.

Harch PG, Kriedt C, Van Meter KW, Sutherland RJ (2007) Hyperbaric oxygen therapy improves spatial learning and memory in a rat model of chronic traumatic brain injury. *Brain Res* 1174: 120–129.

Harch PG, Van Meter KW, Gottlieb SF *et al* (1993) Delayed treatment of of type II DCS: the importance of low pressure HMPAO-SPECT brain imaging in its diagnosis and management. *Undersea Hyperbaric Med* 20(suppl): 51 (abstract).

Harch PG, Van Meter KW, Gottlieb SF *et al* (1994a) The effect of HBO tailing treatment on neurological residual and spect brain images in type II (cerebral) DCI/CAGE. *Undersea Hyperbaric Med* 21(suppl): (abstract).

Harch PG, Van Meter KW, Gottlieb SF *et al* (1994b) HMPAO SPECT brain imaging of acute CO poisoning and delayed neuropsychological sequelae. *Undersea hyperbaric Med* 21(suppl): 15.

Hardenbergh E, Buckies RG, Mils JA *et al* (1973) Cardiovascular changes in anesthetized dogs at 3 and 5 atmospheres absolute pressure. *Aerospace Med* 44: 1231–1235.

Harding SA, Hodder SC, Courtney DJ, Bryson PJ (2008) Impact of perioperative hyperbaric oxygen therapy on the quality of life of maxillofacial patients who undergo surgery in irradiated fields. *Int J Oral Maxillofac Surg* 37: 617–624.

Hardy P, Collet JP, Goldberg J *et al* (2002) Neuropsychological effects of hyperbaric oxygen therapy in cerebral palsy. *Dev Med Child Neurol* 44: 436–46.

Harel D, Obrist WD, Saltman HA *et al* (1974) Cerebral circulatory and metabolic responses to hyperbaric oxygenation in normal subjects and in patients suffering from organic dementias. In Trapp Wg, Banister EW, Davison AJ (Eds.) *Proceedings of the 5th international congress on hyperbaric medicine.* Simon Fraser University, Burnaby, Canada.

Harman D (1999) Free radical theory of aging: increasing the average life expectancy at birth and the maximum life span. *Journal of Anti-Aging Medicine* 2: 199–208.

Harper AM, Ledingham IM, McDowall DG (1965) The influence of hyperbaric oxygen on the blood flow and oxygen uptake of the cerebral cortex in hypovolemic shock. In Ledingham IM (Ed.) *Proceedings of the 2nd international congress on clinical applications of hyperbaric medicine.* Livingstone, Edinburgh, pp 342–346.

Harrison LB, Chadha M, Hill RJ *et al* (2002) Impact of tumor hypoxia and anemia on radiation therapy outcomes. *Oncologist* 7(6): 492–508

Hart GB (1974) Exceptional blood loss anemia. Treatment with hyperbaric oxygen. *JAMA* 288: 1028–1029.

Hart GB *et al* (1983) Gas gangrene – a collective review. *J Trauma* 23: 991–1000.

Hart GB, Grossman (1988) Thermal burns. In Kindwall EP, Goldman RW (eds) *Hyperbaric Medicine Powers*, St. Luke's Medical Center, Milwaukee, pp 98–109.

Hart GB, Lennon PA, Strauss MB (1987) Hyperbaric oxygen in exceptional acute blood-loss anemia. *J Hyperbaric Med* 2: 205–210.

Hart GB, O'Reilly RR, Bronssand ND *et al* (1974) Treatment of burns with hyperbaric oxygen. *Surg Gynecol Obstet* 139: 693–696.

Hart GB, Strauss MB (1979) Responses of ischemic ulcerative conditions to OHP. In Smith G (Ed.) *Hyperbaric medicine*. Aberdeen University Press, Aberdeen, pp 312–314.

Hart GB, Strauss MB (1984) Vital capacity of quadriplegic patients treated with hyperbaric oxygenation. *J Am Paraplegia Soc* 7: 113–114.

Hart GB, Strauss MB (1986) Hyperbaric oxygen in the management of radiation injury. In Schmutz J (Ed.) *Proceedings 1st Swiss symposium on hyperbaric medicine*. Stiftung für Hyperbare Medizin, Basel, pp 31–51.

Hart GB, Thompson RE (1971) The treatment of cerebral ischemia with hyperbaric oxygen therapy. *Stroke* 2: 247.

Hartzog JI, Fisher RG, Snow C (1969) Spinal cord trauma: effect of hyperbaric oxygen therapy. *Proc Ann Clin Spinal Cord Injury Conf* 17: 70–71.

Hashikawa K, Matsumoto M, Moriwaki H *et al* (1994) Split dose iodine-123-IMP SPECT: sequential quantitative regional cerebral blood flow change with pharmacological intervention. *J Nucl Med* 35: 1226–1233.

Hasselbach HC, Ruefer F, Feltgen *et al* (2007) Treatment of central retinal vein occlusion by radial optic neurotomy in 107 cases. *Graefes Arch Clin Exp Ophthalmol* 245: 1145–1156.

Haug H (1985) Are neurons of the human cerebral cortex really lost during aging? A morphologic examination. In Traber J, Gispen WH (Eds.) *Senile dementias of the Alzheimer type*. Springer, Berlin, Heidelberg, New York, pp 150–163.

Hauss J, Spiegel HV (1987) Registration of hyperoxia damages by monitoring of tissue PO2 with surface electrodes (clinical and experimental). In Okyayuz-Baklonti I, Hudlicka O (Eds.) *Muscle ischemia – functional and metabolic aspects*. Wolff, Munich, pp 23–46.

Hayakawa T (1974) Hyperbaric oxygen treatment in neurology and neurosurgery. *J Life Sci* 4: 1–25.

Hayakawa T, Kanai N, Kuroda R *et al* (1971) Response of cerebrospinal fluid pressure to hyperbaric oxygenation. *Neurol Neurosurg Psychiatry* 34: 580–586.

Hayreh SS (1983). Classification of central retinal vein occlusion. *Ophthalmology* 90: 458–474.

Hayreh SS (2003a) Management of central retinal vein occlusion. *Ophthalmologica* 217: 167–188.

Hayreh SS, Kolder HE, Weingeist TA (1980) Central retinal artery occlusion and retinal tolerance time. *Ophthalmology* 87: 75–78.

Hayreh SS, Podhajsky P (1982) Ocular neovascularization with retinal vascular occlusion: II. Occurrence in central retinal and branch retinal artery occlusion. *Arch Ophthalmol* 100: 1581–1596.

Hayreh SS, Podhajsky PA, Zimmerman B (1998) Ocular manifestations of giant cell arteritis. *Am J Ophthalmol* 125: 509–520.

Hayreh SS, Zimmerman B (2003b) Management of giant cell arteritis. Our 27-year clinical study: new light on old controversies. *Ophthalmologica* 217: 239–259.

Hayreh SS, Zimmerman B (2008) Nonarteritic anterior ischemic optic neuropathy. *Ophthalmology* 115: 298–305.

Hayreh SS, Zimmerman MB (2005) Central retinal artery occlusion: Visual outcome. *Am J Ophthalmol* 140: 376–391.

Hayreh SS, Zimmerman MB (2007) Incipient nonarteritic anterior ischemic optic neuropathy. *Ophthalmology* 114: 1763–1772.

Headley DB, Gapany M, Dawson DE *et al* (1991) The effect of hyperbaric oxygen on growth of human squamous cell carcinoma xenografts. *Arch Otolarngol Head Neck Surg* 117: 1269–1272.

Heller MB (1990) Open-chest cardiac massage, a possible rebirth of an old procedure. 87: 189–194.

Helps SC, Gorman DF (1991) Air embolism of the brain in rabbits pretreated with mechlorethamine *Stroke* 22: 351–354.

Henderson LT, Slade JB (2004) Central retinal artery occlusion and hyperbaric oxygen therapy. *Undersea Hyperb Med* 31: 309. (abstract)

Henk JM (1986) Late results of a trial of hyperbaric oxygen and radiotherapy in head and neck cancer: a rationale for hypoxic cell sensitizers? *Int J Radiat Oncol Biol Phys* 12: 1339–1341.

Henriksson J, Nygaard E, Andersson J *et al* (1980) Enzyme activities, fibre types and capillarization in calf muscles of patients with intermittent claudication. *Scand J Clin Lab Invest* 40: 361–369.

Herbstein K, Murchland JB (1984) Retinal vascular changes after treatment with hyperbaric oxygen. *Med J Aust* 6: 728–829.

Hertzog LM, Meyer GW, Carson S, Strauss MB, Hart GB (1992) Central retinal artery occlusion treated with hyperbaric oxygen. *J Hyperbaric Medicine* 7: 33–42.

Heuser G, Uszler JM (2001) Hyperbaric oxygenation for cerebral palsy. *Lancet* 357: 2053–4.

Heyman A, Saltzman HA, Whalen RE (1966) Use of HBO in treatment of cerebral ischemia and infarction. *Circulation* (Suppl II) 33–34: II-20-II-27.

Heyndrickx A, Scheiris C, Vercruysse A *et al* (1970) Gas chromatographic determination of carbon monoxide in blood and the hyperbaric oxygen treatment in carbon monoxide poisoning cases. *J Pharm Belg* 247–258.

Hickey RF, Visick WD, Fairley HB *et al* (1973) Effects of halothane anesthesia on the functional residual capacity and alveolar arterial oxygen tension tension difference. *Anesthesiology* 38: 521–529.

Hiess WD, Graf R, Grond M, Rudolf J (1998) Quantitative neuroimaging for the evaluation of the effect of stroke treatment. *Cerebrovasc Dis* 8(Suppl 2): 23–29.

Hiess WD, Herholz K, Podreka I, Neubauer I, Pietrzyk U (1990) Comparison of [99mTc]HMPAO SPECT with [18F]fluoromethane PET in cerebrovascular disease. *J Cereb Blood Flow Metab* 10: 687–697.

Higgins AC, Pearlstein RD, Mullen JB *et al* (1981) Effect of hyperbaric therapy on long tract neuronal conduction in acute phase of spinal cord injury. *J Neurosurg* 55: 501–510.

Higuchi T, Oto T, Millar IL, Levvey BJ, Williams TJ, Snell GI (2006) Preliminary report of the safety and efficacy of hyperbaric oxygen therapy for specific complications of lung transplantation. *J Heart Lung Transplant* 25(11): 1302–1309.

Hill GB (1976) Hyperbaric oxygen exposures for intrahepatic abscesses produced in mice by nonsporeforming anaerobic bacteria. *Antimicrob Agents Chemother* 9: 312–317.

Hillard JR (1990) Severe claustrophobia in a patient requiring hyperbaric oxygen treatment. *Psychosomatics* 31: 107–108.

Hill RK (1992) A blinded, crossover controlled study of the use of

538 Bibliography

hyperbaric oxygen in the treatment of migraine headache. *Undersea Hyperb Med* 19[suppl]: 106.

Hills BA (1979a) Mechanical vs ischemic mechanisms for decompression sickness. *Aviat Space Environ Med* 50: 363–367.

Hills BA (1979b) Intermittent flow in tendon capillary bundles. *J Appl Physiol* 46: 696–702.

Hills BA, James PB (1982) Spinal decompression sickness; mechanical studies and a model. *Undersea Biomed Res* 9: 185–201.

Hills BA, James PB (1991) Microbubble damage to the blood-brain barrier. *Undersea Biomed Res* 18: 111–116.

Hilpert P, Bähr R, Junger H *et al* (1973) CO-Diffusionskapazität, Compliance und Lungenvolumina nach hyperbarer Oxygenierung (3 ata über 3 std) bei Lungengesunden. *Pneumonologie* 149: 75–81.

Hirakawa W (1996) Hyperbaric oxygen enhances the cytotoxicity of anticancer drugs. *Jpn J Hyperbaric Med* 31: 205–214.

Hiramitsu T, Hasegawa Y, Hirata K *et al* (1976) Formation of lipoperoxide in the retina of rabbit exposed to high concentration of oxygen. *Experientia* 32: 622–623.

Hirayama Y, Matsunaga N, Tashiro J, Amemlya T, Iwasaki M (1990) Bifemelane in the treatment of central retinal artery or vein obstruction. *Clin Ther* 12: 230–235.

Hirn M, Niinikoski J (1988) Hyperbaric oxygen in the treatment of clostridial gas gangrene. *Ann Chir Gynaecol* 77: 37–40.

Hirn M, Niinikoski J (1989) Management of perineal necrotizing fasciitis (Fournier's gangrene). *Ann Chirur Gynacol* 78: 277–281.

Hirn M, Niinikoski J, Lehtonen OP (1993) The effect of hyperbaric oxygen and surgery on experimental multimicrobial gas gangrene. *Eur Surg Res* 25: 265–269.

Hirotani H, Kuyama T (1974) Hyperbaric oxygen therapy for muscular dystrophy. *Arch Jpn Chir* 43: 161–167.

Hitchcock CR (1987) Overwhelming infections in trauma. *Postgrad Med* 82: 77–79.

Hjelde A, Hjelstuen M, Haraldseth O *et al* (2002) Hyperbaric oxygen and neutrophil accumulation/tissue damage during permanent focal cerebral ischaemia in rats. *Eur J Appl Physiol* 86: 401–5.

Hlozek J, Slapak I, Kucera P (1989) Rational treatment of external otitis. *Cas Lek Cesk* 128: 1594–1596.

Hodics T, Linfante I (2003) Cerebral air embolism. *Neurology* 60: 112–45.

Hogan J, Ellison EH (1966) Low molecular weight dextran and high pressure oxygen in the treatment of ligation of the hepatic artery. *Am J Surg* 111: 873–876.

Holbach KH, Caroli A (1974) Oxygen tolerance and the oxygenation state of the injured human brain In Trapp WG *et al* (Eds.) *Procedures of the 5th international congress on hyperbaric medicine.* Simon Fraser University, Burnaby 2, BC, Canada 350–361.

Holbach KH, Caroli A, Wassmann ZH (1977) Cerebral energy metabolism in patients with brain lesions at normo- and hyperbaric oxygen pressure. *J Neurol* 217: 17–30.

Holbach KH, Gött U (1969a) Cerebrale Durchblutungsstörungen und hyperbare Sauerstoff Therapie. *Radiologie* 9: 453–458.

Holbach KH, Gött U (1969b) Beobachtungen und Erfahrungen mit der hyperbaren Sauerstofftherapie bei Hirngeschädigten. *DVL Research Report* 69–78, Bad Godesberg, pp 91–109.

Holbach KH, Schröder FK, Köster S (1972) Alterations of cerebral metabolisms in cases with acute brain injuries during spontaneous respiration of air, oxygen and hyperbaric oxygen. *Eur Neurol* 8: 158–160.

Holbach KH, Wassmann H (1979) Neurochirurgische Therapie der zerebralen Mangeldurchblutung. *Neurol Psychiat (Bucur)* 5: 347.

Holbach KH, Wassmann H, Caroli A (1977a) Continuous rCBF measurements during hyperbaric oxygenation. In *Procedures of the 6th International congress on hyperbaric medicine. Aberdeen University Press* 104–111.

Holbach KH, Wassmann H, Caroli A (1977b) Correlation between electroencephalographical and rCBF changes during hyperbaric oxygenation. In *Procedures of the 6th International congress on hyperbaric medicine. Aberdeen University Press* 112–117.

Holbach KH, Wassmann H, Hohelochter KL (1976) Reversibility of the chronic post-stroke state. *Stroke* 7(3): 297–300.

Holbach KH, Wassmann H, Hohelochter KL, Jain KK (1977) Differentiation between reversible and irreversible poststroke changes in brain tissue. *Surg Neurol* 7: 325.

Holbach KH, Wassmann H, Hoheluchter KL, Linke D, Ziemann B (1975) Clinical course of spinal lesions treated with hyperbaric oxygenation (HO). *Acta Neurochir (Wien)* 31(3-4): 297–298.

Holbach KH, Wassmann H, Kolberg T (1974) Verbesserte Reversibilität des traumatischen Mittelhirnsyndromes bei Anwendung der hyperbaren Oxygenierung. *Acta Neurochir* 30: 247–256.

Holbach KH, Wassmann H, Linke D (1978) The use of hyperbaric oxygenation in the treatment of spinal cord lesions. *Eur Neurol* 16: 213–221.

Hollabaugh RS Jr, Dmochowski RR, Hickerson WL *et al* (1998) Fournier's gangrene: Therapeutic impact of hyperbaric oxygen. *Plast Reconstr Surg* 101: 94–100.

Hollin SA, Espinosa OE, Sukoff MH *et al* (1968) The effect of hyperbaric oxygenation on cerebrospinal fluid oxygen. *J Neurosurg* 29: 229–235.

Hollmann W (1987) Hirndurchblutung und Körperarbeit. *Herz Sport Gesund* 4: 61–65.

Holloway HD, Whalen RW, Saltzman HA *et al* (1965) Hyperbaric oxygenation in treatment of acute coronary artery embolization. *J Lab Clin Med* 66: 596–603.

Holman BL, Devous MD (1992) Functional brain SPECT: The emergence of a powerful clinical method. *J Nucl Med* 33: 1888–1904.

Holman BL, Hill TC, Lee RGL *et al* (1983) Brain imaging with radio-labeled amines. In Freeman LM, Weissmann HS (Eds.) *Nuclear Medicine Annual* 1983. Raven, New York, pp 131–165.

Holmes C, Gargas L (1987) Effects of hyperbaric oxygen. *J Infect Dis* 155: 1084.

Holohan TV (1990) Extracranial-intracranial bypass to reduce the risk of ischemic stroke. *AHCPR Health Technology Assessment Report* Publ No. 91–3473. U. S. Department of Health & Human Services, Washington.

Honda Y, Hata N, Sakakibara Y *et al* (1985) Central hypoxic-hypercapnic in mild hypoxia in man. *Pflugers Arch* 391: 289–295.

Hopkinson BR, Schenk WG (1969) Effect of hyperbaric oxygen on experimental intestinal obstruction. *Arch Surg* 98: 228–232.

Horowitz MD, Portogues CG, Matos LA *et al* (1992) Hyperbaric oxygen: value in the management of non-healing saphenectomy wounds. *Ann Thorac Surg* 54: 782–783.

Hoskin PJ, Saunders MI, Dische S (1999) Hypoxic radiosensitizers in radical radiotherapy for patients with bladder carcinoma: hyperbaric oxygen, misonidazole, and accelerated radiotherapy, carbogen, and nicotinamide. *Cancer* 86: 1322–1328.

Hou H, Grinberg O, Williams B *et al* (2007) The effect of oxygen therapy on brain damage and cerebral pO(2) in transient focal cerebral ischemia in the rat. *Physiol Meas* 28: 963–976.

Hsu AA, Wong TM, How J *et al* (1992) Retinal artery occlusion in a diver. *Singapore Med J* 33: 299–301.

Hsu P, Li H-W, Lin Y-T (1987) Acute hydrogen sulfide poisoning treated with hyperbaric oxygen. *J Hyperbaric Med* 2(4): 215–221.

Hsu YC, Lee KW, Ho KY *et al* (2005) Treatment of laryngeal radionecrosis with hyperbaric oxygen therapy: a case report. *Kaohsiung J Med Sci* 21: 88–92.

Hu ZY, Shi XF, Liang ZF, Tang ZW, Jin XQ (1991) the protective effect of hyperbaric oxygen on hearing during chronic noise exposure. *Aviat Space Environ Med* 62: 403–406.

Huang KL, Wu JN, Lin HC *et al* (2000) Prolonged exposure to hyperbaric oxygen induces neuronal damage in primary rat cortical cultures. *Neurosci Lett* 293: 159–162.

Huang KL, Kang BH, Wan FJ (2002) Treatment of pulmonary air embolism with hyperbaric oxygen and isoproterenol in rats. *Aviat Space Environ Med* 73: 373–378.

Huber S, Rigler B, Machler HE *et al* (2000) Successful treatment of massive arterial air embolism during open heart surgery. *Ann Thorac Surg* 69: 931–933.

Hutchinson JH, Ker MM, Williams KG, Hopkinson WI (1963) Hyperbaric oxygen in the resuscitation of the newborn. *Lancet* 2: 1019–1022.

I

Iazzetti PE, Maciel RE (1988) Effects of hyperbaric oxygen on the rat neurogenic pulmonary edema. *Braz J Med Biol Res* 21: 153–156.

Ignacio DR, Pavot AP, Nevell M *et al* (1984) Treatment of extensive limb ulcers with the use of topical hyperbaric oxygen therapy. *Adv Ther* 1: 55–61.

Ihde DC, Bostick FW, Devite VT (1975) Cytokinetic effect of hyperbaric oxygen in two murine tumors. *Proc Am Assoc Cancer Res* 16: 183.

Iimura M, Iizuka B, Kishino M *et al* (2000) A case of chronic idiopathic intestinal pseudo-obstruction and pneumatosis cystoides intestinalis with pneumatoperitoneum, improved by the hyperbaric oxygen therapy. *Nippon Shokakibyo Gakkai Zasshi* 97: 199–203.

Iitsuka T, Kobayashi M, Izumi Y *et al* (1993) *Nippon Jiinzo Gakkai Shi* 35: 293–297.

Illingworth CFW (1962) Treatment of arterial occlusion under oxygen at two atmospheres pressure. *Br Med J* 2: 1272.

Illingworth CFW, Smith G, Lawson DD *et al* (1961) Surgical and physiological observations in an experimental pressure chamber. *Br J Surg* 49: 22.

Imai E, Kunikata H, Udono T, Nakagawa Y *et al* (2004) Branch retinal artery occlusion: a complication of iron-deficiency anemia in a young adult with a rectal carcinoid. *Tohuko J Exper Med* 203: 141–144.

Imai K, Mori T, Izumoto H *et al* (2006) Hyperbaric oxygen combined with intravenous edaravone for treatment of acute embolic stroke: a pilot clinical trial. *Neurol Med Chir (Tokyo)* 46: 373–378.

Imai T (1974) HBO therapy on the memory disturbances. In Trapp WG *et al* (Eds.) *Proceedings of the 5th international congress on hyperbaric medicine.* Simon Fraser University, Burnaby, Canada, pp 402–408.

Inci E, Erisir F, Ada M *et al* (2002) Hyperbaric oxygen treatment in sudden hearing loss after unsuccessful medical treatment. *Kulak Burun Bogaz Ihtis Derg* 9: 337–341.

Ingvar D, Lassen NA (1965) Treatment of focal cerebral ischemia with hyperbaric oxygen. *Acta Neurol Scand* 41: 92.

Inuzuka K, Unno N, Yamamoto N, Sagara D, Suzuki M, Nishiyama M, Konno H (2007) Effect of hyperbarically oxygenated-perfluorochemical with University of Wisconsin solution on preservation of rat small intestine using an original pressure resistant portable apparatus. *Surgery* 142(1): 57–66.

Isakov IV, Ananev GV, Romasensko MV, Ajde K (1982a) Hyperbaric oxygenation in the acute period of craniocerebral injuries. *Zh Nevropatol Psikhiatr* 82: 7–12.

Isakov IV, Golikov AP, Ustinova EZ *et al* (1981b) Hyperbaric oxygenation in the combined treatment of paroxysmal tachyarrhythmias in ischemic heart disease. *Kardiologiia* 21: 42–45.

Isakov IV, Romasenko MV (1985) Effect of hyperbaric oxygenation on the water content of brain tissue in experimental toxic cerebral edema. *Zh Nevropatol Psikhiatr* 85: 1786–1789.

Isakov YV, Atroschenko ZB, Yufit IS *et al* (1979) Hyperbaric oxygenation in the severe compound trauma of the extremities. *Ortop Traumatol Protez* 9: 34–36.

Isakov YV, Pravdenkova GV, Ananiev IS *et al* (1981a) Hyperbaric oxygenation in acute period of cerebral stroke and craniocerebral injury. In *Abstracts of the 7th international congress of hyperbaric medicine*, Moscow, 2–6 Sept, pp 295–296.

Isakov YV, Pravdenkova SV *et al* (1982b) Effect of hyperbaric oxygenation (HBO) on external respiration in acute cerebral circulatory disorder. *Zh Vopr Neirokhir* (1 Jan-Feb): 34–39.

Isakov YV, Pravdenkova SV, Shchelkovski VN (1985) Hyperbaric oxygenation in ruptured cerebral aneurysms during the postoperative period. *Zh Vopr Neirokhir* 46: 34–39.

Ishida K, Suzuki A, Ogino N (1989) Oxygenation under hyperbaric pressure for cystoid macular edema. *Jpn J Clin Ophthalmol* 43: 1171–1174. (Japanese)

Ishida S, Usui T, Yamashiro K *et al* (2003) VEGF 164 is proinflammatory in the diabetic retina. *Invest Ophthalmol Vis Sci* 44: 2155–2162.

Ishihara H, Matsui H, Kitagawa H *et al* (1997) Prediction of the surgical outcome for the treatment of cervical myelopathy by using hyperbaric oxygen therapy. *Spinal Cord* 35: 763–767.

Ishii Y, Deie M, Adachi N *et al* (2005) Hyperbaric oxygen as an adjuvant for athletes. *Sports Med* 35: 739–746.

Isom GE, Burrows GE, Way GI (1982) Effect of oxygen on the antagonism of cyanide intoxication – cytochrome oxidase, in vivo. *Toxicol Appl Pharmacol* 65: 250–256.

Iturralde D, Spaide RF, Meyerle CB *et al* (2006) Intravitreal bevacizumab (Avastin) treatment of macular edema in central retinal vein occlusion: a short-term study. *Retina* 26: 279–284.

Ivanov KP (1959) The effect of elevated oxygen pressure on animals poisoned with potassium cyanide. *Pharmacol Toxicol* 22: 176–179.

Iwase T, Hasegawa Y, Ito T *et al* (1996) Bone composition and metabolism after hyperbaric oxygenation in rats with 1-hydroxyethylidene-1,1 biphosphonate-induced rickets. *Undersea Hyperbaric Med* 23: 5–9.

Iwatsuki N, Takahashi M *et al* (1994) Hyperbaric oxygen combined with nicardipine administration accelerates neurologic recovery after cerebral ischemia in a canine model. *Crit Care Med* 22(5): 858–863.

Izawa K, Tsunoda T, Ura K *et al* (1993) Hyperbaric oxygen therapy in the treatment of refractory peripancreatic abscess associated with severe acute pancreatitis. *Gastroenterologia Japonica* 28: 284–291.

J

Jackman SV, Thompson JT (1995) Effects of hyperbaric exposure on eyes with intraocular gas bubbles. *Retina* 15: 160–166.

Jackson BT, Piasecki GJ, Novy MJ (1987) Fetal responses to altered maternal oxygenation in rhesus monkey. *Am J Physiol* 252(1 Pt 2): R94–R101.

Jacobs BB, Thuning CA, Sacksteder MR, Warren J (1979) Extended skin allograft survival in mice during prolonged exposure to hyperbaric oxygen. *Transplantation* 28: 70–72.

Jacobs EA, Alvis HJ, Small SM (1972) Hyperoxygenation: a central nervous system activator? *J Geriatr Psychiatry* 5: 107–121.

Jacobs EA, Winter JPM, Alvis HJ, Small SM (1969) Hyperoxygenation effect on cognitive functioning in the aged. *N Engl J Med* 281: 753–757.

Jacobson I, Bloor K, McDowell DG *et al* (1963a) Internal carotid endarterectomy at two atmospheres of pressure. *Lancet* 1: 546–549.

Jacobson I, Harper AM, McDowall DG (1963) The effects of oxygen under pressure on cerebral blood flow and cerebral venous oxygen tension. *Lancet* ii: 549.

Jacobson I, Lawson DD (1963) The effect of hyperbaric oxygen on experimental cerebral infarction in the dog. *J Neursurg* 20: 849.

Jacobson JH, Wang MCH, Yamaki T *et al* (1964) Hyperbaric oxygenation in diffuse myocardial infarction. *Arch Surg* 89: 905.

Jaeger K, Juttner B, Sommer C *et al* (2002) Effects of Repetitive Exposure to Hyperbaric Oxygen (HBO) on Leukocyte Function. *Anasthesiol Intensivmed Notfallmed Schmerzther* 37: 24–8.

Jaeger M, Schuhmann MU, Soehle M, Meixensberger J (2006) Continuous assessment of cerebrovascular autoregulation after traumatic brain injury using brain tissue oxygen pressure reactivity. *Crit Care Med* 34: 1783–1788.

Jain KK (1984) Sutureless extra-intracranial anastomosis using Nd: YAG laser-clinical application. *Lancet* ii: 816–817.

Jain KK (1989a) Effect of hyperbaric oxygenation on spasticity in stroke patients. *J Hyperbaric Med* 4: 55–61.

Jain KK (1989b) *Oxygen in Physiology and Medicine*. Thomas, Springfield.

Jain KK (1990) *Carbon monoxide poisoning*. St. Louis, Green.

Jain KK (1994) High pressure neurological syndrome (HPNS). *Acta Neurologica Scandinavica* 90: 45–50.

Jain KK (1998b) *Textbook of gene therapy*. Hogrefe & Huber, Göttingen-Toronto.

Jain KK (1998c) Pharmacotherapy of chronic venous insufficiency: A critical review. *J Clin Res* 1: 269–288.

Jain KK (2001) *Ageing*. Informa Publications, London (available from Jain PharmaBiotech, Basel, Switzerland).

Jain KK (2002) Personalised medicine. *Curr Opinion Mol Ther* 4: 548–558.

Jain KK (2004) Angiogenesis in brain tumors. In Black PM & Loeffler J (Eds.) *Cancer of the Nervous System*, 2nd ed. Williams & Wilkins, Lippincott, Philadelphia.

Jain KK (2004h) Hyperbaric oxygen in acute ischemic stroke. *Stroke* 34: e9 (letter).

Jain KK (2008) Neuroprotection in traumatic brain injury. *Drug Discovery Today* 12: 1082–1089.

Jain KK (2009) *Textbook of Personalized Medicine*. Springer/Humana, Totowa, NJ.

Jain KK (2009a) High pressure neurological syndrome. *Medlink Neurology*. Medlink Corporation, San Diego.

Jain KK (2009b) Hyperbaric oxygenation for treatment of stroke. *Medlink Neurology*. Medlink Corporation, San Diego, California.

Jain KK (2009c) Neurologic aspects of carbon monoxide poisoning. *Medlink Neurology*. Medlink Corporation, San Diego, California.

Jain KK (2009d) *Neuroprotection*. Basel, Jain PharmaBiotech Publications.

Jain KK (2009e) *Cell Therapy*. Basel, Jain PharmaBiotech Publications.

Jain KK (2009f) Susac syndrome. *Medlink Neurology*. Medlink Corporation, San Diego.

Jain KK (2009g) Neurologic disorders of aging. *Medlink Neurology*. Medlink Corporation, San Diego.

Jain KK (2009h) *Gene Therapy*. Basel, Jain PharmaBiotech Publications.

Jain KK (2009i) Neurologic complications of decompression. *Medlink Neurology*. Medlink Corporation, San Diego.

Jain KK (2009j) *Personalized Medicine*. Jain PharmaBiotech Publications, Basel, pp 300.

Jain KK, Fischer B (1988) New aspects of the use of hyperbaric oxygenation for rehabilitation of stroke patients. *Geriatr Rehabil* 1: 45.

Jain KK, Fischer B, Lehrl S (1988) Mentaltraining: Grundlegende Prinzipien und Anwendungen. *Natur Ganzheit Med 2*: 45–48.

Jain KK, Toole JF (1998a) *Hyperacute Hyperbaric Oxygen Therapy for Cerebral Ischemia* (Edited Proceedings of a Conference, Winston-Salem, NC, November 1997). Undersea Hyperbaric Medical Society, Bethesda, Maryland.

James PB (1981) Problem areas in the therapy of neurological decompression sickness. In James PB (1982a) *The size distribution of gas emboli arising during decompression: A review of the concept of critical diameter*. Proc XIII Annual Congress of EUBS. Dragerwerke, Travemunde, pp 481–486.

James PB (1985) Hyperbaric oxygen and retinal vascular changes: Hyperbaric oxygen and retinal vascular changes. *Med J Aust* 142: 163–164.

James PB (1987) *Hyperbaric oxygen in the therapy of aphonia associated with chronic laryngitis*. Presented at the 9th international congress on hyperbaric medicine, Sydney, Australia, March 1–4.

James PB (1987) The scientific basis for hyperbaric oxygen therapy in focal oedema. In Rose FC, Jones R (Eds.) *Multiple sclerosis*. Libbey, London, pp 223–228.

James PB (1988a) Helium and oxygen mixtures in the treatment of compressed-air illness. *Undersea Biomed Res* 15: 321.

James PB (1988b) Hyperbaric oxygen in neonatal care. *Lancet* 1: 764–765.

James PB (1997) Multiple sclerosis as a diagnosis. *Lancet* 350: 1178.

James PB (2007) Hyperbaric oxygenation in fluid microembolism. *Neurol Res* 29: 156–161.

Jamieson D, Van Den Brenk HAS (1963) Measurement of tension in cerebral tissues of rats exposed to high pressures of oxygen. *J Appl Physiol* 18: 869–876.

Jampol LM (1987) Oxygen therapy and intraocular oxygenation. *Trans Am Ophthalmol Soc* 85: 407–437.

Jampol LM, Orlin C, Cohen SB *et al* (1988) Hyperbaric and transcorneal delivery of oxygen to the rabbit and monkey anterior segment. *Arch Ophthalmol* 106: 825–829.

Jan MH, Jankosky CJ (2003) Multiple sclerosis presenting as neurological decompression sickness in a U. S. navy diver. *Aviat Space Environ Med* 74: 184–6.

Jansen EC, Nielsen NV (2004) Promising visual improvement of cystoid macular edema by hyperbaric oxygen therapy. *Acta Ophthalmol Scand* 82: 485–486.

Jansen HM, Zuurmond WW, Roos CM *et al* (1987) Whole-lung lavage under hyperbaric oxygen conditions for alveolar proteinosis with respiratory failure. *Chest* 91: 829–832.

Jansen T, Barnung S, Mortensen CR, Jansen EC (2003) Isobutyl-nitrite-induced methemoglobinemia; treatment with an exchange blood transfusion during hyperbaric oxygenation. *Acta Anaesthesiol Scand* 47: 1300–1301.

Jarvis RM, Neufeld MV, Westfall CT (2000) Brown recluse spider bite to the eyelid. *Ophthalmology* 107: 1492–6.

Jeffrey M, Wells GAH (1986) Multifocal ischaemic encephalomyelopathy associated with fibrocartilaginous emboli in the lamb. Neuropathol *Appl Neurobiol* 12: 415–24.

Jerrett SA, Jefferson D, Mengel SE (1973) Seizures, H_2O_2 formation, and lipid peroxides in brain during exposure to oxygen under high pressure. *Aerosp Med* 44: 40–44.

Jia SJ, Zhang JD, Qu ZK (1986) *Experience on the clinical use of HBO treatment in cerebral thrombosis: a report of 104 cases.* Presented at the 5th Chinese conference on hyperbaric medicine, Fuzhou, China, Sept 26–29.

Jiang J, Tyssebotn I (1997) Normobaric and hyperbaric oxygen treatment of acute carbon monoxide poisoning in rats. *Undersea Hyperbaric Med* 24: 107–116.

Jiang MY (1986) *Effect of contractility of the myocardium and hemodynamics under 2 ATA combining with external counterpulsation.* Presented at the 5th Chinese conference on hyperbaric medicine. Fuzhow, China, Sept. 26–29.

Jinnai D, Mogami H, Ioko M *et al* (1967) Effect of hyperbaric oxygenation on cereberal edema. *Neurol Med Clin* 9: 260–261.

Jirsa M (1990) Influence of hyperbaric oxygenation on bilirubin and ditaurobilirubin auto-oxidation and porphyrin-sensitized photo-oxidation. *J Photochem Photobiol* 5: 295–302.

Johnson GP (1990) A navigator with non-ischemic central retinal vein occlusion progressing to ischemic central retinal vein occlusion. *Aviat Space Environ Med* 61: 962–965.

Johnson JE, Walford R, Harman D *et al* (1986) *Free radicals, aging, and degenerative diseases.* Liss, New York.

Johnson R (1965) Preliminary observations and results with the use of hyperbaric oxygen and cobalt teletherapy in the treatment of carcinoma of the cervix. *NCI Monogr* 24: 83–91.

Johnson RA, Johnson FK (2000) The effects of carbon monoxide as a neurotransmitter. *Curr Opin Neurol* 13: 709–13.

Jonas JB, Akkoyun I, Kreissig I, Degenring RF (2005) Diffuse diabetic macular edema treated by intravitreal triamcinolone acetonide: a comparative, non-randomized study. *Br J Ophthalmol* 89: 321–326.

Jonas JB, Kreissig I, Degenring RF (2002) Intravitreal triamcinolone acetonide as treatment of macular edema in central retinal vein occlusion. *Graefes Archh Clin Exp Ophthalmol* 240: 782–783.

Jones DP (1985) The role of oxygen concentration in oxidative stress, hypoxic and hyperoxic models. In Sies H (Ed.) *Oxidative stress.* Academic, London.

Jones JP, Ramirez S, Doty SB (1993) The pathophysiologic role of fat in dysbaric osteonecrosis. *Clin Orthop* 296: 256–264.

Jones RF, Unsworth IP, Marosszeky JE (1978) Hyperbaric oxygen and acute spinal cord injuries in humans. *Med J Aust* 2: 573–575.

Jordan WD Jr, Schroeder PT, Fisher WS, McDowell HA (1997) A comparison of angioplasty with stenting versus endarterectomy for the treatment of carotid artery stenosis. *Ann Vasc Surg* 11: 2–8.

Jørgensen TB, Sørensen AM, Jansen EC (2008) Iatrogenic systemic air embolism treated with hyperbaric oxygen therapy. *Acta Anaesthesiol Scand* 52: 566–568.

Juang JH, Hsu BR, Kuo CH, Uengt SW (2002) Beneficial effects of hyperbaric oxygen therapy on islet transplantation. *Cell Transplant* 11: 95–101.

Junod VT (1834) Recherches physiologiques et thérapeutiques sur les effets de la compression et de la rarefaction de l'air, tant sur le corps que sur les membres isoles *Rev Med Fr Etrange* 3: 350.

Jurrell G, Kaisjer L (1973) The influence of varying pressure and duration of treatment with hyperbaric oxygen on the survival of skin flaps. *Scand J Plast Reconstr Surg* 7: 25–58.

K

Kaasik AE, Dmitriev KK, Tomberg TA (1988) Hyperbaric oxygenation in the treatment of patients with ischemic stroke. *Zh Nevropatol Psikhiatr Im S S Korsakova* 88: 38–43.

Kaelin CM, Im MJ, Myers RAM *et al* (1990) The effects of hyperbaric oxygen on free flaps in rats. *Arch Surg* 125: 607–609.

Kahraman S, Düz B, Kayali H *et al* (2007) Effects of methylprednisolone and hyperbaric oxygen on oxidative status after experimental spinal cord injury: a comparative study in rats. *Neurochem Res* 32: 1547–1551.

Kaide CG, Khandelwal S (2008) Hyperbaric oxygen: applications in infectious disease. *Emerg Med Clin North Am* 26: 571–595.

Kaizu T, Ikeda A, Nakao A, Tsung A, Toyokawa H, Ueki S, Geller DA, Murase N (2007) Protection of transplant-induced hepatic ischemia/reperfusion injury with carbon monoxide via MEK/ERK1/2 pathway downregulation. *Am J Physiol Gastrointest Liver Physiol* 294: G236–G244.

Kakhnovskii IM, Efuni SN, Gitel EP (1980a) Effects of hyperbaric oxygenation on the dynamics of the phase structure of right ventricular systole in diabetics. *Ter Arkh* 52: 88–91.

Kakhnovskii IM, Efuni SN, Grishina I (1980c) Electrocardiographic changes during hyperbaric oxygenation in diabetes mellitus. *Kardiologii* 20: 90–94.

Kakhnovskii IM, Efuni SN, Sokolovskaya MV (1982) Correlation of respiratory and pulmonary circulatory oxygenation on the enzyme activity of tissue metabolism in diabetes mellitus. *Probl Endokrinol (Mosk)* 28: 11–17.

Kakhnovskii IM, Pgosbekian LM, Bokaneva IA, Novikova LL, Fedorova EV (1980b) Biochemical indices in diabetes mellitus patients undergoing hyperbaric oxygenation. *Sov Med* 10: 33–37.

Kalani M, Jorneskog G, Naderi N, Lind F, Brismar K (2002) Hyperbaric oxygen (HBO) therapy in treatment of diabetic foot ulcers. Long-term follow-up. *J Diabetes Complications* 16: 153–8.

Kalns J, Krock L, Piepmeier E Jr (1998) The effect of hyperbaric oxygen on growth and chemosensitivity of metastatic prostrate cancer. *Anticancer Res* 18(1A): 363–367.

Kamada T (1985) Superoxide dismutase and hyperbaric oxygen therapy of the patient with rheumatoid arthritis. *Nippon-Seikeigeka Gakkai Zasshi* 59: 17–26.

Kaminski HJ, Ruff RL (1991) Treatment of the elderly patient with headache or trigeminal neuralgia. *Drugs & Aging* 1: 48–56.

Kanno T, Nagata J, Nonomura K et al (1993) New approaches to the treatment of hypertensive intracerebral hemorrhage. *Stroke* 24 (Suppl 12): I96-I100.

Kanno T, Nonomura K (1996) Hyperbaric oxygen therapy to determine the surgical indication for moderate hypertensive intracerebral hemorrhage. *Min Invas Neurosurg* 39: 56–59.

Kapp JP (1979) Hyperbaric oxygen as an adjunct to acute revascularization of the brain. *Surg Neurol* 12: 457–462.

Kapp JP (1980) Neurological response to hyperbaric oxygen – criterion for cerebral revascularization. *Surg Neurol* 15: 43.

Kapp JP, Phillips M et al (1982) Hyperbaric oxygen after circulatory arrest: modification of postischemic encephalopathy. *Neurosurgery* 11: 496–499.

Karagoz B, Suleymanoglu S, Uzun G et al (2008) Hyperbaric oxygen therapy does not potentiate doxorubicin-induced cardiotoxicity in rats. *Basic Clin Pharmacol Toxicol* 102: 287–192.

Karapetian TS, Volozhin AT, Oleinik NN (1985) Treatment of mandibular fractures using hyperbaric oxygenation. *Stomatologiia* (Mosk) 64: 33–38.

Kariakin AM, Kucher VV, Kirienko IV (1992) The pathogenetic and clinical grounds for the advantages of nondrug procedures in the preoperative preparation of patients with diffuse toxic goiter. *Vestn Khir Im I I Grek* 148: 216–20.

Katsenelson K, Arieli Y, Abramovich A, Feinsod M, Arieli R (2007) Hyperbaric oxygen pretreatment reduces the incidence of decompression sickness in rats. *Eur J Appl Physiol* 101: 571–576.

Kau RJ, Sendtner-Gress K, Ganzer U, Arnold W (1997) Effectiveness of hyperbaric oxygen therapy in patients with acute and chronic cochlear disorders. *ORL J Otorhinolaryngol Relat Spec* 59: 79–83.

Kaufman T, Hirshowitz B, Monies-Chass I (1979) Hyperbaric oxygen for postirradiation osteomyelitis of the chest wall. *Harefuah* 97: 220–222, 271.

Kawamura MK, Sakakibara K, Sasakibara B (1976) Protective effect of hyperbaric oxygen for the temporary ischemic myocardium. Macroscopic and histologic data. *Cardiovasc Res* 10: 599–601.

Kawamura MK, Sakakibara K, Yusa T (1978) Effect of increased oxygen on peripheral circulation in acute, temporary limb hypoxia. *J Cardiovasc Surg* 19: 161–168.

Kawamura S, Ohta H, Yasui N et al (1988) Effect of hyperbaric oxygenation in patients with subarachnoid hemorrhage. *J Hyperbaric Med* 3: 243–256.

Kawamura S, Yasui N, Shirasawa M et al (1990) Therapeutic effects of hyperbaric oxygenation on acute focal cerebral ischemia in rats. *Surg Neurol* 34: 101–106.

Kayser B, Jean D, Herry JP et al (1993) Pressurization and acute mountain illness. *Aviat Space Environ Med* 64: 928–931.

Kazantseva NV (1986) Mechanism of action of hyperbaric oxygenation in ischemic stroke. *Zh Nevropatol Psikhiatr* 86: 1315–1320.

Kearney KR, Smith MD, Xie GY et al (1997) Massive air embolus to the left ventricle: Diagnosis and monitoring by serial echocardiography. *J Am Soc Echocardiogr* 10: 982–987.

Keenan HT, Bratton SL, Norkool DM et al (1998) Delivery of hyperbaric oxygen therapy to critically ill, mechanically ventilated children. *J Crit Care* 13: 7–12.

Kei PL, Choong CT, Young T, Lee SH, Lim CC (2007) Decompression sickness: MRI of the spinal cord. *J Neuroimaging* 17: 378–380.

Keim L et al (1997) Quantitative SPECT scanning in the assessment of patients with ischemic/traumatic brain injury treated with HBO-preliminary observations. *Am Coll Chest Phys Annual Meeting.*

Kelly DL, Lassiter KRL, Vongsvivut A, Smith JM et al (1972) Effects of hyperbaric oxygenation and tissue oxygen studies in experimental paraplegia. *Neurosurg* 36: 425–429.

Kendig JJ, Cohen EN (1977) Pressure antagonism to nerve conduction block by anesthetic agents. *Anesthesiology* 228: 6–10.

Kenmure ACF, Murdock WR, Hutton I et al (1972) Hemodynamic effects of oxygen at 1 and 2 atmosphere pressure in healthy subjects. *J Appl Physiol* 32: 223–225.

Kenney RA (1985) Physiology of aging. *Clin Geriatr Med* 1: 37–59.

Kerns W, Isom G, Kirk M (2002) Cyanide and hydrogen sulfide. In Goldfrank LR et al (Eds.) *Goldfrank's Toxicologic Emergencies* pp 1498–1510.

Kestler M, Strutz J, Heiden C (2001) Hyperbaric oxygenation in early treatment of sudden deafness. *HNO* 49: 719–23.

Kern M, Sommerauer P, Wochesländer E et al (1986) Application of hyperbaric oxygen therapy in patients with toxic ambyopia. *Ophthalmologie* 83: 312–314.

Kerwin SC, Hosgood G, Strain GM et al (1992) The effect of hyperbaric oxygen treatment on a compromised axial pattern flap in the cat. *Veterinary Surgery* 22: 31–36.

Kety SS, Schmidt CF (1948) The effects of altered arterial tensions of carbon dioxide and oxygen on cerebral blood flow and cerebral oxygen consumption of normal young men. *J Clin Invest* 27: 484–492.

Keynan Y, Yanir Y, Shupak A (2006) Hyperbaric therapy for bilateral visual loss during hemodialysis. *Clin Exp Nephrol* 10: 82–84.

Kharchenko NM, Boikova SP, Drozdova GA, Demurov EA (1986) Structural changes in the lungs induced by different levels of hyperbaric oxygenation. *Biull Eksp Biol Med* 102: 604–606.

Khiabani KT, Nataraj C, Gabriel A, Stephenson LL, Zamboni WA (2001) Effects of hyperbaric oxygen on ischemia reperfusion induced pmnCD18 polarization. *Undersea Hyperbaric Med* 28(Suppl): 29–30.

Kidokoro M, Sakakibara K, Rakako T, Nimei M, Hibi Y et al (1969) Experimental and clinical studies upon hyperbaric oxygen therapy for peripheral vascular disorders. In Wada J, Iwa T (Eds.) *Hyperbaric Medicine.* Williams and Wilkins, Baltimore, pp 462–468.

Kiene H, von Schön-Angerer (1998) Single-case causality assessment as a basis for clinical judgment. *Alt Ther* 4(1): 41–47.

Kienle GS, Kiene H (1996) Placebo effect and placebo concept: a critical methodological and conceptual analysis of reports on the magnitude of the placebo effect. *Alt Ther* 2(6): 39–54.

Kienlen J, Alardo JP, Dimeglio G et al (1974) Traitement de l'intoxication oxycarbonée par l'oxygène hyperbare – propos de 370 observations. *J Méd Montpellier* 9: 237–243.

Kieper NR (1987) The use of hyperbaric oxygen in the rehabilitation of spinal cord injured patients due to decompression sickness. In Kindwall EP (Ed.) *Proceedings of the 8th international congress on hyperbaric medicine.* Best, San Pedro.

Kim CH, Choi H, Chun YS et al (2001) Hyperbaric oxygenation pretreatment induces catalase and reduces infarct size in ischemic rat myocardium. *Pflugers Arch* 442: 519–25.

Kindwall EP (1992) Creating hyperbaric oxygen unit in a major medical center: a personal experience. *Ann Plast Surg* 29: 543–549.

Kindwall EP (1993) Hyperbaric oxygen. *BMJ* 307: 515–516.

Kindwall EP (1993) Hyperbaric oxygen treatment of radiation cystitis. *Clinics in Plast Surg* 20: 589–592.

Kindwall EP, Goldmann RW (1988) *Hyperbaric medicine procedures.* St. Luke's Medical Center, Milwaukee.

Kindwall EP, Gottlieb LJ, Larson DL (1991a) Hyperbaric oxygen therapy in plastic surgery: A review article. *Plastic Reconstruct Surg* 1991: 898–908.

Kindwall EP, McQuillen MP, Khatri BO *et al* (1991b) Treatment of multiple sclerosis with hyperbaric oxygen. Results of a national registry. *Arch Neurol* 48: 195–199.

Kinney JA, Hammond R, Gelfand R *et al* (1978) Visual evoked cortical potentials in men during compression and saturation in He-O2 equivalent to 400, 800, 1200 and 1600 feet of sea water. *Electroencephalogr Clin Neurophysiol* 44: 157–171.

Kinney JS (1985) Human Underwater Vision: Physiology and Physics. *Bethesda: Undersea and Hyperbaric Society:* 158.

Kirk J, Wingate GW, Watson ER (1976) High-dose effects in the treatment of carcinoma of the bladder under air and hyperbaric oxygen conditions. *Clin Radiol* 27: 137–144.

Kiryu J, Ogura Y (1996) Hyperbaric oxygen treatment for macular edema in retinal vein occlusion: relation to severity of retinal leakage. *Ophthalmologica* 210: 168–170.

Kislyakov YY, Kopyltsov AV (1988) The rate of gas-bubble growth in tissue under decompression. Mathematical modeling. *Respir Physiol* 71: 299–306.

Kitani Y, Miura K, Uchihashi *et al* (1987) *Hyperbaric oxygen therapy for central nervous system disorders and PET (positron emission tomography).* Presented at the 9th international congress on hyperbaric medicine, 1–4 March, Sydney, Australia.

Kitaoka K, Nakagawa Y, Abe H *et al* (1983) Hyperbaric oxygen treatment in patients with the postoperative mental signs after direct operations of ruptured anterior communicating aneurysms. *Hokkaido Igaku Zasshi* 58: 154–161.

Kiuchi T, Oike F, Yamamoto H (2003) Small for size graft in liver transplantation. *Nagoya J Med. Sci.* 66(3–4): 95–102.

Kivisaari J, Niinikoski J (1975) Effects of hyperbaric oxygenation and prolonged hypoxia on the healing of open wounds. *Acta Chir Scand* 141: 14–19.

Kizer KW (1982) Delayed treatment of dysbarism. *JAMA* 247: 2555–2558.

Klebanoff S (1980) Oxygen metabolism and the toxic properties of phagocytes. *Ann Intern Med* 93: 480–489.

Klebs D (1865) Ueber die Wirkung des Kohlenoxyds auf den tierischen Organismus. *Arch Path Anat Physiol Klin Med* 32: 450–517.

Kleep G (1977) Additive Wirkung von hyperbarem Sauerstoff und intraaortaler Ballonpumpe bei der Therapie des akuten Koronarverschlusses im Experiment. *Wien Med Wochenschr* 127: 35.

Klempner Ms, Hu LT, Evans J *et al* (2001) Two controlled trials of antibiotic treatment in patients with persistent symptoms and a history of Lyme disease. *New Engl J Med* 345: 85–92.

Kline HJ, Marano AJ, Johnson CD *et al* (1979) Hemodynamics and metabolic effects of hyperbaric oxygenation in myocardial infarction. *J Appl Physiol* 28: 256–263.

Knighton D, Silver I, Hunt TK (1981) Regulation of wound healing angiogenesis: effect of oxygen gradients and inspired oxygen concentration. *Surg* 90: 262–270.

Koch A, Vermeulen-Cranch DME (1962) The use of hyperbaric oxygen following cardiac arrest. *Brit J Anaesth* 34: 738–740.

Koch AE, Kähler W, Wegner-Bröse H *et al* (2008) Monitoring of CBFV and time characteristics of oxygen-induced acute CNS toxicity in humans. *Eur J Neurol* 15: 746–748.

Koerner SK (1971) Oxygen in ischemic heart disease. *Am Heart J* 82: 269–274.

Kohshi K, Imada H, Nomoto S *et al* (2003) Successful treatment of radiation-induced brain necrosis by hyperbaric oxygen therapy. *J Neurol Sci* 209: 115–7.

Kohshi K, Kinoshita Y, Terashima H *et al* (1996) Radiotherapy after hyperbaric oxygenation for malignant gliomas: a pilot study. *J Cancer Res Clin Oncol* 122: 676–678.

Kohshi K, Wong RM, Abe H *et al* (2005) Neurological manifestations in Japanese Ama divers. *Undersea Hyperb Med* 32: 11–20.

Kohshi K, Yokota A, Konda N *et al* (1993) Hyperbaric oxygen therapy adjunctive to mild hypertensive hypervolumia for symptomatic vasospasm. *Neurol Med Chir (Tokyo)* 33: 92–99.

Kokame GT, Ing MR (1994) Intraocular gas and low-altitude air flight. *Retina* 14: 356–358.

Kol S, Adir Y, Gordon CR *et al* (1993) Oxy-helium treatment of severe spinal cord decompression sickness after air diving. *Undersea Hyperbaric Med* 20: 147–154.

Kol S, Ammar R, Weisz G *et al* (1993a) Hyperbaric oxygenation for arterial air embolism during cardiopulmonary bypass. *Ann Thorac Surg* 55: 401–403.

Kolontai YU, Smirnova LA, Kondrashov AN (1976) Treatment of open fractures in long tubular bones. *Sov Med* 39: 94–100.

Koloskow JB, Dumurow JA (1986) The influence of hyperbaric oxygen in the treatment of gastric and duodenal ulcers. In Schmutz J (Ed.) *Proceedings of the 1st Swiss symposium on hyperbaric medicine.* Foundation for Hyperbaric Medicine, Basel, pp 212–221.

Komarov FI, Pogronov AP, Egorov AP *et al* (1985) Treatment of gastric and intestinal ulcers by hyperbaric oxygen. *Hyperbaric Oxygen Rev* 6: 227–230.

Kohmoto J, Nakao A, Kaizu T, Tsung A, Ikeda A, Tomiyama K, Billiar TR, Choi AM, Murase N, McCurry KR (2006) Low-dose carbon monoxide inhalation prevents ischemia/reperfusion injury of transplanted rat lung grafts. *Surgery* 140(2): 179–185.

Kondo A, Baba S, Iwaki T *et al* (1996) Hyperbaric oxygenation prevents delayed neuronal death following transient ischaemia in the gerbil hippocampus. *Neuropathol App Neurobiol* 22: 350–360.

Kondrashenko VT (1980) Hypoxia in acute exogenous psychoses and its treatment. *Zh Nevropatol Psikhiatr* 80: 898–904.

Koren G, Sharav T, Pastuszak A *et al* (1991) A multicenter, prospective study of fetal outcome following accidental carbon monoxide poisoning in pregnancy. *Reprod Toxicol* 5: 397–403.

Korhonen K, Klossner J, Hirn M, Niinikoski J (1999) Management of clostridial gas gangrene and the role of hyperbaric oxygen. *Ann Chir Gynaecol* 88: 139–42.

Korhonen K (2000) Hyperbaric oxygen therapy in acute necrotizing infections. With a special reference to the effects on tissue gas tensions. *Ann Chir Gynaecol* 89 (Suppl 214): 7–36.

Korkhov SI, Kilchevsky GS, Shiryaev II *et al* (1981) Hyperbaric oxygenation in complex treatment of hypoxic status of the liver. In Yefuny SN (Ed.) *Proceedings of the 7th international congress on hyperbaric medicine.* USSR Academy of Sciences, Moscow, p 354.

Korn HN, Wheeler ES, Miller TA (1977) Effect of hyperbaric oxygen on second degree burn wound healing. *Arch Surg* 122: 732–737.

Korobova LN, Kabakhbaseheva IK, Khodakova AA *et al* (1981) Dynamics of histamine in the blood of pregnant women receiving hyperbaric therapy fordiabetes mellitus. In Yefuny SN (Ed.) *Proceedings of the 7th international congress for hyperbaric medicine. USSR Academy of Sciences, Moscow, p 362.

Korotaev GM, Zavarzin YA, Mamorov SD (1981) Hyperbaric treatment of patients with bronchial asthma. In Yefuni SN (Ed.) Proceedings of the 7th international congress on hyperbaric medicine. USSR Academy of Sciences, Moscow, p 291.

Kosonogov LF, Leonov AN, Shapovalova NV (1978) Extracorporeal perfusion and hyperbaric oxygenation in the treatment of severe traumatic shock. Anesteziol Reanimatol 6: 24–29.

Kostiunin VN, Pahkomov VI, Feoktistov PL et al (1985) Increasing the effectiveness of hyperbaric oxygenation in the treatment of patients with stage IV arterial occlusive disease of the lower limbs. Vestn Khir 135: 48–51.

Kot J, Desola J, Simao AG et al (2004) A European code of good practice for hyperbaric oxygen therapy. Int Marit Health 55: 121–130.

Kothari R, Barsan W, Brott T et al (1995) Frequency and accuracy of prehospital diagnosis of acute stroke. Stroke 26: 937–941.

Kovacevic H (1992) The Investigation of Hyperbaric Oxygen Influence in the Patients with Second Degree of Atherosclerotic Insufficiency of Lower Extremities, Doctoral Dissertation, University of Rijeka, Croatia.

Koyama K (1976) Acute experimental carbon monoxide poisoning and hyperbaric oxygenation (HBO). Tokyo Jikeikai Med J 91: 195–215.

Koziner VB, Yarochkin VS, Fedorov NA, Kolonina IR (1981) Life support by oxygen breathing after total blood replacement by dextran. Exp Biol Med 91: 444–446.

Kozyro VI, Matskevich MV (1981) Clinical aspects of using hyperbaric oxygenation in the treatment of different forms of neurosensory hypoacusis. In Yefuny SN (Ed.) Abstracts of the 7th international congress on HBO medicine. USSR Academy of Sciences, Moscow, pp 306–307.

Krabbe AA (1986) Cluster headache: a review. Acta Neurologica Scandinavica 74: 1–9.

Krakovsky M, Rogatsky G, Zarchin N et al (1998) Effect of hyperbaric oxygen therapy on survival after global cerebral ischemia in rats. Surgical Neurology 49: 412–416.

Kramer WG, Welch DW, Fife WP et al (1983a) Salicylate pharmacokinetics in the dog at 6 ATA in air and at 2.8 ATA in 100% oxygen. Aviat Space Environ Med 54: 682–684.

Kramer WG, Welch DW, Fife WP et al (1983b) Pharmacokinetics of pentobarbital under hyperbaric and hyperoxic conditions in the dog. Aviat Space Environ Med 54: 1005–1008.

Krasnov MM, Kharlap SI, Pereverzina OK et al (1981) Hyperbaric oxygenation in the treatment of vascular diseases of retina. In Yefuny SN (Ed.) Abstracts of the 7th international congress on hyperbaric medicine. USSR Academy of Sciences, Moscow, p 304.

Krill AE, Archer D, Newell FW (1971) Photocoagulation in complications secondary to branch vein occlusion. Arch Ophthalmol 85: 48–60.

Kron RER, Garfinkel SL, Pfeffer SL, Gordon JE, Abraham A (1981) Hyperbaric oxygen therapy in senile dementia: a review. In Yefuni SN (Ed.) Abstracts of the 7th international congress of HBO medicine. USSR Academy of Sciences, Moscow, pp 301–302.

Krott R, Heller S, Aisenbrey S, Bartz-Schmidt KU (2000) Adjunctive hyperbaric oxygenation in macular edema of vascular origin. Undersea Hyperb Med 27: 195–204.

Krupka M, Raska M, Belakova J, Horynova M, Novotny R, Weigl E (2007) Biological aspects of Lyme disease spirochetes: unique bac-

teria of the Borrelia burgdorferi species group. Biomed Pap Med Fac Univ Palacky Olomouc Czech Repub 151: 175–186.

Krupp LB, Hyman LG, Grimson R et al (2003) Study and treatment of post Lyme disease (STOP-LD: a randomized double-masked clinical trial. Neurology 60: 1923–1930.

Kudchodkar BJ, Pierce A, Dory L (2007) Chronic hyperbaric oxygen treatment elicits an anti-oxidant response and attenuates atherosclerosis in apoE knockout mice. Atherosclerosis 193: 28–35.

Kudrow L (1981) Response of cluster headache attacks to oxygen inhalation. Headache 21: 1–4.

Kuhl DE, Phelps ME, Kowell AP, Metter EJ, Selin C, Winter J (1980). Effects of Stroke on Local Cerebral Metabolism and Perfusion: Mapping by Emission Computed Tomography of 18FDG and 13NH3. Ann Neurol 8: 47–60.

Kuhn LA (1974) Clinical management of cardiogenic shock. Bull NY Acad Med 50: 366–390.

Kulak RG, Friedman B, Gelernt IM, Jacobson JH (1978) The entrapped intestinal balloon colon deflation by hyperbaric therapy. Ann Surg 187: 309–312.

Kuleshova MP, Flora AA (1981) Physical rehabilitation of patients with ischemic heart disease using hyperbaric oxygen. In Yefuny SN (Ed.) Proceedings of the 7th international congress of hyperbaric medicine, USSR Academy of Sciences, Moscow, p 268.

Kumagai K, Furukawa M, Ogino N, Larson E, Uemura A (2007) Long-term visual outcomes after vitrectomy for macular edema with foveal hemorrhage in branch retinal vein occlusion. Retina 27: 584–588.

Kuokkanen J, Aarnisalo AA, Ylikoski J (2000) Efficiency of hyperbaric oxygen therapy in experimental acute acoustic trauma from firearms. Acta Otolaryngol Suppl 543: 132–4.

Kurir TT, Markotic A, Katalinic V, Bozanic D, Cikes V, Zemunik T, Modun D, Rincic J, Boraska V, Bota B, Salamunic I, Radic S (2004) Effect of hyperbaric oxygenation on the regeneration of the liver after partial hepatectomy in rats. Braz J Med Biol Res 37(8): 1231–1237.

Kurita A, Nagayoshi H, Okamoto Y et al (2002) Effects of severe hyperbaric pressure on autonomic nerve functions. Mil Med 167: 934–8.

Kurok AM, Kitaoka T, Taniguchi H, Amemiya T (2002) Hyperbaric oxygen therapy reduces visual field defect after macular hole surgery. Ophthalmic Surg Lasers 33: 200–6.

Kuroki K, Masuda A, Uehara H, Kuroki A (1998) A new treatment for toxic megacolon. Lancet 352: 782.

Kurschel S, Mohia A, Weigl V, Eder HG (2006) Hyperbaric oxygen therapy for the treatment of brain abscess in children. Childs Nerv Syst 22(1): 38–42.

Kurtzke JF (1961) On the evaluation of disability in multiple sclerosis. Neurology 11: 686–94.

Kurusz M, Roach JD, Vertrees RA, Girouard MK, Lick SD (2002) Leukocyte filtration in lung transplantation. Perfusion 17(Suppl 2): 63–67.

Kuyama T, Umemura H, Sudo T et al (1988) Clinical studies on various therapy for the intractable trauma of toes and fingers in cases of diabetes mellitus and peripheral ischemic diseases. Nippon Geka Gakkai Zasshi 89: 763–770.

Kuzemko JA, Loder RE (1970) Purpura fulminans treated with hyperbaric oxygen. Br Med J 4: 157.

L

Laloux P, Richelle F, Meurice H, De Coster P (1995) Cerebral blood flow and perfusion reserve capacity in hemodynamic carotid transient ischemic attacks due to innominate artery stenosis. *J Nucl Med* 36: 1286–1271.

Lambertsen CJ (1988) *Physiologic factors in human organ oxygen tolerance extension.* XIVth annual meeting of the European Undersea Biomedical Society, Aberdeen, Scotland, 5–9 September, 1988.

Lamm CH, Walliser U, Schumann K, Lamm K (1988) Sauerstoffpartialdruck-Messungen in der Perilymphe der Scala tympani unter normo- und hyperbaren Bedingungen. *HNO* 36: 363–366.

Lamm H (1969) *Klinische Ergebnisse nach Behandlung von Innenohrschwerhörigkeiten mit hyperbarem Sauerstoff.* Contribution at the HNO Annual Congress of the DDR, Halle/Saale.

Lamm K, Arnold W (1999) Successful treatment of noise-induced cochlear ischemia, hypoxia, and hearing loss. *Ann N Y Acad Sci* 884: 233–48.

Lamm H, Dahl D, Gerstmann W (1977) Die Wirkung von hyperbarem Sauerstoff (OHP) auf die hypoxisch geschädigte Cochlea des Meerschweinchens. *Arch Otorhinolaryngol* 217: 415–421.

Lamm H, Gerstmann W (1974) Erste Erfahrungen mit der hyperbaren Oxygenation in der Otologie. *Wochenschr Ohrenheilk (Wien)* 108: 6–11.

Lamm H, Klimpel L (1971) Hyperbare Sauerstofftherapie bei Innenohr- und Vestibularisstörungen. *HNO* 19: 363–369.

Lamm H, Lamm K (1987) The effect of hyperbaric oxygen on the inner ear. In Kindwall EP (Ed.) *Proceedings of the 8th international congress on hyperbaric medicine.* Best, San Pedro, p 35.

Lamm K, Lamm H, Arnold W (1998) Effect of hyperbaric oxygen therapy in comparison to conventional or placebo therapy or no treatment in idiopathic sudden hearing loss, acoustic trauma, noise-induced hearing loss and tinnitus. A literature survey. *Adv Otorhinolaryngol* 54: 86–99.

Lamm K, Lamm CH, Lamm H, Schumann K (1989a) The effect of hyperbaric oxygen on noise-induced hearing loss. An experimental study using simultaneous measurements of oxygen partial pressure in the inner ear, hearing potentials, arterial blood pressure and blood gas analyses. In Schmutz J, Bakker D (Eds.) *Proceedings of the joint meeting: 2nd Swiss symposium on hyperbaric medicine and 2nd European conference on hyperbaric medicine,* Basel, Switzerland, Sept 22–24.

Lamm K, Lamm CH, Lamm H, Schumann K (1989b) *Simultane Laser-Doppler-Flow Metrie zur Bestimmung des kochleären Blutflusses, Sauerstoffpartialdruckmessungen und Elektrokochleographie während Hämootilution.* 60th annual meeting, Deutsche Gesellschaft HNO Heilkunde, Kiel.

Lamm H, Lamm K, Zimmermann W (1982) The effects of hyperbaric oxygen on experimental noise damage to the ears. *Arch Otorhinolaryngol* 236: 237–244.

Lampl LA, Frey G, Dietze T et al (1989) Hyperbaric oxygen in intracranial abscesses. *J Hyperbaric Med* 4: 111–126.

Landau Z, Schattner A (2001) Topical hyperbaric oxygen and low energy laser therapy for chronic diabetic foot ulcers resistant to conventional treatment. *Yale J Biol Med* 74: 95–100.

Landaw SA, Leon HA, Winchell HS (1979) Effects of hyperoxia on red blood cell survival in the normal rat. *Aerospace Med* 41: 48–55.

Landers MB (1978) Retinal oxygenation via the choroidal circulation. *Trans Am Ophthalmol Soc* 76: 528–556.

Lang GE, Kuba GB (1997) High altitude retinopathy. *Am J Ophthalmol* 123: 418–420.

Larcan A, Laprevote-Heully MC, Lambert H et al (1977) Indications des thrombolytiques au cours des accidents vasculaires cérébraux thrombosants traités par ailleurs. *Thérapie* 32: 259.

Larcan V, Laprevote-Heully MC, Lambert H et al (1973) Intoxication and ingestion of a massive dose of CCl4. Recovery probably related to early hyperbaric oxygen therapy. *Eur J Toxicol* 5: 286–289.

Lareng L, Brouchet A, Plat JJ (1973) Experience of hyperbaric oxygen therapy in 2 cases of traumatic coma. *Anesth Reanim* 30: 525–532.

Larsen PE, Stronczek MJ, Beck FM et al (1993) Osteointegration of implants in radiated bones with and without adjunctive hyperbaric oxygen. *J Oral Maxillofac Surg* 51: 280–287.

Larsson A, Engstrom M, Uusijarvi J et al (2002) Hyperbaric oxygen treatment of postoperative neurosurgical infections. *Neurosurgery* 50: 287–296.

Lassen NA, Palvölgyi R (1968) Cerebral steal during hypercapnia observed by the 133-xenon technique in man. *Scand J Clin Lab Invest {Suppl}* 102: XIII-D.

Lautin EM, Scheinbaum KR (1987) Hyperbaric therapy for the removal of an obstructing intestinal tube balloon. *Gastrointest Radio* 12: 243–244.

LaVan FB, Hunt TK (1990) Oxygen and wound healing. *Clinics Plastic Surg* 17: 463–472.

Laverdant C, Molinie C, Poujol C et al (1971) Résultats comparés du traitement de deux groupes l'hepatites virales graves. *Ann Med Interne* 122: 85–91.

Laverdant C, Poujol C, Lombard E et al (1973) A further comparative study of the treatment of two groups of patients suffering from malignant viral hepatitis. *Lyon Med* 230(20): 767–771.

Lavoisier and Seguin (1789) Traité élémentaire de chimie. *Ouvres de Lavoisier, Vol I.* Imprimerie Impériale, Paris.

Lavoute C, Weiss M, Sainty JM et al (2008) Post effect of repetitive exposures to pressure nitrogen-induced narcosis on the dopaminergic activity at atmospheric pressure. *Undersea Hyperb Med* 35: 21–25.

Lawrence DA, Luskutoff DJ (1986) Inactivation of plasminogen inhibitor by oxidants, *Biochemistry* 25(21): 6351–6355.

Lebedov VV, Isakov IV, Pravdenkova SV (1983) Effect of hyperbaric oxygenation on the clinical course and complications of the acute period of ischemic strokes. *Zh Vopr Neikrohik* 3: 37.

Leber KA, Eder HG, Kovac H et al (1998) Treatment of cerebral radionecrosis by hyperbaric oxygen therapy. *Stereotact Funct Neurosurg* 70 Suppl 1: 229–36.

Ledingham IM, McBride TI, Jennett WB, Adams JH (1968). Fatal brain damage associated with cardiomyopathy of pregnancy, with notes on Caesarean section in a hyperbaric chamber. *Br Med J* 4: 285–7.

Ledingham IMA (1969) Hyperbaric oxygen in shock. *Int Anesthesiol Clin* 7: 819–839.

Lee DJ, Moini M, Giuliano J, Westra WH (1996) Hypoxic sensitizer and cytotoxin for head and neck cancer. *Ann Acad Med Singapore* 25: 397–404.

Lee HC, Niu KC, Chen HC et al (1988) Therapeutic effect on type II decompression sickness. *J Hyperbaric Med* 3: 235–242.

Lee HC, Niu KC, Chen SH, Chang LP, Huang KL, Tsai JD, Chan LS (1991) Therapeutic effects of different tables on type II decompression sickness, *J Hyperbaric Med,* 6(1): 11–17.

Lee YH, Lee JY, Kim YS, Kim DH, Kim J (2006) Successful anticoagulation for bilateral central retinal vein occlusions accompanied by cerebral venous thrombosis. *Arch Neurol* 63: 1648–1651.

Leifer G (2001) Hyperbaric oxygen therapy. *Am J Nurs* 101: 26–34.

Leitch DR, Green RD (1986) Pulmonary barotrauma in divers and the treatment of cerebral arterial gas embolism. *Aviat Space Environ Med* 57: 931–938.

Leitch DR, Greenbaum LJJ, Hallenbeck JM (1984a) Cerebral arterial air embolism: 1. Is there benefit in beginning HBO treatment at 6 bar? *Undersea Biomed Res* 11: 221–235.

Leitch DR, Greenbaum LJJ, Hallenbeck JM (1984b) Cerebral arterial air embolism: II. Effect of pressure and time on cortical evoked potential recovery. *Undersea Biomed Res* 11: 237–248.

Leitch DR, Greenbaum LJJ, Hallenbeck JM (1984c) Cerebral arterial air embolism: III. Cerebral blood flow after decompression from various pressure treatments. *Undersea Biomed Res* 11: 249–263.

Leitch DR, Greenbaum LJJ, Hallenbeck JM (1984d) Cerebral arterial air embolism: IV. Failure to recover with treatment, and secondary deterioration. *Undersea Biomed Res* 11: 265–274.

Leitch DR, Hallenbeck JM (1984) Remote monitoring of neuroaxial function in anesthetized dogs in compression chambers. *Electroencephalog Clin Neurophysiol*, 57: 548–560.

Le Mouel C, Renon P, Asperge SUC, Asperge A (1981) Hyperbaric treatment of dive-induced inner ear accidents. *Med Subaquat Hyperbare* 79: 242–246.

Leninger-Follert E, Hossmann KA (1977) Microflow and cortical oxygen pressure during and after prolonged cerebral ischemia. *Brain Res* 124: 158–161.

Lepawsky M, Tredwall SJ, Kirenman DS (1983) *Avascular osteonecrosis ameliorated by hyperbaric oxygen*. Paper presented at the Ist European conference on hyperbaric medicine. Amsterdam, Sept 7–9.

Leplow B, Tetzlaff K, Holl D, Zeng L, Spatial orientation in construction divers – are there associations with diving experience? (2001) *Int Arch Occup Environ Health* 74: 189–98.

Lepoire J, Larcan A, Fiévé et al (1972) Les occlusions carotidiennes aigues posttraumatiques. Diagnostic et thérapeutique. *J Chir (Paris)* 104: 129–142.

Lerman S (1992) Free radical damage and defence mechanisms in the ocular lens. *Lens Eye Toxicol Res* 9: 9–24.

LeRouic JF, Beggani RA, Rumen F et al (2001) Adventitial sheathotomy for decompression of recent onset branch retinal vein occlusion. *Graefes Arch Clin Exp Ophthalmol* 239: 747–751.

Levitt M (1971) Volume and composition of human intestinal gas determined by means of an intestinal washout technique. *N Engl J Med* 284: 1394–1398.

Levy A, Ngai SH, Finck AD et al (1976) Disposition of propanolol isomers in mice. *Eur J Pharmacol*: 93–100.

Lewis G, Mervin K, Valter K et al (1999) Limiting the proliferation and reactivity of retinal Muller cells during experimental retinal detachment: the value of oxygen supplementation. *Am J Ophthalmol* 128: 165–172.

Li HK, Dejean BJ, Tang RA (1996) Reversal of visual loss with hyperbaric oxygen treatment in a patient with Susac syndrome. *Ophthalmology* 103: 2091–2098.

Li P, Nighawan D, Budihardjo I, Srinivasulas SM, Ahmed M, Alenari ES, Warg X (1997) Cytochrome C and dATP-dependent formation of Apaf-1/caspase-9 complex initiates an apoptotic protease cascade. *Cell*: 91, 479–489.

Li W (1987) *Myasthenia gravis treated by hyperbaric oxygenation. A report of 40 cases*. Presented at the 9th international congress on hyperbaric medicine. Sydney, Australia, March 1–4.

Li XL, Li WR, Lin HY (1986) *Effect of hyperbaric oxygen therapy on the patients' blood rheology*. Presented at the 5th Chinese conference on hyperbaric medicine, Fuzhow, China, Sept. 26–29.

Li Y, Zhou C, Calvert JW, Colohan AR, Zhang JH (2005) Multiple effects of hyperbaric oxygen on the expression of HIF-1 alpha and apoptotic genes in a global ischemia-hypotension rat model. *Exp Neurol* 191(1): 198–210.

Liboni W, Molinari F, Allais G, Mana O, Negri E, Grippi G, Benedetto C, D'Andrea G, Bussone G (2007) Why do we need NIRS in migraine? *Neurol Sci* 28(Suppl 2): S222–S224.

Lilienthal JL, Fugitt CH (1946) The effect of low concentrations of carboxyhemoglobin on the "altitude tolerance" of man. *Am J Physiol* 145: 359–364.

Lim M, Jackson TA, Anfinrud PA (1995) Binding of CO to myoglobin from a heme pocket docking site to form nearly linear Fe-C-O. *Science* 269: 962–966.

Lin Y, Jamieson D (1993) Are leukotrienes or PAF involved in hyperbaric oxygen toxicity. *Agents Actions* 38: 66–75.

Lin S, Shyu KG, Lee CC et al (2002) Hyperbaric oxygen selectively induces angiopoietin-2 in human umbilical vein endothelial cells. *Biochem Biophys Res Commun* 296: 710–5.

Lincoff H, Weinburger D, Stergiu P (1989) Air travel with intraocular gas II – clinical considerations. *Arch Ophthalmol* 107: 907.

Lindenmann J, Matzi V, Kaufmann P et al (2006) Hyperbaric oxygenation in the treatment of life-threatening isobutyl nitrite-induced methemoglobinemia – a case report. *Inhal Toxicol* 18: 1047–1049.

Ling SS, Sader C (2008) Fungal malignant otitis externa treated with hyperbaric oxygen. *Int J Infect Dis* 12: 550–552.

Lischak MW, Fanton JW, Hubbard GH et al (1987) *Hyperbaric oxygen 100% therapy as an adjuvant in the treatment of resuscitated (Brooke formula) guinea pig burn* (3°m 50% BSA) *shock*. Presented at the 9th international congress on hyperbaric medicine, Sydney, Australia, March 1–4.

Litavrin AF, Platonova GB, Gribanov VA (1985) Hyperbaric oxygenation in the treatment of facial neuritis. *Zh Nevropatol Psikhiatr* 85: 528–531.

Litovitz TL, Larkin RF, Myers RAM (1983) Cyanide poisoning treated with hyperbaric oxygen. *Am J Emerg Med* 1: 94–101.

Little T, Butler BD (2008) Pharmacological intervention to the inflammatory response from decompression sickness in rats. *Aviat Space Environ Med* 79: 87–93.

Liu JL (1992) Clinical analysis of radiation optic neuropathy. *Chung Hua Yen Ko Tsa Chih* 28: 86–88.

Liu M-N, Zhuang S-Q, Zhang H-Y, Qin Z-Y, Li X-Y (2006) Long-term effects of early hyperbaric oxygen therapy on neonatal rats with hypoxic-ischemic brain damage. *Zhongguo Dang Dai Er Ke Za Zhi* 8(3): 216–220.

Liu X-h, Zhao Y-l, Ma Q-m, Zhou X-h, Wang Y (2006) Optimal therapeutic window of hyperbaric oxygenation in neonatal rat with hypoxic-ischemic brain damage. *Zhonghua Er Ke Za Zhi* 44(3): 177–181.

Liu Z, Xiong T, Meads C (2006) Clinical effectiveness of treatment with hyperbaric oxygen for neonatal hypoxic-ischaemic encephalopathy: systematic review of Chinese literature. *BMJ* 333 (7564): 374 epub 2006, May 11.

Liu Z, Xiong T, Meads C (2006) Clinical effectiveness of treatment with hyperbaric oxygen for neonatal hypoxic-ischaemic encephalopathy: systematic review of Chinese literature. *BMJ* 333: 374.

Liu ZF, Zhi Y (1986) *Application of HBO in the treatment of 387 cases of bronchial asthma*. Presented at the 5th Chinese congress on hyperbaric medicine. Fuzhow, China, Sept 26–29.

Liu ZJ, Velazquez OC (2008) Hyperoxia, Endothelial Progenitor Cell Mobilization, and Diabetic Wound Healing. *Antioxid Redox Signal* 10: 1869–1882.

Lo WD, Wolny A, Boesel C (1994) Blood-brain barrier permeability in the staphylococcal cerebritis and early brain abscess. *J Neurosurg* 80: 897–905.

Locher DH, Adesina A, Wolf TC *et al* (1996) Postoperative Rhizopus scleritis in a diabetic man. *J Cataract Refract Surg* 24: 562–565.

Locke GE, Yashon D, Feldman RA *et al* (1971) Ischemia in primate spinal cord injury. *J Neurosurg* 34: 614.

Locket S (1973) Clinical toxicology. IV. The treatment of poisoning. What do I do first? Part 2. *Practitioner* 210: 575–579.

Loder R (1977) Use of hyperbaric oxygen in paralytic ileus. *Br Med J* 1: 1448–1449.

Longoni C, Ferani R, Agliati G *et al* (1987) *Hyperbaric oxygen therapy and glucose metabolism in patients with diabetic vasculopathic lesions.* Presented at the European Undersea and Biomedical Society meeting, Palermo, Italy, Sept 9–12.

Lotovin AP, Morozov VG, Khavinson VK *et al* (1981) On the problem of cellular and humoral activity under conditions of hyperoxia. In Yefuni SN (Ed.) *Proceedings of the 7th international congress on hyperbaric medicine.* USSR Academy of Sciences, Moscow, p 399.

Low PA, Schmelzer JD, Ward KK *et al* (1988) Effect of hyperbaric oxygenation on normal and chronic streptozocin diabetic peripheral nerves. *Exp Neurol* 99: 201–212.

Lowe KC (1987) Perfluorochemicals and hyperbaric oxygen in radiation therapy: a cautionary note. *Int J Radiat Oncol Biol Phys* 13: 291–292.

Lowry OH, Passonneau JV, Hasselberger FX *et al* (1984) Effect of ischemia on known substrates and cofactors of the glycolytic pathway in the brain. *J Biol Chem* 239: 18–30.

Lucente RG, Parisier SC, Sone PM (1983) Complications of the treatment of malignant external otitis. *Laryngoscope* 93: 279.

Lukich VL, Filimonova MV, Bazarova VS (1978) Gas exchange in patients with chronic cardiac and pulmonary insufficiency in hyperbaric oxygenation. *Klin Med (Mosk)* 56: 74–83.

Lukich VL, Filimonova MV, Folina TS *et al* (1976) Employment of hyperbaric oxygenation in outpatients (in Russian). *Khirurgiia (Mosk)* 52: 82–86.

Lukich VL, Poliakova LV, Sotnikova TI, Belokrinitskii DV (1991) Hyperbaric oxygenation in the comprehensive therapy of patients with rheumatoid arthritis (clinico-immunologic study). *Fiziol Zh* 37: 55–60.

Lukich VL, Shirokova KI, Matrinitskaya NA *et al* (1981) The results of the use of hyperbaric oxygen in the treatment of peptic ulcer. In Yefuny SN (Ed.) *Proceedings of the 7th international congress on hyperbaric medicine.* USSR Academy of Sciences, Moscow, p 357.

Lumsden CE (1970) Pathogenetic mechanisms in the leuco-encephalopathies in anoxic-ischaemic processes in disorders of the blood and in intoxications. In Vinken PJ, Bruyn GW, (Eds.) *Handbook of clinical neurology: Vol 9.* North-Holland, Amsterdam.

Lumsden CE (1970) The neuropathology of multiple sclerosis. In Vinken PJ, Bruyn GW, (eds.) *Handbook of clinical neurology: Vol 9.* Amsterdam: pp 296–298.

Lund V, Kentala E, Scheinin H *et al* (2000) Hyperbaric oxygen increases parasympathetic activity in professional divers. *Acta Physiol Scand* 170: 39–44.

Lund V, Kentala E, Scheinin H *et al* (1999) Effect of hyperbaric conditions on plasma stress hormone levels and endothelin-1. *Undersea Hyperb Med* 26: 87–92.

Lundgren F, Zachrisson H, Emery P *et al* (1988) Less exchange of amino acids during exercise in patients with arterial insufficiency. *Clin Physiol* 8: 227–241.

Luongo C, Mignini R, Vicario C *et al* (1992) Hyperbaric oxygen therapy in the treatment of benign intracranial hypertension. Follow-up of a preliminary study. *Minerva Anestesiol* 58 (suppl 1): 97–98.

Lutsep HL, Albers GW, DeCrespigny A *et al* (1997) Clinical utility of diffusion-weighted magnetic resonance imaging in the assessment of ischemic stroke. *Ann Neurol* 41: 574–580.

Lusiani L, Visona A, Nicolin P *et al* (1988) Transcutaneous oxygen tension (TcPO2) measurement as a diagnostic tool in patients with peripheral vascular disease. *Angiology* 39: 873–880.

Lynch PR, Brigham M, Tuma R *et al* (1985) Origin and time course of gas bubbles following rapid decompression in the hamster. *Undersea Biomed Res* 12: 105–114.

Lyne AJ (1978) Ocular effects of hyperbaric oxygen. *Trans Ophthalmol Soc* (UK) 98: 66–68.

Lyskin GI, Lebshova AS (1981) Hyperbaric oxygenation in the treatment of labyrinthopathies of vascular genesis. In Yefuny SN (Ed.) *Abstracts of the 7th international congress on hyperbaric medicine.* USSR Academy of Sciences, Moscow, p 307.

M

Machado J (1989) Clinically observed reduction of spasticity in patients with neurological diseases and in children with cerebral palsy from hyperbaric oxygen therapy. *Proceedings of "New Horizons in Hyperbaric Medicine"* American College of Hyperbaric Medicine.

Machin D, Stenning SP, Parmar MK (1997) Thirty years of Medical Research Council randomized trials in solid tumours. *Clin Oncol (R Coll Radiol)* 9: 100–114.

Mader JT, Adams KR, Couch LA, Sutton TE (1978) Potentiation of tobramycin by hyperbaric oxygen in experimental osteomyelitis due to *Staphylococcus aureus* in rabbits. *J Infect Dis* 138: 312–328.

Mader JT, Love JT (1982) Malignant external otitis. Cure with adjunctive hyperbaric oxygen therapy. *Arch Otolaryngol* 108: 38–40.

Madhusudhana KC, Newsom RSB (2007) Central retinal vein occlusion: the therapeutic options. *Can J Ophthalmol* 42: 193–195.

Maeda N (1965) Experimental studies on the effect of decompression procedures and hyperbaric oxygenation for the treatment of spinal cord injury. *J Natl Med Assoc* 16: 429–447.

Magendie F (1821) Sur l'entrée accidentelle de l'air dans les veines, sur la mort subite, qui en est l'effet sur le moyens de prévenir cet accident et d'y remédier. *J Physiol Exp (Paris)* 1: 190–196.

Maguire D, McCabe M, Piva T (1988) The effects of hypo- and hyperthermia on the oxygen profile of a tumor spheroid. *Adv Erp Med Biol* 222: 741–745.

Maillot K, Brather R, Deeg KH (1979) Plazenta-Insuffizienz und intermittierende hyperbare Oxygenation. Ein Tierversuchsmodell. *Arch Gynecol* 228: 223–224.

Mainous EG, Boyne PJ, Hart GB (1973) Hyperbaric oxygen treatment of mandibular osteomyelitis: report of three cases. *J Am Dent Assoc* 87: 1426–1430.

Makhihara N, Hasegawa Y, Sakano S *et al* (1996) Effect of hyperbaric oxygenation on bone in HEBP-induced rachitic rats. *Undersea Hyperbaric Med* 23: 1–4.

Makishima K, Yoshida M, Kuroda Y *et al* (1998) Hyperbaric oxygenation as a treatment for facial palsy. *Adv Otorhinolaryngol* 54: 110–118.

Mäkitie J, Teräväinen H (1977) Histochemical changes in striated muscle in patients with intermittent claudication. *Arch Pathol Lab Med* 101: 658–663.

Mallett-Guy P, Debiec T, Yoshitomi G *et al* (1977) Effets de l'hyperoxie sur le parenchyme hépatique. *Ann Gastroenterol Hepatol (Paris)* 6: 283–305.

Mamistov VA, Dildin AS (1976) Employment of hyperbaric oxygenation in the treatment of patients with acute generalized peritonitis. *Khirurgiia (Mosk)* 2: 89–92.

Mandai M, Ogura Y, Honda Y (1990) Effects of hyperbaric oxygen treatment on macular edema. *Folia Ophthalmol Jpn* 41: 578–583.

Mangat HS (1995) Retinal artery occlusion. *Surv Ophthalmol* 40: 145–156.

Marabotti C, Scalzini A, Cialoni D *et al* (2008) Cardiac changes induced by immersion and breath-hold diving in humans. *J Appl Physiol* doi:00126.2008v1.

Margolis G (1966) Hyperbaric oxygenation: the eye as a limiting factor. *Science* 151: 466–468.

Marmo M, Contaldi G, Luongo C *et al* (1986) Effects of hyperbaric oxygenation in skin and pulmonary infections caused by Pseudomonas aeruginosa. *Minerva Anestesiol* 62: 281–287.

Marmor MF, Maack T (1982) Enhancement of retinal adhesion and subretinal fluid resorption by acetazolamide. *Invest Ophthalmol Vis Sci* 23: 121–124.

Marques AM (2008) Chronic Lyme disease: a review. *Infect Dis Clin North Am* 22: 341–360.

Martel J, Duclos JY, Darrouzet V *et al* (2000) Malignant or necrotizing otitis externa: experience in 22 cases. *Ann Otolaryngol Chir Cervicofac* 117: 291.

Martin DF, Porter EA, Rockwell S, Fischer JJ (1987) Enhancement of tumor radiation response by the combination of a perfluorochemical emulsion and hyperbaric oxygen. *Int J Radiat Oncol Biol Phys* 13: 747–751.

Martindale LG, Milligan M, Fries P (1987) Test of an R-2 defibrillation adapter in hyperbaric chamber. *J Hyperbaric Med* 2: 15–25.

Marx RE, Ehler WJ, Tayapongsak P, Pierce LW (1990) Relationship of oxygen dose to angiogenesis induction in irradiated tissue. *Am J Surgery* 160: 519–524.

Marx RE, Johnson RP (1988) Problem wounds in oral and maxillofacial surgery: The role of hyperbaric oxygen, In Davis JC, Hunt TK (eds) *Problem wounds, the role of oxygen.* Elsevier, New York, NY, pp 65–123.

Marx RE, Johnson RP, Kline SN (1985) Prevention of osteoradionecrosis: a randomized prospective clinical trial of hyperbaric oxygen versus penicillin. *J Am Dent Assoc* 111: 49–54.

Mason J, Feist R, White M Jr, Swanner J, McGwin G Jr, Emond T (2004) Sheathotomy to decompress branch retinal vein occlusion: a matched control study. *Ophthalmology* 111: 540–545.

Mason JO, Nixon PA, Albert MA (2007) Trans-luminal nd:YAG laser embolysis for branch retinal artery occlusion. *Retina* 27: 573–577.

Masterson JST, Fratkin LB, Osler TR, Trapp WG (1978) Treatment of pneumatosis cystoides intestinalis with hyperbaric oxygen. *Ann Surg* 187: 245–247.

Mathieu D, Bocquillon N, Charre S, Wattel F (2000) Hyperbaric oxygenation in acute ischemic encephalopathy (near-hanging). *Eur J Neurol* 7(Suppl 3): 151.

Mathieu D, Nolf M, Durocher A *et al* (1985) Acute carbon monoxide poisoning risk of late sequelae and treatment by hyperbaric oxygen. *Clin Toxicol* 23: 315–324.

Mathieu D, Wattle F, Gosselin B *et al* (1987) Hyperbaric oxygen in the treatment of posthanging cerebral anoxia. *J Hyperbaric Med* 2: 63–67.

Mathus-Vliegen L, Tijtgat GNJ, Bakker DJ (1983) *Pneumatosis cystoides intestinalis and HBO therapy.* Paper presented at the 1st European conference on hyperbaric medicine, Amsterdam, Sept 7–9.

Matsuo T (2001) Multiple occlusive retinal arteritis in both eyes of a patient with rheumatoid arthritis. *Jpn J Ophthalmol* 45: 662–664. (Japanese)

Matsuoka S, Tokuda H (1983) EEG analysis for evaluating chronic cerebral ischemia treated by hyperbaric oxygenation and microsurgery. In Shiraki K, Matsuoka S (Eds.) *Hyperbaric medicine and underwater physiology.* Fukuoka, Kitakyushu, pp 303–314.

Matthews MK (2005) Nonarteritic anterior ischemic optic neuropathy. *Curr Opin Ophthalmol* 16: 341–345.

Mattle H (1963) Elimination of ethanol in rats and in vitro at different oxygen pressures. *Acta Physiol Pharmacol* 12: 1–11.

Maulana O, Djonhar D (1987) *Some experience in hyperbaric oxygenation therapy for dermatological cases in Naval Hospital Jakarta.* Presented at the 9th international congress on hyperbaric medicine. Sydney, Australia, March 1–4.

Maynor ML, Moon RE, Klitzman B *et al* (1997). Brown recluse spider envenomation: A prospective trial of hyperbaric oxygen therapy. *Acad Emerg Med* 4: 184–192.

McCarty DJ (1981) Hyperbaric oxygen therapy for arthritis. *Hyperbaric Oxygen Review* 2: 55–62.

McCormack M, Nias AHW, Smith E (1990) Chronic anemia, hyperbaric oxygen and tumor radiosensitivity. *Brit J Radiol* 63: 752–759.

McCulloch J, Harper AM (1977) Phenylethylamine and cerebral blood flow. Possible involvement of phenylethylamine in migraine. *Neurology* 27: 817–821.

McDermott JJ, Dutka AJ, Koller WA *et al* (1992) effects of an increased PO_2 during recompression therapy for the treatment of experimental cerebral arterial gas embolism. *Undersea Biomed Res* 19: 403–413.

McDonald AB (1989) Gestational Lyme borreliosis. Implications for the fetus. *Rheum Dis Clin North Am* 15: 657–677.

McDonald KR, Bradfield JJ, Kinsella JK *et al* (1996) Effect of hyperbaric oxygenation on existing oral mucosal carcinoma. *Laryngoscope* 106: 957–9.

McDonald WI (1986) Pathogenesis of optic neuritis. In Hess RF, Plant GT (Eds.) *Optic Neuritis.* Cambridge University Press, Cambridge.

McDowell DG (1987) Anesthesia in the pressure chamber. *Anesthesia* 19: 321–336.

McDowell DG, Jennett WB, Bloor K *et al* (1966) The effect of hyperbaric oxygen on oxygen tension of the brain during chloroform anesthesia. *Surg Gynecol Obstet* 122: 545–549.

McDowell F, Flamm ES (1986) EC/IC bypass study. *Stroke* 17: 1–2.

McFarland RA (1963) Experimental evidence of relationship between aging and oxygen want. *Ergonomics* 6: 339–366.

McFarland RA, Roughton FJW, Halperin MH *et al* (1944) The effects of carbon monoxide and altitude on visual thresholds. *J Aviat Med* 15: 381–394.

McGough EK, Gallagher TJ, Hart J *et al* (1989) *Hyperbaric oxygen as an adjuvant in penile re-implantation: a case report.* Paper presented at the annual meeting of the Undersea and Hyperbaric Medical Society, Honolulu, June 10.

McMillan T, Calhoun KH, Mader JT *et al* (1989) The effect of hyperbaric oxygen on oral mucosal carcinoma. *Laryngoscope* 99: 241–244.

McNulty JA, Maher BA, Chu M *et al* (1997) Relationship of short-term verbal memory to the need for hyperbaric oxygen treatment after carbon monoxide poisoning. *Neuropsychiatry Neuropsychol Behav Neurol* 10: 174–179.

McNally VA, Patterson AV, Williams KJ *et al* (2002) Antiangiogenic, bioreductive and gene therapy approaches to the treatment of hypoxic tumours. *Curr Pharm Des* 8: 1319–33.

Meca-Lallana JE, Martin JJ, Lucas C *et al* (1999) Susac syndrome: clinical and diagnostic approach. A new case report. *Rev Neuro* 29: 1027–1032.

Mei-Dan O, Hetsroni I, Mann G *et al* (2008) Prevention of avascular necrosis in displaced talar neck fractures by hyperbaric oxygenation therapy: A dual case report. *J Postgrad Med* 54: 140–143.

Meijne NG, Mellink HM, Kox C (1973) The main present-day indications for clinical treatment in a hyperbaric chamber. *Pneumologie* 149: 173–180.

Meijne NG, Shoemaker G, Bulterijs AB (1963) The treatment of cerebral gas embolism in a high pressure chamber. *J Cardiovasc Surg* 4: 757.

Meirovithz E, Sonn J, Mayevsky A (2007) Effect of hyperbaric oxygenation on brain hemodynamics, hemoglobin oxygenation and mitochondrial NADH. *Brain Res Rev* 54: 294–304.

Meleney FL (1924) Hemolytic streptococcus gangrene. *Arch Surg* 9: 31.

Mendel V, Reichert B, Simanowski HJ, Scholz HC (1999) Therapy with hyperbaric oxygen and cefazolin for experimental osteonyelitis due to staphylococcus auerus in rats. *Undersea Hyperbaric Med* 26: 169–174.

Mengel CE, Kann HE, Heyman A *et al* (1965) Effects of in vivo hyperoxia on erythrocyte II: hemolysis in a human after exposure to oxygen under high pressure. *Blood* 25: 822–829.

Merrick J, Gufler K, Jacobsen E (1978) Ergotism treated with hyperbaric oxygen and continuous epidural analgesia. *Acta Anaesthesiol Scand {Suppl}* 67: 87–90.

Mervin K, Valter K, Maslim J *et al* (1999) Limiting photoreceptor death and deconstruction during experimental retinal detachment: the value of oxygen supplementation. *Am J Ophthalmol* 128: 155–164.

Messier LD, Myers RAM (1991) A neuropsychological screening battery for emergency assessment of carbon-monoxide-poisoned patients. *J Clin Psychology* 47: 675–684.

Mester U, Dillinger P (2002) Vitrectomy with arteriovenous decompression and internal limiting membrane dissection in branch retinal vein occlusion. *Retina* 22: 740–746.

Mestrovic J (1996) Does hyperbaric oxygen have a cancer-causing or -promoting effect? *Undersea Hyperbaric Med* 23: 55–56 (letter).

Mestrovic J, Kosuta D, Gosovic S *et al* (1996) Suppression of rat tumour colonies in the lung by oxygen at high pressure is a local effect. *Clin Exp Metastasis* 8: 113–119.

Meyer GW, Hart GB, Strauss MB (1990) Non invasive blood pressure monitoring in the hyperbaric monoplace chamber: a new technique, *J Hyperbaric Med* 4(4): 211–216.

Meyer JS, Toyoda M, Ryu T *et al* (1968) Evidence for a Pasteur effect on cerebral oxygen and carbohydrate metabolism in cerebrovascular disease. *Circulation* 7: 138.

Meyerstein N, Mazor D, Tsach T *et al* (1989) Resistance of human red cells to hyperbaric oxygen under therapeutic conditions. *J Hyperbaric Med* 4: 1–5.

Meyer-Witting M, Helps S, Gorman SF (1991) Acute carbon monoxide exposure and cerebral blood flow in rabbits. *Anaesth Intensive Care* 19: 373–377.

Mialon P, Barthelemy L (1993) Effect of hyperbaric oxygenation on prostaglandin and thromboxane synthesis in the cortex and the striatum of rat brain. *Mol Chem Neuropathol* 20: 181–189.

Mialon P, Barthelemy L, Michaud A, Lacour JM (2001) Pulmonary function in men after repeated sessions of oxygen breathing at 0.25 MPa for 90 min. *Aviat Space Environ Med* 72: 215–218.

Mialon P, Gibey R, Bigot JC *et al* (1992) Changes in striatal and cortical amino acid and ammonia levels of rat brain after one hyperbaric oxygen-induced seizure. *Aviat Space Environ Med* 63: 287–291.

Michaud A, Mongredien-Taburet H, Barthelemy L *et al* (1989) Traitment par oxygenotherapie Hyperbare (OHB). *Medsubhyp* 8: 139–149.

Mickel HS, Kempski O *et al* (1990) Prominent white matter lesions develop in Mongolian gerbils treated with 100% normobaric oxygen after global brain ischemia. *Acta Neuropathol* 79: 465–72.

Mickel HS, Yashesh N, Vaishnav N *et al* (1987) Breathing 100% oxygen after global brain ischemia in Mongolian gerbils results in increased lipid peroxidation and increased mortality. *Stroke* 18: 426–430.

Mikhailov AM (1982) Correction of glucocorticoid metabolism disorders in patients with bronchial asthma treated by hyperbaric oxygenation. *Klin Med* 60: 52–56.

Mikulka P, O'Donnell R, Heinig P *et al* (1973) The effect of carbon monoxide on human performance. *Ann NY Acad Sci* 174: 409–420.

Milas L, Hunter NM, Ito H *et al* (1985) Increase in radiosensitivity of lung micrometastases by hyperbaric oxygen. *Clin Exp Metastasis* 3: 21–27.

Miller BL (1993) The ethics of cardiac arrest research. *Ann Emerg Med* 22: 118–124.

Miller DH, Austin SJ, Connelly A *et al* (1991) Proton magnetic resonance spectroscopy of an acute and chronic lesion in multiple sclerosis. *Lancet* 337: 58–59.

Miller EF (1958) Effect of breathing 100 % oxygen upon visual fields and visual acuity. *J Aviation Med* 29: 598–602.

Miller JD (1973) The effects of hyperbaric oxygen at 2 and 3 atmospheres: absolute and intravenous mannitol on experimentally increased intracranial pressure. *Eur Neurol* 10: 1–10.

Miller JD (1979) The management of cerebral oedema. *Br J Hosp Med* 21: 152–166.

Miller JD, Ledingham IM (1970) The effect of hyperbaric oxygen on intracranial pressure in experimental cerebral edema. In Wada J, Takashi IWA (Eds.) *Proceedings of the 4th International Congress on Hyperbaric Medicine*. Wilkins and Wilkins, Baltimore, pp 543–556.

Miller JD, Ledingham IM (1971) Reduction of increased intracranial pressure: Comparison between hyperbaric oxygen and hyperventilation. *Arch Neurol* 24: 210.

Miller WC, Suich DM, Unger KM (1987) Hyperbaric environment for chronic hypoxemia. *J Hyperbaric Med* 2: 211–214.

Mills C, Bryson P (2006) The role of hyperbaric oxygen therapy in the treatment of sternal infection. *Eur J Cardiothorac Surgery* 30(1): 153–159.

Mills MD, Devenyi RG, Lam WC, Berger AR, Beijer CD, Lam SR (2001) An assessment of intraocular pressure rise in patients with gas-filled eyes during simulated air flight. *Ophthalmology* 108: 40.

Min L, Jian-xing X (2007) Detoxifying function of cytochrome c against oxygen toxicity. *Mitochondrion* 7(1–2): 13–16.

Mininberg ES, Kvetnoy IM (1974) Hyperbaric oxygenation in the prophylaxis and treatment of acute hepatic insufficiency. *Anesteziol Reanimatol* 4: 46–49.

Mink RB, Dutka AJ (1995a) Hyperbaric oxygen after global cerebral ischemia in rabbits does not promote brain lipid peroxidation. *Crit Care Med* 23(8): 1398–1404.

Mink RB, Dutka AJ (1995b) Hyperbaric oxygen after global cerebral ischemia in rabbits reduces brain vascular permeability and blood flow. *Stroke* 26: 2307–2312.

Miroshnichenko VP, Demurov EA, Koloskow YB *et al* (1983) Effect of guanine nucleotides and hyperbaric oxygenation on cardiac adenylate cyclase activity in rabbits with myocardial hypertrophy. *Bull Exp Biol Med* 95: 179–181.

Mitchell S, Gorman D (2002) The pathophysiology of cerebral arterial gas embolism. *J Extra Corpor Technol* 34: 18–23.

Miura S, Ohyagi Y, Ohno M, Inoue I, Ochi H, Murai H, Furuya H, Yamada T, Kira J (2002) A patient with delayed posthypoxic demyelination: a case report of hyperbaric oxygen treatment. *Clinical Neurology and Neurosurgery* 104: 311–314.

Miyake H, Yanagita N, Niwa H *et al* (1972) Hyperbaric oxygen therapy for sudden deafness. *Jpn J Hyperbaric Med* 7: 6–7.

Miyake Y (1974) Electro-oculographic change in retinal arterial occlusion and its analysis. *Acta Soc Ophthalmol Jpn* 78: 311–323.

Miyake Y, Awaya S, Takahashi H *et al* (1993) Hyperbaric oxygen and acetazolamide improve visual acuity in patients with cystoid macular edema by different mechanisms. *Arch Ophthalmol* 111: 1605–1606.

Miyake Y, Horiguchi M, Matsuura M *et al* (1987) Hyperbaric oxygen therapy in 72 eyes with retinal arterial occlusion. In Bove AA, Bachrach AJ, Greenbaum LJ (Eds.) *Ninth International Symposium on Underwater and Hyperbaric physiology.* Bethesda: Undersea and Hyperbaric Medical Society, pp 949–953.

Miyamoto H, Ogura Y, Honda Y (1995) Hyperbaric oxygen treatment for macular edema after retinal vein occlusion – fluorescein angiographic findings and visual prognosis. *Nippon Ganka Gakkai Zasshi* 99: 220–225. (Japanese)

Miyamoto H, Ogura Y, Wakano Y *et al* (1993) The long term results of hyperbaric oxygen treatment for macular edema with retinal vein occlusion. *Nippon Ganka Gakkai Zasshi* 97: 1065–1069.

Mizoguchi F, Nanki T, Miyasaka N (2008) Pneumatosis cystoides intestinalis following lupus enteritis and peritonitis. *Intern Med* 47: 1267–1271.

Mogami H, Hayakawa T, Kanai N *et al* (1969) Clinical application of hyperbaric oxygenation in the treatment of acute cerebral damage. *J Neurosurg* 31: 636–643.

Mohamed Q, McIntosh RL, Saw SM, Wong TY (2007) Interventions for central retinal vein occlusion. *Ophthalmology* 114: 507–519.

Molnar I, Poitry S, Tsacopoulos M *et al* (1985) Effect of laser photocoagulation on oxygenation of the retina in miniature pigs. *Invest Ophthalmol Vis Sci* 26: 1410–1414.

Molzhaninov Ev, Chaika VK, Domanova AI *et al* (1981) Experiences and prospects of using hyperbaric oxygen in obstetrics. In Yefuny SN (Ed.) *Proceedings of the 7th international congress on hyperbaric medicine.* USSR Academy of Sciences, Moscow, p 360.

Money KE, Buckingham IP, Calder IM *et al* (1985) Damage to the middle ear and the inner ear in underwater divers. *Undersea Biomed Res* 12: 77–84.

Monies-Chass I, Herer D, Alon U, Birkhahn HJ (1976) Hyperbaric oxygen in acute ischaemia due to allergic vasculitis. *Anaesthesia* 31: 1221–1224.

Montani S, Perret C (1967) HBO during experimental intoxication with carbon tetrachloride. *Rev Fr Etud Clin Biol* 12: 274–278.

Montgomery D, Goldberg J, Amar M *et al* (1999) Effects of hyperbaric oxygen therapy on children with spastic diplegic cerebral palsy: a pilot project. *Undersea Hyperb Med* 26: 235–42.

Moody RA, Mead CO, Ruamsuke S, Mullan S (1970) Therapeutic value of oxygen at normal and hyperbaric pressure in experimental head injury. *J Neurosurg* 32: 51–54.

Moon AJ, Williams KG, Hopkinson WI (1964) A patient with coronary thrombosis treated with hyperbaric oxygen, *Lancet* 1: 18–20.

Moon RE (1988) Monoplace chamber use in the treatment of diving accidents. *J Hyperbaric Med* 3: 1–3.

Moon RE, Bergquist LV, Conklin B *et al* (1986) Monaghan 225 ventilator under hyperbaric conditions. *Chest* 89: 846–851.

Moon RE, Camporesi EM (1991) Operational use and patient monitoring in a multiplace hyperbaric chamber. In Moon RE, Camporesi EM (Eds.) *Problems in Respiratory Care: Clinical Applications of Hyperbaric Oxygen.* Lippencott, Philadelphia.

Moon RE, Camporesi EM, Kisslo JA (1989) Patent foramen ovale and decompression sickness in divers. *Lancet* 1: 513–514.

Moore GF, Fuson RL, Margolis G *et al* (1966) An evaluation of the protective effect of hyperbaric oxygenation on the central nervous system during circulatory arrest. *J Thorac Cardiovasc Surg* 52: 618.

Morales-Buenrostro LE, Alberu J (2008) Anti-major histocompatibility class 1-related chain A antibodies in organ transplantation. *Transplant Rev (Orlando)* 22(1): 27–38.

Morgagni J (1769) *The seats and causes of disease.* Translated from the Latin, Benjamin, London.

Mori K, Ohta K, Nagano S *et al* (2007) A case of ophthalmic artery obstruction following autologous fat injection in the glabellar area. *Nippon Ganka Gakkai Zasshi* 111: 22–25. (Japanese)

Morin FC, Egan EA, Norfleet WT (1988) Indomethacin does not diminish the pulmonary vascular response of the fetus to increased oxygen tension. *Pediatr Res* 24: 696–700.

Morita T, Takahashi K, Kitani Y *et al* (1994) Treatment of radiation cystitis wwith hyperbaric oxygen. In *Proceedings of the XI International Congress on Hyperbaric Medicine.* Best, San Pedro.

Morris LE (1952) A new vaporizer for liquid anesthetic agents. *Anesthesiology* 13: 587–593.

Moskowitz MA (1984) The neurobiology of vascular head pain. *Ann Neurol* 16: 157–168.

Mounsey RA, Brown DH, O'Dwyer TP *et al* (1993) Role of oxygen therapy in the management of mandibular osteoradionecrosis. *Laryngoscope* 103: 605–608.

Mrsic-Pelcic J, Pelcic G, Peternel S *et al* (2004) Effects of the hyperbaric oxygen treatment on the Na+, K+ -ATPase and superoxide dismutase activities in the optic nerves of global cerebral ischemia-exposed rats. *Prog Neuropsychopharmacol Biol Psychiatry* 28(4): 667–676.

Mrsic-Pelcic J, Pelcic G, Vitezie D *et al* (2004) Hyperbaric oxygen treatment: the influence on the hippocampal superoxide dismutase and Na+, K+-ATPase activities in global cerebral ischemia-exposed rats. *Neurochem Int* 44(8): 585–594.

Mukoyama M, Tida M, Sobve I (1975) Hyperbaric oxygen therapy. *Exp Neurol* 47: 371–380.

Mullins ME, Beltran JT (1998) Acute cerebral gas embolism from hydrogen peroxide ingestion successfully treated with hyperbaric oxygen. *J Toxicol Clin Toxicol* 36: 253–256.

Muminov AI, Khatamov ZhA, Masharipov RR (2002) Antioxidants and hyperbaric oxygenation in the treatment of sensorineural hearing loss in children. *Vestn Otorinolaringol* 5: 33–34.

Murakawa T, Kosaka M, Mori Y *et al* (2000) Treatment of 522 patients with sudden deafness performed oxygenation at high pressure. *Nippon Jibiinkoka Gakkai Kaiho* 103: 506–515.

Muralidharan V, Christophi C (2007) Hyperbaric oxygen therapy and liver transplantation. *HPB* 9(3): 174–182.

Murdock TJ, Kushner BJ (2001) Anterior segment ischemia after surgery on 2 vertical rectus muscles augmented with lateral fixation sutures. *J AAPOS* 5: 323–324.

Murphy DG, Sloan EP, Hart RG *et al* (1991) Tension pneumothorax associated wilth hyperbaric oxygen therapy. *Am J Emerg Med* 9: 176–179.

Murphy JV, Banwell PE, Roberts AH, McGrouther DA (2000) Frostbite: pathogenesis and treatment. *J Trauma* 48: 171–178.

Murphy-Lavoie H, Butler FK, Hagan C (2008) *Central Retinal Artery Occlusion in Hyperbaric Oxygen 2003: Indications and Results – The Hyperbaric Oxygen Therapy Committee Report.* Dunkirk, Undersea and Hyperbaric Medical Society (in press).

Murphy-Lavoie, H, Harch, P, VanMeter, K (2004) *Effect of hyperbaric oxygen on central retinal artery occlusion.* UHMS Scientific Assembly, Australia.

Murrison AW (1989) The contribution of neurophysiologic techniques to the investigation of diving-related illness. *Undersea Hyperbaric Med* 20: 347–373.

Myers DE, Myers RA (1995) A preliminary report on hyperbaric oxygen in the relief of migraine headache. *Headache* 35: 197–199.

Myers RAM (1985) Delayed treatment of serious decompression sickness, *Ann of Emerg Med* 14: 254–257.

N

Nabeshima T, Katoh A, Ishimaru H *et al* (1991) Carbon monoxide-induced delayed amnesia, delayed neuronal death and change in acetylcholine concentration in mice. *J Pharmacol Exp Ther* 256: 378–384.

Nagakawa Y, Kinomoto H, Mabuchi S *et al* (1982) Significance of oxygenation at high pressure (OHP) as a therapeutic method for occlusive cerebrovascular disease. *No Shinkei Geka* 10: 1067–1074.

Nagao S, Okmura S, Nishimoto A (1975) Effect of hyperbaric oxygenation on vasomotor tone in acute intracranial hypertension: anexperimental study. *Resuscitation* 4: 51–59.

Naiman JL, Donohue WL, Prichard JS (1961) Fatal nucleus pulposus embolism of spinal cord after trauma. *Neurology* 11: 83–87.

Nair S, Nair K, Imbuche R (1973) Treatment of chronic vertigo with hyperbaric oxygen. *Lancet* I: 184–185.

Nakada T (1988) Hyperbaric oxygenation for experimental bladder tumor. *Eur Urol* 14: 145–149.

Nakada T, Koike H, Katayama T *et al* (1984) Increased adrenal epinephrine and norepinephrine in spontaneously hypertensive rats treated with hyperbaric oxygen. *Hinyokika Kiyo* 30: 1357–1366.

Nakada T, Saito H, Ota K (1986) Serum testosterone, testicular connective tissue protein and testicular histology in rats treated with hyperbaric oxygen. *Int Urol Nephrol* 18: 439–447.

Nakada T, Yamaguchi T, Sasagawa I *et al* (1992) Successful hyperbaric oxygenation for radiation cystitis due to excessive irradiation to uterus cancer. *Eur Urol* 22: 294–298.

Nakashima T, Fukuta S, Yanagita N (1998) Hyperbaric oxygen therapy for sudden deafness. *Acta Otorhinolaryngol* (Basel) 54: 100–109.

Nakata M (1976) Hyperbaric oxygen therapy for facial palsy. *Jp J Hyperbaric Med* 10: 99–103.

Narozny W, Sicko Z, Kot J *et al* (2005) Hyperbaric oxygen therapy in the treatment of complications of irradiation in head and neck area. *Undersea Hyperb Med* 32: 103–110.

Narozny W, Sicko Z, Przewozny T *et al* (2004) Sudden sensorineural hearing loss: a treatment protocol including glucocorticoids and hyperbaric oxygen therapy. *Otolaryngol Pol* 58: 821–830.

National Fire Protection Association (1966) *Standard for Health Care Facilities. NFPA 99, Chapter 19, Hyperbaric Facilities.* National Fire Protection Association, Boston.

Nauck M, Karakiulakis S, Perruchoud A, Papakonstantinou E, Roth M (1998a) Corticosteroids inhibit the expression of the vascular endothelial growth factor gene in human vascular smooth muscle cells. *Euro J Pharmacol* 341: 309–315.

Nauck M, Roth M, Tamm M, Eickelberg O *et al* (1998b) Induction of vascular endothelial growth factor by platelet-activating factor and platelet-derived growth factor is down-regulated by corticosteroids. *Am J Resp Cell Mol Biol* 16: 398–406.

Neiman J, Nilsson BY, Barr PO, Perrins DJ (1985) Hyperbaric oxygen in chronic progressive multiple sclerosis: visual evoked potentials and clinical effects. *J Neurol Neurosurg Psychiatry* 48: 497–500.

Nelson AJ, Holt J A (1978) Combined microwave therapy. *Med J Aust* 2: 88–90.

Nelson EW, Bright DE, Viller LF (1990) Closure of refractory perineal Crohn's lesion. *Digestive Diseases and Sciences* 35: 1561–1565.

Neovius EB, Lind MG, Lind FG (1997) Hyperbaric oxygen therapy for wound complications after surgery in the irradiated head, and neck: A review of the literature and a report of 15 consecutive patients. *Head Neck* 19: 315–322.

Neretin VI, Kirjakov Va, Lobov MA, Kiselev SO (1985) Hyperbaric oxygenation in dyscirculatory myelopathies. *Sov Med* 3: 42–44.

Neretin VI, Kirjakov Va, Kotov SV *et al* (1988) Hyperbaric oxygenation in the combined treatment of patients with polyradiculoneuritis. *Zh Nevropatol Psikkiatr* 88: 61–64.

Neretin VI, Lobov MA, Kiselev SO, Lagutina TS, Kirjakov VA (1985) Effect of hyperbaric oxygenation on the recovery of motor functions in vertebrogenic myelopathies. *Zh Nevropatol Psikhiatr* 85: 1774–1778.

Neto JS, Nakao A, Kimizuka K, Romanosky AJ, Stolz DB, Uchiyama T, Nalesnik MA, Otterbein LE, Murase N (2004) Protection of transplant-induced renal ischemia-reperfusion injury with carbon monoxide. *Am J Physiol Renal Physiol* 287(5): F979–F989.

Neubauer AS, Mueller AJ, Schriever S, Gruterich M, Ulbig M, Kampik A (2000) Minimally invasive therapy for clinically complete central retinal artery occlusion-results and meta-analysis of literature. *Klin Monatsbl Augenheilkd* 217: 30–36. (German)

Neubauer RA (1978) Treatment of multiple sclerosis with monoplace hyperbaric chamber. *J Fl Med Soc* 65: 101.

Neubauer RA (1979) Carbon monoxide and hyperbaric oxygen. *Arch of Intern Med* 139: 829–832.

Neubauer RA (1981) Hyperbaric oxygen treatment and stroke (letter). *JAMA* 248: 2574.

Neubauer RA (1983) *Hyperhalic oxygen therapy of stroke; a review.* Ocean Medical Center, Lauderdale-by-the-Sea, Florida.

Neubauer RA (1983a) Generalized small vessel stenosis in the brain. *Minerva Med* 74: 2051–2055.

Neubauer RA (1983b) *Regional cerebral blood flow studies of the effect of hyperbaric oxygen in acute stroke and chronic neurologic deficits of stroke.* Paper presented at the 1st European conference on hyperbaric medicine. Amsterdam, Sept 7–9.

Neubauer RA (1985a) The effect of hyperbaric oxygen in prolonged coma. Possible identification of marginally functioning brain zones. *Minerva Med Subaecquea ed Iperbarica* 5: 75.

Neubauer RA (1986) Hyperbaric oxygen in vegetative coma. In Schmutz J (Ed.) *Proceedings of the 1st Swiss symposium on hyperbaric medicine.* Foundation for hyperbaric medicine, Basel p 116.

Neubauer RA (1988) *Certain neurological indications for hyperbaric oxygen.* Presented at the meeting of the International Society of Hyperbaric Medicine, Oxford, 1–3 Sept.

Neubauer RA (1995) *Interventional brain scanning in neurologic dysfunction*, Ocean Hyperbaric Center, Lauderdale-by-the-Sea, Florida, p 22.

Neubauer RA (2001) Hyperbaric oxygenation for cerebral palsy. *Lancet* 357: 2052–2053.

Neubauer RA, End E (1980) Hyperbaric oxygenation as an adjunct therapy in strokes due to thrombosis. *Stroke* 11: 297.

Neubauer RA, Gottlieb SF (1992c) Reversal of a dense persistent, holohemispheric neurological deficit after an endarterectomy of the carotid artery: Case report. *Neurosurgery* 30: 301–302.

Neubauer RA, Gottlieb SF, Kagan RL (1986) *Magnetic resonance imaging in multiple sclerosis following hyperbaric oxygen.* First Swiss Symposium on Hyperbaric Medicine, Foundation for Hyperbaric Medicine, Basel.

Neubauer RA, Gottlieb SF, Kagan RL (1990) Enhancing "idling" neurons. *Lancet* 335: 542.

Neubauer RA, Gottlieb SF, Miale A (1992) Identification of hypometabolic areas in the brain using brain imaging and hyperbaric oxygen. *Clin Nucl Med* 17: 477–481.

Neubauer RA, Gottlieb SF, Pevsner NH (1998) Long-term anoxic ischemic encephalopathy: predictability of recovery. In Oriani G, Wattel F (Eds.) *Proceedings of the Twelfth International Congress on Hyperbaric Medicine.* Best, Flagstaff, AZ, pp 417–429.

Neubauer RA, James P (1998) Cerebral oxygenation and the recoverable brain. *Neurol Res* 20(Suppl 1): S33-S36.

Neubauer RA, Kagan RL, Gottleib SF (1989a) Use of hyperbaric oxygen for the treatment of aseptic bone necrosis: a case study. *J Hyperbaric Med* 4: 69–76.

Neubauer RA, Kagan RL, Gottlieb SF, James P (1989b) Delayed metabolism, reperfusion or redistribution in iofetamine brain imaging after exposure to hyperbaric oxygen, clinical correlations. *Proceedings of the XV Annual Meeting of the European Undersea Biomedical Society, EUBS,* Eilat, Israel, pp 237–243.

Neubauer RA, Pinella J, Hill RK et al (1988) *The use of hyperbaric oxygen in the successful reanastomosis of the severed ear: three cases.* Presented at the 14th annual meeting of the European Undersea Biomedical Society, Aberdeen, Scotland, Sept 5–9.

Neubauer RA, Walker M (1998) *Hyperbaric Oxygen Therapy*, Avery Publishing Group, Garden City Park, NY.

Neurath MF, Branbrink A, Meyer zum Büschenfelde KH et al (1996) A new treatment for severe malabsorption due to radiation enteritis. *Lancet* 347: 1302.

New P (2001) Radiation injury to the nervous system. *Curr Opin Neurol* 14: 725–34.

Newman NJ, Scherer R, Langenberg P, Kelman S, Feldon S, Kaufman D, Dickersin K (2002) Ischemic Optic Neuropathy Decompression Trial Study Group. *Am J Ophthalmol* 134: 317–328.

Newman RP, Manning EJ (1980) Hyperbaric chamber treatment for "locked-in" syndrome. *Arch Neurol* 37: 529.

Newman WD, Frank HJ (1993) Pyoderma gangrenosa of the orbit. *Eye* 7: 89–94.

Nias AH, Perry PM, Photiou AR (1988) Modulating the oxygen tension in tumors by hypothermia and hyperbaric oxygen. *J R Soc Med* 81: 633–666.

Nichols CW, Lambertsen CJ, Clark JM (1969) Transient unilateral loss of vision associated with oxygen at high pressure. *Arch Ophthalmol* 81: 548–552.

Nichter LS, Morwood DT, Williams GS et al (1991) Expanding the limits of composite grafting: a case report of successful nose reimplantation assisted by hyperbaric oxygen therapy. *Plast Reconstruct Surg* 87: 337–340.

Nida TY, Biros MH, Pheley AM et al (1995) Effect of hypoxia or hyperbaric oxygen on cerebral edema following moderate fluid percussion or cortical impact injury in rats. *J Neurotrauma* 12: 77–85.

Niess AM, Simon P (2007) Response and adaptation of skeletal muscle to exercise – the role of reactive oxygen species. *Front Biosci* 12: 4826–4838.

Niezgoda JA, Cianci P, Folden BW et al (1997) The effect of hyperbaric oxygen therapy on a burn wound model in human volunteers. *Plast Reconstr Surg* 99: 1620–1625.

Nighogossian N, Trouillas P (1997) Hyperbaric oxygen in the treatment of acute ischemic stroke: an unsettled issue. *J Neurol Sci* 150: 27–31.

Nighogossian N, Trouillas P, Adeleine P et al (1995) Hyperbaric oxygen in the treatment of acute ischemic stroke, a double-blind study. *Stroke* 26: 1369–1372.

Niinikoski JR, Pentinnen R, Kulonen E (1970) Effects of hyperbaric oxygen on fracture healing in the rat: a biochemical study. *Calcif Tissues Res* 4: 115–116.

Nilsson B, Nordstrom CH (1977) Experimental head injury in the rat: Part 3. Cerebral blood flow and oxygen consumption after concussive impact acceleration. *J Neurosurg* 47: 262.

Nilsson LP (1989) Effects of hyperbaric oxygen treatment on bone repair. *Swedish Dental J* 64(suppl): 1–33.

Nilsson Remahl AI, Ansjon R, Lind F, Waldenlind E (2002). Hyperbaric oxygen treatment of active cluster headache: a double-blind placebo-controlled cross-over study. *Cephalalgia* 22: 730–739.

Niu AKC, Yang C, Lee HC et al (1987) Burns treated with adjunctive hyperbaric oxygen therapy: a comparative study in humans. *J Hyperbaric Med* 2: 75–85.

Noel WK (1958) Differentiation, metabolic organization, and viability of the visual cell. *Arch Ophthalmol* 60: 702–733.

Noell WK (1962) Effect of high and low oxygen tension on the visual system. In Schaeffer KE (Ed.) *Environmental effects on consciousness.* New York: MacMillan, pp 3–18

Nori H, Shinohara H, Arakawa Y, Kanemura H, Ikemoto T, Imura S, Morine Y, Ikegami T, Yoshizumi T, Shimada M (2007) Beneficial effects of hyperbaric oxygen pretreatment on massive hepatectomy model in rats. *Transplantation* 84(12): 1656–1661.

Norkool DM, Hampson NB, Gibbons RP et al (1993) Hyperbaric

oxygen therapy for radiation-induced hemorrhagic cystitis. *J Urology* 150: 332–334.

Norkool DM, Kirkpatrick JN (1985) Treatment of acute carbon monoxide poisoning with hyperbaric oxygen: a review of 115 cases. *Ann Emerg Med* 14: 1168–1171.

Novikova OA, Klyavinsh YA (1981) Effectiveness of hyperbaric oxygen in severe forms of virus hepatitis of hepatic coma in children. In Yefuny SN (Ed.) *Proceedings of the 7th international congress of hyperbaric medicine.* USSR Academy of Sciences, Moscow, pp 350–351.

Noyer CM, Brandt LJ (1999) Hyperbaric oxygen therapy for perineal Crohn's disease. *Am J Gastroenterol* 94: 318–21.

Nylander G, Lewis D, Nordstrom H, Larsson J (1985) Reduction of postischemic edema with hyperbaric oxygen. *Plast Reconstr Surg* 76: 596–603.

Nylander G, Nordstrom H, Franzen L *et al* (1988) Effects of hyperbaric oxygen treatment in post-ischemic muscle. *Scand J Plast Reconstr Surg* 22: 31–39.

Nylander G, Nordstrom H, Lewis D, Larsson J (1987) Metabolic effects of hyperbaric oxygen treatment in postischemic muscle. *Plast Reconstr Surg* 79: 91–97.

Nylander G, Otamiri DH, Larsson J (1989) Lipid products in postischemic skeletal muscle and after treatment with hyperbaric oxygen. *Scand J Plast Reconstr Surg* 23: 97–103.

O

O'Riordan TC, Zhdanov AV, Ponomarev GV, Papkovsky DB (2007) Analysis of intracellular oxygen and metabolic responses of mammalian cells by time-resolved fluorometry. *Anal Chem* 79: 9414–9419.

Obrist WD, Langfitt TW, Jaggi JL, Cruz J, Gennarelli TA (1984). Cerebral Blood Flow and Metabolism in Comatose Patients with Acute Head Injury. *J Neurosurg* 61: 241–253.

Ogawa M, Katsurada K, Sugimoto T *et al* (1974) Pulmonary edema in acute carbon monoxide poisoning. *Int Arch Arbeitsmed* 33: 131–138.

Ogura Y, Kiryu J, Takahashi K, Honda Y (1988) Visual improvement in diabetic macular edema by hyperbaric oxygen treatment. *Nippon Ganka Gakkai Zasshi* 92: 1456–1460.

Ogura Y, Takahashi M, Ueno S, Honda Y (1987) Hyperbaric oxygen treatment for chronic cystoid macular edema after branch retinal vein occlusion. *Am J Ophthalmol* 104: 301–302.

Ohresser P, Jean C, Alessandrini G *et al* (1980) Treatment by hyperbaric oxygen of sudden deafness: study of 160 cases. *Med Aeronaut Sport Med Subaquatique Hyperbare* 19: (73) 58–60.

Ohta H, Yasui N, Kawamura S *et al* (1985) Choice of EIAB operation candidates by topographic evaluation of EEG and SSEP with concomitant RCBF studies under hyperbaric oxygenation. In Spetzier RF, Carter LP, Selman WR, Martin NA (Eds.) *Cerebral revascularization for stroke.* Thieme Stratton, New York, pp 208–216.

Okihama Y, Umehara M, Naitoh Z *et al* (1987) A successful treatment with hyperbaric oxygenation therapy for a cirrhotic patient with hyperbilirubinemia. *Jpn J Hyperbaric Med* 22: 77–82.

Okinami S, Nihira M, Iwaki M, Sunakawa M, Arai I (1992) Hyperbaric oxygen therapy for cystoid macular edema in uveitis. *Jpn J Clin Ophthalmol* 46: 199–201.

Olesen J (1986) Beta-adrenergic effects on cerebral circulation. *Cephalalgia* 6 (Suppl 5): 41–46.

Ol'mezov VV, Ostanin VV, Borisov IuP *et al* (2001) Use of hyperbaric oxygenation and methylene blue in the treatment of a 10-year-old child with methemoglobin producer poisoning. *Anesteziol Reanimatol* Jan-Feb (1): 69.

Olszanski R, Konarski M, Kierznikowicz B (2002) Changes of selected morphotic parameters and blood plasma proteins in blood of divers after a single short-time operational heliox exposure. *Int Marit Health* 53(1–4): 111–121.

Olver JM, Spalton DJ, McCartney ACE (1990) Microvasculature study of the retrolaminar optic nerve in man: the possible significance in anterior ischemic optic neuropathy. *Eye* 4: 7–24.

Omae T, Ibayashi S, Kusuda K *et al* (1998) Effects of high atmospheric pressure and oxygen on middle cerebral blood flow velocity in humans measured by transcranial Doppler. *Stroke* 29: 94–97.

Ong M (2008) Hyperbaric oxygen therapy in the management of diabetic lower limb wounds. *Singapore Med J* 49: 105–109.

Opremack EM, Bruce RA (1999) Surgical decompression of branch retinal vein occlusion via arteriovenous crossing sheathotomy: a prospective review of 15 cases. *Retina* 19: 1–5.

Orgogozo NM, Dartigues JF (1991) Methodology of clinical trials in acute cerebral ischemia. *Cerebrovasc Dis* 1 (suppl 1): 100–111.

Oriani G, Barnini C *et al* (1982) Hyperbaric oxygen therapy in the treatment of various orthopedic disorders. *Minerva Med* 73: 2983–2988.

Oriani G, Michael M, Meazza D *et al* (1992) Diabetic foot and hyperbaric oxygen therapy: a ten year experience. *J Hyperbaric Med* 7: 213–222.

Orynbaev TO, Myrzaliev VA (1981) Hyperbaric oxygenation in the therapy of viral hepatitis in children. In Yefuny SN (Ed.) *Proceedings of the 7th international congress of hyperbaric medicine.* USSR Academy of Sciences, Moscow, p 35.

Ostashevskaia MI, Afanas-Eva NB, Valuiskova RP *et al* (1986) Experience in the use of hyperbaric oxygenation to treat diabetes mellitus in children. *Probl Endokrinol* 32: 16–19.

Osterloh MD, Charles S (1988) Surgical decompression of branch retinal vein occlusions. *Arch Ophthalmol* 106: 1469–1471.

Ouda M, Moriyama Y, Haibara T *et al* (1977) The therapeutic effect of hyperbaric oxygen in the "shock lung." In Smith G (Ed.) *Proceedings of the 6th international congress on hyperbaric medicine.* University of Aberdeen Press, Aberdeen, pp 82–83.

Oury TD, Ho YS, Piantadosi CA *et al* (1992) Extracellular superoxide dismutase, nitric oxide, and central nervous system oxygen toxicity. *Proc Natl Acad Sci USA* 89: 9715–9719.

Ozkiris A, Evereklioglu C, Erkilic K, Ilhan O (2005) The efficacy of intravitreal triamcinolone acetonide on macular edema in branch retinal vein occlusion. *Eur J Ophthalmol* 15: 96–101.

Ozorio de Almeida A, Costa HM (1938) Treatment of leprosy by oxygen at high pressure associated with methylene blue. *Rev Bras Leprol* 6: 237–265.

Oztas E, Kilic A, Ozyurt M *et al* (2001) Effect of hyperbaric oxygen and penicillin in a murine model of streptococcal myositis. *Undersea Hyperb Med* 28: 181–186.

P

Pace N, Strajman E, Walker EL (1950) Acceleration of carbon monoxide elimination in man by high pressure oxygen. *Science* 111: 652–654.

Padaonkar V, Giblin FJ, Reddan JR *et al* (1993) Hyperbaric oxygen inhibits the growth of cultured rabbit lens epithelial cells without affecting glutathione level. *Exp Eye Res* 56: 443–452.

Padgaonkar V, Giblin FJ, Reddy VN (1989) Disulfide cross-linking of urea-insoluble proteins in rabbit lenses treated with hyperbaric oxygen. *Exp Eye Res* 49: 887–899.

Pallota R, Anceschi S, Costagliola N (1980) Therapy with hyperbaric oxygen of acute pancreatitis. *Ann Med Nav* 85: 27–34.

Pallota R, Anceschi S, Costagliola N *et al* (1978) Recovery from blindness through hyperbaric oxygen in a case of thrombosis on the central retinal artery. *Ann Med Nav* 83: 591–592.

Pallota R, Anceschi S, Costilgliola N *et al* (1980a) Prospettive di terapia iperbarica nella sclerosi a placche. *Ann Med Nav* 85: 57–62.

Pallota R, Longobardi G, Fabbrocini G (1986) Experience in protracted follow-up on a group of multiple sclerosis patients treated with hyperbaric oxygen therapy. In Baixe JH (Ed.) *Symposium sur le traitment de la sclerose multiple par l'oxyene hyperbare*, Paris.

Palmquist BM (1986) Ophthalmological effects of hyperbaric oxygen therapy in the elderly. *Geriatr Med Today* 5: 135–137.

Palmquist BM, Philipson B, Barr PO (1984) Nuclear cataract and myopia during hyperbaric oxygen therapy. *Br J Ophthalmol* 68: 113–117.

Park CH, Jaffe GJ, Fekrat S (2003) Intravitreal triamcinolone acetonide in eyes with cystoid macular edema associated with retinal vein occlusion. *Am J Ophthalmol* 136: 419–425.

Parkinson RB, Hopkins RO, Cleavinger HB *et al* (2002) White matter hyperintensities and neuropsychological outcome following carbon monoxide poisoning. *Neurology* 58: 1525–1532.

Pascual J, Peralta G, Sanchez U (1995) Preventive effects of hyperbaric oxygen in cluster headache. *Headache* 35: 260–261.

Patel P, Raybould T, Maryama Y (1989) Osteoradionecrosis of the jaw bones at the University of Kentucky Medical Center. *J Kentucky Med Assoc* 87: 327–331.

Paty DW, Li DKB *et al* (1993) Interferon-beta 1b is effective in relapsing remitting multiple sclerosis.2. MRI analysis results of a multicenter, randomized double-blind, placebo-controlled trial. *Neurology* 43: 662–667.

Patz A (1955) Oxygen inhalation in retinal arterial occlusion. *Am J Ophthalmol* 40: 789–795.

Patz A (1965) Effect of oxygen on immature retinal vessels. *Invest Ophth* 4: 988–999.

Pavlik L (1976) Hyperbaric oxygen therapy in Meniere's disease. *Cesk Otolaryngol* 25: 160–163.

Paw HGW, Reed PN (1996) Pneumatosis cystoides intestinalis confined to the small intestine treated with hyperbaric oxygen. *Undersea Hyperbaric Med* 23: 115–117.

Pearson RRP, Pezeshkpour GH, Dutka AJ (1992) Cerebral involvement in decompression sickness. *Undersea Biomedical Res* 19: 39–40.

Pellitteri PK, Kennedy TL, Youn BA (1992) The influence of intensive hyperbaric oxygen therapy on skin survival in a swine model. *Arch Otolaryngol Head Neck Surg* 118: 1050–1054.

Peloso OA (1982) Hyperbaric oxygen treatment of intestinal obstruction and other related conditions. *Hyperbaric Oxygen Rev* 3: 103–119.

Pepe P, Zackariah BS, Sayer MR, Floccare D (1998) Ensuring the chain of recovery for stroke in your community. *Acad Emer Med* 5(4): 352–358.

Perkins SA, Magargal LE, Augsburger JJ, Sanborn GE (1987) The idling retina: Reversible visual loss in central retinal artery obstruction. *Ann Ophthalmol* 19: 3–6.

Perrins DJ, James PB (2002) Hyperbaric oxygen therapy and multiple sclerosis. *Undersea and Hyperb Med* 29: 236–238.

Perrins DJ, James PB (2005) Long-term hyperbaric oxygenation retards progression in multiple sclerosis patients. *IJNN* 2: 45–48.

Perrin DSD (1967) Influence of hyperbaric oxygen on split thickness grafts, *Lancet* 1: 868–871.

Perrins D (1977) Hyperbaric oxygenation in paralyticileus. *Br Med J* 1: 1602.

Perrins DJ, Kindwall E, Sukoff MH (1977) Promising research areas. In Davis JC, Hunt TK (Eds.) *Hyperbaric oxygen therapy*. Undersea Medical Society, Bethesda, p 310.

Perrins DJD (1966) Hyperbaric oxygenation of ischemic skin flaps and pedicles. In Brown IW, Cox BG (Eds.) *Proceedings of the 3rd international congress on HBO medicine*. Duke University Press, Durham NC, pp 613–620.

Perrins DJD (1970) The influence of hyperbaric oxygen on the survival of split skin grafts. In Wada J, Iwa T (Eds.) *Proceedings of the 4th international congress on HBO medicine*. Baillere, London, pp 369–376.

Perrins DJD, James PB (1994) The treatment of Multiple Sclerosis with prolonged courses of hyperbaric oxygen. *Proceedings of the 1st European Consensus Conference on Hyperbaric Medicine*. ille: 245–263.

Perrins JD, Barr PO (1986) Hyperbaric oxygenation and wound healing. In Schmutz J (Ed.) *Proceedings of the 1st Swiss symposium on HBO* Foundation for Hyperbaric Medicine, Basel, pp 119–132.

Persel J (1989) Hyperbaric medicine – tools of the trade. *J Hyperbaric Med* 4: 89–93.

Petre PM, Baciewicz FA Jr, Tigan S, Spears JR (2003) Hyperbaric oxygen as a chemotherapy adjuvant in the treatment of metastatic lung tumors in a rat model. *J Thorac Cardiovasc Surg* 125: 85–95.

Petterson JA, Hill MD, Demchuk AM *et al* (2005) Intra-arterial thrombolysis for retinal artery occlusion: The Calgary experience. *Can J Neurol Sci* 32: 507–511.

Pfister RR (1991) The intraocular changes of anterior segment necrosis. *Eye* 5: 214–221.

Pfoff D, Thom SR (1986) Preliminary report on the effect of hyperbaric oxygen on cystoid macular edema. *Cataract Refract Surg* 13: 136–140.

Pfoff DS, Thom SR (1987) Preliminary report on the effect of hyperbaric oxygen on cystoid macular edema. *J Cataract Refract Surg* 13: 136–140.

Phillips D, Diaz C, Atwell G, Chimiak J, Ullman S *et al* (1999) Care of sudden blindness: A case report of acute central retinal artery occlusion reversed with hyperbaric oxygen therapy. *Undersea Hyperbaric Med* 26(supp): 23–24 (abstract).

Piantadosi CA (1987) Carbon monoxide, oxygen transport, and oxygen metabolism. *J Hyperbaric Med* 2: 27–44.

Pierce EC, Jacobson JH (1977) Cerebral edema. In Davis JC, Hunt TK (Eds.) *Hyperbaric oxygen therapy*. Undersea Medical Society, Bethesda, pp 287–302.

Pierre RV (1964) Effects of hyperbaric hyperoxia on erythropoiesis. *Clin Res* 12: 348.

Pilgramm H (1991) *Klinische, hämoreologische und tierexperimentelle Untersuchungen zur Therapieoptierung des akuten Knalltraumas*. Certificate of Habilitation (Thesis), University of Greifswald, Germany.

Pilgramm M, Fischer B, Frey G, Roth M (1986) *Change in rheological parameters under hyperbaric oxygen therapy in patients with inner ear damage.* Ninth international symposium on underwater and hyperbaric physiology, Kobe, Japan.

Pilgramm M, Lamm H, Schumann K (1985) Zur hyperbaren Sauerstofftherapie beim Hörsturz. *Larngologie Rhinol Otol* 64: 351–354.

Pilgramm M, Schumann K (1985) Hyperbaric oxygen therapy for acute acoustic trauma. *Arch Otorhinolaryngol* 241: 246–257.

Pineas H (1924) Klinischer und anatomischer Befund eines Falles von CO-Vergiftung. *Z Neur* 93: 36–38.

Plafki C, Peters P, Almeling M, Welslau W, Busch R (2000). Complications and side effects of hyperbaric oxygen therapy. *Aviat Space Environ Med* 71: 119–24.

Plum F, Pulsinelli WA (1992) Cerebral metabolism and hypoxic-ischemic brain injury. In Asbury AK *et al* (Eds.) *Diseases of the Nervous System: Clinical Neurobiology,* Chap 77, Philadelphia, Saunders, pp 1002–1015.

Pobedinsky ANM, Proshina IV, Fanchenko ND (1981) Hyperbaric oxygenation in treating disorders of the reproductive function in women. In Yefuny SN: *Proceedings of the 7th international congress on hyperbaric medicine.* USSR Academy of Sciences, Moscow, p 359.

Pogorelova TN, Dluzhevskaya TS, Drukker NA (1983) Composition of placental membrane proteins in feto-placental insufficiency treated by means of hyperbaric oxygenation. *Probl Med Chem* 29: 57–61.

Polk JD, Rugaber C, Kohn G, Arenstein R, Fallon WF (2002) Central retinal artery occlusion by proxy: a cause for sudden blindness in an airline passenger. *Aviat Space Environ Med* 73: 385.

Polkinghorne PJ, Bird AC, Cross MR (1989) Retinal vessel construction under hyperbaric conditions. *Lancet* 2: 1099.

Polse KA, Mandell RB (1976) Etiology of corneal striae accompanying hydrogel lens wear. *Invest Ophthalmol* 15: 553–556.

Ponikvar R, Buturovic J, Cizman M *et al* (1998) Hyperbaric oxygenation, plasma exchange, and hemodialysis for treatment of acute liver failure in a 3-year-old child. *Artif Organs* 22: 952–7.

Pontani BA, Warriner RA, Newman RK *et al* (1998) Delayed neurologic sequelae after hydrogen sulfide poisoning treated with hyperbaric oxygen therapy. *Undersea Hyperbaric Med* 25: 10 (abstract).

Poole DC, Barstow TJ, McDonough P, Jones AM (2008) Control of oxygen uptake during exercise. *Med Sci Sports Exerc* 40: 462–474.

Popova ZS, Kuz'minov OD (1996) Treatment of primary open-angle glaucoma by the method of combined use of hyperbaric oxygenation and antioxidants. *Vestn Oftalmol* 112): 4–6.

Porcellini M, Bernardo B, Capasso R (1997) Combined vascular injuries and limb fractures. *Minerva Cardioangiol* 45: 131–138.

Potchen EJ, Potchen MJ (1991) The imaging of brain function. Positron emission tomography, single-photon emission computed tomography, and some prospects for magnetic resonance. *Invest radiol* 26: 258–265.

Poulton TJ, Witcofski RL (1985) HBO therapy for exprmtl. radiation myelitis. *Undersea Biomed Res* 12: 453–458.

Pound MW, May DB (2005) Proposed mechanisms and preventative options of Jarisch-Herxheimer reactions. *J Clin Pharm Ther* 30: 291–295.

Powell MR, Thoma W, Fust HD *et al* (1983) Gas phase formation and Doppler monitoring during decompression with elevated oxygen. *Undersea Biomed Res* 10: 217–224.

Prabhu SS, Sharma RR, Gurusinghe N *et al* (1993) Acute transient

hydrocephalus in carbon monoxide poisoning: a case report. *JNNP* 56: 567–568.

Prass K, Wiegand F, Schumann P *et al* (2000) Hyperbaric oxygenation induced tolerance against focal cerebral ischemia in mice is strain dependent. *Brain Res* 871: 146–50.

Pravaz (1837/38) Mémoire sur l'application du bain d'air comprimé au traitement des affections tuberculeuses, des hémorragies capillaires et des surdies catarrhales. *Bull Acad Natl Med (Paris)* 2: 985.

Prewitt ZP, Peltier GL, Adkinson CD (1989) External replantation. *J Hyperbaric Med* 4: 127–130.

Price ME, Davis MG, Hammett-Stabler C *et al* (1995) Evaluation of glucose monitoring devices in the hyperbaric chamber. *Military Medicine* 160: 143–146.

Priestley J (1775) The discovery of oxygen, part 1. In Faulconer A, Keys TC (Eds.) *Foundations of anesthesiology, Vol. 1.* Thomas, Springfield, 1965, pp 39–70.

Prockop LD, Chichkova RI (2007) Carbon monoxide intoxication: an updated review. *J Neurol Sci* 262: 122–130.

Prockop LD, Grasso RJ (1978) Ameliorating effects of HBO on exptl. allergic encephalomyelitis. *Brain Res Bull* 3: 221–225.

Putnam T, Alexander L (1947) Loss of axis cylinders in sclerotic plaques and similar lesions. *Arch Neurol* 57: 661–672.

Putnam TJ, McKenna JB, Morrison LR (1931) Studies in multiple sclerosis. I. The histogenesis of experimental sclerotic plaques and their relation to multiple sclerosis. *JAMA* 97: 1591–1596.

Q

Qu Zhan-Kui (1986) A brief introduction to the HBO Dept. In *Hospital of YangShang petrochemical corporation paper* presented at the 5th congress of hyperbaric medicine, Fuzhow, China.

Qin Z, Karabiyikoglu M, Hua Y *et al* (2007) Hyperbaric oxygen-induced attenuation of hemorrhagic transformation after experimental focal transient cerebral ischemia. *Stroke* 38: 1362–1367.

Quinlan PM, Elman MJ, Bhatt AK, Mardesich P, Engel C (1990) The natural course of central retinal vein occlusion. *Am J Ophthalmol* 110: 118–123.

R

Rabena MD, Pieramici DJ, Castellarin AA, Nasir MA, Avery RL (2007) Intravitreal bevacizumab (Avastin) in the treatment of macular edema secondary to branch retinal vein occlusion. *Retina* 27: 419–425.

Racic G, Denoble PJ, Sprem N *et al* (1997) Hyperbaric oxygen as a therapy of Bell's palsy. *Undersea Hyperbaric Med* 24: 35–38.

Racic G, Petri NM, Andric D (2001) Hyperbaric oxygen as a method of therapy of sudden sensorineural hearing loss. *Int Marit Health* 52: 74–84.

Radonic V, Baric D, Giunio L *et al* (1997) War injuries of the femoral artery and vein: a report on 67 cases. *Cardiovasc Surg* 5: 641–647.

Rahmani M, Bennani M, Benabdeljlil M *et al* (2006) Neuropsychological and magnetic resonance imaging findings in five patients after carbon monoxide poisoning. *Rev Neurol (Paris)* 162: 1240–1247.

Raju GS, Bendixen BH, Khan J *et al* (1998) Cerebrovascular accident during endoscopy: Consider cerebral air embolism, a rapidly reversible event with hyperbaric oxygen therapy. *Gastrointest Endosc* 47(1): 70–73.

Rakhmatullin IG, Hallev MA (1981) Hyperbaric oxygen in pre- and post-operative periods of patients with thyrotoxic goiter. In Yefuny SN (Ed.) *Proceedings of the 7th international congress on hyperbaric medicine.* USSR Academy of Sciences, Moscow p 373.

Ramaiah SK, Jaeschke H (2007) Role of neutrophils in the pathogenesis of acute inflammatory liver injury. *Toxicol Pathol* 35(6): 757–766.

Ramsden RT, Bulman CH, Lorigan BP (1975) Osteoradionecrosis of the temporal bone. *Otolaryngol Head Neck Surg* 89: 941–955.

Raphael JC, Elkharrat D, Jars-Guincestre MC *et al* (1989) Trial of normobaric and hyperbaric oxygen for acute carbon monoxide intoxication. *Lancet* ii: 414–419.

Raphael JC, Jars-Guincestre MC, Gajdos P (1993) Prise en charge des intoxications oxycarbonées aigues. *Rev Prat (Paris)* 43: 604–607.

Raskin A, Genshon S, Crook TH etal. (1978) Effects of hyperbaric and normobaric oxygen on cognitive impairment in the elderly. *Arch Gen Psychiatry* 35: 50–56.

Rathat C, Gratt MI, Pourriat JL *et al* (1979) Post-operative necrotizing enterocolitis. One case cured by hyperbaric oxygen therapy. *Anaes Analg Reanim* 36: 71–74.

Ratner GL, Kaluzhskikh VN, Dildin AS *et al* (1978) Hyperbaric oxygenation in intensive therapy of automotor disorders of intestinal function. *Anesteziol Reanimatol* 4: 64–68.

Ravicovitch MA, Spalline A (1982) Spinal epidural abscesses. Surgical and parasurgical management. *Eur Neurol* 21: 347–357.

Ravina A, Minuchin O, Kehrmann H (1983) A simple, disposable, hyperbaric oxygen device for treatment. *Isr J Med Sci* 19: 845–847.

Ray DE, Hawgood BJ (1977) Influence of systemic factors on hyperbaric oxygen toxicity in the rat visual system. *Aviat Space Environ Med* 48: 1046–1050.

Raynaud C, Rancurel G, Samson Y *et al* (1987) Pathophysiologic study of chronic infarcts with I-123 isopropyl iodo-amphetamine (IMP): the importance of periinfarct area. *Stroke* 18: 21–29.

Raynaud C, Rancurel G, Tzourio N *et al* (1989) SPECT analysis of recent cerebral infarction. *Stroke* 20: 192–204.

Rebello G, Mason KJ (1978) Pulmonary histological appearances in fatal paraquat poisoning. *Histopathology* 2: 53–66.

Recupero SM, Cruciani F, Picardo V *et al* (1992) Hyperbaric oxygen therapy in the treatment of secondary keratoendotheliosis. *Ann of Opthalmolplain* 24: 448–452.

Regge D, Gallo T, Galli J *et al* (1997) Systemic arterial air embolism and tension pneumothorax: Two complications of transthoracic percutaneous thin-needle biopsy in the same patient. *Eur Radiol* 7: 173–175.

Regillo C, Chang TS, Johnson MW, Kaiser PK, Scott IU, Spaide R, Griggs PB (2007) *Retina and Vitreous: American Academy of Ophthalmology Basic and Clinical Science Course – Section 12.* San Francisco: American Acadeny of Ophthalmology.

Reichardt KA, Nabavi A, Barth H *et al* (2003) Barotrauma as a possible cause of aneurysmal subarachnoid hemorrhage. Case report. *J Neurosurg* 98: 180–182.

Reillo MR (1997) *AIDS under pressure.* Hogrefe & Huber, Toronto-Bern-Göttingen.

Reillo MR, Altieri RJ (1996). HIV antiviral effects of hyperbaric oxygen therapy. *J Assoc Nurses AIDS Care* 7: 43–45.

Reitan JA, Kien ND, Thorup S *et al* (1990) Hyperbaric oxygen increases survival following carotid ligation in gerbils. *Stroke* 21: 119–123.

Ren H, Wang W, Zhaoming CE (2001) Glasgow Coma Scale, brain electric activity mapping and Glasgow Outcome Scale after hyperbaric oxygen treatment of severe brain injury. *Chinese J of Traumatology (English Edition)* 4(4): 239–241.

Resch H, Zawinka C, Weigert G, Schmetterer L, Garhofer G (2005) Inhaled carbon monoxide increases retinal and choroidal blood flow in healthy humans. *Invest Ophthalmol Vis Sci* 46: 4275–4280.

Reshef A, Bitterman N, Kerem D (1991) The effect of carbamazepine and ethosuximide on hyperbaric seizures. *Epilepsy Res* 8: 117–121.

Reul J, Weiss J, Jung A *et al* (1995) Central nervous system lesions and cervical disc herniations in amateur drivers. *Lancet* 345: 1403–1405.

Ricci B, Calogero G, Lepore D (1989) Variations in the severity of retinopathy seen in newborn rats supplemented with oxygen under different conditions of hyperbarism. *Exp Eye Res* 49: 789–797.

Ricci B, Minicucci G, et al. (1995) Oxygen induced retinopathy in the newborn rat: Effects of hyperbarism and topical administration of timolol maleate. *Graefes Arch Clin Exp Ophthalmol* 233: 226–230.

Richards V, Pinto D, Coombs P (1963) Studies in suspended animation by hypothermia combined with hyperbaric oxygenation. *Ann Surg* 158: 349–362.

Richter K, Löblich HJ, Wyllie JW (1978) Ultrastructural aspects of bubble formation in human fatal accidents after exposure to compressed air. *Virchows Arch* 380: 261–272.

Rider SP, Jackson SB, Rusyniak DE (2008 Apr 8) Cerebral air gas embolism from concentrated hydrogen peroxide ingestion. *Clin Toxicol (Phila)* doi:10.1080/15563650701725136.

Rijkmans BG, Bakker DJ, Dabhoiwala NF *et al* (1989) Successful treatment of radiation cystitis with hypealianic oxygenation. *Eur Urol* 16: 354–356.

Riordan SM, Williams R (1997) Treatment of hepatic encephalopathy. *NEJM* 337: 473–479.

Rios-Tejada F, Azofra-Garcia J, Valle-Garrido J (1997) Neurological manifestation of arterial gas embolism following standard altitude chamber flight: A case report. *Aviat Space Environ Med* 68: 1025–1028.

Rioux JP, Myers RAM (1989) Hyperbaric oxygen for methylene chloride poisoning? A report of two cases. *Ann Emerg Med* 18: 691–695.

Riva CE, Pournaras CJ, Tsacopoulos M (1986) Regulation of local oxygen tension and blood flow of the inner retina during hyperoxia. *J Appl Physiol* 51: 592–598.

Rivers EP, Martin GB, Smithline H *et al* (1992) The clinical implications of continuous central venous oxygen saturation during human CPR. *Ann Emerg Med* 21: 1094–1101.

Robbins L (1996) Menstrual migraine with features of cluster headache. A report of 10 cases. *Headache* 36: 166–167.

Röckert HOE, Haglid K (1983) Reversible changes in the rate of DNS synthesis in the testes of rats after daily exposure to a hyperbaric environment of air. *IRCS Med Sci Biochem* 11: 531.

Rockswald GL, Ford SE, Anderson DC *et al* (1992) Results of a prospective randomized trial for the treatment of severely brain-injured patients with hyperbaric oxygen. *J Neurosurg* 76: 929–934.

Rockswold SB, Rockswold GL, Defillo A (2007) Hyperbaric oxygen in traumatic brain injury. *Neurol Res* 29: 162–172.

Rockwell S, Kelley M, Irvin CG *et al* (1992) Preclinical Evaluation of Oxydent as an adjuvant to radiotherapy. *Biomater Artif Cells Immobilization Biotechnol* 20: 883–893.

Rockswold SB, Rockswold GL, Vargo JM *et al* (2001) Effects of hyperbaric oxygenation therapy on cerebral metabolism and intracranial pressure in severely brain injured patients. *J Neurosurg* 95: 544–546.

Roden D, Bostley TM, Fowble B *et al* (1990) Delayed radiation injury to the retrobulbar optic nerves and chiasm. *Ophthalmology* 97: 346–351.

Rogatsky GG, Kamenir Y, Mayevsky A (2005) Effect of hyperbaric oxygenation on intracranial pressure elevation rate in rats during the early phase of severe traumatic brain injury. *Brain Res* 1047: 131–136.

Rogatsky GG, Shifrin EG, Mayevsky A (2003) Optimal dosing as a necessary condition for the efficacy of hyperbaric oxygen therapy in acute ischemic stroke: a critical review. *Neurol Res* 25: 95–98.

Rogatsky GG, Vainshtein MB, Sevostianova TV (1988) Use of hyperbaric oxygenation to correct an acute experimental respiratory insufficiency syndrome. *Biull Eksp Biol Med* 105: 410–411.

Rojas A, Carl U, Reghebii K (1990) Effect of normobaric oxygen on tumor radiosensitivity: fractionated studies. *Int J Radiation Oncol Biol Phys* 18: 547–553.

Rojas A, Stewart FA, Smith KA, Soranson JA, Randhawa VS, Straford MR, Denekamp J (1987) Effect of anemia on tumor radiosensitivity under normo- and hyperbaric conditions. *Int J Radiat Oncol Biol Phys* 13: 1681–1689.

Roman H, Saint-Hillier S, Dick Harms J *et al* (2002) Gas embolism and hyperbaric oxygen treatment during pregnancy: a case report and a review of the literature. *J Gynecol Obstet Biol Reprod (Paris)* 31: 663–667.

Roos JA, Jackson Friedman C, Lyden P (1998). Effects of hyperbaric oxygen on neurologic outcome for cerebral ischemia in rats. *Acad Emerg Med* 5: 18–24.

Ros MA, Magargal LE, Uram M (1989) Branch retinal artery obstruction: a review of 201 eyes. *Ann Ophthalmol* 21: 103–107.

Rosasco SA (1974) Hyperbaric oxygen treatment of patients during resistant leprosy. In Trapp WG, Banister EW, Davison AJ (Eds.) *Proceedings of the 5th international congress on hyperbaric medicine.* Simon Fraser University, Burnaby.

Rosasco SA, Calori B, Cabrini M, Rubio R (1972) Caisson hyperbare et chirurgie des nouveau-nés nourrissons. *Ann Chir Infant* 13: 23–27.

Rosenfeld PJ, Fung AE, Puliafito CA (2005) Optical coherence tomography findings after an intravitreal injection of bevacizumab (avastin) for macular edema from central retinal vein occlusion. *Ophthalmic Surg Lasers Imaging* 36: 336–339.

Rosenthal E, Benderly A, Monies-Chass I *et al* (1985) Hyperbaric oxygenation in peripheral ischaemic lesions in infants. *Arch Dis Child* 60: 372–374.

Rosenthal RE, Silbergleit R, Hof PR, Haywood Y, Fiskum G (2003) Hyperbaric oxygen reduces neuronal death and improves neurological outcome after canine cardiac arrest. *Stroke* 34(5): 1311–1316.

Ross JAS, Manson HJ, Shearer A *et al* (1977) Some aspects of anesthesia in high pressure environments. *Proc Int Congress Hyperbaric Med*, Aberdeen University Press, pp 449–452.

Ross ME, Yolton DP, Yolton RL *et al* (1996) Myopia associated with hyperbaric oxygen therapy. *Optom Vis Sci* 73: 487–494.

Rossi GF, Maira G, Vignati A *et al* (1987) Neurological improvement in chronic ischemic stroke following surgical brain revascularization. *Ital J Neurol Sci* 8: 464–475.

Rossor MN (1993) Headache, stupor and coma. In Walton J (Ed.)

Brain's Diseases of the Nervous System, Tenth Edition, Oxford, Oxford University Press, pp 127–143.

Rothfuss A, Speit G (2002) Overexpression of heme oxygenase-1 (HO-1) in V79 cells results in increased resistance to hyperbaric oxygen (HBO)-induced DNA damage. *Environ Mol Mutagen* 40: 258–265.

Roy M, Bartow W, Ambrus J, Fauci A, Collier B, Titus J (1989) Retinal leakage in retinal vein occlusion: reduction after hyperbaric oxygen. *Ophthalmologica* 198: 78–83.

Rozenek R, Fobel BF, Banks JC *et al* (2007) Does hyperbaric oxygen exposure affect high-intensity, short-duration exercise performance? *J Strength Cond Res* 21(4): 1037–1041.

Rubbini M, Longobardi P, Rimessi A, Pinton P, Morri A, Semprini G, Pistone P, Volpinari L (2007) [A new transportable machine for the preservation of livers to be transplanted by means of hyperbaric oxygenation perfusion] *Chir Ital* 59(5): 723–734.

Rudge FW (1990a) A case of decompression sickness at 2,432 meters (8,000 feet) *Aviat Space Environ Med* 61: 1026–1027.

Rudge FW (1990c) treatment of methylene chloride induced carbon monoxide poisoning with hyperbaric oxygenation. *Mil Med* 155: 570–572.

Rudge FW (1991) Decompression sickness presenting as viral syndrome. *Aviat Space Environ Med* 62: 60–61.

Rudge FW (1992) altitude-induced arterial gas embolism: a case report. *Aviat Space Environment Med* 63: 203–205.

Rudge FW (1993) Osteoradionecrosis of the temporal bone: treatment with hyperbgaric oxygen therapy. *Military Med* 158: 196–198.

Rudge FW, Shafer MR (1991) The effect of delay on treatment outcome in altitude-induced decompression sickness. *Aviat Space Environ Med* 62: 687–690.

Rui-Chang Y (1994) Rhematoid arthritis treated with hyperbaric oxygen. In *Proceedings of the XI International Congress of Hyperbaric Medicine.* Best, San Pedro.

Ruiz E, Brunette DD, Robinson EP *et al* (1986) Cerebral resuscitation after cardiac arrest using hetastarch hemodilution, hyperbaric oxygenation and magnesium ions. *Resuscitation* 14: 213–223.

Ruocco V, Bimonte D, Luongo C, Florio M (1986) Hyperbaric oxygen treatment of toxic epidermal necrolysis. *Cutis* 38: 267–271.

Rusyniak DE, Kirk MA, May JD *et al* (2003) Hyperbaric oxygen therapy in acute ischemic stroke: results of the Hyperbaric Oxygen in Acute Ischemic Stroke Trial Pilot Study. *Stroke* 34: 571–574.

Rzayev RM (1981) Role of hypoxia in pathogenesis of occupational hypoacusis and normalizing action of hyperbaric oxygenation on saturation of arterial blood with oxygen. *Zh Ushn Nos Gorl Bolez* 41: 22–25.

S

Sadan O, Adler M, Ezra S *et al* (1991) Air embolism due to pulmonary barotrauma in a patient undergoing cesarilan section. *Acta Obstet Gynecol Scand* 70: 511–513.

Safar P (1986) Cerebral resuscitation after cardiac arrest: a review. *Circulation* 74(suppl IV): IV-138-IV-153.

Saikovsky RS, Alekberova ZS, Dmitriev AA (1986) The role of hemocarboperfusion and hyperbaric oxygenation in the treatment of patients with rheumatoid arthritis with systemic symptoms. *Ter Arkh* 58: 105–109.

Sainty JM, Aubert L, Conti V, Allessandrini G (1980) Place de l'oxygénothérapie hyperbare dans le traitement de l'ostéonécrose aseptique de la hanche. *Med Aeronaut Spat Med Subaquat Hyperbare* 19(75): 215–217.

Saito H, Ota K, Sageusa T *et al* (1977) Clinical and experimental studies of hyperbaric oxygen treatment of postoperative ileus. In Smith G (Ed.) *Proceedings of the 6th international congress on hyperbaric medicine*. University of Aberdeen Press, Aberdeen, pp 333–337.

Sakakibara K (1986) The history and future prospects of hyperbaric oxygen therapy in japan. *Jpn J Hyperbaric Med* 21: 21–40.

Saltzman HA (1981) Acute hepatic injury due to carbon tetrachloride poisoning and use of hyperbaric oxygen therapy. *Hyperbaric Oxygen Rev* 2: 171–174.

Saltzman HA, Anderson B, Whalen RE *et al* (1966) Hyperbaric oxygen therapy of acute cerebral vascular insufficiency. In Brown IW, Cox BG (Eds.) *Hyperbaric medicine*. National Research Council, Washington D.C.

Saltzman HA, Hart L, Sieker HO *et al* (1965) Retinal vascular response to hyperbaric oxygenation. *JAMA* 191: 114–116.

Salzano JV, Camporesi EM, Stolp BW *et al* (1984) Physiological responses to exercise at 47 and 66 ATA. *J Appl Physiol* 57: 1055–1068.

Samuels AH, Vamos MJ, Taikato MLR (1992) Carbon monoxide, amnesia and hyperbaric oxygen therapy. *Aust NZ J Psychiatry* 26: 316–319.

Sanchez EC, Montes G, Oroz G, Garcia L (1999) Management of intestinal ischaemia, necrotizing enterocolitis and anoxic encephalopathies of neonates with hyperbaric oxygen therapy. *Undersea and Hyperbaric Medicine* 26(Suppl): 22.

Santos PM, Zamboni WA, Williams SL (1996) Hyperbaric oxygen treatment after rat peroneal nerve transection and entubulation. *Otolaryngol Head Neck Surg* 114: 424–434.

Sapunar D, Saraga-Babic M, Peruzovic M *et al* (1993) Effects of hyperbaric oxygen on rat embryos. *Biol Neonate* 63: 360–369.

Sarno JE, Rusk HA, Diller L *et al* (1972) The effect of hyperbaric oxygen on the mental and verbal ability of stroke patients. *Stroke* 2: 10.

Sasaki K, Fukuda M, Otani S *et al* (1978) High pressure oxygen therapy in ocular diseases: with special reference to the effect of concomitantly used stellate ganglion block. *Jpn J Anesth* 27: 170–176.

Sasaki M, Joh T (2007) Oxidative stress and ischemia-reperfusion injury in the gastrointestinal tract and antioxidant, protective agents. *J Clin Biochem Nutr* 40(1): 1–12.

Sasaki T (1975) One-half clearance time of carbon monoxide hemoglobin in blood during hyperbaric oxygen therapy (OHP). *Bull Tokyo Dent Univ* 22: 63–77.

Satoh J, Murase H, Tukagoshi H (1989) Hanging survivor showing alpha coma–a case report. *Rinsho shinkeigaku* 29(5): 612–6.

Saunders RA, Bluestein EC, Wilson ME, Berland JE (1994) Anterior segment ischemia after strabismus surgery. *Surv Ophthalmol* 38: 456–466.

Sause WT, Plenk HP (1979) Radiation therapy of head and neck tumours: a randomized study of treatment in air vs. treatment in hyperbaric oxygen. *Int J Radiat Oncol Biol Phys* 5: 1833–1836.

Savitt MA, Elbeery JR, Owen CH *et al* (1994) Mechanism of decreased coronary and systemic blood flow during hyperbaric oxygenation *Undersea Hyperbaric Med* 21: (in press).

Schaad G, Kleinhanss G, Piekarski C (1983) Zum Einfluss von Kohlenmonoxid in der Atemluft auf die psychophysische Leistungsfähigkeit. *Wehrmed Mschr* 27: 423–430.

Schaffner F, Roberts DK, Ginn FL, Ulvedal F (1966) Electron micros-

copy of monkey liver after exposure of animals to pure oxygen atmosphere. *Pro Soc Exp Biol Med* 121: 1200–1203.

Schaal KB, Hoh AE, Scheuerle A, Schutt F, Dithmar S (2007) Bevacizumab for the treatment of macular edema secondary to retinal vein occlusion. *Ophthalmologe* 104: 285–289.

Schechter Y, Pelled B, Alroy G *et al* (1975) Deleterious effects of hyperbaric oxygen treatment on mortality and pathological changes in nitrogen dioxide poisoned dogs. *Respiration* 32: 210–216.

Scheidt S, Wilner G, Fillmore S, Shapiro M, Killip T (1973) Objective haemodynamic assessment after acute myocardial infarction. *Br Heart J* 35: 908–916.

Scheinker M (1943) Formation of demyelinated plaques associated with cerebral fat embolism in man. *Arch Neurol Psychiatry* 49: 754–764.

Scheinkestel CD, Bailey M, Myles PS *et al* (1999) Hyperbaric or normobaric oxygen for acute carbon monoxide poisoning: a randomised controlled clinical trial. *Med J Aust* 170: 203–210.

Scherer A, Engelbrecht V, Bernbeck B *et al* (2000) MRI evaluation of aseptic osteonecrosis in children over the course of hyperbaric oxygen therapy. *Rofo Fortschr Geb Rontgenstr Neuen Bildgeb Verfahr* 172: 798–801.

Schlaepfer TE, Bärtsch P, Fisch HU (1992) Paradoxical effect of mild hypoxia and moderate altitude on human visual perception. *Clinical Science* 83: 633–636.

Schmitz G (1977) Cognitive function: a review of the problems of research on senility. In Davis JC, Hunt TK (Eds.) *Hyperbaric oxygen therapy*. Undersea Medical Society, Bethesda, pp 329–341.

Schmitz G (1981) Evaluation of hyperbaric oxygen therapy for senility. *HBO Rev* 2: 231.

Schnabel A, Bennet M, Schuster F, Roewer N, Kranke P (2008) [Hyper- or normobaric oxygen therapy to treat migraine and cluster headache pain: Cochrane Review] [Article in German] *Schmerz* 22: 129–136.

Schoenrock GJ, Cianci P (1986) Treatment of radiation cystitis with hyperbaric oxygen. *Urology* 27: 271–272.

Schraibman IG, Ledingham IM (1969) Hyperbaric oxygen and local vasodilatation in peripheral vascular disease. *Brit J Surg* 56: 295–299.

Schramek A, Hashmonai M (1978) Vascular injuries in the extremities in battle injuries. *Br J Surg* 64: 644–648.

Schrot J, Thomas JR, Robertson RF (1984) Temporal changes in repeated acquisition behavior after carbon monoxide exposure. *Neurobehav Toxicol Teratol* 6: 23–28.

Schürks M, Kurth T, Geissler I, Tessmann G, Diener HC, Rosskopf D (2007b) The G1246A polymorphism in the hypocretin receptor 2 gene is not associated with treatment response in cluster headache. *Cephalalgia* 27: 363–367.

Schürks M, Rosskopf D, de Jesus J, Jonjic M, Diener HC, Kurth T (2007a) Predictors of acute treatment response among patients with cluster headache. *Headache* 47: 1079–1084.

Schulte JH (1963) Effects of mild carbon monoxide intoxication. *Arch Environ Health* 7: 524–530.

Schulze G, Jänicke B (1986) Effects of chronic hypoxia on behavioral and physiological parameters. *Neurobiol Aging* 7: 199–203.

Schumacher GA (1974) Critique of experimental trials in multiple sclerosis. *Neurology* 24: 1010–1014.

Schutzer SE, Coyle PK, Belman AL, Golightly MG, Drulle J (1990) Sequestration of antibody to Borrelia burgdorferi in immune complexes in seronegative Lyme disease. *Lancet* 335: 312–315.

Schwerzmann M, Seiler C (2001) Recreational scuba diving, patent foramen ovale and their associated risks. *Swiss Med Wkly* 131: 365–74.

Scolnick B, Hamel D, Woolf AD (1993) The successful treatment of life-threatening prpionnitrile exposure with sodium nitrite/sodium thiosulfate followed by hyperbaric oxygen. *J Occup Med* 35: 577–580.

Sealy R (1991) Hyperbaric oxygen in the radiation treatment of head and neck cancers. *Radiother Oncol* 20(suppl 1): 75–79.

Sealy R, Berry RJ, Ryall RDH et al (1977) The treatment of carcinoma of the nasopharynx in hyperbaric oxygen: an outside assessment. *Int J Radiat Oncol Biol Phys* 2: 711–714.

Sealy R, Harrison GG, Morrell D, Korrubel J et al (1986) A feasibility study of a new approach to clinical radiosensitization: hypothermia and hyperbaric oxygen in combination with pharmacological vasodilatation. *Br J Radiol* 59: 1093–1098.

Sealy R, Hockly J, Shepstone B (1974) The treatment of malignant melanoma with cobalt and hyperbaric oxygen. *Clin Radiol* 25: 211–215.

Sealy R, Jacobs P, Wood L et al (1989) The treatment of tumors by induction of anemia and irradiation in hyperbaric oxygen. *Cancer* 64: 646–652.

Sebban A, Hirst LW (1991) Pterygium recurrence rate at the Princess Alexandra Hospital. *Aust N Z J Ophthalmol* 19: 203–206.

Segal P. *Hyperbaric oxygen and hypothermia improves revival of Hextend-resuscitated hemorrhagic, apneic rats.* Presented at the Experimental Biology 2003 conference in San Diego, California on 15 April 2003.

Seiler WO, Chapius A, Stahelin, Dollfus P (1984) Better prevention of bedsores in the light of current physiopathological findings. *Rev Med Suisse Romande* 104: 949–954.

Sellers LM (1965) The fallibility of Forrestian principle. *Anesth Analg* 44: 39.

Senechal C, Larivee S, Engelbert R, Marois P (2007) Hyperbaric oxygenation therapy in the treatment of cerebral palsy: A review and comparison to currently accepted therapies. *J American Physicians and Surgeons* 12: 109–113.

Senechal C, Larivee S, Richard E, Marois P (2007) Hyperbaric oxygenation therapy in the treatment of cerebral palsy: a review and comparison to currently accepted therapies. *J of Amer Phys and Surgeons* 12(4): 109–113.

Serebrianskaia MV, Masenko VP (1993) Dynamics of prostaglandin E content in patients with duodenal ulcer during various treatment regimens. *Klin Med Mosk* 71: 45–47.

Sergeev SI, Darialova SL, Lavnikova GA (1977) Hyperbaric oxygenation in the preoperative radiotherapy of soft tissue sarcomas. *Copr Onkol* 23: 17–27.

Sethi A, Mukherjee A (2003) Study of the efficacy of hyperbaric oxygen therapy in gross motor abilities of cerebral palasy children of 2–5 years, given initially as an adjunct to occupational therapy. *Indian Journal of Occupational Therapy* 35: 7–11.

Severinghaus J (1965) Hyperbaric oxygenation: anesthesia and drug effects. A committee report. *Anesthesiology* 26: 812–824.

Sevitt S (1962) *Fat embolism.* Butterworths, London, p 59.

Shah GK (2000) Adventitial sheathotomy for treatment of macular edema associated with branch retinal vein occlusion. *Curr Opin Ophthalmol* 11: 171–174.

Shah GK, Sharma S, Fineman MS et al (2000) Arteriovenous adventitial sheathotomy for the treatmet of macular edema associated with branch retinal vein occlusion. *Am J Ophthalmol* 129: 104–106.

Shahid H, Hossain P, Amoaku WM (2006) The management of retinal vein occlusion: is interventional ophthalmology the way forward? *Br J Ophthalmol* 90: 627–639.

Shakarashvilli NV, Gankin EK, Uskov IA (1981) Normalizing effect of hyperbaric oxygen on the production of hormones by thyroid gland. In Yefuny SN (Ed.) *Proceedings of the 7th international congress on hyperbaric medicine.* USSR Academy of Sciences, Moscow, p 371.

Shakhbazyan IE, Lukich VL, Madzhidov VV (1988) Effect of hyperbaric oxygenation on the development of adjuvant arthritis in C57BL/6 strain mice. *Rheumatology (USSR)* 3: 44–50.

Shakhtmeister IA, Savrasov VP (1987) Experience with the photochemotherapy of psoriasis combined with hyperbaric oxygenation. *Vestn Dermatol Venerol* 7: 35–36.

Shalkevich VB (1981) Use of hyperbaric oxygenation in the therapy of transient cerebral circulatory disturbances in the vertebro-basilar system. In Yefuni SN (Ed.) *Abstracts of the 7th international congress on HBO medicine.* USSR Academy of Sciences, Moscow, pp 294–295.

Shameem IA, Shimabukuro T, Shirataki S et al (1992) Hyperbaric oxygen therapy for the control of intractable cyclophosphamide-induced hemorrhagic cystitis. *Eur Urol* 22: 263–264.

Shandling AH, Ellestad MH, Hart GB et al (1997) Hyperbaric oxygen and thrombolysis in myocardial infarction: the "hot MI" pilot study. *Am Heart J* 134: 544–550.

Shannon TM, Celli B (1991) Oxygen therapy. *Emergency Medicine* (Dec 15): 63–70.

Sharp GR, Ledingham IM, Norman JN (1962) The application of oxygen at 2 atmospheres pressure in the treatment of acute anoxia. *Anaesthesia* 17: 136–144.

Shauly Y, Nachum Z, Gdal OM et al (1993) Adjunctive hyperbaric oxygen therapy for actinomycotic lacrimal canaliculitis. *Graef Arch Clin Exp Ophthalmol* 231: 429–431.

Shaw FL, Handy RD, Bryson P et al (2005) A single exposure to hyperbaric oxygen does not cause oxidative stress in isolated platelets: no effect on superoxide dismutase, catalase, or cellular ATP. *Clin Biochem* 38: 722–726.

Sheffield PJ, Davis JC (1976) Application of hyperbaric oxygen therapy in a case of prolonged cerebral hypoxia following rapid decompression. *Aviat Space Environ Med* 47: 759–762.

Sheffield PJ, Desautels DA (1997). Hyperbaric and hypobaric chamber fires: a 73-year analysis. *Undersea Hyperbaric Med* 24: 153–164.

Sheffield PJ, Desautels DA (1998). Hyperbaric chamber fires: an update. *Undersea Hyperbaric Med* 25: p 26 (abstract).

Sheffield PJ, Heimbach RD (1985) Respiratory physiology. In Dehart RL (Ed.) *Fundamentals of aerospace medicine.* Lea and Febiger, Philadelphia, p 87.

Sheffield PJ, Piwinski SE (1983) *Hyperbaric chamber equipment: a consolidated equipment list from selected multiplace hyperbaric facilities.* Report USAF SAM-TR-83–34, USAF School of Aerospace Medicine, Brooks Air Force Base, San Antonio, pp 1–22.

Sheftel TG, Mader JT, Pennick JJ, Cierny G (1985) Methicillin-resistant staphylococcus aureus osteomyelitis. *Cli Orthop* 198: 231–239.

Sheth SG, LaMont JT (1998) Toxic megacolon. *Lancet* 351: 509–513.

Shilling JS, Jones CA (1984) Retinal branch vein occlusion: a study of argon laser photocoagulation in the treatment of macular edema. *Br J Ophthalmol* 68: 196–198.

Shimada H, Morita T, Kunimoto F *et al* (1996) Immediate application of hyperbaric oxygen therapy using a newly devised transportable chamber. *Am J Emerg Med* 14: 412–415.

Shimada M, Ina K, Takahashi H *et al* (2001) Pneumatosis cystoides intestinalis treated with hyperbaric oxygen therapy: usefulness of an endoscopic ultrasonic catheter probe for diagnosis. *Intern Med* 40: 896–900.

Shimosegawa E, Hatazawa J, Nagata K *et al* (1992) Cerebral blood flow and glucose metabolism measurements in a patient surviving one year after carbon monoxide intoxication. *J Nuclear Medicine* 33: 1696–1698.

Shiokawa D, Fujishima M, Yanai T *et al* (1986) Hyperbaric oxygen therapy in experimentally induced acute cerebral ischemia. *Undersea Biomed Res* 13: 337.

Shiraishi T, Satou Y, Makishima K (1998) Hyperbaric oxygenation therapy in idiopathic sudden sensory neural hearing loss. *Nippon Jibiinkoka Gakkai Kaiho* 101: 1380–1384.

Shn-Rong Z (1995) Hyperbaric oxygen therapy for coma (a report of 336 cases). In *Proceedings of the International Congress of Hyperbaric Medicine*, pp 279–285.

Shoemaker WC, Appel PL, Kram HB (1988) Tissue oxygen debt as a determinant of lethal and nonlethal post-operative organ failure. *Crit Care Med* 16: 1117–1120.

Shu-Dong Y (1987) *The treatment of sudden deafness with HBO.* Paper presented at the 9th international congress of hyperbaric medicine, Sydney, Australia, March 1–4.

Shupak A, Gozal D, Ariel A (1987) Hyperbaric oxygenation in acute peripheral posttraumatic ischemia. *J Hyperbaric Med* 2: 7–14.

Shupak A, Greenberg E, Hardoff R *et al* (1989) Hyperbaric oxygenation for necrotizing (malignant) otitis externa. *Arch Otolaryngol Head Neck Surg* 115: 1470–1475.

Shyu KG, Hung HF, Wang BW, Chang H (2008) Hyperbaric oxygen induces placental growth factor expression in bone marrow-derived mesenchymal stem cells. *Life Sci* 83(1–2): 65–73.

Siddiqui A, Davidson JD, Mustoe TA (1995) Ischemic tissue oxygen capacitance after hyperbaric oxygen therapy: a new physiologic concept. *Plast Reconstr Surg* 99: 148–155.

Siegelman S (1992) Unraveling the Mysteries of Migraine. *Business & Health* (Special Issue): 12–19.

Siesjö BK (1981) Cell damage in the brain: a speculative synthesis *J Cereb Blood Flow and Metabol* 1: 155–185.

Siesjö BK, Johannson H, Ljunggren B, Norberg K (1974) Brain dysfunction in cerebral hypoxia and ischemia. *Nerv Ment Dis* 53: 75–105.

Siesjö BK, Katsura K-I, Zhao QI *et al* (1995) Mechanisms of secondary brain damage in global and focal ischemia: a speculative synthesis *J Neurotrauma* 12(5): 943–956.

Silver IA (1973) Local and systemic factors which affect the proliferation of fibroblasts. In Kulonen E, Pikkarainen J (Eds.), *Biology of Fibroblast*, Academic Press, New York, pp 507–520.

Simmons S (1998) Review of permanent pacemakers in hyperbaric chambers. *Undersea Hyper Med* 25: 14 (abstract).

Singhal AB (2007) A review of oxygen therapy in ischemic stroke. *Neurol Res* 29: 173–183.

Sinha AK, Klein J, Schultze P, Weiss J, Weiss HR (1991) Cerebral regional capillary perfusion and blood flow after carbon monoxide exposure. *J Appl Physiol* 71: 1196–1200.

Sirsjo A, Lehr HA, Nolte D *et al* (1993) Hyperbaric oxygen treatment enhances the recovery of blood flow in the postischemic striated muscle. *Circ Shock* 40: 9–13.

Sjöstrand J (1964) The effect of oxygen at high pressure on thyroid function in the rat. *Acta Physiol Scand* 62: 91–100.

Sjöström M, Neglen P, Friden J, Eklof B (1982) Human skeletal muscle metabolism and morphology after temporary incomplete ischaemia. *Eur J Clin Invest* 12: 69–79.

Skene WG, Norman JN, Smith G (1966) Effect of oxygen in cyanide poisoning. In Brown I, Cox B (Eds.) *Proceedings of the 3rd international congress on hyperbaric medicine.* National academy of Sciences, Washington DC, pp 705–710.

Sklizovic D, Sanger J, Kindwall EP *et al* (1993)Hyperbaric oxygen therapy and squamous cell carcinoma cell line growth. *Head & Neck* 15: 236–240.

Skogstad M, Bast-Pettersen R, Tynes T, Bjørnsen D, Aaserud O (1994) Treatment with hyperbaric oxygen: illustrated by the treatment of a patient with retinitis pigmentosa. *JOURNAL??* 114: 2480–2483. (Norwegian)

Skyhar MJ, Hargens AR, Strauss MB *et al* (1986) Hyperbaric oxygen reduces edema and necrosis of skeletal muscle in compartment syndromes associated with hemorrhagic hypotension. *J Bone Joint Surg (Am)* 68A: 1218–1224.

Slack WK, Thomas DA, Dejode LRJ (1966) Hyperbaric oxygen in treatment of trauma, ischemic disease of limbs and varicose ulcerations. In Brown IW, Cox B (eds) *Proceedings of the 3rd international congress on hyperbaric medicine.* National Academy of Sciences – National Research Council, Washington D.C., pp 621–624.

Slade B, Cianci P (1998) Outcomes in 124 patients after monoplace hyperbaric oxygen therapy for radiation tissue damage – a 14 year experience. *Undersea Hyperbaric Med* 25: 9 (abstract).

Sloan EP, Murphy DG, Hart R *et al* (1989) Complications and protocol considerations in carbon monoxide poisoned patients who require hyperbaric oxygen therapy. *Ann Emerg Med* 18: 629–634.

Slosman DO, De Ribaupierre S, Chicherio C *et al* (2004) Negative neurofunctional effects of frequency, depth and environment in recreational scuba diving: the Geneva "memory dive" study. *Br J Sports Med* 38: 108–114.

Sluitjer ME (1963) *The treatment of carbon monoxide poisoning by the administration of oxygen at high pressure.* Thomas, Springfield.

Small A (1984) New perspectives on hyperoxic pulmonary toxicity – a review. *Undersea Biomed Res*, 11: 1–24.

Smet MD, Carruthers J, Lepawsky M (1987) Anterior segment ischemia treated with hyperbaric oxygen. *Can J Ophthalmol* 22: 381–383.

Smetnev AS, Efuni SN, Rodionov VV, Ashurova LD, Aslibekian IS (1979) Hyperbaric oxygenation in the overall therapy of chronic ischemic heart disease. *Kardiologiia* 19: 41–46.

Smilkstein MJ, Bronstein AC, Pickett HM, Rumack BH (1985) Hyperbaric oxygen therapy for severe hydrogen sulfide poisoning. *J Emerg Med* 3: 27–30.

Smith EB (1986) Priestley lecture: on the science of deep sea diving – observations of the respiration of different kinds of air. *Chem Soc Rev* 15: 503–522.

Smith G (1961) Near avulsion of fort treated by replacement and subsequent prolonged exposure of patient to oxygen at two atmospheres pressure. *Lancet* 2: 1122.

Smith G (1962) The treatment of carbon monoxide poisoning with oxygen at two atmospheres absolute, *Ann Occup Hyg* 5: 259–263.

Smith G, Lawson DD, Renfrew S *et al* (1961) Preservation of cerebral cortical activity by breathing oxygen at 2 ATA pressure during cerebral ischemia. *Surg Gynecol Obstet* 113: 13.

Smith G, Ledingham IM, Sharp GR *et al* (1962) Treatment of coal-gas poisoning with oxygen at 2 atmospheres pressure. *Lancet* i: 816–818.

Smith RM (1965) Anesthesia during hyperbaric oxygenation. *Ann NY Acad Sci* 117: 768–773.

Smith RM, Neuman TS (1994) Elevation of serum creatine kinase in divers with arterial gas embolization. *NEJM* 330: 19–24.

Smith RP, Schoen RT, Rahn DW *et al* (2002) Clinical characteristics and treatment outcome of early Lyme disease in patients with microbiologically confirmed erythema migrans. *Ann Intern Med* 136: 421–428.

Smith WDA, Mapleson WW, Siebold K *et al* (1974) Nitrous oxide anesthesia induced at atmospheric and hyperbaric pressures. Parts I and II. *Br J Anaesth* 46: 3–28.

Snyder AAB, Salloum LJ, Barone JE *et al* (1991) Predicting short-term outcome of cardiopulmonary resuscitation using central venous oxygen tension measurements. *Crit Care Med* 19: 111–112.

Snyder JW, Safir EF, Summerville, GP, Midleberg RA (1995) Occupational fatality and persistent neurological sequelae after mass exposure to hydrogen sulfide. *Am J Emerg Med* 13: 199–203.

Snyder RD (1970) Carbon monoxide Intoxication with peripheral neuropathy. *Neurology* 20: 177–180.

Sohn YH, Jeong Y, Kim HS *et al* (2000) The brain lesion responsible for parkinsonism after carbon monoxide poisoning. *Arch Neurol* 57: 1214–1218.

Sokoloff L (1966) Cerebral circulation and metabolic changes associated with aging. *Assoc Res Nerv Ment Dis* 41: 237–254.

Spandau UH, Ihioff AK, Jonas JB (2006). Intraviteal bevacizumab treatment of macular edema due to central retinal vein occlusion. *Acta Ophthlamol Scand* 84: 555–556.

Spandau UH, Wickenhauser A, Rensch F, Jonas JB (2007) Intraviteal bevacizumab for branch retinal vein occlusion. *Acta Ophthlamol Scand* 85: 118–119.

Sparacia G, Banco A, Sparacia B *et al* (1997) Magnetic resonance findings in scuba diving-related spinal cord decompression sickness. *MAGMA* 5: 111–115.

Spears JR, Henney C, Prcevski P *et al* (2002) Aqueous oxygen hyperbaric reperfusion in a porcine model of myocardial infarction. *J Invasive Cardiol* 14: 160–166.

Speit G, Dennog C, Lampl L (1998) Biological significance of damage induced by hyperbaric oxygen. *Mutagenesis* 13: 85–87.

Speit G, Dennog C, Radermacher P, Rothfuss A (2002) Genotoxicity of hyperbaric oxygen. *Mutat Res* 512: 111–119.

Spencer MP (1976) Decompression limits for compressed air determined by ultrasonically detected blood bubbles. *J Appl Physiol* 40: 229–235.

Stalker CG, Ledingham IM (1973) The effect of increased oxygen in prolonged acute ölimb ischaemia. *Br J Surg* 60: 959–963.

Stanford MR (1984) Retinopathy after irradiation and hyperbaric oxygen. *JR Soc Med* 77: 1041–1043.

Stanley FJ, Blair E, Alberman E (2000) *Cerebral palsies: epidemiology and causal pathways.* MacKeith, *London.*

Staples J, Clement D (1996) Hyperbaric oxygen chambers and the treatment of sports injuries. *Sports Med* 22: 219–227.

Starr C (1992) New interest in old drug benefits migraine sufferers. *Drug Topics* 136: 32–35.

Stassano P, Cammarota A, De Martino G *et al* (1989) Hyperbaric oxygen in the treatment of sternal infections. *J Hyperbaric Med* 4: 17–21.

Stefansson E, Landers MB, Wolbarsht ML (1982) The role of oxygen and vasodilatation in diabetic retinopathy. In Friedmann EA, I'Esperance FA (Eds.) *Diabetic renal-retinal syndrome, Vol 2.* Grune and Stratton, New York, pp 117–150.

Sterling DL, Thornton JD, Swafford A *et al* (1993) Hyperbaric oxygen limits infarct size in ischemic rabbit myocardium in vivo. *Circulation* 88: 1931–1936.

Stewart JSS, Meddie NC, Middleton MD *et al* (1974) Gut decompression with hyperbaric oxygen (Letter to the editor). *Lancet* 1: 669.

Stewart KJ, Hiatt WR, Regensteiner JG, Hirsch AT (2002) Exercise training for claudication. *N Engl J Med* 347(24): 1941–1951.

Stoller KP (2007) Hyperbaric oxygen and carbon monoxide poisoning: a critical review. *Neurol Res* 29(2): 146–155.

Stone JA, Scott R, Brill RL *et al* (1995). The role of hyperbaric oxygen in the treatment of diabetic foot wounds. *Diabetes* 44 (suppl 1): 71A.

Stone R, Zink H, Klingele T, Burde R (1977) Visual recovery after central retinal artery occlusion: Two cases. *Ann Ophthalmol* 9: 445–450.

Strain GM, Snider TG, Tedford BL *et al* (1991) Hyperbaric oxygen effects on brown recluse spider (Loxosceles reclusa) envenomation in rabbits. *Toxicon* 29: 989–996.

Strauss MB (1987) Refractory osteomyelitis. *J Hyperbaric Med* 2: 147–159.

Strauss MB, Hargens AR, Gershuni DH *et al* (1986) Delayed use of hyperbaric oxygen for treatment of a model anterior compartment syndrome. *J Orthop Res* 4: 108–111.

Strauss MB, Hart GB (1977) Clinical experiences with HBO in fracture healing. In Smith G (Ed.) *Proceedings of the 7th international congress on hyperbaric medicine.* University of Aberdeen Press, Aberdeen, pp 329–332.

Strauss MB, Snow K, Greenberg D *et al* (1987) *Hyperbaric oxygen in the management of skeletal muscle compartment syndrome.* Presented at the 9th international congress on hyperbaric medicine, Sydney, Australia, March 1–4.

Strauss MB, Winant DM (1998) Femoral head necrosis: a meta-analysis comparing HBO with other interventions. *Undersea Hyperbaric Med* 25: 16 (abstract).

Stravinsky Y, Shandling AH, Ellestad MH *et al* (1998) Hyperbaric oxygen and thrombolysis in myocardial infarction: the 'HOT MI' randomized multicenter study. *Cardiology* 90: 131–136.

Stricker RB (2007). Counterpoint: long-term antibiotic therapy improves persistent symptoms associated with Lyme disease. *Clin Infect Dis* 45: 149–157.

Stricker RB, Phillips SE (2003) Lyme disease without erythema migrans: cause for concern? *Am J Med* 115: 72.

Stillman RM (1983) Effects of hypoxia and hyperoxia on progression of intimal healing. *Arch Surg* 118: 732–737.

Stucker M, Struk A, Altmeyer P *et al* (2002) The cutaneous uptake of atmospheric oxygen contributes significantly to the oxygen supply of human dermis and epidermis. *J Physiol* 538: 985–994.

Sugawa N, Sekimoto T, Ueda S (1988) Oxygenation under hyperbaric pressure (OHP) therapy for the patient with deep coma caused by cerebellar hemorrhage: a case report. *J Kyoto Perfect Univ Med* 97: 1091–1096.

Sugiyama H, Kamiyama K (1987) *The effectiveness of hyperbaric oxy-*

genation on cerebral ischemia. Presented at the 9th international congress on hyperbaric medicine, Sydney, Australia, 1–4 March.

Sukoff MH (1982) Use of hyperbaric oxygenation for spinal cord injury. *Neurochirurgia* 24: 19.

Sukoff MH (1984) Update on the use of HBO for diseases of the central nervous system. *Hyperbaric Oxygen Rev* 5: 35–47.

Sukoff MH (1986) *Update on the use of hyperbaric oxygenation for acute cerebral trauma*. Presented at the 5th Chinese conference on hyperbaric medicine, Fuzhow, China, Sept. 26–29.

Sukoff MH (1986b) *Use of hyperbaric oxygenation in spinal injury*. Presented at the 5th Chinese conference on hyperbaric medicine, Fuzhow, China Sept. 26–29 (Abstract).

Sukoff MH (2001) Effects of hyperbaric oxygenation. *J Neurosurg* 95: 544–546.

Sukoff MH, Gottlieb SF (1989) Chapter 22. In Nussbaum E (Ed.) *Hyperbaric oxygen therapy in the pediatric intensive care* (2nd ed). Futura, New York, p 25.

Sukoff MH, Gottlieb SF (1989) Chapter 26. In Nussbaum E (Ed.) *Hyperbaric oxygen therapy in the pediatric intensive care* (2nd ed). Futura, New York, pp 483–507.

Sukoff MH, Hollin SA, Espinosa OE, Jacobson JH (1968) The protective effect of hyperbaric oxygenation in experimental cerebral edema. *J Neurosurg* 29: 236–241.

Sukoff MH, Hollin SA, Jacobson JH (1967) The protective effect of hyperbaric oxygen in experimentally produced cerebral edema and compression. *Surgery* 62: 40–46.

Sukoff MH, Ragatz RE (1982) Hyperbaric oxygenation for the treatment of acute cerebral edema. *Neurosurg* 10(1): 29–38.

Sun L, Marti HH, Veltkamp R (2008) Hyperbaric oxygen reduces tissue hypoxia and hypoxia-inducible factor-1 alpha expression in focal cerebral ischemia. *Stroke* 39: 1000–1006.

Sunami K, Takeda Y, Hashimoto M, Hirakawa M (2000) Hyperbaric oxygen reduces infarct volume in rats by increasing oxygen supply to the ischemic periphery. *Crit Care Med* 28: 2831–2836.

Sutkovoi DA, Baraboi VA (1985) Oxidative phosphorylation in the rat liver mitochondria under activation of lipid peroxidation. *Ukr Biokhim Zh* 57: 79–81.

Suttorp-Schulten MS, Riemslag FC, Rothova A, van der Kley AJ, Riemslag FC (1997) Long-term effect of repeated hyperbaric oxygen therapy on visual acuity in inflammatory cystold macular oedema. *Br J Ophthalmol* 81: 329.

Svendsen FJ (1986) Treatment of clinically diagnosed brown recluse spider bites with hyperbaric oxygen: a clinical observation. *J Arkansas Med Soc* 83: 199–204.

Swift PC, Turner JH, Oxer HF *et al* (1992) Myocardial hibernation identified by hyperbaric oxygen treatment and echocardiography in postinfarction patients: comparison with exercise thallium scintigraphy. *Am Heart J* 124: 1151–1158.

Symon L (1976) The concept of threshold of ischemia in relation to brain structure and function. *J Clin Pathol {Suppl}* 11: 149–154.

Szewczyk TS (1951) Retrolental fibroplasia; etiology and prophylaxis. *Amer J Ophthalmol* 34: 1609.

Szuki H, Inie J, Horiuchi T (1980) Hyperbaric oxygenation therapy in ophthalmology. Part I: Incipient insufficiency of the retinal circulation. J Clin Ophthalmol 34: 335–343.

T

Tai YJ, Birely BC, Im MJ *et al* (1992) The use of hyperbaric oxygen for preservation of skin flaps. *Ann Plast Surg* 28: 284–287.

Takada C, Kaneko H, Tomomasa T *et al* (2002) Endosonographic diagnosis of pneumatosis cystoides intestinalis in infancy. *Tech Coloproctol* 6: 121–123.

Takahashi M, Iwatsuki N *et al* (1992) Hyperbaric oxygen therapy accelerates neurologic recovery after 15-minute complete global cerebral ischemia in dogs *Crit Care Med* 20(11): 1588–1594.

Takahashi H, Kobayashi S, Hayase H, Sakakirbara K *et al* (1987) Effect of HBO upon experimental thrombosis of mesenteric artery. *Presented at the 9th international congress on hyperbaric medicine*, Sydney, Australia, March 1–4.

Takahashi H, Sakakibara K, Murahashi K, Yanagita N (1989) HBO for sudden deafness – a statistical survey over 907 ears. In Schmutz J, Bakker D (Eds.) *Proceedings of the 2nd Swiss symposium on hyperbaric medicine.* Foundation for Hyperbaric Medicine, Basel.

Takahashi K, Shima T, Yamamuro M (1977) Hyperbaric oxygenation following stellate ganglion block in patients with retinal occlusion. In Smith G (Ed.) *Proceedings of the 6th international congress on hyperbaric medicine.* University of Aberdeen Press, Aberdeen, p 211–215.

Takano T, Miyazaki Y, Nashimoto I *et al* (1980) Effect of hyperbaric oxygen on cyanide intoxication: in situ changes in intracellular oxidation reduction. *Undersea Biomed Res* 7: 191–197.

Takemura K, Aoyagi K, Nagase S *et al* (1990) Urinary excretion rate of methylguanidine as a new marker of active oxygen in vivo: demonstration in hyperbaric oxygen therapy. *Nippon Jinzo Gakkai* 32: 1195–1201.

Takeuchi M, Morita K, Nakatsuka H *et al* (2001) A case of central retinal artery occlusion after anterior posterior fusion of the lumbar spine. *Masui* 50: 899–901. (Japanese)

Takiguchi N, Saito N, Nunomura M *et al* (2001) Use of 5-FU plus hyperbaric oxygen for treating malignant tumors: evaluation of antitumor effect and measurement of 5-FU in individual organs. *Cancer Chemother Pharmacol* 47: 11–14.

Talmage DW, Dart GA (1978) Effect of oxygen pressure during culture on the survival of mouse thyroid allografts. *Science* 200: 1066–1067.

Talmi YP, Finkelstein Y, Zohar Y (1991) Decompression sickness induced hearing loss. A review. *Scand Audiol* 20: 25–28.

Talpalar AE, Grossman Y (2006) CNS manifestations of HPNS: revisited. *Undersea Hyperb Med* 33: 205–210.

Talton IH, Thompson LW, Dent SJ *et al* (1970) Investigation of changes in blood gases, EEG and vigilance behavior during increased oxygen pressure in old and young community volunteers. *Anaesthesist* 19: 241–244.

Tamura H, Miyamoto K, Kiryu J *et al* (2005) Intravitreal injection of corticosteroid attenuates leukostasis and vascular leakage in experimental diabetic retina. *Ophthalmol Vis Sci* 46: 1440–1444.

Tan CM, Im MJ, Myers RAM, Hoopes JE (1984) Hyperbaric oxygen therapy and hyperbaric air on the survival of island skin flaps. *Plast Reconstr Surg* 73: 27–30.

Tan J, Tange RA, Dreschler WA *et al* (1999) Long-term effect of hyperbaric oxygenation treatment on chronic distressing tinnitus. *Scand Audiol* 28: 91–6.

Tang WM, Han DP (2000) A study of surgical approaches to retinal vascular occlusions. *Arch Ophthalmol* 118: 138–143.

Tacquet A, Voisin C, Lelievre G, Mouton Y (1970) Treatment of acute hepatic insufficiency by hyperbaric oxygen therapy. *Lille Med* 15: 1066–1069.

Taylor MD, O'Toole KS, Auble TE *et al* (2000) The Psychometric and

Cardiac Effects of Dimenhydrinate in the Hyperbaric Environment. *Pharmacotherapy* 20: 1051–1054.

Teasdale G, Jennett B (1974) Assessment of coma and impaired consciousness. A practical scale. *Lancet* 2: 81–84.

Teicher BA, Herman TS, Rose CM (1988) Effect of fluosol-Da on the response of intracranial 9L tumors to X-rays and BCNU. *Int J Radiat Oncol Biol Phys* 15: 1187–1192.

Tempel R, Severance HW (2006) Proposing short-term observation units for the management of decompression illness. *Undersea Hyperb Med* 33: 89–94.

Terajima K, Igarashi H, Hirose M *et al* (2008) Serial assessments of delayed encephalopathy after carbon monoxide poisoning using magnetic resonance spectroscopy and diffusion tensor imaging on 3.0T system. *Eur Neurol* 59: 55–61.

Tereshin PI, Charushnikova GA (1985) The effect of high-pressure oxygenation on lipid metabolism of pregnant patients with late gestosis. *Akush Ginekol (Mosk)* 5: 34–35.

Tetzlaff K, Friege L, Theysohn J *et al* (2005) Lung function in military oxygen divers: a longitudinal study. *Aviat Space Environ Med* 76: 974–977.

Thalmann ED (1990) Principles of US navy recompression treatments for decompression sickness. In *Diving Accident Management*, 41st Undersea and Hyperbaric Medical Society Workshop. Undersea and Hyperbaric Medical Society publication 78 (DIVACC), 12/1/90: 194–221.

Thiede WG, Manley J (1976) Cerebral air embolism and cerebral edema: one regiment of treatment. *Aviat Space Environ Med* 47: 553–555.

Thom SR (1990) Antagonism of carbon monoxide-mediated brain, lipid peroxidation by hyperbaric oxygen. *Toxicol Appl Pharmacol* 105: 340–344.

Thom SR (1992) Dehydrogenase conversion to oxidase and lipid peroxidation in the brain after CO poisoning. *J Appl Physiol* 73: 1584–1589.

Thom SR (1993a) Leukocytes in carbon monoxide-mediated brain oxidative injury *Toxicol App Pharmacol* Sept 20: 1–14.

Thom SR (1993b) Functional inhibition of leukocyte B_2 integrins by hyperbaric oxygen in carbon monoxide-mediated brain injury in rats. *Toxicol App Pharmacol* 123: 248–256.

Thom SR (2002) Hyperbaric-oxygen therapy for acute carbon monoxide poisoning. *N Engl J Med* 347: 1105–1106.

Thom SR, Bhopale V, Fisher D *et al* (2002) Stimulation of nitric oxide synthase in cerebral cortex due to elevated partial pressures of oxygen: an oxidative stress response. *J Neurobiol* 51: 85–100.

Thom SR, Bhopale VM, Fisher D (2006) Hyperbaric oxygen reduces delayed immune-mediated neuropathology in experimental carbon monoxide toxicity. *Toxicol Appl Pharmacol* 213: 152–159.

Thom SR, Bhopale VM, Velazquez OC *et al* (2006) Stem cell mobilization by hyperbaric oxygen. *Am J Physiol Heart Circ Physiol* 290: H1378–H1386.

Thom SR, Clark JM (1997) The toxicity of oxygen, carbon monoxide, and carbon dioxide. In Bove AA, Davis JC (Eds.) *Diving Medicine*. Philadelphia: WB Saunders, pp 131–145.

Thom SR, Elbuken ME (1991) Oxygen-dependent antagonism of lipid peroxidation, *Free Radical Biol Med* 10: 413–426.

Thom SR, Fisher D, Zhang J *et al* (2003) Stimulation of perivascular nitric oxide synthesis by oxygen. *Am J Physiol Heart Circ Physiol* 284: H1230–H1239.

Thom SR, Mendiguren I, Fisher D (2001) Smoke inhalation-induced alveolar lung injury is inhibited by hyperbaric oxygen. *Undersea Hyperb Med* 28(4): 175–179.

Thom SR, Taber RL, Mendiguren I *et al* (1992) Delayed neuropsychiatric sequelae following CO poisoning and the role of treatment with 100% O_2 or hyperbaric O_2-a prospective randomized clinical study. *Undersea Biomed Res* 19(suppl): 47.

Thom SR, Taber RL, Mendiguren II *et al* (1995) Delayed neuropsychologic sequelae after carbon monoxide poisoning: Prevention by treatment with hyperbaric oxygen [see comments]. *Ann Emerg Med* 25: 474–480.

Thomas JR, Burch LS, Brandvard RA (1976) Interaction of hyperbaric nitrogen and oxygen effects on behavior. *Aviat Space Environ Med* 47: 965–968.

Thomas MP, Brown LA, Sponseller DR *et al* (1990) Myocardial infarct size reduction by the synergistic effect of hyperbaric oxygen and recombinant tissue plasminogen activator. *Am Heart J* 120: 791–800.

Thomlinson KH, Gray LH (1955) The histological structure of some human lung cancers and the possible implications for radiotherapy. *Br J Cancer* 9: 539–549.

Thomson LF, Mardel SN *et al* (1992) Management of the moribund carbon monoxide victim. *Arch Emerg Med* 9: 208–213.

Thomsen LL, Iversen HK, Olesen J (1995) Cerebral blood flow velocities are reduced during attacks of unilateral migraine without aura. *Cephalalgia* 15: 77–78.

Thorsen E, Haave H, Hofso D, Ulvik RJ (2001) Exposure to hyperoxia in diving and hyperbaric medicine – effects on blood cell counts and serum ferritin. *Undersea Hyperbaric Med* 28: 57–62.

Thurston JG, Greenwood TW, Bending MR, Connor H, Curwen MP (1973) A controlled investigation into the effects of hyperbaric oxygen on mortality following acute myocardial infarction. *Q J Med* 42: 751–770.

Till JS (1984) Ophthalmic aspects of cerebrovascular disease. In Toole JF (Ed.) *Cerebrovascular disorders*. Raven, New York, p 237.

Tilley BC, Lyden PD, Brott TG *et al* (1997) Total quality improvement method for reduction of delays between emergency department admission and treatment of acute ischemic stroke. *Arch Neurol* 54: 1466–1474.

Timchuk LD, Luchko AS, Palamarchok VN *et al* (1981) Hyperbaric oxygen in complex treatment of acute poisoning. In Yefuny SN (Ed.) *Proceedings of the 7th international congress on hyperbaric medicine*. USSR Academy of Sciences, Moscow, pp 333–334.

Tindal A (1941) The perfect anesthetic. Anesthesia by the method of Paul Bert. *Surgery* 7: 33.

Tindall GT, Wilkins RH, Odom GL (1965) Effect of hyperbaric oxygenation on cerebral blood flow. *Surg Forum* 16: 414–416.

Tirpitz D (1986) The value of hyperbaric oxygenation in treatment of gas gangrene. In Schmutz J (Ed.) *Proceedings of the 1st Swiss symposium on hyperbaric medicine*. Foundation for Hyperbaric Medicine, Basel, pp 169–193.

Tirpitz D, Bakyara T (1988) Hyperbare Oxygen bei CO-Intoxikationen. *Der Informierte Arzt* 8: 51–54.

Tisch M, Maier H (2006) Malignant external otitis. *Laryngorhinootologie* 85: 763–769.

Tjarnstrom J, Wikstrom T, Bagge U *et al* (1999) Effects of hyperbaric oxygen treatment on neutrophil activation and pulmonary sequestration in intestinal ischemia-reperfusion in rats. *Eur Surg Res* 31: 147–154.

Tjernström Ö, Casselbrant M, Harris S, Ivarsson A (1980) Current status of pressure chamber treatment. *Otolaryngol Clin North Am* 13: 723–729.

Tkachenko SS, Ruskii VV, Tikhilov RM, Vovchenko VI (1988) Normalization of bone regeneration by oxygen barotherapy. *Vestn Khir* 140: 97–100.

Tobin DA (1978) Explosive decompression in a hyperbaric oxygen chamber. *AJR* 111: 622–624.

Todo K, Nakae S, Wada J (1974) Heart preservstion with metabolic inhibitor, hypothermia, and hyperbaric oxygenation. *Jpn J Surg* 4: 29–36.

Togawa S, Yamami N, Nakayama H *et al* (2004) Evaluation of HBO2 therapy in pneumatosis cystoides intestinalis. *Undersea Hyperb Med* 31: 387–393.

Toklu AS, Korpinar S, Erelel M *et al* (2008 Jun 19) Are pulmonary bleb and bullae a contraindication for hyperbaric oxygen treatment? *Respir Med* doi:10.1016/j.rmed.2008.03.012.

Tolias CM, Reinert M, Seiler R *et al* (2004) Normobaric hyperoxia – induced improvement in cerebral metabolism and reduction in intracranial pressure in patients with severe head injury: a prospective historical cohort-matched study. *J Neurosurg* 101: 435–444.

Tomaszewski C (2002) Carbon monoxide. In Goldfrank LR *et al* (Eds.) *Goldfrank's Toxicologic Emergencies*, pp 1478–1491.

Tomiyama R, Kinjo F, Hokama A *et al* (2003) A case of pneumatosis cystoides intestinalis with diabetes mellitus successfully treated by hyperbaric oxygen therapy. *Nippon Shokakibyo Gakkai Zasshi* 100: 212–214.

Torbati D, Sherpa AK, Lahiri S *et al* (1993) Hyperbaric oxygenation alters carotid body ultrastructure and function. *Respiration Physiology* 92: 183–196.

Toro-Gonzalez G, Navarro-Roman L, Roman GC *et al* (1993) Acute ischemic stroke from fibrocartilagenous embolism to the middle cerebral artery. *Stroke* 24: 730–740.

Torubarov FS, Pakhomov VI, Krylova IV *et al* (1983) Changes in cerebral hemodynamics in patients with vascular pathology in the late stages of radiation sickness treated with hyperbaric oxygenation. *Zh Nevropatol Psikhiatr* 83: 28–33.

Tranos PG, Wickremasinghe SS, Stangoes NT *et al* (2004) Macular edema. *Surv Ophthalmol* 49: 470–490.

Trapp WG, Creighton R (1964) Experimental studies of increased atmospheric pressure on myocardial ischemia after coronary ligation. *J Thorac Cardiovasc Surg* 47: 687–692.

Trefny Z, Svacinka J (1969) Effect of hypoxia and hyperoxia on the quantitative ballistocardiogram. *Bibl Cardiol* 26: 119–124.

Trimble VH (1974) *The uncertain miracle – hyperbaric oxygen*. Doubleday, New York.

Troop BR, Majerus T, Bernacchi A *et al* (1986) Hyperbaric oxygenation improves survival in rats poisoned with carbon tetrachloride. *J Hyperbaric Med* 1: 157–161.

Trouton D, Eysenck HJ (1961) The effects of drugs on behavior. In Eysenck HJ (Ed.) *Handbook of abnormal psychology*. Basic Books, New York, pp 634–696.

Truss CD, Killenberg PG (1982) Treatment of CCl4 poisoning with hyperbaric oxygen. *Gastroenterology* 82: 767–769.

Trytyshnikov IM (1986) Dynamics of the plastic processes in the liver during the use of hyperbaric oxygenation in the recovery period following acute massive blood loss. *Biull Eksp Biol Med* 101: 154–156.

Tsan MF (2001) Superoxide dismutase and pulmonary oxygen toxic-ity: lessons from transgenic and knockout mice (Review). *Int J Mol Med* 7: 13–19.

Tsuji Y (1992). Surgical results of hypospadias by Belt-Fuqua method. Presented at *1st Scientific Meeting of the Japanese Society for Pediatric Urology*. 10 July 1992.

Tsuru M, Nakagawa Y, Kitaoka K, Kawahigashi H (1983) Treatment of cerebral ischemia by hyperbaric oxygenation. In Shiraki K, Matsuoka S (Eds.) *Hyperbaric medicine and underwater physiology*. Fukuoka, Kitakyushu, pp 315–328.

Tsygankova ST, Ashurova LD, Sultanova BG (1986) Hyperbaric oxygenation in the combined therapy of acute hepatitis in patients before and after renal allotransplantation. *Anesteziol Reanimatol* 3: 64.

Turle-Lorenzo N, Zouani B, Risso JJ (1999) Narcotic effects produced by nitrous oxide and hyperbaric nitrogen narcosis in rats performing a fixed-ratio test. *Physiol Behav* 67: 321–325.

Tzuk ST, Bitterman N, Harel D (1991) The effect of vigabatrin on central nervous system toxicity in rats. *Eur J Pharmacol* 202: 171–175.

U

Ubels JL, Hoffert JR (1981) Ocular oxygen toxicity: the effect of hyperbaric oxygen on retinal Na+-K+ ATPase. *Exp Eye Res* 32: 77–84.

Ueda H, Shien CW, Miyazawa T *et al* (1998) Otological complications of hyperbaric oxygen therapy. *Adv Otorhinolaryngol* 54: 119–126.

Ueda M, Kaneda T, Takahashi M *et al* (1993) Effect of hyperbaric oxygen therapy on osseointegration of titanium implants in irradiated bone: a preliminary report. *Int J Oral Maxillofac Implants* 8: 41–44.

Ueng SW, Lee SS, Lin SS *et al* (1998) Bone healing of tibial lengthening is enhanced by hyperbaric oxygen therapy: a study of bone mineral density and torsional strength on rabbits. *J Trauma* 1998 44: 676–481.

Ugrimov VM, Eliniskii MP, Rafikov AM *et al* (1980) Hyperbaric oxygenation in the complex treatment of patients with aneurysms of the cerebral vessels. *Anesthesiology* 28: 675–678.

Ulewicz K, Zannini D (1986) On the possibility of hyperbaric oxygen therapy in some pathological reactions of immunological hypersensitivity. *Bull Inst Maritime Tropical Medicine* (Gdynia) 37: 71–79.

Urano M, Kenton LA, Kahn J (1988) The effect of hyperthermia on the early and late appearing mouse foot reactions and on the radiation carcinogenesis: effect on the early and late appearing reactions. *Int J Radiat Oncol Biol Phys* 15: 159–166.

Urayama H, Takemura H, Kasajima F *et al* (1992) Hyperbaric oxygen therapy for chronic occlusive disease of the extremities. *Nippon Geka Gakkai Zasshi* 93: 429–433.

V

Vahidova D, Sen P, Papesch M *et al* (2006) Does the slow compression technique of hyperbaric oxygen therapy decrease the incidence of middle-ear barotrauma? *J Laryngol Otol* 120: 446–449.

Valentine V, Harch PG (2005) Personal communication.

van Gulik TM, Hullett DA, Boudjema K *et al* (1990) Prolonged survival of murine thyroid allografts after 7 days of hyperbaric organic culturein the UW preservation solution at hypothermia. *Transplantation* 49: 971–975.

van Hoesen KB, Camporesi EM, Moon RE (1989) Should hyperbaric oxygen be used to treat the pregnant patient for acute carbon monoxide poisoning? *JAMA* 261: 1039–1043.

Van Meter K (1991) Field management of the injured diver, In Moon RE, Camporesi EM (Eds.) *Problems in respiratory care: Clinical Applications of Hyperbaric Oxygen,* Lippencott, Philadelphia. Respiratory Care Clinicof North America, 4(2): 189–214.

Van Meter K (1996) Treatment of decompression illness (DCI) and arterial gas embolism (AGE): US experience, New Orleans practice protocols for DCI and AGE. In Moon R, Sheffield PJ (Eds.) *45th UHMS Workshop, Treatment of decompression illness.* Kensington MD, pp 203–243.

Van Meter K (1997) Systemic hyperbaric oxygen therapy as an aid in resolution of selected chronic problem wounds. In Krasner D, Kane D (Eds.) *Chronic Wound Care: A Clinical Source Book for Health Care Professionals* Health Management Pubs, Wayne, pp 260–275.

Van Meter K (1999) Medical field management of the injured diver. *Resp Care Clin North Am* 5(1): 137–177.

Van Meter K (2004) A systemic review of the literature reporting the application of hyperbaric oxygen in the tratment of exceptional blood loss anemia: an evidence-based approach. *Undersea Hyperbaric Med* (in press).

Van Meter K, Gottlieb SF, Whidden SJ (1988) Hyperbaric oxygen as an adjunct in ACLS in guinea pigs after 15 minutes of cardiopulmonary arrest. *UBR* (suppl 15): 55.

Van Meter K, Sheps S, Kriedt F *et al* (2008) Hyperbaric oxygen improves rate of return of spontaneous circulation after prolonged normothermic porcine cardiopulmonary arrest. *Resuscitation* 78(2): 200–214.

Van Meter KW, Harch PG, Andrews LC, Simanonok JP, Staab PK, Gottlieb SF (1994) Should the pressure be off or on in the use of oxygen in treatment of carbon monoxide-poisoned patients. *Ann of Emerg Med* 24: 283–288.

Van Meter KW, Moises J, Marcheselli V, Murphy-Lavoie H, Barton C, Harch PG, Bazaan N (2001a) Attenuation of lipid peroxidation in porcine cerebral cortex after a prolonged 25-minute cardiopulmonary arrest by high-dose hyperbaric oxygen (HBO). *Undersea Hyperbaric Med* 28(sup): 83–84.

Van Meter KW, Sheps SS, Swanson HT, Wilson JP, Barratt DM, Kodu U, Roycraft EL, Moises JP, Nolan TA, Harch PG (1999) A controlled prospective randomized pilot open chest cardiopulmonary resuscitation (CPR) comparing use of 100% oxygen in mechanical ventilation of swine at one, two, and four atmospheres ambient pressure after a 25 minute normothermic cardiopulmonary arrest at one atmosphere. *J of Academic Emergency Medicine* 6(5): 428.

Van Meter KW, Swanson HT, Sheps SS, Barratt DM, Roycraft EL, Moises J, Killeen J, Harch PG (1992) Oxygen dose response in open-chest ACLS in swine after a 25-minute cardiopulmonary arrest. *Ann Emerg Med* 34(4): S11.

Van Meter K, Xiao F, Moises J, Barratt D, Harch P, Murphy-Lavoie H, Bazan N (2001) No difference in leukocyte adherence in the microvasculature in a porcine cerebral cortex by use of normobaric oxygen or low or high-dose hyperbaric oxygen in resuscitation after a prolonged 25 minute cardiopulmonary arrest. *Annals of Emergency Medicine* 38(4): S39.

Van Rynen JL, Taha AM, Ehrlich R, Parlette DM (1987) Treatment of cerebral air embolism in the pediatric patients. *J Hyperbaric Med* 2: 199–204.

Van Slyke DD, Neill JM (1924) The determination of gases in the

blood and other solutions by vacuum extraction and manometric measurement. *J Biol Chem* 61: 523–573.

Van Zyl JJW (1966) *Hyperbaric oxygenation with special consideration of the surgical applications.* Doctoral thesis, University of Stellenbosch, South Africa.

Vandegriff KD, Olson JS (1984) Morphological and physiological factors affecting oxygen uptake and release by red blood cells. *J Biol Chem* 259: 12619–12627.

Vanina LV, Efuni SN, Beilin AL *et al* (1977) Labour in patient with acute myocardial infarction under hyperbaric oxygenation. *Anesteziol Reanimatol* 5: 72–76.

Vanina LV, Efuni SN, Beilin AL *et al* (1981) Obstetrics aid under conditions of hyperbaric oxygenation. In Yefuny SN (Ed.) *Proceedings of the 7th international congress on hyperbaric medicine.* USSR Academy of Sciences, Moscow, p 358.

Varma SD (1991) Scientific basis for medical therapy of cataracts by antioxidants. *Am J Clin Nutr* 53: 335S-345S.

Varma SD, Richards RD (1988) Ascorbic acid and the eye lens. *Ophthalmic Res* 20: 164–173.

Vaupel P, Kallinowski F, Groebe K (1988) Evaluation of oxygen diffusion distances in human breast cancer using cell line specific in vivo data: role of various pathogenetic mechanisms in the development of tumor hypoxia. *Arch Exp Med Biol* 222: 719–726.

Vavrina J, Muller W (1995) Therapeutic effect of hyperbaric oxygenation in acute acoustic trauma. *Rev Laryngol Otol Rhinol (Bord)* 116: 377–380.

Vazquez RL, Spahr RC (1990) Hyperbaric oxygen use in neonates: a report of four patients. *Am J Dis Child* 144: 1022–1024.

Veltkamp R, Siebing DA, Sun L *et al* (2005) Hyperbaric oxygen reduces blood-brain barrier damage and edema after transient focal cerebral ischemia. *Stroke* 36: 1679–1683.

Veltkamp R, Warner DS, Domoki F *et al* (2000) Hyperbaric oxygen decreases infarct size and behavioral deficit after transient focal cerebral ischemia in rats. *Brain Res* 853: 68–73.

Velu SS, Myers RAM (1992) Hyperbaric oxygen treatment of radiation induced hemorrhagic cystitis (abstract). *Undersea Biomed Res* 19 (suppl): 85.

Verma A, Hirsch DJ, Glatt CE *et al* (1993) Carbon monoxide: a putative messenger. *Science* 259: 381–384.

Verweij BH, Amelink GJ, Muizelaar JP (2007) Current concepts of cerebral oxygen transport and energy metabolism after severe traumatic brain injury. *Prog Brain Res* 161: 111–124.

Vila JF, Balcarce PE, Abiusi GR *et al* (2005) Improvement in motor and cognitive impairment after hyperbaric oxygen therapy in a selected group of patients with cerebrovascular disease: a prospective single-blind controlled trial. *Undersea Hyperb Med* 32: 341–349.

Vila JF, Meli FJ, Serqueira OE, Pisarello J, Lylyk P (2005) Diffusion tensor magnetic resonance imaging: a promising technique to characterize and track delayed encephalopathy after acute carbon monoxide poisoning. *Undersea Hyperb Med* 32(3): 151–156.

Vincey P (1978) Application and use of hyperbaric oxygen in ENT. *Laryngol Otol Rhinol* 99: 619–634.

Vingolo EM, Pelaia P, Forte R *et al* (1997) Does hyperbaric oxygen (HBO) delivery rescue retinal photoreceptors in retinitis pigmentosa? *Investigative Ophthalmology* 38: ARVO Abstracts, Number 3296.

Vingolo EM, Pelaia P, Forte R *et al* (1999) Does hyperbaric oxygen (HBO) delivery rescue retinal photoreceptors in retinitis pigmentosa? *Doc Ophthalmol* 97: 33–39.

Vinores SA, Youssri AI, Luna JD *et al* (1997) Upregulation of vascular endothelial growth factor in ischemic and non-ischemic human and experimental retinal disease. *Histol Histopathol* 12: 99–109.

Visona A, Lusiani L, Rusca F *et al* (1989) Therapeutic, hemodynamic, and metabolic effects of hyperbaric oxygenation in peripheral vascular disease. *Angiology* 40: 994–1000.

Vitullo V, Venuti P, Di Marzio GE *et al* (1987) HBO and corneal pathology: clinical evaluations. In EUBS 87, *Proceedings of the 13th annual meeting of the European Undersea Biomedical Society*, Palermo, Italy, Sept 9–12, pp 296–300.

Voitkevich VI, Volzhskaya AM, Korchinskii LA (1979) Effect of hyperbaric hyperoxia on human plasma erythropoiesis inhibitors. *Biull Eksp Biol Med* 87: 96–98.

Voitkevich VI, Volzhskaya AM, Myasnikos AP (1975) Erythropoietic function of the kidneys during exposure to increased oxygen pressure. *Biull Eksp Biol Med* 79: 394–395.

von Heimburg D, Noah EM, Sieckmann UP, Pallua N (2001) Hyperbaric oxygen treatment in deep frostbite of both hands in a boy. *Burns* 27: 404–408.

von Kummer R, Weber J (1197) Brain and vascular imaging in acute ischemic stroke: the potential of computed tomography. *Neurology* 49(5 Suppl 4): S52–S55: 404–408.

Von Lackum K, Babb K, Riley SP, Wattier RL, Bykowski T, Stevenson B (2006) Functionality of Borrelia burgdorferi LuxS: the Lyme disease spirochete produces and responds to the pheromone autoinducer-2 and lacks a complete activated-methyl cycle. *Int J Med Microbiol* 296(Suppl 40): 92–102.

Vucetic M, Jensen PK, Jansen EC (2004) Diameter variations of retinal blood vessels during and after treatment with hyperbaric oxygen. *Br J Ophthalmol* 88: 771–775.

W

Waalkes P, Fitzpatrick DT, Stankus S, Topolski R (2002) Adjunctive HBO treatment of children with cerebral anoxic injury. *US Army Medical Journal* April-June: 13–21.

Wada J, Ikeda T, Kamada K *et al* (1965) Oxygen hyperbaric treatment for severe CO poisoning and severe burns in coal mines (Hokutan-Yubari) gas explosion. *Igaku Jpn* 54: 68.

Wada K, Ito M, Miyazawa T *et al* (1996) Repeated hyperbaric oxygen induces ischemic tolerance in gerbil hippocampus. *Brain Res* 740: 15–20.

Waddell W, Saltzman HA, Fuson RL *et al* (1965) Purpura gangrenosa treated with hyperbaric oxygenation. *JAMA* 191: 971–974.

Walker BR, Attallah AA, Lee JB *et al* (1980) Antidiuresis and inhibition of PGE excretion by hyperoxia in the conscious dog. *Undersea Biomed Res* 7: 113–126.

Walker KJ, Millar IL, Fock A (2006) The performance and safety of a pleural drainage unit under hyperbaric conditions. *Anaesth Intensive Care* 34: 61–67.

Wallyn CR, Jampol LM, Goldberg MF *et al* (1985) The use of hyperbaric oxygen therapy in the treatment of sickle cell hyphema. *Invest Ophthalmol Vis Sci* 26: 1155–1158.

Walsh CA, Mayer EW, Baxi LV (2007) Lyme disease in pregnancy: case report and review of the literature. *Obstet Gynecol Surv* 62: 41–50.

Wan J, Sukoff MH (1992) *The use of HBO in experimental brain injury and its metabolic sequela*. Regional HBO conference, Shanghai Hosp No. 5, Shanghai, China.

Wang C, Schwaitzberg S, Berliner E *et al* (2003) Hyperbaric oxygen for treating wounds: a systematic review of the literature. *Arch Surg* 138: 272–280.

Wang WZ, Olsson T, Kostulas V *et al* (1992) Myelin antigen reactive T cells in cerebrovascular diseases. *Clin Exp Immunol* 88: 157–162.

Wang X, Ding I, Xie H *et al* (1998) Hyperbaric oxygen and basic fibroblast growth factor promote growth of irradiated bone. *Int J Radiat Oncol Biol Phys* 40(1): 189–196.

Ward JA, Roberts RJ (1984) Effect of hyperoxia on phosphatidylcholine synthesis, secretion, uptake and stability in the newborn rabbit lung. *Biochem Biophys Acta* 796: 42–50.

Warren DC, Feehan P, Slade JB *et al* (1997) Chronic radiation proctitis treated with hyperbaric oxygen. *Undersea Hyperbaric Med* 24: 181–184.

Warren J, Sacksteder MR, Thuning CA (1978) Oxygen immunosuppression: modification of experimental allergic encephalomyelitis in rodents. *J Immunol* 121: 315–320.

Warren J, Sacksteder MR, Thuning CA (1979) Therapeutic effect of prolonged hyperbaric oxygen in adjuvant arthritis of the rat. *Arthritis Rheum* 22: 334–339.

Wassman H, Holbach KH (1988) Zerebrale Insuffizienz durch ischsche Hypoxie unter hyperbarer Sauerstoff-Behandlung. *Geriatr Rehahil* 1: 143–150.

Wassmann W (1980) Quantitative Indikatoren des hirnelektrischen Wirkungsverlaufs bei hyperbarer Oxygenierung. *EEG EMG* 11: 97–101.

Watanuki T, Istubo K, Fumoto T (1970) Study on the effects of hyperbaric oxygenation upon intestinal peristalsis. In Wada J, Iwa T (Eds.) *Proceedings of the 4th international congress on hyperbaric medicine*, Baillere, London, pp 395–399.

Watson ER, Halnan KE, Dische S *et al* (1978) Hyperbaric oxygen and radiotherapy: a Medical Research Council report. *Br JRadiol* 51: 879–887.

Wattel F, Mathieu D, Nevier RR (1991) Transcutaneous oxygen pressure measurements. *J Hyperbaric Med* 6: 269–282.

Wattel F, Mathieu D, Neviere R *et al* (1996) L'intoxication au monoxyde de carbone. *Presse Med* 25: 1425–1429.

Wattel FE, Mathieu MD, Fossati P *et al* (1991). Hyperbaric oxygen in the treatment fo diabetic foot lesions- search for healing predictive factors. *J Hyperbaric Med* 6: 263–268.

Way JL, End E, Sheehy M *et al* (1972) Effect of oxygen on cyanide intoxication IV. Hyperbaric oxygen. *Toxicol Appl Pharmacol* 22: 415–421.

Weaver LK (1991) Clinical applications of hyperbaric oxygen – monoplace chamber use. In Moon RE, Camporesi EM (Eds.) *Problems in Respiratory Care: Clinical Applications of Hyperbaric Oxygen*. Lippencott, Philadelphia, PA. *Respiratory Care Clinic of North America* 4(2): 189–214.

Weaver LK, Churchill S (2001) Pulmonary edema associated with hyperbaric oxygen therapy. *Chest* 120: 1407–1409.

Weaver LK, Hopkins RO, Chan KJ *et al* (2002) Hyperbaric oxygen for acute carbon monoxide poisoning. *N Engl J Med* 347: 1057–1067.

Webb JT, Kannan N, Pilmanis AA (2003) Gender not a factor for altitude decompression sickness risk. *Aviat Space Environ Med* 74: 2–10.

Weber J, Remonda L, Mattle HP *et al* (1998) Selective intra-arterial fibrinolysis of acute central retinal artery occlusion. *Stroke* 29: 2076–2079.

Weiland DE (2007) Fasciotomy closure using simultaneous vacuum-assisted closure and hyperbaric oxygen. *Am Surg* 73: 261–266.

Weinberger AWA, Siekmann UPF, Wolf S *et al* (2002) Treatment of acute central retinal artery occlusion (CRAO) by hyperbaric oxygenation therapy (HBO)-a pilot study with 21 patients. *Klin Monatsbl Augenheilkd* 219: 728–734. (German)

Weinstein PR, Hameroff SR, Johnson PC *et al* (1986) Effect of hyperbaric oxygen therapy or dimethyl sulfoxide on cerebral ischemia in unanesthetized gerbils. *Neurosurg* 18(5): 528.

Weiss JP, Neville EC (1989) Hyperbaric oxygen: primary treatment of radiation-induced hemorrhagic cystitis. *J Urol* 142: 43–45.

Weiss LD, Ramasastry SS, Eidelman BH (1989) Treatment of cluster headaches in a hyperbaric chamber. *Headache* 29: 109–110.

Weiss SJ (1989) Tissue destruction by neutrophils. *NEJM* 320: 365–376.

Weissman A, Peretz BA, Michaelson M *et al* (1989) Air embolism following intra-uterine hypertonic saline instillation: treatment in a high pressure chamber; a case report. *Eur J Obstet Gynecol Reprod Biol* 33: 271–274.

Weisz G, Lavy A, Adir Y (1997) Modification of in vivo and in vitro TNF-alpha, IL-1, and IL-6 secretion by circulating monocytes during hyperbaric oxygen treatment in patients with perianal Crohn's disease. *J Clin Immunol* 17: 154–159.

Weisz G, Ramon Y, Waisman D *et al* (1993) Treatment of necrobiosis lipoidica diabeticorum by hyperbaric oxygen. *Acta Derm Venereol (Stockh)* 73: 447–448.

Weizer JS, Stinnett SS, Fekrat S (2003) Radial optic neurotomy as treatment for central retinal vein occlusion. *Am J Ophthalmol* 136: 814–819.

Welch HG (1982) Hyperoxia and human performance; a brief review. *Med Sci Sports Exer* 14: 253–262.

Welch KMA, Barkley GL (1986) Biochemistry and pharmacology of cerebral ischemia. In Barnett HJM *et al* (Eds.) *Stroke*. Churchill-Livingston, New York, pp 75–90.

Wells CH, Hilton JG (1977) Effect of hyperbaric oxygenation on host burn plasma extravasation. In Davis JE, Hunt TK (eds) *Hyperbaric oxygen therapy*. Undersea Medical Society, Bethesda, pp 259–265.

Wells M, Foroozan (2004) Transient visual loss may anticipate occipital infarction from hemodialysis. *Am J Kidney Dis* 43: 29–33.

Wetzig PC (1979) The treatment of acute branch vein occlusion by photocoagulation. *Am J Ophthalmol* 87: 65–73.

Whalen R, Heyman A, Saltzman H (1966) The protective effect of hyperbaric oxygen in cerebral ischemia. *Arch Neurol* 14: 15.

Wherrett CG, Mehran RJ, Beaulieu MA (2002) Cerebral arterial gas embolism following diagnostic bronchoscopy: delayed treatment with hyperbaric oxygen. *Can J Anaesth* 49: 96–99.

Wight JP, Chilcott JB, Holmes MW, Brewer N (2003) Pulsatile machine perfusion vs. cold storage of kidneys for transplantation: a rapid and systematic review. *Clin Transplant* 17(4): 293–307.

Williamson TH, O'Donnell A (2005) Intravitreal triamcinolone acetonide for cystoid macular edema in non-ischemic central retinal vein occlusion. *Am J Ophthalmol* 139: 860–866.

Wilson JR, Hagood CO Jr, Prather ID (2005) Brown recluse spider bites: a complex problem wound. A brief review and case study. *Ostomy Wound Manage* 51: 59–66.

Whitecraft DD III, Bailey TD, Hart GB (1985) Hydrogen sulfide poisoning treated with hyperbaric oxygen. *J Emerg Med* 3: 23–25.

Whittle RJ, Fuller AP, Foley RR (1990) Glottic cancer: results of treatment with radiotherapy in air and hyperbaric oxygen. *Clin Oncol Royal Coll Radiol* 2: 214–219.

Wiernick G, Perrins D (1975) The radiosensitivity of a mesenchymal tissue. The pericryptal fibroblasts sheath in the human mucosa. *Br J Radiol* 48: 382–389.

Wiles CM, Clarke CRA, Irwin HP *et al* (1986) Hyperbaric oxygen in multiple sclerosis: a double-blind study. *Br Med J* 292: 367–371.

Wilkes MK, Palmer AC, Pearce PC *et al* (1989) Cochlear degeneration in minipigs after repeated hyperbaric exposures. *Undersea Biomed Res* 16: 139–152.

Williams JA, Clark D, Dennis WA *et al* (1992) The treatment of pelvic soft tissue radiation necrosis with hyperbaric oxygen. *Am J Obstet Gynecol* 167: 412–415.

Wilkinson FF, Rosasco Sa, Calori BA *et al* (1970) Conclusiones preliminares sobre el uso del oxigeno hiperbaro en lepra lepromatosa. *Rev Leprol* 7: 459–479.

Wilson AT, Channer KS (1997) Hypoxemia and supplemental oxygen therapy in the first 24 hours after myocardial infarction: the role of pulse oximetry. *J Roy Coll Phys Lond* 31: 657–661.

Wilson JR, Foresman BH, Gamber RG *et al* (1998) Hyperbaric oxygen in the treatment of migraine with aura. *Headache* 38: 112–115.

Winstanley J (1963) Treatment of neo-vascularization with oxygen at high pressure. *Br J Ophthalmol* 47: 542–546.

Winter GD, Perrins DJD (1970) Effects of hyperbaric oxygen treatment on epidermal regeneration. In Wada J, Iwa T (Eds.) *Proceedings of the 4th international congress on hyperbaric medicine*. Baillere, London, pp 363–368.

Winter PM, Smith RA, Smith M *et al* (1976) Pressure antagonism of barbiturate anesthesia. *Anesthesiology* 44: 416–419.

Wirjosemito SA, Touhey JE (1988) Hyperbaric oxygen therapy and hereditary spherocytosis: report of 2 cases. *J Hyperbaric Med* 3: 45–50.

Wirjosemito SA, Touhey JE, Workman WT (1989) Type II altitude decompression sickness (DCS): US Air Force experience with 133 cases. *Aviat Space Environ Med* 60: 256–262.

Wityk RJ, Pessin MS, Kaplan RF *et al* (1994) Serial assessment of acute stroke using the NIH stroke scale. *Stroke* 25: 362–365.

Wolf HK, Moon RE, Mitchell PR *et al* (1990) Barotrauma and air embolism in hyperbaric oxygen therapy. *Am J Forensic Med Path* 11: 149–153.

Wolff RS, Wirtschafter D, Adkinson C (1997) Ocular quinine toxicity treated with hyperbaric oxygen. *Undersea Hyperbaric Med* 24: 131–134.

Wong QB, Zhou I (1994) Hyperbaric oxygen treatment in children's epilepsy. *Proc XI International Congress on Hyperbaric Medicine*. Best, San Pedro.

Woo TC, Joseph D, Oxer H (1997) Hyperbaric oxygen treatment for radiation proctitis. *Int J Radiat Oncol Biol Phys* 38: 619–622.

Workman WT, Calcote RD (1989) Hyperbaric oxygen therapy and combat casualty care: a viable potential. *Military Med* 154: 111–115.

World Health Organization Monica Project (1990) *MONICA Manual* (revised edition). Cardiovascular Diseases Unit WHO, Geneva, 1990.

Wormser GP, Dattwyler RJ, Shapiro ED *et al* (2006) The clinical assessment, treatment, and prevention of lyme disease, human granulocytic anaplasmosis, and babesiosis: clinical practice guidelines by the Infectious Diseases Society of America. *Clin Infect Dis* 43: 1089–1134.

Wright JK, Ehler W, McGlasson DL, Thompson W (2002) Facilitation of recovery from acute blood loss with hyperbaric oxygen. *Arch Surg* 137: 850–853.

Wright JK, Franklin B, Zant E (2007) Clinical case report: treatment of a central retinal vein occlusion with hyperbaric oxygen. *Undersea Hyperb Med* 34: 315–319.

Wu L, Mustoe TA (1995) Effect of ischemia on growth factor enhancement of incisional wound healing. *Surgery* 117: 570–576.

Wu Y, Shen Q, Zhang Q (1992) The effect of acupuncture on high oxygen pressure-induced convulsions and its relationship to brain GABA concentration in mice. *Chen Tzu Yen Chiu* 17: 104–109.

Wuellenweber R, Gött U, Holbach KH (1969) RCBF during hyperbaric oxygenation In Brock M, Fieschi C, Ingvar DH, Lassen NA, Schürman K (eds) *Cerebral blood flow*. Springer, Berlin Heidelberg New York, pp 271–272.

X

Xu K, Lamanna JC (2006) Chronic hypoxia and the cerebral circulation. *J Appl Physiol* 100: 725–730.

Xu YN, Huang JG (1991) Hyperbaric oxygen treatment for cystoid macular edema secondary to retinal vein occlusion. *Chung Hua Yen Ko Tsa Chih* 27: 216–218.

Xuejun S, Han C, Lin L et al (2008, August 14) Hyperbaric oxygen preconditioning alleviates myocardial ischemic injury in rats. *Exp Biol Med (Maywood)* doi: 10.3181/0801-RM-8.

Y

Yablon IG, Cruess RL (1968) The effect of hyperbaric oxygen on fracture healing in rats. *J Trauma* 8: 186.

Yadav JS, Roubin GS, Iyer S et al (1997) Elective stenting of extracranial carotid arteries. *Circulation* 95: 376–381.

Yagi H (1987) On the hyperbaric oxygen therapy for severe infected granulation wounds (ulcers) of upper and lower extremities. *Jpn J Hyperbaric Med* 22: 27–40.

Yamami N, Shimaya K, Sera AM et al (1996) Alterations of fibrinolytic activity in human during and after hyperbaric oxygen exposure. *Appl Human Sci* 15: 239–242.

Yamamoto K, Tsujikawa A, Hangai M et al (2005) Neovascular glaucoma after branch retinal artery occlusion. *Jpn J Ophthalmol* 49: 388–390.

Yamamoto S, Saito W, Yagi F, Takeuchi S, Sato E, Mizunoya S (2004) Vitrectomy with or without arteriovenous adventitial sheathotomy for macular edema associated with branch retinal vein occlusion. *Am J Ophthalmol* 138: 907–914.

Yan B, Kong W, Shi H et al (2006) Idiopathic sudden deafness: the therapeutic evaluation of hyperbaric oxygen treatment. *Lin Chuang Er Bi Yan Hou Ke Za Zhi* 20: 309–311.

Yang YJ, Wang XL, Yu XH et al (2008) Hyperbaric oxygen induces endogenous neural stem cells to proliferate and differentiate in hypoxic-ischemic brain damage in neonatal rats. *Undersea Hyperb Med* 35(2): 113–129.

Yang ZJ, Camporesi C, Yang X et al (2002) Hyperbaric oxygenation mitigates focal cerebral injury and reduces striatal dopamine release in a rat model of transient middle cerebral artery occlusion. *Eur J Appl Physiol* 87: 101–107.

Yangsheng, T et al (1995) Hyperbaric oxygen treatment of acute ischemic and anoxic cerebral injury. *Proceedings of the 11th International Congress on Hyperbaric Medicine*. Best, Flagstaff, AZ, pp 218–222.

Yastrebov VE, Kustov VV, Razinkin SM (1987) Effect of a short-term exposure to carbon monoxide high concentrations on man's psychophysiological functions. *Kosm Biol Aviakosm Med* 21: 47–50.

Yatsuzuka H (1991) Effects of hyperbaric oxygen therapy on ischemic brain injury in dogs. *Masui* 40: 208–223 (Japanese).

Yawalkar SJ (2002) *Leprosy for medical practitioners and paramedical workers, 7th ed.* Novartis, Basel.

Yaxi Q, Anquan Y, Guangkai G, Yansheng T (1995) The study of the effect of hyperbaric oxygen on cerebral metabolic enzymes and cAMP during acute cerebral ischemia in rabbits. *Proceedings of the 11th International Congress on Hyperbaric Medicine*. Best, Flagstaff, AZ, pp 194–197.

Yeo JD (1976) Treatment of paraplegic sheep with hyperbaric oxygen. *Med J Aust* 1: 538–540.

Yeo, Stabbach S, McKenzie B (1977) A study of the effects of HBO on experimental spinal cord injury. *Med J Austr* 2: 145–147.

Yildiz S, Aktas S, Cimsit M et al (2004) Seizure incidence in 80,000 patient treatments with hyperbaric oxygen. *Aviat Space Environ Med* 75: 992–994.

Yilmaz MI, Korkmaz A, Kaya A et al (2006). Hyperbaric oxygen treatment augments the efficacy of a losartan regime in an experimental nephrotic syndrome model. *Nephron Exp Nephrol* 104: e15–22.

Yin W, Badr AE, Mychaskiw G, Zhang JH (2002) Down regulation of COX-2 is involved in hyperbaric oxygen treatment in a rat transient focal cerebral ischemia model. *Brain Res* 926: 165–171.

Yiqun F, Jingchang L, Weiguang T, Haihong J, Peizhu X, Shilong L, Fenzhou S (1995) Effect of hyperbaric oxygen on brain Na, K-AT-Pase and ultrastructure of cerebral ischemia gerbils. *Proceedings of the Eleventh International Congress on Hyperbaric Medicine*. Best, Flagstaff, AZ, pp 269–278.

Ylikoski J, Mrena R, Makitie A et al (2008) Hyperbaric oxygen therapy seems to enhance recovery from acute acoustic trauma. *Acta Otolaryngol* 128: 1110–1115.

Yogaratnam JZ, Laden G, Guvendik L et al (2007) Can hyperbaric oxygen be used as adjunctive heart failure therapy through the induction of endogenous heat shock proteins? *Adv Ther* 24: 106–118.

Yogaratnam JZ, Laden G, Guvendik L et al (2008) Pharmacological preconditioning with hyperbaric oxygen: can this therapy attenuate myocardial ischemic reperfusion injury and induce myocardial protection via nitric oxide? *J Surg Res* 149: 155–164.

Yokota T, Suda T, Tsukioka S et al (2000) The striking effect of hyperbaric oxygenation therapy in the management of chronic idiopathic intestinal pseudo-obstruction. *Am J Gastroenterol* 95: 285–288.

Yoshino M, Murakami K, Katsumata et al (2000) Stimulation of glycolysis with hyperglycemia in rats at high altitude hypoxia. *Biomed Res* 7: 113–117.

Yoshiyama M, Asamoto S, Kobayashi N et al (2007) Spinal cord decompression sickness associated with scuba diving: correlation of immediate and delayed magnetic resonance imaging findings with severity of neurologic impairment – a report on 3 cases. *Surg Neurol* 67: 283-287.

Yotsukura J, Adachi-Usami E (1993) Correlation of electroretinographic changes with visual prognosis in central retinal artery occlusion. *Ophthalmologica* 207: 13–18.

Youn BA, Kozikowski RJ, Myers RAM (1989) The development of treatment algorithm in methylene chloride poisoning based on a multicase experience. *Undersea Biomed Res 12 (Suppl)*: 20 Abstract #16.

Young DB, Van Vliet BN (1992) Migraine with aura: a vicious cycle perpetuated by potassium-induced vasoconstriction. *Headache* 32: 24–34.

Young, WB (1997) Jefferson Headache Center, Philadelphia. Personal Communication.

Youngblood DA (1984) Hyperbaric oxygen in the treatment of Hansen's disease. *Hyperbaric Oxygen Rev* 5: 244–250.

Yu DY, Cringle SJ (2005) Retinal degeneration and local oxygen metabolism. *Exp Eye Res* 80: 745–751.

Yu DY, Cringle SJ, Yu PK, Su EN (2007) Intraretinal oxygen distribution and consumption during retinal artery occlusion and graded hyperoxic ventilation in the rat. *Invest Ophthalmol Vis Sci* 48: 2290–2296.

Yu X-H, Yang Y-J, Wang X *et al* (2006) Effect of hyperbaric oxygenation on neural stem cells and myelin in neonatal rats with hypoxic-ischemic brain damage. *Zhongguo Dang Dai Er Ke Za Zhi* 8(1): 33–37.

Yu YL, Farell CL, Mustoe TA (1996) Effects of PDGF-BB with hyperbaric oxygen therapy on PDGF receptor gene expression in rabbit ischemic wounds, *2nd Joint meeting of the Wound Healing Society and the European Tissue Repair Society*, Boston MA, Abstract #93.

Yufu K, Itoh T, Edamatsu R *et al* (1993) Effect of hyperbaric oxygenation on the Na$^+$, K$^+$, ATPase and membrane fluidity of cerebrocortical membranes after experimental subarachnoid hemorrhage. *Neurochem Res* 18: 1033–1039.

Yun DR, Cho SH (1983) Hyperbaric oxygen treatment in acute CO poisoning. *Korean J Prev Med* 16: 153–156.

Yusa T (1981) Chromosomal and teratogenic effects of oxygen in the mouse. *Br J Anaesth* 53: 505–510.

Yusa T, Beckman JS, Crapo JD, Freeman BA (1987) Hyperoxia increases H$_2$O$_2$ production by brain *in vivo*. *J Appl Physiol* 63: 353–358.

Yuzurihara D, Ijima H (2004) Visual outcome in central retinal and branch retinal artery occlusion. *Jpn J Ophthalmol* 48: 490–492. (Japanese).

Z

Zamboni WA, Browder LK, Martinez J (2003) Hyperbaric oxygen and wound healing. *Clin Plast Surg* 30: 67–75.

Zamboni WA, Roth AC, Russel RC *et al* (1992) The effect of hyperbaric oxygen on reperfusion of ischemic axial skin flaps: a laser doppler analysis. *Ann Plast Surg* 28: 339–341.

Zamboni WA, Roth AC, Russel RC *et al* (1993) Morphologic analysis of the microcirculation during reperfusion of ischemic skeletal muscle and the effect of hyperbaric oxygenation. *Plas Reconstr Surg* 91: 1110–1123.

Zarchin N, Meilin S, Rifkind J, Mayevsky A (2002) Effect of aging on brain energy-metabolism. *Comp Biochem Physiol A Mol Integr Physiol* 132(1): 117–120.

Zhang J, Piantadosi C (1992) Mitochondrial oxidative stress after carbon monoxide hypoxia in the rat brain. *J Clin Invest* 90: 1193–1199.

Zhang J, Su Y, Oury TD *et al* (1993) Cerebral amino acid, norepinephrine and nitric oxide metabolism in CNS oxygen toxicity. *Brain Res* 606: 56–62.

Zhang Q, Chang Q, Cox RA *et al* (2008) Hyperbaric oxygen attenuates apoptosis and decreases inflammation in an ischemic wound model. *J Invest Dermatol* 128: 2102–2112.

Zhang XZ, Cao JQ (1986) *Observations on therapeutic results in 80 cases of central serous retinopathy treated with hyperbaric oxygenation*. Presented at the 5th Chinese conference on hyperbaric medicine, Fuzhow, China, Sept 26–29.

Zhao DW (1991) Therapeutic effect of hyperbaric oxygen on recovery of surgically repaired peripheral nerve injury. *Chung Hua Wai Ko Tsa Chih* 29: 118–120.

Zhao LL, Davidson JD, Wee SC, Roth SL, Mustoe TA (1994) Effect of hyperbaric oxygen and growth factors on rabbit ear ischemic ulcers. *Arch Surg* 129; 1043–1049.

Zhdanov GG, Nechaev VN, Alipov PA (1991) Hyperbaric oxygenation and antioxidants in the complex intensive therapy of severe forms of pneumonia in children. *Anesteziol Reanimatol* 2: 54–58.

Zhdanov GG, Rymashevsky VK, Khabakhleashevy K *et al* (1981) Hyperbaric oxygen therapy in pregnant women with diabetes mellitus. In Yefuny SN (Ed.) *Proceedings of the 7th international congress on hyperbaric medicine*. USSR Academy of Sciences, Moscow, p 360.

Zhivoderov VM, Doshchitsin VL, Dunaeva ZI *et al* (1980) Late arrhythmias in myocardial infarct. *Kardiologiia* 20: 22–25.

Zhivoderov VM, Zakharov VN, Doshchitsin VL *et al* (1982) Use of hyperbaric oxygenation for treating arrhythmias ijn ischemic heart disease. *Klin Med (Mosk)* 60: 51–55.

Zhiyong Q, Shuijiang S, Guohua X *et al* (2007) Preconditioning with hyperbaric oxygen attenuates brain edema after experimental intracerebral hemorrhage. *Neurosurg Focus* 22(5): E13.

Zhou BY, Lu GJ, Huang YQ *et al* (2008) Efficacy of hyperbaric oxygen therapy under different pressures on neonatal hypoxic-ischemic encephalopathy. *Zhongguo Dang Dai Er Ke Za Zhi* 10: 133–135.

Zhou C, Li Y, Nanda A, Zhang JH 2003 HBO suppresses Nogo-A, Ng-R, or RhoA expression in the cerebral cortex after global ischemia. *Biochem Biophys Res Commun* 309(2): 368–376.

Zhou LS (1986) *Hyperbaric oxygen in treatment of diffusing scleroderma: report of 5 cases*. Presented at the 5th Chinese conference on hyperbaric medicine, Fuzhow, China, Sept 26–29.

Zirkle LG, Mengel CE, Horton BD *et al* (1965) Studies of oxygen toxicity in the central nervous system. *Aerospace Med* 36: 1027–1032.

Zwacka RM, Zhou W, Zhang Y, Darby CJ, Dudus L, Halldorson J, Oberley L, Engelhardt JF (1998) Redox gene therapy for ischemia/reperfusion injury of the liver reduces AP1 and NF-kB activation. *Nature Medicine* 4: 698–704.

46 Index